DOUG MORRIS

Canine
and Feline
Cardiology

Canine and Feline Cardiology

Edited by

Philip R. Fox, D.V.M., M.S.

Diplomate
American College of Veterinary
 Internal Medicine (Cardiology)
Director of Clinics and Staff Cardiologist
The Animal Medical Center
New York, New York

Churchill Livingstone
New York, Edinburgh, London, Melbourne   1988

Library of Congress Cataloging in Publication Data

Canine and feline cardiology/edited by Philip R. Fox.
    p.   cm.
  Includes bibliographies and index.
  ISBN 0-443-08482-3
  1. Dogs—Diseases. 2. Cats—Diseases. 3. Veterinary cardiology.
I. Fox, Philip R.
  [DNLM: 1. Cardiovascular Diseases—veterinary. 2. Cat Diseases.
3. Dog Diseases. SF 992.C37 C223]
SF992.C37C36 1988
636.7′ 089612—dc 19
DNLM/DLC   88-7264
for Library of Congress   CIP

© **Churchill Livingstone Inc. 1988**

Distributed in the United Kingdom by Churchill Livingstone, Robert Stevenson House, 1–3 Baxter's Place, Leith Walk, Edinburgh EH1 3AF, and by associated companies, branches, and representatives throughout the world.

Accurate indications, adverse reactions, and dosage schedules for drugs are provided in this book, but it is possible that they may change. The reader is urged to review the package information data of the manufacturers of the medications mentioned.

The Publishers have made every effort to trace the copyright holders for borrowed material. If they have inadvertently overlooked any, they will be pleased to make the necessary arrangements at the first opportunity.

Acquisitions Editor: *Linda Panzarella*
Copy Editor: *Margot Otway*
Production Supervisor: *Sharon Tuder*

Printed in the United States of America

First published in 1988

To my parents,
and in memory of my mother

Contributors

Sanford P. Bishop, D.V.M., Ph.D.
Diplomate, American College of Veterinary Internal Medicine (Cardiology); Diplomate, American College of Veterinary Pathology; Professor, Department of Pathology, University of Alabama at Birmingham, Birmingham, Alabama

John D. Bonagura, D.V.M., M.S.
Diplomate, American College of Veterinary Internal Medicine (Cardiology and Internal Medicine); Associate Professor, Department of Veterinary Clinical Sciences, and Staff Cardiologist, Veterinary Teaching Hospital, Ohio State University, Columbus, Ohio

Betsy R. Bond, D.V.M.
Diplomate, American College of Veterinary Internal Medicine (Cardiology); Staff Cardiologist, The Animal Medical Center, New York, New York

Penelope A. Boyden, Ph.D.
Assistant Professor, Department of Pharmacology, Columbia University College of Physicians and Surgeons, New York, New York

Clay A. Calvert, D.V.M.
Diplomate, American College of Veterinary Internal Medicine; Associate Professor, Department of Small Animal Medicine, University of Georgia College of Veterinary Medicine, Athens, Georgia

Kenneth H. Dangman, Ph.D.
Assistant Professor, Department of Pharmacology, Columbia University College of Physicians and Surgeons, New York, New York

Stephen J. Ettinger, D.V.M., F.A.C.C.
Diplomate, American College of Veterinary Internal Medicine (Cardiology and Internal Medicine); California Animal Hospital, Los Angeles, California

A. Thomas Evans, D.V.M.
Diplomate, American College of Veterinary Anesthesiologists; Associate Professor, Department of Small Animal Clinical Sciences, Michigan State University College of Veterinary Medicine, East Lansing, Michigan

George E. Eyster, V.M.D.
Diplomate, American College of Veterinary Surgeons; Professor, Department of Small Animal Clinical Sciences, Michigan State University College of Veterinary Medicine, East Lansing, Michigan

Philip R. Fox, D.V.M., M.S.
Diplomate, American College of Veterinary Internal Medicine (Cardiology); Director of Clinics and Staff Cardiologist, The Animal Medical Center, New York, New York

Rebecca E. Gompf, D.V.M.
Diplomate, American College of Veterinary Internal Medicine (Cardiology); Associate Professor of Cardiology, Department of Urban Practice, University of Tennessee College of Veterinary Medicine, Knoxville, Tennessee

Robert L. Hamlin, D.V.M., Ph.D.
Diplomate, American College of Veterinary Internal Medicine (Cardiology and Internal Medicine); Professor, Department of Veterinary Physiology and Pharmacology, Ohio State University, Columbus, Ohio

Steve C. Haskins, D.V.M.
Diplomate, American College of Veterinary Anesthesiologists; Associate Professor, Department of Surgery, University of California, Davis, School of Veterinary Medicine, Davis, California

John A. E. Hubbell, D.V.M.
Diplomate, American College of Veterinary Anesthesiologists; Associate Professor, Department of Veterinary Clinical Sciences, Ohio State University, Columbus, Ohio

Bruce W. Keene, D.V.M., M.S.
Diplomate, American College of Veterinary Internal Medicine (Cardiology); Assistant Professor, Department of Medical Sciences, University of Wisconsin–Madison School of Veterinary Medicine, Madison, Wisconsin

Mark D. Kittleson, D.V.M., Ph.D.
Diplomate, American College of Veterinary Internal Medicine (Cardiology); Assistant Professor, Department of Medicine, University of California, Davis, School of Veterinary Medicine, Davis, California

Si-Kwang Liu, D.V.M., Ph.D.
Senior Staff, The Animal Medical Center, New York, New York; Consultant Pathologist, New York Zoological Society, Bronx, New York; Consultant, Pig Research Institute, Taiwan, Republic of China

Peter F. Lord, B.V.Sc., D.V.R., F.R.C.V.S.
Diplomate, American College of Veterinary Radiology; Assistant Professor, Department of Surgical Sciences, University of Wisconsin School of Veterinary Medicine, Madison, Wisconsin

Robert H. Lusk, Jr., D.V.M.
Staff Doctor, California Animal Hospital, Los Angeles, California

Diane E. Mason, D.V.M.
Assistant Professor, Department of Surgical Sciences, University of Wisconsin School of Veterinary Medicine, Madison, Wisconsin

Michael S. Miller, V.M.D.
Diplomate, American Board of Veterinary Practitioners; Vice President, Professional Operations of Cardiopet, Division of Animed, Inc., Roslyn, New York; Staff Clinician, A & A Veterinary Hospital, New York, New York

N. Sydney Moise, D.V.M.
Diplomate, American College of Veterinary Internal Medicine (Internal Medicine and Cardiology); Assistant Professor, Department of Clinical Sciences, New York State College of Veterinary Medicine, Cornell University, Ithaca, New York

William W. Muir III, D.V.M., Ph.D.
Diplomate, American College of Veterinary Anesthesiologists; Professor and Chairman, Department of Veterinary Clinical Sciences, and Professor, Department of Medicine, Ohio State University, Columbus, Ohio

C. E. Rhett Nichols, D.V.M.
Diplomate, American College of Veterinary Internal Medicine; Staff Internist, The Animal Medical Center, New York, New York

N. Bari Olivier, D.V.M.
Diplomate, American College of Veterinary Internal Medicine (Cardiology); Assistant Professor, Department of Physiology, Michigan State University College of Osteopathic Medicine; Staff Cardiologist, Department of Small Animal Clinical Sciences, Michigan State University College of Veterinary Medicine, East Lansing, Michigan

Maralyn R. Probst
Cardiology Technician, Department of Small Animal Clinical Sciences, Michigan State University College of Veterinary Medicine, East Lansing, Michigan

Sarah L. Ralston, V.M.D., Ph.D.
Assistant Professor, Mark Morris Chair of Clinical Nutrition, Department of Clinical Sciences, Colorado State University College of Veterinary Medicine and Biomedical Sciences, Fort Collins, Colorado

Clarence A. Rawlings, D.V.M., Ph.D.
Diplomate, American College of Veterinary Surgeons; Professor and Chief of Surgery, Department of Surgery, University of Georgia College of Veterinary Medicine, Athens, Georgia

John R. Reed, D.V.M.
Diplomate, American College of Veterinary Internal Medicine (Cardiology); Staff Cardiologist, Sacramento Animal Medical Group, Carmichael, California

Richard A. Sams, Ph.D.
Associate Professor, Department of Veterinary Clinical Sciences, Ohio State University, Columbus, Ohio

Michael Schollmeyer, D.V.M.
Manager of Clinical Programs, Bradyarrhythmia Products, Cardiac Pacemakers, Inc., St. Paul, Minnesota

D. David Sisson, D.V.M.
Diplomate, American College of Veterinary Internal Medicine (Cardiology); Assistant Professor of Medicine and Staff Cardiologist, Department of Veterinary Clinical Medicine, University of Illinois at Urbana-Champagne College of Veterinary Medicine, Urbana, Illinois

Larry Patrick Tilley, D.V.M.
Diplomate, American College of Veterinary Internal Medicine (Internal Medicine); President, Cardiopet Transtelephonic Electrocardiography, Division of Animed, Inc., and Vice Chairman, Animed Inc., Roslyn, New York; Staff Consultant, Department of Medicine (Cardiology), The Animal Medical Center, New York, New York

Wendy A. Ware, D.V.M., M.S.
Diplomate, American College of Veterinary Internal Medicine (Cardiology); Assistant Professor, Department of Veterinary Clinical Sciences, and Staff Cardiologist, Veterinary Teaching Hospital, Iowa State University College of Veterinary Medicine, Ames, Iowa

Preface

The field of veterinary cardiology has made explosive progress over the past two decades. Major advances have occurred in all areas. These have been fueled by an extensive research effort and by technical innovations, especially in diagnostic modalities such as echocardiography. As a result, the standards of clinical practice and patient care have improved remarkably. Electrocardiography is now widely available, thanks to commercial transtelephonic services; heart failure is managed with potent new drugs that often supplement or replace digitalis glycosides; and vast strides have been made in the understanding and treatment of feline heart disease, a subject little emphasized 10 years ago. The burgeoning literature reporting basic research and clinical advances makes it increasingly difficult to stay abreast of recent changes and developments.

This textbook attempts to bring together in one practical source the current salient information on canine and feline heart disease. The fundamental principles of cardiology are reviewed, and physiology, pathophysiology, diagnosis, pharmacology, and therapy are discussed in depth. The contributors who present this comprehensive range of topics are some of the most knowledgeable experts in their fields; many are among the founding fathers of veterinary cardiology.

I have intended *Canine and Feline Cardiology* to serve a wide range of readers, including students and veterinarians in formal training and clinicians in the continuous training of private practice. It is meant to serve as both a clinical guide to diagnosis and treatment and a resource on cardiovascular disease. Chapters are arranged in sections that encompass related aspects of cardiology. Information is presented in a manner designed to reflect the actual process of clinical problem solving. Care has been taken to minimize both repetition in different chapters and omissions associated with a complex topic. Where issues are controversial, an attempt has been made to present alternative views.

I am indebted to the contributing specialists, whose efforts and time have ensured that this textbook is both comprehensive and up-to-date. I am appreciative of Dr. Betsy R. Bond for her support throughout the arduous task of preparing this manuscript, and of Dr. Si-Kwang Liu for his steadfast, contagious enthusiasm and collaboration in the study of cardiovascular diseases.

Importantly, I wish to acknowledge the Animal Medical Center, its many nurses, interns, residents, and faculty. They have provided academic stimulation, innovative ideas, and dedication to the highest standards of postgraduate education and pet care. This environment has been a great stimulus to the conception and writing of this book. To the many AMC patients whom I have treated and from whom I have learned, I am especially grateful.

Philip R. Fox, D.V.M., M.S.

Contents

Section 1

THE NORMAL HEART AND BLOOD VESSELS

1

Developmental Anatomy of the Heart and Great Vessels

Sanford P. Bishop

A thorough anatomic knowledge of the normal and pathologic heart during development and normal growth and in the adult animal is required for competent evaluation of the cardiovascular system. Detailed reviews of embryologic development[1-3] and an excellent description of cardiac morphogenesis have appeared in the literature.[4]

EMBRYOLOGY

Early Formation of the Heart

In all vertebrates, the heart takes its origin as paired structures in the splanchnic mesoderm, first appearing at about the three- to four-somite stage. This mesodermal tissue eventually becomes the myocardium. Shortly afterward, endocardial tissue from the endoderm combines bilaterally with the mesodermal tissue to form paired *endocardial tubes*. These paired endocardial tubes migrate centrally and fuse to form a single straight *cardiac tube* consisting of mesoderm (myocardium), endoderm (en-

docardium), and associated extracellular material. At this stage, interference with fusion of the two paired structures can result in formation of two independent beating hearts, one on each side of the embryonic midline.

Cardiac Loop

The straight cardiac tube has the ventral aorta on its anterior end and the omphalomesenteric veins at the posterior end and is contained in the primitive pericardial cavity. The tube undergoes a series of bends and folds to form the cardiac loop with the various clearly defined structures, the *sinus venosus, atrium, ventricle,* and *bulbus cordis* (Fig. 1-1). The caudally located sinus venosus receives blood from the entire embryo and is separated from the atrium by the *sinoatrial sulcus*, the site of the future sinoatrial node or pacemaker of the heart. During final stages of cardiac loop development, the atrium forms two lateral lobes but is still a single chamber. Caudal to the atrium, the ventricle takes on a saccular shape and is separated from the atrium by a distinct atrio-

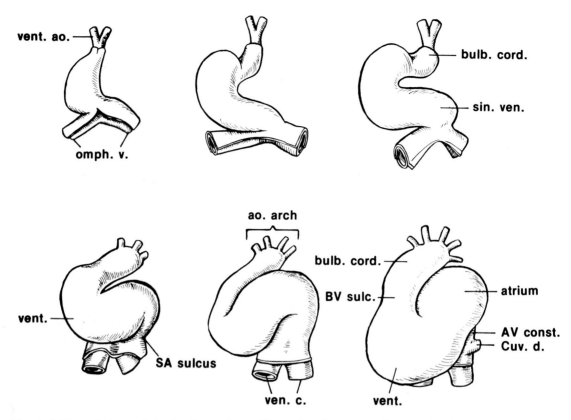

Fig. 1-1 Ventral views of the developing heart, illustrating formation of the cardiac loop from the straight cardiac tube. ao arch, aortic arches; AV const, atrioventricular constriction; bulb cord, bulbus cordis; BV sulc, bulboventricular sulcus; omph v, omphalomesenteric veins; SA sulcus, sinoatrial sulcus; sin ven, sinus venosus; ven c, venae cavae; vent, ventricle; vent ao, ventral aortic roots.

ventricular canal. The bulbus cordis is separated from the ventricle by the bulboventricular sulcus. The part adjacent to the ventricle will become the infundibular region of the adult heart and the most cranial portions will form the aorta and pulmonary artery (Fig. 1-2).

Ventricle Formation

Contractile activity of the heart begins during the early cardiac loop stage, when myocytes have discernible actin and myosin contractile proteins.[5,6] Although valves are not yet formed, forward flow of

Fig. 1-2 Scanning electron micrographs of chick embryo hearts showing modifications of the external form of the heart at postlooping stages (ventral views). (**A**) Third day of incubation. At this stage, the bulbus cordis (T + C) cannot be separated into its two components. Arrows indicate the interatrial (top) and interventricular (bottom) sulci. (**B**) Fourth day of incubation. The bulbus is growing longitudinally and bends around a transverse axis. This is the point at which its two components, truncus and conus, can be distinguished. Compare the size of the two atria. (**C**) Fifth day of incubation. Note the rapid growth of the right atrium. (**D**) Sixth day of incubation. The proximal segments of the aorta and pulmonary artery are already formed. However, there is no external separation. Note the location of the interventricular sulcus (arrowhead). The apex of the heart is already formed by the left ventricle. A, atrium; Ao, aorta; A-Vc, atrioventricular canal; C, conus; LA, left atrium; P, pulmonary artery; RA, right atrium; T, truncus; V, ventricle. (Icardo JM: The growing heart: An anatomical perspective. p. 41. In Zak R (ed): Growth of the Heart in Health and Disease. Raven Press, New York, 1984.)

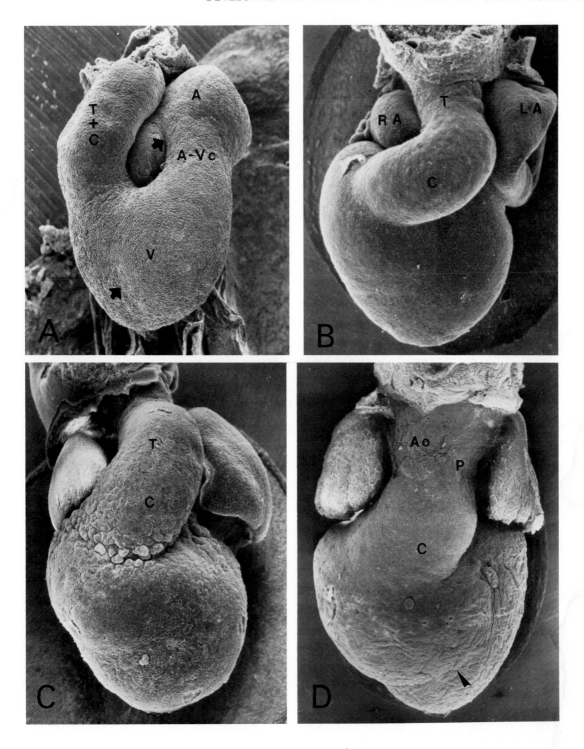

blood is maintained by constriction of the tube at the atrioventricular canal. The endocardium is separated from the myocardium by an extensive extracellular matrix of glycosaminoglycans and glycoproteins, the *cardiac jelly*. The cardiac jelly aids in forming a valvelike action of the primitive heart; once pulsatile forward flow of blood is established during cardiac loop formation, blood pressure of about 1 mmHg may be recorded in the chick embyro.[7] By the time of hatching, blood pressure is reported to reach 30 mmHg.[8]

During formation of the cardiac loop, the endocardium invaginates through the cardiac jelly and into the myocardium, forming trabeculae that persist into adult life and form the papillary muscles. The cardiac jelly disappears from the ventricular portion with the development of trabeculation but persists longer in the atrioventricular canal and bulbus cordis regions. The cardiac jelly is invaded by endocardial cells and in these latter regions form the *endocardial cushions* that participate in cardiac septation.

Septation

After the development of the cardiac loop stage, the heart undergoes a series of septations that divide the left and right sides of the structure. However, openings remain between all chambers resulting in two parallel communicating circulations. The bulbus cordis elongates and separates into two channels, forming the aorta and pulmonary artery. Muscle tissue disappears distal to the tricuspid valve primordia. The proximal portions of the bulbus cordis form the infundibular muscular regions of the ventricles. The sinus venosus becomes separated from the left atrium by deepening of the atrioventricular sulcus and opens only into the right atrium. The caval veins obtain independent openings into the right atrium and part of the sinus venosus becomes the *coronary sinus* (Fig. 1-3A). At the same time, the pulmonary veins connect with the left atrium. In the adult heart, the smooth portions of the left and right atrium are derived from the sinus venosus region of the cardiac loop, while the irregular pectinate portions are derived from the embryonic atria.

Septation of the ventricles begins from the apex

by an extension of the trabeculation process and growth of tissue toward the *atrioventricular canal*, forming the *primary interventricular foramen* (Fig. 1-3B). The primary interventricular foramen partially closes as the ventral septal tissue fuses with the septal portion of the atrioventricular cushion as a connective tissue mass. However, the ventral portion of the primary interventricular foramen remains open, becoming the connection of the aorta with the left ventricle. Various forms of ventricular septal defects result from failure of closure of this ventricular septal partition. They may be located anywhere from the pulmonic infundibular region to the aortic outflow region.

In the atrium, the *septum primum* extends from the dorsal atrial wall toward the atrioventricular canal, forming the *ostium primum*. This opening is normally completely occluded when the septum primum fuses with the dorsal and ventral endocardial cushions (Fig. 1-3C). At the same time, perforations appear in the superior portion of the septum primum and eventually coalesce, forming the *ostium secundum*. Another septum, the *septum secundum*, arises from the dorsal wall of the atrium and descends down over the right side of the septum primum and joins the atrioventricular canal cushion. An opening persists in the septum secundum, which is the *fossa ovalis*. This latter opening is normally covered by the septum primum forming the valve of the fossa ovalis (Fig. 1-3D). Defects in this region include patent *foramen ovale* due to failure of normal postnatal anatomic closure of this opening, ostium primum defects due to incomplete fusion of the septum primum with the atrioventricular cushions, and ostium secundum defects, in which this opening in the septum primum remains unduly large and the septum primum does not cover the fossa ovalis.

The *atrioventricular canal* forms the dorsal and ventral *endocardial cushions*, which fuse together with the atrial and ventricular septae and give rise to the mitral and tricuspid valves (Fig. 1-3C,D). Developmental anomalies in the atrioventricular cushions result in persistence of openings between the chambers, usually accompanied by clefts in the anterior leaflet of the mitral valve and sometimes in the tricuspid valve as well. These are especially common in the cat.

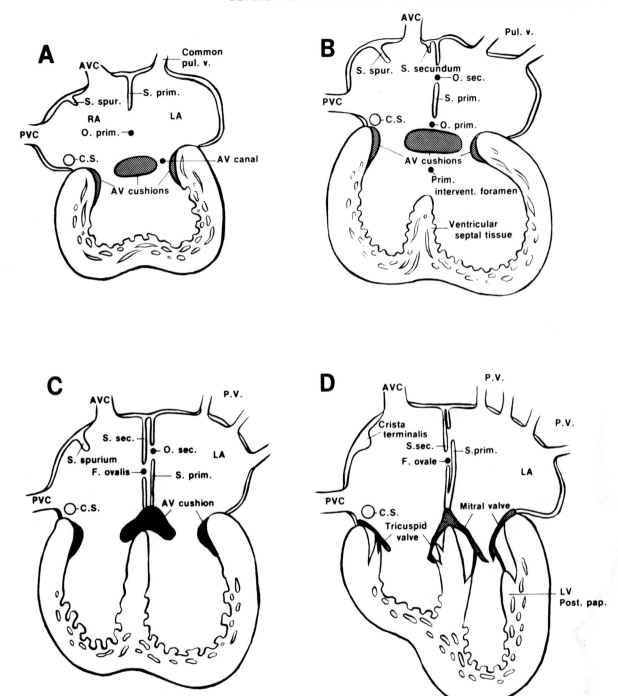

Fig. 1-3 Septal development of the heart. (**A–D**) drawings illustrating development of ventricular and atrial septae and formation of atrioventricular valves by the AV endocardial cushions (from the postloop stage to late fetal development). AVC, anterior vena cava; cs, coronary sinus; f. ovalis, fossa ovalis; f ovale, foramen ovale; LA, left atrium; o sec, ostium secundum; o prim, ostium primum; PV, pulmonary veins; PVC, posterior vena cava; RA, right atrium; s sec, septum secundum; s prim, septum primum; s spur, septum spurium.

Aortic Arches

Six pairs of *aortic arches* develop along with the embryonic heart. The first, second, and fifth pairs regress completely in mammals, and the third pair forms the internal carotid arteries. In mammals, the left fourth arch forms the root of the aorta, joining with the persistent left dorsal aorta. The right fourth arch forms the root of the subclavian artery and the distal right dorsal aorta disappears. The sixth arches form the pulmonary arteries, and the distal portion of the left retains its connection with the dorsal aorta as the *ductus arteriosus* (Fig. 1-4). A large variety of vascular ring anomalies are possible due to malformations in the development of the aortic arches. The most common in dogs is persistence of the right fourth aortic arch, which results in entrapment of the esophagus between the pulmonary artery, trachea, and the ligamentum or patent ductus arteriosus.

Lungs

The lungs develop independent of the heart from primitive foregut and drain during early embryogenesis to the cardinal and umbilicovitelline veins.

The pulmonary veins develop from the left atrium to communicate with pulmonary venous drainage. Anomalous pulmonary venous drainage can result from failure of this system to develop normally.

Specialized Conduction Tissue

Functional specialized conduction tissue may first be recognized at the end of the cardiac loop stage,[9–11] when the heart has already been beating for some time. Although not definitively proved, the specialized conducting tissue including the sinus and atrioventricular nodes and the Purkinje fibers appear to develop from myocardial cells. Cells in the sinus venosus beat at a faster rate than do those of the ventricle even in the cardiac loop stage. These more rapidly beating cells in the sinus venosus presumably become the *sinus node*.

TRANSITION FROM FETAL TO NEONATAL BLOOD FLOW

Fetal Blood Flow

During embryonic to fetal to neonatal circulatory development, transformation occurs from a single circular system to a double parallel circuit to finally,

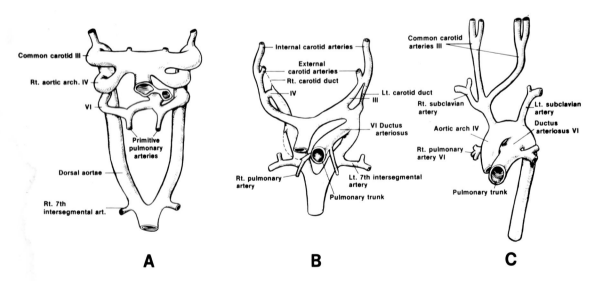

Fig. 1-4 (A–C) Development of the aortic arch system in the dog and cat. Only the third, fourth, and sixth arches are retained, and the seventh intersegmental arteries form the subclavian arteries. (Modified from Van Mierop LHS, Kutsche LM: Embryology of the heart. p. 7. In Hurst JW (ed): The Heart. Vol. 1. 5th Ed. McGraw-Hill, New York, 1982.)

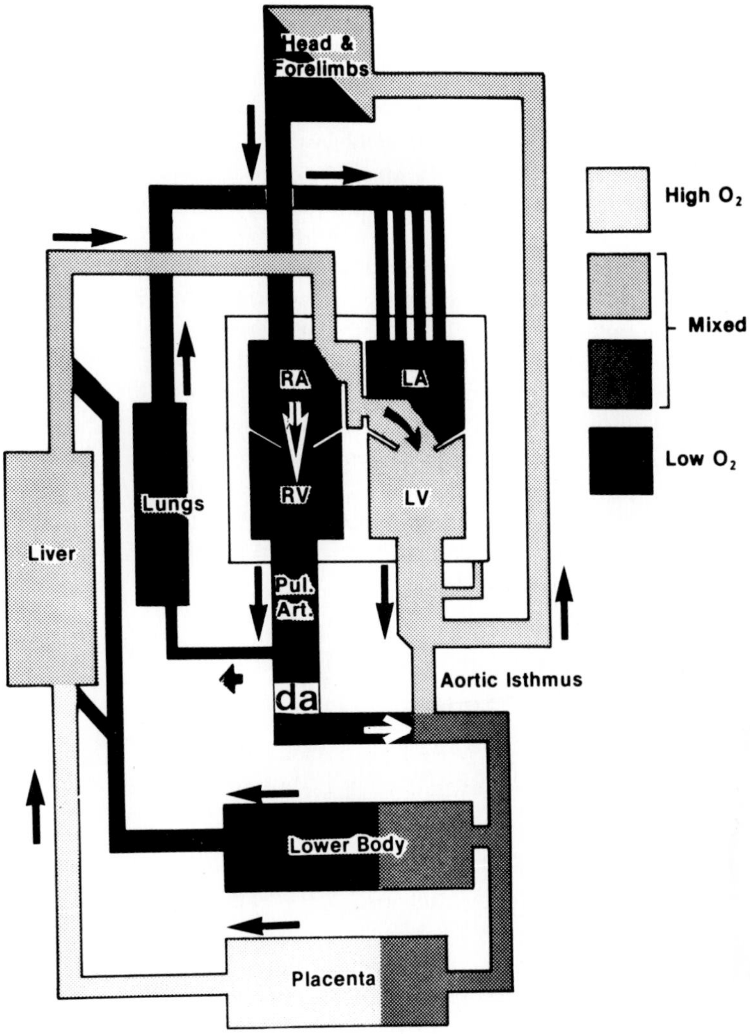

Fig. 1-5 Diagrammatic representation of blood circulation during the late fetal period. Note that the most highly oxygenated blood returning to the heart from the placenta via the posterior vena cava is shunted mainly across the interatrial septum to the left ventricle and that vessels to the heart and head receive this highly oxygenated blood. Oxygen-depleted blood coming from the head is returned to the right ventricle, traverses the ductus arteriosus, and enters the aorta distal to the vessels to the heart and head (white arrow). da, ductus arteriosus.

a double circulation in series[1–3] (Fig. 1-5). In the early embryo, all blood enters the heart through a single venous sinus, traverses straight through the heart and is distributed to the body and placenta by way of the conotruncal bulb and the aortic arches. As partitioning develops, a double circuit is formed with parallel flow and crossover proximal and distal to the ventricles. Virtually all blood entering the right atrium from the head and forepart of the body is shunted by a muscular fold on the atrial septum adjacent to the fossa ovalis directly into the right ventricular cavity. This poorly oxygenated blood is pumped by the right ventricle to the pulmonary artery and across the ductus arteriosus to the descend-

ing thoracic aorta en route to the placenta and lower body. The pulmonary vasculature has very high resistance due to fluid surrounding the vessels and vasoconstriction in response to the low blood oxygen content. Only 5 to 10 percent of right ventricular and pulmonary artery blood traverses the lungs.

Blood returning from the placenta and lower part of the body, on the other hand, has a relatively high oxygen content. The anatomic relationship of the postcava and the fossa ovalis allows it to be shunted directly through the fossa ovalis to the left atrium and ventricle. This highly oxygenated blood then enters the root of the aorta, where most is distributed to the head and heart. The remainder traverses the aortic isthmus to be mixed with poorly oxygenated blood entering the aorta through the ductus arteriosus. Thus, two parallel circuits are present during the fetal period that serve to deliver highly oxygenated blood to the brain and heart and less well-oxygenated blood to the placenta.

Abnormalities of cardiac development do not cause functional abnormality in the fetus as long as there is communication between the right and left sides of the circulatory system. Stenoses and abnormal flow patterns may, however, result in reduced flow in selected areas resulting in underdevelopment or hypoplasia of the affected chamber or vessel. Semilunar valve stenoses (e.g., pulmonic stenosis) may also cause enlargement of a chamber proximal to the stenosis due to the increased work load on the affected ventricle. Experimentally, left ventricular enlargement may be induced by placing a band on the aortic arch in the fetus.[12]

Blood Flow Changes at Birth

At birth and during the subsequent early neonatal period, circulatory changes result in formation of two separate circuits in series. When air is introduced into the lungs, the fluid media surrounding the vasculature is replaced, thus reducing vascular resistance. With this exposure to oxygen, pulmonary vasculature dilates. At the same time, the placental circulation is removed. This increases systemic resistance and prevents right to left blood flow through the ductus arteriosus. The musculature of the ductus arteriosus is highly sensitive to oxygen, and contracts when exposed to the now increased oxygen content of aortic blood coming from the lungs.[13,14] In addition, the ductus arteriosus musculature is responsive to prostaglandins present at birth, and closure may be induced by prostaglandin inhibition.[15,16]

In the fetus, approximately two-thirds of the returning blood enters the right ventricle, causing the right side of the heart to be as large as, or larger than, the left side. With closure of the ductus arteriosus and reduction in pulmonary resistance, a larger volume of blood now enters the left atrium. This increases left atrial pressure and forces the flap of the septum primum against the septum secundum. Effective functional closure of the fossa ovalis

occurs, completing the formation of two circulatory systems in series.

There is very little information concerning fetal cardiovascular blood pressure. In chick embryos, arterial pressure has been reported to be up to 30 mmHg at hatching.[8] In the newborn rat, we have measured femoral artery blood pressure using a servo-null micropressure system. At birth, mean femoral artery pressure was 18 mmHg, increasing to 30 mmHg by 3 days of age, 50 mmHg by 12 days, and 75 mmHg by 21 days of age.[20] In the newborn dog we have measured ventricular pressure by transthoracic puncture of the left and right ventricles with a 21-gauge needle. In newborn puppies, systolic pressure was 35 to 50 mmHg in the left ventricle and 23 to 40 mmHg in the right ventricle. Left ventricular pressure rapidly increased to 75 to 90 mmHg by 3 to 7 days of age and to 120 mmHg by 3 to 4 weeks of age, while right ventricular pressure remained at 20 to 30 mmHg (unpublished data).

FETAL AND NEONATAL MYOCARDIAL CELL GROWTH

In fetal life, right ventricular blood flow is approximately twice that of the left ventricle. As a result, right ventricular muscle mass equals or exceeds that of the left ventricle until the time of birth. Although very few data are available, pressures in both ventricles in utero are presumably nearly equal, since there is large open communication between the two parallel circulatory systems. Following birth, however, left ventricular pressure rapidly increases, while right ventricular pressure remains stable.

Neonatal Ventricular Growth

In the normally growing neonatal dog, right ventricular free-wall weight remains stable for approximately 10 days after birth. Left ventricular weight increases gradually from the time of birth (Fig. 1-6). Right ventricular free wall weight is only slightly less than the combined weights of the left ventricle plus septum (including right ventricular portion of septum) at the time of birth. The relationship rap-

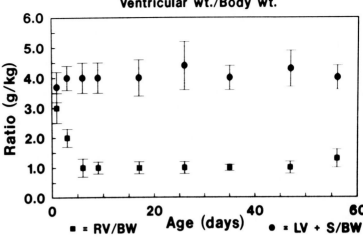

Fig. 1-6 Graph displaying ratios (g/kg) of left ventricle plus septum to body weight (BW) and right ventricular free wall to BW in normal growing neonatal dogs. Values are expressed as mean ± SD for 66 dogs (3 to 17 dogs per sampled time period). LV, left ventricle; S, septum; RV, right ventricle.

idly changes, and by 2 weeks of age, the adult ratio of right to left ventricular weight is obtained. Thereafter, growth is proportionate between left and right ventricles.

Conversion from Hyperplastic to Hypertrophic Myocyte Growth

During the embryonic and fetal growth periods, increase in heart mass is predominantly a result of cell number multiplication (i.e., hyperplasia). Cellular hyperplasia continues into the early neonatal period, when heart growth gradually converts to cellular hypertrophy. In the dog, this conversion occurs at about 2 weeks of age.[17] Thereafter, virtually all increase in cardiac mass is due to increase in myocyte size with addition of other cellular components such as coronary vasculature and connective tissue.

Isolated cardiac myocytes from newborn animals are elongated cells with single nuclei, tapered ends and no clearly defined cell junction areas. Double nucleated cells are first seen at 10 days of age in the dog, are present in 15 percent of cells by 14 days of age, and progressively increase to 85 percent of cells by 6 weeks of age. Binucleation is the result of final DNA synthesis and nuclear mitosis which is not followed by cellular division.[18] This process signals the initiation of hypertrophic cell growth in the cardiac myocyte.

Effect of Work Overload on the Fetal and Neonatal Heart

The type of myocardial cell growth present in the heart when a pressure or volume overload is imposed will determine the cellular response. For example, a tight pulmonic stenosis will produce a load on both ventricles during the fetal period with biventricular enlargement due to an increased number of myocytes. Both ventricles are involved, since there is free communication between cardiac chambers in the fetus, and the massive cardiac enlargement at birth will be due to increased numbers of normal sized cells. On the other hand, canine subaortic fibrous ring stenosis does not typically result in severe outflow tract obstruction until the animal is several months of age. The mechanism of cell growth at this age is hypertrophy and compensatory myocardial thickening will be the result of increased cell size with no increase in cell number. While the clinical significance of these two responses to work overload has received little study, the different mechanisms of cellular response could result in different outcomes to surgical or therapeutic treatment.

MYOCARDIAL ULTRASTRUCTURE

During embryonic and early fetal development cardiac myocytes are poorly differentiated with randomly arranged myofilaments. Cells have a spherical or ovoid shape and intercellular connections are not developed. By the time of birth, myocytes have become elongated and there is a definite longitudinal orientation of myofilaments and organization into myofibrils. This is presumably at least partially a consequence of the molding effects of intraluminal pressure. During the continued postnatal hyperplastic growth phase intercellular connections are very poorly developed and there is an absence of collagenous connective tissue in the interstitium.

Following completion of the last cellular division and the initiation of hypertrophic growth, the cellular ultrastructure rapidly assumes the adult ultrastructural appearance, and all further growth is due to uniform addition of all cellular components.

In the early neonatal period, myocytes have a tapered shape and there is an absence of T tubules in canine myocardium. Myocytes have a cross-sectional area of about 30 μm^2, and the myofibrils are located at the periphery of the cell.[17] Both myofibrils and mitochondria are relatively sparse compared to adult myocardium. Glycogen and ribosomes are abundant. Intercellular junctions are present but do not have the transverse steplike structure present in mature myocardium. Components of the intercalated disc including desmosomes, fil-

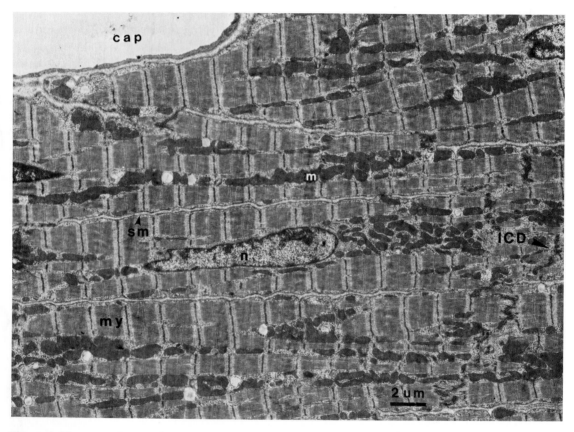

Fig. 1-7 Electron micrograph of the left ventricular myocardium of a normally growing 8-week-old dog. Although myocyte size has not attained that of the adult, internal cell structure is indistinguishable from that of the adult. Note uniform transverse sarcomere alignment of myofibrils (my), central location of nuclei (n), intercalated discs (ICD), mitochondria (m), and distinct sarcolemmal membranes (sm) with very little interstitial space. Cap, capillary. Bar = 2 μm.

ament attachment areas (fascia adherens) and nexus regions are present around the periphery of the cell. Mitoses are frequently evident in neonatal cardiac myocytes. During mitosis there is a dissolution of myofibrillar organization with complete loss of Z-band material.

By 6 weeks of age in the dog, virtually all mitotic activity has ceased and both the few remaining single nucleated cells and double nucleated cells are increased in size. Intercalated discs are well formed, and individual myocytes have the characteristic features of adult heart muscle cells (Fig. 1-7). T tubules are present, providing an extension of the sarcolemmal surface area which penetrates to the deepest part of each cell. The sarcolemma makes intimate contact with the sarcoplasmic reticulum both along the

outer surface and along the T tubules (Fig. 1-8). These junctional areas are the site of calcium and other ion transport into the sarcoplasmic reticulum, an important component of excitation-contraction coupling. Well-organized myofibrils fill the entire cytoplasm and mitochondria are diffusely distributed between myofibrils. Nuclei are centrally located with clusters of mitochondria at their poles. In adult canine myocardium, 80 to 85 percent of myocytes contain two nuclei.[17,19]

The contractile apparatus of cardiac muscle consists of an overlapping arrangement of thin actin and thick myosin filaments together with a variety of other contractile proteins separated into sarcomeres by dense Z bands (Fig. 1-8). The sarcomeres are aligned in series to form myofibrils that have

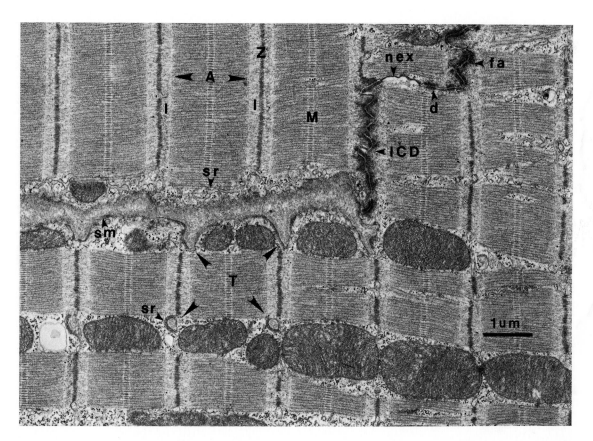

Fig. 1-8 Electron micrograph of normal adult canine left ventricle at higher magnification. Intercalated discs (ICD) have nexuses or gap junctions (nex), desmosomes (d), and filament attachment areas (fa). The sarcolemma (sm) invaginates at the Z-lines (Z) to form the T-tubule system (T). The sarcoplasmic reticulum (sr) is intimately associated with the sarcolemma and T tubules, and surrounds the myofibrils. The sarcomere is composed of myosin-containing A bands (A), central M lines (M), and light I bands (I) flanking the Z lines. Bar = 1 μm.

branching interconnections and extend the entire length of the cell. The myofibrils are surrounded by an intimate network of sarcoplasmic reticulum, which serves as both a source and a sink for calcium during the contraction cycle. Myocardial contraction and relaxation is described later with respect to pathophysiology of heart failure (Ch. 7) and pharmacologic management of the heart failure state (Ch. 8).

REFERENCES

1. Van Mierop LHS, Kutsche LM: Embryology of the heart. p. 7. In Hurst JW (ed): The Heart. Vol 1. 5th Ed. McGraw-Hill Book Co, New York, 1982
2. Los JA: Embryology. p. 1. In Watson H (ed): Paediatric Cardiology. CV Mosby, St Louis, 1968
3. Boyd JD: Development of the heart. p. 2511. In Handbook of Physiology, Sect. 2: Circulation. Vol. 3. American Physiological Society, Washington, DC, 1965
4. Icardo JM: The growing heart: An antomical perspective. p. 41. In Zak R (ed): Growth of the Heart in Health and Disease. Raven Press, New York, 1984
5. Manasek FJ: Embryonic development of the heart. I. A light and electron microscopic study of myocardial development in the early chick embryo. J Morphol 125:329, 1968
6. Lindner E: Myofibrils in the early development of the chick embryo hearts as observed with the electron microscope. Anat Rec 136:234, 1960
7. Van Mierop LHS, Bertuch J Jr: Development of arterial blood pressure in the chick embryo. Am J Physiol 212:43, 1967
8. Girard H: Arterial pressure in the chick embryo. Am J Physiol 224:454, 1973
9. Paff GH, Boucek RJ, Klopfenstein HS: Experimental heart-block in the chick embryo. Anat Rec 149:217, 1964
10. Forsgren S, Thornell LE, Eriksson A: The development of the Purkinje fibre system in the bovine fetal heart. Anat Embryol 159:125, 1980
11. Lieberman M, Paes de Carvalho A: The electrophysiological organization of the embryonic chick heart. J Gen Physiol 49:351, 1965
12. Fishman NH, Hof RB, Rudolph AM, Heymann MA: Models of congenital heart disease in fetal lambs. Circulation 58:354, 1978
13. Born GVR, Dawes GS, Mott JD, Rennick BR: The constriction of the ductus arteriosus caused by oxygen and by asphyxia in newborn lambs. J Physiol (Lond) 132:304, 1956
14. Knight DH, Patterson DF, Melbin J: Constriction of the fetal ductus arteriosus induced by oxygen, acetylcholine, and norepinephrine in normal dogs and those genetically predisposed to persistent patency. Circulation 47:127, 1973
15. Coceani F, Olley PM, Bodach E: Lamb ductus arteriosus: Effect of prostaglandin synthesis inhibitors on the muscle tone and the response to prostaglandin E_2. Prostaglandins 9:299, 1975
16. Friedman WF, Hirschklau MJ, Printz MP, et al: Pharmacologic closure of patent ductus arteriosus in the premature infant. N Engl J Med 295:526, 1976
17. Bishop SP, Hine P: Cardiac muscle cytoplasmic and nuclear development during canine neonatal growth. p. 77. In Roy P (ed): Recent Advances in Studies on Cardiac Structure and Metabolism. Vol. 8: The Cardiac Sarcoplasm. University Park Press, Baltimore, 1975
18. Clubb FJ Jr, Bishop SP: Formation of binucleated myocardial cells in the neonatal rat: An index for growth hypertrophy. Lab Invest 50:571, 1984
19. Vahouny GV, Wei RW, Tamboli A, Albert EN: Adult canine myocytes: Isolation, morphology and biochemical characteristics. J Mol Cell Cardiol 11:339, 1979
20. Clubb FJ Jr, Bell D, Kriseman JD, Bishop SP: Myocardial cell growth and blood pressure development in neonatal spontaneously hypertensive rats. Lab Invest 56:189, 1987

2

Normal Physiology of the Cardiovascular System

Robert L. Hamlin

In order to discuss pathophysiology of heart failure, certain basic principles of normal cardiovascular function must be reviewed. These include (1) heart rate, (2) force of ventricular contraction, (3) interference to blood flow, (4) myocardial stiffness or its reciprocal (i.e., compliance), (5) myocardial oxygen consumption (MVO_2), (6) microcirculation and transcapillary fluid movement into and out of the interstitial compartment, and (7) the cardiac cycle.

HEART RATE

Heart rate[1] (Fig. 2-1) is determined by the rate of discharge of the sinoatrial (SA) node located at the juncture of the cranial vena cava with the right atrium. The SA node has the ability to discharge spontaneously. In dogs, this occurs approximately 100 times per minute. However, depending on the existing balance between parasympathetic nervous impulses (which slow SA nodal discharge) and sympathetic efferent impulses (which speed SA nodal discharge), heart rate may vary from 45 beats/min

at rest to more than 250 beats/min during excitement or peak exertion.

When vagal centers in the medulla oblongata are stimulated, acetylcholine (ACh) binds to its SA nodal receptor sites, decreasing the rate of SA nodal discharge. These receptor sites will be blocked from ACh by administration of a parasympatholytic drug such as atropine. Thus, while vagal stimulation decreases heart rate, vagal blockade by atropine increases it. Atropine administration in dogs will usually increase heart rate to approximately 150 beats/min.

When the sympathetic centers in the medulla are stimulated, norepinephrine binds to its β_1-receptor site on the SA node, and the rate of SA nodal discharge increases. This receptor site will be blocked by administration of adrenergic-blocking agents (e.g., propranolol, atenolol, pindolol, metoprolol). Some of these drugs are specific for the β_1-receptor (e.g., atenolol, metoprolol). Others block both β_1- and β_2-adrenergic receptors (e.g., propranolol, timolol). Thus, while β-adrenergic stimulation may speed the heart rate from a resting value of 60 to a

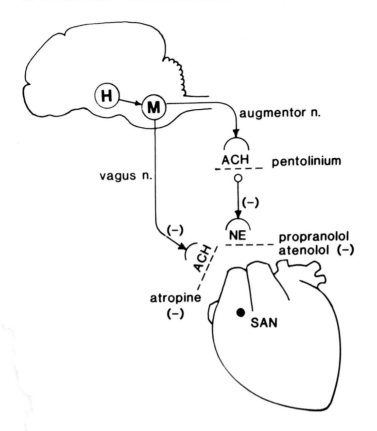

Fig. 2-1 Efferent impulses arising from the medulla oblongata (M) and modulated by the hypothalamus (H) travel to the heart over the vagus (parasympathetic) and augmentor (sympathetic) nerves. Parasympathetic traffic causes the SA node to discharge more slowly, the AV node to conduct more slowly and the myocardium to contract less forcefully. Sympathetic traffic causes opposite responses. Synapses for sympathetic traffic occur in the paravertebral ganglia, whose neurotransmitter is acetylcholine (ACh), which may be blocked by ganglionic blocking agents, such as pentolinium. The postganglionic mediator for the sympathetic efferent traffic is norepinephrine (NE), which may be bllocked by β_1-adrenergic blocking agents such as propranolol (actually a mixed β-blocker) or atenolol. The neurotransmitter for the parasympathetic efferent traffic is acetylcholine, which may be blocked by atropine.

stimulated level of 250 beats/min, β-adrenergic blockade with propranolol may decrease that heart rate to 150 beats/min. Or, if the dog becomes slightly excited, heart rate may not accelerate as much if β-adrenergic receptor blockade is present.

Heart rate therefore depends on the rate of discharge of the SA node. This, in turn, depends on existing autonomic efferent traffic to that structure and the influence of autonomic blocking agents, if administered.

An important modifier of heart rate is mean systemic arterial blood pressure (Fig. 2-2). In general, when systemic arterial pressure is elevated, heart rate slows. Alternatively, when that pressure is reduced, heart rate increases. This protective reflex tends to adjust blood pressure toward normal by changing heart rate, hence cardiac output (e.g., cardiac output equals the product of heart rate multiplied by stroke volume). This reflex depends on pressure sensors within the aortic arch and carotid sinuses, which detect the level of blood pressure.

They send afferent volleys over the vagus and glossopharyngeal nerves to the brain. The brain then sends efferent volleys, predominantly over the vagus nerve, to either increase or slow the heart rate (Fig. 2-3).

FORCE OF VENTRICULAR CONTRACTION

The force[2] with which the ventricle contracts is determined by several factors (Fig. 2-4): (1) the volume of blood within the ventricles just before they begin to contract, that is, end-diastolic volume (EDV) or preload (PL); (2) myocardial contractility, that is, the intrinsic ability of heart muscle contractile elements to generate force (v_m), also called the inotropic state; and (3) resistance to contraction, or afterload (AL).

Preload (Fig. 2-5) is directly related to the forces that distend the ventricle; for example, the end-dias-

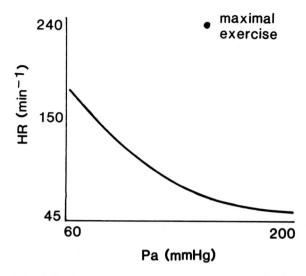

Fig. 2-2 Heart rate (HR) for most mammals varies between 45 and 240 beats/min, and mean systemic arterial blood pressure (Pa) varies between 60 and 200 mmHg. During maximal exertion heart rate is approximately 240 and mean systemic arterial pressure is approximately 150 mmHg. Under nonexercising conditions, as blood pressure elevates, heart rate slows. This is known as the Marey reflex, which is mediated predominantly via the parasympathetic nervous system.

tolic pressure (EDP) minus the intrapleural pressure (P_{pl}). It is inversely related to the stiffness (E_m) of the ventricular wall. Ventricular end-diastolic pressure (EDP) depends on the ratio of the blood volume to the vascular capacity to accommodate the blood volume, the pressures generated by atrial contraction (the atrial "kick"), and the contractile force of the contralateral ventricle (v wave) transmitted through the capillary bed. The P_{pl} depends on lung function.

The functions of the lung and heart are interdependent. The E_m tends to increase, that is, the ventricular myocardium becomes stiffer, in response to most cardiac diseases, dilation, and many drugs.

Myocardial contractility (V_m) is influenced by the state of myocardial health, the balance between sympathetic (β_1-adrenergic) and parasympathetic (vagal) drive, and circulating catecholamine concentration. Both autonomic efferent traffic and adrenal medullary secretion of epinephrine depend on function of the medulla oblongata and hypothalamus and on the afferent impulses to the brain.

Force of ventricular contraction may be measured by peak systolic pressure (see under Cardiac Cycle) or by cardiac ouput; however, these two parameters are also determined by the interference to ejection. In general, the greater the interference to ejection, the greater the peak systolic pressure and the lower the cardiac output. A better measure of force-generating capability of the ventricle is the rate of rise of intraventricular pressure during the period (isovolumetric contraction) when that pressure rises, but the ventricle does not eject. In particular, the maximal rate of rise of intraventricular pressure is a practical and effective means of monitoring force-generating capability. It must be remembered, however, that this capability is increased either by increasing preload (according to the Frank-Starling mechanism) or myocardial contractility (the rate of energy release during the hydrolysis of ATP).

Fig. 2-3 Tension (pressure) receptors at the aortic arch and bifurcation of the carotid artery send afferent impulses along the vagus and glossopharyngeal nerves to the medulla oblongata (M). The intensity of these impulses is directly related to the pressure within the arterial tree. Input from the hypothalamus (H) modulates the afferent impulses from the baroreceptors.

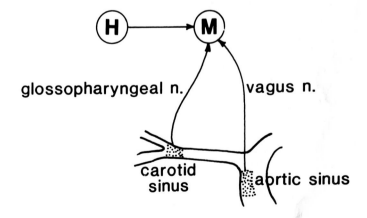

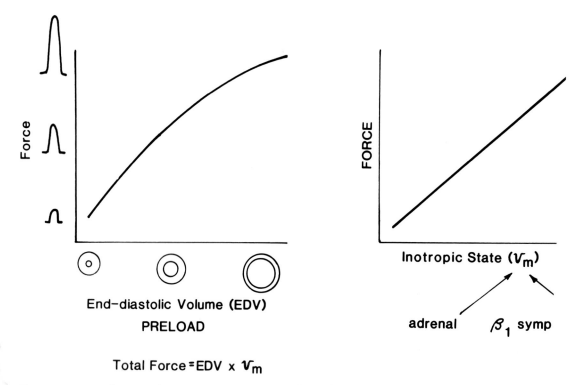

Total Force = EDV x V_m

Fig. 2-4 Force of ventricular contraction (as measured by elevation of ventricular pressure during systole) increases with increase in the volume of blood within the ventricle just before contraction (i.e., EDV, preload). This curvilinear relationship is known as the Frank-Starling law of the heart. Force of contraction also increases linearly with the inotropic state (V_m), which is enhanced with increasing amounts of catecholamines reaching the myocardium (either circulating from the adrenal gland or via β-adrenergic stimulation). The total force of ventricular contraction depends upon end-diastolic volume and myocardial contractility. The resistance against which the heart contracts also determines peak force generated during contraction.

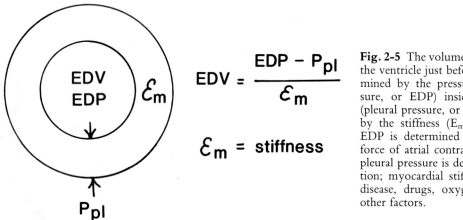

Fig. 2-5 The volume (EDV) of blood within the ventricle just before contraction is determined by the pressure (end-diastolic pressure, or EDP) inside minus the pressure (pleural pressure, or P_{pl}) outside, all divided by the stiffness (E_m) of the myocardium. EDP is determined by blood volume and force of atrial contraction (i.e., atrial kick); pleural pressure is determined by lung function; myocardial stiffness is determined by disease, drugs, oxygen debt, fibrosis, and other factors.

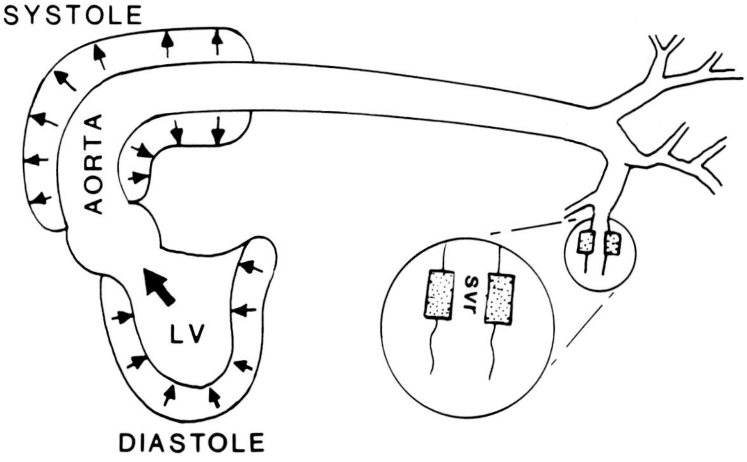

SYSTOLE

AORTA

LV

DIASTOLE

svr

Fig. 2-6 The ventricle (large black arrow) ejects blood into the proximal portion of the aorta. This distends the aorta. The stiffness of this portion of the aorta impedes the flow of blood from the ventricle. Further resistance to the flow of blood occurs at the arterioles (stippled portions of the arterial tree). Both impedance and resistance are increased by α_1 stimulation and $PGF_{2\alpha}$; they are decreased by α_2, β_2, or vagal (V) stimulation, or by prostacyclin (PG_I). svr, systemic vascular resistance.

$$svr = \frac{\alpha_1 + PG_{F2} + O_2}{\alpha_2 + \beta_2 + V + PG_I}$$

INTERFERENCE TO BLOOD FLOW

Interference to flow of blood[3,4] arises from two sources: (1) stiffness of the aorta (impedance) into which the left ventricle must eject blood, and (2) the cross-sectional area of the arterioles (resistance) through which blood must flow before it enters the capillaries (Fig. 2-6).

Normally, most interference to blood flow (e.g., 85 percent) arises from arteriolar resistance; however, up to 15 percent of the interference may occur due to impedance. Both impedance and resistance increase by α_1-efferent traffic to systemic arterioles or the proximal aorta. All autonomic efferent impulses arise in the medulla oblongata and hypothalamus.

With respect to the pulmonary circulation (Fig. 2-7), interference to blood flow is also influenced by lung volume. At lung volumes exceeding or smaller than normal, resistance from pulmonary capillaries might contribute one-half the total pulmonary vascular resistance. Normally, resistance imposed by systemic capillaries is minimal. This emphasizes the interdependence of the heart and lung.

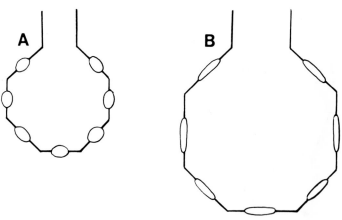

Fig. 2-7 Two alveoli (A and B) are shown, with capillaries within their walls. Note that when the alveolus becomes large, stretching of its wall distorts the capillaries and decreases their lumen. Thus, resistance to blood flow through the lungs is imposed significantly by pulmonary capillaries, and depends on lung volume. Systemic capillaries do not offer significant resistance to flow of blood.

Resistance is usually measured as the ratio of pressure driving blood through a circulation (either pulmonary or systemic) to volume of blood traversing that circulation in a moment's time. Systemic vascular resistance, then, is mean systemic arterial pressure divided by cardiac output.

MYOCARDIAL STIFFNESS AND COMPLIANCE

Myocardial stiffness[5] refers to the ability of the myocardium to resist filling during diastole. Conversely, myocardial compliance refers to the ability of the myocardium to be stretched during diastole. While the physical character of the myocardium causes it to possess stiffness, factors such as the pericardium, fluid within the pericardial sac, and intrapleural pressures contribute to resistance to diastolic filling as well. There are many causes of increased myocardial stiffness (e.g., hypoxia, hypertrophy, most anesthetic agents, myocardial fibrosis). Conversely, there are very few factors that might decrease myocardial stiffness (e.g., catecholamines, possibly digitalis, salbutamide).

Myocardial stiffness can be measured in situ by filling the ventricle to greater and greater volumes and measuring the resultant pressures. The slope of the curve of intraventricular pressure volume during diastole is used to describe diastolic stiffness. The greater the ventricular volume, the stiffer the chamber wall. In a clinical context, increased myocardial stiffness occurs when the ventricle dilates, when the wall hypertrophies, or when myocardial fibrosis is present. It is noteworthy that the ventricular wall is relatively stiff when intramyocardial blood vessels are more full or, at the other extreme, when the myocardium suffers from too little blood supply and is hypoxic.

MYOCARDIAL OXYGEN CONSUMPTION

The amount of oxygen present within the myocardium at any one time results from a balance between the oxygen delivered to the heart minus the oxygen extracted by it[6] (Fig. 2-8). This is termed myocardial oxygen consumption ($M\dot{V}O_2$). Oxygen

$$\text{DELIVERY} \qquad \text{CONSUMPTION } (M\dot{V}O_2)$$

$$\left.\begin{array}{c} \text{LUNG} \\ \\ \text{Hb} \\ \\ \dot{Q}_{cor} \end{array}\right\} \; [O_2] \; \left\{\begin{array}{c} HR = \dfrac{\beta 1}{V} \\[2ex] V_m = \dfrac{\beta 1}{V} \\[2ex] T = \dfrac{EDV \times P_a}{WT} \end{array}\right.$$

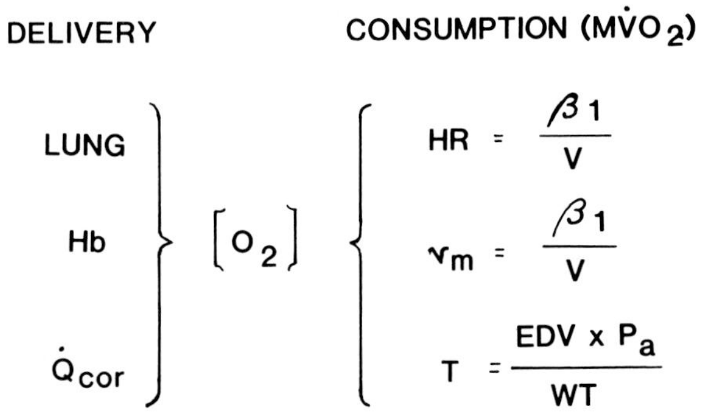

Fig. 2-8 Amount of oxygen (O_2) present in the myocardium depends upon the balance between delivery and consumption ($M\dot{V}O_2$). Oxygen is delivered if the lung functions well, if the blood contains adequate amounts of normal hemoglobin (Hb), and if the coronary blood flow ($\dot{Q}_{cor}$) is sufficient. Oxygen consumption depends mainly on three factors: heart rate (HR), myocardial contractility (V_m) and peak myocardial tension (T) generated during contraction. The former two factors are determined by a balance between β-adrenergic [β_1] (which increase oxygen demand) and vagal [V] (which decrease it) influences. Peak tension (T) is determined by end-diastolic volume (EDV) and diastolic systemic arterial blood pressure (Pa). Peak tension is inversely related with the wall thickness (WT) of the chamber.

delivered to the heart depends on pulmonary function (thus, interdependence of the heart and lung), the amount and quality of hemoglobin that carries oxygen, and the coronary blood flow, which is dependent on forces driving blood through that circulation.

Because of the importance of coronary blood flow, its major determinants must be summarized.[7] As with any tube, the volume of blood flowing through the coronary circulation is a function of the pressure gradient between the two ends (i.e., the aortic pressure minus the right atrial pressure) (Fig. 2-9). However, because the coronary circulation flows through collapsible tubes that traverse the myocardium, ventricular contraction causes their compression and actually interferes with coronary blood flow. Thus, during ventricular systole, intramyocardial tension is great enough to terminate coronary blood flow, even though the pressure gradient between aorta and right atrium is still maintained. During diastole, however, intramyocardial tension falls precipitously, and most of the coronary blood flow occurs during this period. Therefore,

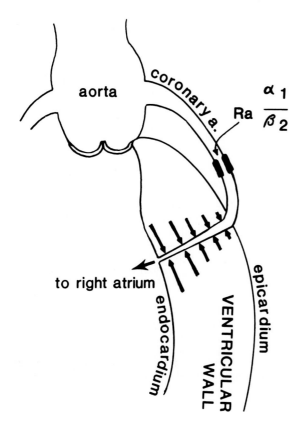

Heart rate and contractility are determined by the balance between β_1-adrenergic and vagal efferent activities. According to the Laplace relationship, peak myocardial tension is directly related to end-diastolic volume (EDV) and aortic diastolic blood pressure (Pa), but is inversely related to ventricular wall thickness (i.e., tension equals the product of intraventricular pressure and internal radius divided by the wall thickness). Thus, events that increase either EDV or Pa or that decrease myocardial wall thickness, increase peak tension, hence $M\dot{V}O_2$. This emphasizes the importance of compensatory responses, which decrease ventricular volume and aortic pressure and keep the ventricular wall thick by establishing concentric hypertrophy.

Two determinants of myocardial oxygen consumption—heart rate and oxygen delivery (the duration of diastole)—can be synthesized in a parameter called percentage diastole (Fig. 2-10). The higher the heart rate, the greater the oxygen consumption and the less time for oxygen delivery. When heart rate speeds, systole shortens, but the

Fig. 2-9 Coronary blood flow ($\dot{Q}$) is equal to the driving force, that is, aortic pressure (Pa) minus right atrial pressure (PRA), divided by the resistance to flow by the coronary arterioles (Ra) plus compression of the coronary vessels by the contracting wall (Rc). Coronary arteriolar resistance (Ra) is increased by α-adrenergic traffic (α_1) while β_2-adrenergic efferent traffic (β_2) decreases that resistance. Note that the compressive forces on the coronary vessel become greater near the endocardium than near the epicardium, since the intramyocardial tension is greater in the deeper regions of the wall than at the more superficial regions. Also, when heart rate becomes more rapid, average ventricular pressure is greater than when heart rate is slower.

coronary blood flow is greatest whenever the heart spends more time in diastole and is least when more time is spent in systole. It follows that when the myocardium requires more oxygen, efforts to slow the heart should improve coronary blood flow by increasing diastole. Oxygen debt could result by increasing heart rate and the time spent in systole.

$M\dot{V}O_2$ is determined primarily by heart rate, myocardial contractility, and myocardial tension.

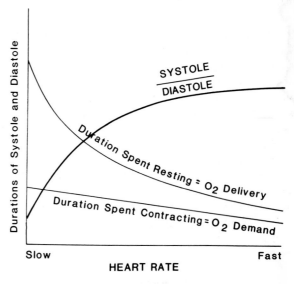

Fig. 2-10 Duration of systole and diastole and the ratio of systole to diastole are plotted against heart rate. Duration in diastole represents the time that coronary blood flows and oxygen is delivered to the myocardium; the duration in systole represents the time that intramyocardial tension obstructs coronary flow and determines the demand of the myocardium for oxygen. Note the distinct advantage for myocardial oxygenation at slower heart rates.

number of systoles increases. Therefore, the time spent in systole increases. However, diastole shortens a disproportionately greater amount, so that the percentage of time spent in diastole falls precipitously.

MICROCIRCULATION

The microcirculation (Fig. 2-11) is a crucial feature of the cardiovascular system because it is at this level that oxygen, carbon dioxide, nutrients, and waste products diffuse between blood and interstitium.[8] Exchange of fluids across either the alveolar-capillary membrane (for the lung) or the systemic cell-capillary membrane (for the systemic tissues) occurs because of a balance between hydrostatic and oncotic pressures on either side of the membrane. Only serum and its solutes could traverse the alveolar-capillary membrane, since proteins are too large to fit through the pores. We shall examine those forces for the alveolar-capillary membrane for which they have been investigated most thoroughly.

The hydrostatic pressure (PHc) within the capillary is approximately 9 mmHg, as a result of the right ventricle pumping blood into the system and the left ventricle sucking blood out of the system. The hydrostatic pressure (PHi) within the interstitial compartment of the lung is approximately −2 mmHg as a result of the elastic recoil of the lung and thoracic wall attempting to move in opposite directions. Thus, there is a hydrostatic pressure gradient of 11 mmHg [9 − (−2)], tending to force fluid out of the capillary into the interstitium of the lung.

Oncotic pressures, contributed by proteins in plasma and interstitial fluid, also influence the transfer of fluid across the alveolar-capillary membrane. These pressures, unlike hydrostatic pressures, tend to hold fluid within a compartment. Because protein concentration is higher in the plasma than within the interstitium, oncotic pressure (POc) of plasma is approximately −24 mmHg and is only −16 mmHg in the interstitium. Thus, there is an oncotic pressure gradient of −8 mmHg [(−24) − (−16)], tending to hold fluid within the capillary. To determine which direction fluid moves across the alveolar-capillary membrane, we merely add these two forces (11 mmHg hydrostatic pressure pushing fluid out and −8 mmHg oncotic retaining fluid within the capillary). Thus, there is a net pressure of 3 mmHg in favor of moving fluid from the capillary into the interstitium. Fluid moves in that direction; however, it does not build up within the

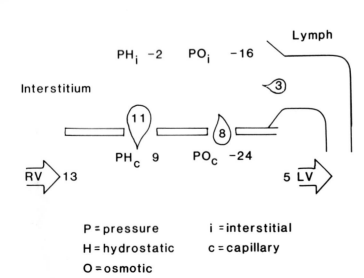

Fig. 2-11 Schematic diagram of a pulmonary capillary wall with two pores. The insterstitium is identified, and the capillary channel has blood forced into it from the right ventricle (RV) and removed from it by the left ventricle (LV). A lymph channel drains excessive interstitial fluid back into the venous circulation. Hydrostatic pressure within the capillary (PHc) forces serum out of the capillary, while hydrostatic interstitial pressure (PHi) sucks fluid out of the capillary. The total hydrostatic force moving fluid out of the capillary is 11 mmHg [9 − (−2)]. Osmotic (i.e., oncotic) pressure within the capillary (POc) tends to hold fluid within the capillary, while osmotic pressure within the interstitium (POi) tends to pull fluid out of the capillary. The total osmotic force moving fluid into the capillary is −8 mmHg [(−24) − (−16)]. The total net pressure moving fluid across the capillary membrane is 3 mmHg (e.g., 11 mmHg pushing it out and 8 mmHg pulling it in).

interstitium, as it is returned by lymphatic channels to the venous circulation.

CARDIAC CYCLE

The sequence of events that occur during contraction and relaxation of the heart is termed the cardiac cycle.[9] Figure 2-12 shows, from top to bottom: aortic flow (AF), aortic pressure (AP), left ventricular pressure (LVP), left atrial pressure (LAP), heart sounds (PCG), left ventricular volume (V), left ventricular wall thickness (WT), intramyocardial tension within the left ventricular wall (T), and an electrocardiogram (ECG). The following description of the cardiac cycle refers to specific periods (I through VI), depicted in Figure 2-12.

Immediately after the P wave (signifying the wave of electric activation traversing the atria), tension builds up in the wall of the left atrium, and that tension is translated into elevation of the pressure (the *a* wave) within that chamber (*I* to *II*). Elevation of atrial pressure forces open the atrioventricular (AV) valve leaflets. Blood is forced from the atria into the ventricles, elevating left ventricular pressure, volume, and tension and decreasing ventricular wall thickness. This is termed the atrial kick, because blood is kicked into the ventricle by the atria. The ventricle has achieved its end-diastolic volume (preload). Blood enters the ventricle during the atrial kick, first rapidly and then at a reduced rate. When this filling changes from rapid to reduced, cardiohemic structures are sent into oscillation, thereby producing the fourth heart sound (S$_4$).

Immediately after the QRS complex (signifying the wave of electric activation traversing the ventricles), tension builds up in the wall of the ventricle (*II* to *III*) and that tension is translated into elevation of pressure within the chamber. The instant (*II*) ventricular pressure exceeds atrial pressure, leaflets of the AV valves are thrown into apposition and forced into the atria until the chordae tendineae and elastic character of the leaflets prohibit further movement. When the leaflets are displaced into the atrium, they elevate the pressure within that chamber—the elevation seen as the *c* wave of the intraatrial pressure curve. As these valves suddenly terminate the motion of blood from the ventricle

toward the atrium, oscillations of cardiohemic structures occur, giving rise to the first heart sound (S$_1$). The interval from *II* to *III* is termed the period of isovolumetric contraction, during which there is constant (iso) volume, although the ventricle is contracting. Constance of volume results from the chamber being closed by the mitral valve on one end, and by the aortic valve on the other. This is the initial period of ventricular systole; it lasts from 40 msec in cats and small dogs to 80 msec in large dogs, and it shortens slightly as heart rate or myocardial contractility increases. The rate of rise of ventricular pressure achieves its maximal value during this interval. The maximal rate of rise is a good measure of the force-generating ability of the ventricle, since it is independent of resistance to ejection.

At the instant (III) ventricular pressure exceeds aortic pressure, the aortic valve opens and blood is ejected into the aorta (III to IV). This is termed the period of isotonic contraction or the ejection time (ET), and lasts from 100 msec in cats and small dogs to more than 250 msec in large dogs. This interval shortens more than isovolumetric contraction time shortens, as heart rate increases. At a heart rate of 60 beats/min, a large dog may have an ET of 250 msec, while when the heart rate reaches 180 beats/min, ET may be abbreviated to only 125 msec. The ejection period is separated into the periods of rapid and reduced ejection. Rapid ejection occurs during the initial third of ET. As ejection occurs, the floor of the atrium is pulled toward the apex of the heart. This enlarges the atrium. Therefore, the pressure within falls, generating the *x* descent of the intraatrial pressure curve. At the end (IV) of ventricular ejection, ventricular pressure falls (IV to V) precipitously; however, pressure within the aorta is sustained by the elastic recoil. The pressure gradient between aorta and ventricle abruptly closes the aortic valve, throwing cardiohemic structures into oscillation. These oscillations generate the second heart sound (S$_2$). Period IV to V is termed the period of isovolumetric relaxation, because the ventricle is relaxing, but there is constancy (iso) of ventricular volume, since that chamber is again closed at both ends by mitral and aortic valves. During the time from reduced ventricular ejection to the end of isovolumetric relaxation (midway between periods II and IV to V), atrial pressure increases as blood from

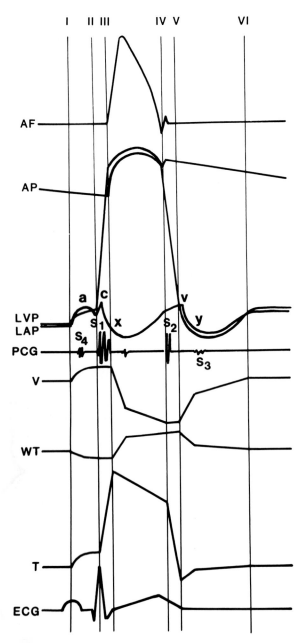

Fig. 2-12 Cardiac cycle curves are (top to bottom): AF, aortic flow; AP, aortic pressure; LVP, left ventricular pressure; LAP, left atrial pressure; PCG, phonocardiogram; V, ventricular volume; WT, ventricular wall thickness; T, intramyocardial tension [=(LVP × V)/WT]; ECG, electrocardiogram. Vertical lines are as follows: I, beginning of atrial contraction; II, end of atrial contraction and beginning of ventricular contraction, closing of atrioventricular valves; III, beginning of ventricular ejection, opening of semilunar valves; IV, end of ventricular ejection, closing of semilunar valves; V, beginning of ventricular filling; VI, end of ventricular filling, beginning of diastasis, Onset of QRS to III: pre-ejection period; I–II, atrial contraction; II–III, isovolumetric contraction; IV–V, isovolumetric relaxation; III–IV, isotonic contraction, ejection period; V–VI, isotonic relaxation period; VI–I of the next cardiac cycle: diastasis; II–IV, systole; IV–II of the next cardiac cycle: diastole.

the contralateral ventricle traverses the capillary bed and veins and enters the atrium. This elevates the atrial pressure and forms the v wave of the atrial pressure pulse. Durations of isovolumetric contraction and relaxation are nearly equal.

At the instant (V) ventricular pressure falls below atrial pressure (period V), leaflets of the AV valve part and blood flows, first quickly, and then at a reduced rate, from atrium into ventricle. Ventricular volume increases from its end-systolic value. When the filling converts from rapid to reduced rate, cardiohemic structures are thrown into oscillation, generating the third heart sound (S_3). This period (V to VI) is termed the period of isotonic relaxation, and it lasts approximately as long as the period of isotonic contraction (ejection).

Following this period and before the next atrial contraction, there is a period of relative quiescence termed the period of diastasis. While no blood moves between ventricle and atrium, the potential energy stored in the elastic deformation of the great arteries squeezes the blood within, holds closed the semilunar valves, and moves blood through the arterioles and capillaries into the veins.

When the heart rate speeds, periods of isovolumetric contraction and relaxation shorten slightly; periods of isotonic contraction and relaxation shorten slightly more; but the period of diastasis shortens the greatest amount. Contrarily, when heart rate slows, periods of isovolumetric contraction and relaxation lengthen slightly; periods of isotonic contraction and relaxation lengthen slightly more, but the period of diastasis lengthens the most.

Although the above discussion and Figure 2-12 illustrate events related to the left side of the heart, nearly identical events occur at the right side of the heart, only slightly out of phase. That is, while left ventricular contraction begins first, right ventricular ejection begins first. In addition, whereas both ventricles eject the same stroke volumes, right ventricular ejection begins first and ends last.

An interesting and clinically important asynchronism between left and right ventricular ejection occurs during ventilation, particularly in dogs. During inspiration, irradiations from the respiratory centers in the medulla produce cardiac acceleration by reducing vagal restraint on the SA node. During exhalation, irradiations from the respiratory centers produce reduction in heart rate by increasing vagal restraint on the SA node. These fluctuations in heart rate attending ventilation (produced by irradiations from medullary centers of respiration to juxtaposed cardioregulatory centers) constitute respiratory sinus arrhythmia. In addition, however, the decrease in intrapleural pressure that causes inspiration tends (1) to pool blood within the right atrium, right ventricle, and all pulmonary vessels, (2) to reduce the return of blood to the left ventricle, and (3) to offer increased impedance to the flow of blood from the right ventricle. This prolongs the period of right ventricular ejection (causing tardy closure of the pulmonic valve at end of right ventricular ejection) and shortens the duration of left ventricular ejection (causing early closure of the aortic valve at the end of left ventricular ejection). During exhalation, when intrapleural pressure swings to a less negative value, the opposite events occur. That is, right ventricular ejection shortens and the pulmonic valve closes earlier, and left ventricular ejection lengthens and the aortic valve closes later. The asynchronous closure of aortic and pulmonic valves and the resultant splitting of S_2 attending ventilation is termed physiologic splitting and represents differences in stroke volumes between the two ventricles. Over a complete respiratory cycle, both ventricles must eject the same volume of blood, or else blood would dam up between the two.

Physiologic splitting is only one clinical example of the importance of committing to memory and understanding all aspects of the cardiac cycle.

REFERENCES

1. Berne RM, Levy MN: Cardiovascular Physiology. CV Mosby, St. Louis, 1967
2. Rushmer RF: Cardiovascular Dynamics. 3rd Ed. WB Saunders, Philadelphia, 1970
3. Folkow B: Role of the nervous system in the control of vascular tone. Circulation 21:706, 1960
4. O'Rourke MF, Taylor MG: Vascular impedance of the femoral bed. Circ Res 18:126, 1966
5. Braunwald E, Ross J, Sonnenblick E: Mechanisms of Contraction of the Normal and Failing Heart. Little, Brown, Boston, 1968
6. Braunwald E: Control of myocardial oxygen consumption. Am J Cardiol 27:416, 1971
7. Gregg DE: Coronary circulation in the ananesthetized dog. p. 54. In Marchette G, Taccardi B (eds): Coronary Circulation and Energetics of the Myocardium. S. Karger, Basel, 1967
8. Duling B: Oxygen, metabolism, and microcirculatory regulation. p. 401. In Kaley G, Altura BM (eds): Microcirculation. Vol. II. University Park Press, Baltimore, 1977
9. Katz AM: Physiology of the Heart. Raven Press, New York, 1977

Section 2

EXAMINATION OF THE DOG AND CAT WITH HEART DISEASE

3

The Clinical Approach to Heart Disease: History and Physical Examination

Rebecca E. Gompf

The most important factors in assessing the patient with heart disease are history and physical examination. The other evaluations only confirm the initial diagnosis. Therefore, the history and physical examination should be done methodically and thoroughly.

HISTORY

The purpose of the history is to collect medical information from the pet owner and establish a doctor-client relationship.[1] The signalment includes the age, breed, and sex of the animal. It may help identify the problem.

The age provides useful information. Congenital heart defects are more likely to be diagnosed in young animals, while older animals usually have acquired defects. In older or geriatric pets, diseases of the liver, kidneys, lungs, or endocrine system may secondarily affect the heart. Thyrotoxicosis, for example, affects older cats, causing various systemic and metabolic alterations, including myocardial hypertrophy and heart failure.

Specific diseases are more prevalent in certain breeds of dogs and cats.[1-8] Congenital heart defects, such as patent ductus arteriosus (PDA), occur more commonly in poodles, collies, and Shetland sheepdogs. Dilated cardiomyopathy develops more frequently in large and giant-breed dogs, such as the Doberman pinscher, German shepherd, and Great Dane and in certain purebred cats, such as the Siamese, Abyssinian, and Burmese (Table 3-1). The clinician should not automatically assume, however, that because the animal is of a particular breed, it must have a specific problem.

The sex of the animal may suggest certain diseases, although very few cardiac defects are sex linked. Females of certain canine breeds are predisposed to congenital defects such as PDA. Male dogs are overrepresented in chronic acquired atrioven-

Table 3-1 Breed and Sex Predispositions for Cardiac Disorders

Disorder	Sex Predispositions	Breed Predispositions
Patent ductus arteriosus	Females	Poodle, Pomeranian, collie, Shetland sheepdog, cocker spaniel, Irish setter, German shepherd
Pulmonic stenosis		English bulldog, terrier, schnauzer, Chihuahua, beagle
Aortic stenosis		Newfoundland, golden retriever, German shepherd, boxer
Tetralogy of Fallot		Keeshond, English bulldog
Persistent right aortic arch		German shepherd, Irish setter
Mitral insufficiency		English bulldog, Chihuahua, Great Dane
Tricuspid insufficiency		Great Dane, Weimaraner
Ventricular septal defect		English bulldog
Atrial septal defect		Samoyed
Dilated (congestive) cardiomyopathy	Males	Large and giant-breed dogs; Burmese, Siamese, Abyssinian cats
Hypertrophic cardiomyopathy	Males	Persian cats
Sick sinus syndrome	Females	Miniature schnauzer
Chronic, acquired atrioventricular valvular disease	Males	Small breed dogs

tricular (AV) valvular insufficiency and dilated cardiomyopathy. Many disorders, however, have no sex predisposition[2,9,10] (Table 3-1).

Other information gained during the signalment includes the diet and weight of the animal. Pretreatment weight is essential in determining the response to diuretic therapy in animals with severe ascites and in measuring the progression of cardiac cachexia. Obese animals often have additional problems, such as respiratory disorders (e.g., chronic obstructive pulmonary disease in dogs), that complicate the treatment of their heart disease. Nutritional abnormalities must be corrected.

Knowledge of the animal's intended function is essential before a prognosis can be made.[3,4] A hunting or racing dog with heart failure may not be able to perform adequately, even after appropriate treatment. Animals with congenital heart defects (whether surgically correctable or uncorrectable) should not be bred. In nonworking animals, heart disease is usually more manageable if the therapeutic end point is to maintain a household pet.

After reviewing the signalment, it is important to obtain a thorough history of all previous medical and surgical problems in addition to the current cardiopulmonary complaint.[1,3,4] Owners should not be asked questions that can be answered with a yes or no response. Instead, they should be asked to describe problems in detail.

The clinician should discuss the following topics with the client during the history-taking process: pet attitude and behavior; appetite; diet; changes in water consumption; respiratory patterns; urinary habits or bowel movements; occurrence of vomiting, coughing, sneezing, pruritus, seizures or syncopal attacks; reproductive status; lamenesses; prior disease or trauma; previous and current environment; immunization status; and current medications or treatments. Once the initial problems have been identified, more detailed questions should be asked. These include the time of onset and duration of the problem, disease progression, compliance, and response to previous and current medications or therapy.

Cardiac diseases often produce clinical signs, such as coughing, dyspnea, ascites, ventral edema, tiring with exercise, episodic weakness, and syncope.[3,4,6–8,11–14] Hemoglobinuria and bilirubinuria occur in dogs with postcaval syndrome due to heartworm disease. An animal may also be presented for signs related to treatment of heart disease, such as polydipsia and polyuria from diuretic therapy or drug-induced vomiting and diarrhea (e.g., digitalis, quinidine, procainamide, aminophylline). Animals with congenital vascular ring anomalies may regurgitate food, which is often mistaken for vomiting.[2] Cats with heartworm disease or congestive heart failure due to dilated cardiomyopathy are also susceptible to vomiting. Vomiting or diarrhea, when exhibited in cardiac patients, may also reflect other diseases (e.g., renal failure, toxemia, gastroenteritis).

Coughing is one of the most common sign of cardiac disease in dogs.[3,4,12,13,15] Dogs in severe heart failure may also present with dyspnea. Stimulation of the pharynx, trachea, bronchi, bronchioli, pleura, pericardium, and diaphragm can induce coughing. However, it should not be automatically assumed that a coughing dog that has a heart murmur has congestive heart failure (i.e., pulmonary edema). Many coughing dogs with heart murmurs have compensated heart disease but are coughing due to collapsing trachea, chronic bronchitis, heartworm disease, or other unrelated problems.

Determination of the characteristics of a cough can sometimes point to a tentative etiology. Most cardiac coughs are loud, harsh, dry, and low pitched. The cardiac cough may be productive with a pinkish-tinged or white fluid if severe pulmonary edema is present. Whenever a dog coughs up non-purulent fluid, pulmonary edema should be suspected. The cardiac cough may be induced by exercise or drinking or may occur spontaneously. Unfortunately, many coughs sound alike, and their characterization is not always dependable.

In contrast to dogs, cats with cardiac disorders generally do not cough.[6] The only exception is cats with feline heartworm disease. In general, cats with congestive heart failure display dyspnea (i.e., difficult, labored, or painful breathing). This can be accompanied by stridor or rhonchi. Dyspnea when exhibited in animals at rest always indicates a severe problem.

Dyspnea may be paroxysmal and induced by mild exercise (exertional dyspnea). If it occurs when an animal is recumbent, it is referred to as orthopnea. Dyspnea can usually be attributed to cardiac or respiratory disease. Occasionally, oxygen-poor environments (e.g., high altitudes) can result in dyspnea in animals that have preexisting cardiopulmonary disease. Increase in the respiratory rate (i.e., polypnea) can be mistaken for dyspnea. However, polypnea can be caused by fever, fear, pain, excitement, or other causes of increased sympathetic tone.

There are three characteristic types of dyspnea: inspiratory, expiratory, and mixed. Inspiratory dyspnea is associated with upper airway disease, while expiratory dyspnea is usually seen with bronchial, interstitial, or alveolar lung disease. Heart failure causing pulmonary edema usually results in expiratory dyspnea. Occasionally, it produces a mixed dyspneic pattern, especially if significant pleural effusion is present, causing expiratory dyspnea.

Ascites is a common clinical sign accompanying right-sided heart failure in dogs but occurs less commonly in cats.[6,12,15] The ascites may be preceded by coughing or dyspnea if left-sided heart failure is present (e.g., pulmonary edema). Ascites can produce dyspnea if the volume of fluid is excessive and restricts diaphragmatic movement. Also, pleural effusion that may be present in association with ascites can contribute to the dyspnea. Ventral or dependent limb edema may occur in animals with ascites and pleural effusion in severe right-sided heart failure patients.

Tiring with exercise is a common early sign of decompensated heart failure. This sign is more commonly noted in dogs, since people play vigorously with these pets and observe them exercising.[3–5,12,15] Exercise intolerance in cats is more subtle and difficult to detect due to the sedentary nature of these pets.[6] A cat will often restrict its exercise when ill. Alteration of a cat's normal behavioral routine may be the only sign it exhibits with early heart failure.

Syncopal episodes occur in both cats and dogs with heart disease but is more common in dogs.[3–8,12,15,16] It can be difficult to differentiate between a syncopal attack and a seizure. Syncope denotes a brief episode; the animal may or may not lose consciousness and exhibit defecation and urination due to autonomic release. Complete recovery occurs within a few minutes or less. Syncope due to heart failure is suspected when dyspnea and coughing are associated with the event; it is a common sign of cardiac decompensation in small-breed dogs with chronic acquired AV valvular disease. Syncope associated with arrhythmias may be difficult to detect without continual electrocardiographic (ECG) (e.g., Holter) monitoring. Arrhythmias are often paroxysmal and the cardiac rhythm may be normal at the time of examination.

PHYSICAL EXAMINATION

After reviewing the signalment and obtaining a thorough history, the next step in the diagnosis of cardiac disease is a complete physical examination. The physical examination should be done in a consistent systematic fashion. No portion should ever be eliminated, even if it appears to be routine or unrewarding.[3–5,17,18]

The clinician should observe the animal on the floor or examining table and observe its posture, rate, rhythm, and depth of respiration. It should be noted whether the animal is dyspneic, polypneic, or coughing. The pet is scrutinized for evidence of ascites or peripheral edema along the neck, head, ventrum, or limbs.

The clinician should begin the physical examination by observing the head and neck. Mucous membrane color and perfusion should be checked. Pallor could indicate decreased cardiac output as well as anemia. Cyanosis is a late change in cardiac disease. Severely decreased cardiac output will prolong the perfusion time to exceed 2 seconds. If the oral mucous membranes are normally black, the ocular conjunctiva can be examined for color.

The mouth should be examined for the presence of severe gingivitis and periodontal disease, which can serve as a nidus for bacterial endocarditis.[19] An elongated soft palate or other pharyngeal abnormalities can cause inspiratory dyspnea. The nose should be evaluated for patency and discharges, which could indicate a complicating upper respiratory problem.

The neck should be examined for abnormal swellings (e.g., thyroid tumors) or for the presence of an abnormal jugular venous pulse. A jugular pulse that extends more than one-third the way up the neck, or persistent jugular distention, is abnormal. These findings suggest right heart failure, advanced AV heart block, arrhythmias, pulmonic stenosis, or pulmonary hypertension. It may be necessary to clip the hair over the jugular vein to visualize a jugular pulse or distended jugular vein.

Tracheal palpation should be postponed until after auscultation has been completed, to avoid paroxysms of coughing. The thorax should be palpated for fractured ribs or tumors. This will also help locate thrills, a palpable sensation from intense vibrations of a loud murmur. The point of maximum intensity (PMI) should be located by thoracic palpation. In the normal cat and dog, the PMI is on the left side between the fourth to sixth intercostal spaces at approximately the level of the costochondral junction. Displacement of the PMI to the right may indicate that the animal was lying on its right side or that it may be due to cardiac enlargement, a mass displacing the heart, or collapsed right lung lobes, allowing the heart to fall to that side.

Decreased intensity of the PMI can be caused by obesity, pericardial or pleural effusion, thoracic masses, severe pneumothorax, myocardial (systolic) failure, or severe hypovolemia. Increased intensity of the PMI can accompany hyperdynamic states (e.g., feline hyperthyroidism), fever, or hypertrophic cardiomyopathy.[3,4,6,14,17,18]

The abdomen should be palpated. Hepatomegaly and splenomegaly may occur secondary to right-heart failure or due to tumors that metastasize to the heart or lungs and occlude venous return. It may be difficult to differentiate abdominal enlargement due to obesity from ascites by palpation alone. If sufficient ascites is present, a fluid wave can be generated by placing one hand on one side of the abdomen and gently pressing the other side. If the clinician is still unsure whether ascites exists, abdominal radiographs can be taken or abdominocentesis performed.

The femoral arteries should then be palpated and arterial pulses compared. A unilateral weak pulse suggests peripheral disease, such as distal aortic thromboembolism. Pulse deficits can be identified by palpating the femoral arteries and auscultating the heart simultaneously. They occur when incomplete cardiac filling is caused by arrhythmias—the heart beats prematurely and insufficient forward stroke volume is produced, so that no pulse is generated. The rhythm of the pulses should be characterized as regular or irregular. If the pulses are irregular, sinus arrhythmia may be present if the heart rate increases with inspiration and decreases with expiration. If the heart rate is erratic, arrhythmias may be the cause.

The pulse rate should be taken and may vary, depending on the breed and the animal's state of relative calm or excitement. Some large dogs have normal resting rates of 60 to 70 beats/min, while small dogs may have normal rates of 160 to 180 beats/min. Normal cats, puppies, and kittens have rates of 160 to 220 beats/min. Excitement, fever, fear, and pain can increase the heart rate. Cardiac disease, especially heart failure, can also produce tachycardia.

The normal character of the femoral arterial pulses should be full, sharply localized, and easily felt with the palpating fingers and should demonstrate a rapid rise and fall in strength. A hyperkinetic (strong) pulse increases quickly in strength, is strong, and loses its strength faster than normal. Hyperkinetic pulses are associated with a large left ventricular volume overload with a rapid diastolic runoff. The pulse duration is short because the blood volume is rapidly drained from the arterial system. These pulses are sometimes called "water-hammer" or "B-B" shot and can occur with fever, hyperthyroidism, patent ductus arteriosus, and aortic insufficiency. A hypokinetic (weak) pulse is difficult to feel. It is caused by poor cardiac output due to myocardial disease (e.g., systolic failure), pericardial disease, arrhythmias, aortic stenosis, systemic hyper-

tension, or severe dehydration (e.g., hypovolemia). Occasionally, pulsus alternans (one weak and one strong pulse) can occur with cardiac failure or severe respiratory disease.[20]

The posterior mucous membranes of the vulva or penis should be examined to identify whether differential cyanosis characteristic of a reverse-shunting patent ductus arteriosus is present. The anterior mucous membranes in this situation are normal, while the mucous membranes in the caudal area are cyanotic. Differential cyanosis is often unrecognized because the posterior mucous membranes are not examined.

The thorax should then be percussed. One of several methods can be used. The thorax can be tapped directly with the fingers. Alternatively, one hand can be placed flat on the thorax, and the fingers of the other hand can be used to tap on the surface of the flat hand (Fig. 3-1). The sound produced (resonance) will be dull over an organ or fluid-filled area. Percussion cannot be mastered without practice but can be useful to detect heart enlargement, thoracic masses, and pleural effusion.

The final and most important part of the cardiac examination is auscultation. It should be done in a quiet room with the animal standing so that the heart lies in a normal position. It may be necessary to hold the dog's mouth shut or close off the nostrils for short periods to reduce respiratory noises superimposed over the cardiac sounds. Respiratory and cardiac sounds should never be auscultated at the same time. Instead, each one should be concentrated on separately.

Thoracic sounds can be generated by noncardiac or nonrespiratory sources. Shivering and twitching may cause rumbles. Movement of the stethoscope across the hair can generate crackles. Incidental sounds must be recognized and disregarded.

The heart should be auscultated in a systematic manner.[20] First, the PMI should be located by careful palpation for left and right cardiac apical impulses. The stethoscope is then placed on the PMI, and the first and second heart sounds, heart rate and rhythm, gallop rhythms, split heart sounds, murmurs, or clicks should be identified. Inspiration may increase and expiration decrease the heart rate through associated decreases and increases in vagal tone, respectively. This respiratory-mediated irreg-

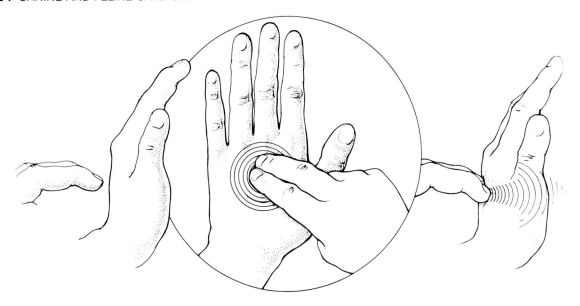

Fig. 3-1 Techniques for percussion of the thorax. One hand is placed flat on the thorax, and two fingers of the other hand are used to tap against that hand. A sound wave is generated that penetrates the thorax. When it is generated over fluid or a solid structure, a dull sound occurs. A higher-pitched sound is generated when the sound wave overlies air.

ular rhythm is called sinus arrhythmia and is much more common in dogs than in cats.[21]

Various heart and lung sounds will produce different sound frequencies. The diaphragm of the stethoscope is used to detect high-frequency sounds, such as the first and second heart sounds, systolic clicks, and high-pitched murmurs. It should be held snugly against the chest. The bell is used for low-frequency sounds, such as the third and fourth heart sounds and diastolic murmurs. It is applied lightly to the chest wall. When applied too tightly, the skin under the bell forms a diaphragm, defeating its purpose. If a sound is difficult to hear, the clinician may need to change from the diaphragm to the bell and to auscultate different locations on the thorax.[20]

The clinician should auscultate all cardiac valve areas because some murmurs are localized. When proceeding cranially from the left apex, the valves encountered are the mitral, aortic, and pulmonic, respectively. The tricuspid valve area may be found at the right hemithorax[22] (Fig. 3-2). The area of each valve sound does not correspond to the anatomic valve location. When initially learning auscultation, it is always a good idea to count the rib spaces and place the stethoscope accordingly, so that each valve

area can be located (it is usually easier to count rib spaces from the back of the rib cage forward).

PMI is usually the mitral area in the dog and cat. In the dog, the mitral area is located at the left fifth intercostal space at the costrochondral junction. In the cat, the mitral area is at the left fifth or sixth intercostal space, one-fourth of the distance from sternum to the vertebrae.

The pulmonic area is at the left second to fourth intercostal space just above the dog's sternum. In the cat, it is at the second or third intercostal space, one-third to one-half the distance from sternum to vertebrae.

The aortic area in the dog is located at the left fourth intercostal space just above the costrochondral junction. In the cat, it is at the left second to third intercostal space, just dorsal to the pulmonic area.

The tricuspid area is the only one located on the right side. In the dog, it is between the third to fifth intercostal space near the costrochondral junction. In the cat, it is at the fourth or fifth intercostal space one-fourth the dorsoventral distance from the sternum and vertebrae.

The clinician should begin auscultation by iden-

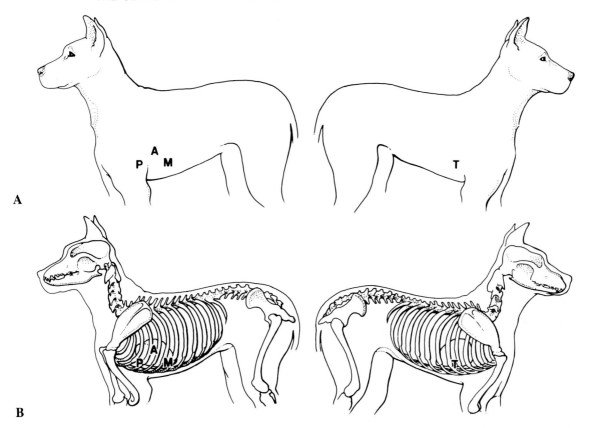

Fig. 3-2 Diagrams illustrating areas for auscultation. (**A**) Relative locations of the four valve areas on the dog thorax. (**B**) Valve locations in relationship to the ribs and the heart. M, mitral area; A, aortic area; P, pulmonic area; T, tricuspid area.

tifying the heart sounds[23] (Fig. 3-3). The first heart sound (S_1) is produced by blood turbulence caused by the closure of the AV valves and vibrations in the great arteries. S_1 is loudest over the mitral area, which is usually the point of maximum intensity. S_1 is louder, longer, and lower pitched than S_2.

The second heart sound is caused by blood turbulence during closure of the semilunar valves and vibrations of the heart and great vessels. It is heard loudest over the left base and is short and high pitched. By moving the stethoscope back and forth between the left base and left apex, the first and second heart sounds can be identified.

Many factors can affect the loudness and quality of the heart sounds.[20,23] S_1 and S_2 may appear louder in thin animals or in animals with a tachycardia. Alternatively, S_1 and S_2 may be hard to detect in obese animals or in those with pleural or pericardial effusion, thoracic masses, diaphragmatic hernias with abdominal viscera in the pericardium or thorax, or bradycardias. Sometimes heart sounds will vary in loudness, especially with atrial fibrillation, ventricular tachycardia, or atrial premature beats.

Since two valves are involved in creating both the first (e.g., mitral and tricuspid valves) and second (e.g., aortic and pulmonic valves) heart sounds, delayed closure of one or the other in each pair can cause splitting of S_1 or S_2.[23] Usually, the valves close almost simultaneously, so that only one sound, either S_1 or S_2, is generated. Splitting of S_2 due to delayed closure of the pulmonic valve is the most common split heart sound in dogs and cats. Diseases that delay closure of the pulmonic valve include pulmonary hypertension, right bundle branch block, ventricular premature beats originat-

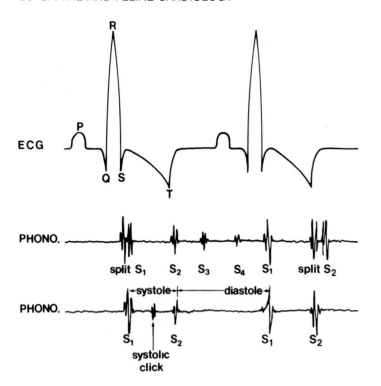

Fig. 3-3 Illustration of relationships between the electrocardiogram (ECG) and timing of heart sounds. Electrical activity depicted on the ECG precedes cardiac mechanical activity shown by the phonocardiogram (phono). The QRS complex represents ventricular activation. The atrioventricular valves close as the ventricles eject blood through the semilunar valves and the first heart sound (S_1) occurs at the R-wave downstroke. The second heart sound (S_2) occurs at the end of ventricular contraction (i.e., ventricular systole), when the semilunar valves close, approximately at the time when ventricular repolarization is at its peak (e.g., peak of the T wave). The third heart sound (S_3) occurs during the first half of diastole, during passive ventricular filling (e.g., between the T wave and ensuing P wave). The fourth heart sound (S_4) occurs late in diastole following atrial activation (P wave) and contraction.

ing from the left ventricle, atrial septal defect, and right heart failure.

Occasionally, splitting of S_2 will occur when there is delayed closure of the aortic valve. This is called paradoxic splitting. It can be caused by ventricular premature beats originating from the right ventricle and left bundle branch block.

Splitting of S_1 is uncommon in dogs and cats. It can occur with right bundle branch block or ventricular premature beats.

The first and second heart sounds should be audible in all normal cats and dogs unless the S_2 is obscured by a murmur or is absent as when premature beats occur. If the heart beats prematurely, such that it contracts close to the previous beat, diastolic ventricular filling is impaired. The mitral and tricuspid valves are forced closed causing S_1, but not enough blood may be present in the ventricles during systole to open the aortic and pulmonic valves. Therefore, S_2 may not be generated. The absence of S_2 can occur with either a supraventricular or ventricular premature beat.

The presence of a third heart sound (S_3) or fourth heart sound (S_4) is a pathologic finding in dogs and cats and constitutes a gallop rhythm. S_3 is generated by termination of rapid diastolic ventricular filling, especially with ventricular dilation and systolic dysfunction (e.g., dilated cardiomyopathy) or chronic volume overloads (e.g., acquired mitral insufficiency). S_3 is lower pitched than S_2 and is heard best in the mitral area. S_4 is generated by atria contracting against stiff, thick ventricles (e.g., hypertrophic cardiomyopathy, restrictive cardiomyopathy), with pressure overloads (e.g., semilunar valvular stenosis) or chronic hypertension. S_4 is usually heard best in the mitral area but can sometimes be more obvious at the left base. Both S_3 and S_4 are heard best with the stethoscope bell (Fig. 3-3).

The presence of a third or fourth heart sound creates the impression of listening to a galloping horse, hence the term gallop rhythm. It may be impossible to tell whether an S_3, S_4, or summation gallop (e.g., superimposition of S_3 and S_4 at high heart rates) is present by auscultation alone. Phonocardiography may be performed to differentiate the gallop rhythms. Gallop rhythms indicate ventricular dysfunction and are useful diagnostic findings indicating organic heart disease or cardiac decompensation.[3,4,6,8,14,17,18,22]

Cardiac murmurs are caused by turbulent blood

flow which develops when flow velocity increases, blood viscosity decreases (e.g., anemia), or flow patterns are disrupted.[5,22–24] They may or may not indicate pathologic heart disease. Functional murmurs can be caused by anemia, which reduces blood viscosity and increases flow velocity, causing turbulence to increase. Fever and hyperthyroidism may also produce murmurs by increasing the rate of blood flow. Large stroke volumes may occur in athletic hearts or with bradycardia and may cause murmurs. Other functional murmurs are classified as innocent murmurs when cardiac disease is absent. Innocent murmurs are usually soft, early systolic, loudest at the left hemithorax, radiate poorly, and wax and wane with changes in heart rate in puppies and kittens. These murmurs may be labile and finally disappear by about 4 to 9 months of age.

Pathologic murmurs are caused by a congenital or acquired structural defect in the heart or great vessels and serve as important diagnostic signs of heart disease. Animals having pathologic murmurs must be evaluated, monitored, and treated if needed.

Murmurs should be described based on timing, loudness, pitch, shape, duration, location, and radiation. The classification of the murmur should be recorded so that progression or changes in the quality of the murmur can be documented (Figs. 3-4 and 3-5).

A murmur is first identified according to its timing and duration relative to the heart sounds. The first and second heart sounds are identified and the murmur's relationship to S_1 and S_2 determined. If the murmur occurs between S_1 and S_2, it is systolic. If it occurs between S_2 of one beat and S_1 of the next beat, it is diastolic. If the murmur starts after S_1, goes through S_2 and ends before the next S_1, it is continuous. A murmur is characterized as being early systolic if it ends by mid-systole, holosystolic if it continues throughout systole but ends before

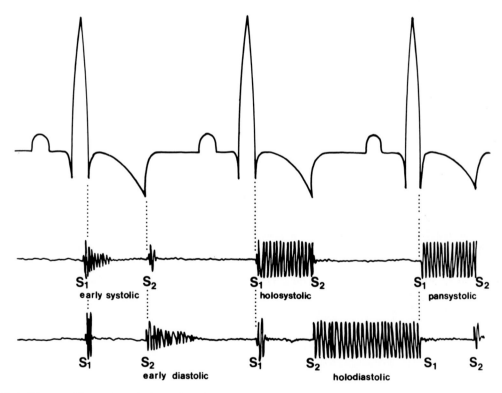

Fig. 3-4 Diagram illustrating timing of cardiac murmurs relative to heart sounds (e.g., S_1, S_2, S_3, S_4) and phase of the cardiac cycle (e.g., systolic, diastolic). S_1, first heart sound; S_2, second heart sound; S_3, third heart sound; S_4, fourth heart sound.

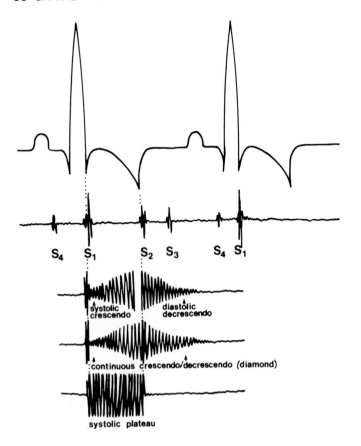

Fig. 3-5 Diagram illustrating classification of cardiac murmurs on the basis of shape or quality. S_1, first heart sound; S_2, second heart sound; S_3, third heart sound; S_4, fourth heart sound.

Table 3-2 Subjective Auscultatory Features of Cardiac Murmurs with Phonocardiographic Correlations

Auscultatory Description	Phonocardiographic Description	Associated Cardiac Anomalies
Systolic		
Ejection	Crescendo-decrescendo (Diamond-shaped)	Aortic, pulmonic stenosis; tetralogy of Fallot; atrial septal defect; functional
Regurgitant	Plateau	Ventricular septal defect; mitral, tricuspid regurgitation
Diastolic		
Decrescendo (blowing)	Decrescendo	Aortic, pulmonic insufficiency; mitral, tricuspid stenosis; heartworm disease
Machinery	Continuous	Patent ductus arteriosus

Table 3-3 Clinical Findings with Common Valvular and Congenital Heart Disease

Lesion	Typical Breeds	Arterial Pulse	Venous Pulse	Precordium	Timing	Cardiac Murmurs PMI	Cardiac Murmurs Configuration
Mitral insufficiency	Acquired, small breeds; congenital, Great Danes, German shepherds	N to ↑	N	↑LAp	Systolic	LAp	Plateau, decrescendo
Tricuspid insufficiency (TI)	Acquired, small breeds; congenital, large breeds	N	↑	↑RAp	Systolic	RAp	Plateau, decrescendo
Ventricular septal defect (VSD)	English bulldog, common in cats	N to ↑	N	↑L + R	Systolic	RSB	Plateau, decrescendo
Pulmonary stenosis (PS)	Beagle, terriers, Chihuahua, English bulldog, schnauzer	N to ↓	N to ↑	↑RAp	Systolic	LB	Ejection
Atrial septal defect (ASD)	Unusual isolated lesion	N	N to ↑	↑RAp	Systolic	LB	Ejection
Tetralogy of Fallot	Keeshond, English bulldog	N to ↓	N to ↑	↑RAp	Systolic	LB	Ejection
Aortic stenosis (AS)	Newfoundland, boxer, German shepherd	↓	N	↑LAp	Systolic	LB, RB, or subaortic	Ejection
Patent ductus arteriosus (PDA)	Many poodles, Pomeranians, collies, German shepherds (female > male)	↑	N to ↑	↑L + RAp	Continuous	LB	Machinery
Aortic insufficiency (AI)	—	↑	N	↑LAp	Diastolic	LB and LAp	Decrescendo

N, normal; ↑, increased; ↓, decreased; R, right; L, left; Ap, apex; B, base; V, variable; PMI, point of maximum intensity. (Bonagura JD, Berkwitt L: Cardiovascular and pulmonary disorders. p. 3. In Fenner WR (ed): Quick Reference to Veterinary Medicine. JB Lippincott, Philadelphia, 1982.)

S_2, and pansystolic if it extends throughout systole and obscures the S_2 (Fig. 3-4). The same timing sequence is applicable to diastolic murmurs, although most do not extend throughout diastole unless tachycardia is present. Continuous murmurs (e.g., patent ductus arteriosus) begin after S_1, peak in intensity at S_2, and end during mid- to late diastole (Fig. 3-4).

The intensity (loudness) of the murmur is arbitrarily graded on a scale of I to VI. A grade I murmur is the softest murmur audible in a quiet room after minutes of listening. A grade II murmur is soft but can be heard readily. A grade III murmur is prominent, of low to moderate intensity, but not loud. A grade IV murmur is loud but is not accompanied by a precordial thrill. A grade V murmur is loud and produces a palpable thrill. A grade VI murmur is so loud that it can be detected without a stethoscope by listening close to the thorax and is accompanied by a precordial thrill.

The murmur should be classified as to its pitch. A high-pitched murmur is one that can be easily heard with the diaphragm of the stethoscope. A low-frequency murmur is heard better with the bell.

Murmurs should also be classified by their shape (Fig. 3-5). A crescendo murmur starts softly and becomes louder before it stops. A decrescendo murmur starts loudly and tapers off. A crescendo-decrescendo or diamond-shaped murmur starts off softly, gets louder, and then tapers softly. A plateau-shaped murmur stays loud throughout. Some heart defects have characteristic murmurs that can aid in diagnosis of the cardiac defect (Table 3-2).

The last part of the scheme for murmur classification is location and radiation. Location refers to the valve area, where the murmur is heard the loud-

Table 3-4 Clinical Findings in Acquired Heart Disease

Lesion	Arterial Pulse	Precordium	Cardiac Auscultation	Other Features
Pericardial disease (effusion)	N, ↓, or changing	↓LAp	Muffled heartsounds	German shepherds, brachycephalic breeds, venous distention—pulsation, hepatomegaly, ascites common; elevated central venous pressure (CVP), $^+$pericardiocentesis
Dirofilariasis	V	↑RAp	V, TI, split or loud S_2	Jugular pulsations, pulmonary adventitial sounds, positive microfilaria, eosinophilia
Canine cardiomyopathy Congestive (dilated) form	N to ↓	V	Atrial fibrillation, V murmur, AV insufficiency, gallop rhythm	Giant to large breeds, males, dyspnea, ascites, often hypothyroid, ↓ serum protein; in puppies, secondary to parvovirus
Feline cardiomyopathy Congestive form	↓	↓LAp	V murmur, AV insufficiency, gallop rhythm	Hypothermia, pallor, cyanosis, dyspnea, aortic thromboembolism, prerenal azotemia
Hypertrophic form	N to ↓	↑LAp	V murmur, AV insufficiency, subaortic stenosis, gallop rhythm	Aortic thromboembolism, dyspnea

N, normal; ↑, increased; ↑, decreased; R, right; L, left; Ap, apex; B, base; TI, tricuspid insufficiency; V, variable. (Modified from Bonagura JD, Berkwitt L: Cardiovascular and pulmonary disorders. p. 3. In Fenner WR (ed): Quick Reference to Veterinary Medicine. JB Lippincott, Philadelphia, 1982.)

est (Fig. 3-2). Each murmur will have a valve area of greatest intensity; however, it may be loud over other areas to which it radiates. Identifying its point of maximum intensity and pattern of radiation is important in identifying the specific cardiac abnormality. Certain defects have characteristic murmurs (Table 3-3).

In addition to murmurs, other sounds can be auscultated. A systolic click may initially sound like a gallop rhythm but, in contrast to a diastolic gallop, the extra heart sound (click) is heard between S_1 and S_2 in systole (Fig. 3-3). They are usually mid- to late systolic sounds, relatively high frequency, and labile. The exact cause of systolic clicks is unknown, but they are attributed to early mitral valve disease and perhaps mitral valve prolapse.

Other auscultatory findings include pleural friction rubs, pericardial friction rubs, pericardial knocks, and ejection sounds.[22] A pleural friction rub is caused by the movement of two relatively dry roughened pleural surfaces over each other. It may sound like squeaky leather and is heard on inspiration and expiration at the same location. Pericardial friction rubs are short scratchy sounds due to diseased pericardium moving over the heart. These rubs will occur with each heart beat. Pericardial knocks can be similar in timing to S_3 and may be heard in animals with constrictive pericarditis when the pericardium suddenly reduces ventricular filling. Ejection sounds are early systolic, high pitched, and heard best at the aortic and pulmonic valve areas (i.e., heart base). They are associated with pulmonic stenosis, dilated great vessels, and severe heartworm disease with pulmonary hypertension. Sometimes they can mimic gallop rhythms.

A list of differential diagnoses is generated after the history and physical examination has been completed (Tables 3-3 and 3-4). Acute medical treatment may be administered if necessary (e.g., intravenous furosemide for fulminating pulmonary edema). Once a differential diagnosis list is completed, further diagnostic and therapeutic strategies are guided by the need to validate or refute the suspected disease processes.

REFERENCES

1. Hurst JW, Morris DC, Crawley IS: The history: Symptoms due to cardiovascular disease. p. 151. In Hurst JW (ed): The Heart. Vol I. 5th Ed. McGraw-Hill, New York, 1982

2. Pyle RL: Congenital heart disease. p. 933. In Ettinger SJ (ed): Textbook of Veterinary Internal Medicine. Vol I. 2nd Ed. WB Saunders, Philadelphia, 1983

3. Gompf RE: History taking and physical examination of the cardiovascular system. p. 3. In Tilley LP, Owens JM (eds): Manual of Small Animal Cardiology. Churchill Livingstone, New York, 1985

4. Gompf RE: Physical examination of the cardiopulmonary system. Vet Clin North Am 13:201, 1983

5. Ettinger SJ, Sutter PF: Canine Cardiology. WB Saunders, Philadelphia, 1970

6. Fox PR: Feline cardiomyopathy. In Bonagura JD (ed): Contemporary Issues in Small Animal Practice: Cardiology. Vol. 9. Churchill Livingstone, New York, 1987

7. Bonagura JD, Hamlin RL: Treatment of heart disease: An overview. p. 310. In Kirk RW (ed): Current Veterinary Therapy. Vol. IX. WB Saunders, Philadelphia, 1986

8. Ware WA, Bonagura JD: Canine myocardial diseases. p. 370. In Kirk RW (ed): Current Veterinary Therapy. Vol. IX WB Saunders, Philadelphia, 1986

9. Mulvihill JJ, Priester WA: Congenital heart disease in dogs: Epidemiologic similarities to man. Teratology 7:73, 1973

10. Patterson DF: Epidemiologic and genetic studies of congenital heart disease in the dog. Circ Res 23:171, 1968

11. Calvert CA, Rawlings CA: Therapy of canine heartworm disease. p. 406. In Kirk RW (ed): Current Veterinary Therapy. Vol. IX. WB Saunders, Philadelphia, 1986

12. Keene BW, Bonagura JD: Valvular heart disease. p. 311. In Kirk RW (ed): Current Veterinary Therapy. Vol. VIII. WB Saunders, Philadelphia, 1983

13. Hamlin RL, Kittleson MD: Clinical experience with hydralazine for treatment of otherwise intractable cough in dogs with apparent left-sided heart failure. J Am Vet Med Assoc 180:1327, 1982

14. Peterson ME, Kintzer PP, Cavanagh PC, et al: Feline hyperthyroidism: Pretreatment and clinical laboratory evaluation of 131 cases. J Am Vet Med Assoc 183:103, 1983

15. Ettinger SJ: Valvular heart disease. p. 959. In Ettinger SJ (ed): Textbook of Veterinary Internal Medicine. Vol. I. 2nd Ed. WB Saunders, Philadelphia, 1983

16. Ettinger SJ: Weakness and syncope. p. 76. In Ettinger SJ (ed): Textbook of Veterinary Internal Medicine. Vol. I. 2nd Ed. WB Saunders, Philadelphia, 1983

17. Fox PR, Tilley LP, Liu SK: The cardiovascular system. p. 249. In Prat PW (ed): Feline Medicine. American Veterinary Publications, Santa Barbara, CA, 1983

18. Harpster NK: The cardiovascular system. p. 820. In

Holzworth J (ed): Diseases of the Cat. Vol. I. WB Saunders, Philadelphia, 1987

19. Black AP, Crichlow AM, Saunders RJ: Bacteremia during ultrasonic teeth cleaning and extraction in the dog. J Am Anim Hosp Assoc 16:611, 1980

20. Braunwald E: The physical examination. p. 13. In Braunwald E (ed): Heart Disease. Vol. 1. 3rd Ed. WB Saunders, Philadelphia, 1988

21. Tilley LP: Essentials of Canine and Feline Electrocardiography. 2nd Ed. Lea & Febiger, Philadelphia, 1985

22. Bonagura JD, Berkwitt L: Cardiovascular and pulmonary disorders. p. 3. In Fenner WR (ed): Quick Reference to Veterinary Medicine. JB Lippincott, Philadelphia, 1982

23. Craig E: Heart sounds. p. 40. In Braunwald E (ed): Heart Disease. Vol. 1. 2nd Ed. WB Saunders, Philadelphia, 1984

24. Reddy PS, Shaver JA, Leonard JJ: Cardiac systolic murmurs: Pathophysiology and differential diagnosis. Prog Cardiovasc Dis 14:1, 1971

4
Electrocardiography

Michael S. Miller
Larry Patrick Tilley

BASIC PRINCIPLES

Definition

The electrocardiogram (ECG) is a record of the average electrical potential generated in the heart muscle, graphed in terms of voltage and time during the different phases of the cardiac cycle. Intracellular and extracellular ionic gradients move across semipermeable membranes and result in cellular transmembrane action potentials. The summation or subtraction of these electric charges generated during the cardiac cycle results in a vector that acts as a dipole. It is measured by the ECG at the body surface. Extracardiac factors may influence the ECG. They include body tissues with different conductive properties and variable body structure.

Normally, each segment of the ECG arises from a specific area of the heart in sequential fashion. The P wave, QRS complex, and T wave are the recognizable deflections of the ECG trace and indicate atrial depolarization (P), ventricular depolarization (QRS), and ventricular repolarization (T) (Fig. 4-1).

Historic Perspectives

The history of electrocardiography as a diagnostic test includes a number of key events. In 1856, Kolliker and Muller[1,2] demonstrated in experiments using a frog nerve-muscle preparation that the beating heart generates electric current. In the experiment, a frog muscle rhythmically twitched when in contact with a contracting ventricle. In 1887, Waller[3] used a capillary electrometer to measure current associated with cardiac electrical activity from the surface of the body. An accurate quantitative measurement of cardiac electric activity measured at the body surface awaited William Einthoven's string galvanometer in 1902.[4] Einthoven also developed the bipolar triaxial lead system and named the specific waveforms produced on the ECG P–QRS–T complexes. Although his 600-lb instrument was used for research, its clinical application as an aid in evaluating cardiac disease developed rapidly. Sir Thomas Lewis used Einthoven's technology and expanded its use in clinical cardiology. Lewis[5] wrote the first authoritative book on clinical electrocardiography in 1913. Frank Wilson developed the concept of a central terminal in 1933 that led to the development of unipolar electrocar-

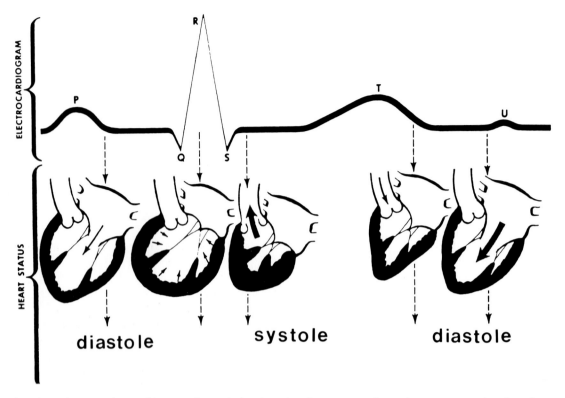

Fig. 4-1 Electrocardiographic waveforms indicating depolarization and repolarization correlated with mechanical events of the cardiac cycle. (Netter F: Clinical Symposia. Vol. 20. CIBA Pharmaceutical Co., 1968.)

diography.[6,7] The central terminal provides an indifferent electrode with small potential change throughout the cardiac cycle. The early recordings of the ECG were not simple and required the patient or animal to place the limbs into large containers filled with saline solution.

Although Waller and Einthoven had recorded canine ECGs, Nürr[8] was the first to approach electrocardiography in the dog clinically. Veterinarians expanded the use of electrocardiography in clinical medicine and research in the 1950s and 1960s.[9-22]

Recording the Electrocardiogram

Electrocardiographic recording paper is usually inscribed with horizontal and vertical lines spaced 1 mm apart. They represent time and amplitude, respectively. The typical ECG examination is performed with electrodes attached at specific body sites. When two electrodes are connected by a conductor (body fluids), current flows and the potential differences are measured by the electrocardiograph (galvanometer). The ECG is a moving record of the deflections generated by the electrocardiograph stylus calibrated in voltage (vertical axis), and time (horizontal axis) and recorded on standardized graph paper (Fig. 4-2).

Electrocardiographic electrodes (leads) sample cardiac potentials at the body surface. The electrocardiograph can combine the electrodes on the body (right and left arms, left leg and exploring electrode) into the specific combinations or leads (Table 4-1). They include bipolar standard limb leads I, II, and III (Fig. 4-3), unipolar limb leads aVR, aVL, and aVF (Fig. 4-4), and unipolar precordial (thoracic) leads CV_6LL, CV_6LU, CV_5RL, and V_{10}. Right lateral recumbency is the standard body position for recording the ECG in the eupneic animal (Fig. 4-5). If respiratory distress is evident, the ECG should be recorded with the animal standing or in a sternal position. Electrodes should be placed just above the olecranons and over the patellar ligaments for bipolar standard and augmented unipolar limb leads.

Precordial leads may be helpful in confirming

Fig. 4-2 Electrocardiographic grid lines. At the standard paper speed of 50 mm/sec, the interval between two heavily drawn vertical lines is 0.10 second and between two fine vertical lines, 0.02 second. At the normal standardization setting, 10 mm (10 small boxes) is equal to 1.0 mV, so each small vertical box is 0.1 mV. (Tilley LP: Essentials of Canine and Feline Electrocardiography. 2nd Ed. Lea & Febiger, Philadelphia, 1985.)

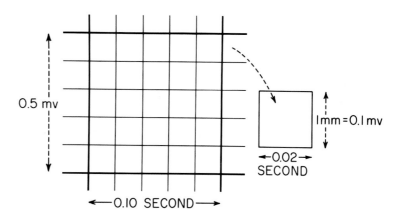

areas of cardiac enlargement, emphasizing the deflections of the standard limb leads (e.g., may be important if P waves are not clearly visible), and for confirming data on the other limb leads. When the ECG lead selector is set to the V position, the exploring electrode is measured against the zero reference equivalent formed by the connected three limb electrodes. The exploring electrode measures potential from its specific location compared with the zero potential at the center of the heart and is the positive pole of each unipolar precordial lead.

Orthogonal leads are oriented perpendicular to each other and view the heart in different planes (leads X, Y, and Z).[22] The X lead measures the frontal plane directed from right to left and is approximated by lead I. The Y lead axis indicates a mid-sagittal plane oriented craniocaudally and is approximated by lead aVF. The Z lead represents the transverse plane directed ventral to dorsal and is approximated by lead V_{10}. The orthogonal leads can be used to generate a vectorcardiogram. Accurate orthogonal lead systems have been introduced (McFee, Schmidt, and Frank lead systems) and require utilization of multiple electrodes at precise locations on the body.

Technical or mechanical problems that are superimposed on or distort the normal P–QRS–T complexes are known as artifact.[22] For accurate ECG interpretation, it is essential to recognize artifact and eliminate the source. Electric 60-cycle artifact may be due to poor electric grounding of the ECG machine, animal, or table on which the animal is positioned. It is recognized on the ECG strip as a regular sequence of fine, sharp, vertical oscillations. Other equipment in the area that uses electric current may cause electric artifact as well. Muscle tremor or body movement may also cause artifact, and efforts should be made to calm the animal and make it comfortable. The placement of a hand on the animal's thorax or blowing into the animal's face may aid in minimizing muscular tremor and res-

Table 4-1 Electrocardiograph Lead System

Bipolar standard leads
Lead I: right arm (−) compared with left arm (+)
Lead II: right arm (−) compared with left leg (+)
Lead III: left arm (−) compared with left leg (+)

Augmented unipolar limb leads
Lead aVR: right arm (+) compared with left arm and left leg (−)
Lead aVL: left arm (+) compared with right arm and left leg (−)
Lead aVF: left leg (+) compared with right and left arms (−)

Special leads
Unipolar precordial chest leads
Lead CV_5RL (rV_2): fifth right intercostal space near edge of sternum
Lead CV_6LL (V_2): sixth left intercostal space near edge of sternum
Lead CV_6LU (V_4): sixth left intercostal space at costochondral junction
Lead V_{10}: over dorsal spinous process of seventh thoracic vertebra
Modified orthogonal lead systems
Lead X: lead I; right (−) to left (+)
Lead Y: lead aVF; cranial (−) to caudal (+)
Lead Z: lead V_{10}; ventral (−) to dorsal (+)

(Tilley LP: Essentials of Canine and Feline Electrocardiography. Interpretation and Management. 2nd Ed. Lea & Febiger, Philadelphia, 1985.)

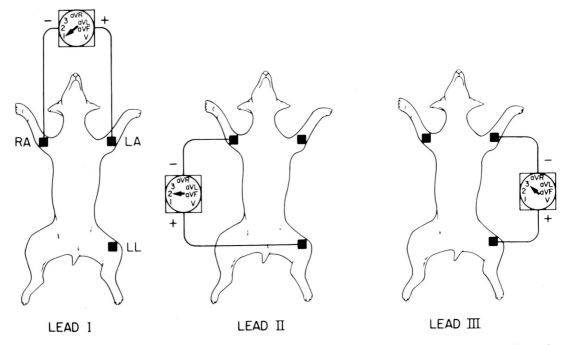

Fig. 4-3 Bipolar standard leads I, II, and III. (Tilley LP: Essentials of Canine and Feline Electrocardiography. 2nd Ed. Lea & Febiger, Philadelphia, 1985.)

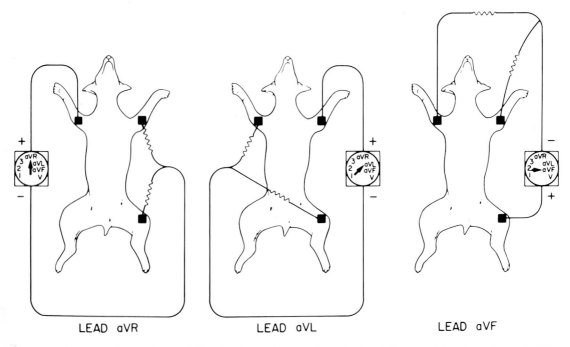

Fig. 4-4 Augmented unipolar limb leads aVR, aVL, and aVF. (Tilley LP: Essentials of Canine and Feline Electrocardiography. 2nd Ed. Lea & Febiger, Philadelphia, 1985.)

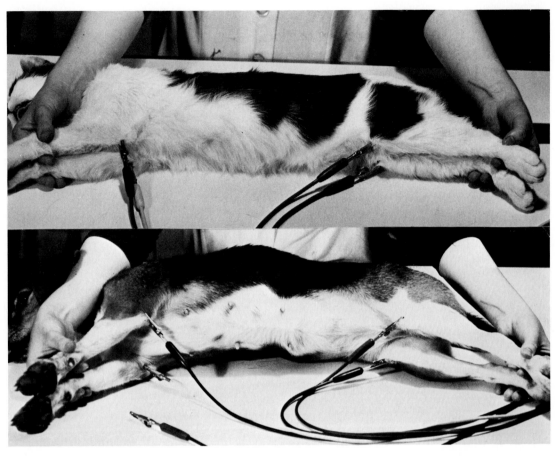

Fig. 4-5 Right lateral recumbency displaying proper electrode placement for recording the ECG in a eupneic animal. (Tilley LP: Essentials of Canine and Feline Electrocardiography. 2nd Ed. Lea & Febiger, Philadelphia, 1985.)

piratory motion. It is important to position the electrode clips correctly and hold the limbs away from the body during the right lateral recumbent position to prevent the electrodes from moving with thoracic respiratory motions (Fig. 4-5).

Vectorcardiography

Another method of recording electric potentials resulting from the cardiac cycle is the vectorcardiogram (Fig. 4-6). Using a cathode ray oscilloscope, it may be projected in the frontal, horizontal, and sagittal planes. In contrast to an ECG lead recording instantaneous vectors (i.e., electric potentials) in a single axis, the vectorcardiogram records electric events simultaneously in two perpendicular axes as a loop recording.[2,19] Vectorcardiography is useful in teaching and research but is rarely used in clinical practice.

BASIC ELECTROPHYSIOLOGIC PRINCIPLES

Each type of cardiac cell has a characteristic transmembrane action potential that is responsible for passing the cardiac impulse from one cell to the next. The summation of these sequential transmembrane action potentials result in the electric activity recorded on the surface ECG. Intracellular properties of automaticity, excitability, conductivity, and refractoriness are important when considering antiarrhythmic drugs (Chs. 13 through 15).

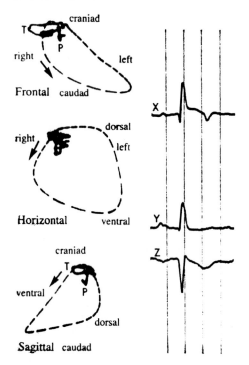

Fig. 4-6 Example of a vectorcardiogram recorded in a dog with right ventricular hypertrophy secondary to heartworm disease. The initial ventricular forces are prolonged and oriented toward the right (0.014 second). Scalar time lines: 0.1 second; teardrops: 0.002 second. (Ettinger SJ, Suter PF: Canine Cardiology. WB Saunders, Philadelphia, 1970.)

Transmembrane Action Potential

A myocardial cell transmembrane action potential may be divided into four recognizable phases[2,22,23] (Fig. 4-7). A negative resting potential, termed phase 4, is characterized by an electrochemical gradient (approximately −90 mV) from intracellular to extracellular. The rapid upstroke of the action potential (phase 0) represents cellular depolarization due to rapid movement of extracellular to intracellular sodium ions (fast sodium channel). Phase 1 is termed the overshoot and is caused by excessive sodium ion entry into the cells. The sodium influx stops and the membrane potential drops toward 0 mV. The slow calcium ion channels open, permitting extracellular to intracellular calcium flow and causing the plateau (phase 2) of the action potential. During the plateau phase, the cardiac cell cannot be restimulated (refractory period). This allows for co-ordination between the electrical and mechanical functions of the cell. At the end of the plateau, the slow intracellular calcium channels close, potassium flow out of the cell persists, and intracellular negativity (phase 3) is re-established. This is termed repolarization. The cardiac cell at the resting potential can then be activated by an electrical or chemical stimulus and is said to be excitable (Ch. 13).

Although the transmembrane action potentials of atrial and ventricular fibers are similar, they differ from pacemaker cell transmembrane potentials (Figs. 13-1,2). Pacemaker cells possess automaticity. They are characterized by a low resting membrane potential, slow activation during phase 0, short action potential duration, no overshoot, and spontaneous depolarization during phase 4, until the threshold potential is reached. Automaticity is the capability of a cell to depolarize spontaneously, reach threshold potential, and initiate an action potential.[23] Such impulses can activate the entire heart. Automaticity is thought to be due to a slow buildup of positive ions (slow calcium channel) inside the cell, resulting in a net inward current during phase 4, until the threshold potential is reached. Pacemaker cells have a slower upstroke and lower amplitude than myocardial cells. Conductivity is the ability of a cell's action potential to produce electric current that stimulates adjacent cell membranes to their threshold potential and depolarize.

Many areas of the heart other than the sinus node have cells that are capable of automaticity, that is, some cells in the atria, mitral and tricuspid valves, distal atrioventricular (AV) nodal and AV junctional tissues, and the His-Purkinje system. Normally, these latent pacemaker cells reach threshold later than do sinus node cells and are thus stimulated before they automatically depolarize. Intracellular properties of automaticity, excitability, conductivity, and refractoriness are extremely important when normal and abnormal cardiac rhythms (arrhythmias) are being considered.

Surface Electrocardiogram

The waveforms of the ECG are scalar records of the electric potentials generated by the heart as projected at the surface of the body.[24] A scalar quantity has magnitude and sense (i.e., positive or negative), but not direction. A vector quantity has mag-

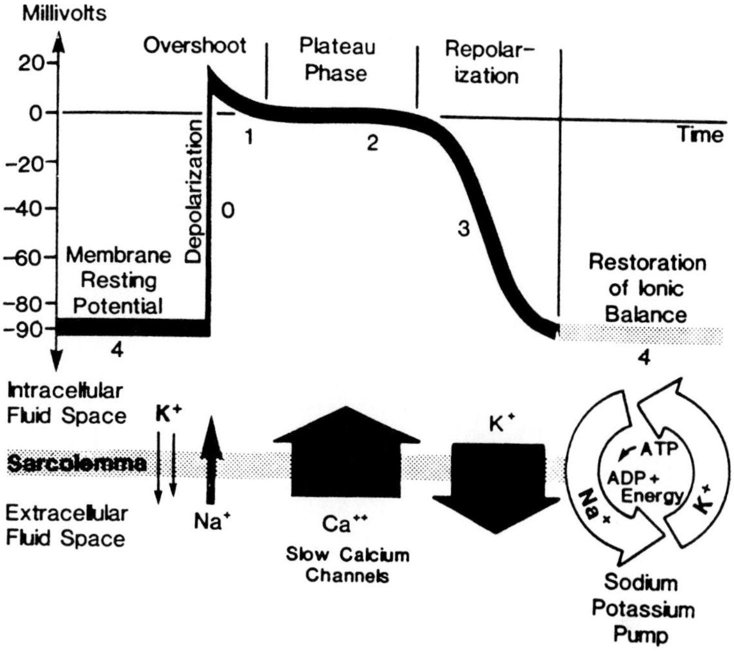

Fig. 4-7 Phases and ionic gradients of the cardiac cell transmembrane action potential. (Lipman BS, Dunn M, Massie E: Clinical Electrocardiography. 7th Ed. Year Book Medical Publishers, Chicago, 1984. Reproduced with permission)

nitude, sense, and direction and may be the result of two or more scalar forces (e.g., two ECG leads) or multiple vector forces. The surface ECG is a recording of the mathematical summation of the electrical activity of all the individual cardiac muscle cells. This electric activity is modified by the spatial relationships of each cardiac cell to all other cardiac cells, the time sequence of activation of the cardiac cells (i.e., they do not all depolarize simultaneously), and the characteristics of the body as an electric field.[25] For example, the first and last ventricular myocardial cells that are stimulated depolarize asynchronously. A difference in electric potential occurs during this depolarization period which results in the QRS complex.

Abnormalities in depolarization result in QRS complex alterations. Disturbances in repolarization are reflected by changes in the ST segment or T wave. These changes may be related to cardiac or extracardiac disorders.

Equivalent Dipole Theory

A review of the dipolar hypothesis can provide a theoretical basis for clinical ECG interpretation. A single pair of equal and opposite charges that are in close proximity to each other constitute an electrical generator, termed a dipole. If the dipole is immersed in a conducting medium (e.g., body fluids), the dipole will generate an electric field throughout the conducting medium.[22,24,26,27] The electric potential measured at any position in the electric field depends on the position of the recording electrode with respect to the positive and negative charges of the dipole. If any two points (electrodes) with a different potential in the electric field are connected by a superior electric conductor (e.g., the ECG lead wires), the potential difference between the electrodes will result in a flow of current through the wires. This electromotive force or voltage is the quantity measured by the surface ECG.

Numerous surface dipoles are formed by the individual myocardial cells and muscle bundles and move during the depolarization-repolarization process (Fig. 4-8). They create an electric field in the surrounding body tissues and fluids and can be represented by vectors that point toward the positive charge. Dipoles differ in orientation and polarity due to their varied spatial relationships in the multidimensional heart. At any given instant during ventricular depolarization or repolarization, all the dipoles can be integrated and a resultant dipole or vector obtained by the ECG.

This equivalent dipole theory assumes that elec-

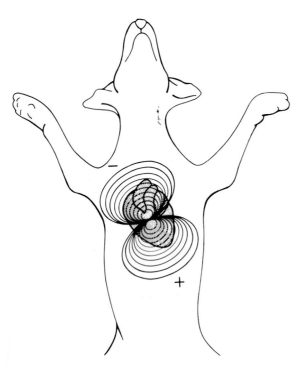

Fig. 4-8 The electric potential of the heart can be determined at an external point and resolved into a single electric force or vector that acts as a dipole. One-half of the dipole or electric field is positive, and the opposite half is negative. When electrodes are attached to the skin on the legs, the electric activity of the heart can be recorded by an electrocardiograph. (Tilley LP: Essentials of Canine and Feline Electrocardiography. 2nd Ed. Lea & Febiger, Philadelphia, 1985.)

tric potentials at the body surface can be represented at any instant by a single resultant dipole vector.[24] Although this concept is oversimplified, it is applicable to surface ECG. The resultant force registered in any given bipolar lead is in direct proportion to the projection of the instantaneous vector on the axis of the lead and is inversely proportional to the cube of the distance between the dipole and each of the lead electrodes. This vector concept was used by Einthoven to determine the mean electric axis of the extremity leads (I, II, and III).

The dipole theory has been criticized because heart muscle is anisotropic (i.e., does not conduct homogeneously in all directions). More accurate analysis of body surface potentials uses the electric field produced from epicardial potentials. Maps de-

scribing potential distribution of the body surface (isopotential lines) can be constructed.[28,29]

THE APPROACH TO THE ELECTROCARDIOGRAM

Indications for Electrocardiography

Electrocardiography is useful in clinical veterinary practice (1) in the definitive diagnosis of cardiac arrhythmias, (2) as an adjunct to determine cardiac enlargement (dilation or hypertrophy), and (3) as an indicator of certain electrolyte, acid-base, systemic, or metabolic disorders (Table 4-2).

Use of the ECG as Part of the Cardiac Data Base

Effective therapeutic management for arrhythmias, heart failure, and a variety of systemic and metabolic disorders is based on an accurate ECG diagnosis. Certain arrhythmias are highly correlated with specific diseases or syndromes (e.g., atrial fi-

Table 4-2 Clinical Indications for Electrocardiography

Arrhythmias
Cardiac monitoring (anesthesia; critical care)
Pacemaker dysfunction
Heart chamber enlargement
Drug effects or toxicities
Myocardial disease
Congenital heart disease
Acquired valvular heart disease
Pericardial disease
Heart failure
Endocrine disorders (e.g., thyrotoxicosis)
Electrolyte imbalance (potassium, calcium)
Acid-base abnormalities
Shock
Dyspnea
Syncope or seizures
Heart murmurs
Gallop rhythms
Cyanosis
Geriatric or presurgical workup
Systemic diseases

brillation and large-breed dog dilated cardiomy-opathy, ventricular arrhythmias and boxer cardio-myopathy, and sick sinus syndrome in schnauzers).

Cardiac lesions do not always correlate with ECG abnormalities. Moreover, a morphologically normal heart may develop lethal arrhythmias in a variety of diseases (e.g., gastric volvulus-dilation-torsion, shock) or with cardiac disorders that become progressively worse.

A large source of confusion involves animals in congestive heart failure with a normal ECG. Abnormalities in cardiac electric activity do not always correlate with cardiac structural or functional derangement during heart failure. For example, myocardial function may be adequate in small-breed dogs with acquired chronic mitral valvular insufficiency. These hearts may be structurally abnormal from a chronic volume overload.[30] Many of these animals have a normal ECG. Other factors may obscure ECG evidence of cardiac chamber enlargement such as body conformation or the dampening effects of pericardial or pleural effusion or obesity.

The ECG may be useful in evaluating animals with metabolic diseases such as endocrinopathies (e.g., hypoadrenocorticism, thyrotoxicosis, pheochromocytoma) or systemic disorders (e.g., shock, neoplasia) (Ch. 27). Severe electrolyte disorders, acid-base disturbances, or metabolic changes may affect electrochemical gradients of myocardial cells and cause ECG changes. In these instances, ECG abnormalities may reflect systemic disease, not organic heart disease. It is therefore essential to correlate the ECG with other diagnostic findings. The ECG should not be used alone without the support of the data base and clinical judgment[31] (Table 4-2).

An ECG is needed to individualize heart failure therapy. Arrhythmias or conduction disturbances with intercurrent heart failure will complicate therapy. *No animal should be given cardiac medication without first evaluating an ECG.* It should be emphasized, however, that *the ECG has limitations and is only a laboratory test that must be interpreted in conjunction with the data base* (i.e., history, physical examination, radiographs, clinical pathology profile). Therefore, the clinician must realize that the ECG has many limitations and may be normal in many clinical syndromes. These include some cases of congestive heart failure, pulmonary thromboembolism, con-genital or acquired valvular disease, and inflammatory heart disease.

Transcription of the Electrocardiogram

The primary function of the heart is to pump blood effectively to the body in an orderly fashion. Atrial and ventricular contractions are preceded by electric activity that initiates excitation-contraction coupling of myocardial cells. The sequence of normal electric activation of the heart is illustrated (Fig. 4-9). The cardiac impulse originates in the pacemaking cells of the sinus node located at the junction of the cranial vena cava and right atrium. A depolarization (activation) wave spreads through specialized internodal tracts to activate first the right and then the left atrium. The cardiac impulse then slows dramatically while traversing the specialized conduction tissue of the AV node and AV junctional tissue. This delay facilitates more effective synchronized atrial and ventricular contractions. When the impulse emerges from the AV junctional tissue, its velocity increases through the bundle of His, right bundle branch, common left bundle branch, anterior and posterior divisions of the common left bundle branch, and Purkinje network. The cardiac impulse emerges from the Purkinje network and then spreads by cell-to-cell conduction through ventricular myocardial cells.

By convention, the Q wave is termed the first negative wave in the ventricular depolarization complex. The R wave is the first positive wave, and the S wave is the first negative wave following the R wave. Collectively, these waves are called the QRS complex. Ventricular recovery (repolarization) is represented as the T wave on the ECG. The Q-T interval is the ventricular depolarization-repolarization time. It has clinical significance in specific disease processes. The sequential depolarization of atrial and ventricular myocardial fibers gives rise to the changing dipoles that result in the P wave and QRS complex, respectively.

Analyzing the Electrocardiogram

Prior to evaluation of the actual ECG strip, familiarization with the ECG machine, proper animal positioning restraint, electrode placement, and min-

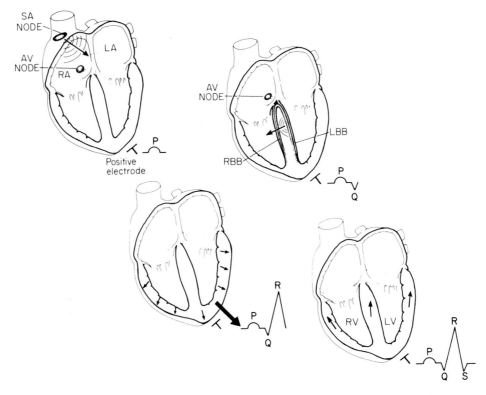

Fig. 4-9 Sequence of electrical impulse conduction and cardiac chamber activation as it relates to the electrocardiogram. (Tilley LP: Essentials of Canine and Feline Electrocardiography. 2nd Ed. Lea & Febiger, Philadelphia, 1985.)

imizing of electric or mechanical artifacts is essential to ensure accurate analysis of the ECG.

A methodical approach to ECG interpretation is mandatory to avoid overlooking vital information. Although many schemes have been advocated, a reasonable approach is as follows. The heart rate should be calculated from the lead II rhythm strip. Both atrial and ventricular rates should be computed, since they may vary in some arrhythmias.[22] When the basic rhythm is irregular, the ventricular rate can be calculated by counting the number of cycles (R–R intervals) within 3 seconds and multiplying by 20. When the rhythm is regular, the following methods to calculate the heart rate may be used (Fig. 4–2):

1. At a paper speed of 50 mm/sec, one small box is 0.02 sec in width. Therefore, the number of small boxes equaling 1 minute is 60 seconds divided by 0.02 sec (or 3,000). Thus, the number of small boxes encompassing one R–R interval divided into 3,000 gives the heart rate per minute.

2. A large box comprises five small boxes and is equal to 0.02 sec times 5, or 0.10 sec. The number of large boxes equaling 1 minute is 60 seconds divided by 0.1 sec (or 600). Therefore, the number of large boxes within one R–R interval divided into 600 gives the heart rate per minute.

3. A heart rate calculator ruler provided by cardiac drug or ECG companies can also be used for rapid determination of the rate. These rulers may be calibrated for the standard human paper speed of 25 mm/sec, necessitating a conversion.

After calculating the heart rate, the heart rhythm should then be evaluated. Calipers are helpful for making measurements. It is important to examine all recorded leads for arrhythmias. The following steps are important in the general evaluation of the cardiac rhythm[2,22]:

1. *General inspection* will show whether the rhythm is characteristic of an arrhythmia or a normal sinus rhythm. If an arrhythmia is present, it should be determined whether it is occasional, frequent, repetitive, regular, or irregular.

2. *Identification* of *P waves* plays a crucial role in the ECG examination. If P waves cannot be found, it is impossible to determine the relationship to QRS complexes. Where present it is important to determine whether the P waves are uniform, multiform, regular, or irregular.

3. *Recognition* of *QRS complexes* and characterization regarding their configuration, uniformity, and regularity should then be performed.

4. *Analysis* of the *P-QRS relationship* is the final step. Recognition of P waves is crucial in determining this relationship. Doubling the sensitivity of the ECG may be helpful in magnifying the P waves. Precordial chest or esophageal leads may demonstrate P waves that are unrecognizable in other leads.

Following the calculation of heart rate and analysis of rhythm, all amplitudes, durations, and intervals of P-QRS-T complexes can be determined on the lead II rhythm strip.

Measuring the Normal Canine and Feline P-QRS-T Complex

Normal ECG values for the dog and cat are listed in Table 4-3. The duration of the P wave is measured from its beginning to the end and its amplitude from the isoelectric line to the maximum height of the P wave (Table 4-3). The P-R interval is measured from the beginning of the P wave to the beginning of the QRS complex. The QRS complex duration is measured from the beginning of the Q wave (if present) or R wave (if no Q wave) to the end of the S wave (if present) or where the R wave deflection crosses the baseline. The amplitude of the QRS complex is the sum of the excursions of the positive R wave and negative S wave. The Q-, R-, and S-wave amplitudes are measured from the baseline to the point of their maximal excursion. The interval between the end of the QRS complex and beginning of the T wave is the S-T segment. The measurement between the beginning of the Q wave and end of the T wave is referred to as the Q-T interval. This time may vary with many factors such as heart rate, cardiac disease and electrolyte disorders. The T wave amplitude and duration is variable and depends on a multitude of factors. Examples of a normal canine and feline ECG are shown in (Figures 4-10 and 4-11).

Mean Electrical Axis

Einthoven introduced the equilateral triangle concept to help analyze the ECG. It is based on three limb extremities forming the apexes of an equilateral triangle with the heart situated in the center. The sides of the triangle are analogous to the standard limb leads. During ventricular depolarization-repolarization, many dipoles contribute to the electric field and may be represented by a single dipole or vector at any given instant. The average of all vectors is termed the mean electrical axis, which can be projected onto Einthoven's triangle. When the three sides of the triangle (leads I, II, and III) are transposed so that their centers are superimposed on one another, the triaxial reference system is formed (Fig. 4-12). The hexaxial reference system (Fig. 4-13) is formed by adding the unipolar limb lead axes to the triaxial system.

The mean electrical axis (MEA) refers to the average direction of the electrical potential generated by the heart during the entire cardiac cycle.[22] It is useful for suggesting chamber enlargement or intraventricular conduction defects. The MEA may be applied to atrial depolarization (P wave) or ventricular repolarization (T wave) but traditionally has been applied to ventricular depolarization (QRS complex). Using the six limb leads and the hexaxial reference system, the MEA in the frontal plane can be calculated. In the normal canine heart, the axis lies between +40 and +100 degrees. In the normal feline heart, the axis lies between 0 and +160 degrees.[22]

There are several methods to determine the MEA. The most accurate (and time-consuming) method involves measuring the net amplitudes in lead I and lead III and plotting these vectors on the triaxial reference system (marked off from the zero point). Perpendicular lines are then drawn from these points

Table 4-3 Normal Values for the Canine and Feline Electrocardiogram

<u>**Rate**</u>
Dog
> 70 to 160 beats/min for adult dogs
> Up to 180 beats/min for toy breeds
> Up to 220 beats/min for puppies

Cat
> Range: 160 to 240 beats/min
> Mean: 197 beats/min

<u>**Rhythm**</u>
Dog
> Normal sinus rhythm
> Sinus arrhythmia
> Wandering SA pacemakeer

Cat
> Normal sinus rhythm
> Sinus tachycardia (physiologic reaction to excitement)

Measurements (lead II, 50 mm/sec, 1 cm = 1 mV)
Dog
> P wave
>> Width: maximum, 0.04 second
>> Height: maximum, 0.4 mV
> P-R interval
>> Width: 0.06 to 0.13 second
> QRS complex
>> Width: maximum, 0.05 second in small breeds
>>> maximum, 0.06 second in large breeds
>> Height of R wave[a]: maximum, 3.0 mV in large breeds
>>> maximum, 2.5 mV in small breeds
> S-T segment
>> No depression: not more than 0.2 mV
>> No elevation: not more than 0.15 mV
> T wave
>> Can be positive, negative, or biphasic
>> Not greater than one fourth amplitude of R wave
> Q-T interval
>> Width: 0.15 to 0.25 second at normal heart rate; varies with heart rate (faster rates have shorter Q-T intervals and vice versa)

Cat
> P wave
>> Width: maximum, 0.04 second
>> Height: maximum, 0.2 mV
> P-R interval
>> Width: 0.05 to 0.09 second
> QRS complex
>> Width: maximum, 0.04 second
>> Height of R wave: maximum, 0.9 mV
> S-T segment
>> No marked depression or elevation
> T wave
>> Can be positive, negative, or biphasic— most often positive
>> Maximum amplitude: 0.3 mV
> Q-T interval
>> Width: 0.12 to 0.18 second at normal heart rate (range 0.07 to 0.20 second); Varies with heart rate (faster rates, shorter Q-T intervals; and vice versa)

<u>**Mean electrical axis**</u> (frontal plane)
Dog
> +40 to +100 degrees
Cat
> 0 to +160 degrees

<u>**Precordial chest leads**</u> (values of special importance)
Dog
> CV_5RL (rV_2): T wave positive
> CV_6LL (V_2): S wave not greater than 0.8 mV, R wave not greater than 2.5 mV[a]
> CV_6LU (V_4): S waves not greater than 0.7 mV, R wave not greater than 3.0 mV[a]
> V_{10}: negative QRS complex, T wave negative except in Chihuahua

Cat
> No well-established normal values to date
> CV_6LU (V_4): R wave not greater than 1.0 mV

[a] Not valid for thin, deep-chested dogs under 2 years of age.
(Tilley LP: Essentials of Canine and Feline Electrocardiography. Interpretation and Management. 2nd Ed. Lea & Febiger, Philadelphia, 1985.)

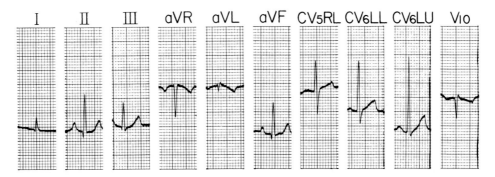

Fig. 4-10 Normal canine electrocardiogram illustrating the bipolar standard leads (I, II, III), augmented unipolar limb leads (aVR, aVL, aVF), and unipolar precordial chest leads (CV$_5$RL, CV$_6$LL, CV$_6$LU, and V$_{10}$). Mean electrical axis, +60 degrees. (Tilley LP: Essentials of Canine and Feline Electrocardiography. 2nd Ed. Lea & Febiger, Philadelphia, 1985.)

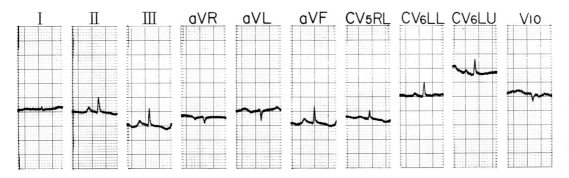

Fig. 4-11 Normal feline electrocardiogram illustrating the bipolar standard leads (I, II, III), the augmented unipolar limb leads (aVR, aVL, aVF), and the unipolar precordial chest leads (CV$_5$RL, CV$_6$LL, CV$_6$LU, and V$_{10}$). Mean electrical axis, +90 degrees (isoelectric lead is I). Note the normal small amplitudes of complexes in all leads. (Tilley LP: Essentials of Canine and Feline Electrocardiography. 2nd Ed. Lea & Febiger, Philadelphia, 1985.)

Fig. 4-12 (A) The equilateral triangle of Einthoven, formed by leads I, II, and III. **(B)** The triaxial lead reference system is produced by transposing the three sides of the triangle (leads I, II, III) to a common central point of zero potential. This triaxial lead system will later be used to formulate the hexaxial lead system. (Tilley LP: Essentials of Canine and Feline Electrocardiography. 2nd Ed. Lea & Febiger, Philadelphia, 1985.)

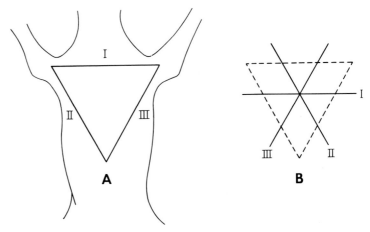

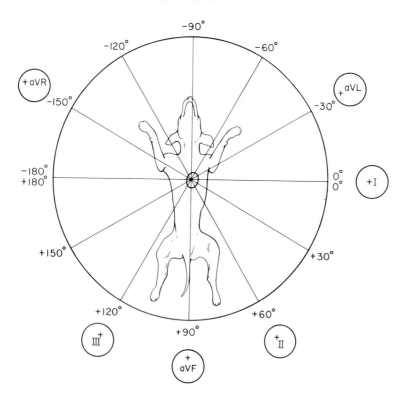

Fig. 4-13 The hexaxial lead system in Figure 4-12 can be enclosed in a circle and used for determining the direction and magnitude of the electrical axis of the heart. The positive pole of each lead is indicated by a small circle. (Tilley LP: Essentials of Canine and Feline Electrocardiography. 2nd Ed. Lea & Febiger, Philadelphia, 1985.)

to their intersection. A line drawn from the center of the axial reference system to this intersection represents the angle (in degrees) of the QRS axis. A more simple (and less accurate) method is to examine all standard and augmented limb leads and identify the one that is isoelectric (algebraic sum of the QRS deflections is zero). The MEA is directed approximately perpendicular to this isoelectric lead in the direction of its net (positive or negative) value.

THE ABNORMAL ELECTROCARDIOGRAM

The first and most important step in ECG interpretation is differentiating between normal and abnormal waveforms. The second step is differentiating between the various abnormal ECG patterns and correlating them with known cardiac entities. ECG abnormalities suggesting cardiac enlargement require further definition with thoracic radiography, echocardiography, or angiocardiography. A simple checklist for this process is provided in Table 4-4.

For further information, ref. 22 is recommended.

All ECGs are *lead II* recorded at a *paper speed of 50 mm/sec* with *amplitude* measured at *1 cm = 1 mV*, unless otherwise noted. Classification of cardiac arrhythmias is listed in Table 4-5.

ATRIAL AND VENTRICULAR ENLARGEMENT

Right Atrial Enlargement

Right atrial enlargement may be determined from the ECG and can be due to hypertrophy or dilation (Fig. 4-14A; see also Fig. 4-16, below). Causes of right atrial enlargement include chronic respiratory disease (e.g., bronchitis, pneumonia, and especially collapsed trachea in the canine), various congenital heart defects (e.g., tricuspid dysplasia), and acquired chronic tricuspid insufficiency. Right atrial enlargement has the following ECG characteristics:

1. The P-wave amplitude is greater than 0.4 mV (greater than 0.2 mV in the cat).

2. The P wave is usually tall, slender, and peaked,

especially in chronic pulmonary disease (often called *P pulmonale*).

3. A slight depression of the baseline following the P wave is sometimes seen in right atrial enlargement. This represents atrial repolarization and is called the T_a wave. The T_a wave can also be seen in very rapid heart rates.

Left Atrial Enlargement

Left atrial enlargement is often found with acquired mitral valvular insufficiency in the canine (Fig. 4-14B; see also Figs. 4-36 and 4-41, below). Other associated conditions include various congenital heart defects, such as mitral valvular mal-

---

Table 4-4 Evaluation of the ECG
for Arrhythmias—A Checklist

1. Are P waves present?
   a. If not, is there other evidence of atrial activity (flutter or fibrillatory waves)?
2. What is the relationship between atrial activity and QRS complexes?
   a. What are the atrial and ventricular rates?
   b. Is a P wave related to each QRS complex?
   c. Does a P wave precede or follow the QRS complex?
   d. Is the P-R or R-R interval constant?
   e. Are the P-R and R-R intervals regular or irregular?
3. Are the P waves and QRS complexes normal and of similar morphology?
4. Are the QRS complexes wide (greater than 0.05 sec) or normal?
5. Is the ventricular rhythm regular or irregular?
6. Are durations and amplitudes of P, P-R, QRS, and Q-T intervals normal?
7. Are there pauses or premature complexes that require explanation?
8. What is the significance of the arrhythmias in context with the clinical setting?
   a. Is there a danger posed by the arrhythmia?
   b. Should attempts be made to directly terminate the arrhythmia?
   c. Can an underlying disorder be corrected, thereby abolishing the arrhythmia?

(Fox PR, Kaplan P: Feline arrhythmias. p. 251. In Bonagura JD (ed): Contemporary Issues Small Animal Medicine. Vol. 7. Cardiology. Churchill Livingstone, New York, 1987.)

Table 4-5 Classification of Cardiac Arrhythmias

Normal sinus impulse formation
   Normal sinus rhythm
   Sinus arrhythmia

Disturbances of sinus impulse formation
   Sinoatrial arrest
   Atrial premature complexes
   Atrial tachycardia
   Atrial flutter
   Atrial fibrillation
   Atrioventricular junctional rhythm

Disturbances of ventricular impulse formation
   Ventricular premature complexes
   Ventricular tachycardia
   Ventricular asystole
   Ventricular fibrillation

Disturbances of impulse conduction
   Sinoatrial block
   Atrial standstill
   First-degree AV block
   Second-degree AV block

Disturbances of both impulse formation and impulse conduction
   Sick sinus syndrome
   Ventricular pre-excitation

(Miller MS: Treatment of cardiac arrhythmias and conduction disturbances. p. 334. In Tilley LP, Owens JM (eds): Manual of Small Animal Cardiology. Churchill Livingstone, New York, 1985.)

---

formation, aortic stenosis, ventricular septal defect, and patent ductus arteriosis. In the cat, left atrial enlargement is often seen with both the hypertrophic and dilated forms of cardiomyopathy. Electrocardiographically, the P wave is of increased duration and is called *P mitrale*. The P wave is often notched from superimposition of asynchronous right and left atrial conduction. Mitral valvular disease can lead to increased left atrial pressure and/or volume, which can result in cellular hypertrophy and atrial dilation. Left atrial enlargement has the following ECG characteristics:

1. The duration of the P wave is greater than 0.04 seconds in both the dog and cat (best visualized in lead II).

2. Notching of the P wave itself is not abnormal unless the wave is wide as well.

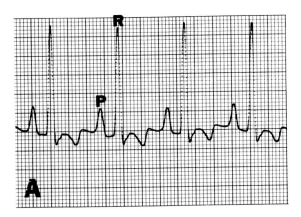

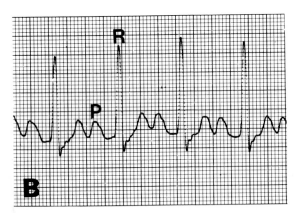

Fig. 4-14 (**A**) Biatrial enlargement in a small-breed dog with a collapsed trachea and compensated mitral insufficiency. The P wave is 0.6 mV tall (P pulmonale) and 0.05 sec wide (P mitrale). (**B**) Left atrial enlargement in a recording from a geriatric small breed dog with chronic acquired mitral insufficiency. P waves are wide (0.075 second) and notched. They are also equivocally tall.

Biatrial Enlargement

In biatrial enlargement, the P wave is of increased amplitude and duration (Fig. 4-14A). These changes could also occur in right atrial enlargement with an intraatrial defect or interatrial conduction defect in the left atria. There is considerable normal variation in the voltage, duration, morphology, and direction of the P wave. For example, giant breeds sometimes have normal P waves that are 0.05 second in duration. The P wave is also very sensitive to autonomic influences. Biatrial enlargement can be caused by chronic mitral and tricuspid valvular in-

sufficiency, dilated and hypertrophic cardiomyopathy, and various congenital heart defects, especially those that occur in combinations. Biatrial enlargement has the following ECG characteristics:

1. The P wave is taller than 0.4 mV (greater than 0.2 mV in the cat) and wider than 0.04 sec in the dog and cat.
2. Notching or slurring of the P wave is often present.

Right Ventricular Enlargement

It is usually not possible to distinguish between ventricular hypertrophy and ventricular dilation on the ECG, so the term enlargement is preferred (Fig. 4-15). The heart is composed mainly of left ventricle. Because of the order of depolarization and the dominance of the left ventricle, the right ventricle must be markedly enlarged to cause changes on the ECG. Associated conditions include certain congenital cardiac defects (pulmonic stenosis, tetralogy of Fallot, reverse-shunting patent ductus arteriosus, and tricuspid dysplasia), severe heartworm disease, mitral and tricuspid valvular insufficiency, acute cor pulmonale secondary to pulmonary embolism, and occasionally, chronic, diffuse, pulmonary disease. Right ventricular enlargement may occur in cats with cardiomyopathy, but this ECG change is uncommon.

In the canine, when any three of the following features are present on the ECG, right ventricular enlargement can be diagnosed with a low incidence of false-positive results:

1. S wave in lead CV_6LL greater than 0.8 mV
2. The MEA of the QRS complex in the frontal plane +103 degrees and clockwise
3. S wave in lead CV_6LU greater than 0.7 mV
4. S wave in lead I greater than 0.05 mV
5. R/S ratio in CV_6LU less than 0.87 mV
6. S wave in lead II greater than 0.35 mV
7. S waves in leads I, II, III, and aVF
8. Positive T wave in lead V_{10} (except in Chihuahua)
9. W-shaped QRS complex in V_{10}

In the feline, ECG criteria for right ventricular enlargement in the cat have not been well estab-

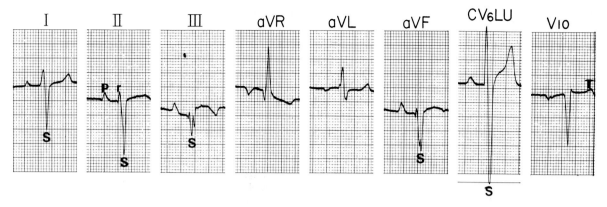

Fig. 4-15 Severe right ventricular enlargement in a dog with pulmonic stenosis. There is a right axis deviation of approximately −110 degrees. Note the large S waves in leads I, II, III, aVF, and CV_6LU. The T wave is positive in V_{10}. (Tilley LP: Essentials of Canine and Feline Electrocardiography. 2nd Ed. Lea & Febiger, Philadelphia, 1985.)

lished. Severe right ventricular enlargement produces some of the same ECG features observed in the dog. The most frequently observed ECG signs include the following:

1. S waves in leads I, II, III, and aVF (usually 0.5 mV or greater)
2. Mean electrical axis of the QRS complex in the frontal plane greater than +160 degrees and clockwise, especially when serial ECGs on the same animal are compared
3. Large S waves in leads CV_6LL and CV_6LU (usually greater than 0.7 mV)
4. Positive T wave in lead V_{10}
5. Right atrial enlargement (tall P waves)

Right bundle branch block (RBBB) in the cat is often difficult to differentiate from right ventricular enlargement. The exclusion of diseases and radiographic signs of right ventricular enlargement supports the diagnosis of a conduction defect.

Left Ventricular Enlargement

Left ventricular enlargement electrocardiographically may indicate dilation and/or hypertrophy (Fig. 4-16; see also Fig. 4-39 below, and Fig. 19-1). The main determinant of ECG voltage measurements is not ventricular wall thickness, but muscle mass. In compensated pressure overload, cavity en-

largement does not occur, and wall thickness is the main dimension contributing to ventricular mass. In volume overload, both wall thickness and cavity size increase. Voltage measurement is greater in animals with volume overload than in those with pressure overload. As a result of the increased muscle mass and hypertrophy, the height of the R wave is increased, the QRS complex is delayed or altered in conduction, the S-T segment is depressed, and the T wave is changed. Prolongation of the QRS complexes occurs only with severe left ventricular enlargement. An abnormal left axis deviation is not diagnostic by itself for left ventricular enlargement. It should also be understood that the voltage criteria for enlargement have some inherent inaccuracy. This is related to the fact that limb, and especially precordial lead voltage, is influenced by the distance between the electrodes and the heart. In young, emaciated, or narrow-chested animals, the criteria for increased voltage are not as valid. Also, conditions such as pericardial and thoracic effusions, pneumothorax, and obesity may reduce the amplitude of QRS deflections recorded at the body surface.

Left ventricular enlargement may be caused by increased ventricular volume (diastolic overload or increased preload) and increased pressure (systolic overload or increased afterload). Associated conditions include mitral insufficiency, aortic insufficiency, ventricular septal defect, patent ductus ar-

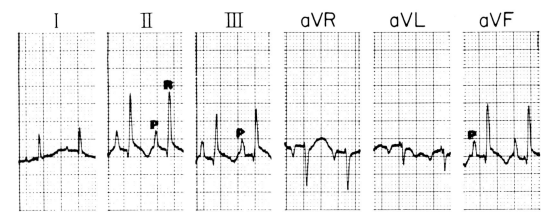

Fig. 4-16 Right atrial enlargement and left ventricular enlargement in a cat with hypertrophic cardiomyopathy. P waves are tall in leads II, III, and aVF. The R waves are abnormally high; 1.6 mV in lead II. (Tilley LP: Essentials of Canine and Feline Electrocardiography. 2nd Ed. Lea & Febiger, Philadelphia, 1985.)

teriosus, aortic stenosis, and primary myocardial disease, especially the dilated form. The ECG pattern for left ventricular enlargement is common in cats with all forms of cardiomyopathy (especially the hypertrophic form), chronic anemia, chronic renal disease (possibly secondary to systemic hypertension), and hyperthyroidism.

Left ventricular enlargement has the following ECG characteristics:

1. In dogs under 2 years of age with narrow chest cavities, the R wave of the QRS complex should not be greater than 3.0 mV in leads II and aVF. In older dogs, the R wave should not exceed 2.5 mV in leads II, III, and aVF. In the feline, the R wave in lead II should not exceed 0.9 mV. The R wave should not exceed 3.0 mV (1.0 mV in the feline) in CV_6LU or 2.5 mV in Cv_6LL.

2. The maximum width of the QRS in small and medium canine breeds is 0.05 second; in large breeds, 0.06 second. In cats, the QRS should not exceed 0.04 second.

3. Displacement of the S-T segment occurs in a direction opposite the main QRS deflection. This causes the S-T segment to sag into the T wave (S-T coving).

4. Repolarization changes cause the T wave to be of increased amplitude.

5. A MEA deviation in the frontal plane of less than +40 degrees may be present (less than 0 degrees in the feline).

Biventricular Enlargement

Simultaneous enlargement of both ventricles is difficult to diagnose accurately by electrocardiography. The diagnosis of left ventricular enlargement is more accurate, whereas the concomitant ECG diagnosis of right ventricular enlargement is less reliable. Associated conditions include mitral and tricuspid valvular insufficiency, certain congenital cardiac defects such as patent ductus arteriosus or mitral insufficiency, and the dilated form of cardiomyopathy. Biventricular enlargement has the following ECG characteristics:

1. Precordial chest leads show changes for both right (deep S waves in CV_6LL and CV_6LU) and left (tall R waves in CV_6LL and CV_6LU) ventricular enlargement.

2. Left ventricular enlargement is seen on the ECG along with a right axis deviation.

3. Left ventricular enlargement changes on the ECG are associated with high-amplitude R waves and increased QRS duration in CV_6LU.

4. A normal ECG in the presence of severe cardiomegaly on thoracic radiographs may indicate biventricular enlargement (unless pericardial effusion is present).

5. Deep Q waves in leads I, II, III, and aVF, along with left ventricular enlargement changes on the ECG, may indicate biventricular enlargement.

6. Left and right atrial enlargement changes often accompany these ECG patterns.

CONDUCTION ABNORMALITIES

Abnormalities of Decreased Conduction

SINOATRIAL BLOCK

Sinoatrial (SA) block is a disturbance of conduction in which the SA nodal impulse is blocked from depolarizing the atria. SA block can be difficult to differentiate from *sinus arrest*, the failure of impulses to be formed within the SA node owing to depressed automaticity (Fig. 4-17. See also Fig. 4-40, below). SA block may be caused by various pathologic conditions affecting the atria: dilation, fibrosis, cardiomyopathy, drug toxicity (e.g., quinidine, propranolol, and especially digitalis), and electrolyte imbalances and is associated with sick sinus syndrome.

Sinoatrial block (or arrest) has the following ECG characteristics:

1. Heart rate can be variable, depending on the underlying mechanism. SA block is suggested when pauses in the rhythm are precise multiples of normal R-R intervals. Junctional or ventricular escape complexes can often occur.
2. P waves are usually of normal configuration.
3. The QRS configuration is normal, unless an intraventricular conduction defect exists.
4. The P-R interval is essentially constant.

PERSISTENT ATRIAL STANDSTILL

Atrial standstill is characterized by an absence of P waves and a regular escape rhythm with supraventricular-type QRS complexes (Fig. 4-18). It may be temporary, terminal, or persistent. Temporary atrial standstill occurs with digitalis toxicity and hyperkalemia. Terminal atrial standstill is associated with cardiac arrest or severe hyperkalemia. Persistent atrial standstill may represent a hereditary disease in the canine (especially in the English springer spaniel), be acquired due to fibrous replacement of atrial muscle cells due to severe volume overload or inflammatory disorders, or occasionally accompany feline dilated cardiomyopathy.

Persistent atrial standstill is characterized by the following ECG changes:

1. The heart rate is slow, usually 60 beats/min or less (less than 160 beats/min in the cat), and the rhythm is regular.
2. No P waves are observed in any lead, including intracardiac ECGs.
3. The QRS is of nearly normal configuration with supraventricular-type escape QRS complexes or of increased duration with bundle branch block pattern.
4. There is no increase in heart rate, nor are P waves evident after administration of atropine sulfate or following exercise.
5. An *a* wave component (caused by atrial systole) on the right atrial pressure tracing is missing.

FIRST-DEGREE AV BLOCK

A delay or interruption in conduction of a supraventricular impulse through the AV junction and bundle of His is called AV block (Fig. 4-19). The

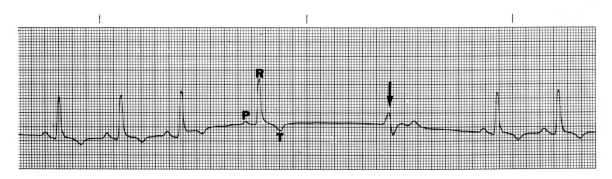

Fig. 4-17 Sinoatrial block or arrest in a female miniature schnauzer with syncope. Note the ventricular escape complex (arrow).

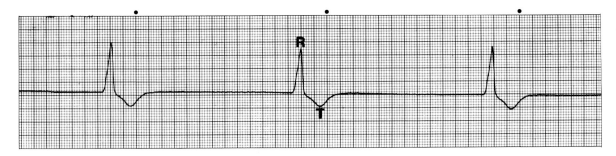

Fig. 4-18 Persistent atrial standstill in a 4-year-old Siamese cat with clinical signs of dyspnea. No P waves are present; the QRS complexes are increased in voltage and duration, indicating left bundle branch block and/or left heart enlargement. The heart rate is only 40 beats/min. (Tilley LP: Essentials of Canine and Feline Electrocardiography. 2nd Ed. Lea & Febiger, Philadelphia, 1985.)

term block should not be used if conduction delay or failure occurs because a supraventricular premature impulse has reached the AV junction or bundle of His too early. The P-R interval represents the total time period of impulse conduction from the atria to the ventricles. The precise site of delay cannot be identified from the ECG. Bundle of His recordings can delineate the precise site of delay or block, but these are not performed on a clinical basis.

First-degree AV block may occur in animals that are clinically normal and healthy. Commonly, a prolonged P-R interval is the result of degenerative changes in the AV conduction system that accompanies aging. The P-R interval tends to lengthen with advancing age and shortens with rapid heart rates. Other associated conditions include drugs (digitalis, propranolol, quinidine, and procainamide), hyperkalemia, hypokalemia, vagotonia asso-

ciated with respiratory sinus arrhythmia (causing a cyclic increase in the P-R interval) and other causes of increased vagal tone.

First-degree AV block is characterized electrocardiographically according to the following criteria:

1. The rate and rhythm depend on the presence of other arrhythmias but the rate is usually normal.

2. The P wave is normal.

3. The configuration of the QRS is usually normal. If bundle branch block is present, first-degree AV block may be caused by the conduction delay in the other bundle branch rather than in the AV junction.

4. The P-R interval in the dog is longer than 0.13 second (>0.09 second in the cat). This is true only in the presence of a regular sinus rhythm.

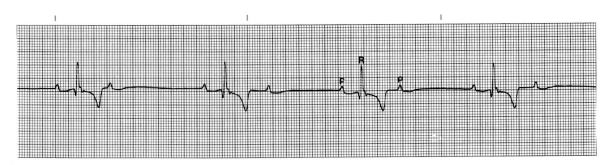

Fig. 4-19 First-degree and second-degree AV block in a dog with syncope. The P-R interval is prolonged (0.14 second). Every other atrial impulse is conducted (2:1 second-degree block).

SECOND-DEGREE AV BLOCK

Second-degree AV block is characterized by an intermittent failure or disturbance of AV conduction (Figs. 4-19, 4-20). One or more P waves are not followed by QRS-T complexes. A proposed classification takes into consideration the width of the QRS complexes: type A block, with a normal QRS duration, and type B, with a wide QRS. In type A block, the site of conduction failure is assumed to be above the bifurcation of the bundle of His. In type B, the site of blockage is assumed to be below the bifurcation.

Second-degree AV block may be a normal finding in dogs, especially in the early years of life. It is often associated with sinus arrhythmia and other causes of increased vagal tone. It can be physiologic when associated with supraventricular tachycardia, due to microscopic idiopathic fibrosis in older dogs, hereditary stenosis of the bundle of His in pugs, result from drug effects (e.g., digitalis, intravenous atropine, xylazine, and quinidine), or be caused by electrolyte imbalances. In the cat, second-degree AV block can occasionally be associated with hypertrophic cardiomyopathy.

Second-degree AV block is characterized by the following ECG criteria:

Mobitz type I (Wenckebach phenomenon), usually type A (Fig. 4-20):
1. The ventricular rate is slower than the atrial rate because of blocked P waves. The rhythm is regularly irregular in the typical form of Wenckebach. The R-R interval becomes progressively shorter as the P-R interval becomes progressively longer until a P wave is blocked.
2. The P wave is usually of normal configuration.
3. The QRS is usually normal, indicating that the bundle branches are also normal.

Mobitz type II, usually type B:
1. The ventricular rate is slower than the atrial rate because of blocked P waves. The rhythm is broken by the absence of one or more QRS complexes.
2. The P waves are usually normal.
3. The QRS complexes are often of abnormal configuration, an indication that the conduction defect involves the bundle of His or proximal bundle branches. Mobitz type II AV block (type B) may progress to higher degrees of AV block.
4. There is a fixed relationship between the atrial and ventricular complexes of 2:1 (two P waves to one QRS), 3:1, 4:1, and so forth. The P-R interval is always constant but may be either normal or longer than normal.

COMPLETE HEART BLOCK

Complete heart block occurs when AV conduction is absent and the ventricles are under the control of pacemakers below the area of the block (Fig. 4-21). No relationship exists between the P waves and the QRS complexes. Clinical signs associated with complete heart block are syncope, sudden death, and congestive heart failure. They may be caused by reduced cardiac output from ventricular asystole

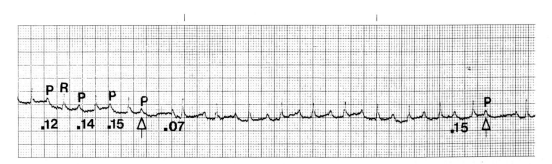

Fig. 4-20 Mobitz type I (Wenckebach phenomenon) in a hyperthyroid cat. The P-R interval progressively lengthens until a P wave is not conducted (arrow). (Modified from Fox PR, Kaplan P: Feline arrhythmias. p. 251. In Bonagura JD (ed): Contemporary Issues in Small Animal Practice. Vol. 9. Cardiology. Churchill Livingstone, New York, 1987.)

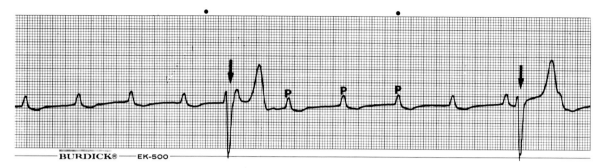

Fig. 4-21 Complete heart block with an idioventricular escape rhythm (arrows) of 30 beats/min, from a dog with syncope and severe ascites. A cardiac neoplasm was found at necropsy. (Tilley LP: Essentials of Canine and Feline Electrocardiography. 2nd Ed. Lea & Febiger, Philadelphia, 1985.)

or the development of ventricular tachyarrhythmias leading to circulatory failure. Physical examination will indicate variation in the intensity of the first heart sound, intermittent cannon *a* waves in the jugular venous pulse, and variable third and fourth heart sounds.

Associated conditions include isolated congenital AV block, congenital defects such as aortic stenosis and ventricular septal defect, severe digitalis toxicity, infiltrative cardiomyopathy, idiopathic fibrosis, hypertrophic cardiomyopathy, bacterial endocarditis, myocardial infarction, and hyperkalemia. Lesions have been found in the bundle of His in Doberman pinschers and pugs. Degeneration or fibrosis of the AV node and bundle branches is often associated with endocardial and myocardial fibrosis in cats with cardiomyopathy.

Complete heart block is characterized electrocardiographically as follows:

1. The ventricular rate is slower than the atrial rate (more P waves than QRS complexes).

2. P waves are usually of normal configuration.

3. The QRS is wide and bizarre when the rescuing pacemaker is located in the ventricle or lower AV junction with bundle branch block. It is normal when the escape pacemaker is located in the lower AV junction (above the His bundle bifurcation).

4. The P waves bear no constant relationship to the QRS complexes. The P-P and R-R intervals are relatively constant.

Intraventricular Conduction Defects

An intraventricular conduction defect results from a delay or block in one or more conduction system pathways below the bundle of His. The intraventricular conduction system is composed of three major conduction pathways: (1) the right bundle branch, (2) the anterior fascicle of the left bundle branch, and (3) the posterior fascicle of the left bundle branch. A block or delay in conduction can occur in one, two, or all three pathways at the same time. The major forms of intraventricular block can be classified as follows:

1. Bundle branch block (RBBB, LBBB)

2. Fascicular block (left anterior, left posterior)

3. Various combinations of block in the three major conduction pathways (e.g., RBBB with anterior or posterior fascicular block)

4. Block in all three conduction pathways, producing complete (third-degree) AV heart block

LEFT BUNDLE BRANCH BLOCK

Left bundle branch block is a delay or block of conduction in the left bundle branch, either in the main branch or at the level of the anterior and posterior fascicles (Fig. 4-22; see also Fig. 4-37 below). This causes a supraventricular impulse to activate the right ventricle first through the right bundle branch. The left ventricle is activated later, having to rely on cardiac impulse transmission through my-

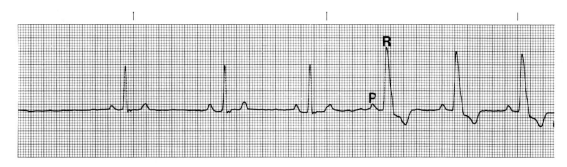

Fig. 4-22 Intermittent left bundle branch block in a dog. The QRS complexes are wider and taller in the fourth, fifth, and sixth complexes.

ocytes instead of Purkinje fibers. This causes the QRS complex to become wide and bizarre. LBBB usually indicates a severe underlying disorder, such as cardiomyopathy, aortic stenosis, or ischemic cardiomyopathy (myocardial infarction, arteriosclerosis).

Left bundle branch block is characterized by the following ECG features:

1. The QRS complex duration is 0.07 second or greater in the dog (or 0.06 second in the cat).
2. The QRS complex is wide and positive in leads I, II, III, and aVF and in leads over the left precordium (CV$_6$LL and CV$_6$LU).
3. The QRS complex is inverted in leads aVR and CV$_5$RL.
4. When the left bundle branch is blocked, the normal initial septal activation is disturbed and the first part of the QRS is altered. The Q wave is often absent in leads that definitely record septal activity in the right-to-left axis (e.g., leads I and CV$_6$LU).
5. LBBB must be differentiated from left ventricular enlargement. The absence of left ventricular enlargement on thoracic radiographs lends support to a diagnosis of isolated LBBB.
6. Intermittent bundle branch block (tachycardia or bradycardia-dependent) or bundle branch block alternans may be present in serial tracings or in the same tracing.

RIGHT BUNDLE BRANCH BLOCK

Right bundle branch block is a delay or block of conduction in the right bundle branch (Fig. 4-23). The right ventricle is depolarized by transmission through myocytes instead of Purkinje fibers by impulses that pass from the left bundle branch to the right side of the septum below the block. It is then activated with delay, causing the QRS complex to become wide and bizarre. The block can be located in the proximal portion of the right bundle branch (complete block) or more peripheral in the right bundle branch (incomplete block). RBBB is occasionally found in normal and healthy dogs and cats. It may be caused by congenital heart disease, chronic valvular fibrosis, surgical correction of a ventricular septal defect, cardiac needle puncture for obtaining blood samples or performing angiography, cardiac neoplasia, trauma, sometimes cardiomyopathy, and after cardiac arrest. Incomplete right bundle branch block has been found in the Beagle as a genetically determined localized variation with right ventricular wall thickness.

Right bundle branch block is characterized by the following ECG features:

1. For complete RBBB, the QRS complex is greater than 0.07-second duration in all dogs (0.07 seconds or greater in toy breeds) and 0.06 seconds or greater in cats.
2. A right axis deviation is usually present.
3. The QRS complex is positive in aVR, aVL, and CV$_5$RL and has a wide RSR' or rsR' pattern (often M shaped) in CV$_5$RL.
4. The QRS complexes have large wide S waves in leads I, II, III, aVF, CV$_6$LL, and CV$_6$LU. An S wave or W pattern is usually seen in lead V$_{10}$.
5. An incomplete RBBB can be diagnosed when any of features listed in 2 to 4 are observed but the QRS duration is within normal limits.

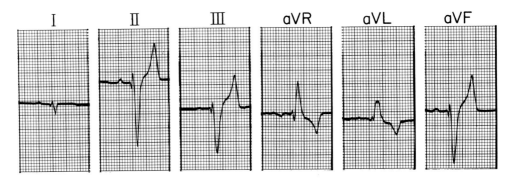

Fig. 4-23 Right bundle branch block in a dog. The QRS duration is 0.09 second. Large and wide S waves are present in leads I, II, III, and aVF. There is a right axis deviation (approximately −90 degrees).

6. Support can be given to the diagnosis of isolated RBBB if diseases causing severe right ventricular enlargement are excluded. For example, in most cases, the thoracic radiograph can be used to evaluate right ventricular enlargement.

7. Intermittent bundle branch block (i.e., tachycardia or bradycardia-dependent) or bundle branch block alternans may be present in serial tracings or in the same tracing.

FASCICULAR BLOCK

A block in either the anterior or posterior fascicle of the left bundle branch causes only a slight prolongation of left ventricular depolarization (Fig. 4-24). The main ECG effect is on the direction of the depolarization. The anterior and posterior fascicles each pass through the base of the corresponding papillary muscle. If the path to one of these papillary muscles is blocked, activation of the left ventricle can begin only at the other papillary muscle. The general direction of left ventricular depolarization is shifted toward the blocked fascicle and corresponding papillary muscle.

Left anterior fascicular block is a common intraventricular conduction defect in the cat and is associated with severe left ventricular hypertrophy (e.g., idiopathic hypertrophic cardiomyopathy or secondary to hyperthyroidism). This pattern is compatible with an actual conduction defect and/or left ventricular hypertrophy.

Left posterior fascicular block is the least common intraventricular conduction defect in both the dog and cat. The posterior fascicle is better protected because of its anatomical position and greater blood supply.

Besides cardiomyopathy, fascicular block is associated with other causes of left ventricular hypertrophy including aortic stenosis, hyperkalemia, and after surgical repair of ventricular septal defect. Fascicular blocks, in and of themselves, do not cause hemodynamic abnormalities.

Left anterior fascicular block can be recognized by the following combination of ECG features:

1. QRS complex duration usually within normal limits

2. Marked left axis deviation in the frontal plane

3. Small Q wave and tall R wave in leads I and aVL

4. Deep S waves in leads II, III, and aVF

Other causes of the left anterior fascicular pattern should be excluded, particularly hyperkalemia, left ventricular hypertrophy, and an altered position of the heart within the thorax.

Right bundle branch block and left anterior fascicular block are recognized by the combination of ECG features for each block:

1. QRS complex duration greater or equal to 0.07 second in the dog, 0.06 second in cat

2. Marked left axis deviation in the frontal plane

3. Wide and deep S waves in leads I, II, III, aVF, and CV_6LU

4. Tall R wave and small Q wave in leads I and aVL

5. QRS complex in CV_5RL with a wide rsR′ or RSR′ pattern (often M shaped)

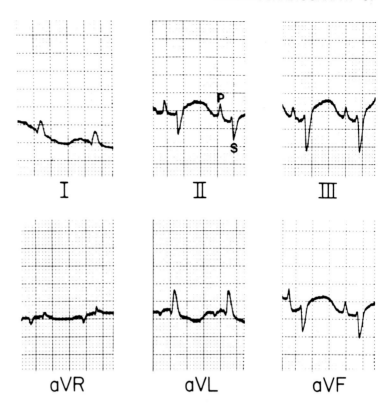

Fig. 4-24 Left anterior fascicular block in a cat with hypertrophic cardiomyopathy. There is a severe left axis deviation (−60 degrees) with a qR pattern in leads I and aVL and an rS pattern in leads II, III, and aVF. (From Tilley LP, et al: Primary myocardial disease in the cat: A model for human cardiomyopathy. Am J Pathol 86:493, 1977.)

Ventricular Pre-excitation and the Wolff-Parkinson-White Syndrome

Ventricular pre-excitation occurs when impulses originating in the SA node or atrium activate a portion of the ventricles prematurely through an accessory pathway (Fig. 4-25). SA impulses are able to reach the ventricles initially without going through the AV node. The Wolff-Parkinson-White (WPW) syndrome consists of ventricular pre-excitation with episodes of paroxysmal supraventricular tachycardia.

The anatomic basis of ventricular pre-excitation is controversial. Three accessory conduction pathways are postulated: bundles of Kent (accessory AV connections), James fibers (AV nodal bypass tracts), and Mahaim fibers (nodoventricular tracts).

The sinus or atrial impulses conducted via the ac-

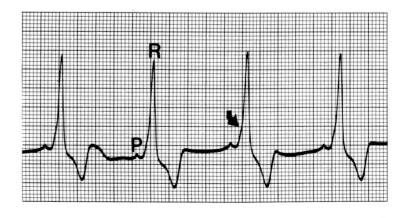

Fig. 4-25 Ventricular pre-excitation in a dog. A short P-R interval and a widened QRS complex with slurring or notching (arrow) of the upstroke (Δ wave) are present.

cessory pathways activate a portion of the ventricles without passing through the bundle of His; the rest of the ventricle is activated via the normal AV pathway. The accessory pathway may go to the left ventricle (left type or type A) or to the right ventricle (right type or type B). This classification is an arbitrary one because some cases cannot be classified clearly into either type A or B. The pre-excitation shortens the P-R interval because the entire impulse is not slowed by normal conduction delay in the AV junction. The QRS complex has a slurred upstroke and is wide because the pre-excitation impulse is conducted through ordinary myocardium without the aid of the specialized conduction system. If the atrial impulse is conducted over the James bypass fibers, a short P-R interval with a QRS complex of normal duration will result (Lown-Ganong-Levine syndrome).

Paroxysmal tachycardia associated with ventricular pre-excitation (WPW syndrome) can be explained by the reentry mechanism. An impulse traveling to the ventricles through the AV junction may turn around and reenter the atria through the accessory pathway. A reciprocal rhythm or electrical circuit is thus established.

This ECG abnormality can be congenital in origin, with no organic heart disease present. Associated conditions include congenital and acquired cardiac defects and hypertrophic cardiomyopathy. Most cats with ventricular pre-excitation have hypertrophic cardiomyopathy.

The following are ECG characteristics of this abnormality:

1. Heart rate and rhythm are normal in ventricular pre-excitation. In the WPW syndrome, the heart rate is extremely rapid, often greater than 300 beats/min (400 to 500 beats/min in the cat).

2. Sinus P waves are normal in ventricular pre-excitation but difficult to recognize in the WPW syndrome.

3. The QRS in ventricular pre-excitation is widened with slurring or notching of the upstroke of the R wave (Δ wave). The left type (type A) has predominantly positive QRS complexes in CV_5RL, whereas the right type (type B) has predominantly negative QRS complexes in CV_5RL. In the WPW syndrome, the configuration of the QRS complexes can be normal, wide with a delta wave, or very wide and bizarre.

4. The P-R interval of the P-QRS in ventricular pre-excitation is short. In the WPW syndrome there is usually 1:1 conduction (P wave for every QRS complex).

S-T SEGMENT, Q-T INTERVAL, AND T WAVE ABNORMALITIES

S-T Segment Abnormalities

The S-T segment represents the time from the end of the QRS interval to the onset of the T wave (Fig. 4-26; see also Fig. 4-39, below). It may be above (elevated), at, or below (depressed) the level of the baseline.

The baseline or the isoelectric line is on the same level as the T-P segment, between the T wave and the P wave. The shape of the S-T segment is significant.

S-T segment changes can represent normal variation. S-T segment depression in leads with dominant R waves can be associated with myocardial ischemia, acute myocardial infarction, electrolyte disturbances, digitalis toxicity, and trauma to the heart. S-T segment elevation (Fig. 4-26) in leads with dominant R waves can be associated with myocardial infarction, pericarditis, and myocardial hypoxia. Hypertrophy, bundle branch block, and ventricular premature complexes can cause secondary S-T segment changes following abnormalities of the QRS complex. Pseudodepression of the S-T segment due to a prominent T_a wave (atrial repolarization) can occur with tachycardia or pathologic atrial changes.

The electrocardiographic features of S-T segment abnormalities are as follows:

1. Abnormal deviations of the S-T segment in the dog include depression equal to or greater than 0.2 mV or elevation of 0.15 mV in leads I through aVF, depression of 0.3 mV in leads CV_6LL, or elevation of 0.3 mV in leads CV_6LL and CV_6LU. Significant S-T segment deviations in the cat must be at least 0.1 mV in amplitude.

2. The S-T segment normally curves gently into the proximal limb of the T wave.

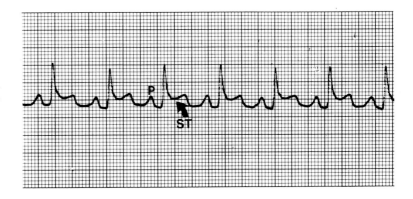

Fig. 4-26 S-T segment elevation (arrow) in a dog with pericardial effusion.

3. It is helpful to compare any S-T segment changes with those seen on previous tracings from the same animal.

Q-T Interval Abnormalities

The Q-T interval is measured from the onset of the Q wave to the end of the T wave (Fig. 4-27). It is the summation of ventricular depolarization and repolarization and represents electrical systole. The Q-T interval varies inversely with the heart rate; the faster the heart rate, the shorter the interval. Various formulas and tables correlate the relationship of Q-T interval to heart rate, age, and sex in humans. In veterinary medicine, the Q-T interval alone is often not helpful in establishing a diagnosis.

Drugs that affect the autonomic nervous system can influence the Q-T interval directly or by changing the heart rate. It has been shown in humans that atropine and propranolol shorten the Q-T interval independent of rate, demonstrating a direct vagal effect on the Q-T interval. Q-T interval deviation is determined chiefly by an interplay of autonomic influences. A *prolonged* Q-T interval can occur with hypocalcemia, hypokalemia, quinidine toxicity, ethylene glycol poisoning, strenuous exercise, hypothermia, and central nervous system (CNS) disorders. A *shortened* Q-T interval can be associated with hypercalcemia, digitalis toxicity, and hyperkalemia.

Electrocardiographic features of Q-T abnormalities include the following:

1. The normal range (sinus rhythm) is 0.15 to 0.25 second in the dog, 0.12 to 0.18 second in the cat.
2. An approximate rule of thumb is that the Q-T interval should be less than one-half the preceding R-R interval for a normal sinus heart rate.

T-Wave Abnormalities

The T wave is the first major deflection following the QRS complex. It represents the ventricular recovery period (repolarization) and may be positive, notched, negative, or biphasic (Fig. 4-28). It is most accurately analyzed when compared with T waves

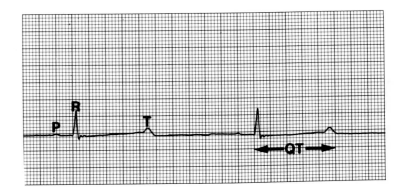

Fig. 4-27 Lead II rhythm strip recorded from a dog with acute pancreatitis. Sinus bradycardia and prolongation of the Q-T interval (0.50 sec) is present. Despite the slow heart rate, the Q-T interval is prolonged. (Tilley LP: Essentials of Canine and Feline Electrocardiography. 2nd Ed. Lea & Febiger, Philadelphia, 1985.)

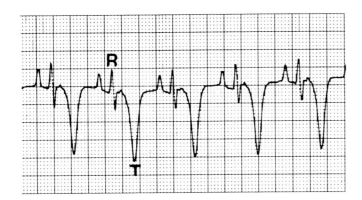

Fig. 4-28 Large negative T waves in a dog with severe heartworm disease.

on previous tracings. The T wave may be of abnormal amplitude, shape, or direction (polarity). Abnormalities can be classified into two general types: (1) primary—changes independent of depolarization, and (2) secondary—changes directly dependent on the depolarization process.

T-wave abnormalities can occur from myocardial hypoxia, anesthetic complications, hyperventilation in heat stroke, in animals with heart disease, during bradycardia (T waves larger), and myocardial infarction (T wave larger with a change in polarity). Intraventricular conduction defects such as RBBB or LBBB are often associated with large T waves secondary to the QRS change. T waves become larger and spiked with hyperkalemia, while smaller and biphasic with hypokalemia. Nonspecific T wave changes are associated with metabolic diseases (e.g., anemia, shock, uremia, and fever), drug toxicity (e.g., digitalis, quinidine, procainamide), and respiratory abnormalities. T-wave alternans can occur from increases in circulatory catecholamines, hypocalcemia, and acute increase in sympathetic discharge.

The ECG features of T-wave abnormalities are as follows:

1. The T-wave amplitude in the dog generally should not be greater than 25 percent of the R-wave amplitude. The T wave rarely exceeds 0.3 mV in the cat.
2. The T wave is normally slightly asymmetric. T waves that are sharply pointed or notched may indicate an underlying abnormality, such as an electrolyte imbalance (e.g., hyperkalemia). A marked change in the shape of the T wave on serial ECGs is usually abnormal.
3. Polarity of secondary T-wave changes is not always equal to that of the QRS complex, as is the case in humans. The T wave should be positive in leads CV_5RL in dogs over 2 months of age. It can normally be biphasic. It should be negative in lead V_{10} in all breeds except the Chihuahua. Reversal in polarity of the T wave on serial ECGs is most often abnormal.
4. Isolated T wave alternans can occur. This phenomenon consists of the rhythmic alteration of the configuration of T wave without any concomitant change in the QRS complex.

EFFECT OF SELECTED DISEASES ON THE ELECTROCARDIOGRAM

Myocardial Infarction

As a naturally occurring disease, myocardial infarction is infrequent in the dog. Most cases involve the left ventricle. Microscopic intramural myocardial infarctions (MIMI) (Fig. 4-29) and focal areas of myocardial fibrosis are common findings in dogs with acquired cardiovascular disease. Consistent ECG patterns diagnostic for precise localization of spontaneous myocardial infarction are not well established. Myocardial infarction can occur from bacterial endocarditis emboli, neoplasia, or generalized septicemia, intramural coronary arteriosclerosis in older dogs, and subvalvular aortic stenosis.

The ECG features of myocardial infarction are as follows:

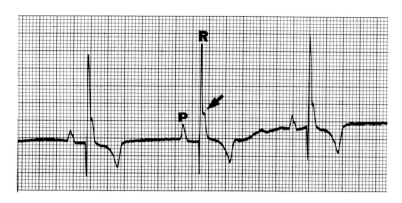

Fig. 4-29 The notched R-wave descent (arrow) in this old dog may indicate a microscopic intramural myocardial infarction (MIMI). (Tilley LP: Essentials of Canine and Feline Electrocardiography. 2nd Ed. Lea & Febiger, Philadelphia, 1985.)

1. If serial tracings with QRS and ST-T wave changes are present, the diagnosis and location of myocardial infarction can be established with a higher degree of accuracy. The zone of ischemia that surrounds the infarcted region accounts for the S-T segment and T-wave abnormalities.
2. Possible ECG indications of infarction include
   a. Sudden deviation of the S-T segment
   b. Tall, peaked T waves (first few hours)
   c. Sudden development of Q waves or a change in direction of the T wave
   d. Axis shift in the frontal plane
   e. Low-voltage QRS complexes
   f. Sudden development of bundle branch block or heart block
   g. Sudden onset of ventricular arrhythmias due to ischemic effects on the ventricular myocardium
   h. Ventricular arrhythmias 12 to 24 hours later due to ischemic effects on the subendocardial Purkinje system
3. A sloppy R-wave descent that may be associated with MIMI

Hyperkalemia

The effects of severe uncorrected hyperkalemia on cardiac conduction and rhythm are often lethal (Fig. 4-30). Resultant wide and bizarre QRS complexes may simulate an idioventricular rhythm but should be termed *sinoventricular*. The SA node continues to fire and its impulses are transmitted via the internodal pathways to the AV junction and ventricles. No P wave is recorded because the atrial myocardium is not activated. ECG changes may not occur until serum potassium concentrations are greatly elevated.

Hyperkalemia is a common clinical problem in cats with urinary obstruction. Addison's disease (adrenocortical insufficiency) is a common cause of hyperkalemia in the dog. Other causes of hyperkalemia include renal insufficiency, untreated diabetic ketoacidosis, excessive potassium infusion, metabolic acidosis, and transfusion of stored blood.

The following ECG changes may be observed without sharp distinctions between serum potassium levels:

1. Serum potassium greater than 5.5 mEq/L (T waves larger and peaked)
2. Serum potassium greater than 6.5 mEq/L (decreased amplitude of the R wave, prolonged QRS and P-R intervals, S-T segment depression)
3. Serum potassium greater than 7 mEq/L (decreased amplitude of the P wave with increased duration, longer QRS and P-R intervals, Q-T interval prolonged)
4. Serum potassium greater than 8.5 mEq/L (disappearance of the P wave with atrial standstill and resultant sinoventricular rhythm)
5. Serum potassium greater than 10.0 mEq/L (increased widening of the QRS complex with eventual replacement by a smooth biphasic curve; final stage is ventricular flutter, ventricular fibrillation, or ventricular asystole)

Pericardial Effusion

Pericardial effusion is often associated with low voltage complexes, S-T segment deviation, and sometimes electrical alternans (Fig. 4-31). The am-

A

B

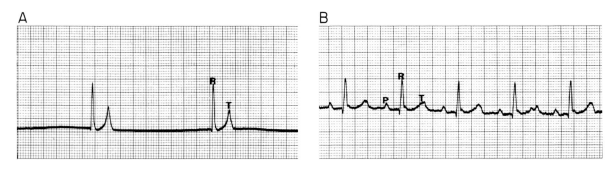

Fig. 4-30 (**A**) Hyperkalemia in a dog presenting with hypovolemic shock due to addisonian crisis. P waves are absent and T waves are tall and peaked. Serum potassium was 8.4 mEq/L. (**B**) After instituion of therapy, P waves are present and the QRS-T complex is of smaller amplitude. Serum potassium was 4.8 mEq/L. (Tilley LP: Essentials of Canine and Feline Electrocardiography. 2nd Ed. Lea & Febiger, Philadelphia, 1985.)

plitude of the QRS complex is dependent on many factors besides the effects of cardiovascular diseases such as the distance of the heart from the recording electrode. This distance can be influenced by the chest size, thickness of the chest wall, and the presence of emphysema, pneumothorax, or pleural effusion.

Pericardial effusion may be associated with the following ECG features:

1. A decreased QRS amplitude in serial ECGs recorded at different time periods (in the dog, R waves may be smaller than 0.5 mV in leads I, II, III, and aVF)

2. S-T segment elevation in leads I, II, III, and aVF, most often seen in acute pericarditis, resulting from subepicardial ischemia due to compression by pericardial fluid

3. P-R segment depression in leads I, II, III, and aVF, probably representing subepicardial atrial injury

4. Electrical alternans

Electrical alternans is diagnosed when the P, QRS, or T complexes (or any combination) alter their configuration on every other, every third, every fourth complex, and so forth. The most common alternating ratio is every other complex and usually involves the QRS complex alone. Cardiac motion is accepted as the cause of electrical alternans in pericardial effusion. The heart position has been recorded by echocardiography to shift in the peri-

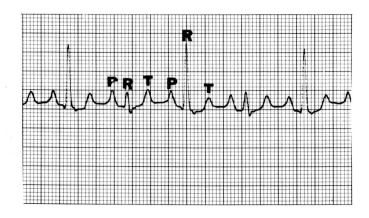

Fig. 4-31 Electrical alternans in a dog with pericardial effusion. Every other R wave alternates in amplitude.

cardium during every other beat. This causes the anatomic relationship of the heart to any given electrode to alternate producing these ECG changes.

Hyperthyroidism

Hyperthyroidism is a common disease in the older cat. Excessive production of the thyroid hormones usually results from a functional adenoma that involves one or both thyroid lobes. Cardiac abnormalities are a common feature of feline hyperthyroidism and include radiographic evidence of mild to severe cardiomegaly, pleural effusion or pulmonary edema, left ventricular hypertrophy, and arrhythmias.

Sinus tachycardia (greater than 240 beats/min) and increased R-wave amplitude in lead II are the most common ECG abnormalities (Fig. 4-32). Atrial and ventricular arrhythmias (e.g., atrial premature complexes, atrial tachycardia, ventricular premature complexes, and ventricular tachycardia) and conduction abnormalities are frequently recorded. Sinus tachycardia, increased R-wave amplitude, and most arrhythmias usually resolve following successful therapy.

ARRHYTHMIAS

An arrhythmia is an abnormality in the rate, regularity, or site of cardiac impulse origin and/or a disturbance of impulse conduction. During normal sinus rhythm, the cardiac impulse originates in the SA node and spreads in an orderly fashion throughout the atria, AV node and His-Purkinje system, and ventricles. Abnormalities of impulse formation or conduction provide a basis for arrhythmia classification (Table 4-5) and treatment (Chs. 14 and 15).

Normal Sinus Rhythm

Sinus rhythm is the normal mechanism for initiating cardiac systole. The SA node normally has an inherent pacemaker rate of 70 to 160 beats/min in the adult dog (Fig. 4-33) The rates can become as high as 180 in toy breeds and up to 220 in puppies. A range of 160 to 240 beats/min occurs in adult cats. A regular sinus rhythm below this rate is sinus bradycardia, whereas above the normal heart rate is sinus tachycardia. An irregular sinus rhythm is called *sinus arrhythmia.*

The ECG features of a sinus rhythm are as follows:

1. The rhythm is regular with less than 10 percent variation in R-R intervals. The difference between the largest and smallest R-R intervals in the dog is less than 0.12 second (0.10 second in the cat).
2. P waves are positive in lead II with a consistent configuration.
3. The QRS complexes are normal, or they may be wide and bizarre, if an intraventricular conduction defect is present.
4. The P-QRS complex is normal with a constant P-R interval.

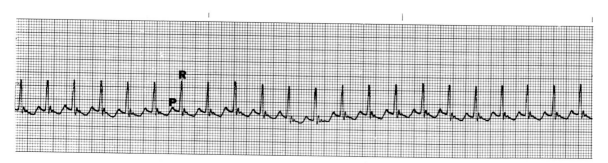

Fig. 4-32 Sinus tachycardia at a rate of 285 beats/min from a cat with hyperthyroidism. The R wave voltage is 1.1 mV, indicating left ventricular enlargement.

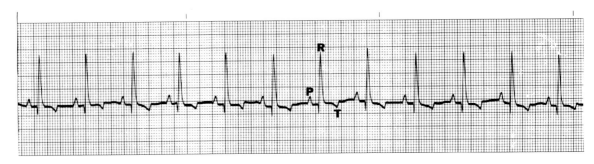

Fig. 4-33 Normal sinus rhythm in a dog. The heart rate is 165 beats/min. (Tilley LP: Essentials of Canine and Feline Electrocardiography. 2nd Ed. Lea & Febiger, Philadelphia, 1985.)

ARRHYTHMIAS ORIGINATING IN THE SINUS NODE

Sinus Tachycardia

Sinus tachycardia can be associated with many conditions: (1) a physiologic mechanism in response to increased body metabolism resulting in a greater demand for oxygenation; (2) a compensatory mechanism to increase cardiac output; (3) underlying cardiac, systemic, or metabolic pathology; or (4) in response to pharmacologic agents. Sinus tachycardia is the most common arrhythmia in the dog and cat (Fig. 4-32).

Examples of physiologic conditions associated with sinus tachycardia include pain, fright, or excitement during restraining procedures. Pathologic conditions include fever, shock, anemia, infection, congestive heart failure, hypoxia, and hyperthyroidism. Drugs that can cause sinus tachycardia include atropine, epinephrine, ketamine, and vasodilators.

This arrhythmia is characterized by the following ECG changes:

1. All criteria of a normal sinus rhythm are met except that the heart rate is above 160 beats/min in the dog (above 180 in toy breeds and above 220 in puppies). For the cat, the heart rate is above 240 beats/min.

2. The rhythm is regular with less than 10 percent variation in R-R intervals and constant P-R intervals. Ocular pressure produces only a gradual, transient slowing of the heart rate, if any change at all.

Sinus Bradycardia

A regular sinus rhythm slower than the normal sinus heart rate is sinus bradycardia (Fig. 4-34). Severe sinus bradycardia may adversely affect cardiac output and/or increase susceptibility to abnormal cardiac impulse formation. Sinus bradycardia can occur from severe systemic disease (e.g., renal failure), from toxicities, with dilated cardiomyopathy in the cat, or during end-stage heart failure. Physiologic causes of sinus bradycardia include increased vagal tone due to carotid sinus pressure, eyeball compression, or elevated intracranial pressure. Hypothermia and hypothyroidism have been associated with sinus bradycardia. Drug-induced causes include tranquilizers, propranolol, digitalis, quinidine, morphine, and various anesthetic agents. Bradycardia may be a normal ECG variation. Many large-breed dogs normally have heart rates of 60 to 70 beats/min.

The ECG features of sinus bradycardia are as follows:

1. All criteria of normal sinus rhythm are met, except that the heart rate is less than 70 beats/min in the dog and below 160 for the cat.

2. The rhythm is usually regular with a slight variation in the P-P interval.

3. The P-R interval is constant.

Sinus Arrhythmia

Sinus arrhythmia is an irregular sinus rhythm originating in the SA node (Fig. 4-35). It is represented by alternating periods of slower and more

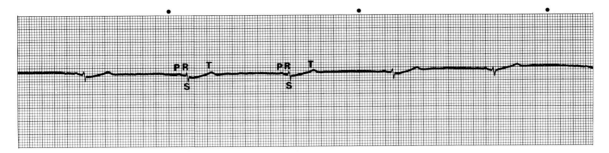

Fig. 4-34 Sinus bradycardia in a cat (75 beats/min) during surgical anesthetic complications. (Tilley LP: Essentials of Canine and Feline Electrocardiography. 2nd Ed. Lea & Febiger, Philadelphia, 1985.)

rapid heart rates which is usually related to respiration. The heart rate increases with inspiration and decreases with expiration. Respiratory sinus arrhythmia is a frequent normal finding in the dog, especially in brachycephalic breeds in which vagal tone is increased by upper airway obstruction. Sinus arrhythmia is accentuated by vagotonic procedures, such as carotid sinus massage and eyeball compression. Atropine will usually eliminate sinus arrhythmia, indicating that its origin is vagal in nature. It is important to differentiate sinus arrhythmia from other dangerous arrhythmias.

Sinus arrhythmia has the following ECG characteristics:

1. All criteria of normal sinus rhythm are met, except that a variability of 0.12 second or more exists between successive P waves, or the R-R interval variation is greater than 10 percent. In the cat, a variability of 0.10 second or more exists between successive P waves.

2. The P wave, QRS complexes, and P-R interval are normal.

3. A *wandering pacemaker* is often present. A wandering sinus pacemaker is a shift of the pacemaker from within the SA node or from the SA node to the AV node. A wandering pacemaker is an irregular, multiform, supraventricular rhythm with changing P-wave morphology.

Sinus Arrest

Sinus arrest is a failure of SA nodal impulse formation caused by depressed automaticity. Differentiating between SA block or arrest is difficult (Fig. 4-17; see also Fig. 4-40, below). Failure of the SA node to fire on time can cause fainting, especially if the lower pacemaker focus fails to take over.

Intermittent sinus arrest can be a normal incidental finding in brachycephalic breeds but is rare in the cat. Inspiration in these breeds causes a reflex

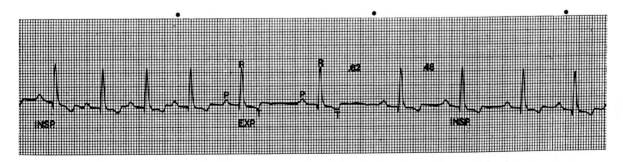

Fig. 4-35 Respiratory sinus arrhythmia in a dog with an average rate of 120/min. The R-R intervals vary more than 0.12 second as the rate changes with inspiration (INSP) and expiration (EXP). (Tilley LP: Essentials of Canine and Feline Electrocardiography. 2nd Ed. Lea & Febiger, Philadelphia, 1985.)

decrease in vagal tone that leads to an exaggerated sinus arrhythmia. Ocular or carotid sinus pressure often produces sinus arrest or block. Possible causes include irritation of the vagal nerve, such as surgical manipulation, thoracic or cervical neoplasms.

Sinus arrest within normal sinus rhythm has the following ECG characteristics:

1. The heart rate can be variable, depending on the underlying mechanism. The rhythm is regularly irregular or irregular with pauses demonstrating a lack of P-QRS-T complexes. The pauses are equal or greater than twice the normal R-R interval.
2. The P waves are usually of normal configuration but may vary in shape if a wandering pacemaker is present.
3. The QRS configuration is normal unless an intraventricular conduction defect exists.
4. The P-R interval is essentially constant.

ARRHYTHMIAS ORIGINATING IN THE ATRIAL MUSCLE

Arrhythmias originating in the atria include atrial premature complexes, atrial tachycardia, atrial flutter, and atrial fibrillation.

Atrial Premature Complexes

Atrial premature complexes (APCs) arise from ectopic atrial foci (Fig. 4-36; see also Fig. 4-47, below). They are frequently caused by cardiac disease and may progress to atrial tachycardia, atrial flutter, or atrial fibrillation. Rare APCs can be a normal finding in very aged dogs and cats. Atrial premature complexes are often caused by atrial enlargement from acquired chronic valvular insufficiency, primary myocardial diseases, congenital heart diseases, right atrial hemangiosarcoma, hyperthyroidism, digitalis toxicity, general anesthesia, and various drug, chemical, or noxious stimuli.

Atrial premature complexes have the following ECG features:

1. The heart rate is usually normal, but the rhythm is irregular due to the premature P wave (called a P′ wave) that disrupts the normal sinus-initiated P-wave rhythm.
2. The ectopic P′ wave is premature, and its configuration is different from that of the sinus P waves. It may be negative, positive, biphasic, or superimposed on the previous T wave.
3. The QRS complex is premature and its configuration is usually the same as the sinus initiated complexes.
4. The QRS is absent when the P′ wave occurs too early for the AV node to completely recover and permit ventricular conduction. A nonconducted P′ wave results.
5. If there is partial recovery in the AV node or the intraventricular conduction system, the P′ wave is conducted with a long P′-R interval or is conducted with a change in the normal QRS configuration (aberrant conduction).
6. The P′-R interval is usually as long as or longer than the P-R interval.
7. A *noncompensatory pause* may result when the

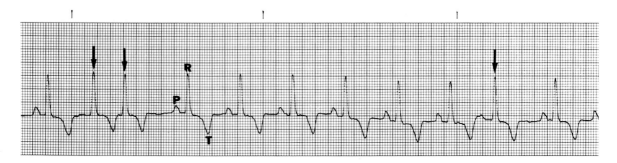

Fig. 4-36 Atrial premature complexes (arrows) and P mitrale in a dog with congestive heart failure.

R-R interval of the two normal sinus complexes enclosing the premature atrial complex is less than the R-R intervals of three consecutive sinus complexes. This is attributable to retrograde conduction of the APC into the SA node which discharges it and resets the timing of the normal sinus rhythm.

Atrial Tachycardia

Atrial tachycardia is a rapid regular rhythm that originates from an ectopic atrial focus (Fig. 4-37). Three or more consecutive APCs are considered atrial tachycardia. It is clinically important to distinguish atrial tachycardia from sinus tachycardia. Atrial tachycardia usually accompanies organic heart disease, may be terminated immediately with ocular pressure, and has P' waves different from sinus P waves. The same conditions that cause APCs are associated with atrial tachycardia. Other predisposing conditions include ventricular pre-excitation, hypertrophic cardiomyopathy in the cat, and cardiac neoplasia. Atrial tachycardia with AV block is often due to digitalis toxicity. Recent studies have established two mechanisms for atrial tachycardia: (1) enhanced automaticity of an ectopic focus, and (2) re-entry.

Atrial tachycardia is characterized by the following ECG features:

1. The heart rate is rapid, above 160 beats/min (above 180 in toy breed dogs) and above 240 in the cat. Rhythm is perfectly regular in most cases, but may be slightly irregular. Atrial tachycardia can be either intermittent (paroxysmal) or continuous.

2. P' waves are usually positive in lead II, with the P'-P' intervals regular. They may not be easily seen because of the fast ventricular rate or a prolonged P'-R' interval. Configuration of the P' waves is generally somewhat different from that of the sinus P waves. If the atrial rhythm is irregular and the P' waves are of varying configuration, the term multifocal atrial tachycardia is used.

3. The QRS configuration is usually normal or wide and bizarre due to bundle branch block, aberrant ventricular conduction, or ventricular pre-excitation.

4. The P'-R interval of the P-QRS is usually constant (1:1 AV conduction). At extremely high heart rates, varying degrees of AV block can occur (e.g., 2:1, 3:1, 4:1).

Atrial Flutter

Atrial flutter is a rapid atrial rhythm at a rate usually greater than 300 to 350 beats/min. The typical form is regular with P waves being replaced by sawtooth waves (called F waves). Varying degrees of

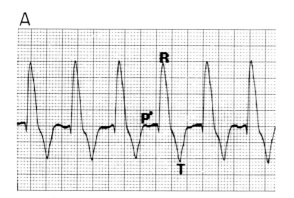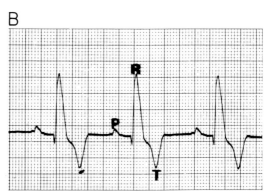

Fig. 4-37 (A) Supraventricular tachycardia, probably atrial tachycardia in a dog. The focus of origin cannot be identified with accuracy in this strip. **(B)** After ocular pressure, the tachycardia has been terminated. The configuration of these sinus QRS complexes is the same as in strip A and represents a left bundle branch block configuration. (Tilley LP: Essentials of Canine and Feline Electrocardiography. 2nd Ed. Lea & Febiger, Philadelphia, 1985.)

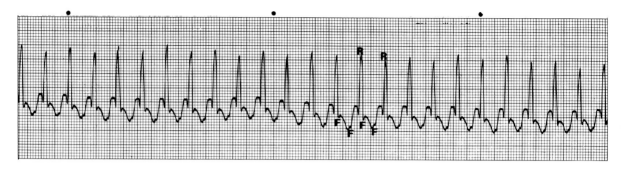

Fig. 4-38 Atrial flutter with 2:1 conduction at a ventricular rate of 330/min in a dog with an atrial septal defect. (Tilley LP: Essentials of Canine and Feline Electrocardiography. 2nd Ed. Lea & Febiger, Philadelphia, 1985.)

AV conduction are usually present. The term supraventricular tachycardia is used when atrial flutter cannot be differentiated from atrial tachycardia (Fig. 4-38).

Atrial flutter is associated with conditions which cause other atrial arrhythmias. Diseases producing atrial enlargement are the most common. Other associated conditions include quinidine therapy for atrial fibrillation, atrial septal defect, tricuspid dysplasia, ventricular pre-excitation (WPW syndrome), and hypertrophic cardiomyopathy in the cat.

Atrial flutter has the following ECG characteristics:

1. The atrial rhythm (F waves) is regular with a rate usually above 300 to 350 beats/min. The ventricular rhythm and rate depend on the atrial rate and the state of AV conduction (e.g., when same as the atrial rate, 1:1 conduction; when one-half the atrial rate, 2:1).

2. Normal P waves are replaced by sawtooth flutter waves (F waves), a combination of ectopic and pronounced atrial repolarization waves.

3. The QRS configuration is normal or wide and bizarre due to bundle branch block, aberrant ventricular conduction, or ventricular pre-excitation.

4. When conduction through the AV node is constant, the interval between the QRS complex and the F wave is of constant duration. This interval may vary based on changing conduction and second-degree AV block.

Atrial Fibrillation

Atrial fibrillation is common in the dog and is usually associated with severe organic heart disease (Fig. 4-39; see also Figs. 14-1 and 23-1). It can be paroxysmal but is usually sustained. The loss of atrial kick combined with the rapid heart rate may substantially reduce cardiac output and cause congestive heart failure. Atrial fibrillation is rare in cats and is primarily associated with hypertrophic or restrictive cardiomyopathy.

Atrial fibrillation results from the same conditions as other atrial arrhythmias with those causing marked atrial enlargement the most common. In the dog, it is usually associated with chronic AV valvular insufficiency in small breeds, dilated cardiomyopathy in large and giant breeds, and congenital heart defects. Digitalis toxicity, heartworm disease, cardiac trauma, and severe metabolic disorders are less common causes. Atrial fibrillation may occasionally occur in the absence of cardiac disease without clinical signs, especially in giant-breed dogs.

Electrocardiographic features of atrial fibrillation include the following:

1. Atrial and ventricular rates are rapid and totally irregular.

2. In coarse atrial fibrillation, large oscillations (f waves) of varying amplitude replace the normal sinus P waves. Sometimes these prominent f waves resemble atrial flutter. The term atrial flutter-fibrillation is then used.

3. The QRS configuration is normal or wide and bizarre owing to bundle branch block or ventricular pre-excitation. Normal QRS complexes sometimes vary in amplitude, especially during fast heart rates.

4. The ventricular rate is irregularly irregular because the AV junction conducts only a limited number of fibrillatory waves to the ventricles in a sporadic fashion.

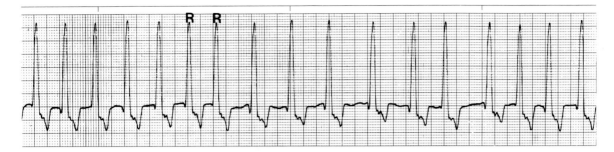

Fig. 4-39 Atrial fibrillation in a dog with congestive heart failure. The heart rate is rapid and irregularly irregular. P waves are absent. The tall and wide QRS complexes indicate left heart enlargement. The S-T segment is depressed.

Sick Sinus Syndrome

Sick sinus syndrome (Fig. 4-40) describes a number of ECG abnormalities of the SA node, including severe sinus bradycardia and severe SA block and/or sinus arrest. Dogs with these abnormalities have recurrent episodes of supraventricular tachycardia in addition to sinus bradycardia and/or bradyarrhythmia. This subset of the sick sinus syndrome is called the bradycardia-tachycardia syndrome.

Most dogs with sick sinus syndrome also have coexisting dysfunction of the AV junction and/or bundle branches. Automaticity of lower pacemakers is often depressed. During long periods of SA block or arrest, the latent AV junctional pacemaker fails to pace the heart and cardiac standstill can result.

The clinical manifestations of sick sinus syndrome are quite variable. Heart rates may be so slow as to reduce cardiac output and cause cardiac failure. The most common signs are syncope and weakness. The female miniature schnauzer is susceptible to this disorder. Sick sinus syndrome is rare in the cat.

Possible causes of sick sinus syndrome include disease affecting the SA node artery or replacement of the SA node with fibrous tissue. Genetic inheritance of this condition is possible. Digitalis toxicity can cause changes consistent with the sick sinus syndrome.

Sick sinus syndrome has the following electrocardiographic characteristics:

1. Severe and persistent sinus bradycardia not induced by drugs

2. Short or long pauses of SA block or arrest with or without escape rhythms

3. Failure of the sinus rhythm to begin after electric cardioversion of tachycardia

4. Atrial fibrillation with a slow ventricular rate in the absence of drugs usually due to accompanying disease of the AV junction

5. In the bradycardia-tachycardia syndrome, periods of severe sinus bradycardia alternating with

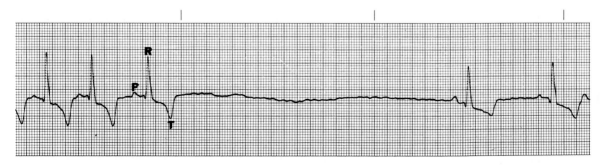

Fig. 4-40 Prolonged ventricular asystole due to sinoatrial block or arrest after ocular pressure in a dog with sick sinus syndrome. No escape beats occur during this interval.

ectopic supraventricular tachycardias (atrial tachycardia, atrial fibrillation, or atrial flutter)

6. Long pause following an atrial premature complex

7. AV junctional escape rhythm (with or without slow and unstable sinus activity)

Tests for SA node dysfunction include the following:

1. Ocular or carotid sinus massage may cause prolonged periods of sinus arrest (e.g., longer than 3 seconds). Increased vagal tone may partially be responsible for this syndrome.

2. Atropine administered intravenously (0.015 mg/ kg body weight) fails to cause a marked increase in heart rate (normally at least a 50 percent increase occurs), indicating that the SA node dysfunction is not due to excessive vagal tone.

3. Simultaneous automatic monitoring with radiotelemetry and time-lapse videorecordings have been used in dogs to correlate syncope with arrhythmias on the ECG.

4. After cessation of rapid right atrial pacing, the atrium can fail to depolarize for as long as 15 seconds (normal in the dog is 1.5 second).

ARRHYTHMIAS ORIGINATING IN THE AV JUNCTION

Atrioventricular Junctional Premature Complexes

Atrioventricular junctional premature complexes are caused by the early firing of an ectopic AV junctional focus (Fig. 4-41; see also Fig. 4-46, below). The impulse spreads backward (retrograde) to the atria as well as forward (anterograde) to the ventricles. The term junctional is more accurate for describing rhythms that arise in the region extending from the atrial fibers approaching the AV junction to the bifurcation of the bundle of His. Junctional premature complexes are often associated with digitalis toxicity. Other causes are the same as those associated with APCs.

The ECG features of AV junctional premature complexes are as follows:

1. The heart rate is usually normal. The rhythm is irregular due to the premature P′ waves that disrupt normal sinus-initiated P-wave rhythm.

2. The P′ wave is almost always negative in lead II.

3. The QRS complex is premature. Its configuration is usually normal but can be wide and bizarre due to bundle branch block, aberrant ventricular conduction, or ventricular pre-excitation.

4. The P′ wave may precede, be superimposed on, or follow the QRS depending on the location of the ectopic focus and on the conduction velocity above and below the AV junctional focus. For example, the negative P′ wave precedes the QRS when retrograde impulse conduction is faster than anterograde conduction.

5. A *noncompensatory pause* is usually present. It is characterized by an R-R interval enclosing the premature complex that is less than twice the normal R-R interval duration.

Atrioventricular Junctional Tachycardia

In AV junctional tachycardia, the ectopic focus in the AV junction acts as a primary pacemaker that discharges faster than the inherent AV junctional rate of 40 to 60 beats/min (in the dog). The term enhanced AV junctional rhythm is used for rates above 60, but less than 100, in the dog. It is usually impossible to differentiate atrial tachycardia from an AV junctional tachycardia, since the inverted P waves are superimposed on the QRS-T complexes. Because the two arrhythmias are electrocardiographically and mechanistically similar, the term supraventricular tachycardia can be used for both.

Associated conditions include those disorders associated with atrial arrhythmias. Digitalis toxicity is often associated with an AV junctional arrhythmia.

An AV junctional tachycardia has the following ECG characteristics:

1. The heart rate is over 60 beats/min in the dog. The rhythm is usually regular. Junctional tachycardia can be either paroxysmal or continuous.

2. P′ waves are negative in lead II and may precede, be superimposed on, or follow the QRS complex.

3. The configuration of the QRS complex is usually

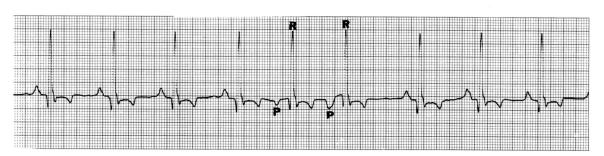

Fig. 4-41 Two junctional premature complexes (fifth and sixth complexes) in a dog with digitalis toxicity. P mitrale is also present.

normal or can be wide and bizarre as a result of bundle branch block, aberrant ventricular conduction, or ventricular pre-excitation.

4. The P′-R interval is constant. The P′-R interval for a high AV junctional focus is normal or longer when there is conduction delay below the AV junctional focus. At higher rates, varying degrees of AV block can occur.

ARRHYTHMIAS ORIGINATING IN THE VENTRICULAR MUSCLE

Ventricular Premature Complexes

Ventricular premature complexes (VPCs) are impulses that arise from an ectopic ventricular focus (Fig. 4-42; see also Figs. 4-45 and 4-46 below, and Fig. 23-6). They spread through both ventricles with delay, causing a bizarre, widened QRS complex. As in the cat, VPCs in the dog comprise the most frequent arrhythmia after sinus tachycardia. Two possible mechanisms for VPCs are reentry and increased automaticity. Occasional VPCs seldom produce clinical signs. A significant reduction in cardiac output is more likely when the animal has pre-existing heart disease.

There are numerous causes of VPCs. Occasionally, they may occur in normal hearts without clinical significance. Cardiac causes of VPCs include congestive heart failure, myocardial infarction, neoplasia, pericarditis, traumatic myocarditis, idiopathic myocarditis in boxers and Doberman pinschers, and bacterial endomyocarditis. Secondary

causes include changes in autonomic tone, hypoxia, anemia, uremia, pyometra, gastric dilation-volvulus, pancreatitis, and parvovirus. Drugs that can cause VPCs include digitalis, epinephrine, anesthetic agents, and atropine.

Ventricular premature complexes have the following ECG characteristics:

1. The heart rate is usually normal. The rhythm is irregular due to the premature QRS complex that disrupts the normal sinus rhythm.

2. P waves are of normal configuration.

3. The ectopic QRS complex is premature, bizarre, and often of large amplitude.

4. The T wave is directed opposite to the QRS deflection.

5. The ventricular origin of the VPCs can be suggested as follows: if the major QRS deflection is negative in lead II, the ectopic focus is in the left ventricle; the reverse is true for right-sided VPCs.

6. VPCs are not associated with the P wave. The independent normal P wave may precede, be within, or follow the VPC.

7. A *compensatory pause* usually follows a VPC because the ectopic impulse generally cannot penetrate retrograde through the AV junction and depolarize the SA node (see Fig. 4-45). The sinus rhythm continues undisturbed and the next sinus impulse after the VPC occurs on time. Thus, the R-R interval of the sinus initiated QRS complexes on either side of the VPC equals twice the normally conducted R-R interval.

8. VPCs of identical shape are called unifocal; when

the QRS is variable, they are termed multiform VPCs.

Ventricular Tachycardia

Ventricular tachycardia is a continuous series of three or more VPCs (Figs. 4-42 and 4-43; see also Figs. 14-1 and 23-7). It may be intermittent (e.g., paroxysmal) or persistent and sustained. Ventricular tachycardia is generally considered a serious and life-threatening tachyarrhythmia. Affected animals often present with concomitant hypotension and congestive heart failure.

The same conditions that cause VPCs also cause ventricular tachycardia. Ventricular tachycardia is usually a manifestation of significant organic heart disease. In various cardiac and noncardiac disorders, ventricular ectopic activity may not occur until 12 to 36 hours after a myocardial ischemic event (e.g., gastric dilatation-volvulus, myocardial infarction, or traumatic myocarditis).

The ECG features of ventricular tachycardia include the following:

1. In the dog, the ventricular rate is usually above 100 beats/min with a regular rhythm. Ventricular tachycardia between 60 and 100 is termed idioventricular tachycardia (also called an enhanced ventricular rhythm). In the cat, the rate is usually above 150 beats/min.

2. P waves that are visible are of normal configuration.

3. QRS complexes are wide and bizarre with T waves directed opposite to the QRS deflection.

4. Fusion complexes may occur implying ventricular activation from two different foci.

5. Capture beats by normal sinus initiated rhythm or complexes may be present.

6. There is no relationship between the QRS complexes and the P waves; the P waves may precede, be hidden within, or follow the QRS complexes.

7. Hallmark features of ventricular tachycardia include *fusion complexes, capture beats,* and *AV dissociation.*

Ventricular Fibrillation

Ventricular fibrillation causes cardiac arrest and is often a terminal event (Fig. 4-44). Ventricular contractions are weak and uncoordinated. Cardiac output is essentially nonexistent. The ECG shows irregular, chaotic, and deformed deflections of varying amplitude, width, and shape. Immediate defibrillation and cardiopulmonary resuscitation must be undertaken. Possible associated conditions include shock, anoxia, myocardial damage, electrolyte and acid-base imbalances, aortic stenosis, drug reactions, cardiac surgery, electric shock, myocarditis, and hypothermia.

Ventricular fibrillation is characterized by the following ECG features:

1. The heart rate is rapid with irregular, chaotic, and bizarre waves. By contrast, *ventricular flutter* is a rhythmic series of bizarre and uniform undulating waves that usually progresses to ventricular fibrillation (Fig. 14-1).

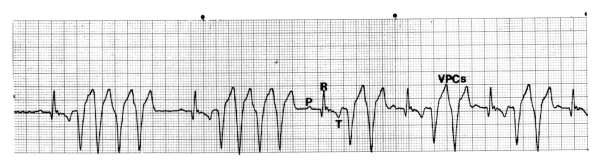

Fig. 4-42 Frequent ventricular premature complexes (VPCs) and paroxysmal ventricular tachycardia in a dog with septicemia-endocarditis. (Tilley LP: Essentials of Canine and Feline Electrocardiography. 2nd Ed. Lea & Febiger, Philadelphia, 1985.)

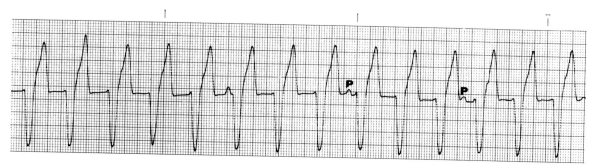

Fig. 4-43 Sustained ventricular tachycardia in a dog with gastric torsion. There is no relationship between the QRS complexes and the P waves.

2. P waves cannot be recognized.
3. QRS and T deflections are not discernible.
4. There are two types of ventricular fibrillation: one with large oscillations termed coarse, and the other with small oscillations termed fine.

Ventricular Asystole

Ventricular asystole is the absence of ventricular complexes. It represents cardiac arrest and carries a grave prognosis. Clinically, a peripheral arterial pulse cannot be palpated during cardiac arrest due to ventricular fibrillation, ventricular asystole, or electromechanical dissociation. An ECG is needed to differentiate these arrhythmias. Ventricular asystole may be caused by severe SA block or sinus arrest, third-degree AV block, severe electrolyte or acid-base disorder, or other terminal systemic diseases.

Electrocardiographic features of ventricular asystole include the following:

1. There is no ventricular rhythm. Normal P waves are present at a regular rhythm if complete AV block exists. With severe SA block or arrest, the faster the original rate, the longer is the period of asystole.
2. No QRS complexes are seen.

ADVANCED ELECTROCARDIOGRAPHIC CONCEPTS AND TECHNIQUES

Ladder Diagrams

The ladder (Lewis) diagram (Figs. 4-45 and 4-46) is a graphic illustration of cardiac impulse formation and conduction that enhances the clinician's understanding of arrhythmias and conduction disorders. These diagrams aid in explaining and illustrating the more complex rhythm disorders.[22,32] The technique illustrating its use is presented in Figure 4-45.

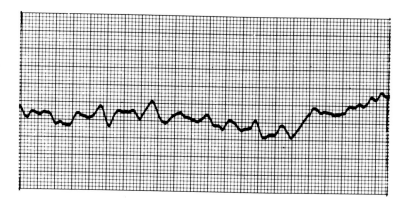

Fig. 4-44 Coarse ventricular fibrillation. Disorganized oscillations without recognizable QRS-T deflections are evident. (Tilley LP: Essentials of Canine and Feline Electrocardiography, 2nd Ed. Lea & Febiger, Philadelphia, 1985.)

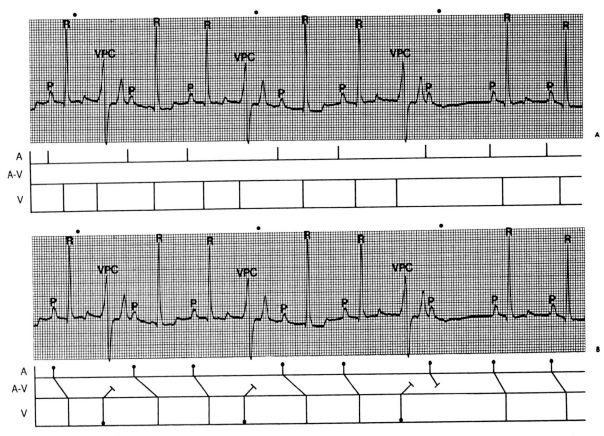

Fig. 4-45 Technique to use the atrioventricular (AV) ladder diagram. (**A**) First use a ruler to line up the beginning of the P waves with a subsequent vertical line drawn at the A (atrial) level. Then line up the beginning of the QRS (Q wave) with the ventricular (V) level and draw a corresponding vertical line. Finally, indicate AV conduction by connecting the bottom of the atrial line with the top of the ventricular line. A dot indicates the site of impulse formation. (**B**) The first two interpolated VPCs have penetrated the AV junction causing the subsequent P-R interval to be prolonged. The third VPC has similarly rendered the AV junction completely refractory preventing conduction of the subsequent sinus P wave. A compensatory pause occurs after the third VPC. (Tilley LP: Essentials of Canine and Feline Electrocardiography. 2nd Ed. Lea & Febiger, Philadelphia, 1985.)

Aberrant Conduction

Aberrant conduction (Figs. 4-46 and 4-47) occurs when a premature impulse conducts through a bundle branch that is in its absolute or relative refractory period.[22,33] The duration of the refractory period of the individual bundle branch cells lengthens with longer cardiac cycles. Aberrant conduction is more likely to occur with slower heart rates or with a prolonged cycle immediately preceding an ectopic beat (*Ashman's phenomenon*). The refractory period of the right bundle branch normally exceeds that of the left bundle branch. Therefore, aberration due to Ashman's phenomenon usually shows a RBBB con-

figuration and these QRS complexes must be differentiated from ventricular premature complexes. A P′ wave with a slightly prolonged P′-R interval preceding the aberrant QRS complex will favor a diagnosis of aberrant conduction of a supraventricular premature complex versus a ventricular premature complex (Fig. 4-47).

Concealed Conduction

Concealed conduction (Figs. 4-45 and 4-46) emphasizes the importance of deductive reasoning in

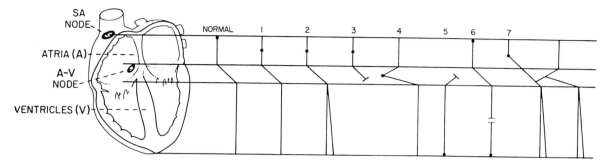

Fig. 4-46 Representative examples of the atrioventricular (AV) ladder diagram: (1) Atrial premature complex (APC) with normal conduction; (2) APC with aberrant ventricular conduction (also used to illustrate left and right bundle branches); (3) APC not conducted; (4) AV junctional premature complex with anterograde ventricular and retrograde atrial conduction; (5) Ventricular premature complex (VPC) with partial penetration of the AV junction; (6) Ventricular fusion complex between a sinus impulse and an ectopic ventricular impulse; (7) APC and one reciprocal complex (re-entry) with aberrant ventricular conduction. (Tilley LP: Essentials of Canine and Feline Electrocardiography. 2nd Ed. Lea & Febiger, Philadelphia, 1985.)

arrhythmia analysis. This term explains the phenomenon of incomplete cardiac impulse conduction in a specialized conduction tissue (e.g., AV node). The effect of this incompletely conducted impulse on the behavior of the subsequent cardiac impulse is manifested in subsequent P-QRS-T complexes.[22,33,34] For example, VPCs can result in retrograde spread of impulses into the AV node. This can result in conduction delay evident in a prolonged P-R interval or complete block of sinus P wave. Altered behavior of impulses that are subsequently affected by concealed conduction can be manifested as delay of conduction, block of conduction, displacement of the pacemaker, enhancement of conduction, or a combination of the above. Although the presence of concealed conduction may be deduced, further studies may be needed to confirm this possibility.

Supernormality

Supernormality is an ECG effect of improved conduction in the presence of depressed conductivity resulting from a supernormal phase of excitability or conduction.[35] It is characterized by an unexpected response to a stimulus or by a response that is less abnormal than expected. Supernormality is often deduced when paradoxic enhancement of depressed AV or intraventricular conduction is evident. However, this concept is controversial and a

Fig. 4-47 Aberrant ventricular conduction in a dog. Atrial tachycardia is initiated by an APC (after the second sinus complex). This first APC contains a long P′-R interval with aberrant ventricular conduction (arrow). This aberrancy is probably secondary to Ashman's phenomenon, owing to the long cardiac cycle preceding the short cycle. Secondary ST-T changes are also noted. (Tilley LP: Essentials of Canine and Feline Electrocardiography. 2nd Ed. Lea & Febiger, Philadelphia, 1985.)

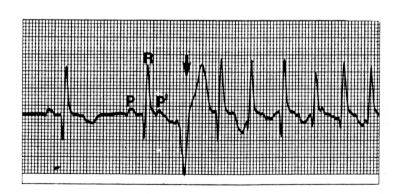

number of alternative explanations have been advanced.

Re-entry

Re-entry (Fig. 4-46; see also Figs. 13-12 and 13-13) is a mechanism for supraventricular and ventricular arrhythmias whereby the electrical impulse that activates a segment of cardiac tissue returns in a different pathway and reactivates the same tissue.[22,36] Arrhythmias have been caused by re-entry in terminal Purkinje fibers, ischemic myocardial tissue, bundle branches and His bundle, AV nodal tissue, and accessory AV pathways (WPW syndrome). Concealed re-entry occurs when an impulse makes a circus movement through a loop of depressed fibers but does not re-excite the heart. The pathway becomes refractory prior to the impulse returning to the site of origin. Concealed re-entry is only deduced because of its effect on the next impulse that traverses the same route.[36]

Holter Monitor Electrocardiography

The resting ECG usually demonstrates only a short period of the cardiac rhythm. When wishing to evaluate the cardiac rhythm for prolonged periods or during normal activities, the veterinarian can use the technique of long-term ECG (Holter) monitoring.[22,32] This technique employs a precordial lead system (two or three electrodes positioned on the chest wall), connected to a portable ECG monitor. The ECG signal is recorded on magnetic tape for 10 to 24 hours. The tape can be rapidly analyzed on a special scanner (Fig. 4-48) or by computerized techniques.

Long-term ECG monitoring can be performed to obtain a diagnosis of paroxysmal tachyarrhythmias, bradyarrhythmias, or conduction disorders (especially when the routine ECG fails to record an arrhythmia), to evaluate the frequency of premature atrial or premature ventricular complexes, to determine the etiology of syncope when a cardiac origin is suspected, to assess the effectiveness of antiarrhythmic therapy or a permanent cardiac pacemaker, and to evaluate an asymptomatic animal with complete heart block or bifascicular block for life-threatening arrhythmias.

Transtelephonic Electrocardiography

The system of transtelephonic electrocardiography can accurately characterize rhythm disturbances and conduction abnormalities. It involves the use of

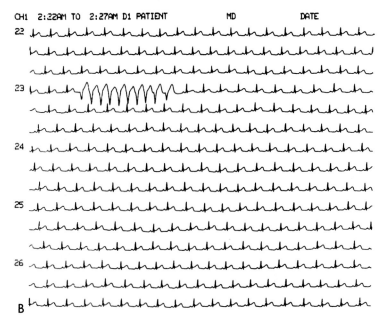

CH1 2:22AM TO 2:27AM D1 PATIENT   MD   DATE

B

Fig. 4-48 Printouts of a displayed time segment from a Holter monitor system. A period of paroxysmal ventricular tachycardia can be easily recognized and correlated with the time of occurrence by referring to digital time entries displayed adjacent to the ECG data. By this technique, arrhythmias can be efficiently recognized and graphically enlarged for complete analysis and documentation. (Courtesy of Del Mar Avionics, Irvine, California.)

a small, portable, battery-powered, transistorized, ECG preamplifier that converts ECG signals into tones that can be transmitted over the telephone line.[22,37] Transtelephonic electrocardiography is well established in veterinary and human medicine.

The technique is simple. The animal is positioned in right lateral recumbency (the sternal position can also be employed) and electrode clips from the transmitter are attached to the limbs in a similar manner as used in routine electrocardiography. The ECG data center is then contacted by telephone, and relevant historical, physical examination, radiographic, and laboratory findings are communicated to a technician. The veterinarian supervising the transmission places the telephone mouthpiece on the transmitter and a standard six limb-lead ECG with amplitude calibration is recorded.

In a clinical review of 2,000 consecutive transte-

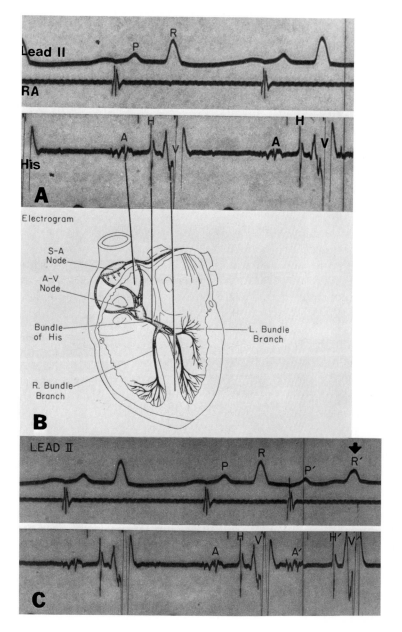

Fig. 4-49 (**A**) Canine bundle of His (His) electrogram (bottom) recorded simultaneously with a right atrial (RA) electrogram (middle) and lead II electrocardiogram (top). (P, P wave; R, R wave; A, atrial deflection; H, His bundle deflection; V, ventricular deflection.) (**B**) His bundle electrogram (from Fig. A above) related to the corresponding conduction system sites illustrated in the in-situ heart. (**C**) Same scheme as in Fig. A. Origin of the third complex from left (arrow) in the lead II ECG is supraventricular. P′ wave is premature and the His bundle electrogram displays a lengthened A′-H′ interval due to prolonged conduction through the AV node which has not fully recovered from the previous impulse. The third complex (R′) represents aberrant conduction. (Tilley LP: Essentials of Canine and Feline Electrocardiography. 2nd Ed. Lea & Febiger, Philadelphia, 1985, with permission.)

lephonic canine ECGs, 18 types of arrhythmias were detected in 20 percent (396) of dogs. Atrial arrhythmias included atrial premature complexes, atrial tachycardia, atrial fibrillation, and atrial flutter. Ventricular arrhythmias included ventricular premature complexes and ventricular tachycardia-fibrillation. Conduction disorders visualized included first-degree, second-degree, and third-degree AV block, SA block and/or arrest, atrial standstill, and ventricular pre-excitation. Although technical limitations of transtelephonic electrocardiography include attenuation of recorded voltages, and inadequate frequency response of the mechanical system (recorder stylus), they do not provide a major problem in the interpretation of the clinical ECG.

Computerized Electrocardiography

Computerized electrocardiograpic interpretation is an emerging field in veterinary medicine.[22,32] In human medicine,[38] it has contributed to improved technical quality of the ECG, technician efficiency (i.e., no need to cut, mount, or store the ECG), improved diagnostic criteria, stimulated teaching, and reduced the time needed for analysis and interpretation of the ECG.

It is mandatory that all ECGs be reviewed by an electrocardiographer and that the computer analysis not be the final assessment. Currently available programs cannot accurately interpret most complex arrhythmias, although they are effective in diagnosing common problems. Most human computer programs can analyze abnormal ECGs with 80 to 90 percent accuracy. Inherent variations in knowledge and interpretation by the electrocardiographer designing the program contributes to inaccuracies. Although numerous ECGs must be recorded for computed electrocardiography to be cost effective, it may one day play a significant role in veterinary medicine.

Intracavitary Electrocardiography

A routine ECG does not provide detailed information about conduction system activation and may not provide evidence of atrial activity (P waves). This information can be obtained by inserting catheter electrodes transvenously into the heart.[22,32,39]

Intracardiac electrocardiography may thus demonstrate atrial activity in complex tachyarrhythmias, distinguish aberrant ventricular conduction from ventricular arrhythmias, localize the site of AV block, determine conduction intervals between the atrium and His bundle and between His bundle and ventricles, and facilitate therapeutic cardiac pacing (Fig. 4-49).

Intracavitary recordings can generate a cardiac electrogram using uni-, bi-, tri-, quadri-, or hexapolar catheters inserted in the right atrium or ventricle. These cardiac ECGs can be further defined according to the electrode recording position. Special His bundle catheters can provide a His bundle ECG that records atrial and ventricular activity, atrium to His bundle conduction, His bundle to ventricle conduction, and other information.

ACKNOWLEDGMENT

We thank Mrs. Eileen Willis for her excellent assistance in the preparation of this chapter.

REFERENCES

1. Kolliker A, Muller H: Nockweis der Negativen Schwankung des Muskelstrom am Naurlich sich contrahireiden Muskel. Verh Phys Med Ges 6:528, 1856
2. Lipman BS, Dunn M, Massie E: Clinical Electrocardiography. 7th Ed. Year Book Medical Publishers, Chicago, 1984
3. Waller AD: A demonstration on man of electromotive changes accompanying the heart's beat. J Physiol (Lond) 8:229, 1887
4. Burch GE, DePasquale NP: A History of Electrocardiography. Year Book Medical Publishers, Chicago, 1964
5. Lewis T: Clinical Electrocardiography. Shaw & Sons, New York, 1913
6. Wilson FN, Johnston FD, Macleond AG, et al: Electrocardiograms that represent the potential variations of a single electrode. Am Heart J 9:477, 1934.
7. Wilson FN, Johnston FD, Rosenbaum FF, et al: On Einthoven's triangle, the theory of unipolar electrocardiographic leads and the interpretation of the precordial electrocardiogram. Am Heart J 32:279, 1946
8. Lannek N: A clinical and experimental study of the electrocardiogram in dogs (thesis). Stockholm, 1949

9. Detweiler DK: Electrocardiographic and clinical features of spontaneous auricular fibrillation and flutter (tachycardia) in dogs. Zentralbl Veterinaermed 4:509, 1957

10. Detweiler DK, Patterson DF: The prevalence and types of heart disease in dogs. Ann NY Acad Sci 127:481, 1965

11. Patterson DF, Detweiler DK, Hubben K, et al: Spontaneous abnormal cardiac arrhythmias and conduction disturbances in the dog (a clinical and pathologic study of 3,000 dogs). Am J Vet Res 22:355, 1961

12. Hamlin RL, Smith CR: Anatomical and physiological basis for interpretation of the electrocardiogram. Am J Vet Res 21:701, 1960

13. Hamlin RL, Smetzer DL, Smith CR: The electrocardiogram, phonocardiogram and derived ventricular activation process of domestic cats. Am J Vet Res 24:792, 1960

14. Hamlin RL: Electrocardiographic detection of ventricular enlargement in the dog. J Am Vet Med Assoc 153:1461, 1968

15. Hill JD: The electrocardiogram in dogs with standardized body and limb positions. J Electrocardiol 1:175, 1968

16. Moore EN, Morse HT, Price AC: Cardiac arrhythmias produced by catecholamines in anesthetized dogs. Circ Res 15:77, 1964

17. Moore EN: Microelectrode studies on concealment of multiple premature atrial responses. Circ Res 18:660, 1966

18. Moore EN, Jomain SL, Stuckey JH, et al: Studies on ectopic atrial rhythms in dogs. Am J Cardiol 19:676, 1967

19. Ettinger SJ, Suter PF: Canine Cardiology. WB Saunders Co, Philadelphia, 1970

20. Bolton GR: Handbook of Canine Electrocardiography. WB Saunders, Philadelphia, 1975

21. Tilley LP: Essentials of Canine and Feline Electrocardiography. CV Mosby, St. Louis, 1979

22. Tilley LP: Essentials of Canine and Feline Electrocardiography. Interpretation and Management. 2nd Ed. Lea & Febiger, Philadelphia, 1985

23. Lazzara R: Basic electrophysiology. p. 16. In Helfant R (ed): Bellet's Essentials of Cardiac Arrhythmias. WB Saunders, Philadelphia, 1979

24. Silber EN, Katz LN: Electrocardiography and vectorcardiography. p. 294. In Heart Disease. Macmillan, New York, 1975

25. Greenspan K: Cardiac excitation, conduction and the electrocardiogram. p. 311. In Selkurt EE (ed): Physiology. 4th Ed. Little, Brown, Boston, 1976

26. Horan LG, Flowers NC: Electrocardiography and vectorcardiography. p. 198. In Braunwald E (ed): Heart Disease. WB Saunders, Philadelphia, 1980

27. Castellanos A, Myerburg R: The resting electrocardiogram. p. 206. In Hurst JW (ed): The Heart. 6th Ed. McGraw-Hill, New York, 1986

28. Wallace AG: Electrical activity of the heart. p. 115. In Hurst JW (ed): The Heart. 5th Ed. McGraw-Hill, New York, 1982

29. Abildskov JA: The electrocardiogram. p. 312. In Sodeman WA (ed): Pathologic Physiology, Mechanisms of Disease. 5th Ed. WB Saunders, Philadelphia, 1974

30. Kittleson MD, Eyster GE, Knowlen GG, et al: Myocardial function in small dogs with chronic mitral regurgitation and severe congestive heart failure. J Am Vet Med Assoc 184:455, 1984

31. Stang JM, Ryan JM: The magic of the electrocardiogram (ECG)—Diagnostic utility of the scalar and vector ECG in the 1980's: A perspective. p. 51. In Warren JV, Lewis RP (eds): Diagnostic Procedures in Cardiology: A Clinician's Guide. Year Book Medical Publishers, Chicago, 1985

32. Tilley LP: Advanced electrocardiographic techniques. Vet Clin North Am 13:365, 1983

33. Fisch C: Electrocardiography of arrhythmias: From deductive analysis to laboratory confirmation—Twenty-five years of progress. J Am Coll Cardiol 1:306, 1983

34. Fisch C: Concealed conduction. p. 63. In Zipes DP (ed): Cardiology Clinics. Vol. 1. WB Saunders, Philadelphia, 1983

35. Rosenbaum MB, Levi RJ, Elizar MV, et al: Supernormal excitability and conduction. p. 75. In Zipes DP (ed): Cardiology Clinics. Vol. 1. WB Saunders, Philadelphia, 1983

36. Marriott HJL, Conover MH: Advanced Concepts in Arrhythmias. CV Mosby, St. Louis, 1979

37. Tilley LP: Transtelephonic analysis of cardiac arrhythmias in the dog. Vet Clin North Am 13:63, 1983

38. Sridharan MR, Flowers NC: Computerized electrocardiographic analysis. Modern Concepts of Cardiovascular Disease 53(7):37, 1984

39. Chung EK: Principles of Cardiac Arrhythmias, 3rd Ed. Williams & Wilkins, Baltimore, 1983

5
Radiologic Examination

Peter F. Lord

THE ROLE OF RADIOLOGY IN HEART DISEASE

Thoracic radiographs are a cornerstone in the evaluation of animals with suspected heart disease. The cardiac silhouette and lung field provide direct information regarding the size of the heart and condition of the lungs and circulation, reflecting the degree of heart failure. A careful and systematic radiographic examination of the thorax may facilitate or confirm a clinical diagnosis suspected on the basis of physical examination. It also aids in assessing the severity and significance of known heart disease and helps in evaluating the effectiveness of treatment.

Many clinical signs of heart disease or failure, such as coughing, dyspnea, fainting, and cyanosis, may be caused by other diseases. In patients whose history, clinical signs, and physical examination are not specific enough to confer a definitive diagnosis, the radiologic examination may make the diagnosis possible. Radiologic information may also lead to other diagnostic tests not previously considered (e.g., echocardiography). It may suggest certain treatments that may not be specific for a disease (e.g., diuretics for pulmonary edema) but will help a patient improve and assist in diagnosis by evaluating response to therapy.

Thoracic radiology is an essential part of the examination of patients with suspected heart disease.

However, contrast studies (angiocardiography, pericardiography) have declined in importance with the use of echocardiography for the diagnosis of congenital malformations, assessment of pericardial effusion and evaluation of cardiac function.

This chapter describes principles of radiologic evaluation of heart disease. Using the radiologist's approach of looking for radiologic signs and ascribing conditions or diseases to them, differential diagnoses can be generated based on the significance and reliability of radiologic signs in conjunction with clinical signs.

RADIOGRAPHIC EVALUATION

Image Quality

The veterinarian must be familiar with the technical factors that produce a good image of the thoracic organs. Time and effort spent in accomplishing this results in the security of knowing that the diagnosis is based on accurate information. Poor image quality leads to frustration, no diagnosis, or—worse—misdiagnosis.

Technical factors must be standardized. A technique chart that uses high kilovoltage and low milliamp-seconds is best for thoracic radiography because it minimizes exposure time, reduces motion unsharpness, and produces a low-contrast high-latitide image that is ideal for the thorax. The natural contrast provided by the air in the lungs outlines the heart, mediastinum, thoracic wall, diaphragm, and pulmonary structures. The density of the ribs, spine, and muscle masses is minimized, while the lungs and airways are optimally exposed. Because most of the thorax contains air, fogging caused by scattered radiation is not a great problem and is less important than stopping motion by using a short exposure time. For this reason, a grid should not be used (even on fairly large dogs), if it increases exposure times so much that a blurred image would result. Good quality fast screens are essential. Rare earth screens are 50 to 200 percent faster than standard high-speed screens with little or no decrease in resolution. Their use combined with an accurate electronic timer will usually ensure acceptable films from a low-power machine.

Standard development (either by the time-temperature method using fresh developer and fixer or an automatic film processor) is another essential element for reproducible diagnostic films. Old developer and fixer mars image quality.

Radiographic Positioning

The animal must be positioned straight. Slight obliquity in either lateral, ventrodorsal (VD) or dorsoventral (DV) views distorts the cardiac silhouette and displaces the positions of the bronchi and pulmonary vessels. This makes it impossible to distinguish normal from abnormal structures. In the lateral view, obliquity makes the heart appear rounder. The mainstem bronchi, instead of being superimposed on each other, are tilted, giving the impression of left atrial enlargement. When the thorax is straight in the lateral view, the dorsal arches of the ribs on each side will line up with each other. In the DV and VD views, the tips of the spinous processes should be within the bounds of the vertebral bodies.[1]

Problems in taking whole-body radiographs of animals larger than cats are (1) resolving the difference in density between the thorax and abdomen, and (2) distorting the diaphragmatic[2] and cardiac silhouettes by oblique radiographs. The tube should be centered at the fifth or sixth ribs to minimize distortion.

Radiographic positioning should be standardized. Either the right or left lateral view, or the DV or VD view, should be used routinely. Slight differences in shape of the heart between left and right lateral and DV and VD views may be mistaken for pathologic changes in the cardiac silhouette.[3,4] The heart is more elongated in the VD than in the DV view. Sternal contact may be greater in the left than the right lateral view. Consistency with follow-up examinations is more important than which view is chosen initially.[3,5]

Some special conditions may affect the choice of DV or VD views to be used. The animal may be uncomfortable or dyspneic, for example, and may not tolerate certain positions. It may be more difficult to pull the forelegs forward in the DV view. In addition, certain structures are better highlighted in different views. In the dog, the hilar area and the pulmonary arteries in the caudal lobes are more sharply delineated in the DV view because the dorsal lung is better inflated with the animal in the prone position,[5] making subtle signs of heartworm disease and peribronchial lesions more likely to be diagnosed. In the cat, the lungs are normally better inflated in the VD views because the thorax is more expanded. The suspicion of pleural effusion requires that a VD view be taken if possible, because fluid is less likely to obscure the cardiac silhouette in this view than in the DV view.[4,6]

Tranquilization should be used judiciously if necessary to achieve a diagnostic image. Many animals radiographed for heart disease are dyspneic, tachypneic, and distressed, and the radiographs may be of poor quality. The risk to the patient of sedation should be weighed against the loss of diagnostic information from a distorted image, motion unsharpness, underinflated lungs in an uncooperative animal.

Ideally, the radiograph should be exposed at the peak of natural inspiration.[4,7] Poorly inflated lungs are a major source of misdiagnosis. At expiration, the heart appears relatively larger. Inadequately inflated lungs are denser and vessels and small lesions poorly defined. The diaphragm may also overlap the caudal heart border during expiration. If tidal volume is poor in conditions restricting lung inflation, particularly obesity, the clinician must recognize the cause of the increased lung density and take it into consideration during radiographic evaluation. Increased abdominal pressure, due to hepatomegaly, obesity, large masses, or ascites, may displace the diaphragm cranially, compressing the lungs and preventing good inflation. The thick thoracic walls of an obese animal impart a uniform gray density (scattered radiation) to the films which further decreases diagnostic quality, particularly in the lateral view of small, round-chested dogs.

One must be particularly cautious in interpreting films made under general anesthesia. The dependent lung or both lungs may be underinflated, creating false density after only a few minutes of lateral recumbency. Conversely, overinflation of the lungs by mechanical ventilation may eliminate pulmonary infiltrates, such as pulmonary edema, by creating artificial pulmonary lucency.

Conformation

Normal variations in the conformation of dogs can cause greater differences in relative heart size and shape than is caused by heart disease within a particular breed. It is essential to consider cardiac size and contour within the context of the particular conformation of the dog.[4] Deep- and narrow-chested dogs have an elongated, more vertically oriented heart that appears almost circular in the DV view. The other extreme is the very rounded thoracic cage. Dogs with this conformation have hearts that appear rounder and larger in the lateral view with greater sternal contact. These hearts appear ovoid on the DV or VD views. Puppies normally have slightly larger hearts than do adult dogs. Fat around the heart can create the impression of a large heart, particularly in the VD or DV view. Cats have far less variation, which is individual rather than breed related. The angle of the long axis of the heart is more variable than the shape of the heart. The degree of extension of the neck and forelimbs influences the shape of the thorax in the lateral view.

EVALUATING CARDIAC SIZE AND CONTOUR

When evaluating the heart the reader must determine whether the heart is normal or abnormal in both size and shape. Variations in conformation, po-

sitioning, and technique may create a false appearance of cardiac enlargement in animals suspected of having heart disease. Physiologic rather than pathologic conditions may affect heart size. The stage of respiration has been mentioned as a factor.

The stage of the cardiac cycle has a slight effect on size and shape.[8] External transverse diameter changes only 7 percent to make a volume change from diastole to systole of 50 percent in the normal heart[9] because (1) the linear dimensions are cubed to give a volume, and (2) most of the change in internal volume (stroke volume) is caused by the ventricular walls thickening in systole. Similarly, proportionately large increases in internal volume will cause a relatively small increase in external dimensions. Knowledge of cardiac anatomy (Fig. 5-1) is essential.

Changes in circulating blood volume can change cardiac size. Congestive heart failure increases blood volume, increasing the size of the heart. Shock and hypovolemia decrease circulating blood volume, decreasing heart size and lung density. Dehydration, often caused by overdiuresis, may mask cardiac enlargement and congestive heart failure.

The precise difference between a normal and abnormal heart is difficult to determine. Mild heart enlargement that is only suspected should be evaluated within the context of other findings and should not be weighted heavily in the assessment. Cardiac shape changes are usually easier to detect than are small changes in cardiac size. Size determination is often unreliable for several reasons: (1) conformation (species and breed differences—es-

Table 5-1 Cardiac Diseases That May Present with a Normal Cardiac Silhouette

Small atrial and ventricular septal defects
Mild aortic and pulmonic stenosis
Functional murmurs
Bacterial endocarditis
Myocarditis
Hypertrophic cardiomyopathy
Early mitral regurgitation
Conduction disturbances
Constrictive pericarditis
Neoplasia
Congestive failure overtreated with diuretic and/or
  vasodilator drugs

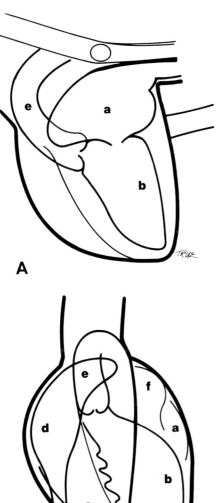

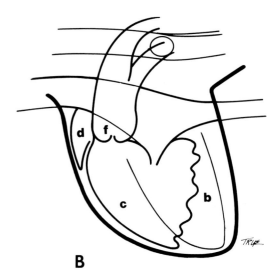

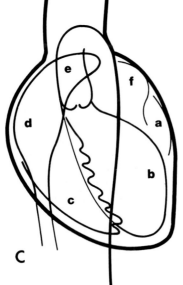

Fig. 5-1. Schematic diagrams of the normal canine silhouette illustrating radiographic anatomy. (**A,B**) Right lateral view; (**C**) dorsoventral view. a, left atrium; b, left ventricle; c, right ventricle; d, right atrium; e, aorta; f, pulmonary trunk.

pecially dogs, deformity, age), (2) obesity, (3) stage of respiration, (4) stage of cardiac cycle, (5) change in blood volume (e.g., dehydration, overhydration), (6) positioning errors, (7) pleural effusion, and (8) acquired or congenital heart disease.

Many cardiovascular disorders, with or without clinical signs, may have a normal cardiac silhouette (Table 5-1). Therefore, absence of cardiac enlargement does not always suggest benign or insignificant disease.

Criteria for a Small Heart

In the lateral view, the long cardiac axis is shorter with a small heart, making the trachea appear farther away from the spine than normal. The apex may be displaced dorsally from the sternum, creating a gap that may be mistaken for pneumothorax. The apex is more pointed, and transverse dimension of the heart is narrower. In the DV or VD view, the cardiothoracic ratio is decreased. A small heart is a result of decreased venous return. Causes of poor venous return include dehydration, overinflated lungs (physiologic, e.g., hyperpnea or upper airway obstruction, or pathologic, e.g., emphysema), shock, pneumothorax, and obstructed inflow (Fig. 5-2).

Criteria for Cardiac Enlargement

The heart enlarges in response to volume overload or myocardial failure. Volume overload may be caused by valvular incompetence, central or peripheral arteriovenous shunts (e.g., ventricular septal defect, patent ductus arteriosus, or arteriovenous fistula), or severe bradycardia (e.g., complete heart block). Myocardial failure may be primary (e.g.,

congestive cardiomyopathy), or secondary to the chronic high wall stress of severe pressure or volume overload. Myocardial failure cannot be evaluated by radiography but requires echocardiography, contrast angiocardiography, or radionuclide angiocardiography. A pressure overload will cause wall thickening rather than dilation and enlargement. The thick wall encroaches on the lumen, especially in systole. The pressure overloaded ventricle will dilate if it fails. The left ventricular wall is also thickened in hypertrophic cardiomyopathy, and this is not apparent on radiographs. Echocardiography is the best method to evaluate wall thickness.

The generally enlarged heart has a more rounded silhouette than the normal heart, in both views (Fig.

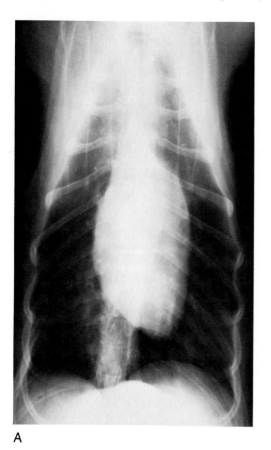

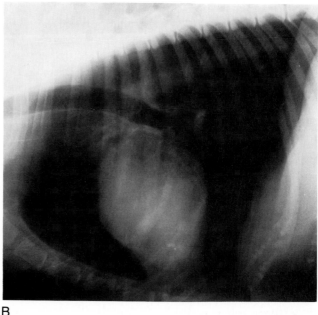

A   B

Fig. 5-2. Microcardia in a 6-year-old female mix-breed dog due to hypovolemia associated with adrenocortical insufficiency (Addison's disease). (**A**) Dorsoventral view illustrates an oblong heart shape due to reduction in width. There is increased lung inflation, reduced pulmonary vessel size, and a pointed left apex. (**B**) Right lateral view shows increased lung inflation, reduced cardiac caudal vena caval and pulmonary vessel size. (Courtesy of Dr. Philip Fox.)

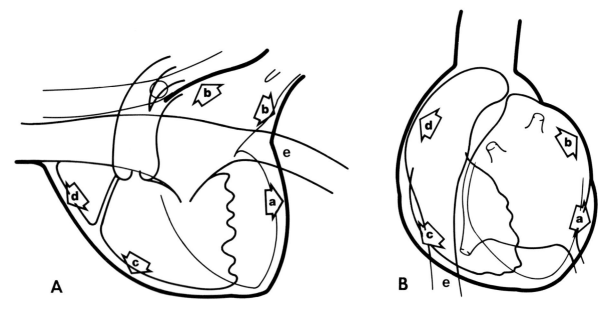

Fig. 5-3. Schematic diagrams of the canine cardiac silhouette showing enlargement of all chambers due to volume overload and/or myocardial failure. (**A**) Right lateral view; (**B**) dorsoventral view. The left ventricular border (a) is prominent; the left atrium (b) bulges dorsally, caudally, and laterally; the right ventricular border (c) is more convex and the right atrium (d) more prominent; the caudal vena cava (e) is often widened.

5-3). In the DV or VD view, the cardiothoracic ratio is increased. This ratio of the width of the heart to the width of the thorax is usually about 0.6[10,11] but varies with the stage of respiration and is affected by pulmonary and pleural diseases. In the lateral view, the long axis is increased, pushing the trachea dorsally towards the spine. A large cardiac silhouette may indicate either severe chronic volume overload or myocardial failure, or both. However, it may also indicate pericardial effusion or congenital peritoneopericardial diaphragmmatic hernia; the heart itself is normal. This may occasionally be differentiated from chronic volume overload by determining whether the left atrium is prominent. If it is, a disease causing volume overload is more likely. A large rounded heart without a prominent left atrium indicates pericardial effusion. As approximately one-fourth of pericardial effusions in one series[12] and more than three-fourths of hemorrhagic effusions in another[13] were benign, diagnosis of the cause is important. Pericardiography[4,12,14] and two-dimensional echocardiography[12] are diagnostic methods that should precede exploratory pericardiotomy (Ch. 6 and 24).

Severe right atrial and ventricular enlargement in congenital tricuspid valve malformation may resemble severe generalized cardiac enlargement or pericardial effusion.[4,15] However, the apex of the heart is usually still apparent with tricuspid valve malformation.

Many attempts have been made to evaluate cardiac enlargement objectively by measuring dimensions, ratios, and areas. These efforts have been defeated by variations in conformation, positioning, and radiographic technique. The best method is a comparative one evaluating heart enlargement using previous films of the same animal or films of an animal of the same breed.[16]

The ability to evaluate chamber enlargement accurately by radiography in humans is probably overrated,[17] and the same would be at least as likely in animals. A range of normal variations in cardiac size and shape overlaps pathologic enlargement. The heart is enclosed in the pericardium, which tends to minimize local protrusion of individual chambers. In most heart diseases, more than one chamber is affected by a volume or pressure load. For example, if the left ventricle fails, the resulting high diastolic (filling) pressure is transmitted back through the lungs, loading the right ventricle, which then hypertrophies. It may dilate and eventually fail, followed by right atrial dilation. Thus, all chambers may be enlarged by a lesion affecting the left ventricle.

Left Ventricular Enlargement

In the lateral view, the caudal cardiac border usually becomes convex, rather than maintaining its normally straight or nearly straight contour, and the caudal vena cava is elevated (Fig. 5-4). In the VD or DV view, part of the left heart border (between approximately 2 and 5 o'clock) is more convex than normal (Figs. 5-3B; 18-2,10) In most heart diseases of the dog or cat, left ventricular enlargement is accompanied by left atrial enlargement, and it is often difficult to differentiate the two. Disappearance of the caudal cardiac waist (an indentation in the caudal border at the atrioventricular groove) is supposed to indicate left heart enlargement. However, if left atrial enlargement greatly exceeds left ventricular enlargement (e.g., chronic mitral insufficiency in small- and toy-breed dogs and hypertrophic cardiomyopathy of cats), the caudal waist is accentuated by the bulging left atrium (Figs. 5-4 through 5-6).

The left ventricle responds to volume overload by dilating to increase the force of contraction through the Frank-Starling mechanism. With chronic volume overload, the wall thickens in response to increased tension (law of LaPlace), and so-called eccentric hypertrophy results (i.e., ventricular hypertrophy with dilation).

Left Atrial Enlargement

In the lateral view, the angle between the trachea and the caudal border of the left atrium (dorsal to the caudal vena cava) changes with progressive left atrial enlargement from obtuse, to a right angle, and then to an acute angle. The left mainstem bronchus in the dog or the entire trachea and both bronchi are displaced dorsally (Figs. 5-4,5 and 9-2,3). Small dogs with severe, chronic mitral regurgitation may have a large left atrium which compresses the left mainstem bronchus (Fig. 5-5). The lumen may be compressed at expiration only. Lateral films may

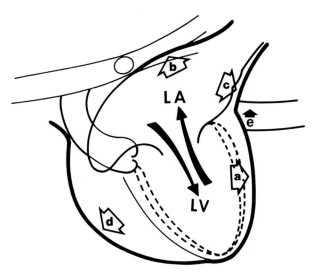

Fig. 5-4. Schematic diagram showing cardiac changes associated with chronic volume overload due to mitral regurgitation (long arrows). The inner broken line indicates the left ventricular chamber (LV) with associated dilation (eccentric hypertrophy). The outer broken line represents the left ventricle with myocardial failure. The chamber is dilated, and the wall is thinner than normal. These differences in internal dimension and wall thickness are not detected on plain radiographs. Radiographic changes with chronic volume overload: the left ventricular border (a) becomes convex; the left atrium (LA) enlarges and displaces the left mainstem bronchus (b); the LA bulges caudally (c); the right ventricular border becomes more convex (d) in response to an increased work load or myocardial failure; the caudal vena cava (e) is elevated (small arrow).

have to be taken at inspiration and expiration to confirm this bronchial collapse. Mechanical impingement of the bronchus by the left atrium may induce coughing even in the absence of congestive heart failure.

In the VD or DV views, the left atrium may bulge beyond the left ventricular border at the 2 to 3 o'clock position (Figs. 5-3B and 9-4; see also Fig. 12-2). With extreme left atrial enlargement, in congenital or longstanding mitral regurgitation or feline hypertrophic cardiomyopathy, the left atrium may be outlined as a distinct mass superimposed on the heart.[18,19] In cats with hypertrophic cardiomyopathy, the left atrium is disproportionately larger than the left ventricle. The cardiac waist will be accentuated, creating a bean-shaped heart in the lateral view, and a prominent left auricle at 2 to 3 o'clock

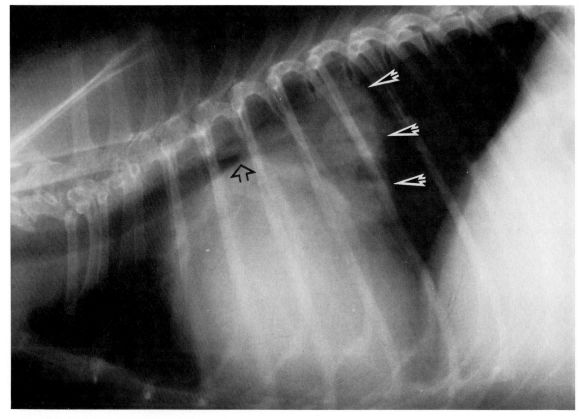

Fig. 5-5. Right lateral radiograph of an 11-year-old, 5-kg poodle with chronic mitral regurgitation. A very large left atrium is present (outlined by three arrows), compressing the left mainstem bronchus (open arrow). (Courtesy of Dr. Philip Fox.)

in the DV (or VD) view. Cats with advanced myocardial disease or atrioventricular valvular dysplasia may display biatrial enlargement in the DV (VD) view (Fig. 5-6B; see also 12-2). The term "valentine-shaped" heart is thus characteristic of many diseases.

There is no relationship between the size of the left atrium and the degree of left ventricular failure. Often the left atrium is severely enlarged before heart failure becomes apparent[18,19] (Fig. 5-6), unless left ventricular failure is the cause of secondary mitral regurgitation. In chronic mitral regurgitation, the large compliant left atrium buffers the lungs from the regurgitated blood. End-diastolic (filling) pressure does not increase initially because the ventricle maintains its compliance as it enlarges.[20] As the regurgitant volume increases and forward volume (true cardiac output) falls, blood volume increases. Increasing volume and pressure in the pulmonary venous capacitance bed incites compensatory mechanisms of proximal venodilation, peripheral vasoconstriction and increased lymphatic drainage to protect the lungs from pulmonary edema. Because there is little reserve capacity, the balance of these factors may be upset acutely, precipitating alveolar pulmonary edema.[4]

A contrasting situation exists in the case of acute aortic[21] or mitral regurgitation secondary to bacterial endocarditis. The left ventricle responds to the acute volume overload by dilating. As it approaches the limits of distention imposed by the myocardium and pericardium, the end-diastolic pressure increases. These limits are reached with a small increase in volume because the structures have not had time to adapt to the sudden load. Also, the left

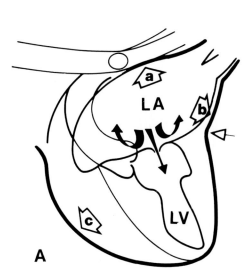 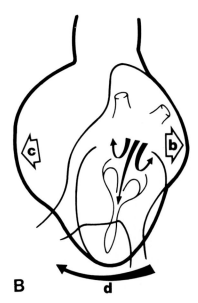

Fig. 5-6. Schematic diagrams of a heart with diastolic dysfunction (e.g., hypertrophic cardiomyopathy) illustrating left atrial enlargement. The thickened, stiff, noncompliant left ventricle (LV) causes diastolic resistance to ventricular filling (curved arrows). Increased left atrial end-diastolic pressure results. Combined with secondary mitral regurgitation (due to conformational changes in the annulus fibrosus), left atrial enlargement occurs. (**A**) In the right lateral view, the large left atrium (LA) displaces the trachea dorsally (a) and bulges caudally and laterally (b), creating a notch (open arrow) in the caudal heart border. (**B**) In the dorsoventral (DV) (or VD) view, the large left atrium causes a prominent bulge (b) at 2 to 3 o'clock. The right ventricle usually enlarges secondarily (c). The cardiac apex may be pushed to the right (d) by the enlarged left atrium.

atrium has not had time to compensate by enlarging. Pulmonary edema can result. Rapidly progressing congestive cardiomyopathy may also develop pulmonary edema with only moderate cardiac enlargement for similar reasons of diastolic dysfunction. The ejection fraction decreases and the ventricle dilates; end-diastolic pressure rapidly increases, and pulmonary edema occurs with less radiographic cardiomegaly than with diseases causing chronic volume overload (e.g., patent ductus arteriosus or chronic mitral regurgitation[20,22]).

In feline hypertrophic and restrictive cardiomyopathies, the thick left ventricular wall becomes stiff and indistensible in diastole, causing a rise in diastolic pressure. The left atrium enlarges and becomes a reservoir that protects the lungs from acute pulmonary edema due to elevated filling pressures.[18] The left atrium can become huge while the external left ventricular contour remains normal. The heart commonly rotates clockwise on the DV or VD view, so that the apex appears on the right side[11] (Fig. 5-6).

Right Ventricular Enlargement

On the lateral view, right ventricular enlargement is determined by increased convexity of the heart cranial to the apex, causing increased sternal contact (Fig. 5-7). If severe right ventricular enlargement is present without an enlarged left heart, it may push the apex dorsally off the sternum (apex tipping) (Fig. 26-2A). The trachea is usually elevated where it passes over the cranial heart.

In some cases of pure right ventricular enlargement, the right ventricle may be almost normal on the lateral view, yet grossly enlarged on the DV or VD view. This occurs because the heart rotates to the left as it enlarges, and the cranial bulge is not apparent.

On the DV or VD view, right ventricular en-

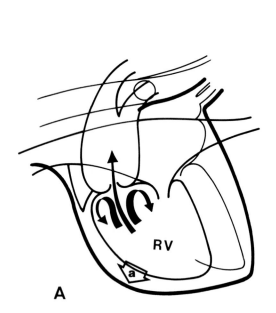

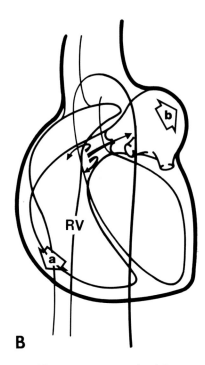

Fig. 5-7. Schematic diagrams of right ventricular enlargement caused by a pressure overload (e.g., pulmonic stenosis). Because of the fixed outflow obstruction, right ventricular emptying is reduced (curved arrows), and systolic pressure rises. Right ventricular wall hypertrophy occurs secondarily; the right ventricle becomes more rounded and the border more convex (a). (**A**) In the lateral view, sternal contact increases (a), which may push the apex dorsally off of the sternum (apex tipping). (**B**) The main pulmonary artery (pulmonary trunk) (b) bulges at the 2 o'clock position on the dorsoventral (DV) (VD) view. The heart is rotated counterclockwise due to the large right ventricle (RV).

largement creates a more convex border to the right of the apex (which is normally at the 5 o'clock position). The convexity extends clockwise to about the 10 o'clock position (see Fig. 19-10B). If there is no left heart enlargement, the large right ventricle will create a reverse-D contour (Fig. 5-7B; see also Figs. 18-6 and 25-9). Rather than bulging out toward the right thoracic wall, the heart often rotates counterclockwise (as shown in Fig. 5-7B) to move the apex farther to the left. An enlarged main pulmonary artery will accompany it, except in tetralogy of Fallot, in which the pulmonary trunk is hypoplastic because of the right to left shunt.

A prominent right ventricle may result from high pulmonary vascular resistance with chronic lung disease (cor pulmonale), or hypertensive patent ductus or ventricular septal defect,[23-26] and by fixed ventricular outflow obstruction in pulmonic stenosis. Although dirofilariasis is the most common

cause of cor pulmonale, the latter is present in many small dogs with chronic airway obstruction due to stenoses in the nasal cavity and pharynx, collapsing trachea, or bronchi and chronic bronchitis.[4] Under these conditions, the large caudal pulmonary arteries are usually dilated.

Right ventricular volume overload is caused by large ventricular and atrial septal defects, congenital or acquired tricuspid insufficiency, or congestive heart failure (Fig. 5-3). Myocardial failure may accompany severe volume overload or dilated cardiomyopathy.

The effects of these loads on the right ventricle is different from those on the left. The low pressure at which the right ventricle normally operates permits it to have a thin wall and a large radius of curvature. A volume overload (e.g., tricuspid regurgitation) or acute pressure overload (e.g., massive pulmonary thromboembolism) will cause the chamber to dilate. By contrast, a chronic pressure load from pulmonic stenosis, cor pulmonale, or left ventricular disease will cause concentric hypertrophy, which thickens the right ventricular wall and makes the chamber resemble the left ventricle.[27,28] On cross section, these changes will confer a figure-eight appearance to both ventricles. Thus, both pressure and volume overload on the right ventricle will produce an enlarged contour on the radiograph.

Right Atrial Enlargement

On the lateral view, the cardiac silhouette may bulge cranially due to right atrial enlargement (Fig. 5-3A; see also Fig. 18-20). The angle formed by the cranial vena cava and the cranial heart border will be filled in, and the transverse (craniocaudal) cardiac axis will be increased or enlarged. In the DV or VD views, a large right atrium causes a bulge at 9 to 11 o'clock on the cardiac silhouette (Fig. 5-3B). The trachea will be elevated as it passes over the cranial part of the heart.

The right atrium dilates in response to a chronic volume and pressure overload in a manner similar to the left atrium. The overload may be caused by either a failing right ventricle or tricuspid regurgitation. In congenital tricuspid regurgitation, the right atrium may become huge before congestive heart failure ensues.[4,15] Gross right atrial enlargement may be difficult to distinguish from pericardial effusion. Localizing the apex of a severely enlarged heart is the best way to separate right from left heart enlargement. If an apex is still apparent, and the heart is ovoid, severe right heart disease should be more strongly considered than pericardial effusion.

Right atrial neoplasia, usually hemangiosarcoma, may cause this chamber to bulge slightly, but the pericardium tends to smooth out the radiographic contours. Pericardial effusion, commonly present with this tumor, may make the cardiac silhouette large and rounded[29] (see Fig. 24-7A). Two-dimensional echocardiography is the best method to diagnose this neoplasm[12,30] (see Figs. 6-50 and 24-9). A nonselective angiocardiogram may demonstrate an intraluminal mass or a pneumopericardiogram may outline the right atrial tumor[12,14] (see Fig. 24-12).

GREAT VESSELS AND MEDIASTINAL STRUCTURES

Since the great vessels entering and leaving the heart are enclosed within the mediastinum, they are considered together.

Great Vessels

The great vessels enlarge in response to either an increased pressure load or turbulence. Semilunar valvular stenoses cause poststenotic enlargement of the pulmonary trunk and aortic arch. The pathophysiology of enlargement is complex and is related to the turbulence causing the murmur[4] and is not proportional to the pressure.

When flow in a vessel is reduced by an intracardiac shunt, the vessel may be small or hypoplastic. This occurs with tetralogy of Fallot, since pulmonic stenosis causes high right ventricular pressure with right to left shunting through the ventricular septal defect.

The absence of detectable enlargement does not mean that poststenotic dilation and semilunar valve stenosis can be excluded from the differential diagnosis of a congenital disease with a systolic murmur. It only means that stenosis, if present, is probably not severe.

Enlarged Pulmonary Trunk

In the lateral view, the pulmonary trunk is not projected outward from the heart and thus is not visible on plain radiographs unless enlarged. When grossly enlarged, a bulge or cap may be seen superimposed on the trachea[31] (see Fig. 18-8). In the DV or VD view, the main pulmonary trunk normally fills the cardiac border at the 1 to 2 o'clock position, at the junction with the cranial mediastinum (see Fig. 5-1). A prominent bulge at this point most likely represents an enlarged pulmonary trunk (see Fig. 18-6) caused by pulmonic stenosis or pulmonary hypertension (see Fig. 25-9). Dirofilariasis in the cat does not cause this enlargement.[32,33]

Enlarged Aortic Arch

In the lateral view, poststenotic dilation due to aortic stenosis extends into the cranial mediastinum, filling in the angle formed by the cranial vena cava and the cranial heart border (see Fig. 18-13). It increases the cranial mediastinal density in both views (see Figs. 18-10 and 18-13).

In the DV or VD view, it may fill the angle formed by the right atrial appendage and the cranial vena cava at 11 o'clock, bulging into the mediastinum and filling the angle between the cranial mediastinum and the pulmonary trunk at the 1 o'clock position (see Fig. 18-10). A bulging pulmonary trunk can be differentiated from the enlarged aortic arch here; the lateral border of the aortic arch continues down the mediastinum just to the left of the spine. There is considerable variation in the normal curve of the aortic arch to the left side of the dog.[16] Old cats sometimes have a prominent bump on the left border of the cranial mediastinum formed by the aortic arch viewed end-on. This represents a variation of normal.

In a patent ductus, the aorta is dilated at the point of exit of the ductus. The dilation is better seen on a DV view, which must be perfectly straight. It appears as a slight bulge on the left side of the border of the aorta just caudal to the arch (see Fig. 18-2).

Caudal Vena Cava

In the lateral view, the position of this vessel provides a clue to the size of the heart. It is elevated if either ventricle is enlarged (see Figs. 5-3,4).

Because the diameter of the caudal vena cava fluctuates with respiration, a single film cannot be used to evaluate it. A persistently full and wide caudal vena cava is evidence of right ventricular failure, pericardial tamponade, constrictive pericarditis, or right atrial obstruction by an intracavity neoplasm or thrombus.[34] However, it is a relatively insensitive sign of venous hypertension.[16,35] A persistently thin cava is associated with poor venous return, hypovolemia, and increased pleural pressure caused by air trapping (overinflation, asthma, bronchitis, emphysema). It is seen with either underperfused or overinflated lungs, or both.

Perihilar and Heart Base Masses

Opacities in this region are usually poorly defined because the many vessels and mediastinal structures are superimposed on each other. Hilar lymphade-

nopathy from fungal pneumonia or lymphosarcoma increases the soft tissue density around the carina and left atrium, and in the lateral view can be mistaken for left atrial enlargement. A significant difference between hilar lymphadenopathy and left atrial enlargement, however, is that the former density lies dorsal to the mainstem bronchi, which are not elevated; left atrial enlargement lies ventral to the carina and elevates the mainstem bronchi (Figs. 5-3A,4,5). Just cranial to this area, a dilated right main pulmonary artery from severe dirofilariasis causes an increased density over the aortic arch in the lateral view.

Heart base tumors (chemodectoma, aortic body tumors), infiltrating primary bronchogenic carcinoma and right atrial hemangiosarcomas, can displace the great vessels and trachea and cause protrusions or densities around the heart base (Figs. 24-11,12). They may cause pericardial effusion and tamponade with right heart failure or may obstruct the cranial or caudal vena cava.[4] A vena cavagram[34] is a simple method of outlining intracavitary obstructions in this region. Selective angiocardiography may be necessary[36] (Fig. 24-15). Pericardiography is the recommended contrast study to evaluate pericardial effusion suspected to be caused by neoplastic masses[12,14,29] (see Figs. 24-11 and 24-12). Two-dimensional echocardiography[12,30,37] is the preferred noninvasive method for evaluating cardiac masses and pericardial effusion (Figs. 6-42,45-48,50; 24-6,9,10). Magnetic resonance imaging (MRI) is a new, sensitive, and costly technique for assessing cardiovascular structures (see Fig. 24-8).

The Esophagus

Air throughout the esophagus or in the cranial thoracic part of a slightly dilated esophagus is a common finding in dyspneic animals. The esophagus will be displaced dorsally and slightly compressed by an enlarged heart. Vascular ring anomalies may compress the esophagus and dilate it in the cranial mediastinum (see Fig. 19-12). Signs of aspiration pneumonia are common in puppies and kittens with this condition. The spectrum of vascular ring anomalies is wide and complex (see Fig. 1-4). Persistent right aortic arch (PRAA), also called dextroaorta with left-sided ligamentum arteriosum, is the most prevalent type in dogs and cats (see Fig. 19-13). It is correctable by surgery, although complications caused by the dilated esophagus are common.[38] Severe tracheal compression and malformed tracheal rings are evidence of double aortic arch.[39] Persistent left cranial vena cava also may be present to complicate surgery.[4]

The Trachea and Bronchi

The position of the caudal trachea in the lateral view provides a guide to the size of the heart. A trachea displaced toward the spine suggests a large heart. In particular, dorsal displacement and compression of the left mainstem bronchus indicates left atrial enlargement. Perihilar density caused by enlarged lymph nodes in canine lymphosarcoma or fungal infection resembles left atrial enlargement. The position of the trachea and mainstem bronchi helps differentiate these conditions.

Tracheal collapse is often present in conjunction with a murmur of mitral regurgitation in small coughing dogs. Radiologic examination helps resolve the cause of the coughing (Fig. 5-8). The trachea may be collapsing in either the cervical or the thoracic sections, or both. Upper airway obstruction by an elongated or swollen soft palate will exaggerate the collapse. Lateral films should be taken during expiration and inspiration to confirm tracheal collapse.[4] The differences in pleural and airway pressures will cause a change in tracheal width.

Another cause of coughing similar to that caused by collapsed trachea, is compression of the left

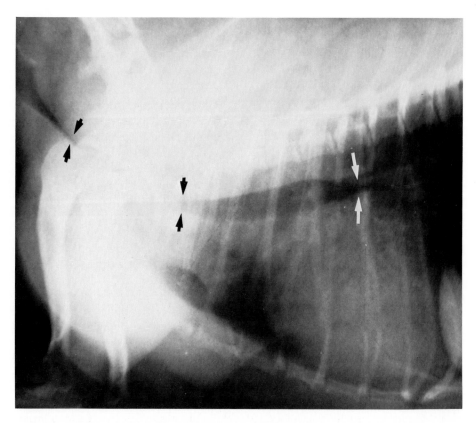

Fig. 5-8. Right lateral thoracic radiograph of a 9-year-old female poodle with mitral regurgitation and a chronic cough. Tracheal collapse is evident at the cervical region (black arrows) and at the heart base (white arrows). (Courtesy of Dr. Philip Fox.)

mainstem bronchus (see Fig. 5-5). This is caused or exacerbated by a very large left atrium from chronic mitral valve endocardiosis. Thus, the cough caused by a collapsed bronchus is easily mistaken for a cardiac cough.

THE LUNG FIELD IN HEART DISEASE

The pulmonary radiograph has been likened to a window for cardiac function reflecting the underlying pathophysiology of the heart. Air in the small airways and alveoli acts as a contrast medium outlining the pulmonary vessels and parenchyma. This makes radiography a more sensitive and specific method of assessing the pulmonary vascular circulation than auscultation. The amount of this contrast medium fluctuates with respiration. In the assessment of heart disease, evaluation of the lung fields may provide more useful information than the determination of cardiac chamber size. It helps in assessing the severity of the hemodynamic disturbance (i.e., congestive heart failure), and the effects of therapy.

Hyperperfusion (Overcirculation)

In this pattern, best appreciated in the lateral view, the arteries and veins are prominent and widened (Fig. 5-9). The hypervascular appearance is the result of significantly increased pulmonary blood flow (two or more times normal). Causes include left to right shunts (central or peripheral), hyperdynamic states such as chronic, severe anemia, fluid overload, pregnancy, or thyrotoxicosis. Hyperdynamic states cause relatively mild overcirculation, which may not be apparent on radiographs.

Normally, only a small proportion of the pulmonary capillary bed is perfused. Greater flow causes more capillaries to open up. The large number of perfused vessels reduces the contrast of the lung parenchyma against the vessels and creates a hazy increase in interstitial density resembling interstitial pulmonary edema (Ch. 9). These are indistinguishable, but the distribution of hypervascularity is more widespread. It extends to the periphery of the lungs as opposed to cardiac interstitial edema, which is more central in distribution.

The location of the cardiovascular shunt may be suggested by radiographic changes in the heart. The degree of enlargement is variable, depending on the size of the shunt. Large left to right atrial shunts will overload the right ventricle, enlarging it and the pulmonary artery. Large ventricular septal defects will overload the left ventricle, the left atrium and the main pulmonary artery, which may be prominent at the 1 o'clock position on the DV (VD) film. Peripheral shunts (patent ductus arteriosus, arteriovenous malformations) primarily overload the left ventricle. Large shunts may eventually cause a pressure load on the right ventricle (and enlargement) if pulmonary vascular resistance rises.[23-26]

Hypoperfusion (Undercirculation)

Thin pulmonary arteries and veins and a relatively radiolucent interstitium characterize this pattern (see Fig. 5-2). Causes of generalized hypoperfusion include right to left shunts or low cardiac output, such as shock, severe dehydration, acute adrenocortical insufficiency, restrictive pericarditis, caval or right atrial obstruction, cardiac tamponade, right heart failure, complete heart block, severe emphysema.

Technical faults during radiography or processing may create images that resemble this condition. Examples are overexposure, overdevelopment, or overinflation due to struggling or upper airway obstruction. Overinflation can be recognized by the appearance of a flat diaphragm on the lateral view, and wide costodiaphragmatic angles in the VD or DV views. Overexposed pneumothorax may also resemble undercirculation.

Various clinical and radiographic findings may be helpful in the diagnosis of causes contributing to hypoperfusion. Right ventricular enlargement without an enlarged main pulmonary artery suggests tetralogy of Fallot (see Fig. 19-11) or Ebstein's anomaly; the right atrium and ventricle will be enlarged in right ventricular failure; a rounded cardiac silhouette will be present in pericardial effusion and cardiac tamponade; and in Eisenmenger's syndrome, the pulmonary arteries will be wide and tortuous and the peripheral lung field will be hypovascular.

Isolated pulmonic stenosis has been reported to

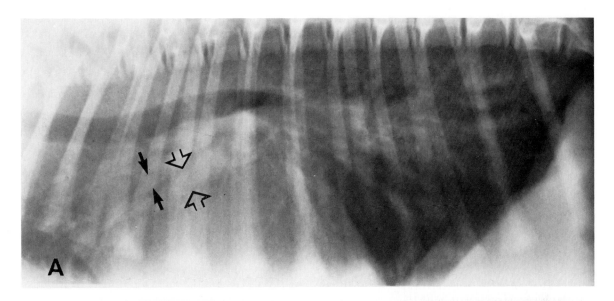

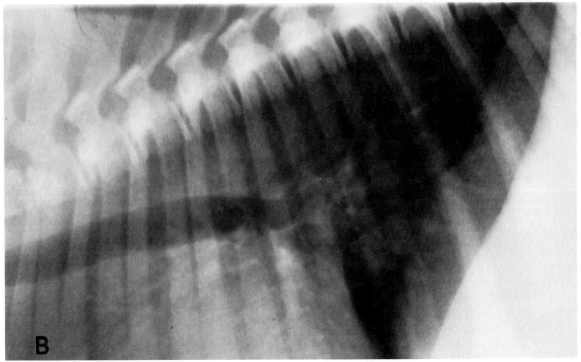

Fig. 5-9. Right lateral thoracic radiograph of a pair of 2-month-old golden retriever littermates. (**A**) Hyper-perfused (over-circulated lungs are caused by a left-to-right shunting patent ductus arteriosus. Note the engorged distended pulmonary veins (open arrows) overlying the cardiac silhouette. Pulmonary arteries (closed arrows) are also abnormally wide and are best visualized in the cranial lung lobes. There is a diffuse interstitial pulmonary density, especially evident in the perihilar region, due to overcirculation. The left atrium is enlarged and elevates the trachea. Compare these changes with those in the normal littermate (**B**).

cause an underperfused lung field, even in clinically normal dogs. The question of whether the appearance reflects true hypoperfusion, hyperlucency due to other causes, or overreading the films because of bias (belief that pulmonic stenosis should cause hypoperfusion) is not resolved. Pulmonary perfusion should be normal until the ventricle fails.

Lobar hypoperfusion is a sign of pulmonary thromboembolism.[40] It may be associated with alveolar infiltrates, pleural effusion, proximally dilated pulmonary artery, and an enlarged right ventricle.

Prominent Pulmonary Arteries

Prominent pulmonary arteries are a sign of pulmonary arterial hypertension. The proximal arteries become wide and the middle portions become tortuous (see Fig. 18-4). The peripheral sections are usually thin. The most common cause is canine heartworm disease (see Figs. 25-5, 25-6, and 25-9). In the lateral view, the cranial arteries lie dorsal to the veins and can usually be seen even when the caudal vessels are obscured by perivascular inflammatory infiltration. Hypertension can be determined by evaluation of the relative size of the right cranial pulmonary artery in the lateral view. The upper limit of normal is 1.2 times the width of the right fourth rib at a point just below the spine.[41]

Slight irregularities and tortuosity of the right main caudal artery are the most sensitive signs of mild early dirofilariasis. At this stage, the heart is normal, and there is no visible perivascular reaction.[42,43] Arterial signs of dirofilariasis have been described as dilation, indentation or scalloping, tortuosity, disappearance, pruning, and serration.[4] To maximize the chance of recognizing these subtle changes in pulmonary artery morphology, particularly in vessels which overlie the liver, a DV view with good lung inflation rather than a VD view is necessary.[43] Periarterial inflammatory lesions and edema[44] often make the vessels difficult to identify, particularly in the lateral view. The classic signs of enlarged right ventricle and main pulmonary artery may be obscured. Under these conditions severe heartworm lesions may be confused with pulmonary neoplasia because the grossly enlarged and distorted arteries, partially obscured by pulmonary inflammatory infiltrates, resemble lung masses. This error is particularly likely if only a lateral view is

taken on which the main caudal arteries are superimposed. The accompanying changes in the right ventricle and pulmonary trunk are less likely to be visible than on the DV view.

In the cat, diagnosis of heartworms requires careful inspection of the main caudal pulmonary arteries, seen best in the DV or DV oblique views[32,33] (see Figs. 26-2B, and 26-4B). They may be obscured by interstitial inflammatory infiltrate.[33] The cat is an aberrant host for *Dirofilaria immitis*. Fewer and smaller worms are present and the arteritis is less severe. Typically, pulmonary hypertension is not severe enough to cause a prominent pulmonary trunk. The eosinophilic inflammatory reaction is not specific, and microfilaremia is only occasionally present.[45] Nonselective angiography and serology are the best methods to confirm feline dirofilariasis[32,46] (see Figs. 26-2 and 26-3).

Other causes of chronic pulmonary hypertension include left to right shunts that develop pulmonary hypertension[4,25,26] (Eisenmenger's syndrome), chronic obstructive pulmonary disease, and chronic hypoxia. Radiologic signs of pulmonary hypertension may be present in dogs with chronic upper airway obstruction, particularly collapsed trachea and elongated soft palate in brachycephalic dogs.

Acute pulmonary hypertension can result from severe pulmonary thromboembolism.[4,40] The proximal part of the affected lobar or main pulmonary artery is wide and truncated but not tortuous. A variety of concurrent radiologic lesions may be present, such as lung consolidation due to infarction, regional hyperlucency due to oligemia distal to the obstruction, and pleural effusion.

Prominent Pulmonary Veins

Chronic pulmonary venous hypertension results in distended and tortuous pulmonary veins. They can best be identified on a DV view with the lungs well inflated. The veins lie medial to the arteries. They may also be visible in the lateral view in the perihilar region. Distention is greatest in the perihilar area, where the veins are widest and wall tension (according to the Law of Laplace) is greatest at any venous pressure. Therefore, lung periphery is spared.

Pulmonary venous hypertension is caused by chronically elevated left ventricular filling pressure as with left ventricular failure in dogs with chronic valvular disease (i.e., mitral insufficiency) (see Fig. 9-2) or hypertrophic cardiomyopathy in cats (see Fig. 9-4) or dogs. These changes are always associated with a large left atrium. Because long duration is required for the vessels to adapt, the signs are not always present. They may be obscured by pulmonary edema.

PULMONARY PARENCHYMA

Interstitial Pulmonary Edema

The normal, faint, interstitial density of the lungs is created by the supporting structures of the parenchyma which carry the small airways and vessels (see Fig. 9-1). The interstitium is regarded as an extravascular tissue compartment. It expands to accommodate excess transudated fluid, which is then drained by pulmonary lymphatics. Interstitial pulmonary edema appears as a uniform, poorly defined increase in density. This interstitial veil will partially obscure the vascular markings (see Figs. 9-3 through 9-5). Whether it can be diagnosed radiographically depends on the uniformity of radiographic technical factors, including lung inflation. The latter is rarely well controlled and is difficult to standardize in dyspneic animals. These variables make comparisons between sets of radiographs dependent on standardization of image quality when evaluating effects of treatment in the same patient. Evaluation of a single film with a mental range of normal is more difficult and less accurate.

Alveolar Pulmonary Edema

Alveolar pulmonary edema is a more advanced state of left ventricular failure than is interstitial edema (see Figs. 9-2 through 9-5). It is characterized by absence of pulmonary air contrast, the air being replaced by edema fluid in the alveoli. If sufficiently severe, the edema obscures vascular markings. The bronchi are not flooded and show up as radiolucent air bronchograms. In the lateral view, air bronchograms appear as tapering and branching radiolucent lines surrounded by opacity, obscuring the adjacent vessels[4] (see Figs. 9-3 and 9-5). In the DV (VD) views the air bronchograms are often shorter or even round because the bronchi are foreshortened or appear end-on in this view (see Fig. 9-4A).

An alternative appearance for acute pulmonary edema is one of a finely stippled or fine nodular pattern. This air alveologram pattern is caused by groups of fluid-filled acini mixed with air-filled acini.

Many other conditions besides left ventricular failure cause an acute alveolar pattern. The distribution of the infiltrates is helpful.[4,47] The most common distribution of cardiogenic pulmonary edema in dogs is dorsal, perihilar, and symmetric. By contrast, pneumonia is typically peribronchial, lobar, cranial, ventral, and asymmetric in distribution. Therefore, it is usually possible to differentiate these two common causes of dyspnea by radiology. Sometimes the edema will be accentuated in the right caudal lobe rather than symmetric.[4] The reason is not known. The dorsal location and the presence of an enlarged left atrium are supporting evidence for edema rather than pneumonia. Bronchopneumonia in cats appears similar to dogs but is less common.

In cats with hypertrophic cardiomyopathy, pulmonary edema is usually patchy and asymmetrically distributed and the air alveologram pattern predominates (see Fig. 9-4). This is because the edema is usually acute or paroxysmal in onset, and patterns of lymphatic drainage and reflex vasoconstriction have not developed. The perihilar distribution is rare.

Pulmonary edema as a sign of left ventricular failure may be masked. Overinflation by a forced inspiration due to stress on the radiographic table, or if the animal is ventilated while under general anesthesia, will reduce the density of pulmonary edema. Right ventricular failure accompanying left ventricular failure may decrease pulmonary perfusion pressure sufficiently to prevent edema formation. Diuretic therapy may reduce blood volume sufficiently to eliminate pulmonary edema and reduce the size of the heart. This radiologic evidence is deceptive, as cardiac output is subnormal.

Pulmonary Fibrosis

Pulmonary fibrosis causes a diffuse interstitial opacity that may be indistinguishable from poor lung inflation or pulmonary edema.[4] As pulmonary fibrosis is associated with chronic obstructive pulmonary disease caused by chronic bronchitis and tracheal and bronchial collapse, the differential diagnosis in small dogs with chronic cough and concurrent mitral regurgitation may be difficult to make.

Focal Pulmonary Lesions Associated with Heart Disease

A variety of focal lesions may occur in the lungs in association with cardiovascular disorders. The most common cause is dirofilariasis.[4,44,48] Distribution of lesions may range from a patchy or diffuse interstitial pattern in occult heartworm disease (see Fig. 25-11) to lung consolidations caused by thromboembolisation following adulticidal treatment in dogs. Pulmonary granulomas may be present (see Fig. 25-12). The pulmonary pattern in cats with dirofilariasis is usually much milder. Patchy interstitial and alveolar densities have been reported[32,33,45,49] (see Figs 26-5 and 26-6).

Acute pulmonary thromboembolism in dogs as a complication of systemic diseases is manifested in a variety of focal pulmonary lesions. They include single or multiple alveolar opacities, lobar collapse, and asymmetric lucency because of oligemia in the affected lung or lobe.[40]

Bacterial endocarditis may cause septic pneumonia as well as pulmonary edema. The pulmonary lesions may be difficult to differentiate. Embolic pneumonia is usually more irregular in density and distribution than cardiogenic pulmonary edema. Consolidated areas may be present due to embolization.[4]

Pulmonary metastases may be associated with cardiac neoplasia. The most common cardiac tumor in the dog is right atrial hemangiosarcoma. Pulmonary metastases from this tumor may cause a fine, nodular, interstitial pattern, sometimes with superimposed alveolar infiltrates caused by hemorrhage.

THE PLEURAL CAVITY AND ABDOMEN

Two radiographic signs of pleural involvement may be seen in heart failure. The least common is pleural thickening or pleural edema. This is caused by acute, severe, left ventricular failure, which overwhelms the pulmonary lymphatic drainage. Therefore, it is seen always with acute alveolar edema.

Left ventricular failure does not produce pleural effusion unless it is associated with generalized congestive heart failure.

The radiographic signs of pleural effusion have been described in detail.[4] In the DV view, even small amounts of pleural effusion may obscure the cardiac silhouette and diaphragm (see Fig. 22-1). Therefore, a VD view should be taken if possible, since in the supine position, fluid gravitates away from the heart and diaphragm to the dorsal regions of the pleural cavity.[4,6] Alternatively, radiographing the thorax after thoracocentesis will provide relief from dyspnea and ensure a good outline of the thoracic organs.

Pleural effusion is a sign of congestive heart failure (right ventricular failure). It is also formed with constrictive pericarditis and tamponade from pericardial effusion.[12,50] In the former disease, the heart is not usually enlarged.[50] In the dog, pleural effusion usually follows liver congestion and ascites in the progression of signs of right ventricular failure. In the cat, pleural effusion is a common finding with congestive failure, whether due to myocardial disease or severe congenital malformation. A wide variety of cardiac and noncardiac diseases can cause pleural effusion and a complete data base may be required to facilitate diagnosis.

If possible, thoracic radiographs should include the cranial abdomen. Liver enlargement and ascites are evidence of congestive heart failure. When congenital peritonoediaphragmatic pericardial hernia is suspected, an enlarged, rounded cardiac silhouette, missing or cranially displaced abdominal organs can support the diagnosis.

Liver enlargement is overdiagnosed on radiographs. Standard criteria for normal liver size state that the caudoventral tip should lie within the costal arch. However, the liver moves with the diaphragm in respiration, so some projection beyond the arch is common. This is particularly true if the thorax is expanded and the diaphragm is flat, as occurs during dyspnea or when pleural effusion is present.

DIAGNOSIS OF CONGENITAL HEART DISEASE

The heart and lungs should always be interpreted together. A scheme for their evaluation in congenital heart disease shows how diagnoses of common specific disorders can be made from plain films (Table 5-2). The addition of clinical signs often enables a specific diagnosis to be made.

In addition to assisting in the diagnosis of a particular congenital anomaly, the radiologic examination offers a prognostic guide by revealing the severity of cardiomegaly and its hemodynamic consequences. This is more important than diagnosis of the actual defect to the new pet owner whose young animal has a murmur. Patent ductus arteriosus should be diagnosed clinically and confirmed by radiology, because it is correctable by surgery. If a specific diagnosis is required, nonselective angiocardiography may sometimes be performed in a clinical practice setting, or the patient can be referred for echocardiography, cardiac catheterization and selective angiocardiography. When discussing invasive diagnostic methods (e.g., angiocardiography) with the owner, the veterinarian must realize

that the knowledge attained by this procedure must be able to influence therapeutic management favorably to offset its risk to the animal and cost to the owner.

Knowledge of the prevalence of different diseases within particular breeds helps in deciding the most likely diagnosis, especially in congenital heart diseases of dogs that have a hereditary basis.[51] This does not hold true, however, for cat breeds.

Angiocardiography

Cardiac catheterization and selective angiocardiography are necessary for a complete evaluation of the cardiac anatomy (Chs. 18 and 19). Of the cardiac anomalies commonly treated by surgery (e.g., pulmonic stenosis, patent ductus arteriosus), cardiac catheterization should not be required to diagnose patent ductus unless pulmonary hyperten-

Table 5-2 Diagnostic Scheme for Congenital Heart Diseases

Lung Field	Congenital Cardiac Anomaly	Cardiac Silhouette
Underperfused	Severe pulmonic stenosis Tricuspid dysplasia Tetralogy of Fallot Pulmonic stenosis with atrial septal defect (R → L shunt)	Right side enlarged (or usually enlarged)
Prominent pulmonary veins	Aortic stenosis in left ventricular failure Mitral valve malformation	Left side enlarged
Prominent arteries and veins (overperfused)	Atrial septal defects (L → R shunt) Ventricular septal defects (L → R shunt) Patent ductus arteriosus (L → R shunt) Arteriovenous shunts (L → R shunt)	Generally enlarged
Prominent pulmonary arteries	Eisenmenger's syndrome (hypertensive, R → L shunting, VSD, PDA, ASD)	Variable cardiac enlargement
Normal	Pulmonic stenosis Pulmonic or tricuspid incompetence Small ventricular septal defect	Right side enlarged
	Aortic stenosis (severe) Compensated congenital mitral valve malformation	Left side enlarged
	Multiple defects Peritoneodiaphragmatic pericardial hernia	General enlargement
Edema	Left ventricular failure Biventricular failure	Variable cardiac enlargement

sion is suspected. Also, since about 10 percent of animals with congenital anomaly have multiple cardiac defects, angiocardiography may be needed.[23,51] Pulmonic stenosis requires cardiac catheterization to determine the transvalvular gradient and to exclude other anomalies that would contraindicate surgery.[31] Pressures and gradients are a better guide to prognosis in pulmonic and aortic stenosis than is the degree of abnormality seen on the angiocardiogram (see Figs. 18-5, 18-9, and 18-12).

Nonselective angiocardiography[52-56] and left ventriculography by direct transthoracic puncture[57] can be performed in private practice. Large valvular stenoses, tetralogy of Fallot, and feline myocardial diseases can often be diagnosed with nonselective angiocardiography, most reliably in cats and in dogs less than 15 kg (Chs. 18, 19, and 22). It is essential to inject a bolus of contrast medium rapidly that will pass as a bolus through the right and then left cardiac chambers, permitting clear visualization of these structures. If the injection is protracted or continuous, all chambers will be simultaneously opacified. This will obscure some lesions and make interpretation inaccurate. To facilitate injection of a large contrast bolus the largest cannula possible should be used. Injections are best made in the jugular vein. Ventricular septal and atrial septal defects are unlikely to be diagnosed by nonselective angiocardiography. However, pulmonic and aortic stenosis, tetralogy of Fallot and patent ductus arteriosus may be demonstrated in cats and dogs less than 15 kg in weight. Evaluation of feline myocardial disease is also enhanced. Although echocardiography is more accurate for the characterization of myocardial structure and function,[58] nonselective angiocardiography can more clearly define certain diseases (e.g., restrictive cardiomyopathy) than M-mode echocardiography and is useful for demonstrating vascular thromboemboli and cardiac chamber thrombi.[52,54] Feline dirofilariasis may often be best diagnosed with nonselective angiocardiography[32] (Figs. 26-2,3), since serologic tests lack specificity.[46]

CONCLUSIONS FROM THE RADIOGRAPHIC EXAMINATION

The astute clinician will evaluate radiologic signs of cardiopulmonary disease within the context of clinical and electrocardiographic (ECG) findings.

Mental point scores may be assigned for each sign, based on its reliability and severity, weighing information suggested by each radiologic sign against other radiologic and clinical data. Computer algorithms have not yet replaced the educated and prepared mind. The sensitivity and reliability of each type of diagnostic modality evaluated should be considered for each structure or function being assessed. For example, radiography is more sensitive for left atrial and right ventricular enlargement than the ECG,[59,60] but even severe conduction disturbances may not affect heart size.

The reading of the films should be done as objectively as possible to take advantage of all information available. Human factors causing errors of diagnosis (visual psychophysics, commitment, complacency, and faulty reasoning)[4] can be reduced by systematic methods of reading films. Normal or negative findings should be assessed, as they may support or refute other radiologic or clinical evidence. One should work with clinical and radiologic lists of differential diagnosis in order to avoid faulty reasoning. For example, an open mind will allow the possibilities that the presence of a heart murmur does not automatically mean that the cause of coughing is left ventricular failure, or that pulmonary density is always edema. Evaluation of all radiologic signs relating to the heart and lungs will complement information from the history and physical examination and help formulate a correct diagnosis.

Although criteria for the diagnosis of specific chamber enlargement are used routinely, the accuracy of assessing minor degrees of enlargement of individual chambers is questionable.[16,17] Studies comparing radiologic with echocardiographic assessment[59,60] do not correlate closely but there is no gold standard to determine which method is most accurate. The more sensitive a test is made (i.e., the looser the criteria for abnormality), the more false-positive diagnoses will be made.[61] It is more important to evaluate the heart in relationship to the history, physical examination, and radiologic signs in the lung fields than to try and determine degrees of specific chamber enlargement or minor degrees of general cardiac enlargement. The lung field should be used in evaluating the cardiopulmonary hemodynamic status and to determine the presence of other diseases likely to cause similar clinical signs. If the cause of an abnormality in the lung is in doubt, it is often useful to treat the diseases suspected to be responsible for these radiographic changes and repeat the radiograph later to assess response to therapy. The lability of pulmonary edema to diuretics and other cardiac drug therapy, for example, may be useful as a retrospective guide to a diagnosis of edema. Pneumonia usually takes longer to regress and does not respond to the aforementioned drugs. Lack of abnormal radiologic signs may not rule out certain diseases.

REFERENCES

1. Holmes RA, Smith GF, Lewis RE, Kern EM: The effects of rotation on the radiographic appearance of the canine cardiac silhouette in dorsal recumbency. Vet Radiol 26:98, 1985
2. Grandage J: The radiology of the dog's diaphragm. J Small Anim Pract 14:89, 1974
3. Ruehl WW, Thrall DE: The effect of dorsal versus ventral recumbency on the radiographic appearance of the canine thorax. Vet Radiol 22:10, 1981
4. Suter PF, Lord PF: Thoracic Radiography: Thoracic Diseases of the Dog and Cat. PF Suter, Wettswil, Switzerland, 1984
5. Carlisle CH, Thrall DE: A comparison of normal feline thoracic radiographs made in dorsal versus ventral recumbency. Vet Radiol 23:3, 1982
6. Groves TF, Ticer JW: Pleural fluid movement: Its effect on appearance of ventrodorsal and dorsoventral radiographic projections. Vet Radiol 24:99, 1983
7. Silverman S, Suter PF: Influence of inspiration and expiration on canine thoracic radiographs. J Am Vet Med Assoc 166:502, 1975
8. Toal RL, Losonsky JM, Coulter DB, De Novellis R: Influence of cardiac cycle on the radiographic appearance of the feline heart. Vet Radiol 26:63, 1985
9. Rankin JS, McHale PA, Arentzen CE, et al: The three-dimensional dynamic geometry of the left ventricle in the conscious dog. Circ Res 39:304, 1976
10. Hamlin RL: Analysis of the cardiac silhouette in dorsoventral radiographs from dogs with heart disease. J Am Vet Med Assoc 153:1446, 1968
11. Lord PF, Zontine WJ: Radiologic examination of the feline cardiovascular system. Vet Clin North Am 7:291, 1977
12. Berg RJ, Wingfield W: Pericardial effusion in the dog: A review of 42 cases. J Am Anim Hosp Ass 20:721, 1983
13. Gibbs C, Gaskell CJ, Darke PGG, Wotton PR: Id-

iopathic pericardial hemorrhage in dogs: A review of 14 cases. J Small Anim Pract 23:483, 1982
14. Thomas WP, Reed JR, Gomez JA: Diagnostic pneumo-pericardiography in dogs with spontaneous pericardial effusion. Vet Radiol 25:2, 1984
15. Liu S-K, Tilley LP: Dysplasia of the tricuspid valve in the dog and cat. J Am Vet Med Assoc 169:623, 1976
16. Suter PF, Lord, PF: A critical evaluation of the radiographic findings in canine cardiovascular diseases. J Am Vet Med Assoc 158:358, 1971
17. Murphy ML, Blue LR, Thenabada PN, et al: The reliability of the routine chest roentgenogram for determination of heart size based on specific ventricular chamber evaluation at postmortem. Invest Radiol 20:21, 1985
18. Lord PF, Wood A, Tilley LP, Liu SK: Radiographic and hemodynamic evaluation of cardiomyopathy and thromboembolism in the cat. J Am Vet Med Assoc 164:154, 1974
19. Lord PF, Wood A, Liu SK, Tilley LP: Left ventricular angiocardiography in congenital mitral valve insufficiency of the dog. J Am Vet Med Assoc 166:1069, 1975
20. Lord PF: Left ventricular diastolic stiffness in dogs with congestive cardiomyopathy and volume overload. Am J Vet Res 37:953, 1976
21. Sisson D, Thomas WP: Endocarditis of the aortic valve in the dog. J Am Vet Med Assoc 184:570, 1984
22. Lord PF: Ventricular volumes of the diseased canine heart, congestive cardiomyopathy and volume overload (patent ductus arteriosus and primary mitral valvular insufficiency). Am J Vet Res 35:493, 1974
23. Patterson OF, Pyle RL, Buchanan JW, et al: Hereditary patent ductus arteriosus and its sequelae in the dog. Circ Res 29:1, 1971
24. Ackerman N, Burk R, Hahn, AW, Hayes HM Jr: Patent ductus arteriosus in the dog: a retrospective study of radiographic, epidemiologic, and clinical findings. Am J Vet Res 39:1805, 1978
25. Weirich WE, Blevins WE, Rebar AH; Late consequences of patent ductus arteriosus in the dog: A report of six cases. J Am Anim Hosp Assoc 14:40, 1978
26. Feldman EC, Nimmo-Wilki JS, Pharr JW: Eisenmenger's syndrome in the dog: Case reports. J Am Anim Hosp Assoc 17:477, 1981
27. Laks MM, Morady T, Garner D, Swan HJC: Relation of ventricular volume, compliance and mass in the normal and pulmonary artery banded heart. Cardiovasc Res 6:187, 1982
28. Weber KT, Janicki JS, Shroff SG: The right ventricle: Physiologic and pathophysiologic considerations. Crit Care Med 11:323, 1983

29. Lombard CE: Pericardial disease. Vet Clin North Am 13:337, 1983

30. Thomas WP, Sisson D, Bauer TG, Reed JR: Detection of cardiac masses by two dimensional echocardiography. Vet Radiol 25:50, 1984

31. Fingland RB, Bonagura JD, Myer CW: Pulmonic stenosis in the dog: 29 cases (1975–1984). J Am Vet Med Assoc 189:218, 1986

32. Green BJ, Lord PF, Grieve RB: Occult feline dirofilariasis confirmed by angiography and serology. J Am Anim Hosp Assoc 19:847, 1983

33. Dillon R: Feline dirofilariasis. Vet Clin North Am 14:1185, 1984

34. Edwards DF, Bahr RJ, Suter PF, et al: Portal hypertension secondary to a right atrial tumor in a dog. J Am Vet Med Assoc 173:750, 1978

35. Thrall DE, Calvert CA: Radiographic evaluation of canine heartworm disease coexisting with right heart failure. Vet Radiol 24:124, 1983

36. Cantwell HD, Blevins WE, Weirich WE: Angiographic diagnosis of heartbase tumor in the dog. J Am Anim Hosp Assoc 18:83, 1982

37. Atkins, CE, Badertscher RR, Greenlee P, Nash S: Diagnosis of an intracardiac fibrosarcoma using two-dimensional echocardiography. J Am Anim Hosp Assoc 20:131, 1984

38. Shires PK, Liu WI: Persistent right aortic arch in dogs: A long term follow-up after surgical correction. J Am Anim Hosp Assoc 17:773, 1981

39. Martin DG, Ferguson EW, Gunnels RD, et al: Double aortic arch in a dog. J Am Vet Med Assoc 183:697, 1983

40. Flukiger M, Gomez J: Radiographic findings in dogs with spontaneous pulmonary thrombosis or embolism. Vet Radiol 25:124, 1984

41. Thrall DE, Losonsky JM: A method for evaluating canine pulmonary circulatory dynamics from survey radiographs. J Am Anim Hosp Assoc 12:457, 1976

42. Losonsky JR, Thrall DE, Lewis RE: Thoracic radiographic abnormalities in 200 dogs with spontaneous heartworm infestation. Vet Radiol 24:120, 1983

43. Holmes RA: Techniques to aid in the radiographic diagnosis of heartworm disease. J Am Vet Med Assoc 186:1063, 1985

44. Calvert CA, Rawlings CA: Pulmonary manifestations of heartworm disease. Vet Clin North Am 15:991, 1985

45. Donahue JMR, Kneller SK, Lewis RE: Hematologic and radiographic changes in cats after inoculation with infective larvae of *Dirofilaria immitis*. J Am Vet Med Assoc 168:413, 1976

46. Wong MM, Pederson NC, Cullen J: Dirofilariasis in cats. J Am Anim Hosp Assoc 19:855, 1983

47. Burk RL: Radiographic examination of the cardiopulmonary system. Vet Clin North Am 13:241, 1983

48. Ackerman N: Radiographic aspects of heartworm disease. Sem Vet Med Surg (Small Anim) 2:15, 1987

49. Hoskins JD, Root CR: What is your diagnosis? J Am Vet Med Assoc 179:489, 1981

50. Thomas WP, Reed JR, Bauer TG, Bresnock EM: Constrictive pericardial disease in the dog. J Am Vet Med Assoc 184:546, 1984.

51. Patterson DF: Congenital defects of the cardiovascular system of dogs. Studies in comparative cardiology. Adv Vet Sci Comp Med 20:1, 1976

52. Owens JM, Twedt DC: Non-selective angiocardiography in the cat. Vet Clin North Am 7:309, 1977

53. Bonagura JD, Myer CW, Pensinger RD: Angiocardiography. Vet Clin North Am 12:239, 1982

54. Fox PR, Bond BR: Nonselective and selective angiocardiography. Vet Clin North Am 13:259, 1983

55. Childers HE, Bazar N: What is your diagnosis? J Am Vet Med Assoc 188:195, 1986

56. Stickle RL, Anderson LK: Diagnosis of common congenital heart anomalies in the dog using survey and nonselective contrast radiography. Vet Radiol 28:6, 1987

57. Wood S: What is your diagnosis? J Am Vet Med Assoc 182:529, 1983

58. Fox PR: Feline cardiomyopathy. p. 157. In Bonagura JB (ed): Contemporary Issues Small Animal Practice. Vol 7: Cardiology, Churchill Livingstone, New York, 1987

59. Lombard CW, Ackerman N: Right heart enlargement in heartworm-infected dogs: A radiographic, electrocardiographic, and echocardiographic correlation. Vet Radiol 25:210, 1984

60. Lombard CW, Spencer CP: Correlation of radiographic, echocardiographic and electrocardiographic signs of left heart enlargement in dogs with mitral regurgitation. Vet Radiol 26:89, 1985

61. Wortman JA, Chang-Winterkorn P, Knight DH: Receiver operating characteristic curve analysis of the utility of chest radiographs for the diagnosis of feline cardiac disease. Vet Radiol 28:121, 1987

6

Echocardiography

N. Sydney Moise

Echocardiography is an exciting and growing field in which many diagnoses can be made noninvasively and safely. Coupled with a thorough history, physical examination, and data base, echocardiography is a powerful diagnostic tool. Many excellent references are available.[1–9]

BASIC PRINCIPLES OF ULTRASOUND

Ultrasound uses high-frequency sound waves with a frequency of greater than 20,000 cycles/sec (Hz). They are not audible and do not pass through air. Their velocity is equal to the product of the frequency (number of cycles in a given time) and wavelength and is proportional to the density and elastic properties of the media through which it passes.[1,2] The denser the substance, the faster ultrasound waves travel.

Ultrasound is produced with a crystal that has piezoelectric properties; that is, when electricity hits the crystal it expands and contracts producing sound waves. If sound waves hit the crystal (e.g., reflected sound waves), electricity is produced. The crystal is housed in a plastic casing and is called a *transducer*. When the transducer produces a series of waves, an ultrasound beam is generated. This beam leaves the transducer and travels in a straight line without diverging for a distance, determined by the radius of the crystal and the wavelength. The larger the radius and the smaller the wavelength (i.e., higher frequency), the longer the beam travels without divergence. Objects imaged within this distance, termed the *near field*, will be visualized better than will objects outside this distance, termed the *far field*. Higher-frequency transducers will produce a better near field. The amount of divergence can be reduced with a lens or electronically focused. Many lower-frequency transducers are focused in this fashion.[1,2]

The *acoustic impedance* of a medium describes how sound travels through it. When an ultrasound beam traverses the interface between two media that have different acoustic impedance properties, it is reflected and refracted. Greater differences in acoustic impedance, termed acoustic mismatch, cause higher amounts of reflected and refracted sound waves. Conversely, when an ultrasound beam travels through a homogenous substance it does so in a straight line without reflection and refraction.[1]

Two types of ultrasound waves are reflected at an acoustic interface: specular echoes and scattered echoes. The term echo is used because the sound waves are bounced back, or echoed, from the interface. Specular echoes are ultrasound waves reflected from large objects as the sound beam strikes the interface perpendicularly at a 90-degree angle.

Scattered echoes are the ultrasound waves reflected back from small irregular objects in which reflection is not angle dependent. The scattered echoes are important for visualizing myocardial tissue character. When ultrasound waves strike a structure parallel to the sound beam, they are scattered echoes that permit tissue visualization.[1,2]

Sound-wave reflection depends on the wavelength and frequency of the sound wave and the size of the object. To cause reflection, an object must be at least one-fourth the size of the sound wavelength. Ultrasound with a high-frequency or short wavelength can be reflected from smaller structures, permitting better structural definition and resolution.

Ultrasound transducers are made in different frequencies ranging from 1.6 MHz to 7.5 MHz (1 MHz = 1,000,000 cycles/sec). When more ultrasound is reflected, there is less available for transmission through deeper tissues. Therefore, increase in frequency reduces penetrating power.

Penetration also is influenced by the tissue struck by the beam. Different tissues cause varying amounts of absorption and scatter. Homogenous tissues are easier to penetrate than those that are nonhomogeneous.

Attenuation is the process whereby ultrasound is lost due to tissue absorption and sound-wave scatter. The distance that ultrasound must travel to have one-half its energy attenuated is referred to as its half-power distance (cm). For comparison, the half-power distances are for water, 380 cm; for blood, 15 cm; for soft tissue other than muscle, 1 to 5 cm; for muscle, 0.6 to 1 cm; and for lung, 0.05 cm.[1]

The half-power distance of lung demonstrates that sound waves do not penetrate organs with air. Air is the enemy of ultrasound, and structures below air cannot be imaged well. Ultrasound does not penetrate bone either.

Resolution is the ability of the image to represent individual structural objects. There is axial, lateral, and azimuthal resolution. Axial resolution is the ability to separate objects that are parallel to the ultrasound beam (i.e., one object behind another). Lateral resolution is the ability to separate objects that are perpendicular to the ultrasound beam (i.e., one object beside another). Azimuthal (or elevational) resolution relates to the thickness of the imaging plane. With poor azimuthal resolution, structures are superimposed where superimposition does not exist. The resolution of objects is better if they are situated within the center of the ultrasound beam and if the beam is narrow. The width of the beam can be changed by gain controls. If the gain is increased, the beam width increases, resolution decreases, and artifacts worsen.

When tissue does not reflect ultrasound, it is termed *anechoic* or *sonolucent*. If a tissue reflects ultrasound minimally compared with the surrounding tissues, it is referred to as *hypoechoic*. Conversely, if a tissue is highly reflective, it is said to be *hyperechoic* or to have greater echogenicity. When ultrasound passes through a tissue that is anechoic or hypoechoic, called through-transmission, the next tissue to be struck with the ultrasound beam will appear hyperechoic because of acoustic enhancement. When an ultrasound beam strikes an object that contains calcium or other substances that block through-transmission, that object will be hyperechoic. However, behind it there will be no image. This is referred to as an *acoustic shadow*.

TYPES OF ECHOCARDIOGRAPHY

When ultrasound is used to image the heart, it is called echocardiography, and the ultrasound unit instrument or machine is called an echocardiograph. Medical ultrasound transducers send and receive ultrasound waves. The transducers act principally as receivers because sound waves are transmitted less than 1 percent of the time; therefore, the amount of energy transmitted to the body is low. The ultrasound wave information received by the transducer is processed by the echocardiograph and displayed on an oscilloscope. Depending on the type of unit, the images are recorded on either videotape or paper, or both.[1,2]

There are basically three types of echocardiography: M-mode, two-dimensional, and Doppler. *M-mode* (motion-mode) echocardiography was the first type used for examining the heart. It employs a single icepick ultrasound beam that focuses on a very small portion of the heart. Because the heart moves back and forth from the transducer with each cardiac cycle, sound waves are reflected from different points. The echocardiograph oscilloscope sweeps from right to left, adding the dimension of time to the received image, and displaying the structure and motion of the heart. M-mode echocardiography has a high sampling rate (pulse repetition rate, 1,000 to 2,000/sec), facilitating visual appreciation of rapidly moving structures such as cardiac valves. Thus, cardiac structure and motion are imaged[5-7] (Fig. 6-1).

Information from M-mode echocardiography is valuable, particularly the ability to assess quantitatively the cardiac dimensions and contractile indices rapidly and easily. Shortcomings of this technique are principally due to the lack of consistent and accurate spatial orientations. Two-dimensional echo-

cardiography confers the ability to assess spatial orientation. Most cardiologists prefer to use both modes for a complete examination.

Two-dimensional echocardiography provides a more realistic, understandable, and complete image of the heart.[1-5] Mistakes made with M-mode echocardiograms, especially with morphologic orientation, may be circumvented with the two-dimensional examination. Mechanical scanners and phased array scanners represent the types of two-dimensional units currently available. For several years, debate has raged as to which type is better. Each type has its advantages and disadvantages.[3,4]

Mechanical scanners have a single crystal element that rapidly oscillates or several crystals that rapidly

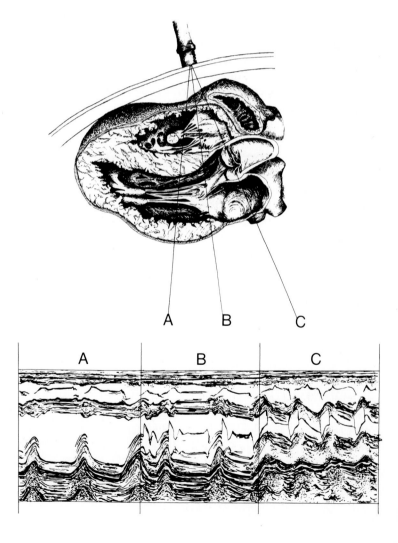

Fig. 6-1 Standard icepick cardiac ultrasound views imaged by M-mode echocardiography as the transducer is directed over different areas of the heart. (**A**) Transducer sends ultrasound waves (in sequence) through the right chest wall, right ventricular wall and chamber, interventricular septum, left ventricular chamber, chordae tendineae, and free wall. (**B**) Sound beam traverses the right heart and, depending on the angle of the transducer, may intersect the tricuspid valve, the most basilar portion of the interventricular septum, the anterior and posterior mitral valve leaflets, and the left ventricular free wall. (**C**) Sound beam traverses the right heart, aortic root, and aortic valve, and left atrium. (See Figs. 6-9 and 6-10).

rotate. Each scanner sends fan-shaped ultrasound beams toward the heart. Instead of only an icepick transection, as with M-mode, a large slice of the heart, similar to a tomogram, is captured, producing a more complete cardiac image.

Linear or phased-array echocardiographs have transducers with crystal elements in series that do not move mechanically. Rather, they are electronically fired multiply for a fanlike two-dimensional image, or one element may be fired to produce an M-mode image. Phased-array transducers permit simultaneous two-dimensional and M-mode studies. In addition, simultaneous Doppler examinations are possible. Linear scanners are usually less well suited to echocardiography than are mechanical scanners because the crystal elements are lined up like a bar. This orientation causes ultrasound beams to be sent along the length of the bar-shaped transducer, making it difficult to image the heart without rib interference. This type of ultrasound unit is relatively inexpensive and is more useful for abdominal ultrasound imaging and for equine reproductive work.

The newest advance in cardiac ultrasound is *Doppler* echocardiography, which permits evaluation of the velocity and character of blood flow within the cardiovascular system. Valvular stenoses, insufficiencies, and intracardiac and extracardiac shunts can be qualified and quantified.[8,9] By listening to the audible signals received, one can guide the ultrasound beam to determine peak velocity.

The Doppler principle is based on the change in reflected sound-wave frequency that occurs when sound waves hit a moving object. Ultrasound waves are transmitted from a transducer at a specified frequency. If the sound waves strike an object, such as red blood cells (RBCs), moving toward the transducer, the frequency of the sound waves reflected is increased and the wavelength decreased. Conversely, if sound waves strike RBCs moving away from the transducer, the frequency of the sound waves reflected is decreased, and the wavelength is increased. The difference in the frequency transmitted, and the frequency received is called the Doppler shift. The magnitude of this shift in frequency is proportional to the velocity of the RBC; therefore, the direction and speed of blood flow can be determined. The Doppler equation for calculating *blood flow velocity* is as follows:

$$V = \frac{(\Delta f) \times (C)}{(2) \times (f_0) \times \cos \theta}$$

where:

V = flow velocity of blood cells in m/sec
C = the speed of ultrasound in blood
f_0 = the transmitted frequency
θ = the intercept angle

One of the important determinants of accuracy in Doppler examination is the intercept angle (θ) between the ultrasound beam and the moving RBCs. In contrast to other types of echocardiography in which the ultrasound beam is ideally oriented perpendicular to the object imaged, the ideal situation with Doppler is for the sound waves to strike the RBCs parallel so that the angle of intercept is close to 0 degrees. With an angle of at least less than 20 degrees, the percent error in velocity determination is less than 6 percent. The cosine of angles of less than 20 degrees is close to one for calculation of the velocity using the Doppler equation.

In addition to velocity determinations, pressure gradients can be calculated from Doppler echocardiography using a modified Bernoulli equation:

$$P_1 - P_2 = 4V^2$$

where $P_1 - P_2$ is the pressure gradient across an obstruction and V is the maximum velocity distal to the obstruction. Cardiac output may also be estimated from Doppler studies. These calculations can be performed by the ultrasound unit computer.

There are currently three types of Doppler echocardiography: pulsed, continuous-wave, and high pulsed repetition frequency. All have their advantages and disadvantages.

Pulsed Doppler echocardiography uses the same transducer as the sender and receiver of ultrasound waves. It has a pulse-repetition frequency (i.e., the frequency at which sound waves are emitted) for a given depth and a range resolution (i.e., the blood flow at a specific point within the heart or vessel can be measured by adjusting the time-gate delay). With this adjustment, only ultrasound waves reflecting from RBCs at that particular point are received by the transducer for analysis. Range resolution makes it possible, for example, to localize an obstruction specific to the valvular or subvalvular area.

The disadvantage of pulsed Doppler echocardiography is that it is limited in its ability to measure high velocities, especially when increasing examination depth. In order to measure the velocity of blood flow accurately, the pulse repetition frequency must be at least twice the unknown frequency rate. This is called the Nyquist limit. If blood flow velocities are too high, the pulsed Doppler cannot accurately measure the speed of flow or determine its direction. On the spectral display, the band of high frequency goes beyond the pulsed Doppler limit and appears to wrap around the baseline. This distortion of the Doppler wave is called *aliasing* (Fig. 6-2), whereby the observed frequency of a periodically varying quantity is distorted when it exceeds one-half the sampling frequency. The lower the frequency of the Doppler transducer, the higher are the blood flow velocities that can be determined.

Continuous-wave Doppler echocardiography uses separate transmitting and receiving crystals within a transducer. Because of the independent crystals, ultrasound waves can be continuously transmitted and received. Continuous-wave Doppler does not permit range resolution. The receiving crystal analyzes the flow along the entire depth range of received Doppler shifts. Because there is no range resolution, pinpointing the location of a defect is difficult with continuous-wave Doppler alone. The advantage of this type of Doppler is that there is no limit to the velocities of blood flow that can be measured.

With high pulse-repetition Doppler the frequency of transmitted and therefore, received ultrasound waves, is so rapid that higher velocities can be measured with some degree of range resolution. It is not as accurate as pulsed Doppler in locating lesions and it cannot measure velocities as high as does continuous wave Doppler; however, it is a good compromise.

At present, cardiologists use both pulsed and continuous-wave Doppler for examination. For example, a lesion is localized with the pulsed-wave Doppler and the maximum velocity measured with the continuous wave Doppler.

Spectral analysis of normal mitral valve flow and

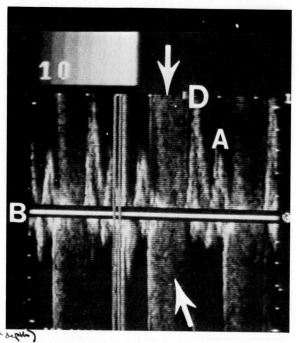

Fig. 6-2 Pulsed Doppler echocardiographic examination of the left atrium of a dog with mitral regurgitation. The gate for sampling the Doppler shift is at the left atrial side of the mitral valve. The velocity of blood flow is so high that aliasing occurs (arrows). This distortion of the Doppler wave makes it unable to determine the direction of flow and true peak velocity. Despite this artifact, however, pulsed Doppler echocardiography can still accurately diagnose mitral regurgitation. D, D wave for rapid diastolic ventricular filling; A, A wave for ventricular filling occurring during atrial contraction; B, baseline.

mitral regurgitation for the pulsed wave Doppler examination is contrasted (Fig. 6-3). The shape of the blood flow through the mitral valve is similar to the shape of mitral valve motion on the M-mode echocardiogram. The Doppler wave corresponding to rapid diastolic filling is called the D wave; the peak of this wave coincides with point E of the mitral valve on the M-mode display. The Doppler wave corresponding to ventricular filling due to atrial contraction is called the A wave; the peak of this wave coincides with point A on the M-mode mitral valve display. With mitral regurgitation, blood flow is detected within the left atrium during systole. The blood flow velocity is so rapid that the pulsed Doppler cannot determine the direction of

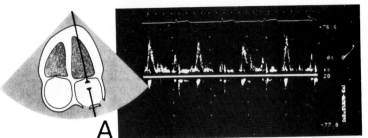

Normal Flow Pattern
PW Doppler

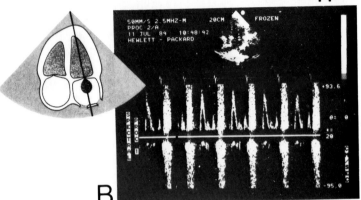

Mitral Regurgitation
PW Doppler

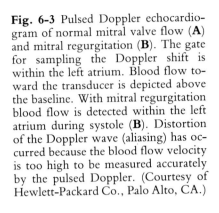

Fig. 6-3 Pulsed Doppler echocardiogram of normal mitral valve flow (**A**) and mitral regurgitation (**B**). The gate for sampling the Doppler shift is within the left atrium. Blood flow toward the transducer is depicted above the baseline. With mitral regurgitation blood flow is detected within the left atrium during systole (**B**). Distortion of the Doppler wave (aliasing) has occurred because the blood flow velocity is too high to be measured accurately by the pulsed Doppler. (Courtesy of Hewlett-Packard Co., Palo Alto, CA.)

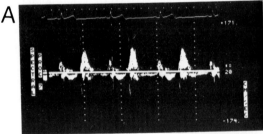

Normal Flow Pattern
CW Doppler

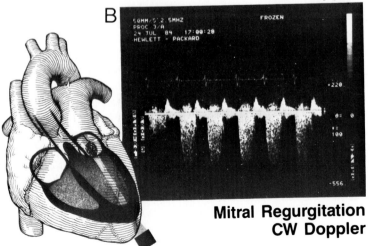

Mitral Regurgitation
CW Doppler

Fig. 6-4 Continuous-wave (CW) Doppler echocardiogram of normal mitral valve flow (**A**) and mitral regurgitation (**B**). The left atrial regurgitant high-velocity blood flow is seen during systole below the baseline. (Courtesy of Hewlett-Packard Co., Palo Alto, CA.)

flow or the maximum flow velocity. Aliasing results. In this situation, continuous Doppler echocardiography can determine these variables, although the diagnosis of mitral regurgitation is still apparent from the pulsed Doppler echocardiogram. Continuous-wave Doppler examination of normal mitral valve flow and of mitral regurgitation is illustrated in Figure 6-4. The regurgitated left atrial high-velocity jet is seen during systole below the baseline.

In addition to the direction and velocity of blood flow, turbulent blood flow is also detectable with Doppler echocardiography. Turbulence causes a spectral broadening of many frequencies because the velocities are of multiple magnitudes and directions. The flow disturbance is audibly dissonant and harsh. Thus, Doppler echocardiography promises to become one of the most helpful noninvasive diagnostic aids in clinical cardiology.

PERFORMING THE M-MODE AND TWO-DIMENSIONAL ECHOCARDIOGRAPHIC EXAMINATION

The first step in learning how to perform echocardiography is knowing what you are looking for and understanding what represents a good or bad image. High-quality normal M-mode and two-dimensional echocardiograms should be closely studied. Normal parameters must be learned. Familiarization with instrumentation is a necessity.

To perform an M-mode examination, the dog or cat is restrained in left lateral recumbency. Most animals do not require chemical restraint, but if needed, light tranquilization is advocated. Most drugs will affect echocardiographic measurements. Dogs can usually be muzzled, eliminating the need for chemical immobilization. For cats that cannot be held in place quietly, ketamine hydrochloride may be judiciously administered (2 to 10 mg IM or IV). With M-mode echocardiography, clipping the hair is not usually necessary. A generous quantity of coupling gel is applied on the thorax over the heart to eliminate air that may be present between the skin and transducer. The transducer frequency should be appropriately chosen for optimal resolution and penetration. For smaller animals, less penetration is required and more resolution is needed. Therefore, a higher-frequency transducer is best. Conversely, as the size of the animal increases, lower-frequency transducers will be needed. M-mode transducers are usually supplied as 7.5-, 5.0-, 3.5-, 2.25-, or 1.6-MHz and may or may not be focused. For small to medium-size cats, small puppies and toy breed dogs, a 7.5-MHz transducer is usually adequate. Large cats and small to medium sized dogs may require a 5-MHz transducer, and a 3.5-MHz transducer is used in some medium-size, large, and giant-breed dogs. A large dog might require a 2.25-MHz transducer for optimal examination.

The transducer is placed between the fourth or fifth intercostal space on the right hemithorax. An acoustic window is sought that permits the heart to be imaged without interference from ribs and lungs. Occasionally, the animal's position may need to be manipulated to orient the heart closer to the thoracic wall. If an acoustic window is still lacking, one or both forelimbs may be positioned more forward or a towel wedged under the ventral or dorsal thorax. The transducer angle with the thorax should be perpendicular when the mitral valve is imaged, rather than angled. While directing the transducer toward the heart the instrument controls are adjusted to enhance image quality.

The first controls to regulate are depth and gain. Initially, the depth is set based on an estimate of how deep the sound waves must travel to image the left ventricular pericardium. Once the heart is visualized, the depth compensation or time gain control is adjusted to compensate for loss of ultrasonic energy as the beam enters and traverses the thorax. Some units have levers, slide-pods, or knobs that adjust a certain portion of the overall depth gain; other units (particularly dedicated M-mode echocardiographs) have an additional near field gain control. The gain determines the amount of energy (i.e., ultrasound) sent.[1] If too much gain is used, the image is obscured by excessive return of echoes and resolution is lessened. Conversely, if gain is inadequate, information is lost because too few sound waves are available to be reflected back for an image. Ultrasound is attenuated as it travels through the body. Mechanisms are needed for reducing proximal and enhancing distal echoes. Visualization of structures in the far field requires a considerable ultrasound (i.e., gain); however, structures in the near field are seen with minimal ultrasound. Therefore, ultrasound gain can be damped to the near field and relatively enhanced in the far field. The reject control does not affect the amount of ultrasound sent; instead, it eliminates from the image miscellaneous, weak echoes. The ideal echocardiographic settings call for minimal gain and minimal reject. With this attempt for proper settings, artifacts can be avoided and the most informative image achieved.

Once the proper depth and gain settings are found, the echocardiographer can concentrate on scanning the heart. At least the three individual cardiac views should be standardly recorded (Fig. 6-1). In addition, a continuous sweep of the heart from base to apex or vice versa should be done to verify continuity of the structures. This can be achieved by moving from the ventricular apex, where the transducer is angled caudoventrally to the mitral valve by angling the transducer craniodorsally, and then to the aorta by angling more craniodorsal and medially. Using a cadaver specimen to study the

heart in the thorax and the relative positions of the chambers and valves is beneficial for the beginner.

An understanding of three-dimensional cardiovascular spatial orientation is especially important for two-dimensional echocardiographic conception.[10] Two-dimensional echocardiographic technique is more dependent on close airtight contact between the skin and transducer. Shaving is usually required. In addition, because a wider fan of ultrasound is transmitted, a larger acoustic window is needed. In dogs and cats, the best way to achieve this is to position the animal on a table with a hole cut in it. The animal's thorax in lateral recumbency is positioned over the hole such that the heart is scanned from below. Principles of gain control for M-mode echocardiography also apply to the two-dimensional examination.

The American Society of Echocardiography (ASE) has made recommendations for the plans of two-dimensional study and the terminology to be used.[11] The ASE has recommended that the transducer location be named suprasternal (transducer in

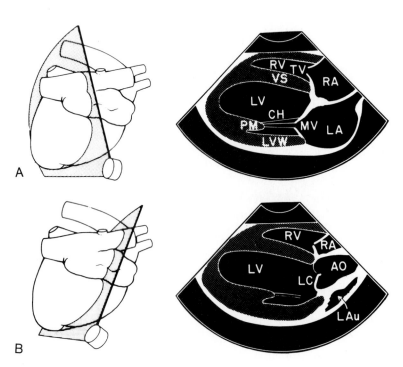

Fig. 6-5 Two-dimensional echocardiographic long-axis views obtained from the right intercostal transducer location. The diagrams on the left illustrate the heart viewed from the right side, the cylindrical transducer, and the orientation of the fan-shaped beam transecting the heart. The diagrams on the right illustrate the echotomographic images corresponding to the imaging planes showing on the left. (**A**) Long-axis four-chamber view. (**B**) Long-axis view of left ventricular outflow region. Note that the body of the left atrium, the left ventricle, and aorta usually cannot be imaged in a single plane from this location. RV, right ventricle; TV, tricuspid valve; VS, ventricular septum; RA, right atrium; LV, left ventricle; CH, chordae tendineae; PM, papillary muscle; MV, mitral valve; LA, left atrium; LVW, left ventricular wall; AO, aorta; LC, left cusp (aortic valve): LAu, left auricle. (Thomas WP: Two-dimensional, real-time echocardiography in the dog: Technique and anatomic validation. Vet Radiol 25:50, 1984.)

the suprasternal notch), subcostal (transducer located near the midline of the body and beneath the lowest ribs), apical (transducer over the apex impulse), and parasternal (transducer to the side of the sternum and above the apex impulse). Imaging planes are described as long-axis view (transection parallel to the long axis of the heart), short-axis view (transection perpendicular to the long axis of the heart), and four-chamber view (transection parallel to the dorsal and ventral surfaces of the body). Two-dimensional images are then identified by the transducer location and the imaging plane (e.g., parasternal long-axis view).

The problem with applying this human terminology to veterinary echocardiography is that some of the images studied in humans are not obtainable in animals because of different thoracic confirmations.[10] Thomas made terminology recommendations for veterinary echocardiography (Figs. 6-5 through 6-8). Some of the imaging identification

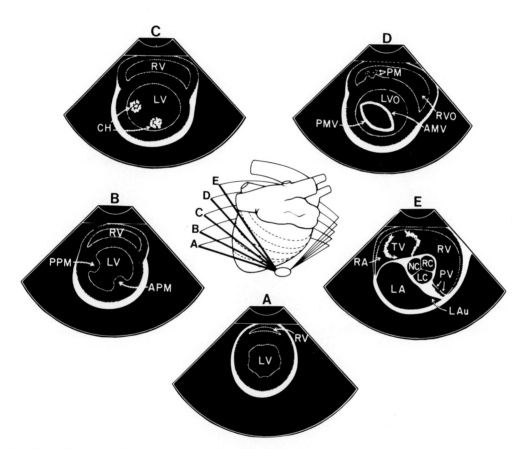

Fig. 6-6 Two-dimensional echocardiograpic short-axis views obtained from the right intercostal location. The diagram in the center illustrates the beam orientations used to obtain images at five levels of the left ventricle. The corresponding images are shown clockwise from the bottom. (**A**) Apical level. (**B**) Papillary muscle level. (**C**) Chordal level. (**D**) Mitral valve level (diastole). (**E**) Aortic valve level (diastole). RV, right ventricle; LV, left ventricle; CH, chordae tendineae; PM, papillary muscle; LVO, left ventricular outflow tract; PMV, posterior (parietal) mitral valve cusp; RVO, right ventricular outflow tract; AMV, anterior (septal) mitral valve cusp; PPM, posteromedial (dorsal) papillary muscle; APM, anterolateral (ventral) papillary muscle; PV, pulmonary valve; RA, right atrium; TV, tricuspid valve; LA, left atrium; NC, noncoronary or septal cusp (aortic valve); RC, right cusp (aortic valve); LC, left cusp (aortic valve): LAu, left auricle. (Thomas WP: Two-dimensional, real-time echocardiography in the dog: Technique and anatomic validation. Vet Radiol 25:50, 1984.)

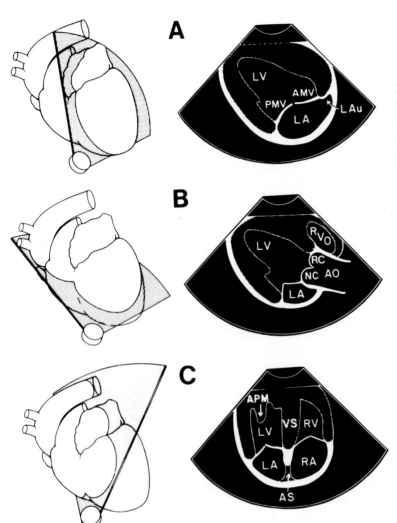

Fig. 6-7 Two-dimensional echocardiographic views obtained from the left caudal (apical) intercostal location. Note that the echo window is not at the true left ventricular apex. The diagrams on the left illustrate the heart viewed from the left side with the approximate transducer and echo-beam orientations. The corresponding echotomographic images are shown on the right. (**A**) Long-axis two-chamber view of the left atrium and ventricle. (**B**) Long-axis view of the left ventricular outflow region. (**C**) Four-chamber view. LV, left ventricle; AMV, anterior (septal) mitral valve cusp; PMV, posterior (parietal) mitral valve cusp; LA, left atrium; LAu, left auricle; RVO, right ventricular outflow tract; RC, right cusp (aortic valve); NC, noncoronary or septal cusp (aortic valve); AO, aorta; APM, anterolateral (ventral) papillary muscle; VS, ventricular septum; RV, right ventricle; RA, right atrium; AS, atrial septum. (Thomas WP: Two-dimensional, real-time echocardiography in the dog: Technique and anatomic validation. Vet Radiol 25:50, 1984.)

corresponds to that used in humans. Thomas's nomenclature is not universally used, however, as some veterinary echocardiographers prefer the terminology of the ASE where applicable.[12] Suprasternal and subcostal views have not yet been adequately studied in animals.

Two-dimensional echocardiographs have an indicator knob on the transducer to indicate left and right orientation on the monitor screen. This knob should always be pointed toward the animal's head for standard orientation. Some echocardiographs have a control that permits the operator to turn an image 180 degrees without moving the transducer.

INTERPRETATION OF THE ECHOCARDIOGRAM

M-mode echocardiograms of a normal dog (Fig. 6-9) and cat (Fig. 6-10) with structures commonly measured are illustrated. Standards for measuring the M-mode echocardiogram have been set by the ASE.[13] These recommendations are generally accepted, although variations are still reported.[1] The echocardiogram to be measured should be of a quality that permits clear delineation of walls, chambers, and valves. Measuring poor-quality echocardiograms predisposes to diagnostic error and should be avoided.

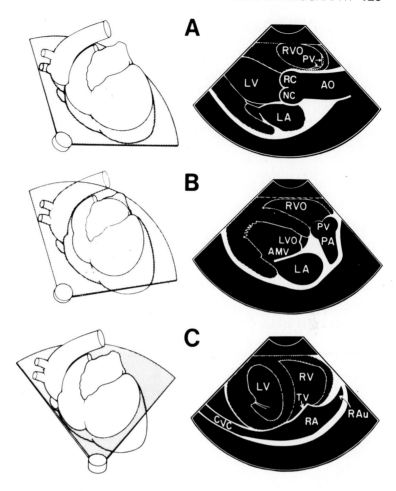

Fig. 6-8 Two-dimensional echocardiographic views obtained from the left cranial intercostal location. (**A**) Long-axis view of the left ventricular outflow region. (**B**) Long-axis view of the right ventricular outflow region. (**C**) Oblique view of the heart with a long-axis view of the right atrium and caudal vena cava. The transducer is shown in the caudal location; however, this view is often obtainable in either location. RVO, right ventricular outflow tract; PV, pulmonary valve; LV, left ventricle; RC, right cusp (aortic valve); NC, noncoronary or septal cusp (aortic valve); AO, aorta; LA, left atrium; PA, pulmonary artery; LVO, left ventricular outflow tract; AMV, anterior (septal) mitral valve cusp; RV, right ventricle; TV, tricuspid valve; CVC, caudal vena cava; RA, right atrium; RAu, right auricle. (Thomas WP: Two-dimensional, real-time echocardiography in the dog: Technique and anatomic validation. Vet Radiol 25:50, 1984.)

At each acoustic interface (e.g., blood to muscle), lines appear, and the thickness of a line will vary with gain control. The leading edge is the part of the line closest to the transducer. The part of the line farthest from the transducer is the trailing edge. Structures are more accurately measured from leading edge to leading edge because it denotes the location of a specific interface.[13] This recommendation is also true for two-dimensional images, for which axial measurements have better resolution and are more accurate than lateral measurement.[1]

Diastolic dimensions are measured at the Q or R wave of a simultaneously recorded electrocardiogram (ECG). In viewing the left ventricular diameter in diastole, it will be noted that atrial contraction can add a significant dimension to this measurement. Atrial contraction may also produce

significant thinning of the walls. Therefore, some echocardiographers prefer to measure the left ventricle before measuring atrial contraction.

The left ventricular systolic dimension is measured from the peak downward motion of the interventricular septum to the echocardial surface of the left ventriculaar free wall. Normally the interventricular septum and left ventricular free wall move toward each other in systole and away from each other during diastole, but the peak motions may not correspond exactly because of slight differences in myocardial depolarization. The septum is usually depolarized a few milliseconds before the free wall, causing it to contract that much sooner.

At the beginning of diastole, there normally may be a diastolic dip of the interventricular septum toward the left ventricular chamber. Right ventricular

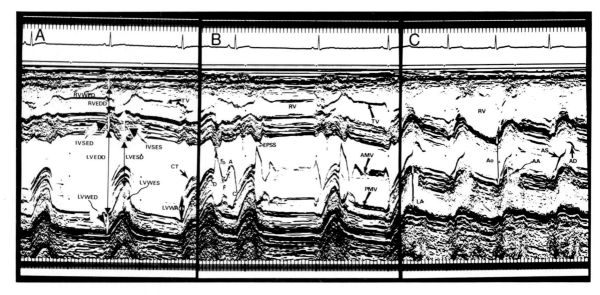

Fig. 6-9 M-mode echocardiogram recorded from a normal dog demonstrating structures that are measured. *Frame A:* RVWED, right ventricular wall at end-diastole; RVEDD, right ventricular end-diastolic diameter; TV, tricuspid valve; IVSED, interventricular septum at end-diastole; IVSES, interventricular septum at end-systole; LVEDD, left ventricular end-diastolic diameter; LVESD, left ventricular end-systolic diameter; LVWED, left ventricular wall at end-diastole; LVWES, left ventricular wall at end-systole; LVWA, left ventricular wall amplitude; CT, chordae tendineae. *Frame B:* RV, right ventricle; D, initial opening of mitral valve; E, maximum early diastolic opening of mitral valve; F, closure of leaflets after early diastolic filling; the slope from E to F is the velocity of diastolic closure (and if this is not a straight line, point F_0 is also used); C, closure of mitral leaflets just before systole; EPSS, E point septal separation; AMV = anterior mitral valve; PMV, posterior mitral valve. *Frame C:* RV, right ventricle; Ao, aortic root; AS, aortic valve during systole; AD, aortic valve during diastole; AA, aortic amplitude; LA, left atrium. An electrocardiogram is recorded at the top of each echogram.

filling momentarily precedes left ventricular filling, briefly causing the septum to expand from right to left.

Measurements of right and left ventricular chamber and walls should be made at the level of the chordae tendineae, not at the level of the ventricular apex or papillary muscle. Right ventricular structures are often inadequately imaged and cannot be accurately measured. In the healthy animal, the left ventricular chamber is three to four times larger than the right. Other measurements that can be made at the chordae level include amplitudes of motion (left septal echo or left ventricular free wall echo) or the rate of rise of the left ventricular free-wall echo.

Early reports of echocardiography proposed conversion of chamber dimensions to volume, ejection fraction, and cardiac output. Because of geometric assumptions and inaccuracies, this extrapolation of measurements is not recommended.

Indices of cardiac function calculated at the chordae level are the percentage of left ventricular wall thickening, percentage of ventricular septal thickening, fractional shortening, and circumferential shortening. The percentage thickening of the ventricular free wall and the septum are calculated as the systolic thickness minus the diastolic thickness divided by the systolic thickness times 100. The fractional shortening is calculated by

$$100 \times \frac{\substack{\text{left ventricular chamber end-diastolic dimension}\\ -\text{ left ventricular chamber end-systolic dimension}}}{\text{left ventricular chamber end-diastolic dimension}}$$

The circumferential shortening is calculated by

$$\frac{\substack{\text{left ventricular chamber end-diastolic dimension}\\ -\text{ left ventricular chamber end-systolic dimension}}}{\substack{\text{left ventricular chamber end-diastolic dimension}\\ \times\text{ left ventricular ejection time}}}$$

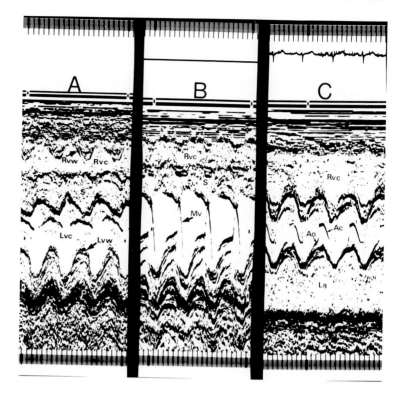

Fig. 6-10 M-mode echocardiogram of a normal cat recorded with a 7.5-MHz transducer. Rvw, right ventricular wall; Rvc, right ventricular chamber; s, interventricular septum; Lvc, left ventricular chamber; Lvw, left ventricular wall; Mv, mitral valve; Ao, aortic valve open; Ac, aortic valve closed; La, left atrium.

Fractional shortening is a commonly used index of cardiac performance. However, there are certain limitations in its clinical application (e.g., mitral insufficiency). In assessing cardiac function by the M-mode echocardiogram, an assumption is made of uniform wall motion. Moreover, the whole heart is not seen, and akinetic, hypokinetic, or dyskinetic areas may be overlooked. This problem, for the most part, is solved by two-dimensional imaging. Another erroneous assumption made with the M-mode imaging is that the measurements represent the minor (i.e., craniocaudal) cardiac dimension. This may not be true if the heart is viewed at an angle instead of perpendicularly to the ultrasound beam. This problem also can be solved with two-dimensional imaging.

The M-mode scan is next evaluated at the level of the mitral valve.[1] It normally has a biphasic opening and closing pattern, as does the tricuspid valve. Peak opening and closing points are identified by letters (see Fig. 6-9). At rapid heart rates (Fig. 6-11), the points of the mitral valve may not be distinctly identifiable at the usual recording speed of 50 mm/sec. Point D on the mitral valve corresponds

to the initial rapid opening of the leaflets at early diastole, and point E is the maximum opening during this phase of ventricular filling. The slope of a line from D to E indicates the velocity of blood flow (decreased flow with a decreased slope) between the left atrium and left ventricle. This measure is more flow related than pressure related. Point F is the end of rapid ventricular filling, and the slope of a line from point E to point F (E to F slope) indicates the diastolic closure rate of the mitral valve (Fig. 6-9). This may be altered in selected diseases. A decrease in the E to F slope may be found with mitral stenosis, decreased left ventricular compliance, or pulmonary hypertension without left ventricular compliance abnormalities. There is a technical problem with the E to F slope because the mitral valve descent is not always straight and a point (F_0) between the E and F points may interrupt the straight descent. In this situation, the true closing rate is questionable. After the early diastolic filling of the ventricle, atrial contraction occurs forcing the mitral leaflets to open again, and the maximum opening point is point A. In the normal animal, the excursion of point E is greater than point A. In situations in

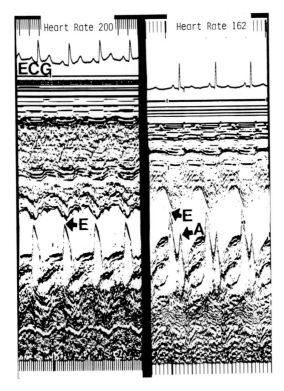

which atrial contraction is significant and vital to ventricular filling (e.g., reduced ventricular compliance), the excursion of the leaflet to point A may be greater than to point E. Point C is the point of valve coaptation during ventricular systole. Normally there is a straight line between point A and C, but in situations of elevated left ventricular end-diastolic pressure there may be an interruption in

Fig. 6-11 M-mode echocardiogram contrasting the different mitral valve leaflet appearances in a cat due to heart rate variation. *Left frame:* heart rate = 200; the A point cannot be identified. *Right frame:* heart rate = 162. Both E and A points are visualized. Paper speed, 50 mm/sec. ECG, electrocardiogram.

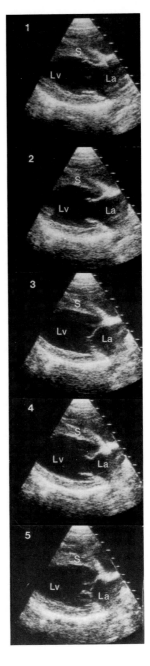

Fig. 6-12 Two-dimensional frames recorded from a normal dog (right intercostal position) showing the left heart in long axis. In *frame 1* the mitral valve leaflets are wide open and would correspond to M-mode point E, the maximum opening during rapid ventricular filling. In *frame 2* the mitral valve is beginning to close, and in *frame 3* the leaflets meet at the end of rapid ventricular filling. In *frame 4* the atrium contracts and the mitral valve opens again, but not as widely as in frame 1. The mitral valve here corresponds to M-mode point A, the maximum excursion of the mitral valve with atrial systole. In *frame 5* the mitral valve has closed at end-diastole. Note the progressive decrease in the left atrial size from frames 1 to 5. Lv, left ventricle; S, interventricular septum; La, left atrium.

the descent causing a bump (called the B bump). The presence of the B bump may indicate elevated diastolic pressures, but it is an insensitive criteria. The distance separating the left ventricular septal echo from the mitral valve point E is another measure of ventricular function. If this distance (E point to septal separation) is great, poor contractility is indicated. Although significant cardiac dysfunction is evidenced by a large E point to septal separation (except in certain situations such as mitral stenosis), it is an insensitive indicator of contractility. The mitral valve opening and closing sequence as seen in two-dimensional echocardiography is illustrated for contrast (Fig. 6-12).

The aorta and left atrium are also evaluated (see Fig. 6-9). Aortic diameter is measured at end-diastole at the Q or R wave and the left atrium at the maximal systolic excursion.[13] The leading edge method is preferred. The ratio of left atrial to aortic diameter is helpful in judging the size of these structures. This ratio should be approximately 1:1 in the normal dog and cat. The amplitude of the aorta may also be determined (i.e., the aortic excursion from diastole to systole). This may be measured from the anterior aortic wall (closest to the transducer) or from the posterior aortic wall (farthest from the transducer). Aortic root motion is affected by forward stroke volume and left atrial filling. A low aortic amplitude may indicate poor cardiac output. If the aortic valve is clearly seen, the opening amplitude or systolic time intervals can be calculated. The aortic valve should look like an angled rectangle in the normal animal (see Fig. 6-1). In the M-mode echocardiogram, it is usually the right coronary cusp and the noncoronary cusp that are imaged.

Systolic time intervals can be used as indices of car-

Table 6-1 Normal Echocardiographic Values in Cats

Mensural	$(N = 11)^{22}$	$(N = 25)^{23}$	$(N = 30)^{24}$	NG[6]	$(N = 30)^{25,c}$	$(N = 16)^{26,c}$
LVEDD (cm)	1.51 ± 0.21[a]	1.48 ± 0.26[a]	1.59 ± 0.19[a]	1.10–1.60[b]	1.40 ± 0.13[a]	1.28 ± 0.17[a]
LVESD (cm)	0.69 ± 0.22	0.88 ± 0.24	0.80 ± 0.14	0.60–1.00	0.81 ± 0.16	0.83 ± 0.15
Ao (cm)	0.95 ± 0.15	0.75 ± 0.18	0.95 ± 0.11	0.65–1.10	0.94 ± 0.11	0.94 ± 0.14
LA (cm)	1.21 ± 0.18	0.74 ± 0.17	1.23 ± 0.14	0.85–1.25	1.03 ± 0.14	0.98 ± 0.17
LA/Ao (cm)	1.29 ± 0.23	—	1.30 ± 0.17	0.80–1.30	1.10 ± 0.18	1.09 ± 0.27
IVSED (cm)	0.50 ± 0.07	0.45 ± 0.09	0.31 ± 0.04	0.25–0.50	0.36 ± 0.08	—
IVSES (cm)	0.76 ± 0.12	—	0.58 ± 0.06	0.50–0.90	—	—
LVWED (cm)	0.46 ± 0.05	0.37 ± 0.08	0.33 ± 0.06	0.25–0.50	0.35 ± 0.05	0.31 ± 0.11
LVWES (cm)	0.78 ± 0.10	—	0.68 ± 0.07	0.40–0.90	—	0.55 ± 0.88
RVED (cm)	0.54 ± 0.10	—	0.60 ± 0.15	—	0.50 ± 0.21	—
LVWA (cm)	0.50 ± 0.07	—	—	—	—	0.32 ± 0.11
EPSS (cm)	0.04 ± 0.07	—	0.02 ± 0.09	—	—	—
AA (cm)	0.36 ± 0.10	—	—	—	—	—
MVEFS (mm/sec)	54.4 ± 13.4	—	87.2 ± 25.9	—	—	83.78 ± 23.81
ΔD% (%)	55.0 ± 10.2	41.0 ± 7.3	49.8 ± 5.3	29–35	42.7 ± 8.1	34.5 ± 12.6
LVWT (%)	39.5 ± 7.6	—	—	—	—	—
IVST (%)	33.5 ± 8.2	—	—	—	—	—
HR (beats/min)	182 ± 22	167 ± 29	194 ± 23	—	255 ± 36	—
WT (kg)	4.3 ± 0.5	4.7 ± 1.2	4.1 ± 1.1	—	3.91 ± 1.2	—

[a] Mean ± SD.
[b] Usual range.
[c] Cats anesthetized with ketamine.
NG, information not given; LVEDD, left ventricular end-diastolic diameter; LVESD, left ventricular end-systolic diameter; Ao, aorta; LA, left atrium; LA/Ao, left atrium to aortic root ratio; IVSED, interventricular septum at end-diastole; IVSES, interventricular septum at end-systole; LVWED, left ventricular wall at end-diastole; LVWES, left ventricular wall at end-systole; RVED, right ventricular diameter at end-diastole; LVWA, left ventricular wall amplitude; EPSS, E point-septal separation; AA, aortic amplitude; MVEFS, mitral valve E-F slope; ΔD%, fractional shortening; LVWT, left ventricular wall thickening; IVST, interventricular septal thickening; HR, heart rate; WT, weight.

diac function but, because the opening and closing of the aortic valve are not always clearly seen, these calculations cannot always be performed. The left ventricular ejection time is a systolic time interval measured as the duration of time which the aortic valve is open during systole. Other systolic intervals that can be determined with the echocardiogram are the pre-ejection period (measured as the time from the Q wave on the ECG to the opening of the aortic valve) and electromechanical systole (left ventricular ejection time plus the preinjection period).

Measurements of cardiac structures can be made from either the M-mode or the two-dimensional echocardiogram. Studies have demonstrated a high correlation between measurements made using these two different techniques.[12] Normal values for cardiac mensurals have been published for the dog[6,14-21] (Figs. 6-13 through 6-16) and cat[6,12,22-28] (Table 6-1). There is greater variation in canine cardiac mensurals due to breed differences than between cat breeds.

Once the echocardiogram has been measured, it is assessed to identify abnormalities in chamber size, wall thickness, valve motion, and indices of cardiac function. In addition, other evaluations of cardiac structure and motion can be made.

The left ventricle is studied for evidence of abnormalities in chamber size, wall thickness, or mo-

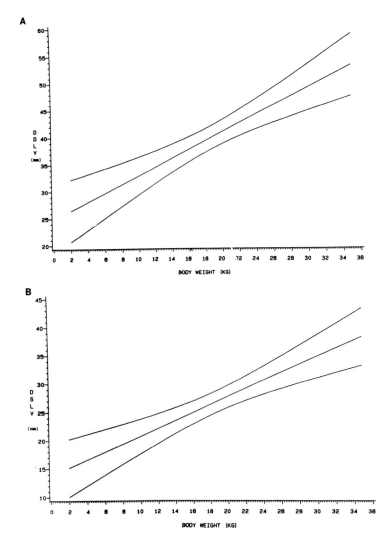

Fig. 6-13 Graphic representation of normal values for (**A**) left ventricular internal dimension during diastole (DDLV) and (**B**) systole (DSLV) in the dog. Predicted value ±95 percent confidence interval are displayed. (Bonagura JD, O'Grady MR, Herring DS: Echocardiography: Principles of interpretation. Vet Clin North Am 15:1177, 1985. Reprinted with permission from WB Saunders Co.)

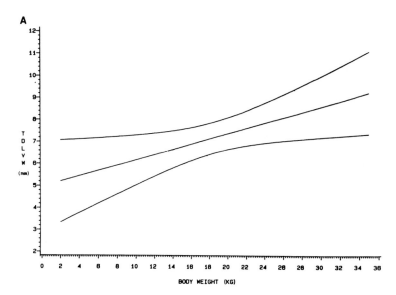

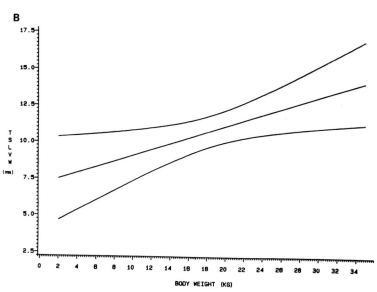

Fig. 6-14 Graphic representation of the normal left ventricular wall thickness during (**A**) diastole (TDLVW) and (**B**) systole (TSLVW) in the dog. (Bonagura JD, O'Grady MR, Herring DS: Echocardiography: Principles of interpretation. Vet Clin North Am 15:1177, 1985. Reprinted with permission from WB Saunders Co.)

tion.[6] Diseases that cause dilation because of volume overload may include mitral insufficiency, aortic insufficiency, left-to-right shunts, cardiomyopathy, and anemia. The left ventricular chamber may be reduced in size in states of volume depletion (e.g., hypoadrenocorticism, severe dehydration, hypovolemic shock) or inadequate return of blood to the left atrium and ventricle (e.g., heartworm disease, tetralogy of Fallot). The left ventricular wall may be thickened due to hypertrophic cardiomyopathy, subaortic stenosis, hyperthyroidism, systemic hypertension, and infiltrative myocardial disease. *Hy-perkinesis* of the left ventricle may be seen in mitral or aortic insufficiency, certain volume overload states (e.g., anemia), hyperthyroidism, sympathetic stimulation, or hypertrophic cardiomyopathy. With dilated cardiomyopathy or diseases resulting in myocardial failure (e.g., doxorubicin cardiotoxicity, end-stage mitral insufficiency), *hypokinesis* will be seen.

The right ventricle will be dilated with tricuspid insufficiency, chronic pulmonic stenosis, cor pulmonale, atrial septal defect, or heartworm disease. Pulmonic stenosis, tetralogy of Fallot, and heart-

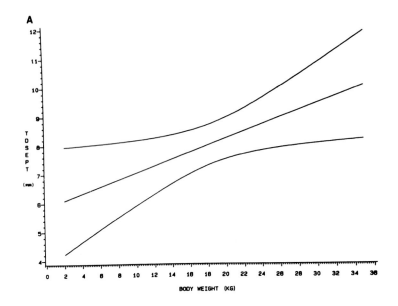

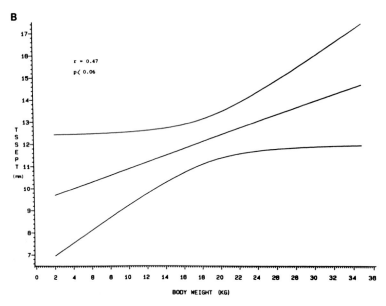

Fig. 6-15 Graph showing the normal ventricular septal thickness in (**A**) diastole (TDSEPT) and (**B**) systole (TSSEPT) in the dog. (Bonagura JD, O'Grady MR, Herring DS: Echocardiography: Principles of interpretation. Vet Clin North Am 15:1177, 1985. Reprinted with permission from WB Saunders Co.)

worm disease will result in right ventricular wall hypertrophy.

The interventricular septum may be hypertrophied by diseases affecting the left or right heart. In some disorders (e.g., hypertrophic cardiomyopathy), the septum may hypertrophy more than the free wall (e.g., asymmetric septal hypertrophy). When scanning the ventricular septum by M-mode or two-dimensional echocardiography, continuity of the septum must be assessed to detect ventricular septal defects or abnormal relationships between the septum and other cardiac structures (e.g., overriding aorta in tetralogy of Fallot).

Septal motion reflects filling and depolarization patterns of the left and right ventricles.[1] In left ventricular volume overload (e.g., aortic or mitral regurgitation), the septal motion may be hyperkinetic; during early diastole, marked anterior (i.e., toward the transducer) movement may occur due to excessive inflow of blood. Conversely, in right ventric-

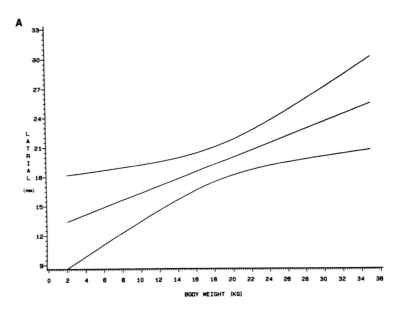

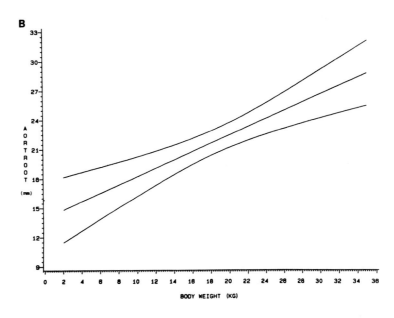

Fig. 6-16 Graphic representation of (**A**) left atrial (LATRIAL) and (**B**) aortic root (AORTROOT) dimensions in the dog. (Bonagura JD, O'Grady MR, Herring DS: Echocardiography: Principles of interpretation. Vet Clin North Am 15:1177, 1985. Reproduced with permission from WB Saunders Co.)

ular pressure or volume overload, the interventricular septal motion may be reduced in amplitude or may be paradoxic. Paradoxic septal motion is recognized echocardiographically as rapid anterior septal movement during systole and is seen with advanced diseases (Fig. 6-17). The two-dimensional examination facilitates appreciation of paradoxic interventricular septal motion. In pure right ventricular volume overload (e.g., tricuspid insufficiency), septal flattening and paradoxic motion occur during diastole; during systole, the left ventricle resumes a normal circular appearance. However, with pure right ventricular pressure overload or in right ventricular pressure and volume overload, the left ventricle never attains a circular shape. This is because the septum moves toward the left ventricle and remains flattened, giving the left ventricle the shape of a half-moon (Fig. 6-18).

The left and right atria are evaluated for evidence of dilation.[6] Left atrial enlargement is seen with congenital left-to-right shunts, cardiomyopathies, mitral stenosis, and mitral insufficiency.[1,6] Right atrial enlargement may occur with cardiomyopathy, tricuspid regurgitation or stenosis, heartworm disease, atrial septal defect, or hyperthyroidism. The atrial septum may bulge away from the atrium in which a volume overload is present. An intact atrial septum should be verified during two-dimensional scanning.

Identification of the pulmonary artery is usually possible only with a two-dimensional echocardiogram. Its normal spiral relationship to the aorta should be demonstrated.[4] The pulmonary trunk may be dilated with congenital left-to-right shunts, pulmonic stenosis, heartworm disease, or cor pulmonale. The aorta will be reduced in size when forward cardiac output is reduced and dilated with sub-

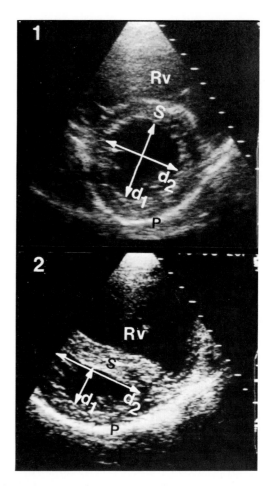

Fig. 6-18 Two-dimensional echocardiographic short-axis views recorded at the level of the chordae tendineae in diastole. *Frame 1* is from a healthy 35-kg Chesapeake Bay retriever demonstrating normal circular left ventricular geometry. The two perpendicular left ventricular minor axis dimensions (d_1 and d_2) were equal in both systole and diastole. *Frame 2* is from a 6-year-old 32-kg German shepherd with heartworm disease and associated pressure and volume overload. The two dimensions are unequal during systole and diastole. Note the flattened interventricular septum (S). Rv, right ventricle; P, pericardium.

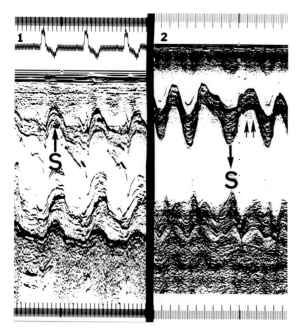

Fig. 6-17 M-mode echocardiograms comparing effects of right ventricular (*frame 1*) and left ventricular (*frame 2*) volume overloads in two dogs on interventricular septal (S) motion. In right ventricular volume overload (frame 1), there is a rapid anterior motion of the septum (arrow) with the onset of systole (i.e., paradoxic septal motion). In overload of the left ventricle (frame 2), septal motion is exaggerated toward the left ventricular posterior wall in systole (single arrow). Marked anterior septal motion occurs (double arrows) during early diastole. Paper speed = 50 mm/sec.

aortic stenosis, tetralogy of Fallot, patent ductus arteriosus, or systemic hypertension.

The *cardiac valves* are studied with respect to their motion and structure.[1,6] The valve leaflets should appear as smooth, echodense, fine lines. Irregularities, masses, or thickening may indicate endocardiosis or vegetative endocarditis. The atrioventricular valves may demonstrate fine diastolic fluttering, suggesting insufficiency of the corresponding semilunar valve. Atrioventricular insufficiency, when severe, may cause systolic fluttering of the respective valve. The atrioventricular valves should not be seen within the corresponding atria. If they are, this may indicate valve prolapse or rupture of the chordae tendineae.

The aortic and pulmonic valves should also be fine and smooth. Three leaflets may be identified on a two-dimensional echogram. Diastolic fluttering may indicate semilunar valvular insufficiency. Systolic fluttering may be normal or occur with high blood flow. The semilunar valves should not prolapse into the ventricle; this may indicate endocarditis with valvular thickening. If the semilunar valves close prematurely, ventricular outflow obstruction may be present. Early valve closure may also occur with low-flow states and poor cardiac output. During systole, the leaflets should open very close to the vessel wall. If doming of the valve is seen, valvular stenosis may be present.

Evaluation for *pericardial effusion*, extracardiac *masses* (e.g., heart base tumor), and *pleural fluid* should be performed. Ultrasonic examination of the cardiac patient need not stop at the diaphragm. Di-

lated caudal vena cava, dilated hepatic veins, enlarged round liver, or ascites may provide further useful information (Fig. 6-19).

Arrhythmias can alter the cardiac contractile sequence and distort the motion of heart chambers and valves.[1,29] Figures 6-20 through 6-23 provide examples of dynamic alteration in cardiac structure and function from rhythm disturbances.

Understanding and recognizing artifacts is important in echocardiographic interpretation.[1,5] Artifacts may exist because of the properties of ultrasound, transducer or ultrasound equipment qualities, improper scanning technique, or instrument control adjustments. Improper preparation of the skin (e.g., poor clipping or inadequate quantity of coupling gel) may cause horizontal lines to appear over the two-dimensional image. Excessive gain will decrease lateral resolution, causing some distinct objects to appear fused. Hypoechoic or anechoic areas may be obscured when the gain is too high. Conversely, when the gain is too low, cardiac structures may not be detected. Lung artifact may interfere with obtaining a readable echocardiogram if the acoustic window is inadequate. Static echoes and poor near-field resolution in small animals (i.e., less than 5 kg) are also problems. Attainable near-

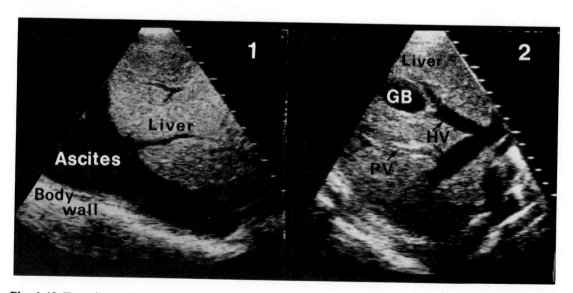

Fig. 6-19 Two-dimensional abdominal sonograms recorded from two different dogs with hepatomegaly. *Frame 1* is from a dog with severe mitral and tricuspid insufficiency. Ascites and an enlarged liver with rounded edges is evident. *Frame 2* was recorded from a dog with passive hepatic congestion. The hepatic veins (HV) are markedly enlarged compared with the portal veins (PV). GB, gallbladder.

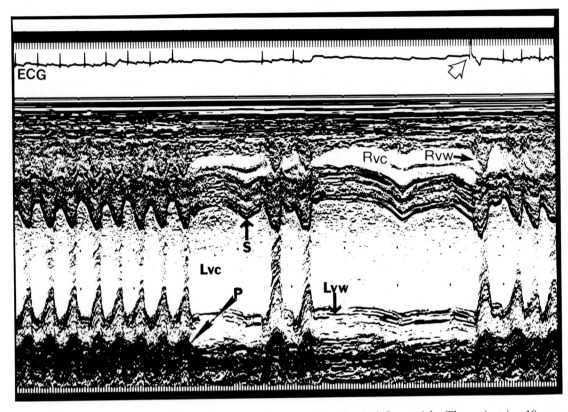

Fig. 6-20 M-mode echocardiogram at the chordae tendineae level in the left ventricle. The patient is a 10-year-old miniature schnauzer with syncope due to sick sinus syndrome. Supraventricular tachycardia is evident in the beginning one-third of this tracing and reduces the time for ventricular diastolic filling. The relatively flat septum (S) and left ventricular free wall (Lvw) reflect lack of ventricular systole during sinoatrial arrest. The open arrow on the electrocardiogram (ECG) points to a ventricular escape beat. P, pericardium; Lvc, left ventricular chamber; Rvc, right ventricular chamber; Rvw, right ventricular wall.

field resolution is variable between different ultrasound units. For the small or young patient, the use of a standoff may aid in obtaining a higher-quality image (Fig. 6-24).

Side lobes constitute another artifact. They are caused by beams of ultrasound generated from the edges of a transducer crystal that are not oriented in the direction of the main beam.[1] Side lobes may generate faint bands of echoes that reflect off of echogenic structures and interfere with the cardiac image. They are commonly located within dilated left atria and at the atrioventricular groove (Fig. 6-25). In the normal heart, side lobe echoes are not seen because they fall just outside the left atrial border; however, with left atrial enlargement, this ane-

choic chamber beside the atrioventricular groove creates a place for side lobes to be seen, especially with two-dimensional echoes.

Another artifact that may occur is reverberations.[1,5] Reverberations may be seen when using transducers with standoffs but can occur with transducers by themselves. They result when sound waves are reflected off intracardiac structures. The reverberation does not have to be the same structure seen in the primary image, and the sound waves may reverberate back and forth until the ultrasound signal is attenuated (Fig. 6-25). Increasing gain will increase reverberations. Alternately, mirror images of echoed structures may result (e.g., two-beating hearts). Increasing the gain will enhance the rever-

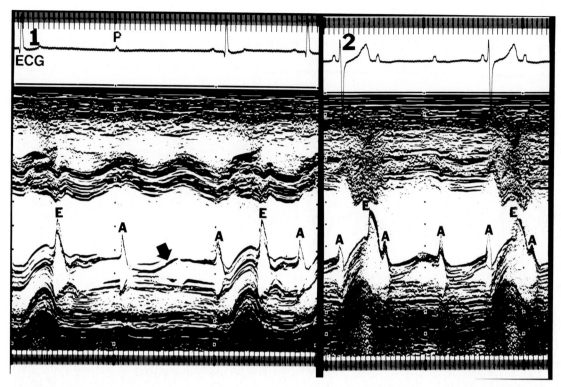

Fig. 6-21 M-mode echocardiograms at the mitral valve level from dogs with atrioventricular (AV) block. In *frame 1,* a P wave (P) results from atrial systole but is not conducted through the atrioventricular node (second degree AV block). Atrial contraction causes diastolic mitral valve opening (point A). There is no early, rapid diastolic filling (or point E) but instead, gradual opening of the mitral valve is recorded (arrow). In *frame 2,* atrial systoles (P waves) are not associated with ventricular contractions (ventricular escape rhythm) due to third-degree AV block. This is reflected in irregular peaks and valleys of the anterior mitral valve leaflet. ECG, electrocardiogram.

berations. To avoid the reverberation artifact, the depth of field should not exceed the limits of the echoed structure. Artifacts also may be caused by breathing. Undulations of cardiac structures can result and simulate abnormal conditions (Fig. 6-26).

Contrast echocardiography is a helpful and sensitive diagnostic technique used to identify and verify cardiac chambers and intracardiac shunts.[1,31] It is performed by agitating a fluid substance, such as 0.9 percent saline, 5 percent dextrose and water (D_5W), indocyanine green, or the animal's own blood, eliminating macroscopic bubbles, and then rapidly injected 3 to 5 ml into a blood vessel or cardiac chamber. Selective or nonselective studies may be performed. Ultrasound waves are then re-

flected off of these microbubbles (Figs. 6-27 and 6-28).

Injection of contrast into a cardiac chamber that has a shunt (e.g., ventricular septal defect) may show a positive contrast effect in that chamber or microbubbles will be detected in the chamber into which blood is shunting. In addition, a negative contrast effect may be detected if a shunt exists seen as dilution of the microbubble contrast in the chamber into which blood is shunting. One should not confuse this with normal dilution of a chamber's blood volume; for example, right atrial contrast could be normally diluted by blood returning from the coronary sinus and caudal vena cava.[1] The negative contrast effect may be difficult to detect. A

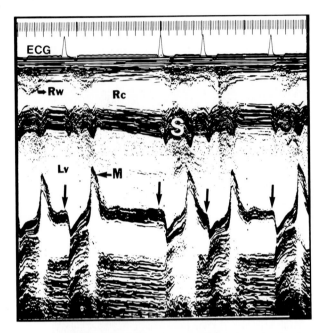

Fig. 6-22 M-mode echocardiogram at the mitral valve level recorded from a 1-year-old golden retriever with a patent ductus arteriosus. Because of atrial fibrillation, there are no organized atrial contractions. Therefore, biphasic valve opening is absent (i.e., arrows illustrate lack of mitral valve point A—compare with Figs. 6-9, 6-11, 6-21). Fine undulations of the mitral leaflets may be seen rarely in dogs with atrial fibrillation. The left ventricle is dilated, and the E-point septal separation is increased. Rw, right ventricular wall; Rc, right ventricular chamber; S, interventricular septum; Lv, left ventricular chamber; M, mitral valve; ECG, electrocardiogram.

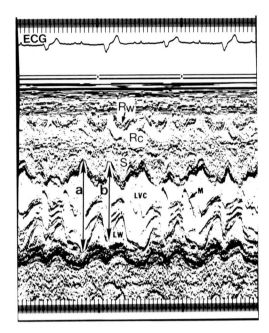

Fig. 6-23 M-mode echocardiogram at the mitral valve level of a cat with ventricular bigeminy. The ventricular premature contractions reduce the end-diastolic dimension; for example, compare dimension a (normal) with b (abnormal). The mitral valve motion is disturbed, and premature closure of the leaflets occurs. RW, right ventricular wall; RC, right ventricular chamber, S, interventricular septum; LVC, left ventricular chamber; M, mitral valve; LW, left ventricular free wall.

positive contrast result represents stronger evidence for a defect. Regurgitation and turbulence may also be detected with contrast echocardiography.

Spontaneous contrast may occasionally be seen due to sluggish blood flow. This has been identified in the cranial vena cava in dogs with right heart failure and in cats with cardiomyopathy. At times, the blood may appear to stand still, which may be confused with a mass or organized blood clot. This spontaneous contrast effect has not been observed in normal dogs and cats.

Contrast echocardiography may also aid other diagnostic procedures such as pericardiocentesis. A needle positioned within the pericardial sac may be imaged by the echocardiogram and its precise location detected after injection of saline.

ECHOCARDIOGRAPHY AND THE DIAGNOSIS OF CONGENITAL HEART DISEASE

Many congenital heart defects may be specifically diagnosed or strongly suspected on the basis of echocardiographic examination.[1,4,30–32] Two-dimensional echocardiography is superior to the M-mode technique for this purpose. Doppler echocardiography should aid in the diagnosis and characterization of congenital heart disease.[1] When evaluating echocardiograms of animals with congenital heart disease, it is important to have a sound knowledge of normal cardiac anatomy and respective structural spatial relationships.

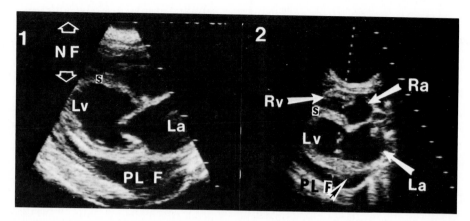

Fig. 6-24 Two-dimensional echocardiograms. Long-axis views were both recorded from the right intercostal transducer position in a 13-year-old cat with dilated cardiomyopathy. *Frame 1* was imaged using a 5-MHz transducer. The near field (NF) is not clear, and right heart structures cannot be visualized. *Frame 2* was imaged using a 7.5-MHz transducer with a standoff. The picture is smaller, and the cardiac image is farther away from the transducer crystal, but the right heart structures are easily seen. The dotted line is the M-mode cursor directed through the tricuspid and mitral valves. Lv, left ventricle; La, left atrium; PL F, pleural fluid; Rv, right ventricle; Ra, right atrium; S, interventricular septum; NF, near field.

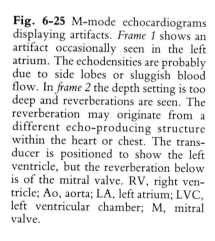

Fig. 6-25 M-mode echocardiograms displaying artifacts. *Frame 1* shows an artifact occasionally seen in the left atrium. The echodensities are probably due to side lobes or sluggish blood flow. In *frame 2* the depth setting is too deep and reverberations are seen. The reverberation may originate from a different echo-producing structure within the heart or chest. The transducer is positioned to show the left ventricle, but the reverberation below is of the mitral valve. RV, right ventricle; Ao, aorta; LA, left atrium; LVC, left ventricular chamber; M, mitral valve.

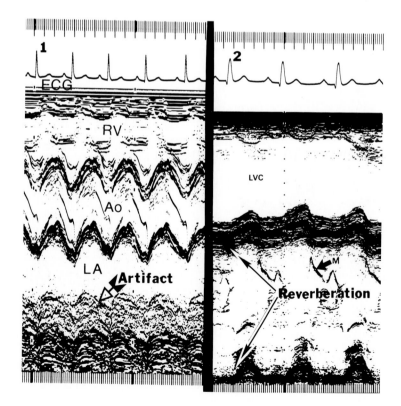

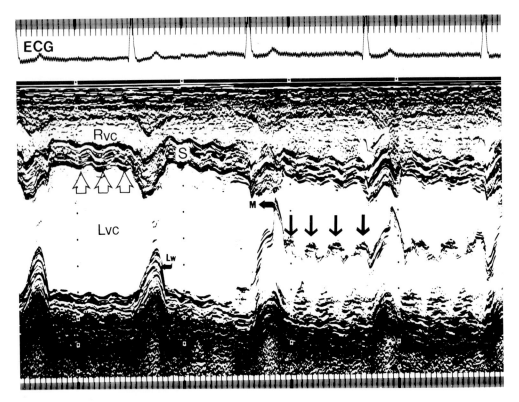

Fig. 6-26 M-mode echocardiogram recorded from a 2-year-old 32-kg female Labrador retriever with atrial standstill. During the study the dog constantly panted at a very rapid rate (250/min). The motion of the dog's chest moving up and down created an artifact in wall movement (open arrows) and valve motion (solid arrows). This artifact could be mistaken for the abnormal motion seen with atrial flutter and fibrillation. Rvc, right ventricular chamber; S, interventricular septum; Lw, left ventricular free wall; M, mitral valve; Lvc, left ventricular chamber; ECG, electrocardiogram.

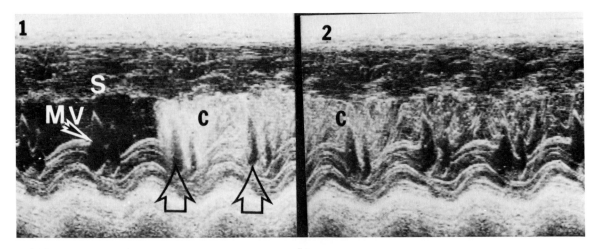

Fig. 6-27 Contrast M-mode echocardiogram of a normal dog at the mitral valve level. A catheter was placed in the left ventricle and 0.9 percent saline injected. The microbubbles cause a cloud of dense echogenic reflections which opacify this chamber. Note that the mitral valve orifice in *frame 1* does not opacify during diastole (open arrows), since it contains blood from the left atrium. In *frame 2* the microbubbles are gradually cleared from the left ventricle due to the dilution of ventricular blood with that from the left atrium as the left ventricle ejects blood into the aorta. C, contrast; MV, mitral valve; S, septum.

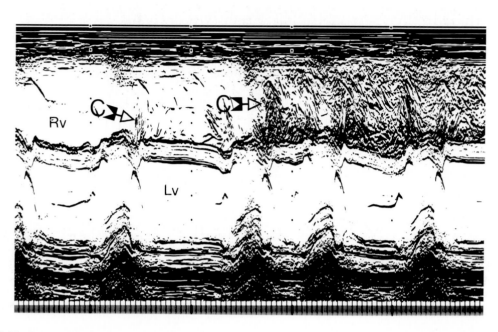

Fig. 6-28 Contrast M-mode echocardiogram made by injection of 0.9 percent saline into the cephalic vein of a dog. The right ventricle is opacified, but the left heart is not. This indicates lack of right-to-left shunting at the ventricular or atrial level (microbubbles do not pass through the lungs into the left ventricle). The right ventricle is greatly enlarged. C, contrast; Rv, right ventricle; Lv, left ventricle.

PATENT DUCTUS ARTERIOSUS

Patent ductus arteriosus (PDA) is difficult to image. In humans, a suprasternal approach is usually preferred to visualize this congenital defect.[1,4] Although the diagnosis of PDA is usually straightforward based on its characteristic continuous heart murmur, echocardiography provides a noninvasive means to assess for concurrent congenital defects. Also, the degree of cardiac chamber dilatation and myocardial function can be assessed for therapeutic and prognostic purposes (Figs. 6-29 and 6-30).

Most dogs with PDA have a reduced fractional shortening or a value in the low-normal range. The left ventricular wall and interventricular septum will usually have a normal thickness. Dilation of the atria and ventricles, especially of the left heart, are often dramatic. Exaggerated septal motion may be present. Mitral valve excursions range from normal to exaggerated, although the E point to septal separation is frequently greatly elevated. Biventricular and biatrial dilatation is often dramatic. The aortic amplitude may be reduced (Fig. 6-29). A dilated aorta may be detected, especially by two-dimensional echocardiography. Occasionally, the descending aorta may be seen behind the left atrium (Fig. 6-30). This echolucent structure may be mistaken for a dilated coronary sinus.[32] Contrast echocardiography may be helpful in identifying this structure. Injection of a contrast solution into the jugular vein of a dog with dilated coronary sinus will result in opacification of this structure, but not the descending aorta. On the other hand, contrast solution injected into the aortic root or left ventricle of a dog with PDA will cause opacification of the pulmonary trunk which is usually dilated.

After surgical ligation of the ductus arteriosus, the shunt-induced volume overload is eliminated. Reduction of cardiac chamber size will be appreciated on the echocardiogram.

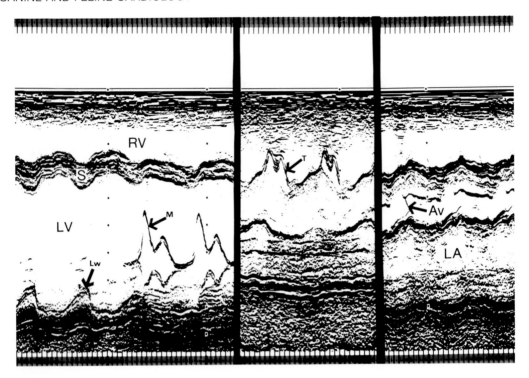

Fig. 6-29 M-mode echocardiogram of a 4-month-old Australian shepherd with patent ductus arteriosus (PDA). The fractional shortening is low (24 percent), the E point to septal separation is high, and the aortic amplitude reduced. Left and right heart volume overload is present. RV, right ventricular chamber; LV, left ventricular chamber; S, interventricular septum; M, mitral valve; T, tricuspid valve; Av, aortic valve in diastole; LA, left atrium.

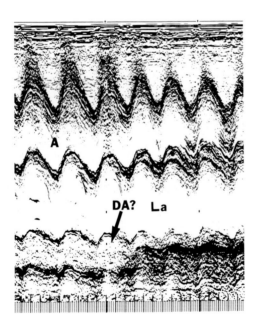

Fig. 6-30 M-mode echocardiogram at the aorta-left atrium level from a golden retriever puppy with patent ductus arteriosus. An echo-free space is seen below the left atrium which is probably the descending aorta. Other possible differentials for this finding would include dilated coronary sinus or cor triatriatum. A, aorta; La, left atrium; DA, descending aorta.

VENTRICULAR SEPTAL DEFECTS

Ventricular septal defect (VSD) may be diagnosed more easily with two-dimensional echocardiography than with M-mode echocardiographs (Figs. 6-31; see also 18-14 and 18-17). It most commonly occurs at the heart base, where the thin membranous septum may be mistaken for a septal defect. To diagnose a VSD reliably, the lesion should be observed in several imaging planes and a T sign should be seen.[1] This is an effect in which the edge of a VSD elongates the echo due to a beam-width artifact. It delineates the VSD edge rather than displaying just an imprecise dropout of echoes. Echocardiographic evidence of volume overload may be present and include a dilated left ventricle and left atrium. The right heart may also be enlarged. Indices of cardiac function (e.g., fractional shortening, mitral valve excursions, aortic root amplitude) may indicate a hypercontractile state. Three echocardiographic contrast patterns are diagnostic of a VSD: (1) movement of contrast material from the right ventricle across the defect to the left ventricle during systole, (2) appearance of contrast in the left ventricle during diastole without its appearance in the left atrium, and (3) negative contrast effect in the right ventricle. However, a small VSD can be missed, even with good echocardiographic technique.

ATRIAL SEPTAL DEFECTS

Atrial septal defect (ASD) (e.g., ostium primum, ostium secundum, sinus venosus) may be detected echocardiographically.[1,4,30] Because the foramen ovale is covered only by a thin membrane and the normal atrial septum thins as it approaches the foramen ovale, echo dropout at this point may be misdiagnosed as a defect, especially in the left intercostal four-chamber view. As with a VSD, the T sign is helpful in making an accurate diagnosis, and the defect should be seen in several imaging planes (Fig. 6-32; see also 18-7 and 18-16).

With an atrial septal defect, the blood shunts from the left to right atrium unless another defect or pulmonary hypertension exists. The right ventricle and right atrium are dilated due to this volume overload. The left heart and pulmonary trunk also may be dilated. With ostium primum defects, abnormalities of the atrioventricular valves may be detected. The tricuspid valve excursion may be increased in an animal with an ASD.

Contrast echocardiography may be helpful in confirming the diagnosis (Fig. 6-32). With an ASD that shunts from right to left, contrast will appear in the left atrium before the left ventricle. The septal defect must therefore be located at the atrial level. It is possible that some shunting of blood from the right atrium to left atrium will occur through a small patent foramen ovale with concurrent pulmonary

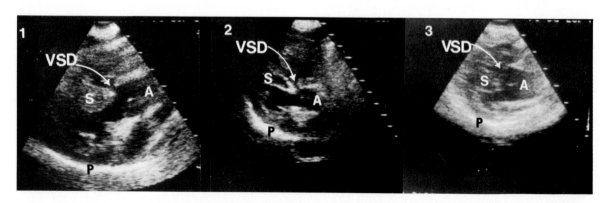

Fig. 6-31 Two-dimensional echocardiograms recorded from the right intercostal position showing a long-axis view of the left ventricular outflow tract. *Frame 1* was recording from a basset hound puppy with a ventricular septal defect (VSD). *Frame 2* was recording from a 7-year-old Border terrier with a pulmonic stenosis and a VSD. In *frame 3* a large aortic root (A) overrides the interventricular septum (S), and a large VSD is seen. This keeshond also had a pulmonic stenosis and right ventricular hypertrophy, components of tetralogy of Fallot. P, pericardium.

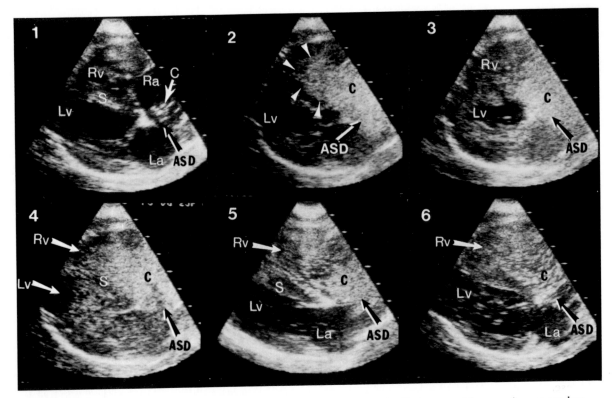

Fig. 6-32 Contrast two-dimensional echocardiogram (long-axis view) of a boxer with an ostium secundum defect shown in frame 2 of Fig. 18-7. *Frame 1* shows the first appearance of contrast (C) in the right atrium. In *frame 2* the contrast has filled the right atrium and right ventricle (white arrows) and has crossed the atrial septal defect (ASD) into the left atrium. In *frame 3* the left atrium is filled with contrast, and in *frame 4,* all chambers have contrast within them. The echogenicity of the contrast bubbles is greater in the right heart. Contrast is still being injected and therefore continues to fill the right atrium. In *frame 5,* contrast has been cleared from the left heart. In *frame 6,* remaining contrast in the right heart continues to the ASD and bubbles are still seen in the left ventricle. RV, right ventricle; S, interventricular septum; LV, left ventricle; Ra, right atrium; La, left atrium.

hypertension. Negative contrast echo effects may also demonstrate an ASD as well. Many septal defects permit bidirectional shunting of blood. Even if the shunting is primarily left to right, enough right-to-left shunting may occur to make a nonselective contrast injection diagnostic.

TETRALOGY OF FALLOT

Tetralogy of Fallot is another congenital heart defect readily diagnosed with echocardiography.[1,4,30] Each of the features of this complex anomaly can be imaged: (1) ventricular septal defect, (2) pulmonic stenosis, (3) overriding aorta, and (4) right ventricular hypertrophy. A decrease in the size of the left ventricle and left atrium may also be seen. Septal hypertrophy and paradoxic or flattened motion will be present (see Fig. 18-17). Carefully sweeping the heart from apex to base with M-mode echocardiography permits visualization of an overriding aorta; however, with improper transducer angling, false-positive and false-negative results may occur. Using two-dimensional echocardiography, the pulmonary trunk and pulmonic valve should be examined carefully at their sites of origin to differentiate tetralogy of Fallot from truncus arteriosus or pulmonic atresia. Contrast echocardiography shows right-to-left shunting in animals with a tetralogy of Fallot (see Fig. 18-18). If palliative surgery is performed in an effort to increase blood to the pulmonary circulation (e.g., Blalock-Taussig or Waterson-Cooley procedure), the left atrial size relative to the aorta can be examined as an indicator of surgical success. The left atrium should increase in size due to additional blood going to and returning from the lungs.

SUBAORTIC STENOSIS

Subaortic stenosis is relatively common in the dog, and a subaortic fibrous band may be identified echocardiographically (see Fig. 18-11). Qualitative and quantitative evaluations of this defect, however, can be difficult without Doppler echocardiography. Dogs uncommonly have valvular aortic stenosis and in cats, aortic stenosis is rare.

Occasionally, premature aortic valve closure or coarse systolic fluttering of the aortic valve may be noted. Mild aortic valve systolic fluttering may be normal or increased with high blood flow. Discrete premature closure of the aortic valve may accompany left ventricular outflow obstruction. In this disease, a dynamic obstruction to left ventricular outflow may occur due to systolic anterior motion of the mitral valve.[1] The anterior mitral valve leaflet may encroach on the outflow of blood during systole by moving toward the interventricular septum. True anterior motion of the mitral valve causes it to have a flat echocardiographic appearance during systole, which then returns to normal before the onset of diastole (Fig. 6-33). With rapid heart rates or improper transducer angling, pseudosystolic anterior motion may occur. Dogs at rest may not exhibit left ventricular outflow obstruction, and provocative testing may be necessary for its detection with isoproterenol or exercise. The presence of systolic anterior motion is not pathognomonic of subaortic stenosis and may be present in other conditions, including hypertrophic cardiomyopathy, left ventricular hypertrophy, and hypercontractile states. Propranolol may decrease left ventricular obstruction and eliminate the systolic anterior motion of the mitral valve.

Aortic stenosis has been studied echocardiographically in the dog.[33] The aortic diameter at diastole and systole is usually greater than normal and post-stenotic aortic dilatation may be seen. The left

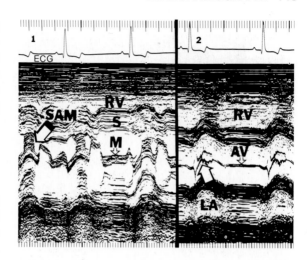

Fig. 6-33 M-mode echocardiogram from a 1-year-old German shepherd with congenital subaortic stenosis. In *frame 1* systolic anterior motion (SAM) of the mitral valves is evident. The anterior leaflet appears flattened and abuts the interventricular septum (open arrow), causing a dynamic left ventricular outflow obstruction to ejection of blood. In *frame 2,* premature aortic valve closure (large open arrow) results from the outflow obstruction. RV, right ventricular chamber; S, interventricular septum; M, mitral valve; AV, aortic valve; LA, left atrium; ECG, electrocardiogram.

atrium and left atrium/aortic ratio are increased. Left ventricular posterior wall and interventricular septal hypertrophy are detectable (Fig. 6-34). The fractional shortening may be normal or increased. However, mild cases of aortic stenosis can be difficult to detect on the echocardiogram.

PULMONIC STENOSIS

Pulmonic stenosis may be deteced or its diagnosis supported by the echocardiogram.[1,4,30] Abnormal thickening and doming of the pulmonic valve leaflets may be seen by the two-dimensional examination. Identification of abnormal pulmonic valve motion by the M-mode echocardiogram is difficult and unreliable. Post-stenotic dilatation of the main pulmonary artery is usually seen in the parasternal, short axis, two-dimensional view (see Fig. 18-7). Secondary findings caused by the right ventricular outflow obstruction of pulmonic stenosis can be identified and include right ventricular wall hyper-

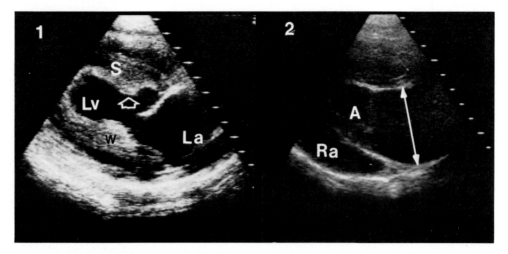

Fig. 6-34 *Frame 1* is a two-dimensional echocardiogram recorded from the right intercostal position. This long-axis view of the left heart is from a 6-month-old German shepherd with subaortic stenosis and mitral insufficiency. Myocardial hypertrophy is evident by thickening of the interventricular septum (S) and left ventricular posterior wall (W). The left atrium (La) is extremely dilated. Hypertrophied septum (open arrow) bulges into the left ventricular cavity (Lv). *Frame 2* is a two-dimensional echocardiogram recorded from a left intercostal position from a 2-year-old Newfoundland with subaortic stenosis. The arrow delineates a dilated aortic arch. A, aorta; Ra, right atrium;

trophy, interventricular septal hypertrophy, enlargement of the right ventricular chamber, reduction of the left ventricular chamber, and flattened or paradoxic septal motion[34] (Fig. 6-35; see also Fig. 18-7). Doppler echocardiography facilitates the diagnosis and allows grading of valvular stenosis lesions. Echocardiographic changes in the pulmonary artery of dogs with various congenital lesions are illustrated (Fig. 6-35).

CONGENITAL VALVULAR INSUFFICIENCIES

Congenital insufficiencies of the mitral or tricuspid valves may be diagnosed directly with selective echocontrast studies or indirectly from functional or structural changes (e.g., chamber dilation) (Fig. 6-36). Wide excursions of affected valves, high fractional shortening, and exaggerated septal motion may occur with mitral regurgitation; flattened or paradoxic interventricular septal motion may occur with tricuspid insufficiency. Ebstein's anomaly constitutes a rare form of tricuspid dysplasia in which the tricuspid valve is displaced toward the cardiac apex causing atrialization of the right ventricle.

Congenital aortic insufficiency is characterized by fine, rapid fluttering of the mitral valve leaflets.[1] The jet of blood regurgitating from the aorta back into the left ventricle during diastole hits the mitral valve leaflet, causing these vibrations. Fluttering of the interventricular septum due to a similar mechanism may also be detected. Left atrial and ventricular dilatation are usually present. Occasionally, diastolic fluttering of the aortic valve and exaggerated septal motion may occur.

Other congenital defects are also detectable by echocardiography, including tricuspid atresia, common atrioventricular canal, mitral or tricuspid stenosis, transposition of the great vessels, double-outlet right ventricle, pulmonic insufficiency, or aorticopulmonary window.[4]

ECHOCARDIOGRAPHIC EVALUATION OF ACQUIRED CARDIAC DISEASE

Chronic Atrioventricular Valvular Disease

Two-dimensional and M-mode echocardiography does not directly quantitate the degree of mitral or tricuspid insufficiency associated with chronic

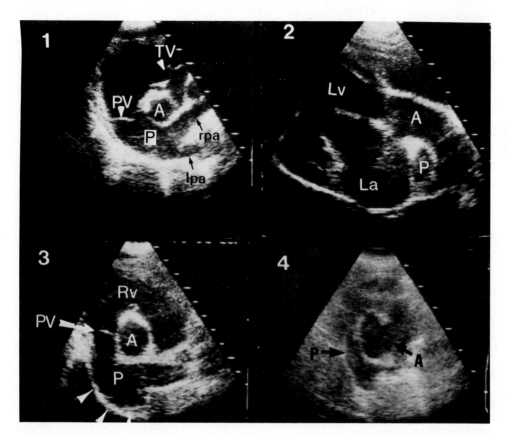

Fig. 6-35 Two-dimensional echocardiograms illustrating pulmonary artery changes due to various congenital heart defects. *Frame 1* was recorded from the right intercostal position, shows a short-axis view of the heart base from a 4-month-old Australian shepherd with volume overload secondary to patent ductus arteriosus (PDA). The pulmonary artery (P) is dilated. In *frame 2*, a long-axis view of the heart base from a golden retriever with PDA shows an enlarged left atrium (La). The aortic arch (A) is evident and a portion of the pulmonary artery (P) can be seen. *Frame 3*, recorded from a right intercostal position, shows the post-stenotic dilation (i.e., three white arrowheads) of the pulmonary artery (P) associated with valvular pulmonic stenosis. In *frame 4*, the aorta (A) is greatly enlarged compared with the pulmonary trunk (P) in a Keeshond with tetralogy of Fallot. TV, tricuspid valve; PV, pulmonic valve; rpa, right pulmonary artery; lpa, left pulmonary artery.

Fig. 6-36 M-mode echocardiograms from a 9-month-old Labrador retriever with congenital tricuspid dysplasia. *Frame 1* is at the ventricular level just below the mitral valve. Severe right ventricular enlargement is evident. *Frame 2* is at the aortic root position. A large right ventricle is obvious and the tricuspid valves (TV) are clearly imaged. RV, right ventricle; LV, left ventricle; A, aorta; LA, left atrium; ECG, electrocardiogram.

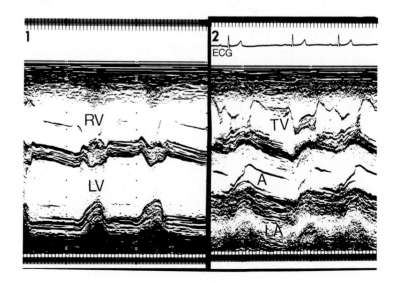

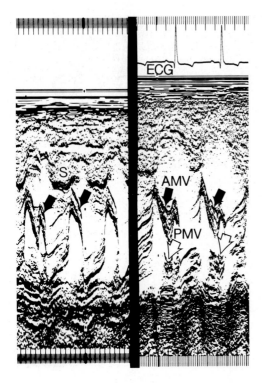

Fig. 6-37 M-mode echocardiograms from two dogs with mitral insufficiency from chronic acquired atrioventricular valve disease (endocardiosis). Thickening of the anterior (black arrows) and posterior (open arrows) mitral valves is evident. AMV, anterior mitral valve; PMV, posterior mitral valve; S, interventricular septum; ECG, electrocardiogram.

atrioventricular valvular diseases, or endocardiosis. Doppler echocardiography, however, does permit quantitative assessment of the degree of regurgitation.

Cardiac structural and functional changes secondary to mitral regurgitation may include atrial and ventricular dilation, exaggerated interventricular septal motion, absence of early diastolic septal dip, increased fractional shortening, high mitral valve excursions, fluttering of mitral valve during systole, decreased left ventricular chamber diameter during the pre-ejection period, or early aortic valve closure. The presence of each of the above depends on the severity of the insufficiency. Thickened valve leaflets are detectable with both M-mode and two-dimensional scanning (Figs. 6-37 through 6-39).

Most animals with acquired chronic atrioventricular insufficiency do not have myocardial failure until late in the disease process. Because of the mitral insufficiency, the left ventricle is able to unload part of its blood volume into a low-resistance chamber (left atrium). The ventricle does not have to work as hard as it would if it ejected all the blood into the systemic circulation through the aorta. In addition, there is an exaggerated motion of the septum toward the right ventricle during diastole. These two factors contribute to the high fractional shortening present in mitral insufficiency (Fig. 6-39). However, if fractional shortening is recorded in the low-normal range, this may be suggestive of myocardial failure, since normal to supranormal fractional shortening usually occurs with mitral regurgitation. With tricuspid insufficiency, right atrial and ventricular dilation are present. Septal motion may be flattened or paradoxic[34] and, if a pure volume overload exists, the flattened septal motion occurs only during diastole. If tricuspid regurgitation is severe and unaccompanied by mitral regurgitation, the left heart chambers may be reduced in size. When tricuspid and mitral insufficiency are present simultaneously various combinations of the above finding will be present (see Figs. 6-39 and 6-47).

Rupture of a *chordae tendineae* can be detected echocardiographically by chaotic diastolic motion of the mitral leaflets, systolic fluttering of the mitral valve, the presence of left atrial echoes during ventricular systole, evidence of a mobile echo in diastole situated between the anterior and posterior mitral leaflets, prolapse of the mitral valve into the left atrium during systole, or paradoxic posterior mitral valve movement.[1] Other signs compatible with severe mitral regurgitation will be observed.

Myocardial Diseases

Echocardiography has greatly improved characterization of myocardial disorders. In the dog[35,36] and cat,[22,26] dilated and hypertrophic cardiomyopathy can be readily differentiated by this technique.

In *dilated (congestive) cardiomyopathy,* the following echocardiographic findings may be recorded:[22,26,35,36] dilated left and right ventricles, dilated left and right atria, hypokinetic and paradoxic septal motion, reduced fractional shortening (less than 25 percent) and velocity of circumferential fiber shortening, reduced left ventricular free wall

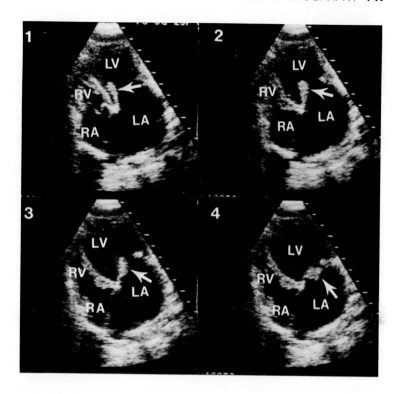

Fig. 6-38 Two-dimensional echocardiogram showing the four-chamber view obtained from the left caudal intercostal location of a 13-year-old poodle–cross with endocardiosis. Frames 1–4 demonstrate the thickened mitral valve leaflets. The early diastolic (*frames 1 and 2*) and end-diastolic motion (*frame 3*) of the anterior mitral valve leaflet (arrows) may be seen. In *frame 4,* the thickened leaflet prolapses into the left atrium. The left atrium and left ventricle are dilated. LV, left ventricle; RV, right ventricle; LA, left atrium; RA, right atrium.

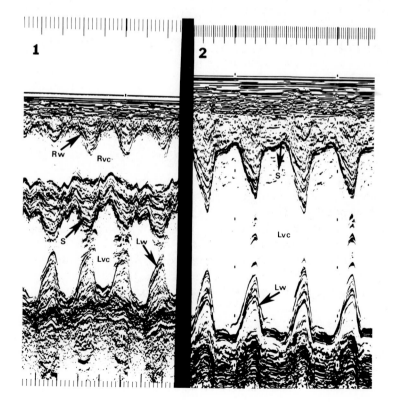

Fig. 6-39 M-mode echocardiograms at the ventricular level just below the mitral valve. *Frame 1* was recorded from a 2-kg poodle with mitral and tricuspid insufficiency. The right ventricle is dilated. Fractional shortening is elevated (67 percent). *Frame 2* was recorded from a mixed-breed dog with mitral insufficiency. Exaggerated septal motion is seen. The fractional shortening is high (55 percent). Rvc, right ventricular chamber; s, interventricular septum; Lvc, left ventricular chamber; Lw, left ventricular wall; Rw, right ventricular wall.

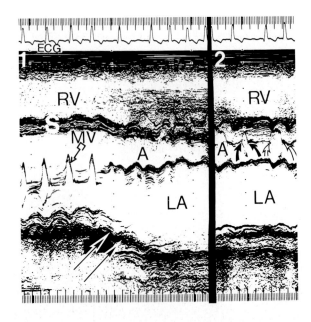

Fig. 6-40 M-mode echocardiogram recorded from a Great Dane with dilated cardiomyopathy and atrial fibrillation. In *frame 1*, the right ventricle is dilated. A large distance between the anterior mitral valve and interventricular septum indicates left ventricular dilation. As the ultrasound beam is swept from the mitral valve level to the aorta and left atrium at the heart base, the cardiac contour enlarges sharply (double arrow) because of the severely enlarged left atrium. In *frame 2,* the aortic root amplitude is reduced. The amount of aortic blood flow determines the duration of time the aortic valve is open. When atrial fibrillation shortens diastolic filling time, the aortic valve closes quickly (black arrows) and when filling time is longer, the valves stay open longer (white arrows). RV, right ventricular chamber; S, interventricular septum; MV, mitral valve; A, aorta; LA, left atrium.

amplitude, normal to thin myocardial wall thickness, increased E point to septal separation, decreased excursions of the mitral valve, abnormal delayed closure of the mitral valve resulting in a visible hump (B shoulder), dilated left ventricular outflow tract, decreased aortic amplitude, decreased aortic root diameter, decreased ejection period, and prolonged pre-ejection period (see Figs. 22-3; 23-2-4). Dilated cardiomyopathy in dogs is frequently associated with atrial fibrillation and this arrhythmia

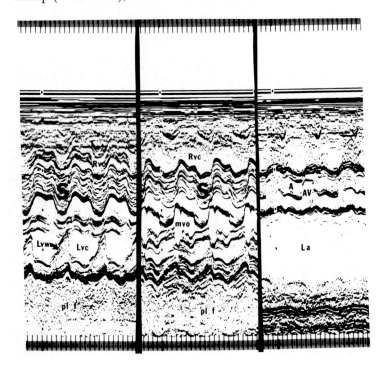

Fig. 6-41 M-mode echocardiogram of a 15-year-old hyperthyroid cat with asymmetric septal hypertrophy. The interventricular septum is thicker than the left ventricular free wall. Note pleural fluid, abnormal mitral valve motion, decreased aortic root motion, and enlarged left atrium. Rvc, right ventricular chamber; S, interventricular septum; Lvw, left ventricular free wall; Lvc, left ventricular chamber; pl f, pleural fluid; mvo, mitral valve orifice; A, aorta; AV, aortic valve; La, left atrium.

will also affect the echocardiogram[37] (Fig. 6-40; Fig. 23-2).

Hypertrophic cardiomyopathy commonly occurs in the cat. Echocardiography is a sensitive indicator of left ventricular hypertrophy.[1,22,26] A left ventricular free wall or interventricular septum that measures greater than 0.56 cm at end-diastole is a reliable change,[22] although these measurements may be influenced by body weight and body surface area.[25] Asymmetric septal hypertrophy is occasionally noted. The left atrium is usually greatly enlarged. Left ventricular internal dimensions are normal or decreased, and fractional shortening is usually normal to increased (Fig. 22-6). The echocardiogram

of cats with hyperthyroidism frequently display left ventricular hypertrophy and left and right atrial enlargement and echocardiographic indices of cardiac function are increased, indicating a hypercontractile state[38,39] (Fig. 6-41). Uncommonly, contractility will be reduced.[40]

In hypertrophic cardiomyopathic dogs, similar changes may be recorded. Endomyocardial fibrosis may sometimes cause increased echogenicity (Fig. 6-42).

Infiltrative cardiac disease such as amyloidosis in man, may cause myocardial hypertrophy.[1] Lymphosarcoma may rarely infiltrate the dog or cat heart.[35] Inflammatory myocardial disease will oc-

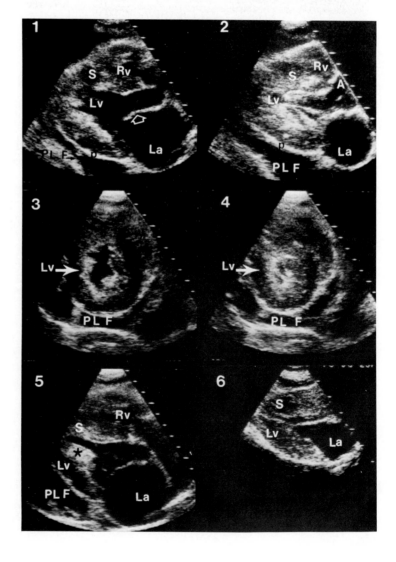

Fig. 6-42 Two-dimensional echocardiograms recorded from a 2-year-old Rhodesian ridgeback with hypertrophic cardiomyopathy (frames 1–5). Left ventricular hypertrophy, left atrial enlargement, and pleural fluid are seen. In *frame 1,* a long-axis view was recorded during mid-diastole from the right intercostal position. In *frame 2,* from the same position, the heart is seen just after aortic valve closure at end-systole. The left ventricular internal dimension is greatly reduced. *Frames 3* and *4* are short-axis views at the papillary muscle level. Reduction of the left ventricular chamber is seen in diastole in frame 3 and during systole (frame 4), the cavity is obliterated. In each echocardiogram, the endocardial surface is hyperechoic and in *frame 5,* the papillary muscle has a prominent hyperechoic appearance (star). Necropsy demonstrated extensive myocardial fibrosis, especially in the papillary muscles, endocardial surface, and myocardium closest to the endocardium. *Frame 6* was recorded from a cat with hypertrophic cardiomyopathy, showing marked left ventricular hypertrophy and left atrial enlargement. S, interventricular septum; Rv, right ventricle; Lv, left ventricle; arrow, anterior mitral valve leaflet; La, left atrium; P, pericardium; PL F, pleural fluid; A, aorta.

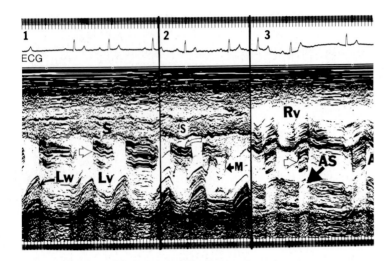

Fig. 6-43 M-mode echocardiogram from a 9-year-old English setter with a calcified aortic valvular mass. *Frames 1* and *2* show a mass in the left ventricular outflow tract (open arrow) during diastole. In *frame 3,* this mass (open arrow) appears in the aortic root during systole, where it causes an acoustic shadow (AS) as it blocks ultrasound transmission. For a two-dimensional characterization of this mass, see Figure 6-44. S, interventricular septum; Lw, left ventricular free wall; Lv, left ventricular chamber; M, mitral valve, Rv, right ventricular chamber; A, aorta; ECG, electrocardiogram.

casionally cause a cellular infiltrate of neutrophils and macrophages with myocardial swelling.

Bacterial Endocarditis

Vegetative endocarditis can be detected with the M-mode or two-dimensional echocardiogram.[1,4,41–44] The mitral and aortic valves are most frequently involved (Figs. 6-43, 44; 21-3-5). Even if vegetative lesions are not seen, however, a diagnosis of myocarditis cannot be excluded. Vegetative lesions may calcify, become hyperechoic, and cast an acoustic shadow (Figs. 6-43 and 6-44). Abscesses within the myocardium will appear as hypoechoic areas.

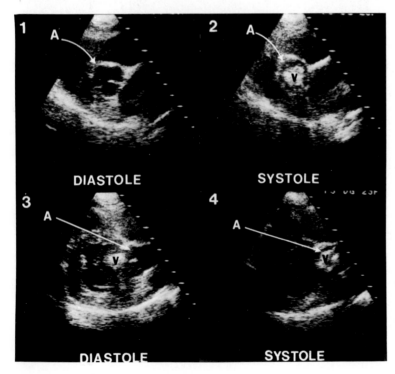

Fig. 6-44 Two-dimensional echocardiogram from a 9-year-old English setter with a history of syncope. *Frames 1* and *2* are short-axis views at the level of the aortic valve. During diastole (frame 1) the three aortic cusps can be seen. A large, hyperechoic, vegetative mass occupies the aortic orifice during systole (frame 2). *Frames 3* and *4* are longitudinal views of the aortic root. During diastole (frame 3) the hyperechoic mass is situated in the left ventricular outflow tract, but during systole (frame 4), it enters the aortic root. The mass was believed to be a vegetative endocarditis lesion attached to the aortic valve. A, aortic root; v, vegetative mass.

Fig. 6-45 Two-dimensional echocardiograms demonstrating pleural and pericardial effusions. *Frame 1* is a cross-sectional view of the left and right ventricle at the papillary level from a cat with pleural fluid. The appearance of the pericardiodiaphragmatic ligament (arrow) and lung (L) indicate that the effusion is of pleural rather than pericardial origin. *Frame 2* is a similar view during systole of another cat with pleural fluid. The dotted line is the M-mode cursor. *Frame 3* is a long-axis view recorded from the right intercostal position from a Great Dane with pericardial effusion. *Frame 4* was recorded from a German shepherd with pericardial and pleural effusion. The pericardium (P) is outlined forming a circular sac around the heart. The right ventricle and atrium are transected in this view, note the erratic contour of the right heart walls (arrowheads) associated with cardiac tamponade. Pl F, pleural fluid; L, lung; Rv, right ventricle; RA, right atrium; Lv, left ventricle; PE, pericardial effusion; ct, chordae tendineae; L, left heart; R, right heart; P, pericardium.

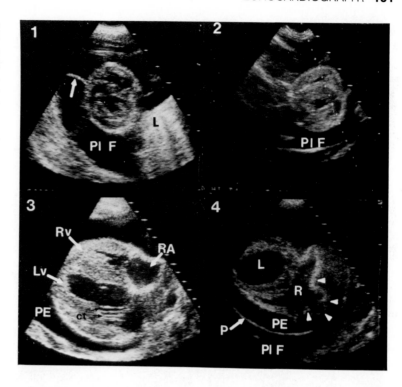

Fig. 6-46 M-mode echocardiogram recorded at the three standard levels from a 19-year-old cat with pleural effusion. Note that in *frames 1* and *2*, there is no separation of the left ventricular epicardium and parietal pericardium by a sonolucent space, as would occur if pericardial effusion were present (see Figs. 6-45 and 6-47). Also, pleural effusion is located behind the left atrium (*frame 3*), a feature that does not occur with pericardial effusion. S, interventricular septum; Lc, left ventricular chamber; Lw, left ventricular free wall; CW, chest wall; M, mitral valve; Av, aortic valve; A, aorta; LA, left atrium; Rc right ventricular cavity; P, pericardium; PL F, pleural fluid.

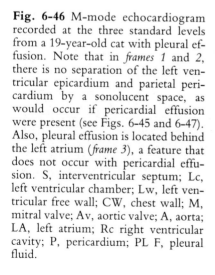

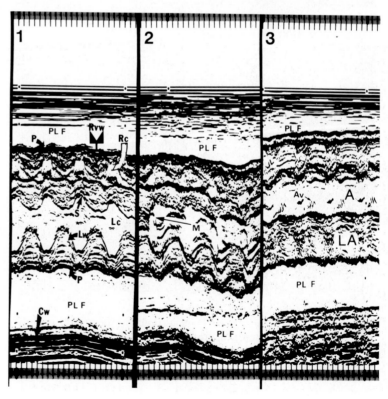

Pericardial Effusion

Echocardiography provides a sensitive technique with which to diagnose pericardial effusion.[1,4,35,45,46] Pericardial effusion is identifiable as a relatively anechoic (black) or hypoechoic (dark) area between the epicardium and pericardium. If pleural fluid is also present, the pericardium can be distinctly outlined. It is important that pericardial fluid not be mistaken for epicardial fat, descending aorta, or other structures. *Pleural effusion* must be carefully differentiated from pericardial effusion (Figs. 6-45–48, 50). Several echocardiographic observations assist in this differentiation.[1] The quantity of pleural fluid is usually much greater than pericardial fluid; therefore, the echo-free space is larger with pleural effusion. Delineation of collapsed lung lobes, the pericardiodiaphragmatic ligament (caudal mediastinum), and the cranial mediastinum is possible with pleural but not pericardial fluid. With pleural fluid, the descending aorta is situated next to the left atrium, whereas with pericardial effusion, the descending aorta is separated from the left atrium. Pericardial effusion will be most abundant at the cardiac apex, decreases toward the heart base, and is virtually absent behind the left atrium (Figs. 6-45 and 6-47). With large amounts of pericardial

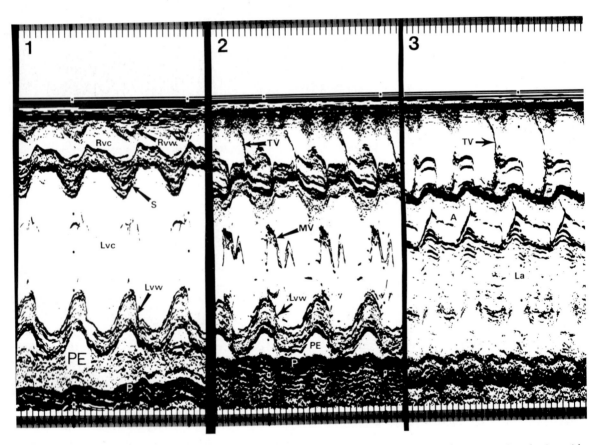

Fig. 6-47 M-mode echocardiogram recorded at the three standard levels of a dog with mitral and tricuspid insufficiency and pericardial effusion. An echo-free space represents pericardial effusion (PE) in *frames 1* and *2*. The distance between the pericardium and the epicardium is greatest near the cardiac apex and least at the heart base. Pericardial effusion is characteristically absent behind the left atrium (*frame 3*). Dilated left ventricle and left atrium are present as well as thickening of the mitral valve leaflet. Rvc, right ventricular chamber; Rvw, right ventricular wall; Lvc, left ventricular chamber; S, interventricular septum; Lvw, left ventricular free wall; P, pericardium; TV, tricuspid valve; MV, mitral valve; A, aorta; La, left atrium.

Fig. 6-48 *Frame 1* is a two-dimensional echocardiogram showing a long-axis view recorded from the right intercostal space of a beagle-cross dog with heartworm disease. The adult worms are seen as echogenic specs (arrows) within the right heart. The right ventricle is dilated, whereas the left ventricle and atrium are reduced in size. The interventricular septum is flattened in this view and in the cross-sectional view shown in *frame 2. Frame 3* is an M-mode echocardiogram from this dog at the level of the right ventricle and aorta. Normally, the aortic valve leaflets remain open during systole and close abruptly at end-systole. With decreased forward stroke volume due to heartworm disease in this dog, however, the leaflets gradually close during systole (arrows). Right ventricular enlargement is present. *Frame 4* is a Two-dimensional echocardiogram recorded from the left intercostal space 2 days after *frames 1–3* were recorded. Pleural effusion has developed. Pulmonary artery enlargement is evident and heartworms are seen (arrow) in the right atrium. Rv, right ventricle; RA, right atrium; S, interventricular septum; LA, left atrium; LVW, left ventricular wall; P, pericardium; Lv, left ventricle; A, aorta; PA, pulmonary artery; Pl F, pleural fluid.

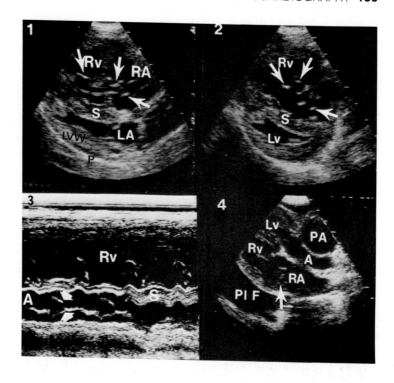

effusion, cardiac motion is disturbed. The heart may move back and forth within the sac with alternate beats to produce electric alternans on the ECG.[46] With cardiac tamponade, collapse or compression of the cardiac chambers can occur, and indentation of the right heart walls can be seen (Fig. 6-45).[1]

Intracardiac and Extracardiac Masses

Echocardiography, especially two-dimensional ultrasound, can be diagnostically useful in identifying intracardiac and extracardiac masses.[1,47] *Heartworms* within the right heart or pulmonary artery can be seen as fine irregular threads or as a large irregular dense mass, when the worms are incorporated into a thrombus.[48] Echocardiographic changes associated with heartworm disease include right ventricular and atrial dilation, flattened or paradoxic septal motion, reduced left ventricular and atrial chamber dimensions, pulmonary artery enlargement, and pleural or pericardial effusion (Fig. 6-48).

Intracardiac thrombi can be identified echocardiographically (Fig. 6-49). Stagnant blood should not be confused with an organized clot. The later will be more echodense, but differentiation can sometimes be difficult.

Heart-base tumors (e.g., chemodectoma, hemangiosarcoma, ectopic thyroid adenocarcinoma, lymphosarcoma) can be identified with echocardiography.[47] Two-dimensional ultrasound permits a more complete assessment of mass lesions. When a mass is detected, its origin and orientation should be defined to aid in diagnostic and therapeutic strategies.[47] For example, a mass involving only the right

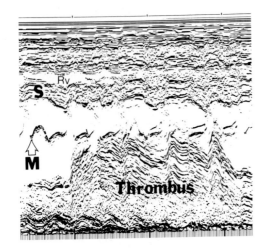

Fig. 6-49 M-mode echocardiogram at the mitral valve level from a cat with hypertrophic cardiomyopathy. A large organized thrombus in the left ventricular inflow tract is evident. S, interventricular septum; M, mitral valve; Rv, right ventricular chamber.

Fig. 6-50 Two-dimensional echocardiograms from dogs with various heart-base tumors. *Frame 1* is a short-axis view at the aortic level recorded from the right side of a mixed-breed dog. The tumor surrounds the aorta and the right and left pulmonary arteries. RA, right atrium; A, aorta; PT, pulmonary trunk; M, tumor mass. *Frame 2* is a short-axis view at the atrioventricular level recorded from the right intercostal position from a miniature poodle with a chemodectoma. A mass (arrowheads) protrudes into the left atrium and is of different echogenicity from the myocardium. Pericardial effusion (PE) is also seen. S, interventricular septum; MV, mitral valve; P, pericardium. Frame 3 is a long-axis view of the left ventricular outflow and inflow tract recorded from the right side of an English bulldog with a chemodectoma. The tumor is large and encroaches on the left atrium. LVOT, left ventricular outflow tract; MV, mitral valve. *Frame 4* is a short-axis view at the level of the papillary muscle recorded from the right intercostal position of a 10-year-old golden retriever. A mass is apparent within the pericardial effusion next to the right heart. Right atrial hemangiosarcoma was found at surgery. M, tumor mass; RV, right ventricle; S, interventricular septum; LV, left ventricle; PE, pericardial effusion; P, pericardium.

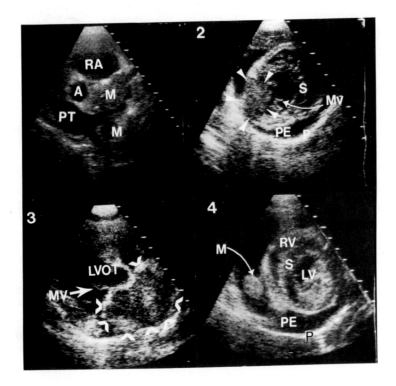

atrium is more likely to be a hemangiosarcoma than a chemodectoma. Also, hemangiosarcoma is more likely to have hypoechoic or anechoic areas than a chemodectoma. Various heart-base tumors are shown in Figure 6-50.

REFERENCES

1. Feigenbaum H: Echocardiography. 4th Ed. Lea & Febiger, Philadelphia, 1986
2. Feigenbaum H: Echocardiography. p. 83. In Braunwald E (ed): Heart Disease: A Textbook of Cardiovascular Medicine. 3rd Ed. WB Saunders, Philadelphia, 1988
3. Weyman AE: Cross-Sectional Echocardiography. Lea & Febiger, Philadelphia, 1982
4. Sahn DJ, Anderson F: An Atlas for Echocardiography: Two-Dimensional Anatomy of the Heart. John Wiley & Sons, New York, 1982
5. Herring DS, Bjornton G: Physics, facts, and artifacts of diagnostic ultrasound. Vet Clin North Am 15:1107, 1985
6. Bonagura JD, O'Grady MR, Herring DS: Echocardiography: Principles of interpretation. Vet Clin North Am 15:1177, 1985
7. Bonagura JC: M-mode echocardiography; Basic principles, cardiopulmonary diagnostic techniques. Vet Clin North Am 13:299, 1983
8. Goldberg SJ, Allen HD, Marx GR, et al: Doppler Echocardiography. Lea & Febiger, Philadelphia, 1985
9. Hatle L, Angelsen B: Doppler Ultrasound in Cardiology. Lea & Febiger, Philadelphia, 1985
10. Thomas WP: Two-dimensional, real-time echocardiography in the dog: Technique and anatomic validation. Vet Radiol 25:50, 1984
11. Henry WL, DeMaria A, Gramiak R, et al: Report of the American Society of Echocardiography Committee on nomenclature and standards in two-dimensional echocardiography. Circulation 62:212, 1980
12. DeMadron E, Bonagura JC, Herring DS: Two-dimensional echocardiography in the normal cat. Vet Radiol 26:149, 1985
13. Sahn DJ, DeMaria A, Kisslo J, et al: Recommendations regarding quantitation in M-mode echocardiography: Results of a survey of echocardiographic measurements. Circulation 58:1072, 1980
14. Lombard CW: Normal values of the canine M-mode echocardiogram. Am J Vet Res 45:2015, 1984
15. Boon J, Wingfield WE, Miller CW: Echocardiographic indices in the normal dog. Vet Radiol 24:214, 1983
16. Dennis MO, Nealeigh RC, Pyle RL, et al: Echocardiographic assessment of normal and abnormal valvular function in beagle dogs. Am J Vet Res 39:1591, 1978
17. Baylen BG, Garrer DJ, Laks MM, et al: Improved echocardiographic evaluation of the closed-chest canine: Methods and anatomic observations. J Clin Ultrasound 8:335, 1980
18. Franklin TD Jr, Weyman AE, Egenes KM: Closed-chest canine model for cross-sectional echocardiography study. Am J Physiol 233:H417, 1977
19. Mashiro I, Nelson RR, Cohn JN, et al: Ventricular dimensions measured noninvasively by echocardiography in the awake dog. J Appl Physiol 41:953, 1976
20. Eaton LW, Maughan WL, Shovkas AA, et al: Accurate volume determination in the isolated ejecting canine left ventricle by two dimensional echocardiography. Circulation 60:320, 1979
21. Pipers FS, Andrysco RM, Hamlin RL: A totally noninvasive method for obtaining systolic time intervals in the dog. Am J Vet Res 39:1822, 1978
22. Moise NS, Dietze AE, Mezza LE, et al: Echocardiography, electrocardiography, and radiography of cats with dilatation cardiomyopathy, hypertrophic cardiomyopathy, and hyperthyroidism. Am J Vet Res 47:1476, 1986
23. Pipers FS, Reef V, Hamlin RL: Echocardiography in the domestic cat. Am J Vet Res 40:882, 1979
24. Jacobs G, Knight DV: M-mode echocardiographic measurements in nonanesthetized healthy cats: Effects of body weight, heart rate, and other variables. Am J Vet Res 46:1705, 1985
25. Fox PR, Bond BR, Peterson ME: Echocardiographic reference values in healthy cats sedated with ketamine hydrochloride. Am J Vet Res 46:1479, 1985
26. Soderberg SF, Boon JA, Wingfield WE, et al: M-mode echocardiography as a diagnostic aid for feline cardiomyopathy. Vet Radiol 24:66, 1983
27. Allen DG: Echocardiographic study of the anesthetized cat. Can J Comp Med 46:115, 1982
28. Jacobs G, Knight DH: Changes in M-mode echocardiographic values in cats given ketamine. Am J Vet Res 46:712, 1985
29. Drinkovic N: Use of echocardiography in the diagnosis of cardiac arrhythmias. Pract Cardiol 11:124, 1985
30. Bonagura JD, Herring DS: Echocardiography: Congenital heart disease. Vet Clin North Am 15:1195, 1985
31. Bonagura JD, Pipers FS: Diagnosis of cardiac lesions by contrast echocardiography. J Am Vet Med Assoc 182:396, 1983

32. Jacobs G, Bolton GR, Watrous BJ: Echocardiographic features of dilated coronary sinus in a dog with persistent left cranial vena cava. J Am Vet Med Assoc 182:407, 1983

33. Wingfield WE, Boon JA, Miller CW: Echocardiographic assessment of congenital aortic stenosis in dogs. J Am Vet Med Assoc 183:673, 1983

34. DeMadron E, Bonagura JD, O'Grady MR: Normal and paradoxical ventricular septal motion in the dog. Am J Vet Res 46:1832, 1985

35. Bonagura JD, Herring DS: Echocardiography acquired heart disease. Vet Clin North Am 15:1209, 1985

36. Lombard CW: Echocardiographic and clinical signs of canine dilated cardiomyopathy. J Small Anim Pract 25:59, 1984

37. Wingfield WE, Boon J, Miller CW: Echocardiogenic assessment of mitral valve motion, cardiac structures, and ventricular function in dogs with atrial fibrillation. J Am Vet Med Assoc 181:46, 1982

38. Moise NS, Deitze AE: Echocardiographic, electrocardiographic, and radiographic detection of cardiomegaly in hyperthyroid cats. Am J Vet Res 47:1487, 1986

39. Bond B, Fox PR, Peterson ME: Echocardiographic evaluation of 45 cats with hyperthyroidism. J Ultrasound Med 2:184, 1983

40. Jacobs G, Hutson C, Daugherty J, et al: Congestive heart failure associated with hyperthyroidism in cats. J Am Vet Med Assoc 118:52, 1986

41. Bonagura JD, Pipers FS: Echocardiographic features of aortic valve endocarditis in a dog, a cow, and a horse. J Am Vet Med Assoc 182:595, 1983

42. Lombard CW, Buergelt CD: Vegetative bacterial endocarditis in dogs: Echocardiographic diagnosis and clinical signs. J Small Anim Pract 24:325, 1983

43. Pipers FS, Bonagura JD, Hamlin RL, et al: Echocardiographic abnormalities of the mitral valve associated with left-sided heart diseases in the dog. J Am Vet Med Assoc 179:580, 1981

44. Yamaguchi RA, Pipers FS, Gamble DA: Echocardiographic evaluation of a cat with bacterial vegetative endocarditis. J Am Vet Med Assoc 183:118, 1983

45. Bonagura JD, Pipers FS: Echocardiographic features of pericardial effusion in dogs. J Am Vet Med Assoc 179:49, 1981

46. Bonagura JD: Electrical alternans associated with pericardial effusion in the dog. J Am Vet Med Assoc 178:574, 1981

47. Thomas WP, Sisson D, Bauer TG, et al: Detection of cardiac masses in dogs by two-dimensional echocardiography. Vet Radiol 25:65, 1984

48. Lombard CW, Buergelt CD: Echocardiographic and clinical findings in dogs with heartworm-induced cor pulmonale. Comp Cont Educ 5:971, 1983

Section 3

ABNORMALITIES OF CIRCULATION AND CARDIOVASCULAR FUNCTION

7

Pathophysiology of Heart Failure

Robert L. Hamlin

When the cardiovascular system fails to circulate enough blood to meet the metabolic demands of the body for nutrients or when blood backs up within a venous or capillary bed,[1] the patient manifests a complex of clinical signs and symptoms and may suffer a reduced quality or duration of life.[2] This condition, in which clinical signs and symptoms result from the inability of the cardiovascular system to maintain normal circulation, is called either *heart failure* or *congestive heart failure*. If signs and symptoms result from blood damming up in a venous or capillary bed, the engorgement constitutes the entity of congestive heart failure. Alternatively, if signs and symptoms result from a reduced forward flow of blood into the systemic circulation, the clinical entity is called heart failure, since circulatory engorgement is not present. Both entities (engorgement and underperfusion) may occur concurrently. Many authorities refer to all failure as congestive heart failure, whether or not a regional circulation is congested.

Causes of cardiovascular failure can be grouped according to those related primarily with the heart (e.g., structural, biochemical or electrophysiological) or those related primarily with the vasculature (e.g., increased or decreased vascular resistance).

Most often, it is an interaction between the heart and peripheral vasculature that results in abnormal cardiovascular function.[3]

Abnormal functions of the heart can be grouped according to abnormalities of contraction (systolic) or relaxation (diastolic) function. Examples of diseases leading to abnormal systolic function are stenosis or regurgitation of atrioventricular or semilunar valves, myocardial power failure, or chronic distention, as may result from left to right cardiac shunts. Examples of diseases leading to abnormal diastolic function are increased myocardial stiffness, pericardial effusion with tamponade, constrictive pericarditis, and elevation of interpleural pressure.

As with most elastic containers, as ventricular volume increases, the walls become stiffer. Therefore, abnormal systolic function leading to increased ventricular dilation may result in abnormal diastolic function. Similarly, an abnormally stiff ventricle may not fill to a normal end-diastolic volume. Therefore, force of ventricular contraction (i.e., systolic function) may be decreased according to the Frank-Starling mechanism.

Abnormal cardiac function is caused by an interaction between a specific etiologic agent or lesion and associated compensatory or homeostatic responses (e.g., myocardial hypertrophy, increased autonomic efferent traffic). For example, myocarditis due to *Trypanosoma cruzi* may reduce the ability of the myocardium to generate a normal forceful contraction. This may cause systemic arterial pressure to fall. Baroreceptors then become stimulated and send afferent volleys to the brain over the vagus and glossopharyngeal nerves. The brain increases sympathetic and decreases parasympathetic efferent volleys that speed the heart, constrict systemic arterioles, make the aorta stiffer, increase thirst and water intake, and decrease urine output. These com-

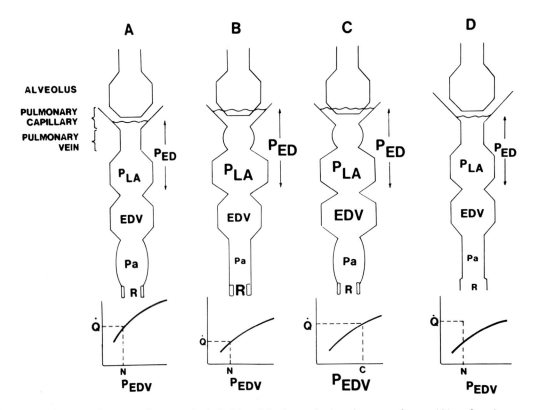

Fig. 7-1 Schematic diagrams showing the left side of the heart during the normal state (**A**) and various stages of failure (**B,C**) and in response to afterload reduction (**D**). From top to bottom: an alveolus, a funnel representing pulmonary capillaries surrounding the alveolus, the relative fullness with blood of pulmonary capillaries shown by the wavy line, left atrial pressure (P_{LA}) for any given end-diastolic pressure (P_{ED}), end-diastolic left ventricular volume (EDV), aortic pressure (Pa), systemic vascular resistance (R), a Frank-Starling curve in which cardiac output ($\dot{Q}$) is plotted against left ventricular preload (P_{EDV}), where N represents normal load and C represents preload during the congested (C) state. During the normal state (**A**), the alveoli are not congested and the Frank-Starling curve is relatively steep, showing a fairly great cardiac output for the particular preload. (**B**) When myocardial contractility is decreased, cardiac output is reduced for the same preload (depicted by a more gradual slope of the Frank-Starling curve). Thus, systemic arterial pressure is reduced, peripheral resistance is increased by reflex vasoconstriction, and blood dams up in the pulmonary capillaries. (**C**) As a result of blood having dammed up in the pulmonary capillaries, the increased left atrial pressure forces the left ventricle to a larger preload; even though contractility is reduced, cardiac output, systemic arterial pressure and systemic vascular resistance return toward normal. Note that the Frank-Starling curve still shows the reduction in contractility by the slope of the cardiac output-preload relationship being less than for the normal state. (**D**) In response to a systemic arterial vasodilator, systemic vascular resistance is reduced pharmacologically. The left ventricle can move blood more easily from pulmonary to systemic circulation; thus, even though systemic arterial pressure is reduced, cardiac output is normal. The Frank-Starling curve still shows reduced contractility (i.e., reduced slope), yet pulmonary congestion is reduced and intracardiac pressures and volumes return toward normal.

pensatory responses exact a further toll by producing a state of overhydration (i.e., increased thirst with decreased urine output) and increased interference to ventricular ejection (i.e., increased afterload against which the ventricles must eject). Of course, these compensatory physiologic responses initially serve a useful purpose when increased arterial stiffness and decreased urine production help sustain blood pressure under certain circumstances (e.g., dehydration, hemorrhage). From this example, both the *T. cruzi* infection and the homeostatic mechanisms impede the ability of the cardiovascular system to sustain circulation within normal limits.

The ventricle both sucks blood from the veins in diastole and pumps it into the arteries during systole; these two functions are inextricable. Nonetheless, it is still possible to have abnormal cardiovascular function so that (1) venous circuit is overdistended (elevated venous pressure), but cardiac output is normal; (2) venous circuit is not overdistended (normal venous pressure), yet cardiac output is reduced, or (3) venous circuit is overdistended (elevated venous pressure) and cardiac output is low.[4] Examples of each possibility include the following (Fig. 7-1):

1. With reduced myocardial contractility (Fig. 7-1B), cardiac output $\dot{Q}$ will decrease and mean systemic arterial pressure Pa will decrease, but there will be a reflex increase in systemic vascular resistance R. The reduction in myocardial contractility is reflected on the Frank-Starling curve (Fig. 7-1B), which shows that for any given end-diastolic pressure P_{ED}, cardiac output Q is lower than for the normal curve (Fig. 7-1A). Because of decreased cardiac output, blood backs up within the left atrium, left atrial pressure P_{LA} increases, and pulmonary veins and capillaries become congested with blood. During the next diastole (Fig. 7-1C), the increased left atrial pressure forces the left ventricle to a larger-than-normal end-diastolic volume (EDV). Even though the ventricle is weaker than normal, the force of contraction and cardiac output return to normal as a consequence of the Frank-Starling mechanism. The return of cardiac output toward normal causes the return of systemic vascular resistance toward normal. As discussed in chapters 8–9, if systemic vascular resistance can be artificially lowered (Fig. 7-1D), even the weakened myocardium can maintain a normal cardiac output without increased preload. Thus, increased preload might cause pulmonary congestion, but it permits sustenance of cardiac output, even with a weakened myocardium. With decreased systemic vascular resistance, cardiac output can be sustained without need for pulmonary congestion.

2. Cardiac output may be reduced without the venous and capillary circulation upstream from the failing ventricle being congested. If both left and right ventricles reduce their outputs simultaneously, the decrease in left ventricular output will be matched by a decrease in right ventricular output. Although blood is not removed adequately by one ventricle, it is not pumped adequately by the contralateral one. Therefore, blood will not back up in any of the venous or capillary compartments. This occurs with combined aortic and pulmonic stenosis and with atrial fibrillation.

3. When only one ventricle reduces its output, both reduction in cardiac output and venous congestion may occur. This is because the blood not ejected by one ventricle must accumulate between the failing ventricle and the normal contralateral one. This cannot continue indefinitely because a lethal amount of blood would accumulate between the failing and normal ventricles. Instead, a new equilibrium develops with venous pressure elevated and cardiac output reduced.

HEART FAILURE AND THE AUTONOMIC NERVOUS SYSTEM

The precise role of the autonomic nervous system in the pathogenesis of heart failure, especially the postganglionic mediator, norepinephrine, is poorly understood. However, alterations in autonomic function are common in heart failure. It is not known whether these are a cause or a consequence of heart failure. Circulating concentrations of norepinephrine and urinary concentrations of its metabolites are increased in proportion to the severity of clinical signs. Paradoxically, stores of norepinephrine in myocardium and ganglia are decreased, and contractile response to exogenous catecholamines is reduced.[5] Depletion is thought to arise from reduction in norepinephrine production and storing capacity. Production is apparently reduced due to tyrosine hydroxylase deficiency, the enzyme that catalyzes tyrosine to DOPA (the initial step in norepinephrine synthesis). Reduction in contractile response is thought to arise from downregulation of adrenergic receptors (adenylate cyclase) due to prolonged elevation of circulating catecholamines. While these changes in norepinephrine sensitivity do not alter cardiac function at rest, they become more important during exercise when norepinehrine normally mediates both increase in heart rate and force of myocardial contraction. The sustained high levels of circulating catecholamines contribute to the increased systemic vascular resistance and aortic stiffness (i.e., increased impedance) characteristic of heart failure.

RENAL CONSEQUENCES IN HEART FAILURE

Edema is an important sequela of congestive heart failure.[6] Edematous tissues frequently cause clinical signs leading to the diagnosis of heart disease and decrease duration and quality of life. Distribution of edema fluid depends on capillary dynamics. Edema can develop without renal fluid retention or excessive water consumption. However, animals with congestive heart failure frequently retain excess quantities of water and consume greater volumes due to homeostatic mechanisms that normally protect against dehydration, hypovolemia, or electrolyte imbalance.

The normal response to hypovolemia is as follows. Because of decreasing cardiac output (which may result from heart disease or inadequate return of blood to the heart due to hypovolemia), mean systemic arterial pressure and renal plasma flow fall. The decrease in mean systemic arterial pressure is sensed by baroreceptors in the aortic and carotid sinus, which transmit that information to the medulla oblongata and hypothalamus. These central structures send efferent impulses to the heart (usually decreasing vagal traffic) and to systemic arterioles and venules (usually increasing adrenergic traffic). Decreased vagal traffic causes increased

heart rate; increased adrenergic traffic causes vascular constriction and increased vascular stiffness.

The kidneys response to decreased renal plasma flow results in its attempt to expand blood volume to return renal plasma flow toward normal (Fig. 7-2). When renal plasma flow falls, less sodium is presented to the juxtaglomerular apparatus (JGA), located at the point at which afferent and efferent glomerular arterioles come into apposition. In response to decreased sodium delivery, or possibly, to decreased blood flow or pressure, the JGA secretes renin. This substance activates the inactive polypeptide, angiotensin I. Angiotensin I circulates to the lung, where it is converted by angiotensin converting enzyme (ACE) to angiotensin II, the biologically active polypeptide. This peptide has three profound actions: it causes arteriolar vasoconstriction, increases thirst, and increases renal sodium chloride and water retention.[7]

Vasoconstriction caused by angiotensin II increases systemic vascular resistance and stiffness of the great arteries. This tends to return systemic arterial pressure toward normal. Increased thirst results from a direct action of angiotensin II on the central nervous system (CNS) thirst centers. Antidiuretic hormone (ADH) is released in direct response to angiotensin II. The adrenal cortex accelerates production of aldosterone in response to angiotensin II. Aldosterone is the final messenger that causes more vigorous renal reabsorption of sodium chloride (and with it, water) from the renal tubules. Thus, increased water intake (by increasing thirst) and water conservation (by decreasing urine output), causes blood volume to return toward normal in states of hypovolemia. This compensatory response may be elicited by a relatively minute reduction in blood volume. The opposite response occurs when blood volume is expanded, as by drinking excessive water.

The precise mechanism(s) by which this homeostatic response is triggered are not known. It has been proposed that volume receptors in the relatively low-pressure veins or atria (in particular, the left atrium) send appropriate signals to the brain, which then sends efferent neural traffic to the kidneys and blood vessels. Recently, atrial natriuretic factor (ANF) has been identified. This substance is produced in the atria in response to stretch by increased left atrial (or total) blood volume. ANF

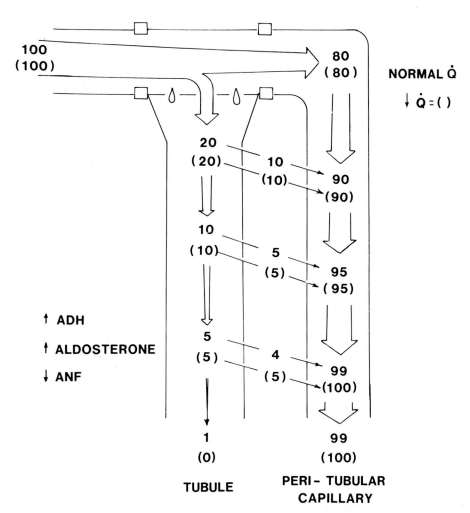

Fig. 7-2 Schematic diagram of a single giant nephron representing the entire kidney during normal function or during alterations in factors (e.g., increased ADH, increased aldosterone, decreased ANF) that might result from a reduction in cardiac output (Q). Renal plasma flow entering the nephron at the top left is 100 ml/min. In the glomerulus, 20 ml/min continues into the peritubular capillary surrounding the proximal convoluted tubule. From the proximal tubule, 10 ml/min is reabsorbed into the peritubular capillary, bringing the flow through the capillary to 90 ml/min and presenting the loop of Henle with 10 ml provisional urine. From the loop of Henle, 5 ml/min is reabsorbed into the peritubular capillary, bringing the flow through the capillary to 95 ml/min and presenting 5 ml/min of provisional urine to the distal convoluted tubule. From the distal convoluted tubule, different volumes of provisional urine are reabsorbed depending on whether there is a low blood flow state (↓ Q) or normal cardiac output. With a low-flow state, because of increases in ADH and aldosterone and decrease in ANF, nearly all (5 ml/min.) of the provisional urine presented to the distal tubule is reabsorbed into the peritubular capillary; plasma volume leaving the kidney equals plasma entering the kidney, and no urine is produced. Thus, if fluid intake remains constant, body water must increase since loss in urine is reduced drastically. Q, total blood flow (i.e., cardiac output); parentheses, disease state; ADH, antidiuretic hormone; ANF, atrial natriuretic factor.

stimulates the kidney to lose salt and water, thereby returning blood volume toward normal. Conversely, decreased atrial stretch would reduce ANF production, decrease urine production, and restore blood (and intraatrial) volume toward normal. Thus, ANF antagonizes actions of angiotensin II.

Another homeostatic mechanism that tends to balance blood volume uses ADH as a messenger. When blood volume decreases or when blood osmotic concentration increases, the posterior pituitary gland secretes ADH. ADH circulates to the renal distal convoluted and collecting tubules and increases their permeability to water. These tubules traverse a medullary region that is hyperosmotic with respect to fluid in the distal and collecting tubules. Therefore, that fluid is attracted by the osmotic particles in the peritubular milieu and leaves the tubules and collecting ducts. This causes water conservation by reducing urine output.

It is believed that increased aldosterone, increased ADH, decreased ANF, and increased angiotensin II all tend to reduce urine output in response to reduction in cardiac output or due to incorrect interpretation by volume or osmoreceptors of the true status of blood volume. In any case, by injection of large amounts of aldosterone, ADH, or angiotensin II, or by removing ANF, it is impossible to simulate the salt and water conservation occurring at the kidney in patients with heart failure. It is thought that another factor is responsible. This important response is termed increased filtration fraction (FF).

FILTRATION FRACTION AS THIRD FACTOR

Normally, for every 100 ml plasma flowing into the kidney, approximately 20 ml is filtered from the glomerular capillaries into the renal tubules as provisional urine. The glomerular membrane is impermeable to protein. Therefore, the filtrate is relatively low in protein, while the 80 ml nonfiltered plasma that continues on its path in the peritubular capillaries is protein rich. Furthermore, the fluid pressure within the tubules is relatively low, while that within peritubular capillaries is relatively high. The gradient of oncotic pressure is greater in peritubular capillary blood than in provisional urine and favors fluid reabsorption from the tubule to the per-

itubular capillary. The gradient of fluid pressure (greater in the peritubular capillary than in the renal tubule) discourages reabsorption from tubule to peritubular capillary. However, oncotic forces are dominant over those of fluid pressure. Therefore, almost 50 percent of provisional urine is reabsorbed from the proximal convoluted tubule by surrounding peritubular capillaries.

When renal plasma flow decreases and the renin-angiotensin-aldosterone axis is activated, efferent glomerular arterioles constrict and afferent glomerular arterioles dilate. This causes the volume of glomerular filtrate to remain nearly constant despite a fall in renal plasma flow. Thus, filtration fraction—the ratio of volume of glomerular filtration to renal plasma flow—which is normally 0.2, elevates to as high as 0.3 (Fig. 7-3). This means that the volume of renal plasma flow destined for pertibular capillaries (i.e., renal plasma flow minus glomerular filtrate) is diminished. The reduced plasma volume is both richer in protein (i.e., possesses greater oncotic pressure) and is perfusing at a lower fluid pressure (i.e., there is less of it). Thus, a relatively greater amount (both percentage and absolute volume) will be reabsorbed from renal tubule to peritubular capillary. This causes a reduction in urine volume and conservation of water and solutes, at a time when the animal may be manifesting increased water intake due to thirst precipitated by excessive angiotensin II. This sequence accounts for the oliguria and polydypsia observed in animals with congestive heart failure and also presents the circulation with fluid to be distributed, according to hydrostatic and oncotic forces, as ascites, pulmonary edema, or pitting edema stimulated by excessive angiotensin II. Thus, oliguria and polydypsia occur and the circulatory system develops an excess volume of fluid distributed as ascites, pulmonary edema, or peripheral edema, according to prevailing hydrostatic and oncotic forces.

EDEMA FORMATION

Edema occurs when excessive fluid accumulates within interstitial compartments[6] (Fig. 7-4). Excessive fluid accumulation may result from hypoproteinemia and reduced ability of the vascular compartment to hold fluid, from excessive capillary

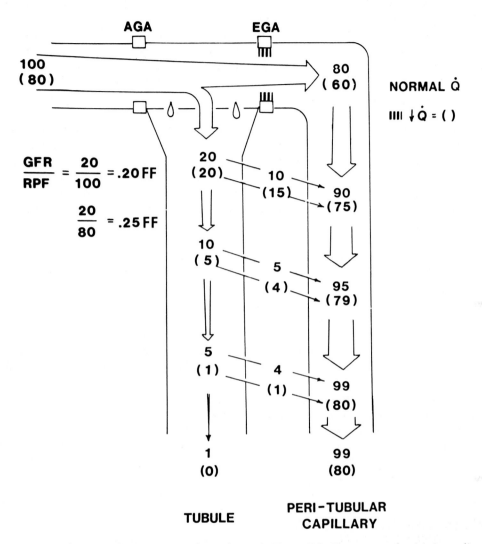

Fig. 7-3 Schematic diagram of same giant nephron shown in Figure 7-2. However, reduction in cardiac output (↓ Q̇) resulted in reduction in renal plasma flow from a normal of 100 to only 80 ml/min (upper left). Because of increased sympathetic efferent activity, efferent glomerular arteriole (EGA) is constricted (shown by vertical lines), thereby increasing resistance to flow through it and sustaining glomerular filtration rate (GFR) 20 ml/min) at normal levels. Note that the filtration fraction (ratio of GFR to renal plasma flow, RPF) increases from 0.20 to 0.25. Since GFR is sustained in the presence of decreased RPF, it follows that the volume of plasma presented to the peritubular capillary around the proximal convoluted tubule is smaller (60 ml/min) than normal (80 ml/min). Because of the constancy of provisional urine with reduction in fluid within the peritubular capillary, there is an increased volume (e.g., 15 ml/min instead of 10 ml/min) of fluid reabsorbed from tubule to capillary. This presents less provisional urine (5 ml/min instead of 10 ml/min) to the loop of Henle and distal tubule and a relatively greater percentage is reabsorbed from tubule to capillary. Thus, because of the increased filtration fraction, urine volume falls to near-zero, while plasma exiting the kidney equals plasma entering the kidney. As in the previous diagram, if water intake remains constant and urine production falls, body water must increase.

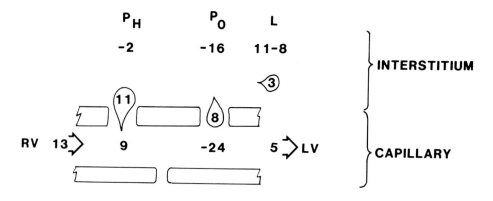

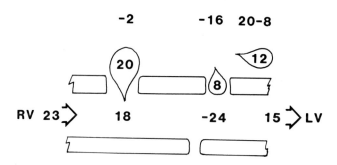

Fig. 7-4 Schematic diagrams of alveolar-capillary dynamics during normal cardiovascular function (top) and during congestion (bottom) (i.e., elevation of capillary hydrostatic pressure) resulting from failure of the left ventricle. Interstitial and capillary compartments are labeled for the normal state (top). Values for osmotic (i.e., oncotic)(P_O) and hydrostatic (P_H) pressures (in mmHg) are displayed. A teardrop containing a number represents the direction fluid would move—either into or out of the capillary—depending on prevailing hydrostatic or osmotic forces. Values for those forces are indicated within each compartment (listed under P_H and P_O at the top). Lymph flow (L) is shown to the right of each state. Note that the lymph flow increases from 3 to 12 during the state of congestion (bottom). This increase results from the elevation of capillary hydrostatic pressure from a normal value of 9 to the increased value of 18. RV, right ventricle; LV, left ventricle.

fluid pressure, or both. Rarely, excessive interstitial fluid accumulation may occur if the interstitial compartment fluid pressure is too negative.

Edema commonly results when capillary fluid pressure is too high (Fig. 7-1B,C). Capillary microvascular fluid pressure elevation results from congestion of veins emptying those capillaries. Both arise from the ventricle in front of those beds failing to remove a normal quantity of venous blood. Such failure may stem from weakened contraction, a stenotic semilunar valve, arterial hypertension that offers too great an interference to ventricular ejection, regurgitation through the atrioventricular

(AV) valve permitting blood to back up in the atrium and vein, or poor ventricular diastolic filling (and sucking from the veins).

If the right atrium-right ventricle fails, fluid pressure in the systemic capillaries is increased; fluid extravasation from those capillaries exceeds lymphatic return to the circulation. The ensuing edema produces clinical signs termed *right-sided congestive heart failure*. The precise location of fluid accumulation depends on which systemic tissues drain into the venous circulations with the greatest fluid pressure—the so-called dependent portions. In a quadruped, those regions are below the level of the heart (e.g., the brisket, limbs, and prepuce). For reasons not clearly understood, hepatic venous and capillary pressure elevates disproportionately, and fluid weeps from the liver into the abdominal cavity as ascites. Ascites is one of the most common manifestations of right-sided heart failure.

If the failing side of the heart is the left atrium-left ventricle, pressures in the pulmonary veins and pulmonary capillaries elevate. Pulmonary veins become engorged and fluid weeps from the pulmonary capillaries into the interstices of the lung faster than it can be returned to the circulation by lymphatics. Fluid accumulation occurs in an ordered fashion, first as a cuff surrounding airways, next within the interstitial tissue widening the alveolar-capillary membrane, then in the angles of the alveoli, and finally as overt alveolar flooding. Pulmonary edema that follows causes clinical signs termed *left-sided congestive heart failure.*

As fluid that is relatively low in protein weeps from the pulmonary capillaries into the interstitium of the lung, that fluid removes proteins from the interstitium and returns them to the blood. Thus, pulmonary edema may be relatively self-limiting since, as oncotic pressure of the interstitium falls and that of the blood increases, the tendency for fluid to leave the circulation for the interstitium will decrease. This explains why pulmonary capillary pressure may remain at rather high levels (up to 40 mmHg) for long periods if the increase occurred slowly enough to permit washing out of protein from the interstitium. However, if pulmonary capillary pressure were elevated acutely (e.g., to only 25 mmHg), the oncotic pressure within the interstitial compartment would still be great enough to result in florid edema and sudden death.

In either right- or left-sided heart failure, hypoproteinemia will exacerbate edema formation. Animals with poor cardiac and hepatic function that develop hypoproteinemia may experience worsened clinical signs caused by edema or effusions.

WHY DOES THE HEART MUSCLE FAIL?

Inability to generate a forceful myocardial contraction may be attributed to failure of any number of steps, from depolarization of the myocardial fibers to contraction and relaxation of myofibrils. These steps are classified as excitation, excitation-contraction coupling, contraction, and relaxation.[8]

Excitation is the process whereby a wave of depolarization traverses the myocardium. This wave occurs as sodium ions enter the cell, causing the polarity to change from the resting value (-80 mV inside) to the excited value (+25 mV inside). Abnormality of the depolarization process from electrolyte imbalance or changes in membrane permeability can result in reduced force of contraction or asynchrony of contraction between the two ventricles. Depolarization of the cell membrane permits calcium ions to enter the cell from their region of higher concentration outside the cell. Also, calcium ions are released from their location of sequestration within the sarcoplasmic reticulum. It is this availability of calcium ions that sustains the process of contraction. Reduction in calcium ion concentration outside the cell or failure of opening of the calcium channels in the cell membrane may weaken force of contraction.

Excitation-contraction coupling (Fig. 7-5A) proceeds when calcium ions made available by excitation bind to troponin (Fig. 7-5B). They cause the tropomyosin (to which troponin is bound) to slide between binding sites on actin filaments and heads of myosin filaments. This generates contraction. Calcium ions may be unavailable for this process, if they are bound too tightly to the sarcoplasmic reticulum, or if as a result of intracellular acidosis, they become bound to mitochondria. When the myosin heads attach to the binding sites on actin, energy is released through the hydrolysis of ATP to ADP by ATPase. The rate of energy release in this process is intimately related to the property termed myocardial contractility. Another reason for reduced myocardial contractility may be reduction in ATPase activity or in stores of ATP.[9] It is the energy made available from this hydrolysis that causes the myosin heads to swing (Fig. 7-5C), causing the actin filaments to slide toward the center of the sarcomere and pull with them the Z bands to which they are tethered. Motion of the Z bands causes shortening of the muscle; if shortening is prevented, tension is developed in isometric contraction. Structural changes in contractile proteins (i.e., actin, myosin) may result in reduced myocardial contractility.

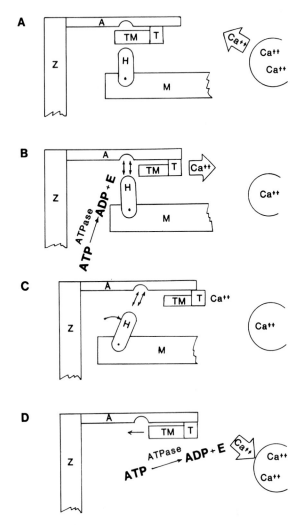

Fig. 7-5 Schematic diagrams depicting mechanisms of myocardial contraction and relaxation. The contractile unit is the sarcomere and is composed of two Z bands (Z) with actin filaments (A) attached at right angles. Only a single Z band and actin filament are shown, although in reality, each Z band has numerous actin filaments. Binding sites (invaginations) are present on actin filaments to which heads of myosin (M) are attached if not obstructed by tropomyosin (TM). Calcium ions (Ca^{2+}) are present in the sarcoplasmic reticulum. Troponin (T) is a protein attached to tropomyosin and represents the binding site for calcium ions. (**A**) During the resting state the myosin head is prevented from contacting the actin binding site by tropomyosin. Following cellular repolarization, Ca^{2+} enters the cell and is released from the sarcoplasmic reticulum. (**B**) Ca^{2+} binds to troponin and the Ca^{2+}-troponin complex causes the tropomyosin to move from its point of obstruction. The myosin head binds to the actin site. Energy (E) is released when ATPase hydrolyzes ATP to ADP. (**C**) The released energy causes

Relaxation of myofilaments occurs when calcium ions are actively displaced (Fig. 7-5D) from the troponin and are either resequestered by the sarcoplasmic reticulum or actively extruded from the cell. As with contraction, this activity derives its energy from high energy stored in ATP. Any of the factors identified as contributing to reduced contraction may also cause relaxation to falter. This, then, causes incomplete or tardy relaxation and leads, ultimately, to failure of contraction.

Energy stored in both ATP and creatine phosphate (CP) as high-energy phosphate bonds is the immediate source of energy for both contraction and relaxation. Most ATP is produced by an aerobic process (Krebs cycle and electron-transport chain) in the mitochondria (Fig. 7-6). However, a smaller but important portion (glycolysis) occurs either aerobically or anaerobically in the cyctoplasm. Anerobic glycolysis[10] may be particularly important in disease states when inadequate amounts of oxygen are available for the electron-transport chain.

In glycolysis, glycogen and glucose are broken down aerobically (if enough oxygen is present) to pyruvate or anaerobically (if oxygen is absent) to lactate. This process requires ATP for energy but produces twice as much ATP as is used. ATP produced in this manner is inadequate to sustain myocardial function for long or at high levels. In the mitochondria, acetyl coenzyme A (produced from glycolysis and especially from fatty acids generated by β-oxidation of fats) enters the Krebs (tricarboxylic acid) cycle. Acetyl coenzyme A enters mitochondria through the action of carnitine. Once within the mitochondria, a series of reactions occurs that feed protons to the electron-transport chain. In the electron-transport chain, a series of reactions occur that consumes oxygen and produces carbon dioxide, water, and the vast majority of ATP used

the myosin head (bound to the actin filament) to swing. This results in contraction of the sarcomere Z bands as the actin and myosin filaments slide over one another. This causes muscle shortening. If shortening is prohibited, tension is generated. (**D**) Relaxation occurs when additional energy drives Ca^{2+} ions from troponin out of the cell and into the sarcoplasmic reticulum. This permits tropomyosin to come between actin and myosin heads and actin to slide back to its resting state and causes the Z bands to return to the resting state.

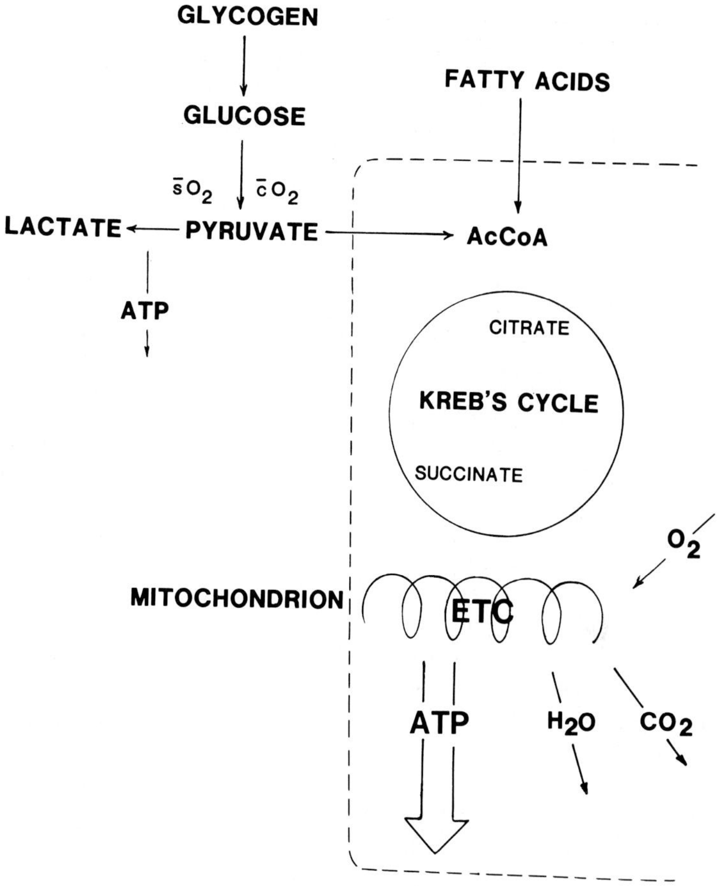

GLYCOGEN

GLUCOSE

FATTY ACIDS

LACTATE ← PYRUVATE → AcCoA

ATP

KREB'S CYCLE

CITRATE

SUCCINATE

MITOCHONDRION

ETC

O_2

ATP H_2O CO_2

Fig. 7-6 Schematic diagram illustrating metabolic sources of ATP for myocardial contraction and relaxation. A small quantity of ATP results from catabolism of glucose (or its precursor, glycogen) to either pyruvate and then acetyl coenzyme A (aerobic glycolysis) or to lactate (anaerobic glycolysis). The major source of ATP is the Krebs cycle and electron-transport chain within the mitochondria. This process requires oxygen and produces ATP, water, and carbon dioxide. Acetyl coenzyme A (AcCoA) is generated predominantly from β-oxidation of fat, although a smaller amount is derived from pyruvate. AcCoA enters the mitochondria due to the action of carnitine.

for muscle function. If too little oxygen is available to react with the hydrogen, or if insufficient quantities of carnitine are available to permit acetyl coenzyme A to enter the mitochondria, too little ATP may be produced and muscle function may deteriorate.

Thus, heart failure may result from any number of physical, chemical or physical-chemical defects in the myocyte. The force of myocardial contraction may be reduced, or relaxation may be inadequate.

Meerson[11] listed three stages that describe the response to chronic volume overload: (1) myocardial damage, (2) hyperfunction, and (3) exhaustion. During the initial stage, clinical signs occur due to heart failure from low cardiac output or due to venous congestion. The ventricle dilates; myocardial fibers swell and separate; stores of high-energy phosphate and glycogen become depleted; lactate production increases; and mitochondrial mass, RNA levels, and protein synthesis increase. These responses appear to represent the consequences of oxygen debt and include a shift toward anaerobic energy production and increased muscle mass.

The second stage usually lasts for a relatively long time and clinical signs abate. Hypertrophy occurs by increased myocardial fiber diameter. The ratio of fiber mass to myocardial mass increases. Glycogen and high-energy phosphate supplies, RNA levels, and protein synthesis return toward normal.

In the third stage, myocardial exhaustion occurs. The myocardium is replaced by fibrous connective tissue that both lacks ability to contract and offers greater resistance to stretch. During this stage, protein synthesis cannot replace myocardial tissue. Since both systolic and diastolic function deteriorates, the patient manifests increased clinical signs associated with heart failure. Death becomes imminent.

The chronology of events starting from the inciting etiologic factors (e.g., mitral regurgitation or reduced myocardial contractility) to cessation of adaptive myocardial hypertrophy may be summarized as follows. Decreased forward left ventricular stroke volume results when a disease process (e.g., mitral regurgitation or systolic failure) becomes severe. Blood dams up in the left atrium and left atrial blood volume increases. This subsequently distends the left ventricle to a greater end-diastolic volume with a thinner ventricular wall. These dimensional changes temporarily permit the ventricle to improve. That is, the augmented preload resulting from added ventricular volume increases muscle stretch prior to its activation, enhancing contractility and stroke volume. However, peak myocardial tension is increased according to the Laplace relation. It predicts that the load on the muscle fibers (wall tension) is the product of pressure and ventricular chamber radius divided by twice the myocardial wall thickness. Since peak myocardial tension is a prime determinant of myocardial oxygen consumption, the latter increases. Increased oxygen demand outstrips the ability of the lung and coronary circulation to meet myocardial oxygen demand. An oxygen debt results. This causes activation of adenylate cyclase which increases production of cyclic adenosine monophosphate (cAMP). Protein kinases are activated by increased cAMP, which catalyzes protein synthesis. Resultant myocardial hypertrophy and increased muscle mass permits that chamber to perform increased work with less tension according to Laplace's law. Reduced myocardial tension reduces myocardial oxygen demand, which equilibrates with oxygen availability, reducing or eliminating the aforementioned steps responsible for hypertrophy. It appears that this sequence permits the ventricle to work at an increased level without outstripping oxygen availability. Thus, the patient benefits from a cardiac output sustained at near-normal levels despite either mitral regurgitation or myocardial disease.

The functional significance of a failing heart[8] must be discussed in terms of immediate and long-term consequences. Immediate consequences of severe heart failure are evident if cardiac output is inadequate to sustain life or if acute fulminating pulmonary edema produces asphyxia. However, if the heart is failing to a lesser degree, myocardial oxygen demands may be reduced due to reduction in the level of one of its prime determinants (e.g., con-

tractility). The long-term consequences, then, are that the myocardium may be protected against ischemic necrosis or fibrosis. Thus, Meerson's third-stage response to chronic volume overload (i.e., myocardial exhaustion) may be delayed by this physiologic (or pathologic) state of putting the heart at rest. Furthermore, if myocardial ATP production can be preserved, myocardial compliance may also be salvaged, since it is ATP that drives calcium from its binding site on troponin back to the sarcoplasmic reticulum, permitting relaxation. Therefore, therapeutic strategies directed at strengthening the weakened myocardium may improve the quality of life in the short term but hasten death in the long term under some circumstances. This remains to be more closely investigated.

REFERENCES

1. Braunwald E, Ross J, Sonnenblick EH: Mechanisms of Contraction of the Normal and Failing Heart. Little, Brown, Boston, 1976
2. Mason DT: Congestive Heart Failure. Yorke Medical Books, New York, 1976
3. Zelis R, Mason DT: Compensatory mechanisms in congestive heart failure—The role of peripheral resistance vessels. N Engl J Med 282:962, 1970
4. Forrester J, Diamond G, Chatterjee K, et al: Medical therapy of acute myocardial infarction by application of hemodynamic subsets. N Engl J Med 295:1356, 1977
5. Spann JF, Chidsey JA, Braunwald E: Reduction of cardiac stores of norepinephrine in experimental heart failure. Science 145:439, 1964
6. Staub NC: Pulmonary edema. Physiol Rev 54:678, 1974
7. Humes HD, Gottlieb MN, Brenner BM: The kidney in congestive heart failure. In Brenner BM, Stein JH (eds): Sodium and Water Homeostasis, Churchill Livingstone, New York, 1978
8. Katz AM: Physiology of the Heart. Raven Press, New York, 1977
9. Pool PE, Spann JF, Buccino RA, et al: Myocardial high-energy phosphate stores in cardiac hypertrophy and heart failure. Circ Res 21:365, 1967
10. Bishop SP, Altshuld R: Evidence for increased glycolytic metabolism in cardiac hypertrophy and congestive heart failure. In Bing OHL (ed): Cardiac Hypertrophy. Academic Press, Orlando, FL, 1971
11. Meerson FZ: The Myocardium in Hyperfunction, Hypertrophy and Heart Failure. American Heart Association Monograph, New York, 1969

8

Management of Heart Failure: Concepts, Therapeutic Strategies, and Drug Pharmacology

Mark D. Kittleson

Heart failure is caused by systolic and/or diastolic cardiac dysfunction and is the end result of many different diseases. Resulting clinical signs may occur with exercise or at rest and are referrable to decreased peripheral perfusion, congestion, or edema. Appropriate and logical therapy of heart failure requires individualized therapy to address the underlying disorder rather than haphazard treatment of every patient in the same manner.

Management of canine and feline heart failure is a common practice for the veterinary clinician. Success requires pharmacologic and physiologic knowledge, clinical judgment, and development of a close client rapport.

CONCEPTS

In order to understand therapeutic strategies for the management of heart failure, useful groupings of clinical signs and disease categories are presented. The groups are based on chronicity (acute versus chronic heart failure), clinical severity (mild to se-

vere), clinical signs (backward versus forward heart failure), and type of failure present (e.g., heart failure due to pressure overload, volume overload, myocardial failure, or diastolic dysfunction).

Heart failure can present as an acute or chronic problem. Acute heart failure can truly be the acute onset of a new disease, or it can represent the exacerbation of an existing chronic disorder. Most commonly, acute heart failure is caused by an acute decrease in myocardial contractility due to an overdose of an anesthetic agent or other drug, by circulating myocardial toxins or depressants, or by myocardial trauma. Clinical signs are generally referrable to poor cardiac output and hypotension, rather than to edema. Edema is generally not present because the body has not had time to compensate for decreased cardiac output with fluid and water retention.

Acute heart failure can also be caused by sudden volume overloads accompanying valvular damage (e.g., ruptured chordae tendineae, acute aortic regurgitation due to bacterial endocarditis). In this case, edema is usually present. Patients display signs of severe heart failure requiring intensive therapy with intravenous drugs, including positive inotropes, diuretics, and vasodilators, depending on the underlying abnormality.

In chronic heart failure, clinical signs referrable to edema and congestion usually predominate. Signs due to poor cardiac output may be present at rest in severe cases or may only become evident during exercise.

Signs of heart failure are divided into those referrable to backward and forward heart failure. Signs of backward heart failure are those referrable to congestion and edema. In left heart backward failure, increased diastolic pressure in the left ventricle and/or high systolic and diastolic pressures in the left atrium and pulmonary veins result in increased pulmonary capillary pressure and pulmonary edema. This results in coughing, dyspnea, orthopnea, and tachypnea. The diagnosis is made on the basis of radiographic identification of pulmonary edema associated with left heart disease; ruling out other causes of pulmonary edema; or measuring elevated pulmonary capillary, left atrial, or left ventricular end-diastolic pressures. In right heart backward failure, increased right ventricular diastolic pressure and/or increased right atrial and systemic venous pressures cause ascites, pleural effusion, or peripheral edema. The diagnosis is made by identifying one of these signs in association with right heart disease or with documentation that the right atrial or central venous pressure is increased.

Poor tissue perfusion due to a decreased cardiac output defines forward failure. Clinical signs include fatigue, weakness, poor exercise tolerance, cold extremities, slow capillary refill time, poor mucous membrane color, and hypothermia. All signs except exercise intolerance will not become evident until forward failure becomes severe. Laboratory documentation of forward failure consists of decreased cardiac output, widened arteriovenous oxygen difference, decreased venous oxygen tension if the patient is not hypoxemic or anemiac[1] (Fig. 8-1), and prerenal azotemia and lactic acidosis if the forward failure is severe.

Decreased cardiac output results in diminished tissue oxygen delivery:

Tissue oxygen delivery =
    arterial oxygen content × cardiac output

At rest, if tissue oxygen consumption remains stable, the actively metabolizing cells must extract more oxygen from the blood stream to meet their metabolic cells needs. This results in a decreased oxygen content and partial pressure of oxygen at end-capillary and venous sites. The oxygen tension at the end of the capillary bed is the critical factor in determining whether enough oxygen will reach mitochondria. In normal animals, the value for end-capillary or venous oxygen tension is 30 to 50 mmHg. If oxygen delivery decreases significantly at rest because of reduced cardiac output, or if exercise increases tissue oxygen consumption in excess of tissue oxygen delivery, end-capillary or venous oxygen tension may decrease below the critical level of 21 to 24 mmHg. When end-capillary PO_2 is <21 to 24 mmHg, cells must start relying on anaerobic metabolism resulting in lactic acid production. During exercise, lactic acid production in skeletal muscle will result in fatigue and force the patient to stop exercising. Therefore, in dogs with mild to moderate forward heart failure signs are best identified by either exercising the patient or obtaining a history of its exercise capabilities. Patients with severe failure often show signs of forward heart failure at rest.

As a general rule, dogs with chronic heart failure first exhibit signs of backward failure. Moreover, signs of forward failure are generally only seen in conjunction with those signs of backward failure for the following reason.

The cardiovascular systems' basic function is to maintain normal systemic arterial pressure, tissue blood flow, and systemic and pulmonary capillary pressures. Elaborate control mechanisms are present to maintain these functions in normal animals. When the cardiovascular system fails, however, all functions cannot be maintained, and it works instead within a framework of priorities.

Maintaining systemic arterial blood pressure is the body's main priority. It will do everything to maintain blood pressure, even at the expense of the other functions. For example, if myocardial contractility is decreased suddenly, reduction in stroke volume and therefore cardiac output results. Decreased blood flow into the arterial system lowers the systemic arterial pressure as long as arteriolar tone remains the same:

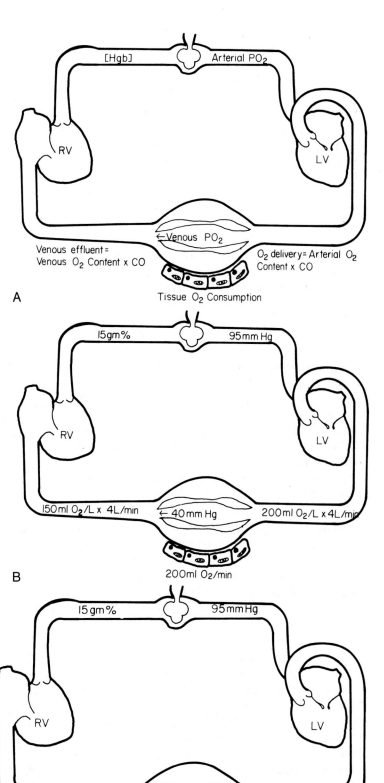

Fig. 8-1 Schematic diagram of the circulation depicting the balance between arterial oxygen content, oxygen delivery, tissue oxygen consumption, and resultant end-capillary or venous oxygen tension (**A**). CO, cardiac output; Hgb, hemoglobin concentration. (**B**) Normal canine values listed for the variables depicted in (**A**). Note that the venous oxygen tension is 40 mmHg. (**C**) Low cardiac output due to heart failure (e.g., 1.5 L/min) results in decreased tissue oxygen delivery and decreased venous oxygen tension.

Blood flow × arteriolar resistance =
arterial pressure

The cardiovascular system must then choose either to increase blood pressure by increasing arteriolar tone and therefore the resistance to blood flow or to decrease arteriolar tone, reducing resistance to blood flow, and improving cardiac output. The cardiovascular system always chooses to increase blood pressure, even though by doing so, cardiac output decreases further.

The second priority of the cardiovascular system is to maintain a normal cardiac output. Its third priority is to maintain normal capillary pressures. For example, a dog with chronic mitral regurgitation and mild heart failure may suffer a ruptured chordae tendineae. This condition worsens the mitral regurgitation, increases left atrial blood volume and pressure, and decreases forward aortic blood flow. The cardiovascular system compensates by retaining salt and water to increase cardiac output rather than decreasing salt and water retention or left atrial pressure.

Because of these physiologic priorities, dogs with chronic heart failure usually present first with signs referable to congestion and edema, since the cardiovascular system permits venous pressures to rise in an attempt to maintain systemic arterial pressure and flow. Later, signs referable to poor tissue perfusion develop. The body continues to try to increase cardiac output by retaining salt and water as long as the cardiac output is decreased, even though this fluid retention aggravates any edema present. Systemic arterial blood pressure is maintained within normal limits until extremely late in the course of heart failure, even though the arteriolar constriction needed to maintain normal pressure contributes to poor tissue perfusion.

The cause of these physiologic responses may be related to the need to maintain adequate perfusion in critical vascular beds requiring mean systemic arterial blood pressure greater than 60 mmHg (i.e., the brain, heart, and kidneys). As all three vascular beds have high innate resistances to blood flow, relatively high pressures are needed to force blood through them. Other vascular beds would function normally with systemic arterial blood pressure well below 60 mmHg. With a decreased cardiac output, the vascular system can compensate for poor blood flow to the critical vascular beds by constricting blood vessels in other regions of the body, shifting blood flow to the brain, heart, and kidneys. If blood flow and oxygen delivery become inadequate to the other regions of the body, however, anaerobic metabolism lactic acidosis, and poor exercise performance result, leading to cell death and eventual patient demise. Ultimately, maintaining blood flow clearly takes priority over maintaining normal capillary pressures.

Elevated capillary pressures cause edema resulting in poor organ function. The rapidity with which this causes mortality depends on the organ involved. Peripheral edema of skin and subcutaneous tissue, for example, usually does not cause death, whereas fulminant pulmonary edema can rapidly kill the patient. Receptors in the left atrium prevent increased atrial pressure in normal animals, but they become desensitized in chronic heart failure, permitting pressure to increase unchecked.[2] However, other receptors in the body that regulate blood pressure and flow remain functional in heart failure, demonstrating relative priorities.

Therapy of chronic heart failure depends on the types of signs present as well as their severity. Patients are generally categorized into one of *four functional heart failure classes* on the basis of ability to exercise and severity of the clinical signs. Signs of heart failure can be detected early in the course of failure if the patient is active and observed to exercise strenuously.

Functional class I is reserved for those patients with cardiac disease but no evidence of heart failure. These patients should not be treated (Fig. 8-2).

If an animal exhibits cardiac-related exercise intolerance, it is placed in New York Heart Association functional class II[3] (Fig. 8-2). Treatment depends on the underlying heart disease but generally includes discontinuation of heavy exercise and low-dose diuretic therapy. Patients in this class with left heart failure generally do not display radiographic evidence of pulmonary edema, although the left heart and pulmonary veins are usually enlarged. Patients with concentric left ventricular hypertrophy, however, may exhibit minimal evidence of left ventricular enlargement, and the left atrium may only be mildly enlarged in this stage of disease.

Patients in functional class III have signs of heart failure during normal activity (Fig. 8-2). Radiographic signs are more apparent. Early perihilar congestion and interstitial edema is generally present in left heart failure. With right heart failure, the liver may be enlarged, but ascites is usually absent. Treatment is generally more aggressive and depends more on the underlying disease. Diuretic administration, salt restriction, and curtailment of physical activity are therapeutic modalities common to almost all patients in this class.

Most patients with heart failure are presented in functional class IV (Fig. 8-3). They show signs of heart failure at rest or with minimal activity. Since most pets are not subjected to strenuous exercise, owners are often unaware of abnormal clinical signs until this stage develops, especially with cats. In late class IV, heart failure is so severe as to constitute a medical emergency. Radiographs demonstrate pulmonary edema with left heart failure and ascites, or hydrothorax with right heart failure. The cardiac silhouette is almost always enlarged. Treatment is predicated on the pathophysiology of the underlying disease and is generally aggressive. Diuretics are indicated, as is salt and exercise restriction. Examples of other therapeutic interventions include the administration of positive inotropes (e.g., digitalis glycosides, sympathomimetics and bipyridine compounds, administration of vasodilators, physical removal of fluid (e.g., pericardiocentesis, thoracocentesis, abdominocentesis), and surgery (e.g., pericardiectomy). Therapy depends on the type of disease that is causing heart failure.

A vast array of cardiac diseases cause signs of heart failure. Appropriate treatment depends on the ability of the clinician to make an accurate diagnosis and understand the pathophysiology of the underlying disease. All patients with a particular disorder may not have the exact same abnormalities contributing to their signs. Most diseases, however, behave in a manner similar enough to make general recommendations regarding therapy. Disorders of cardiac function are broken down into those resulting in systolic and diastolic dysfunction.

Fig. 8-2 Frank-Starling curves (filling pressure of a ventricle or atrial pressure plotted against cardiac index) of functional class I, II, and III heart failure. Class I is normal. Class II is at point E at rest but moves into the right upper quadrant (congestion due to an atrial pressure >18 mmHg) with exercise. Cardiac output is inadequate for an exercising patient. Class III starts at point A at rest but moves to point B with nonstrenuous activity (e.g., walking around the block). The class III patient can move to point C with a positive inotrope or arteriolar dilator if he has myocardial failure or to point E with a positive inotrope, a positive inotrope and diuretic or venodilator, or a balanced vasodilator. A patient with mitral regurgitation can move from point A to E with an arteriolar dilator or balanced vasodilator. (Kittleson M: Concepts and therapeutic strategies in the management of heart failure. p. 279. In Kirk RW (ed): Current Veterinary Therapy. Vol. VIII. WB Saunders, Philadelphia, 1983. Reprinted with permission from WB Saunders Co.)

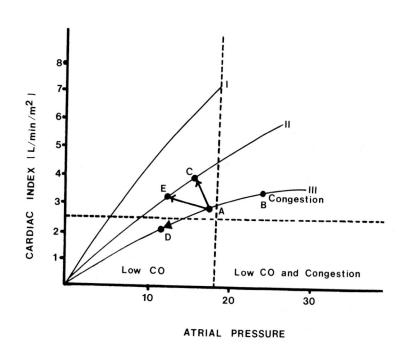

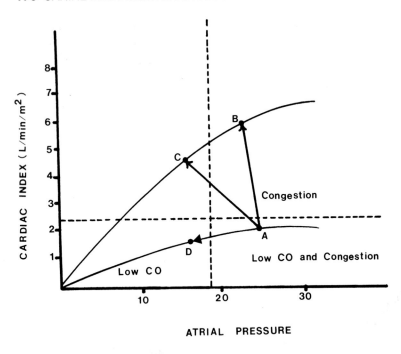

Fig. 8-3 A Frank-Starling curve of a patient in class IV heart failure (point A). With myocardial failure, administration of a positive inotrope or arteriolar dilator causes improvement to point B; with a positive inotrope and diuretic (or venodilator) or balanced vasodilator, improvement occurs to point C. Patients with mitral regurgitation can move from point A to point C with an arteriolar dilator or a balanced vasodilator. Overzealous diuretic administration or dehydration can result in the patient's cardiovascular function moving to point D. Note that little change in cardiac index occurs in this situation. (Kittleson M: Concepts and therapeutic strategies in the management of heart failure. p. 279. In Kirk RW (ed): Current Veterinary Therapy. Vol. VIII. WB Saunders, Philadelphia, 1983. Reprinted with permission from WB Saunders Co.)

Diastolic Dysfunction

Diastolic dysfunction means that a disease has resulted in an inability of the heart to fill properly during diastole. The most common problem is an increase in ventricular stiffness (i.e., a decrease in compliance) (Fig. 8-4). This occurs when the myocardium or endocardium becomes infiltrated with scar tissue, when the myocardium becomes thicker than normal (concentric hypertrophy),[4] or when the pericardium is diseased. Endocardial fibrosis and overt myocardial fibrosis are generally called restrictive cardiomyopathy. Treatment is usually limited to symptomatic therapy and is typically unrewarding.[5] Diuretics and a low-salt diet can be used to control signs of congestion and edema. Systolic function is usually normal. Therefore, administration of positive inotropes may not be beneficial, although their use is not contraindicated.

Hypertrophic cardiomyopathy is a disease in which the left ventricular myocardium loses its ability to control the process of hypertrophy. The net result is left ventricular *concentric hypertrophy* (a thicker than normal wall and a normal chamber size), a stiff chamber, and decreased afterload (see the section on systolic dysfunction).[6] Abnormal papillary muscle orientation and other unexplained factors may also produce mitral regurgitation in this disease. The increased chamber stiffness results in an increased left ventricular diastolic pressure. This, along with the mitral regurgitation, can cause pulmonary edema. Treatment consists of diuretic administration. Propranolol is often given to reduce heart rate and prolong the ventricular filling time in hypertrophic cardiomyopathy. Therapy aimed at decreasing left ventricular stiffness would be helpful and, in humans, calcium-channel blockers can produce this desired effect.[7] The pharmacology of verapamil in cats has been studied recently; the recommended dose is 1 to 2 mg/kg administered every 8 hours.[8] The effects of verapamil on hemodynamics in cats with hypertrophic cardiomyopathy have not been studied. Untoward effects have been reported in some persons with hypertrophic cardiomyopathy following verapamil administration. If verapamil is used in cats to treat hypertrophic cardiomyopathy it should be used cautiously.

Pericardial disease results in diastolic dysfunction and potentially, heart failure. Heart failure due to the accumulation of pericardial fluid is called pericardial tamponade. Acute pericardial tamponade is due to the rapid accumulation of pericardial fluid

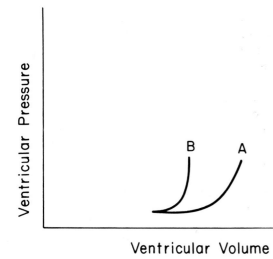

Fig. 8-4 Diastolic pressure-volume relationship in a dog with normal ventricular compliance (curve A), and a dog with a stiff ventricle (curve B). Note that with a stiff ventricle (curve B), ventricular pressure increases dramatically in response to a smaller increase in ventricular volume.

resulting in an acute increase in intrapericardial pressure. This results in both an increase in right ventricular diastolic pressure and a decrease in cardiac output. In chronic tamponade, cardiac output is usually normal, since the body has had time to compensate through salt and water retention. Therefore, these patients present with signs of chronic right heart failure.

Scarring and fibrosis of the pericardium and epicardium (constrictive pericarditis) can also produce diastolic dysfunction and signs of chronic right heart failure. The cause is usually chronic pericarditis and treatment involves surgical removal of the pericardium and portions of the epicardium.

Signs of right heart failure predominate in pericardial disease for two reasons. First, the right ventricular free wall is thinner than the left ventricular free wall, and pressures within the pericardial sac are more easily transmitted to the right ventricular cavity. An increase in intrapericardial pressure, therefore, first causes an increase in right atrial, systemic venous, and systemic capillary pressures. Second, systemic capillaries are more porous than pulmonary capillaries, which normally withstand a hydrostatic pressure of 12 mmHg. Systemic capil-

laries can only withstand a hydrostatic pressure of 5 mmHg. Therefore, for any given intrapericardial pressure, even if transmitted equally to both ventricles, the right side would show signs of backward failure first.

Abnormalities of myocardial relaxation occur in diseases characterized by myocardial failure, such as congestive (dilated) cardiomyopathy.[4] This probably occurs because of cellular calcium overload and contributes to the signs of heart failure. Mitral and tricuspid stenosis also can result in signs of heart failure by producing diastolic dysfunction. Both lesions are rare in veterinary medicine.

Systolic Dysfunction

Systolic dysfunction encompasses a number of different problems including decreased myocardial contractility (myocardial failure), inadequate preload, increased afterload, leaks leading to volume overload, and stenoses leading to pressure overload. To comprehend systolic dysfunction, an understanding of normal systolic function is first required. Wall stress-volume loops will be provided for this purpose.

Definitions of the determinants of systolic function (e.g., contractility, afterload, and preload) contribute to an appreciation of these concepts. *Contractility* is the force, velocity, and extent of contraction independent of the load on the myocardium. As a corollary, contractility of your biceps muscle could be determined by measuring the velocity and the extent of the motion of your hand within a given time period if you were to flex your elbow as rapidly as possible with nothing in your hand. When using wall stress-volume loops only the extent of myocardial contraction will be examined. The extent of contraction is very dependent on afterload but independent of preload.[9]

Afterload (systolic myocardial wall stress) is the force opposing myocardial contraction (Fig. 8-5).[10] Afterload to your biceps muscle would be a weight lifted while flexing the elbow. Wall stress is approximated by the following formula[11]:

$$\text{Wall stress} = \frac{(\text{intraventricular pressure} \times \text{radius})}{\text{wall thickness}}$$

Thus, afterload is not just arterial blood pressure.

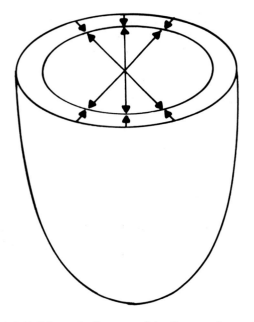

Fig. 8-5 Schematic diagram of the forces acting against the ventricular wall during systole and diastole. During systole, the arrows pointing out toward the ventricular walls represent the force or load against which the walls must contract (i.e., afterload). During diastole, the arrows pointing out also represent the force that stretches the myocardium to a certain end-diastolic point (i.e., preload).

Afterload can be increased by increasing systolic intraventricular pressure, (increasing the weight), increasing the chamber radius or diameter (changing the geometry of elbow flexion), or decreasing wall thickness (making the muscle smaller). Chronic increases in afterload are countered by the myocardium through hypertrophy.

Preload is the force pushing on the myocardium to create a given amount of stretch placed on the sarcomere at end-diastole.[12] The increased stretch results in increased contractile force according to Starling's law. The amount of stretch is determined by multiple variables but for the purposes of this discussion, preload is defined as the force that results in fiber stretching (i.e., end-diastolic wall stress). For the most part, sarcomere stretch plays only a minor role in chronic heart diseases with volume overload, since myocardial fibers or sarcomeres are maximally stretched early on in the course of these cardiac diseases. Increase in preload, however, is

thought to result in eccentric hypertrophy, a major compensatory mechanism for volume overload.

A normal wall stress-volume loop is depicted in Figure 8-6. During diastole, the ventricle fills to a certain end diastolic volume and achieves a certain end-diastolic wall stress. During isovolumic systole, by definition, volume does not change, since the mitral and aortic valves are closed. During this phase, intraventricular pressure increases and chamber diameter and wall thickness do not change. This results in increased wall stress. When the aortic valve opens, ejection begins. During ejection, pressure increases a small amount and then decreases, chamber diameter decreases, and the wall thickens. This results in a decrease in wall stress throughout ejection. During isovolumic relaxation, wall stress decreases while end-systolic volume stays the same.

The relationship among systolic wall stress, contractility, and ventricular volume is illustrated in Figure 8-7. If systolic intraventricular pressure is increased, systolic wall stress (afterload) also increases, resulting in decreased fiber shortening.

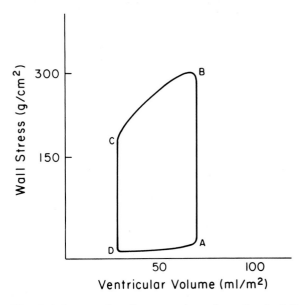

Fig. 8-6 A normal wall stress-volume loop for the left ventricle. A, end-diastole and the point at which the mitral valve closes. A-B, isovolumic systole. B, the onset of ejection and opening of the aortic valve. B-C, ejection; the volume at B minus the volume at C is the stroke volume. C, end-systole and closing of the aortic valve. C-D, isovolumic relaxation. D, opening of the mitral valve. D-A, ventricular filling.

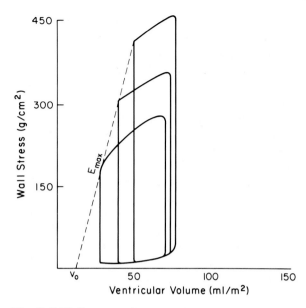

Fig. 8-7 Wall stress-volume loops before and after the administration of an agent that constricts systemic arterioles. As end-systolic pressure (hence wall stress) increases, heart muscle contraction is reduced at end-systole. This causes an increase in end-systolic volume and a decrease in stroke volume. The slope (E_{max}) and x intercept (V_o) of the line connecting the end-systolic wall stress-volume points defines myocardial contractility.

Therefore, end-systolic volume increases because the chamber no longer can empty as completely as it did before. In the earlier example, this would be analogous to increasing the weight that the biceps muscle must lift. As the weight is increased, the velocity and extent of elbow flexion during a given time interval will decrease linearly. In Figure 8-7, a line has been drawn connecting the end-systolic wall stress-volume points from each loop (which is the same as plotting the extent of elbow flexion against the weight of the load). This line has a slope (E_{max}) and x-axis intercept (V_o). These two variables define myocardial contractility.[13] When myocardial contractility is decreased, E_{max} flattens and V_o shifts to the right. Therefore, for any given end-systolic wall stress (i.e., for any given force against which the heart muscle must push), end-systolic volume is increased; the muscle fibers cannot shorten as far because they are weaker.[14] When contractility is increased the slope (E_{max}) increases and V_o shifts to the left or remains stationary.

Myocardial failure (i.e., decreased myocardial

contractility), can be primary or can occur secondary to chronic increases in cardiac workload. Primary myocardial failure is generally called congestive or dilated cardiomyopathy and its cause is usually unknown. A defect in Syrian hamsters with an inherited form of myocardial failure has been identified in the sacroplasmic reticulum of the cell.[15] The sarcoplasmic reticulum is the intracellular structure that binds most of the intracellular calcium during diastole. Myocardial contractility is determined by a number of factors, but one of the major determinants is the number of caclium ions that reach the contractile proteins during systole.[16]

The major determinant of myocardial contractility is the amount of calcium bound to the sarcoplasmic reticulum during diastole (Fig. 8-8). The defect in the sarcoplasmic reticulum in Syrian hamsters results in poor diastolic calcium binding, hence diminished release of calcium during systole. This results in poor contractility. A similar defect may exist in dogs and cats with congestive (dilated) cardiomyopathy. Chronic pressure or volume overloads can result in chronic myocardial hypoxia and resultant intracellular acidosis.[17] Acidosis results in sarcoplasmic reticulum dysfunction, decreasing the sensitivity of troponin for calcium, and thereby decreasing myocardial contractility.

Whichever the mechanism, poor diastolic uptake of calcium by the sarcoplasmic reticulum results in increased diastolic concentrations of calcium. This is harmful in several ways. First, it forces other intracellular structures to bind more calcium, including the mitochondria. The mitochondria can bind up to 28 times their normal amount of calcium. This causes mitochondrial toxicity, resulting in reduced energy production.[18] Second, high diastolic calcium concentrations cause electric instability, which can result in arrhythmias due to abnormal automaticity.[19] Third, calcium is not removed from troponin as rapidly as normal resulting in impaired myocardial relaxation.

In myocardial failure, a series of compensatory mechanisms occurs. Myocardial failure, by definition, results in an increase in end-systolic volume (decreased extent of myocardial contraction during systole). This causes a decrease in stroke volume as long as the end-diastolic volume remains the same:

Stroke volume =
    end-diastolic volume − end-systolic volume

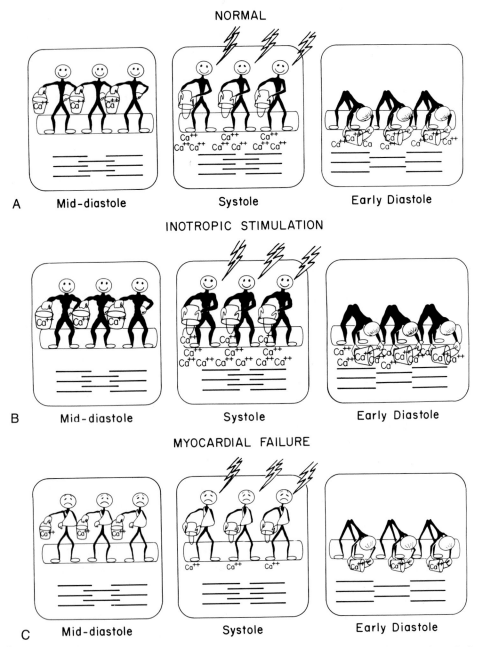

Fig. 8-8 Cartoons depicting the function of the sarcoplasmic reticulum (SR) during systole and diastole in normal cells (**A**), normal cells under the influence of inotropic stimulation (**B**), and cells in myocardial failure (**C**). (**A**) In normal cells, the SR (depicted by the men) binds most of the intracellular calcium during diastole. With electric stimulation during systole, the SR releases the calcium, which interacts with the contractile proteins to produce contraction. During early diastole the SR binds the calcium again resulting in muscle relaxation. (**B**) With inotropic stimulation, the SR binds more calcium during diastole, allowing it to release more during systole. More forceful contraction results. (**C**) In myocardial failure, the dysfunctional SR is unable to bind as much calcium during diastole and so less calcium is available for release during systole. Myocardial contractility is decreased as a result.

The cardiovascular system compensates for decreased stroke volume by increasing heart rate and renal salt and water retention. The increase in heart rate increases cardiac output:

Cardiac output = stroke volume × heart rate

The increase in fluid retention increases end-diastolic volume and thereby increases stroke volume. The increase in end-diastolic volume causes the normal ventricular wall to stretch around a larger than normal chamber; thus, the ventricular wall becomes thinner, increasing end-diastolic wall stress. The myocardium compensates through hypertrophy. In volume overload (increased end-diastolic volume), sarcomeres (i.e., the contractile elements in the myocardium) replicate in series.[20] The end result is a ventricular wall with normal thickness and a larger or dilated ventricular chamber. The increased wall thickness reduces afterload (wall stress) back toward normal and helps maintain systolic function.

The replication of the sarcomeres in series (sarcomere hyperplasia) results in the heart growing larger and is called *eccentric hypertrophy*. The larger heart is then able to pump a greater stroke volume for any given decrease in myocardial contractility.

As an example, let us define contractility as the extent of myocardial contraction and assume that afterload remains constant in this situation. A normal dog whose measured end-systolic volume is 30 ml and end-diastolic volume is 70 ml has a stroke volume of 40 ml and an ejection fraction of 57 percent. The percentage of the end-diastolic volume ejected during systole is calculated as follows:

Ejection fraction =
        stroke volume/end-diastolic volume

The dog then develops a gradual decrease in contractility, resulting in an increase in end-systolic volume to 60 ml. To compensate, the kidneys retain salt and water and blood volume increases, resulting in an increase in left ventricular end-diastolic volume (e.g., to 100 ml) through eccentric hypertrophy. The stroke volume is still 40 ml. However, end-systolic volume has increased and the percentage of blood ejected has diminished to 48 percent. The heart is less efficient now but is still able to eject a normal quantity of blood for that given size of patient. Because of these compensatory changes, the heart in this 60-lb dog has enlarged to a size comparable to that in a 90-lb dog. However, if contractility were normal in the larger dog, its heart would still eject 57 percent of the end-diastolic volume and result in a normal end-systolic volume for its size. The net comparison illustrates that for the same size heart a larger stroke volume occurs for the larger dog (having a normal heart), while a normal stroke volume may result for the smaller dog having myocardial failure but at the expense of a larger less efficient heart. Eventually, eccentric hypertrophy becomes inadequate when myocardial failure becomes severe and stroke volume decreases.

A wall stress-volume loop from a patient with severe myocardial failure typical of congestive (dilated) cardiomyopathy is depicted in Figure 8-9. End-diastolic volume index is increased from <100 ml/m^2 of body surface area (i.e., normal) to 250 ml/m^2. Similarly, end-systolic volume index is increased from a normal value of <30 ml/m^2 to 220 ml/m^2. The mitral valve annulus has been enlarged by left ventricular dilation, resulting in some mitral regurgitation. This patient's total left ventricular stroke volume index (i.e., end-diastolic volume index − end-systolic volume index) is 30 ml/m^2. However, 40 percent of that stroke volume index is ejected into the left atrium due to the mitral regurgitation. Therefore, the forward stroke volume index (that amount ejected into the aorta) is only 18 ml/m^2. Normal stroke volume index = 40 to 50 ml/m^2. I have seen forward stroke volumes as low as 5 ml/m^2 of body surface area in dogs with congestive (dilated) cardiomyopathy. Because of the large end-diastolic volume and a stiffer than normal myocardium, the end-diastolic pressure is increased, causing pulmonary edema. The increased end-diastolic pressure and chamber dilation has increased end-diastolic wall stress, maximally stretching the sarcomeres at end-diastole. However, they were already maximally stretched at a much lower wall stress; thus, the added wall stress only stimulates further sarcomere replication and chamber dilation. Because of the myocardial failure, sarcomeres are unable to respond normally to an increase in end-diastolic sarcomere length. Therefore, this mechanism probably no longer helps increase stroke volume. Compensatory myocardial hypertrophy may not be adequate enough to offset the increase in chamber size. As a result, an increase in systolic wall

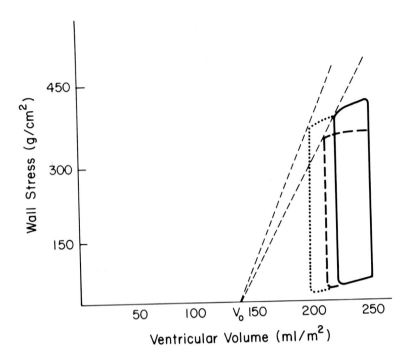

Fig. 8-9 Wall stress-volume loops from a dog with severe myocardial failure. The solid line represents baseline values. End-diastolic ventricular volume is increased because of renal salt and water retention leading to eccentric hypertrophy. End-systolic volume is increased because of decreased myocardial contractility and increased systolic wall stress (afterload). Compared with Fig. 8-7, E_{max} (the slope of the line defining contractility) is flatter than normal and Vo (the x intercept of that line) is shifted to the right (i.e., myocardial contractility is decreased). The dotted line represents a portion of the new loop formed after administration of a positive inotrope. E_{max} becomes steeper resulting in a decrease in end-systolic volume and therefore, increase in stroke volume. The dashed line forms a portion of a new loop that forms after the administration of an arteriolar dilator. E_{max} and Vo do not change, but systolic wall stress decreases because of the resultant decrease in blood pressure. End-systolic volume decreases as a result of increased stroke volume.

stress (afterload) contributes to the poor myocardial contraction.

Mitral, aortic, and tricuspid regurgitation and left-to-right shunts, such as ventricular septal defect (VSD) and patent ductus arteriosus (PDA) are examples of leaks that cause volume overloads of either the left or right heart, or both. The volume overload is there to compensate for the leaks within the cardiovascular system. It results in eccentric hypertrophy of the involved chambers and, if severe, heart failure. Myocardial failure can result from prolonged volume overloading but is usually not severe, except in longstanding PDA and aortic regurgitation.

To contrast with myocardial failure (Fig. 8-9), a wall stress-volume loop for a dog with acute mitral regurgitation is illustrated (Fig. 8-10). Acute mitral regurgitation causes a decrease in forward stroke volume by permitting a certain percentage of the ejected stroke volume to leak from the left ventricle back into the left atrium. The increased left atrial volume increases left atrial pressure and pulmonary

capillary pressure. This causes pulmonary edema. The decreased stroke volume and cardiac output stimulates catecholamine release, thereby increasing heart rate, renin release, and contractility (via β-adrenergic receptor stimulation). Within 2 to 4 days, the β-receptors become desensitized to catecholamine stimulation and contractility returns to normal.[21] Fluid retention then becomes the major compensatory change for the loss of stroke volume by increasing end-diastolic volume through eccentric hypertrophy. Since contractility is normal and systolic wall stress relatively normal, end-systolic volume is normal. The net result is an increase in total left ventricular stroke volume. A variable percentage of the stroke volume, however, is ejected into the left atrium, again causing increased left atrial pressure and a decreased forward stroke volume. Myocardial contractility tends to remain normal for a prolonged period.[22]

The progression from acute pressure overload to myocardial failure is shown in Figure 8-11. Acute aortic stenosis results in increased intraventricular

Fig. 8-10 Wall stress-volume loop from a dog with mitral regurgitation. There is no isovolumic systole because blood is ejected into the left atrium as soon as systole starts. Because the left ventricle is able to unload itself into the left atrium, peak systolic wall stress remains normal. In this case, end-diastolic volume index has increased to 250 ml/m², while end-systolic volume has remained normal at 25 ml/m². The stroke volume index is markedly increased to 225 ml/m², but about 90 percent of that stroke volume index is ejected into the left atrium. Therefore, the regurgitant stroke volume index is 200 ml/m², and the forward stroke volume index (i.e., the amount ejected into the aorta) is 25 ml/m².

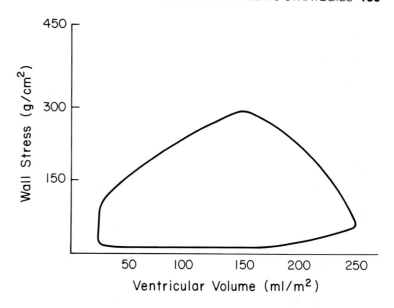

Fig. 8-11 Relationships between ventricular wall stress or tension (T), intraventricular pressure (P), ventricular radius (r), and ventricular wall thickness (h) in aortic stenosis. LaPlace's law predicts that the load on the myocardial fibers (i.e., wall stress or tension) equals (Pxr)/2h. If afterload increases with elevated intraventricular pressure, it follows from this equation that systolic wall stress or tension increases. (**A**) The myocardium must develop greater force to eject the same stroke volume. Concentric hypertrophy occurs as a compensatory response to reduce systolic wall stress. (**B**) If the myocardium fails, renal salt and water retention increases end-diastolic volume and radius. This again increases systolic wall stress and reduces left ventricular performance (**C**). (Modified from Fox PR, Bond BR: Congestive Heart Failure in Dogs. Hoechst-Roussel Agri-Vet Co Monograph, Somerville, NJ, 1985.)

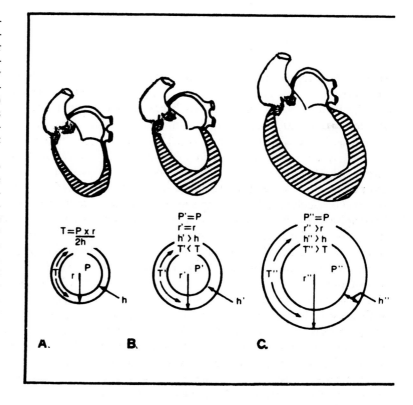

pressure, causing wall tension or stress (afterload) during systole to increase (Fig. 8-11A). This increase in the force against which the ventricle must pump initially results in an increase in end-systolic volume and a decrease in stroke volume. The myocardium responds to this pressure overload through concentric hypertrophy (Fig. 8-11B). In concentric hypertrophy, the sarcomeres are thought to replicate in parallel, causing the muscle to thicken. The heart muscle responds to this increase in systolic force in the same way that skeletal muscle responds to an increased lifting force, as evidenced by the muscular hypertrophy seen in weight lifters. The concentric hypertrophy decreases systolic wall stress back to or toward normal, decreasing end-systolic volume (the bigger muscle can contract further or lift a weight further) and normalizes left ventricular function. Because capillary density does not increase adequately with increased muscle mass, muscle with concentric hypertrophy can become hypoxic, leading to arrhythmias, sudden death, and myocardial failure (Fig. 8-11C). Myocardial failure results in increased end-systolic volume and decreased stroke volume and cardiac output. Compensatory responses include retention of salt and water, resulting in increased end-diastolic volume. This causes an increase in chamber radius and increased wall stress, further increasing end-systolic volume.

Myocardial failure in volume and pressure overloads probably develop because of prolonged increases in myocardial oxygen consumption and resultant myocardial hypoxia. Volume and pressure overloads tend to produce chronic increases in systolic myocardial wall stress, especially if the volume or pressure overloads are severe and the myocardial hypertrophy cannot adequately compensate for the increased wall stress. Systolic wall stress is a major determinant of myocardial oxygen consumption; thus, when wall stress is elevated, myocardial oxygen consumption is increased. Oxygen delivery/consumption at rest is less in the myocardium than in all other organs of the body. Even small increases in oxygen consumption can result in mild myocardial hypoxia.

In mitral regurgitation, about 50 percent of the total left ventricular stroke volume is ejected into the left atrium before the aortic valve opens. This permits the left ventricle to eject a large blood volume at relatively low pressure and with low wall stress. As a result, myocardial oxygen consumption and myocardial contractility remains normal for prolonged periods.[22] Ventricular septal defects cause similar hemodynamic alterations, and myocardial function remains similarly preserved.

By contrast, with aortic regurgitation, the left ventricle must eject all its increased stroke volume into the high-pressure aorta, increasing wall stress and oxygen consumption and resulting in earlier development of myocardial failure. The same is true for PDA.

THERAPEUTIC STRATEGIES

Myocardial Failure

Therapy for myocardial failure at this time involves administration of a positive inotropic agent to improve contractility and diuretics, vasodilators, and sodium-restricted diets to relieve clinical signs (e.g., edema, effusions) resulting from decreased contractility. Antiarrhythmic therapy is crucial for many patients with myocardial failure, especially when atrial fibrillation is present. Response of a failing left ventricle to positive inotropes, diuretics, and vasodilators is illustrated in Figures 8-2, 8-3, and 8-9.

The treatment modality depends on the severity of clinical heart failure signs (functional class I is not treated) as depicted in Figure 8-12. For dogs in functional class II, vigorous exercise should be restricted. Administration of an orally active positive inotrope may be indicated at this stage and a low dose of a diuretic may be helpful. (Fig. 8-12) Patients with functional class III failure should receive an orally active positive inotrope. If they respond well to a positive inotrope and have no extracardiac sign of congestion, no further therapy may be required. If they do not respond, diuretics will be needed to control clinical signs from edema or effusions. A low-salt diet may be beneficial but is not crucial, since signs of backward failure can usually be readily controlled with diuretic administration. Vigorous exercise should be curtailed. Normal exercise should only be curtailed if the patient fails to control its own activity. Patients in functional class IV due to myocardial failure require positive inotropic support. The prognosis depends on the animal's ability

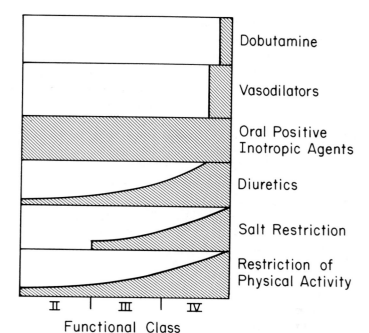

Dobutamine

Vasodilators

Oral Positive
Inotropic Agents

Diuretics

Salt Restriction

Restriction of
Physical Activity

Functional Class

Fig. 8-12. Therapeutic strategy for treating dogs with myocardial failure (e.g., dilated cardiomyopathy) based on functional class of heart failure.

to respond to a positive inotrope; it is much better if the animal does respond.[23] Therefore, prognostication should be withheld until response has been ascertained. Adjunctive therapy with diuretics is almost always needed. A low-salt diet may be beneficial if the response to diuretics is inadequate. Vasodilators may improve clinical signs and generally appear to prolong survival time.

Patients presented with fulminant pulmonary edema require emergency medical therapy. Intravenous administration of dobutamine or amrinone is indicated for inotropic support. The administration of massive doses of furosemide (up to 8 mg/kg every 1 to 2 hours for dogs) may be lifesaving with severe pulmonary edema. Oxygen therapy may be required for survival but should not be administered by mask if the patient struggles. Any type of stress (e.g., restraint for radiographs, restraint for venipuncture) in this situation must be avoided, since it increases tissue oxygen demands and serum catecholamine concentrations, which can result in death.

Volume Overloads

The therapeutic strategy for treating heart failure secondary to volume overload depends on the lesion producing the volume overload. Ideally, every le-

sion would be treted surgically in order to cure the cause of the overload. This is generally not feasible in veterinary medicine. A therapeutic strategy for treating patients with mitral regurgitation is shown in Figure 8-13.

Patients with mitral regurgitation usually respond well to agents that decrease the volume overload (hence signs of backward heart failure) or decrease the degree of mitral regurgitation (and signs of backward and forward heart failure). Positive inotropes, such as digitalis glycosides, may be used but may not produce beneficial effects like other pharmacologic agents. Newer positive inotropes, such as milrinone, also have arteriolar dilating properties and may be efficacious. Response of a failing left ventricle (from chronic mitral regurgitation) to positive inotropes, diuretics, and vasodilators is illustrated in Figures 8-2 and 8-3.

Functional class II patients with mitral regurgitation respond well to exercise restriction. Low-dose diuretic administration is occasionally helpful. Functional class III patients respond well to low to medium doses of a potent diuretic, such as furosemide, or to medium to high doses of a thiazide diuretic. If the patient will eat a commercial low-salt diet or sodium-restricted diet prepared by the owner, either may be instituted. Their use may re-

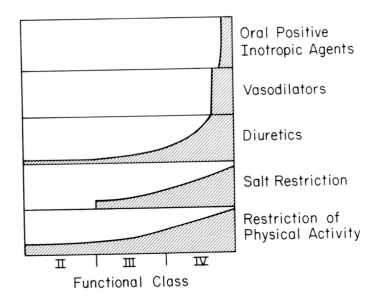

Fig. 8-13. Therapeutic strategy for treating dogs with volume overload from acquired mitral regurgitation based on functional class of heart failure.

duce the required dose of diuretic. A low-salt diet at this time is not critical, however, since the diuretic dose can readily be adjusted to control signs of heart failure. Furosemide may be started at 2 mg/kg given every 8 to 12 hours and adjusted according to the patient's response.

Dogs that first present in function class IV heart failure due to mitral regurgitation may respond to the administration of diuretics but require higher doses (e.g., up to 4 mg/kg every 8 to 12 hours initially for furosemide). Digitalis is often administered at this time as well, but preliminary data suggest that it provides little benefit.[24] Patients in functional class IV failure may become refractory to furosemide. These patients respond well to vasodilators or to the addition of a thiazide diuretic. Hydralazine, an arteriolar dilator, increases forward stroke volume and decreases regurgitant flow, resulting in a decrease in left atrial pressure and reduction in pulmonary edema.[25] Hydralazine also improves renal clearance of furosemide by increasing renal blood flow in patients with heart failure. This increases the effectiveness of furosemide.[26] Some patients experience gastrointestinal (GI) irritation with hydralazine and cannot tolerate its administration. If hydralazine is not efficacious or causes untoward effect, captopril (a balanced vasodilator) may be used as a substitute. It is second choice because not all patients respond well to it.[24] Vasodilators can cause reflex tachycardia necessi-

tating use of a negative chronotropic agent. A digitalis glycoside is generally the first choice for this purpose, since it has no negative inotropic effects (i.e., it does not decrease myocardial contractility). A β-adrenergic blocking agent, such as propranolol, is the second choice but may decrease contractility. Patients refractory to furosemide and a vasodilator should receive a positive inotrope. The clinical response to newer and more powerful positive inotropes, such as milrinone, should be better than the response to the digitalis glycosides.

In patients with aortic regurgitation, generally bacterial endocarditis is the cause. If the patient is in heart failure, onset of clinical signs is often acute or subacute. Diuretics and vasodilators, such as hydralazine, are generally the most effective agents in treating congestive heart failure. Milrinone may be beneficial as well, but studies have not yet been performed to document efficacy in this situation.

Puppies with decompensated congenital heart defects such as PDA may present in heart failure. Myocardial failure is not a prominent feature of this disease in the early stages. Treatment should consist of diuretic administration before surgical closure of the ductus arteriosus is performed. Occasionally, an older dog will present with heart failure due to long-standing PDA. These patients have severe myocardial failure and may be in atrial fibrillation. Treatment is the same as for congestive (dilated) cardiomyopathy, except that the patent ductus should be ligated as soon as the animal is stabilized.

Tricuspid regurgitation results in volume overload of the right heart in the same fashion as described for mitral regurgitation, causing volume overload of the left heart. The function of the right ventricular myocardium in tricuspid regurgitation is unknown; it may be normal or depressed. Therapy of right heart failure due to tricuspid regurgitation generally consists of diuretic and digitalis administration. Milrinone may be beneficial, but its efficacy in this disease is unknown. Captopril may help control ascites in patients refractory to other drugs. Repeated abdominocenteses may be required in patients refractory to drug therapy.

Causes of volume overloads due to left-to-right shunts other than PDA are only rarely treated surgically. Heart failure due to ventricular septal defects alone or in combination with other lesions resulting in left-to-right shunts (e.g., endocardial cushion defects in cats) can be managed medically with diuretics in the early to middle stages. Digitalis may be used but probably is not beneficial enough to result in clinical improvement unless a supraventricular arrhythmia is present as well. Arteriolar dilators decrease the amount of left-to-right shunting across a ventricular septal defect by decreasing left ventricular pressure, hence, the driving force for blood flow across the ventricular septal defect. Hydralazine can be used for this purpose in dogs and cats.

Atrial septal defects cause right heart volume overload. Lesions large enough to produce heart failure are rare. Heart failure can be managed with diuretics, and digitalis may or may not be used. Milrinone may be effective but is currently untested in this situation. Captopril may be used as adjunctive therapy.

Pressure Overloads

Pressure overloads are generally created by stenotic lesions involving the great arteries, valves or outflow tracts of either ventricle (e.g., subvalvular, valvular, and supravalvular aortic or pulmonic stenosis). This condition also can be secondary to systemic or pulmonary hypertension. It is uncommon for systemic hypertension alone to produce signs of heart failure. More commonly, systemic hyperten-

sion complicates mitral regurgitation by exacerbating left heart failure in dogs. Pulmonary hypertension secondary to heartworm disease is a common cause of right heart failure in endemic areas.

Extremely severe pulmonic or aortic stenosis can, by itself, cause signs of heart failure. More commonly, longstanding severe stenotic lesions result in myocardial failure, diastolic dysfunction, and signs of heart failure. These patients should be treated similarly to animals with congestive (dilated) cardiomyopathy. Systolic wall stress in these cases is increased because of elevated left ventricular systolic pressure. End-systolic volume increases because of the reduction in myocardial contractility and elevation in systolic wall stress. The combination of myocardial failure and increased systolic wall stress limits myocardial fiber shortening and makes this problem especially difficult to treat. The prognosis is poorer than for patients with myocardial failure alone.

DRUGS USED IN TREATING HEART FAILURE

Digitalis Glycosides

Since their auspicious beginning in the treatment of dropsy by William Withering[27] in 1785, the digitalis glycosides have been embroiled in controversy regarding their use, mechanism of action, and efficacy. During the nineteenth century, they were regarded only as useful in controlling rapid heart rates and were considered too toxic for the treatment of heart failure in patients with sinus rhythm. Early in the twentieth century, documentation of the positive inotropic effects and efficacy in treating patients with heart failure in sinus rhythm was provided. Since that time, digitalis has become one of the most studied of all cardiac drugs. Still, controversy exists, especially pertaining to its efficacy in treating myocardial failure. The human literature is replete with reports documenting the efficacy[28-31] and lack of efficacy[32-35] of digitalis in the treatment of heart failure patients. The controversy may be partly attributable to the fact that populations are usually heterogeneous (e.g., patients with congestive cardiomyopathy, coronary artery disease, and valvular disease are commonly combined in one study). Also, some patients respond well to the drug, while others do not. Investigators who identify a homogeneous response tend to report their findings more readily, so reports of heterogeneous responses are fewer. Many investigators report their findings according to the group's response; moreover, the variability of individual patient responses is often ignored in the literature.

Pharmacodynamics

The digitalis glycosides increase contractility in normal myocardium and may also do so in failing myocardium. However, their ability to increase contractility in normal myocardium is only about one-third that of the sympathomimetics (e.g., dopamine, dobutamine) and bipyridine compounds (e.g., milrinone).

The positive inotropic effect of digitalis is thought to be caused by the effect of digitalis on the $Na,^+K^+$-ATPase pump located on myocardial cell membranes.[36] Digitalis competitively binds to the site at which potassium normally attaches and effectively stops pump activity.[37] Thus, the cell loses its most effective means of extruding sodium from the intracellular space during diastole, resulting in an increase in intracellular sodium concentration. This leads to increased intracellular osmolality, a potentially lethal situation for the cell. The cell counters by exchanging the intracellular sodium for extracellular calcium. The net result is an increase in the number of calcium ions within the cell. In a normal cell, these excess calcium ions are bound by the sarcoplasmic reticulum during diastole. They are subsequently released onto the contractile proteins during systole, causing increased contractility.[38] This mechanism also works in failing myocardium if the myocytes are able to handle increased calcium or if there is a mixed population of normal with failing cells able to respond to the digitalis. If all or most cells are badly damaged, it seems unreasonable to expect digitalis to cause increased contractility. In cells in a failing myocardium, the sarcoplasmic reticulum is thought to be diseased.[39] As a result, they are unable to bind as much calcium during diastole and so cannot release as much calcium during systole. Poor contractility and elevated diastolic concentrations of calcium result. Digitalis should not be able to force more calcium into the cell in this situation. Even if it did, it is unlikely that this would result in increased contractility. Cells that are overloaded with calcium are thought to be electrically unstable.[19,40] If digitalis did increase intracellular calcium in this situation, further electric instability and arrhythmia formation could occur.

The digitalis glycosides are used as antiarrhythmic agents, mostly for controlling supraventricular tachyarrhythmias. These agents increase parasympathetic nerve activity to the sinus node, atria, and AV node when digitalis serum concentrations are within the therapeutic range.[41] By so doing, they decrease sinus rate, are capable of abolishing supraventricular premature depolarizations and supraventricular tachycardia, and usually slow the ventricular response to atrial flutter and fibrillation. They also produce direct effects that help slow AV nodal conduction and prolong the AV nodal refractory period.

Although digitalis may be effective in controlling some ventricular arrhythmias, other drugs are preferred. Digitalis should be used with extreme caution for this purpose in patients with myocardial failure. The mechanism by which digitalis glycosides suppress ventricular arrhythmias may be related to increased vagal tone. In one study on human subjects, 45 percent of patients had improved rhythms after administration of acetylstrophanthidin, a short-acting cardiac glycoside, while 26 percent showed no change and 28 percent had worse ventricular arrhythmias.[42] There were no clinical or hemodynamic features that predicted which patients would respond to the drug. The antiarrhythmic effect appeared to be separate from any positive inotropic action. Proarrhythmic effects of digitalis in the setting of heart failure and ventricular arrhythmias must always be a clinical concern.

Clinical Uses and Efficacy

The digitalis glycosides are indicated for the treatment of myocardial failure and supraventricular tachyarrhythmias. Myocardial failure is always present in patients with congestive (dilated) cardiomyopathy or longstanding (>5 to 7 years) PDA. It is usually present in patients with heart failure secondary to longstanding pressure overload and with subacute to chronic severe aortic regurgitation. Myocardial failure is usually not severe in dogs with heart failure secondary to chronic volume overloads other than aortic regurgitation and longstanding PDA.

Myocardial failure is never present in hypertrophic cardiomyopathy and pericardial diseases. The use of digitalis for the treatment of heart failure due to chronic volume overload is not contraindicated, but other drugs are more beneficial. Digitalis is usually contraindicated in hypertrophic cardiomyopathy, since increased contractility can worsen outflow tract gradients. In cats with right heart failure secondary to hypertrophic cardiomyopathy, its use has been advocated but efficacy unproved. It is not contraindicated in pericardial diseases, but beneficial effects should not be expected.

In dogs with myocardial failure, digitalis does not routinely result in a clinically significant increase in myocardial contractility. Of 22 dogs with congestive cardiomyopathy in one study, only five responded to digoxin.[23] All five dogs had lived longer than 6 months after their response. Dogs with congestive cardiomyopathy that respond to digoxin live significantly longer than do those that do not respond.[24]

The digitalis glycosides are also used to treat supraventriculr tachyarrhythmias. They are generally regarded as being moderately effective in controlling supraventricular premature depolarization and supraventricular tachycardia and moderately effective for controlling the ventricular rate in atrial fibrillation.

Pharmacokinetics

The pharmacokinetics of the two most commonly used digitalis glycosides, digoxin and digitoxin, are remarkably different despite their similar molecular structures. Digoxin is well absorbed after oral administration. Approximately 60 percent of the tablet is absorbed, while about 75 percent of the elixir is absorbed. There is very little hepatic metabolism, so that almost all of the drug that is absorbed reaches the serum. In the serum, 27 percent of digoxin is bound to albumin.[43]

In the dog, serum half-life is 23 to 39 hours.[44,45] Much interpatient variability exists. With a drug whose half-life exceeds the dosing interval (digoxin is usually administered every 12 hours in the dog), drug accumulation occurs until a steady-state serum

concentration is reached. It takes one half-life to achieve 50 percent of the steady-state serum concentration, two half-lives to reach 75 percent, three half-lives to reach 87.5 percent, and so forth. Theoretically, it takes about five half-lives to reach steady state, and so it is commonly thought that five half-lives are required to achieve therapeutic serum concentrations. However, this is not the case. Serum concentrations of digoxin between 1.0 and 2.5 ng/ml are generally considered to be within the therapeutic range.[46] The canine maintenance dose of digoxin (0.011 mg/kg BID) generally achieves serum concentrations of 1.5 to 2.0 ng/ml. Serum concentrations after two half-lives should be 1.1 to 1.5 ng/ml and after three half-lives, 1.3 to 1.75 ng/ml. Therefore, maintenance doses should achieve therapeutic serum concentrations within 2 to 4.5 days. In one study of dogs given 0.022 mg/kg digoxin every 24 hours, the serum concentration was within therapeutic range by the second day.[47] Based on these data, maintenance doses of digoxin in dogs should be used to achieve therapeutic serum concentrations in almost all situations. Loading doses designed to achieve therapeutic concentrations within a shorter period should only be used for emergencies, and then with great caution. Loading dose schedules routinely produce toxic serum concentrations. Other positive inotropic agents, such as dobutamine and amrinone, are safer and more efficacious and are preferred for acute short-term inotropic support. If digoxin is used parenterally in an emergency situation, it must be given slowly over at least 15 minutes, since rapid intravenous administration results in peripheral vasoconstriction and increased afterload.[48]

Most of a digoxin dose is excreted in the urine via glomerular filtration and renal secretion. About 15 percent is metabolized in the liver. Renal failure reduces renal clearance, body clearance, and volume of distribution, resulting in increased serum digoxin concentrations.[49] Digoxin should generally be avoided in dogs with renal failure and digitoxin used instead. Formulas have been devised to calculate the reduction in digoxin dosage needed to achieve therapeutic serum concentrations in humans with renal failure.[50] There is no correlation between the degree of azotemia and serum digoxin concentrations in the dog, so such formulas cannot be used.[51] Digitoxin is not a viable option for cats due to its long half-life in that species. Therefore, in cats and dogs with renal failure that are given digoxin, the dosage should be markedly reduced and serum concentrations monitored.

The pharmacokinetics of digoxin in the cat are controversial. The half-life is variable from cat to cat, ranging from 25.6 to 50.6 hours in one study (mean = 33.5 hours)[52] and 39.4 to 78.8 hours in another report (mean = 57.8 hours).[45] The first study reported that the half-life of digoxin increased dramatically to an average of 72.7 hours after prolonged oral administration. The elixir formulation results in serum concentrations approximately 50 percent higher than the tablet.[53] However, cats generally dislike the taste of the alcohol-based elixir. When digoxin tablets are administered with food to cats, serum concentrations are reduced by about 50 percent compared to the concentrations without food.[53]

Tincture of digitoxin (Foxalin, Standex Laboratories Inc, Columbus, OH) has superior pharmacokinetic properties in the dog as compared with digoxin.[54] Its half-life is only 8 to 12 hours. Therapeutic serum concentrations can be achieved more rapidly than with digoxin, and serum concentrations decrease more quickly if a dog becomes toxic; 95 to 100 percent of tincture of digitoxin is absorbed. About 90 percent of the drug is bound to serum protein, so a higher dose of digitoxin is needed relative to digoxin. Digitoxin is excreted by the liver and can therefore be used safely in dogs with renal failure.

In cats, the half-life of digitoxin is greater than 100 hours.[55] Therefore, this drug should be avoided in cats. Digoxin is the only recommended digitalis glycoside.[56]

In small dogs weighing less than 22 kg, digoxin may be dosed based on body weight at 0.011 mg/kg given every 12 hours. In dogs weighing more than 22 kg, this dose can not be safely used. Instead, dosage should be based on body surface area (i.e., 0.22 mg/m^2 of body surface area given every 12 hours).[55]

Digoxin is dosed at one-fourth of a 0.125-mg tablet given every other day for cats weighing less than 3 kg; at one-fourth tablet every day for cats weighing 3 to 6 kg; and at one-fourth tablet every day to BID for cats weighing more than 6 kg.[56] Tablets are better tolerated than the elixir.

The dose of digitoxin in dogs is 0.033 mg/kg given every 8 to 12 hours.[54] In general, small dogs should receive the dose every 8 hours and large dogs every 12 hours. The cumulative daily dose in small dogs would be greater than that for large dogs on a per-weight basis but similar on a per-body surface area basis.

Commonly, the dose of a digitalis glycoside needs to be modified because of factors that alter the pharmacokinetics of the drug. In a study in which digoxin dose (0.005 to 0.23 mg/kg/day) was plotted against serum concentration in dogs with heart failure, the correlation coefficient was only 0.39 (1.0 is a perfect correlation).[57] This weak correlation was statistically significant. Drug dosage is therefore a factor determining serum concentration, but it is only one factor among a number of other variables to consider when dosing digoxin.

Because most of the digitalis is bound to skeletal muscle, dogs or cats that have lost a significant muscle mass have increased serum concentrations for any given dose. Therefore, for patients that are cachectic, the dose must be reduced. Older dogs commonly have decreased muscle mass and impaired renal function, so dosing digoxin in these patients must be performed cautiously.

Digoxin is poorly lipid soluble. Therefore, dosing should be based on a lean body weight estimate. Conversely, digitoxin is lipid soluble, so no change in dosage is required for lean or obese dogs.

The administration of other drugs along with digitalis may affect the serum levels. Quinidine displaces digoxin from skeletal muscle binding sites and reduces its renal clearance, resulting in increased serum digoxin concentrations.[58] Quinidine probably also displaces digoxin from myocardial binding sites.[59] This may lessen the direct cardiac toxicity of digoxin and decrease its positive inotropic effect. In general, the combination of digoxin and quinidine should be avoided. If both drugs must be used together, the rule of thumb in human medicine is to reduce the digoxin dosage by 50 percent.[60] No interaction between digitoxin and quinidine exists in the dog. Verapamil also increases serum digoxin concentrations, so they should be administered together cautiously.[61]

Drugs that alter hepatic microsomal enzymes may affect digoxin pharmacokinetics, since about

15 percent of digoxin is metabolized in the liver.[62] Drugs that induce hepatic microsomal enzymes, such as phenylbutazone and the barbiturates, may have a tendency to increase digoxin clearance, while such drugs as chloramphenicol and tetracycline, which inhibit hepatic enzymes, should increase the serum digoxin concentration. However, one study has documented that chloramphenicol decreases serum digoxin concentration in dogs.[63] The effects of these drugs on digitoxin elimination are unknown.

Hypokalemia predisposes to digitalis myocardial toxicity. Digitalis and potassium compete for binding sites on the membrane Na^+, K^+-ATPase pump. Hypokalemia leaves more binding sites available for digitalis. Hyperkalemia displaces digitalis from the myocardium. Hypercalcemia and hypernatremia potentiate the positive inotropic and toxic effects of digitalis, while hypocalcemia and hyponatremia reduce these effects.

Hyperthyroidism increases the myocardial effects of digitalis, while hypothyroidism reduces its clearance.[49] The dose may need to be decreased in both situations.

Myocardial failure increases the sensitivity of the myocardium to the toxic effects of digitalis. Failing myocardial cells are usually thought to be overloaded with calcium. Digitalis may cause further calcium loading. Calcium-overloaded cells may become electrically unstable, resulting in tachyarrhythmias.[64] Digitalis should be administered cautiously in these patients, and loading doses should not be used.

Hypoxia increases the sensitivity of the myocardium to the toxic effects of digitalis. The mechanism is unexplained but digitalis should be used carefully in hypoxemic patients.

In general, patients to receive digitalis should be evaluated carefully before its administration. Factors that alter the dosage should be noted and an initial dose chosen. The patient should be monitored during the initial course of therapy for signs of toxicity or improvement. A decrease in heart rate or resolution of an arrhythmia are documentable benefits in patients with tachycardia or arrhythmia. Clinical responsiveness due to improved hemodynamics in patients with heart failure is the desired endpoint of digitalis administration but can be difficult to identify. First, other drugs are generally given with digitalis, so it may be impossible to identify the beneficial drug. Second, many dogs do not respond to digoxin, so clinical resolution may never occur. The dosage in the latter case should not be increased unless serum concentrations have been measured and documented to be subtherapeutic (i.e., less than 1.0 ng/ml).

Toxicity

Therapeutic end points for digitalis in patients with heart failure include clinical improvement or attainment of therapeutic serum concentration. Progressive dosing until signs of toxicity occur or until the P-R interval is prolonged is not justified.[65] By the time GI signs of toxicity are present in dogs with myocardial failure, myocardial toxicity is usually present and may be fatal. Dogs without myocardial failure (e.g., dogs with mitral regurgitation) tolerate digitalis toxicity much better than do those with myocardial failure (i.e., myocardial toxicity occurs at higher serum concentrations) and generally show signs of anorexia and vomiting before exhibiting electrocardiographic (ECG) evidence of myocardial toxicity.

The incidence of digoxin toxicity in human medicine is estimated to be between 13 and 23 percent.[66] At the same time, 11 to 36 percent of patients have been identified as being underdigitalized. The incidence in veterinary medicine is less clear. In one canine study, 25 percent of dogs receiving digoxin had a serum concentration in the toxic range, while 24 percent had subtherapeutic concentrations. In dogs receiving digitoxin, 5 percent were found to be toxic and 19 percent to be in the subtherapeutic range.[54] In my experience, digitalis toxicity is rare if the drug is used judiciously. It typically occurs if an owner becomes overzealous with drug administration when the patient is not responding and when the pet develops renal failure while on digoxin.

Problems from digitalis intoxication fall into two general classes: those referrable to GI signs and those referrable to myocardial toxicity. Anorexia and vomiting are probably due to the direct effect of the digitalis molecule on chemoreceptors located in the area postrema in the medulla.[67] In dogs without myocardial failure, GI signs of toxicity generally occur well before signs of myocardial toxicity. This may not be true in the patient with myocardial failure. Also, signs of anorexia may go unnoticed in the hospitalized patient, especially if the animal was not eating before digitalis administration.

Myocardial toxicity is the most serious complication of digitalis administration. Toxic serum concentration disrupt the normal electric activity of the heart in several ways. Sympathetic nerve activity to the heart is increased, resulting in increased automaticity.[68] Digitalis slows conduction and alters the refractory period, making it easier for re-entrant arrhythmias to develop. Myocardial cells normally cannot depolarize spontaneously, but digitalis can promote abnormal automaticity by stimulating them to undergo diastolic depolarization.[64] The classic cellular event is the formation of late afterdepolarizations in which the diastolic membrane potential oscillates, eventually reaches threshold potential, and depolarizes the cell. The counterpart of this depolarization would be a premature beat. Late afterpolarizations are attributed to cellular calcium overload and are more easily induced in myocardium that has been stretched (analogous to the dilated heart) and in a hypokalemic environment.

Clinically, myocardial toxicity can take the form of almost every known rhythm disturbance. In the dog, ventricular tachyarrhythmias are most common, consisting of ventricular premature depolarizations, ventricular bigeminy and trigeminy, and ventricular tachycardia. Digitalis, however, can induce supraventricular premature depolarizations and tachycardia, junctional escape rhythms, sinus arrest, Mobitz type-1 second-degree AV block, and other arrhythmias. At times it may be difficult or impossible to distinguish whether an arrhythmia is due to digitalis or to the underlying heart disease. Arrhythmias characterized by tachycardia with impaired conduction are highly suggestive of digitalis-induced problems. Ventricular tachyarrhythmias appearing in a dog taking digitalis should generally be regarded as being digitalis induced until proved otherwise.

Massive digitalis overdose can produce hyperkalemia and possibly hyponatremia.[69] This is probably caused by digitalis inhibition of the $Na,^+K^+$-ATPase pump throughout the body.

Treatment of Digitalis Intoxication

Gastrointestinal signs related to digitalis overdose are treated by drug withdrawal and correction of fluid and electrolyte abnormalities. Conduction disturbances usually require only digitalis withdrawal, although atropine administration is occasionally needed. Ventricular tachyarrhythmias are generally treated aggressively, especially when ventricular tachycardia is present. It is estimated that two-thirds of human patients with ventricular tachycardia secondary to digitalis intoxication will not survive, despite therapy.[70]

Lidocaine is the drug of choice for treating ventricular tachyarrhythmias due to digitalis intoxication. It decreases sympathetic nerve traffic and can abolish re-entrant arrhythmias and late after depolarizations.[19,71] Lidocaine usually has little effect on sinus rate or AV nodal conduction, so it does not exacerbate these problems. It is safe in the dog, can readily be administered intravenously, and has a rapid onset of action. It may be given as an initial bolus (2 to 4 mg/kg IV over 1 to 2 minutes) followed by continuous infusion of 30 to 80 µg/kg/min for arrhythmia control. Cats are more sensitive to the neurotoxic effects of lidocaine, so the dose must be reduced and the drug used with caution (0.25 to 1 mg/kg IV over 5 minutes).

Phenytoin (diphenylhydantoin) is the second drug of choice for the treatment of digitalis-induced toxicity in the dog. It has similar properties to lidocaine. When given intravenously, the drug vehicle can produce hypotension and exert a depressant effect on the myocardium.[72] Total intravenous dose is 10 mg/kg, given in 2-mg/kg increments over 3 to 5 minutes. Phenytoin can also be administered orally either to treat a ventricular tachyarrhythmia or to prevent tachyarrhythmias.[54] Oral dose is 35 mg/kg given every 8 hours.[73]

Serum potassium concentration should always be determined in patients intoxicated with digitalis. If serum potassium is less than 4.0 mEq/L, potassium supplements should be given, preferably in intravenous fluids. Potassium competes with digitalis for binding sites on the $Na,^+K^+$-ATPase pump and provides a more suitable environment for the antiarrhythmic agents to work.

Other drugs may be administered in digitalis intoxication. Propranolol may be useful for digitalis-induced ventricular tachyarrhythmias, but not when the patient exhibits conduction blocks. Quinidine increases the serum concentration of digoxin and should not be used to treat digitalis intoxication. Procainamide is less effective than other drugs in treating digitalis-induced arrhythmias.

Cholestyramine, a steroid-binding resin, may be useful in digitoxin and early digoxin intoxication.[74] Cholestyramine binds digitalis in the intestinal tract. Digitoxin undergoes enterohepatic circulation and so can be bound by this resin. However, digoxin undergoes minimal enterohepatic circulation so cholestyramine administration would only be useful soon after accidental overdose.

Cardiac glycoside-specific antibodies have recently been released for use in humans to bind digitalis glycosides in the bloodstream and thus remove them from myocardial binding sites.[75] This method may be a useful means of treating life-threatening digitalis intoxication in veterinary medicine in the future.

SYMPATHOMIMETICS

Sympathomimetic amines increase contractility by binding to cardiac β-adrenergic receptors. This interaction results in activation of adenyl cyclase within the cell. Adenyl cyclase cleaves adenosine triphosphate (ATP) to cyclic adenosine monophosphate (cAMP), which stimulates a cellular protein kinase system. Protein kinases phosphorylate intracellular proteins, such as the sarcoplasmic reticulum, allowing them to bind more calcium during diastole and thereby release more calcium during systole[76] (Fig. 8-14).

Most sympathomimetics have the ability to increase contractility about 100 percent above baseline, but many are unsuitable for treating heart failure because of other drug properties. Sympathomimetics also stimulate β$_2$- and α-adrenergic receptors. The degree to which each type of receptor is stimulated depends on the specific sympathomimetic.[77] Isoproterenol is a pure β-adrenergic-stimulating agent. It increases contractility but also increases heart rate, stimulates the formation of arrhythmias, and decreases blood pressure. Norepinephrine increases contractility but also stimulates peripheral α-adrenergic receptors, increasing blood pressure. Epinephrine also produces tachycardia and is arrhythmogenic. All three of these drugs are therefore unsuitable for treating heart failure. Newer sympathomimetics, such as dopamine and dobutamine, are less arrhythmogenic, produce less increase in heart rate, and are more suitable for heart failure therapy.[78]

All currently available sympathomimetics have very short half-lives (1 to 2 minutes). When given orally they are metabolized extensively by the liver.[79] Therefore, they must be administered intravenously, usually as a constant rate infusion.

Dopamine

Dopamine is the precursor of norepinephrine. It stimulates cardiac β$_1$-adrenergic receptors as well as peripherally located dopaminergic receptors.[80] The latter appear to be located most prevalently in the renal and mesenteric vascular beds, where they produce vasodilation. Dopamine administration to a patient with acute heart failure should improve contractility and thereby increase cardiac output. The renal and mesenteric vasodilation should cause preferential blood flow to these areas. In humans, dopamine administration to patients with chronic heart failure can cause increased ventricular filling pressures and edema formation.[81] For this reason, dopamine is only recommended for use in animals with acute myocardial failure.

The dosage for dopamine is 1 to 10 μg/kg/min. However, doses higher than 10 μg/kg/min can result in norepinephrine release and increased peripheral vascular resistance and heart rate.[82] An initial dose of 2 μg/kg/min may be started and titrated upward to obtain the desired clinical effect.

Dobutamine

Dobutamine is a synthetic catecholamine. It stimulates β$_1$-adrenergic receptors, increasing myocardial contractility. It also weakly stimulates peripheral β$_2$ and α$_1$-adrenergic receptors. As this response is balanced, systemic arterial blood pressure is usually unchanged after dobutamine administration.[83] Dobutamine is less arrhythmogenic than most of the other sympathomimetics and also produces little increase in heart rate. When administered to a patient

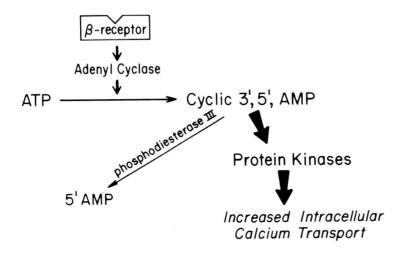

Fig. 8-14 Illustration depicting the cascade of events that results in increased myocardial contractility after myocardial β-adrenergic receptor stimulation. A similar cascade can be induced by phosphodiesterase III inhibition.

with acute or chronic heart failure, it should increase contractility and cardiac output and decrease ventricular diastolic pressures, leading to a decrease in edema formation.

In clinical situations, dobutamine can be used to treat acute heart failure until inotropic support is no longer needed or until other longer acting positive inotropic agents (e.g., digitalis) have taken effect. It can also be used to treat acute exacerbations of chronic heart failure requiring acute inotropic support. There is some evidence in human medicine to suggest that intermittent administration of dobutamine to patients with chronic myocardial failure can result in continued improvement in cardiac function.[84]

The dosage of dobutamine is 5 to 40 μg/kg/min. Doses of 5 to 20 μg/kg/min are generally adequate for dogs. Infusion rates of greater than 20 μg/kg/min may produce tachycardia. Cats may be given 5 to 15 μg/kg/min. The positive inotropic effect is dosage dependent.

Bipyridine Compounds

Amrinone and milrinone are two examples of bipyridine compounds. Amrinone is commercially available for intravenous administration. Milrinone is about 30 to 40 times as potent as amrinone and is currently under investigation for oral use in dogs with heart failure.

Bipyridine compounds primarily act as inhibitors of phosphodiesterase III[85] (Fig. 8-14). Phosphodiesterase III is an intracellular enzyme that specifically breaks down cAMP. When phosphodiesterase III is inhibited, intracellular cAMP concentration increases, resulting in greater calcium availability for contractile proteins and increased contractility. At high doses, alterations in calcium transport may contribute to the increase in contractility seen with amrinone and milrinone.[85] Bipyridine compounds also produce arteriolar dilation, probably mediated by phosphodiesterase inhibition. Increased cAMP decreases calcium uptake in vascular smooth muscle, which results in muscle relaxation and vasodilation.

In normal anesthetized dogs, an intravenous bolus of amrinone (1.0 to 3.0 mg/kg) causes contractility to increase 60 to 100 percent, systemic arterial blood pressure to decrease 10 to 30 percent, and heart rate to increase 5 to 10 percent. Maximal contractility occurs in 5 minutes after injection and decreases 50 percent by 10 minutes. Effects are dissipated within 20 to 30 minutes. This short duration of effect necessitates administering the drug by constant infusion. Infusion rates of 10 to 100 μg/kg/min in the anesthetized dog increases contractility 30 to 90 percent and in the unanesthetized dog, 10 to 80 percent above baseline. In the anesthetized dog, an infusion of 10 μg/kg/min does not decrease blood pressure, whereas 30 μg/kg/min decreases it 10 percent and 100 μg/kg/min decreases it 30 percent. Heart rate does not increase at 10 μg/kg/min but elevates 15 percent at 30 μg/kg/min and increases 20 percent at 100 μg/kg/min. In anesthetized dogs with drug-induced myocardial failure, amrinone infusions increase contractility 40 to 200 percent above baseline and increase cardiac output by 80 percent. Constant infusions in dogs take about 45 minutes to reach peak effect. In cats, amrinone infused at 30 μg/kg/min causes contractility to increase 40 percent above baseline. Peak effect occurs 90 minutes after starting an infusion.[86]

Studies have not been performed to determine the hemodynamic changes brought about by amrinone administration in dogs or cats with naturally occurring heart failure. Based on the information from normal dogs, however, clinical recommendations can be made. The drug has a wide margin of safety, and the risk of toxicity is low. With milrinone (which has similar toxic effects in dogs as amrinone), exacerbation of ventricular arrhythmias may occur in about 5 percent of dogs treated for heart failure. In humans, amrinone can cause thrombocytopenia and flulike symptoms in a small percentage of patients,[87] but these signs have not been noted in drug studies involving amrinone and normal dogs. Amrinone is advocated only for short-term administration. Initial dose should be 1 to 3 mg/kg as a slow intravenous bolus followed by a constant rate infusion of 10 to 100 μg/kg/min. One-half the initial bolus may be administered 20 to 30 minutes after the first bolus. The same regimen may be effective in the cat.

Milrinone is not currently marketed but has undergone testing in normal dogs and in dogs with heart failure. It appears that milrinone may be safe and effective for treating canine heart failure in the future.

In normal anesthetized dogs, milrinone dosed at 30 to 300 μg/kg increases contractility 40 to 120 percent, while decreasing diastolic blood pressure 10 to 30 percent.[88] Peak effect occurs within 1 to 2 minutes and is reduced to 50 percent of maximum in 10 minutes, and effects are essentially gone in 30 minutes. Constant rate intravenous infusions (1 to 10 μg/kg/min) increase contractility 50 to 140 percent, with peak effect in 10 to 30 minutes. In the normal unanesthetized dog, the oral administration of 0.10 mg/kg milrinone increases contractility 30 percent above baseline, 0.30 mg/kg increases contractility 50 percent above baseline, and 1.0 mg/kg increases contractility more than 80 percent above baseline. Systemic arterial blood pressure is essentially unchanged at these doses, while heart rate increases up to 30 percent at the 1.0-mg/kg dose. In

the normal anesthetized cat, a constant rate infusion of 1.0 μg/kg/min increases contractility about 40 percent, with peak effect occurring within 30 minutes.

Dogs with myocardial failure (predominantly from congestive cardiomyopathy) displayed improved echocardiographic parameters with milrinone dosed at 0.5 to 1.0 mg/kg BID during a 4-week treatment regimen. Ventricular arrhythmias worsened in a small percentage of dogs.[89]

In another study of canine congestive cardiomyopathy, cardiac index increased 54 percent, stroke volume index increased 40 percent, and pulmonary capillary pressure (the pressure that determines whether or how much pulmonary edema is produced) decreased 50 percent. Mean arterial blood pressure did not change. Heart rate increased 11 percent. The end-systolic diameter (measured from the M-mode echocardiogram) decreased 9 percent, while blood pressure remained constant. This suggested an increase in E_{max} or a decrease in V_o (i.e., an increase in contractility)[90] (Fig. 8-9).

DIURETICS

Diuretics increase urine flow by increasing renal plasma flow or by altering nephron function. Diuretics that increase renal plasma flow by expanding plasma volume (e.g., mannitol, glucose) are contraindicated in patients with heart failure because they increase venous pressures and edema formation. Agents that alter nephron function increase urine production by interfering with ion transport or the action of antidiuretic hormone (ADH) within the nephron. Since the goal of diuretic therapy in heart failure is promotion of salt and water loss, agents that cause only water loss by interfering with ADH are not indicated for use.

Agents that interfere with ion transport do so by altering (1) intracellular ionic entry, (2) energy generation and utilization for ion transport, or (3) ion transfer from the cell to the peritubular capillaries through the antiluminal membrane.[91] Agents that interfere with ion transport also differ as to their site of action within the nephron. In general, agents that act on the loop of Henle are the most potent.

Three classes of diuretics are used clinically in dogs to treat heart failure: thiazide diuretics, loop diuretics, and potassium-sparing diuretics. They differ in their ability to promote salt and water excretion and in mechanism of action. Thiazide diuretics are mildly to moderately potent agents.[92] Their use is usually reserved for patients with functional class II or III heart failure, but they can be used in conjunction with a loop diuretic in functional class IV patients refractory to loop diuretics. The loop diuretics are the most potent and can be used in small doses in functional class II and III patients and in higher doses in patients in functional class IV heart failure. The use of potassium-sparing diuretics is reserved for those patients that become hypokalemic with other diuretics and for patients refractory to other agents because of elevated plasma aldosterone concentrations. In the latter situation, potassium-sparing diuretics are given in conjunction with another drug, usually a loop diuretic.

Loop diuretics (furosemide) are most commonly used in cats, but thiazides are occasionally employed. Potassium-sparing agents are rarely used in cats.[56]

Thiazide Diuretics

The thiazides act primarily by reducing membrane permeability in the distal convoluted tubule to sodium and chloride.[92] They promote potassium loss at this site and produce large increases in the urine sodium concentration but only mild to moderate increases in urine volume. Therefore, only mild to moderate renal sodium loss is promoted. Thiazides increase renal sodium excretion from a normal of about 1 percent to 5 to 8 percent of the filtered load. However, thiazide-induced renal sodium excretion is only one-third to one-half that achieved with the loop diuretics. The thiazides are ineffective when renal blood flow is low, which may explain their lack of efficacy in patients with severe heart failure. In dogs, the thiazides are well absorbed after oral administration. The action of chlorothiazide begins within 1 hour, peaks at 4 hours, and lasts 6 to 12 hours. Dosage is 20 to 40 mg/kg BID. Hydrochlorothiazide has an onset of action within 2 hours, peaks at 4 hours, and lasts 12 hours. Its oral canine dose is 2 to 4 mg/kg BID; cats are given 1 to 2 mg/kg BID. The newer, more lipid soluble thiazides (trichlormethiazide, cyclothiazide) have not been studied in the dog or cat.

Loop Diuretics

The loop diuretics include furosemide, ethacrynic acid, and bumetanide. Furosemide is the most commonly used diuretic for treating heart failure in the dog and cat. Ethacrynic acid is rarely used. Bumetanide is a new agent that is 40 to 50 times as potent as furosemide and may offer some clinical advantages.[93] All loop diuretics inhibit active sodium, potassium, and chloride reabsorption in the thick portion of the ascending loop of Henle.[94] In so doing, they inhibit sodium and obligatory water reabsorption in the nephron. The loop diuretics are capable of increasing the maximal fractional excretion of sodium to 23 percent of the filtered load, making them the most powerful natriuretic agents available. In addition to their diuretic effects, loop diuretics may act as venodilators, decreasing venous pressures before diuresis takes place (especially after intravenous administration). However, this effect has been strongly challenged.[95]

Furosemide is highly protein bound and not extensively metabolized in the dog and cat. Most is secreted into the proximal tubule, where it acts as a mild carbonic anhydrase inhibitor. Furosemide decreases renal vascular resistance; thus, it acutely increases renal blood flow. Intravenously its onset of action is 5 minutes, peak effects occur within 30 minutes, half life is 15 minutes and duration of effect is 2 hours. After oral administration onset of action occurs within 60 minutes, peak effects occur within 1 to 2 hours and duration of effects last 6 hours. The oral canine dose ranges from 1 mg/kg every other day to 4 mg/kg TID, depending on the severity of the clinical signs associated with backward heart failure. Oral furosemide dose in cats ranges from 1 mg/kg every 2 to 3 days to 2 mg/kg BID. Severe pulmonary edema requires immediate intensive intravenous therapy in dogs using doses up to 8 mg/kg every 1 to 2 hours. Such intensive dosing may result in hyponatremia, hypokalemia, and dehydration, which must be addressed after the life-threatening pulmonary edema has been controlled (e.g., electrolyte disturbances may result in exacerbation of ventricular arrhythmias and hypokalemia may potentiate or even create digitalis intoxication). Electrolyte disturbances and dehydration are rare in the dog unless maximal doses are employed.

Cats are very sensitive to furosemide. They rarely

require more than 1 mg/kg BID or TID for the treatment of pulmonary edema.[56]

Potassium-Sparing Diuretics

This class of diuretics (e.g., spironolactone, triamterene) acts by inhibiting the action of aldosterone on distal tubular cells. In normal animals, plasma aldosterone concentration is relatively low, hence the mild effect of these diuretics. In normal dogs, they can only increase the maximal fractional excretion of sodium to 2 percent of the filtered load.[96] In dogs with heart failure and increased plasma aldosterone concentration the effect of these diuretics may be greater. When potassium-sparing diuretics are administered with other diuretics, potassium loss is decreased. Therefore, they can be administered to patients that become hypokalemic because of other diuretic agent administration.

Spironolactone is structurally similar to aldosterone and binds competitively to aldosterone's binding sites in the distal tubule. Its onset of action is slow and peak effect does not occur until 2 to 3 days after administration commences. The drug is extensively and rapidly metabolized to conrenone in plasma, and it is this metabolite that is pharmacologically active. The dose of spironolactone for dogs is 2 to 4 mg/kg/day.

Triamterene competitively displaces aldosterone from its binding sites but also directly inhibits the distal tubular transport of potassium.[97] Its action begins within 2 hours, peaks at 6 to 8 hours, and lasts 12 to 16 hours. The oral canine dose of triamterene is 2 to 4 mg/kg/day.

LOW-SODIUM DIET

A diet low in sodium is one means of reducing circulating blood volume in the patient with heart failure. Sodium is retained in these patients by a variety of mechanisms including activation of the renin-angiotensin-aldosterone system. Diuretic therapy as a therapeutic modality for reducing total body sodium and blood volume has previously been discussed.

Patients with severe heart failure that are refractory to diuretic administration have the greatest need for a low-sodium diet. Patients with early and mild heart failure generally do not need marked salt restriction. Chapter 10 details the dietary and sodium requirements for canine and feline heart failure.

VASODILATORS

Vasodilators are drugs that act on arteriolar or venous smooth muscle to cause vasodilation. Their effects depend on the vascular beds they influence, as well as relative drug potency. The effect of these drugs on the pulmonary vasculature is erratic or insignificant. The discussion is therefore limited to the systemic vascular beds.

Vasodilators are generally classified as arteriolar dilators, venodilators, or combination (i.e., balanced) arteriolar and venodilators. Arteriolar dilators relax the smooth muscle of systemic arterioles, decreasing peripheral vascular resistance or impedance. This usually results in decreased systemic arterial blood pressure, systolic intraventricular pressure and systolic myocardial wall stress (or afterload). Thus, the force that opposes myocardial fiber shortening is reduced. This allows the heart muscle to shorten further and increase stroke volume (Fig. 8-9). With mitral regurgitation, arteriolar dilators (i.e., afterload reducers) decrease systolic intraventricular pressure, reduce the systolic mitral valvular pressure gradient, decrease the regurgitant flow, and enhance forward flow into the aorta. The decreased regurgitant flow decreases left atrial pressure, pulmonary capillary pressure and pulmonary edema formation (see Figs. 8-2, 8-3 above, and Fig. 8-15).

Venodilators relax systemic venous smooth muscle, effectively redistributing the blood volume into the systemic venous reservoir, decreasing cardiac blood volume, and reducing pulmonary congestion. The net result is reduced ventricular diastolic pressure, decreased pulmonary and systemic pressures, and diminished edema formation. Therefore, venodilators (i.e., preload reducers) are used in the same situations as diuretics and low-sodium diets (see Figs. 8-2 and 8-3 above).

Hydralazine

Hydralazine is a pure arteriolar dilator that probably acts by increasing the prostacyclin concentration in systemic arterioles.[98] It decreases resistance

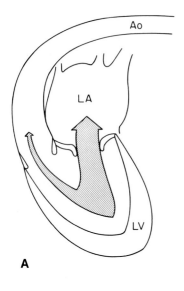

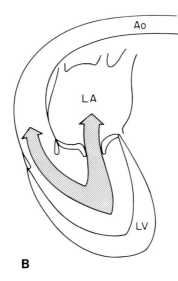

Fig. 8-15 Schematic diagrams of the left ventricle and atrium in a dog with mitral regurgitation before (**A**) and after (**B**) arteriolar dilator therapy with hydralazine. Arteriolar dilation decreases systemic and left ventricular systolic pressure. This decreases the pressure gradient across the mitral valve, decreases left atrial regurgitant flow and increases forward flow into the aorta (**B**).

in renal, coronary, cerebral, and mesenteric vascular beds more than in skeletal muscle beds.[99] Increased renal blood flow can improve renal function (if initially depressed) and thereby enhance digoxin excretion.[100]

In patients with low catecholamine concentrations the decrease in blood pressure resulting from hydralazine may result in reflex tachycardia. Hydralazine directly stimulates histamine release. This causes release of norepinephrine, which can also cause tachycardia. If tachycardia is a clinically significant complication following hydralazine administration, digoxin, digitoxin, or propranolol may be used to counter this effect.

Patients with elevated catecholamine concentrations may not experience tachycardia when given hydralazine. When dogs with congestive heart failure were treated with hydralazine, similar numbers of patients experienced tachycardia, had no change in heart rate, or had a decrease in heart rate.

The oral route of hydralazine administration has been studied in dogs.[101,102] It is well absorbed from the gastrointestinal tract but undergoes first-pass hepatic metabolism by acetylation.[103] Although hydralazine is not excreted by the kidney, its biotransformation is affected by renal failure, which may increase serum concentration.

The vasodilating effect of hydralazine occurs within 1 hour after oral administration and peaks within 3 hours. The effect is then stable for the next 8 to 10 hours, after which it rapidly dissipates. The net duration of effect is about 12 hours.[102]

In small dogs with mitral regurgitation refractory to the administration of furosemide, left atrial regurgitant flow may constitute 80 to 90 percent of cardiac output.[104] Left ventricular contractile function is usually normal or only mildly depressed.[24] Therefore, the major hemodynamic abnormality is caused by marked regurgitant flow through an incompetent mitral valve. The ideal treatment would be mitral valve replacement, but this is not technically feasible at this time. Therefore, the treatment of choice is arteriolar dilator administration. Hydralazine decreases regurgitant flow, increases forward aortic flow and venous oxygen tension, and decreases radiographic evidence of pulmonary edema.[101,105] Therapeutic dosage decreases mean arterial blood pressure from 100 to 110 mmHg to 60 to 80 mmHg. These effects improve the quality of life and seem to prolong survival time. Because of its reliability and potency, hydralazine is the initial vasodilator selected for dogs in congestive heart failure due to mitral regurgitation (Fig. 8-15).

In dogs with congestive (dilated) cardiomyopathy, hydralazine also improves cardiac output and may decrease pulmonary edema. The beneficial effects produced by the drug seem to improve the quality of life for the patient, but in my experience, it does not usually result in appreciable prolongation of life.

The hemodynamic effects of hydralazine are dose dependent. Overdosing can result in hypotension. Therefore, the dose must be clinically titrated, starting low and gradually increasing until clinical or hemodynamic improvement is noted. To start a dog on hydralazine therapy, a baseline clinical assessment should include measurement of capillary refill time, assessment of mucous membrane color, and radiographic evaluation of pulmonary edema. If facilities are available for measuring blood pressure or blood gases, systemic arterial blood pressure and jugular vein oxygen tension may be evaluated. Their measurement is not needed for titration, however. A dose of 1 mg/kg PO should be given initially. If blood pressure or oxygen tension is monitored, they can be repeated in 2 or 3 hours to document whether the dose of hydralazine has had an effect. If clinical signs only are being monitored, the 1-mg/kg dose should be repeated every 12 hours for 1 or 2 days and the patient reassessed as an outpatient at the end of that time. With inpatient treatment, effectiveness can be assessed 5 or 6 hours after drug administration. An effective dose is indicated by reduced capillary refill time, pinker mucous membranes, regression of pulmonary edema (the diuretic dose should not be changed during this time, if possible), or clinical patient improvement. If the initial dose was not effective, it should be increased to 2 mg/kg every 12 hours and the dog reassessed; 3 mg/kg may be given every 12 hours if clinical response is still lacking. When hydralazine is titrated in this manner, adverse effects are infrequent.

Hydralazine causes vomiting in some dogs. Reducing the dose to 0.25 to 0.5 mg/kg BID for 1 to 2 weeks and then increasing the dose to its therapeutic range may be effective in resolving this complication. In other cases, the vomiting may be intractable, necessitating the use of a different vasodilator.

The most serious adverse effect is hypotension, indicated by signs of weakness and depression. In most cases, this does not require treatment and the signs will disappear 10 to 12 hours after the last dose of hydralazine. The dose should then be reduced. Rarely, hypotension may be severe; dopamine may be administered (10 μg/kg/min) in such instances to increase blood pressure.

Captopril

Captopril is an inhibitor of angiotensin-converting enzyme. This enzyme cleaves two peptides off the decapeptide angiotensin I, to create the octapeptide, angiotensin II.[106] Angiotensin II is a potent arteriolar and venoconstrictor and is a stimulus for aldosterone secretion. Therefore, administration of captopril results in arteriolar and venodilation and decreased circulating plasma aldosterone concentration (Fig. 8-16). Decreased arteriolar tone reduces systemic blood pressure and afterload. This permits a greater stroke volume, which increases cardiac output. Decreased venous tone coupled with the reduced aldosterone concentration decreases venous pressure and edema formation in patients with congestive heart failure.

In dogs with experimentally induced myocardial failure and heart failure, captopril produces mild reductions in systemic arterial blood pressure and pulmonary capillary pressure. Its effects last about 4 hours. In dogs with acquired mitral regurgitation, some display marked improvement following captopril administration; others have no change or reduced cardiac output.[24] These variable effects may be explained by differences in baseline aldosterone concentrations, but this remains to be studied. In humans, captopril is thought to be an effective drug for treating all stages of heart failure in which therapy is required. The drug produces mild to moderate reductions in blood pressures,[107] improves exercise tolerance, and may prolong life. Improvement in survival time has not been documented in cats.

In dogs, captopril (0.5 to 2.0 mg/kg) has a short duration of effect. In general 1.0 mg/kg produces a greater effect than does 0.5 mg/kg, but a dose of 2.0 mg/kg usually causes no more improvement than does 1.0 mg/kg. Therefore, 1.0 mg/kg is recommended for most dogs. The drug should be given at least three times per day unless side effects occur (e.g., anorexia, vomiting, diarrhea, hypotension). Doses in excess of 2.0 mg/kg TID can produce renal failure, hence should be avoided. Gastrointestinal side effects are common. Other arteriolar dilators should not be administered concurrently with captopril.

The dose in cats, determined from clinical experience, is 0.5 to 1.5 mg/kg BID to TID Anorexia is a common side effect.[108]

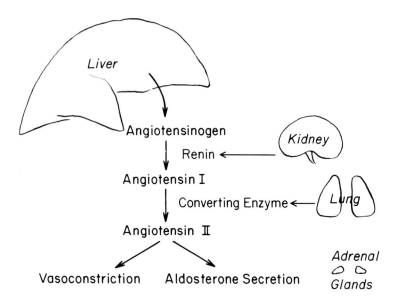

Fig. 8-16 Compensatory homeostatic events during heart failure may overcompensate, resulting in excessive formation of angiotension II (a vasoconstrictor) and aldosterone. This leads to increase in afterload, preload, effusions, or edema. Angiotensin converting enzyme inhibitors (e.g., captopril) decrease plasma angiotensin II concentration, thereby causing vasodilation. Plasma aldosterone concentration is also reduced, resulting in less sodium and water retention, decreasing preload.

Nitrates

No studies have been performed to document the pharmacodynamics or establish therapeutic dosage of the nitrates in dogs or cats. Nitrates act primarily as venodilators. They do have variable arteriolar dilating effects, depending on the agent and route of administration. Intravenous nitroglycerin is a potent venodilator with moderate arteriolar dilating properties. Administration would require hemodynamic monitoring; it has not been used in clinical veterinary practice.

Nitroglycerin ointment is available in a 2 percent formulation to be spread on the skin for absorption into the systemic circulation.[107] It is also supplied in a transdermal patch preparation.[109]

In dogs and cats, 2 percent nitroglycerin cream has been used ($\frac{1}{2}$ to 2 inches every 4 to 6 hours for dogs, $\frac{1}{8}$ to $\frac{1}{4}$ inch every 4 to 6 hours for cats) but efficacy has not been documented. In my experience, topical nitroglycerin produces no harmful effects, but whether it produces benefit is questionable. Dog and cat skin is different from human skin, and it is doubtful that direct comparisons regarding absorption and duration of effect can be made. If transdermal nitroglycerin cream is used, it should be applied on a hairless or shaved area, using gloves, since transdermal absorption will occur in the clinician as well as in the patient.

Isosorbide dinitrate is a nitrate that can be administered orally. Its efficacy in dogs and cats has not been studied. An empirical dose that has been used for dogs is 0.22 to 0.44 mg/kg given every 8 hours (Bond BR, personal communication).

Prazosin

Prazosin is an arteriolar and venodilating agent. It acts primarily by blocking α_1-adrenergic receptors but also peripherally inhibits phosphodiesterase.[110] Since prazosin does not block α_2-adrenergic receptors, norepinephrine release is still controlled via negative feedback. Reflex tachycardia is generally not seen. The vasodilating effects of prazosin become attenuated after the first dose in humans[111] and in rats.[112] In rats, it is thought that this effect is brought about by stimulation of the renin-angiotensin-aldosterone system.

The hemodynamic effects of prazosin have not been documented in the dog or cat. In humans, its administration decreases right and left ventricular filling pressures, edema, and congestion, and increases stroke volume and cardiac output.[113] The starting dose in dogs is 1 mg TID for dogs weighing less than 15 kg and 2 mg TID for dogs weighing more than 15 kg. The dose then needs to be titrated upward if the initial dose is ineffective, or reduced if hypotension occurs. Prazosin is supplied as capsules containing 1, 2, and 5 mg of drug. This preparation is therefore not amenable for use in cats.

β-ADRENOCEPTOR-BLOCKING DRUGS

β-Adrenergic blocking agents are standard therapy for reducing heart rate in dogs with atrial fibrillation secondary to congestive (dilated) cardiomyopathy. Recently, several investigators in human medicine found that the administration of β-adrenergic blocking drugs to patients with chronic myocardial failure has resulted in improvement in left ventricular function and apparent prolongation of survival time.[114,115] In some situations, patients that have been waiting for a heart transplant after failing to respond to all other types of drugs have received β-adrenergic blocking agents and improved enough to be taken off the waiting list. The reason for this apparent paradoxic improvement is unknown but several theories have been proposed.[116] One theory is that the chronic increase in circulating catecholamine concentrations in patients with heart failure could result in myocardial cell death and that by blocking this effect, improvement in myocardial function could result. Another theory is that β-receptors have downregulated (i.e., they are less sensitive or fewer in number) because of the chronically elevated catecholamine concentrations; β-adrenergic blockade may result in upregulation, allowing myocardial function to improve by β-receptor stimulation.

These findings are exciting. However, it is currently unknown whether canine and feline dilated cardiomyopathies respond similar to these results described in humans. The effectiveness of β-adrenoceptor blocking drugs in animal cardiomyopathy remains to be explored.

REFERENCES

1. De La Rocha AG, Edmonds JF, Williams WG, et al: Importance of mixed venous oxygen saturation in the care of critically ill patients. Can J Surg 21:227, 1978
2. Zucker IH, Earle AM, Gilmore JP: The mechanism of adaptation of left atrial stretch receptors in dogs with chronic congestive heart failure. J Clin Invest 60:323, 1977
3. Criteria Committee, New York Heart Association, Inc: Diseases of the Heart and Blood Vessels. Nomenclature and Criteria for Diagnosis. 6th Ed. Little, Brown, Boston, 1964
4. Furubayashi K: Hemodynamic characteristics of hypertrophic and congestive cardiomyopathies. Jpn Circ J 45:1014, 1981
5. Siegel RJ, Shah, PK, Fishbein MC: Idiopathic restrictive cardiomyopathy. Circulation 70:165, 1984
6. Pouleur H, Rousseau M, Van Eyll C, et al: Force-velocity-length relations in hypertropic cardiomyopathy: Evidence of normal or depressed myocardial contractility. Am J Cardiol 52:813, 1983
7. Bonow, RO, Rosing DR, Bacharach SL, et al: Effects of verapamil on left ventricular systolic function and diastolic filling in patients with hypertrophic cardiomyopathy. Circulation 64:787, 1981
8. Pion P, Babish J, Schwark W, et al: Pharmacokinetics and electrocardiographic effects of verapamil in cats. J Vet Intern Med (in press)
9. Suge H: Left ventricular time-varying pressure/volume ratio in systole as an index of myocardial inotropism. Jpn Heart J 12:153, 1971
10. Burns JW: Mechanics of isotonic left ventricular contractions. Am J Physiol 224:725, 1973
11. Yin FCP: Ventricular wall stress. Circ Res 49:829, 1981
12. Starling EH: Linacre Lecture on the Law of the Heart. Longmans, Green, London, 1918
13. Suga H, Sagawa K: Instantaneous pressure-volume relationships and their ratio in the excised, supported canine left ventricle. Circ Res 35:117, 1974
14. Grossman W, Braunwald E, Mann T, et al: Contractile state of the left ventricle in man as evaluated from end-systolic pressure-volume relations. Circulation 56:845, 1977
15. McCollum WB, Crow C, Harigaya S, et al: Calcium binding by cardiac relaxing system isolated from myopathic syrian hamsters (strains 14.6, 82.62 and 40.54). J Mol Cell Cardiol 1:445, 1970
16. Kaztz AM, Brady AJ: Mechanical and biochemical correlates of cardiac contraction. Mod Concepts Cardiovasc Dis 40:45, 1971
17. Nayler WG, Stone J, Carson V, et al: Effect of ischemia on cardiac contractility and calcium exchangeability. J Mol Cell Cardiol 2:125, 1971
18. Lindenmeyer GE, Harigaya S, Bajusz E, et al: Oxidative phosphorylation and calcium transport of mitochondria isolated from cardiomyopathic hamster hearts. J Mol Cell Cardiol 1:249, 1970
19. Hoffman BF, Rosen MR: Cellular mechanisms for cardiac arrhythmias. Circ Res 49:1, 1981
20. Grossman W, Jones D, McLaurin LP: Wall stress and patterns of hypertrophy in the human left ventricle. J Clin Invest 56:56, 1975

21. Drummond GI, Severson DL: Cyclic nucleotides and cardiac function. Circ Res 44:145, 1979

22. Kittleson MD, Eyster GE, Knowlen GG, et al: Myocardial function in small dogs with chronic mitral regurgitation and severe congestive heart failure. J Am Vet Med Assoc 184:455, 1984

23. Kittleson MD, Eyster GE, Knowlen GG, et al: Efficacy of digoxin administration in dogs with idiopathic congestive cardiomyopathy. J Am Vet Med Assoc 186:162, 1985

24. Kittleson MD: Positive inotropic agents and captopril. p. 19. Proceedings of the Ninth Annual Kal Kan Symposium, Kal Kan Foods Inc, Vernon, CA, 1986

25. Kittleson MD, Johnson LE, Olivier NB, et al: Acute hemodynamic effects of hydralazine in dogs with chronic mitral regurgitation. J Am Vet Med Assoc 187:258, 1985

26. Nomura A, Yasuda H, Minami M, et al: Effect of furosemide in congestive heart failure. Clin Pharmacol Ther 30:177, 1981

27. Withering W: An account of the foxglove and some of its medical uses, with practical remarks on dropsy, and other diseases. In Willis FA, Keys TE (eds): Classics of Cardiology. Henry Schuman, New York, 1941

28. Dobbs SM, Kenyon WI, Dobbs RJ: Maintenance digoxin after an episode of heart failure: placebo-controlled trial in outpatients. Br Med J 1:749, 1977

29. Kleiman JH, Ingels NB, Daughters G: Left ventricular dynamics during long-term digoxin treatment in patients with stable coronary artery disease. Am J Cardiol 41:937, 1978

30. Arnold, SB, Byrd RC, Meister W, et al: Long-term digitalis therapy improves left ventricular function in heart failure. N Engl J Med 303:1443, 1980

31. Mulrow, CD, Feussner JR, Velez R: Reevaluation of digitalis efficacy. Ann Intern Med 101:113, 1984

32. Gheorghiade M, Beller G: Effects of discontinuing maintenance digoxin therapy in patients with ischemic heart disease and congestive heart failure in sinus rhythm. Am J Cardiol 51:1243, 1983

33. Taggart AJ, Johnston GD, McDevitt DG: Digoxin withdrawal after cardiac failure in patients with sinus rhythm. J Cardiac Pharm 5:229, 1983

34. McHaffie D, Purcell H, Mitchell-Heggs P, Guz A: The clinical value of digoxin in patients with heart failure and sinus rhythm. Q J Med 188:401, 1978

35. Davidson C, Gibson D: Clinical significance of positive inotropic action of digoxin in patients with left ventricular disease. Br Heart J 35:970, 1973

36. Hougen TJ, Smith TW: Inhibition of myocardial monovalent cation active transport by subtoxic doses of ouabain in the dog. Circ Res 42:856, 1978

37. Caprio A, Farah A: The effect of the ionic milieu on the response of rabbit cardiac muscle to ouabain. J Pharm Exp Ther 155:403, 1967

38. Mason DT, Zelia R, Amsterdam EA (eds). Unified concept of the mechanism of action of digitalis: Influence of ventricular function and cardiac disease on hemodynamic response to fundamental contractile effect. p. 283. In Marks BH, Weissler AM (eds): Basic and Clinical Pharmacology of Digitalis. CV Mosby, Springfield, IL, 1972

39. Chidsey CA (ed): Calcium Metabolism in the Normal and Failing Heart. HP Publishing Co, New York, 1974

40. Ferrier GR, Moe GK: Effect of calcium on acetylstrophanthidin-induced transient depolarization in canine Purkinje tissue. Circ Res 33:508, 1973.

41. Moe GK, Farah AE: Digitalis and allied cardiac glycosides. p. 677. In Goodman LS, Gilman A (eds): Pharmacological Basis of Therapeutics. 4th Ed. Macmillan, New York, 1970

42. Lown B, Graboys TB, Podrid RJ, et al: Effect of a digitalis drug on ventricular premature beats. N Engl J Med 296:301, 1977

43. Baggot JD, Davis LE: Plasma protein binding of digitoxin and digoxin in several mammalian species. Res Vet Sci 15:81, 1973

44. Breznock EM: Application of canine plasma kinetics of digoxin and digitoxin to therapeutic digitalization in the dog. J Am Vet Med Assoc 34:993, 1973

45. Weidler DFJ, Jazllad NS, Movahhed HS, et al: Pharmacokinetics of digoxin in the cat and comparisons with man and the dog. Res Commun Chem Pathol Pharm 19:57, 1987

46. De Rick A, Balpaire FM, Bogaert MG, Mattheuws D: Plasma concentrations of digoxin and digitoxin during digitalization of healthy dogs and dogs with cardiac failure. Am J Vet Res 39:811, 1978

47. Pedersoli WM: Serum digoxin concentrations in healthy dogs treated without a loading dose. J Vet Pharm Ther 1:279, 1978

48. DeMots H, McAnulty JH, Porter GA, et al: Effects of rapid and slow infusion of ouabain on systemic and coronary vascular resistance in patients not in clinical heart failure. Circulation 52:77, 1975

49. Smith TW: Digitalis. III. N Engl J Med 289:1063, 1973

50. Doherty JE: Pharmacokinetics and their clinical implications. Ann Intern Med 79:229, 1973

51. Gierke KD, Perrier D, Mayersohn M, Marcus EL: Digoxin disposition kinetics in dogs before and during azotemia. J Pharm Exp Ther 205:459, 1978

52. Bolton GR: Pharmacokinetics of digoxin in the cat. Preliminary report. Personal communication

53. Erichsen DF, Harris SG, Upson DW: Plasma levels of digoxin in the cat: Some clinical applications. J Am Anim Hosp Assoc 14:734, 1978

54. Hamlin RL: Basis for selection of a cardiac glycoside for dogs. Proceedings of the First Symposium on Veterinary Pharmacology and Therapeutics, Baton Rouge, LA, 1978

55. Kittleson MD: Drugs used in the management of heart failure. p. 285. In Kirk RW (ed): Current Veterinary therapy. Vol. VIII, WB Saunders, Philadelphia, 1983

56. Fox P: Feline myocardial diseases. p. 387. In Kirk RW (ed): Current Veterinary Therapy. Vol. VIII. WB Saunders, Philadelphia, 1983

57. Bonagura JD, Ware WA: Atrial fibrillation in the dog: Clinical findings in 81 cases. J Am Anim Hosp Assoc 22:111, 1986

58. Bigger JT: The quinidine-digoxin interaction. Mod Concepts Cardiovasc Dis 51:73, 1982

59. Warner NJ, Barnard JT, Uhl JT, Bigger Jr: Digoxin, quinidine and monovalent cation transport. Circulation 66:57, 1982

60. Klein HO, Land R, Weiss E, et al: The influence of verapamil on serum digoxin concentration. Circulation 65:998, 1982

61. Zatuchni J: Verapamil-digoxin interaction. Am Heart J 108:412, 1980

62. Breznock EM: Effects of phenobarbital on digitoxin and digoxin elimination in the dog. Am J Vet Res 36:371, 1975

63. Pedersoli WM: Serum digoxin concentration in dogs before and after concomitant treatment with chloramphenicol. J Am Anim Hosp Assoc 16:839, 1980

64. Karagueuzian HS, Katzung BG: Relative inotropic and arrhythmogenic effects of five cardiac steroids in ventricular myocardium: oscillatory afterpotentials and the role of endogenous catecholamines. J Pharm Exp Ther 218:348, 1981

65. Gross DR, Hamlin RL, Pipers FS: Response of P-Q intervals to digitalis glycosides in the dog. J Am Vet Med Assoc 162:888, 1973

66. Smith TW: Digitalis toxicity: Epidemiology and clinical use of serum concentration measurements. Am J Med 58:470, 1975

67. Borison HL, Wang SC: Physiology and pharmacology of vomiting. Pharmacol Rev 5:193, 1953

68. Gillis RA: Digitalis: A neuroexcitatory drug. Circulation 52:739, 1975

69. Citrin D, Stevenson IH, O'Malley K: Massive digoxin overdose: observations on hyperkalemia and plasma digoxin levels. Scott Med J 17:275, 1972

70. Dreifus LS, McKnight EH, Katz M, Likoff W: Digitalis intolerance. Geriatrics 18:494, 1963

71. Peon J, Ferrier GR, Moe GK: The relationship of excitability to conduction velocity in canine Purkinje tissue. Circ Res 43:125, 1978

72. Rall TW, Schleifer LS: Drugs effective in the therapy of the epilepsies. p. 539. In Gilman AG, Goodman LS, Gilman A (eds): The Pharmacological Basis of Therapeutics. 6th Ed. Macmillan, New York, 1980

73. Sanders JE, Yeary RA: Serum concentrations of orally administered diphenylhydantoin in dogs. J Am Vet Assoc 172:153, 1978

74. Caldwell JH, Bush CA, Greenberger NJ: Interruption of the enterohepatic circulation of digitoxin by cholestyramine. Effect on metabolic disposition of tritium-labeled digitoxin and cardiac systolic intervals in man. J Clin Invest 50:2638, 1971

75. Smith TW, Butler VP, Haber E, et al: Treatment of life-threatening digitalis intoxication with digoxin-specific antibody fragments. N Engl J Med 307:1357, 1982

76. Katz A: Congestive heart failure. Role of altered myocardial cellular control. N Engl J Med 293:11284, 1975

77. Adams HR: New perspectives in cardiopulmonary therapeutics: Receptor-selective adrenergic drugs. J Am Vet Med Assoc 85:966, 1984

78. Maekawa K, Liang C, Hood WB: Comparison of dobutamine and dopamine in acute myocardial infarction. Circulation 67:750, 1983

79. Murphy PJ, Williams TL, Kau DLK: Disposition of dobutamine in the dog. J Pharm Exp Ther 199:423, 1976

80. McNay JL, McDonald RH, Goldgern LI: Direct renal vasodilatation produced by dopamine in the dog. Circ Res 16:510, 1965

81. Loeb HS, Bredzakis J, Gunner RM: Superiority of dobutamine over dopamine for augmentation of cardiac ouput in patients with chronic low output cardiac failure. Circulation 5:375, 1977

82. Robie NW, Goldberg LI: Comparative systemic and regional hemodynamic effects of dopamine and dobutamine. Am Heart J 90:340, 1975

83. Vatner SF, McRitchie J, Braunwald E: Effects of dobutamine on left ventricular performance, coronary dynamics, and distribution of cardiac output in conscious dogs. J Clin Invest 53:1265, 1974

84. Unverferth DV, Magorian RD, Lewis RP, Leier CV: Long-term benefit of dobutamine in patients with congestive cardiomyopathy. Am Heart J 100:622, 1980

85. Mancini D, LeJemtel T, Sonnenblick E: Intravenous use of amrinone for the treatment of the failing heart. Am J Cardiol 56:8B, 1985

86. A Summary of Laboratory and Clinical Data on In-

ocor (brand of amrinone). Sterling Winthrop Research Institute, Rensselaer, NY, 1980

87. Treadway G: Clinical safety of intravenus amrinone. A review. Am J Cardiol 56:39B, 1985

88. Alousi AA, Canter JM, Montenaro MJ, et al: Cardiotonic activity of milrinone, a new and potent cardiac bipyridine, on the normal and failing heart of experimental animals. J Cardiovasc Pharm 5:792, 1983

89. Kittleson MD, Pipers FS, Knauer KW, et al: Echocardiographic and clinical effect of milrinone in dogs with myocardial failure. Am J Vet Res 46:1659, 1985

90. Kittleson MD, Johnson LE, Pion PD: The acute hemodynamic effects of milrinone in dogs with severe idiopathic myocardial failure. J Vet Intern Med 1:127, 1987

91. Grantham JJ, Chonko AM: The physiologic basis and clinical use of diuretics. p. 178. In Brenner BM, Steinm JH (eds): Contemporary Issues in Nephrology. Vol. 1: Sodium and Water Homeostasis. Churchill Livingstone, New York, 1978

92. Kunau RT, Weller DR, Webb HL: Clarification of the site of action of chlorothiazide in the rat nephron. J Clin Invest 56:401, 1975

93. Brater DC: Disposition and response to bumetanide and furosemide. Am J Cardiol 57:20A, 1986

94. Puschett JB: Clinical pharmacologic implications in diuretic selection. Am J Cardiol 57:6A, 1986

95. Mukherjea SK, Katz MA, Michael UF, Ogden CA: Mechanisms of hemodynamic actions of furosemide: Differentiation of vascular and renal effects on blood pressure in functionally anephric hypertensive patients. Am Heart J 101:313, 1981

96. Brater DC, Thier SO: Renal Disorders. Macmillan, New York, 1978

97. Crosley AP, Ronquillo LM, Strickland WH, Alexander F: Triameterene, a new natriuretic agent. Ann Intern Med 56:241, 1962

98. Greenwald JE: Modulation of prostaglandin biosynthesis: Proposed mechanism of action of hydralazine. Dissertation, The Ohio State University, Akron, OH, 1981

99. Spokas EG, Wang H: Regional blood flow and cardiac responses to hydralazine. J Pharm Exp Ther 212:294, 1980

100. Cogan JJ, Humphreys MH, Carlson CJ: Acute vasodilator therapy increases renal clearance of digoxin in patients with congestive heart failure. Circulation 64:973, 1981

101. Kittleson MD, Johnson LE, Olivier NB: Acute hemodynamic effects of hydralazine in dogs with chronic mitral regurgitation. J Am Vet Med Assoc 187:258, 1985

102. Kittleson MD, Hamlin RL: Hydralazine pharmacodynamics in the dog. Am J Vet Res 44:1501, 1983

103. Koch-Weser J: Hydralazine. N Engl J Med 295:320, 1976

104. Kittleson MD: Mitral regurgitation in the dog. p. 69. Proceedings of the Ninth Annual Kal Kan Symposium. Kal Kan Foods Inc, Vernon, CA, 1986

105. Kittleson MD, Eyster GE, Olivier NB, Anderson LK: Oral hydralazine therapy for chronic mitral regurgitation in the dog. J Am Vet Med Assoc 182:1205, 1983

106. Vidt DG, Bravo EL, Fouad FM: Captopril. N Engl J Med 306:214, 1982

107. Ader R, Chatterjee K, Ports T, et al: Immediate and sustained hemodynamic and clinical improvement in chronic heart failure by an oral angiotensin-converting enzyme inhibitor. Circulation 61:931, 1980

108. Fox PR: Feline cardiomyopathy. p. 157. In Bonagura JD (ed): Contemporary Issues in Small Animal Practice. Vol. 8: Cardiology. Churchill-Livingstone, New York, 1987

109. Packer M, Medina N, Yusak M, Hung Lee W: Hemodynamic factors limiting the response to transdermal nitroglycerin in severe chronic congestive heart failure. Am J Cardiol 57:260, 1986

110. Lowenstein J, Steele JM: Prazosin. Am Heart J 95:262, 1978

111. Packer M, Meller J, Gorlin R, Herman MV: Hemodynamic and clinical tachyphylaxis to prazosin-mediated afterload reduction in severe chronic congestive heart failure. Circulation 59:531, 1979

112. Smith RD, Tessman DK, Kaplan HR: Acute tolerance to prazosin in conscious hypertensive rats: Involvement of the renin-angiotensin system. J Pharm Exp Ther 217:397, 1981

113. Awan NA, Miller RR, DeMaria AN, et al: Efficacy of ambulatory systemic vasodilator therapy with oral prazosin in chronic refractory heart failure. Circulation 56:346, 1977

114. Swedberg K, Waagstein F, Hjalmarson A, Wallentin I: Beneficial effects of long-term beta blockade in congestive cardiomyopathy. Br Heart J 44:117, 1980

115. Weber KT, Likoff MJ, McCarthy D: Low-dose beta blockade in the treatment of chronic cardiac failure. Am Heart J 104:877, 1982

116. Bristow MR, Kantrowitz NE, Ginsburg R, Fowler MB: Beta-adrenergic function in heart muscle disease and heart failure. J Mol Cell Cardiol 17:41, 1985

9

Pulmonary Edema

Wendy A. Ware
John D. Bonagura

Pulmonary edema, the abnormal accumulation of extravascular pulmonary fluid, occurs when transudation or exudation into the lung exceeds the capacity of lymphatic drainage.[1,2] Normal interstitial and alveolar spaces of the lung are kept relatively fluid free. By disrupting gas exchange and lung mechanics, pulmonary edema can cause disability and death in small animals. This chapter focuses on pulmonary edema that is cardiogenic in origin, although noncardiogenic causes are discussed briefly as well.

THE NORMAL PULMONARY CIRCULATION

The Starling equation describes the net fluid flow out of the capillary in terms of the balance between hydrostatic and osmotic forces and modified by certain membrane characteristics. This flow Q is determined by the difference between capillary P_c and interstitial P_i hydrostatic pressures and the capillary π_c and interstitial π_i colloid osmotic pressure gradient. Thus

$$Q = K[(P_c - P_i) - \sigma(\pi_c - \pi_i)]$$

where K is the filtration coefficient and σ is the re-

flection coefficient, describing how well the membrane prevents protein movement out of the capillary.[1-3] It is evident from this relationship that excess fluid moving into the interstitium results from high capillary hydrostatic pressure, low capillary osmotic pressure (rarely a cause), or increased capillary permeability. Furthermore, decreased lymphatic drainage also can contribute to interstitial fluid accumulation.[4]

The pulmonary alveoli are richly supplied with capillaries (Fig. 9-1). Each capillary is surrounded by an interstitial space. The interstitium on one side of the capillary is very narrow, representing a joining of the capillary basement membrane with that of the alveolar epithelium. This juncture is believed to be the major surface for gas exchange in the lung. The interstitial space on the other side of the capillary, however, is much thicker and contains collagen fibers. Fluid filtered from the capillaries first accumulates in this larger space until it is removed by the lymphatic system.[1,2,5] Pulmonary capillary endothelium is highly permeable to water and small solutes. While movement of proteins across this membrane is somewhat restricted, the pulmonary capillaries are more permeable to proteins than are the systemic capillaries.[1,4] By contrast, the alveolar epithelium is relatively impermeable to most sub-

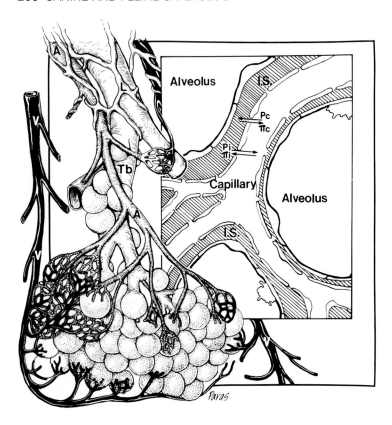

Fig. 9-1 Schematic of a respiratory unit. The arteriole branches into capillary plexes surrounding alveoli. Starling's forces controlling fluid movement into or out of the capillary are indicated. P_c, capillary hydrostatic pressure; π_c, capillary colloid osmotic pressure; P_i, interstitial hydrostatic pressure; π_i, interstitial colloid osmotic pressure. A, arteriole; V, venule; L, lymphatic vessel; Tb, terminal bronchiole. (Inset) IS, interstitial space.

stances except water. This barrier protects the interior of the alveolus from protein and electrolyte accumulation.[4]

The pulmonary capillary circulation differs from the systemic circulation in several ways. Overall pulmonary capillary hydrostatic pressure is low compared with the rest of the body, although gravitational influences within the lung result in greater hydrostatic pressures ventrally. In contrast to the systemic circulation, a major portion of the arterial to venous pressure drop occurs in the alveolar wall capillary rather than in the arteriole.[6] Pulmonary interstitial pressure is lower than systemic pressure and is well below atmospheric pressure.

Net pulmonary fluid flow is directed out of the capillaries and the subsequent lymphatic flow has been estimated to be 4 to 20 ml/hr in normal dogs.[1,7,8] There is a tremendous capacity for lymphatic diameter and flow to increase. Increases in lymphatic flow of 300 to 2,800 percent over control have been demonstrated in a canine model of chronic congestive heart failure.[7] There do not ap-

pear to be alveolar lymphatics. Therefore, fluid must move through the interstitium to adjacent perivascular and peribronchial areas where lymphatics are located.[1,6] From there, lymph flows toward the bronchial and hilar lymph nodes, finally returning to the venous circulation. Movement of lymph most likely results from the pumping action caused by fluctuating pleural pressure as well as intrinsic lymphatic wall contractions.[3,4,9] Free interstitial fluid may also accumulate in peribronchial and perivascular spaces or may drain into the mediastinum to be removed by the mediastinal lymphatics.[6]

Several factors oppose the formation of edema. These include the normal negative value of interstitial fluid pressure, the pumping action of pulmonary lymphatics, and the capacity for increased lymphatic flow. Since lymphatic walls are also very permeable, accumulated interstitial proteins are removed along with fluid. When edema is not caused by increased capillary permeability, lymphatic removal of proteins decreases interstitial osmotic pressure and tends to oppose formation of further edema.[4] Another factor that retards continued formation of edema is the increase in interstitial hydrostatic pressure that occurs as more fluid leaks from the capillaries. This lessens the net filtration pressure.[1] Pulmonary surfactant lines the alveoli, minimizes alveolar surface tension, and impedes the onset of alveolar flooding.[10,11]

CAUSES OF PULMONARY EDEMA

The major clinical cause of pulmonary edema is elevated pulmonary capillary hydrostatic pressure which usually occurs secondary to increased left atrial pressure (Table 9-1). Common causes of left-sided congestive heart failure include cardiomyopathy, mitral valve insufficiency, and aortic valve disease. Severe dysrhythmias also can elevate pulmonary venous pressure. Rarely, obstructive lesions of the left atrium, a major pulmonary vein, or mitral valve orifice produce edema. While excessive pulmonary blood flow secondary to congenital left to right cardiac shunts, anemia, or exercise can promote pulmonary edema, this is more likely to occur when there is marked volume overloading of the left ventricle with left ventricular diastolic dysfunction.[2] Certainly, overzealous intravenous fluid administration (greater than 100 ml/kg/hr in normal dogs) can cause pulmonary edema by increasing capillary hydrostatic pressure and diluting serum proteins. Systemic venous hypertension has experimentally been shown to contribute to increased lung water and edema, presumably by inducing bronchial venous hypertension.[12]

The amount of high-pressure edema formed depends in part on the rate of rise of intravascular pressures and vascular permeability.[1] Normal dogs, subjected to acute increases in left atrial pressure above 23 mmHg, develop lung edema. Conversely, pressure can be chronically elevated to 40 to 45 mmHg without development of significant edema because of gradually increasing lymphatic capacity.[4] Moreover, many causes of so-called high-pressure edema result in intercurrent increases of vascular permeability that further enhance edema formation.

On the basis of the Starling relationship, it is conceivable that low plasma colloid osmotic pressure can induce edema. However, severe hypoprotein-

Table 9-1 Causes of Pulmonary Edema

Increased pulmonary capillary pressure[a]
Cardiogenic: primarily left heart failure
Noncardiogenic: pulmonary veno-occlusive disease; overinfusion of fluids/blood
Decreased plasma osmotic pressure: severe hypoproteinemia
Altered alveolar capillary permeability[a]
Inhaled toxins: smoke and other noxious gases
Aspiration of gastric contents
O_2 toxicity
Circulating exogenous toxins: ANTU, insect and snake venoms, bacterial toxins, monocrotaline
Circulating endogenous toxins: vasoactive compounds (released in disseminated intravascular coagulation, local thrombosis, pancreatitis, immunologic reactions, anaphylaxis or shock), uremia
Other: salt water near drowning, infectious pulmonary disease
Mixed or undetermined causes[a]
Neurogenic: head trauma, seizures, electrocution, cardioversion
Rapid removal of pleural fluid after prolonged atelectasis
Drug induced (?): ketamine HCl, anesthetic agents, narcotic overdosage
Lymphatic insufficiency: neoplastic infiltration

[a] Pulmonary edema often results from both increased pressure and permeability.
(Modified from Bonagura JD: Pulmonary edema. p. 243. In Kirk RW (ed): Current Veterinary Therapy. vol. VII. WB Saunders, Philadelphia, 1980.)

emia is rarely implicated as the sole cause of edema, although it does exacerbate the edema generated by other mechanisms.[1,2] In the dog with normal plasma proteins, it has been shown that edema will not occur until left atrial pressure rises above 23 mm Hg. But when the protein level is decreased by 50 percent, edema forms at a left atrial pressure of only 12 mmHg.[13]

The second major cause of pulmonary edema, increased capillary permeability, causes a condition termed "shock lung" and acute (adult) respiratory distress syndrome (ARDS) in people. This type of lung injury follows inhalation of noxious gases, smoke, gastric secretions, or prolonged exposure to high concentrations of O_2. High-permeability pulmonary edema can also be caused by endotoxic, cardiogenic, or hypovolemic shock, sepsis, pancreatitis, or trauma or can result from pulmonary microemboli, anaphylaxis, or immune complex disease.[2,6,14] Toxic substances, including organophosphates, herbicides, (α-naphthylthiourea) (ANTU), insect and snake venoms, and toxins of uremia can cause permeability edema.[15,16] Drowning can flood alveoli and damage capillaries, causing pulmonary edema.[15,17] Both direct damage to lung tissue and indirect injury mediated by vasoactive components of the clotting cascade, the complement system, the arachidonic cascade, leukotrienes, lysosomal enzymes, and oxygen free radicals participate in the pathogenesis of permeability edema.[6,18-20] It should be recognized that increased vascular pressure may also occur in conjunction with some of the above causes of permeability edema.

The protein exudation associated with high-permeability edema inhibits resorption of fluid from the interstitium. Moreover, following alveolar flooding, this protein-rich fluid tends to coat the alveolus, leaving a hyaline membrane as fluid is resorbed. This type of lesion can reduce gas exchange and alveolar compliance.[2] The protein content of edema fluid in high permeability pulmonary edema has been measured at 70 to 100 percent of plasma protein, whereas the protein level with cardiogenic edema is only 40 to 50 percent that of the plasma.[6,8,21,22]

On occasion, pulmonary edema is neurogenic in origin, resulting from head trauma, seizures, intoxicants such as organophosphates and chlorinated hydrocarbons, other central nervous system (CNS) lesions, or electrocution[23-25] (see Table 9-1). The mechanism for this edema is unknown but is thought to be related to changes in autonomic nerve discharge.[1] Marked increases in pulmonary artery and left atrial pressures occur. Sympathetic-induced transient pressure waves also may cause capillary pore stretching and altered permeability of the vessles. Apparently, this edema can be prevented by sympathetic blockers.[6] Electrocution produces edema secondary to seizure activity.[24] One experimental report noted no change in left atrial pressure but significant pulmonary hypertension when increased intracranial pressures caused lung edema in cats. It was theorized that the surge in sympathetic

nerve discharge was limited to the lung.[26] High-protein levels also have been found in this type of edema fluid.[6]

Uncommon causes of pulmonary edema include obstruction to lymphatic drainage (as might occur secondary to carcinomatosis[1]), systemic venous hypertension, and re-expansion pulmonary edema. The latter occurs when a previously collapsed lung lobe is suddenly inflated. Experimentally, there is a correlation between the vigor of re-expansion, the length of time the lobe was collapsed, and the degree of edema. Recently, the idea that excessive negative interstitial pressure during re-expansion causes the lung edema has been questioned. Damage to capillary endothelium may be involved as studies indicate the protein content of the edema fluid is elevated.[6] Rarely, pulmonary edema has been associated with hypoglycemia[24] and ketamine HCl administration in cats.[16] While pulmonary edema occurs in some people exposed to high altitude, this has not been reproduced in experimental animals.[6]

PATHOPHYSIOLOGIC ALTERATIONS CAUSED BY PULMONARY EDEMA

Once edema begins to form the sequence of accumulation appears to be similar, regardless of cause. However, the venous congestion of cardiogenic edema causes an initial increase in pulmonary blood volume with redistribution of flow, leading to better perfusion in the upper lobes.[8,27] After fluid seeps out of the pulmonary capillaries, it accumulates first on the thick side of the interstitial space where the collagen fibrils are located (Fig. 9-1). Since the capillary endothelium abuts the alveolar epithelium on the thin side of the interstitial space, there is no great increase in the alveolar-capillary membrane thickness during the early stages of cardiogenic edema, and gas exchange is relatively unaffected.[2,5,27] If there is increased capillary permeability, however, this anatomical relationship may be quickly disrupted. There is experimental evidence for degeneration of both endothelium and epithelium in high-permeability edema.[5] Fluid moves from the pericapillary interstitium toward peribronchial and perivascular areas.

The surrounding lymphatics distend with the increased flow. Enlarged lymphatics and free fluid form a cuff around the bronchioles and vessels. This progresses as edema worsens. Later, as interstitial pressure and fluid continue to increase, alveolar flooding begins.[1,4,8] Since there is no evidence that alveolar capillary barrier injury occurs in cardiogenic pulmonary edema, there is speculation that the terminal airway epithelium is the site at which fluid enters the alveoli.[6] This flooding appears to be an all-or-none phenomenon with respect to an individual alveolus. Both flooded and nonflooded alveoli can be identified adjacent to one another.

As more alveoli become fluid filled, total pulmonary gas exchange progressively deteriorates. Flooded alveoli act as regions of pure shunt, since no ventilation occurs; accordingly, the degree of arterial hypoxemia is related to the number of unventilated units.[1,2,8] During the late stages of edema, frothy fluid spills from the alveoli into the airways. Usually, this froth is pink tinged, a result of capillary membrane damage. At this point, hypoxemia is magnified, often to a fatal degree. Flooding prevents alveolar ventilation, and any alveoli remaining open behind a froth-filled airway will be unventilated due to airway obstruction.[1,2]

Lung compliance, or the ease with which the lung can be expanded, is severely impaired in pulmonary edema. Reduced lung compliance is an early feature of pulmonary edema. As lung tissue becomes stiffer, there is an increased tendency for lung collapse.[1,2] With advancing perivascular and peribronchial cuffing, the fluid compresses these structures and isolates them from the normal inspiratory retracting forces of the surrounding lung.[27] Narrowing and premature expiratory closure of small airways are accentuated in older animals and during recumbency. These changes elevate peripheral airway and vascular resistances and promote ventilation-perfusion mismatching at various levels within the lung.[8,27] If fluid enters the alveoli, surface tension increases, causing the flooded units to be smaller. This further contributes to the decrease in lung compliance. Small airway closure throughout the respiratory cycle and alveolar edema result in a true intrapulmonary shunt.

It has been shown that at higher lung volumes these compliance abnormalities and small airway closure are minimized.[27] Thus, if several deep breaths can be stimulated during therapy, ventilation should improve. Gravity causes more marked airway and vascular compression in the dependent areas of the lung. Consequently, there may be intermittent ventilation of these areas.[1] Airway narrowing may also be exacerbated by reflex bronchoconstriction, especially if free fluid within the airway stimulates irritant receptors.[1] Chronic interstitial edema and high pulmonary capillary pressure induce reactive tissue changes and lung fibrosis, which decrease pulmonary compliance as well.[8]

The shallow rapid breathing that occurs with pulmonary edema is related to the increased stiffness of the lungs. This breathing pattern minimizes the work of breathing for the patient. Lowered PO_2 may also be a stimulus for the tachypnea, as may stimulation of J receptors in the alveolar walls.[1]

Arterial PO_2 (PaO_2) decreases from ventilation-perfusion mismatching, yet the PCO_2 tends to remain normal or decline. The shallow rapid breathing seen in patients with edema causes hyperventilation of unaffected alveoli. Since CO_2 diffuses much more rapidly than O_2 and dogs have good collateral ventilation, hypercapnia occurs only with fulminant edema.[1] Animals with heart disease and decreased cardiac output also have a decreased mixed venous PO_2, which leads to decreased PaO_2 for any level of ventilation-perfusion mismatch. Hypoxic pulmonary vasoconstriction is an attempt to minimize this mismatching by redirecting blood flow away from unventilated alveoli and by redistributing flow toward the better ventilated apices of the lung.[27]

CLINICAL FINDINGS

Just as the pathophysiologic disruptions of pulmonary edema differ with stage of severity, so does the spectrum of associated historical and physical findings. With milder accumulations of lung fluid, tachypnea or exertional dyspnea occur. There may be a dry frequent cough of recent onset in dogs. Orthopnea may develop, and affected dogs tend to stand with elbows abducted. Dogs, unlike cats, are reluctant to lie down. Paroxysms of dyspnea and coughing often occur at night or during recumbency as added blood volume is returned from the extremities to the central pool.[6] Hyperpnea or dyspnea is accentuated with hypoxemia, especially at a PaO_2

below 60 mmHg, and with lactic acidosis.[8] With severe edema, Cheyne-Stokes respiration, expectoration of pink foam, and cyanosis may be seen. Cats, unlike dogs, do not often cough due to pulmonary edema. As edema worsens, cats often crouch in a sternal position with elbows abducted and ventilate rapidly and shallowly. Open-mouth breathing in a cat is often a sign of severe respiratory distress.

Auscultatory findings vary as well. There may be no noticeable abnormalities with early interstitial edema. As smaller airways become compressed, fine crackles may be heard on inspiration as previously closed bronchioles snap open. Initially, crackles may only be heard ventrally at end-inspiration after a deep breath. It is helpful to hold off the animal's breath for a short time to stimulate deep inspiration. As edema worsens, wheezes and crackles of varying pitch and more widespread distribution may be heard during both inspiration and expiration. It is important to realize that abnormal respiratory sounds are not specific for pulmonary edema. Other lung diseases, especially pulmonary fibrosis and bronchitis, are associated with loud crackles and wheezes. Thus, the clinician must critically evaluate abnormal lung sounds within the context of history, physical findings, cardiac auscultation, thoracic radiography, and ancillary tests.

RADIOGRAPHY

The early detection of pulmonary edema is difficult. Despite advances in diagnosis with CT scans and double-indicator dilution techniques,[8] radiography remains the most practical diagnostic modality.[28] Measurement of pulmonary capillary wedge pressure is a useful hemodynamic index of the left atrial and left ventricular end-diastolic pressures. For example, correlation between increased pulmonary capillary wedge pressure with edema evident on chest radiographs was good in 90 percent of human myocardial infarction patients. When the pulmonary capillary wedge pressure was less than 18 mmHg, chest radiographs showed minimal left ventricular failure. Moderate to severe failure was diagnosed when the pulmonary capillary wedge pressure was greater than 18 mmHg. Currently, pulmonary capillary wedge pressure is considered the most reliable clinical index of lung water in humans with congestive heart failure.[8]

The characteristic locations of lung infiltrates and the caliber of pulmonary vessels permit radiologic diagnosis of pulmonary edema and may help the clinician distinguish cardiogenic edema from edema attributable to other causes. It is important for the clinician to consider the quality of the chest radiograph, positioning of the animal, phase of respiration, and artifacts, before a diagnosis of lung edema is made. The radiographic diagnosis can be complicated by pre-existing chest pathology and the commonly observed time lag between edema formation and appearance of radiographic abnormalities.[8] The onset of left-sided congestive heart failure is heralded by pulmonary venous congestion. In the dog, this is evidenced radiographically as dilated pulmonary veins and increased symmetrical perihilar interstitial density. On the lateral view, the cranial pulmonary vessels are arranged with the lobar artery dorsal and lobar vein ventral to the accompanying bronchus. Normally, the width of the vein is equal to that of the artery and averages 70 to 75 percent of the diameter of the proximal third of the fourth rib. The lobar artery is craniolateral to the vein and associated bronchus on the dorsoventral or ventrodorsal view. As pulmonary congestion increases, the pulmonary veins dilate and become denser than the arteries (Fig. 9-2). Sometimes on lateral views the cranial vein appears to sag down away from the bronchus. Although pulmonary venous dilation is a significant indicator of left-sided congestive heart failure, it is not always present. Secondary right-sided failure or compensatory venoconstriction will reduce the engorgement of pulmonary veins. Cats with acute pulmonary edema frequently exhibit enlargement of both lobar vein and artery.

Cardiomegaly is common when left heart failure is caused by chronic mitral regurgitation, cardiomyopathy, or congenital left to right shunts (Figs. 9-2 and 9-3). Typical radiographic changes in the cardiac silhouette are described elsewhere.[28,29] However, some cases of left heart failure may not be associated with obvious radiographic signs of heart enlargement. Examples include some cases of hypertrophic cardiomyopathy, acute endocarditis, acute myocardial failure, tachyarrhythmias, ruptured chordae tendineae with acute mitral insufficiency, or constrictive pericarditis.

Pulmonary parenchymal densities increase as pul-

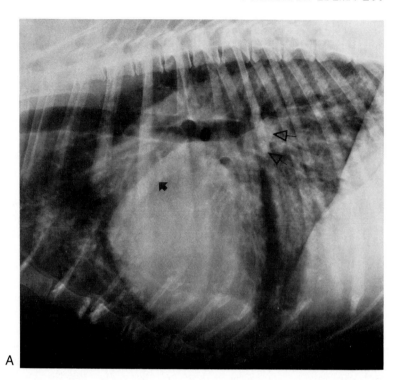

Fig. 9-2 Lateral radiographs from an 11-year-old Afghan hound with dilated cardiomyopathy and mitral insufficiency. (**A**) Marked diffusely increased pulmonary density throughout the lung fields. Air bronchograms are present. A large lobar pulmonary vein is evident (closed arrow); the left atrium is moderately enlarged (open arrows). (**B**) Following heart failure therapy. The lung fields are considerably reduced in density compared with the pretreatment radiograph (**A**). The pulmonary vein is still distended (arrow). The left atrium is prominent, and the cardiac silhouette is mildly enlarged.

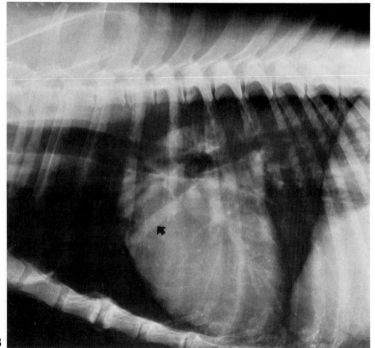

monary edema develops. Increased interstitial fluid density blurs the outline of the pulmonary vessels and cuffs the bronchi, especially in the hilar region. Pleural thickening may be seen but because dogs and cats have little interlobular tissue, Kerley lines—a feature of pulmonary edema in humans—do not appear.[28] Chronic interstitial edema can stimulate interstitial lung fibrosis adding to the overall increase in radiographic density.[28]

When edema enters the alveoli, radiography indicates areas of fluffy or mottled soft tissue density. This represents groups of flooded alveoli intermingled with aerated units.[28] As alveolar fluid continues to increase, these areas become more confluent. A homogeneous density occurs in severely edematous areas, pulmonary vessels are obscured, and air bronchograms are evident (Figs. 9-2 and 9-3). Interlobar borders are commonly visualized and may indicate subpleural edema or pleural fluid.[28]

The limitations of thoracic radiography in detecting and quantifying pulmonary edema must be recognized. There is a time lag between the onset and clearance of pulmonary fluid and its radiographic appearance and disappearance. Thus, the animal may clinically seem better or worse than radiographs indicate. Likewise, if preexisting lung changes are present, identification of pulmonary edema may be complicated. Small changes in interstitial density are difficult to appreciate.[28] Pulmonary edema may be minimal if right-sided heart failure is significant, since less blood is pumped into the pulmonary circuit. Following therapy with diuretics, the radiographic evidence of pulmonary edema may be minimal even though the patient still exhibits significant tachypnea, tiring, or cough.

Cardiogenic edema in dogs accumulates to a greater extent in the hilar area, the reasons for which are not totally clear (Fig. 9-3). This edema is usually symmetric bilaterally, although sometimes the right lobes appear more involved.[28] Hypostatic fluid accumulation can also cause an asymmetric radiographic appearance of pulmonary edema if the animal has been recumbent. Pulmonary edema in dogs with fulminant congestive heart failure (e.g., Doberman Pinscher cardiomyopathy) may be diffuse (Fig. 9-2A).

In contrast to dogs, cardiogenic pulmonary edema in cats is often unevenly distributed, patchy, or concentrated in the middle lung zones (Fig. 9-4; see Fig. 22-4). Differentiation from other infiltrative lung lesions can therefore be more difficult in the cat.

When lung infiltrates are present in a lobar, asymmetric, or otherwise uncharacteristic pattern for car-

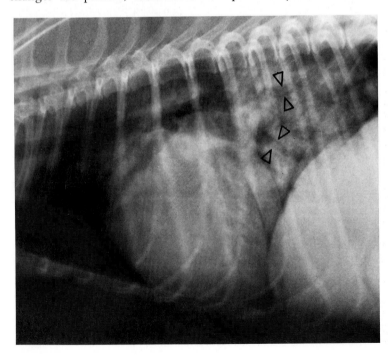

Fig. 9-3 Lateral radiograph from an 11-year-old poodle with congestive heart failure due to mitral regurgitation. Moderate generalized cardiomegaly is present. The left atrium is prominent. Interstitial and alveolar densities compatible with pulmonary edema are evident dorsally, caudally, and in the perihilar region. They result in air bronchograms (arrowheads). Pulmonary interlobar borders are visualized. Diuretic therapy led to prompt radiographic clearing of these pulmonary densities.

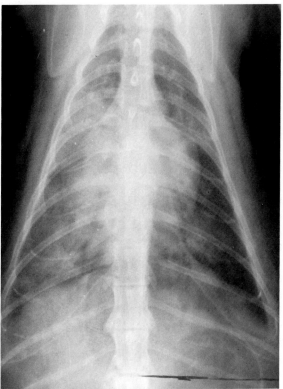

Fig. 9-4 Radiographs from two cats with hypertrophic cardiomyopathy and left-sided congestive heart failure. (**A**) Ventrodorsal view of one cat displaying patchy interstitial and alveolar lung densities, which are most prominent caudal to the heart. (**B**) Lateral view of a different cat, illustrating interstitial and alveolar lung densities. There is a predisposition to the caudal lung lobes, although some patchy densities are also observed cranial to the heart. Moderate cardiomegaly is present in both views. (Fig. A courtesy of Dr. Philip Fox.)

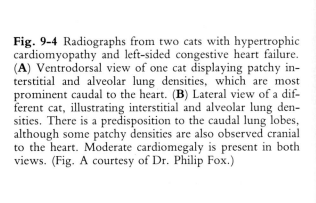

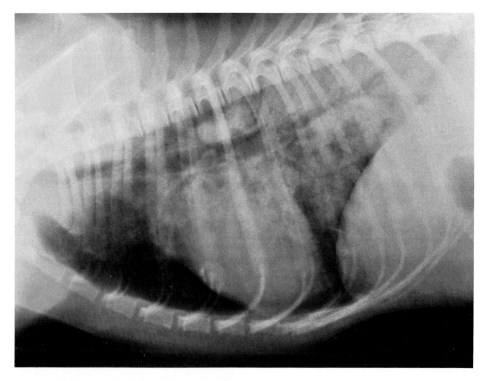

Fig. 9-5 Lateral radiograph from an 18-month-old Siberian husky with noncardiogenic pulmonary edema secondary to seizure. The cardiac silhouette is normal sized (compare with Figs. 9-2 and 9-3). A profound increase in pulmonary interstitial and alveolar densities with air bronchograms is evident in the caudal lung lobes. The dorsocaudal lung fields display particularly increased opacity, typical of neurogenic pulmonary edema.

diogenic edema, it is important to consider alternative etiologies (e.g., pneumonia, thromboembolism, neoplasia, obstructive lung disease) or noncardiogenic edema. Neurogenic edema (Fig. 9-5) tends to be located dorsocaudally in the lung periphery.[23,24] By contrast, emphysema and hyperinflation of the lung decrease the visibility as well as the formation of edema. This may complicate a diagnosis of left-sided heart failure.[28]

THERAPY OF PULMONARY EDEMA

Therapeutic objectives for pulmonary edema of any cause include restoration of arterial oxygenation, removal of alveolar fluid, and correction of the underlying etiology (Table 9-2). Supplemental oxygen, airway suction (if frothing is evident), redistribution of pulmonary blood to the peripheral circulation, rest, and diuresis are the mainstays of therapy. Determination of the severity of edema as well as the cause dictates which therapeutic measures must be employed.

Oxygen can be administered by face mask, nasal catheter, endotracheal tube or O_2 cage. A cage should have temperature and humidity controls—a maximum of 65 degrees in normothermic animals has been recommended.[15] Oxygen flows of 6 to 10 L/min are usually adequate. Initially, concentrations of 50 to 100 percent O_2 may be necessary. When foaming within the airways is evident, nebulization of 20 percent ethanol may break down bubbles in the edema fluid by reducing surface tension.[15,30] In severely affected animals, endotracheal or tracheotomy tube placement and mechanical ventilation

Table 9-2 Therapy of Pulmonary Edema

Do not stress the animal!

Restore oxygenation
　Check airway patency
　Give supplemental O_2 (avoid >50% for >24 hours)
　Provide cage rest
　Intubate and supply positive-pressure ventilation, if
　　needed
　If frothing is evident, suction airways and nebulize
　　with ethanol (20–50%)

Remove alveolar fluid
　Redistribute blood volume:
　　Morphine (0.05–0.5 mg/kg IV, IM, or SC to
　　　effect–dogs *only*)
　　Vasodilators:
　　　2% nitroglycerin ointment ($\frac{1}{4}$–$\frac{3}{4}$ inch topically
　　　　q6h—dogs; $\frac{1}{8}$–$\frac{1}{4}$ inch q6h—cats
　　　Na nitroprusside (5–20 μg/kg/min constant rate
　　　　infusion)
　　Phlebotomy (6–10 ml/kg)
　Initiate diuresis:
　　Furosemide (1–4 mg/kg IV, IM, or PO—dogs; 1–
　　　2 mg/kg IV, IM, PO—cats) can repeat q6–12h

Reduce anxiety
　Morphine (dogs)
　Acepromazine—cats: (0.05–0.2 mg/kg SC)
　Diazepam (2–5 mg IV—cat; 5–10 mg IV–dog)

Reduce bronchoconstriction
　Aminophylline (6–10 mg/kg IV, IM, SC, PO, can
　　repeat q6h–dogs; 4–8 mg/kg IM, SC, PO, can
　　repeat q8–12h—cats)

Administer inotropic support (if myocardial failure is
　present)
　Digoxin (0.01–0.015 mg/kg PO div. BID—dog;
　　0.005 mg/kg IV div. or 0.005–0.01 mg/kg PO–
　　cats)
　Dobutamine (2–10 μg/kg/min constant rate infusion)
　Dopamine (2–8 μg/kg/min constant rate infusion)

Increase cardiac output and reduce afterload[a]
　Na nitroprusside (see above)
　Hydralazine (0.5–3 mg/kg PO, q12h—dogs)

Treat high-permeability edema
　Consider glucocorticoids
　Institute specific measures depending on etiology

Provide ancillary therapy
　Correct acid-base imbalance (e.g., sodium
　　bicarbonate; ventilation)
　Monitor CBC, serum biochemistries, ECG, pulse
　　strength, respiratory rate; arterial, pulmonary
　　capillary wedge, and central venous pressures;
　　hydration, urine output, body weight, etc.

[a] Most useful for severe mitral regurgitation in dogs.

with positive end-expiratory pressure (PEEP) or continuous positive airway pressure (CPAP) can be lifesaving. Salutory effects of PEEP ventilation include clearing of small airways, expanding small volume alveoli, forcing alveolar fluid back into the interstitium, and increasing lung volume to augment the interstitial fluid capacity.[6] High O_2 concentrations (> 70 percent) can injure lung tissue. A formula has been devised for humans that uses an initial FiO_2 (inspired O_2 concentration) of less than 50 percent. Therapy is then adjusted by adding increments of 5 mmHg PEEP until the PaO_2 divided by the FiO_2 is greater than 300.[27] Alternatively, PEEP can be achieved with spontaneous ventilation through a respirator and by exhaling against a 4 to 20 cm H_2O pressure.[15,30] It is essential to have careful and continuous patient and equipment monitoring for intubated animals.

Rapid diuresis can be achieved with intravenous furosemide. This potent loop-acting diuretic promotes rapid and effective diuresis. Experimentally, it has been shown to reduce pulmonary shunting by augmenting perfusion of nonflooded alveoli before diuresis occurs.[31] Other diuretics, such as the thiazides or aldosterone antagonists, can be helpful either alone or in conjunction with oral furosemide in treating chronic edema in dogs. Pulmonary edema in cats is usually responsive to furosemide.

Aminophylline, given intramuscularly or by slow intravenous injection, has mild diuretic and positive inotropic actions as well as a bronchodilating effect. The usual dose is 6 to 10 mg/kg every 6 to 8 hours. Aminophylline can also be given orally.

Dogs with pulmonary edema benefit from morphine sulfate. It may be given intravenously (0.05 to 0.1 mg/kg) every 2 to 3 minutes until the desired clinical response is achieved[30] or administered as a single intramuscular or subcutaneous dose of 0.2 to 0.5 mg/kg.[16] Anxiety is relieved, the respiratory center is depressed so that slower, deeper breaths are taken, and splanchnic blood vessels are dilated leading to decreased cardiac return and redistribution of volume away from the lungs. Morphine can raise intracranial pressure. Therefore, it is contraindicated in neurogenic edema.

Morphine is contraindicated in cats. Cats can potentially receive acepromazine, 0.05 to 0.2 mg/kg subcutaneously, as an alternative. This drug might promote peripheral redistribution of blood. However, it may exacerbate pre-existing hypothermia.

Vasodilating drugs, such as 2 percent nitroglycerin ointment applied cutaneously, or intravenous nitroprusside (used with careful patient monitoring), can be helpful in fulminant cardiogenic edema by virtue of their ability to increase systemic venous capacitance and lower pulmonary venous pressure. Nitroprusside also dilates systemic arterioles and may increase cardiac output. Hydralazine is beneficial in the treatment of refractory pulmonary edema caused by mitral regurgitation. Further information on these and other drugs can be found in Chapter 8.

Care should be exercised when positive inotropic drugs are used. Catecholamines may cause elevations in pulmonary and systemic vascular resistance, potentially exacerbating interstitial fluid accumulatin. Also, acidosis and hypoxemia, both of which are common in severe edema, can increase myocardial sensitivity to digitalis-induced dysrhythmias.[27] Monitoring of electrolyte and acid-base balance is important.

Other techniques that have been used in acute cardiogenic edema include phlebotomy of up to 25 percent of total blood volume and rotating tourniquets (which is probably not very effective in animals). It is important for all treatments to be given with a minimum of stress to the patient.

Noncardiogenic or high-permeability pulmonary edema is difficult to treat, and a detailed discussion of possible therapy is beyond the scope of this textbook. Often this type of edema, as well as its underlying etiology, is progressive. Oxygen therapy is given as outlined above. Diuretics may be helpful, but careful attention should be paid to cardiac output, blood pressure, and hydration. Corticosteroids may or may not be helpful, depending on the etiology of lung edema; their use is still controversial. Corticosteroids have been advocated in the early treatment of smoke inhalation, electric shock, snake bites, septic shock, and anaphylaxis.[27,30,32] Identification of the primary problem, if possible, may suggest further therapeutic measures. For example, neurogenic pulmonary edema secondary to organophosphate intoxication should be treated with atropine as well as basic supportive care. Further information on the therapy of high permeability edema can be found elsewhere.[15,33–35]

REFERENCES

1. West JB: Pulmonary Pathophysiology—The Essentials. 2nd Ed. Williams & Wilkins, Baltimore, 1982
2. Nunn JF: Applied Respiratory Physiology. 2nd Ed. Butterworths, London, 1977
3. Cottrell TS, Levine OR, Senior RM, et al: Electron microscopic alterations at the alveolar level in pulmonary edema. Circ Res 21:783, 1967
4. Guyton AC: Textbook of Medical Physiology. 7th Ed. WB Saunders, Philadelphia, 1985
5. Staub NC: Pulmonary edema. Physiol Rev 54:679, 1974
6. Uhley HN, Leeds SE, Sampson JJ, Friedman M: Role of pulmonary lymphatics in chronic pulmonary edema. Circ Res 11:966, 1962
7. Weaver LJ, Carrico CJ: Congestive heart failure and edema. p. 543, In Staub NC, Taylor AE (eds): Edema. Raven Press, New York, 1984
8. Staub NC: Pathophysiology of pulmonary edema. p. 719. In Staub NC, Taylor AE (eds): Edema. Raven Press, New York, 1984
9. Enderson BL, Rice CL, Beaver CW, et al: High frequency ventilation and the accumulation of extravascular lung water. J Surg Res 36:433, 1984
10. Neiman GF, Brendenberg CE: High surface tension pulmonary edema induced by detergent aerosol. J Appl Physiol 58:129, 1985
11. Seeger W, Stohr G, Wolf HRD, Neuhof H: Alteration of surfactant function due to protein leakage: Special interaction with fibrin nonomer. J Appl Physiol, 58:326, 1985
12. Miller WC, Simi WW, Rice DL: Contribution of systemic venous hypertension to the development of pulmonary edema in dogs. Circ Res 43:598, 1978
13. Guyton AC, Lindsey AW: Effect of elevated left atrial pressure and decreased plasma protein concentration on the development of pulmonary edema. Circ Res 7:649, 1959
14. Kuida H, Hinshaw LB, Gilbert RP, Visscher MB: Effect of gram-negative endotoxin on pulmonary circulation. Am J Physiol 192:335, 1958
15. Suter PF, Ettinger SJ: Pulmonary edema. p. 747. In Ettinger SJ (ed): Textbook of Veterinary Internal Medicine, Diseases of the Dog and Cat. 2nd Ed. WB Saunders, Philadelphia, 1983
16. Bonagura JD: Pulmonary edema. p. 243. In Kirk RW (ed): Current Veterinary Therapy. Vol. VII. Small Animal Practice. WB Saunders, Philadelphia, 1980
17. Modell JH: Drowning. p. 679. In Staub NC, Taylor AE (eds): Edema. Raven Press, New York, 1984
18. Herndon DN, Traber DL, Niehaus GD, et al.: The

pathophysiology of smoke inhalation injury in a sheep model. J Trauma 24:1044, 1984

19. Malik AB, Perlman MB, Cooper JA, et al: Pulmonary microvascular effects of arachidonic acid metabolites and their role in lung vascular injury. Fed Proc 44:36, 1985

20. Brigham KL: Metabolites of arachidonic acid in experimental lung vascular injury. Fed Proc 44:43, 1985

21. Lord PF: Neurogenic pulmonary edema in the dog. J Am Anim Hosp Assoc 11:778, 1975

22. Vreim CE, Snashall PD, Staub NC: Protein composition of lung fluids in anesthetized dogs with acute cardiogenic edema. Am J Physiol 231:1466, 1976

23. Fein A, Grossman RF, Jones JG, et al: The value of edema fluid protein measurement in patients with pulmonary edema. Am J Med 67:32, 1979

24. Newman MM, Kligerman M, Willcox M: Pulmonary hypertension, pulmonary edema, and decreased pulmonary compliance produced by increased intracranial pressure in cats. J Neurosurg 60:1207, 1984

25. Bradley RL, Keating ML: Neurogenic pulmonary edema in a cat. Fel Pract 9:26, 1979

26. Kolata RJ: The clinical features of electrical cord bite injury in dogs. p. 460. In Proceedings of the Forty-first Annual Meeting of the American Animal Hospital Association, 1974

27. Ayres SM: Mechanisms and consequences of pulmonary edema: Cardiac lung, shock lung, and principles of ventilatory therapy in adult respiratory distress syndrome. Am Heart J 103:97, 1982

28. Suter PF: Thoracic Radiography. PF Suter, Wettswil, Switzerland, 1984

29. Davis LE: Management of acute pulmonary edema. J Am Vet Med Assoc 175:97, 1979

30. Hamlin RL: Radiographic diagnosis of heart disease in dogs. J Am Vet Med Assoc 137:458, 1960

31. Ali J, Wood LDH: Pulmonary vascular effects of furosemide on gas exchange in pulmonary edema. J Appl Physiol Respir Environ Exer Physiol 57:160, 1984

32. Bauer TG, Thomas WP: Pulmonary Edema. p. 252. In Kirk RW (ed): Current Veterinary Therapy. Vol. VIII. Small Animal Practice. WB Saunders, Philadelphia, 1983

33. Prewitt RM, McCarthy J, Wood LDH: Treatment of acute low pressure pulmonary edema in dogs. J Clin Invest 67:409, 1981

34. Morgan RV: Respiratory emergencies. Part I. Compend Contin Educ 5:228, 1983

35. Olivier NB: Pulmonary edema. p. 1011. In Veterinary Clinics of North America. Vol. 15: Small Animal Practice. WB Saunders, Philadelphia, 1985

10

Dietary Management, Nutrition, and the Heart

Sarah L. Ralston
Philip R. Fox

OVERVIEW OF NUTRITIONAL MANAGEMENT

Proper nutritional management is an essential factor in the treatment of many diseases.[1,2] It is important for recovery, stabilization and longevity during therapy of chronic heart failure.[1-6] Dietary modification may provide a significant but relatively simple means of treating chronic heart failure[6] and usually accompanies other therapeutic measures (Ch. 8). To be beneficial, nutritional management must take into account the characteristics of nutrients, their required amounts, effects of excesses or deficiencies, the nutrient content of foods (both home prepared and commercial), factors affecting their palatability, and cost.

Alterations in Salt and Water Retention with Heart Failure

When the heart fails, compensatory homeostatic neurohumoral and cardiorenal adjustments occur that assist in supporting circulation and blood pressure. One important adjustment—incresed ventric-

ular filling pressures due to expanded plasma volume—results from renal salt and water retention. This, however, may also contribute to clinical signs through secondary formation of edema or effusions (Chs. 2, 7, and 9).

Patients with advancing heart failure have a significantly reduced ability to excrete a salt or water load, despite marked expansion of blood and interstitial fluid volumes. This progressively worsens as the heart failure state advances.[7] The inability to excrete salt has been suggested as an indicator of heart failure.[8]

Therapeutic goals for heart failure include maintaining tissue oxygenation, controlling rhythm disturbances, improving circulation, modifying fluid compartments and venous pressures to maintain blood flow but prevent congestion (Ch. 8).

Reversibility of myocardial failure has been demonstrated in taurine deficient cats after supplementing oral taurine. These animals had been previously fed commercial diets resulting in taurine depletion.[6]

Dietary sodium restriction has been a basic component in therapeutic strategies of heart failure man-

219

agement in dogs. Appropriate dietary modification in chronic congestive heart failure may help alleviate clinical signs of edema and effusions, improve attitude, and reduce the need for certain pharmacologic therapies.[4,5,7,8–11]

NUTRITIONAL REQUIREMENTS WITH HEART FAILURE

Sodium restriction is not the only concern in dietary selection for animals with advanced cardiac diseases. The effects of chronic congestive heart failure on nutritional needs and the methods of insuring adequate nutritional support must also be considered.[1,2]

Cardiac Cachexia

Cardiac cachexia is common in late stages of chronic, acquired valvular heart diseases (mitral and tricuspid insufficiency) and dilated cardiomyopathy in dogs and cats. Many factors contribute to loss of mean body mass, including reduced caloric intake resulting from poor palatability of low-sodium foods,[5,11] malaise, congestion, effusions, drug toxicity, and anorexia.[7] Gastric compression in states of severe ascites may be contributory, although this has not been clearly documented. Malabsorbtion due to poor splanchnic and gastrointestinal perfusion or villous atrophy secondary to malnutrition and anorexia may exist.[9,12,13] Cellular hypoxia resulting from low cardiac output and poor perfusion, decreased peripheral delivery of cellular nutrients, and removal of metabolic waste products may occur.[12] Hypermetabolism may result from greater energy expenditure by cardiac and respiratory tissues and/or stress.[14]

The state of cardiac cachexia may have certain adaptive consequences, such as reduced demand for oxygen by the lean muscle mass.[11] However, reduced caloric intake and an inappropriate nutritional plane may impair immune competency,[1] contribute to development of hypoalbuminemia, and decrease tissue repair and ability to respond to therapy.[2,16,17] Reduced plasma levels of iron, hemoglobin, thiamine, and folic acid have been documented in humans with heart failure.[9] Severe malnutrition may itself affect the heart adversely.[7]

RELATIONS BETWEEN HEART FAILURE, NUTRITION, AND PHARMACOKINETICS

Drug absorption, distribution, biotransformation, and elimination may be adversely affected by heart failure, subsequent lack of nutritional intake, and cachexia. Hypovolemia (dehydration, vomiting, diarrhea), decresed plasma albumin (hepatic or renal disease, lack of protein intake, protein-losing enteropathy, or malabsorption syndromes), altered organ blood flow, and decreased peripheral tissue binding (circulatory failure, shock) may increase unbound plasma drug concentration, decrease volume of distribution, alter drug elimination, promote lack of efficacy, or cause drug toxicity.[18]

Chronic renal failure (CRF) may be present concomitantly with heart failure, especially in the older pet. Systemic hypertension may be presented in half the canines with chronic renal disease and may contribute to cardiac enlargement, heart failure, and renal failure.[19] Renal insufficiency also alters elimination of many cardiovascular drugs such as digoxin. Therapeutic strategies may need to employ additional dietary modifications in such instances.

Reduced intake of dietary protein may help ameliorate clinical signs of uremia, although the extent and timing of protein restriction are controversial.[20] Diets that are protein deficient or excessive may cause adverse effects in CRF.[21] Dogs with mild to moderate CRF (mean serum creatinine concentration, 1.5 to 4.5 mg/dl) should be fed 1.5 to 3.5 g high-biologic-value protein per kilogram body weight daily. This may be accomplished with home prepared foods or commercial products. Dietary protein intake should be individualized. If hypoalbuminemia or significant weight loss occurs, dietary protein sources with essential amino acids of high biologic value (eggs, chicken, and cottage cheese) may minimize renal excretion of metabolic byproducts from amino acid deamination.[16]

Cats have higher dietary protein needs than dogs, but their requirements with renal failure are not well documented. In states of CRF, cats may be fed diets containing 20 percent of the calories as protein (equivalent to 3.5 to 4.0 g high-biologic-value protein per kilogram body weight) when given 70 to 80 kcal/kg/day.[19,22] There may be a problem with palatability, in which case sufficient protein and fat should be added to ensure intake.

GOALS OF DIETARY MANAGEMENT OF THE CARDIAC PATIENT

The goal of dietary management is to maintain lean body weight while providing adequate levels of protein, vitamins, and minerals in a diet that the animal will consume readily. Characteristics of the recommended diet for chronic heart disease are presented in Table 10-1.

Maintenance of Body Weight

Initial caloric needs for compensated heart failure without cachexia (dogs–60 to 110 kcal/kg body weight; cats–60 to 85 kcal/kg body weight) becomes inadequate later during the disease course. When body weight is lost, daily caloric requirements may need to be increased 25 to 50 percent or more. In general, 6 g protein should be provided for each 150 kcal energy in the diet,[9] unless the animal is in renal or hepatic failure. If renal or hepatic failure is present, dietary protein should be reduced and be from high quality, highly digestible sources (e. g., egg or casien). Red meats should be avoided, especially in cases of hepatic failure. Their high levels of tryptophan and aromatic amino acids have been incriminated in the development of hepatic encephalopathy.

Table 10-1 Dietary Characteristics for Heart Failure Patients (Dry Matter Basis)

Energy—Moderate to High
  20–25% fat

Protein—Moderate to Low
  High-biologic-value
  Dogs: 18–21%
  Cats: >30

NaCl—Low
  Less than 0.3% (cats)
  Less than 0.1% (dogs)

Vitamin B content—High

If malabsorption is documented by the presence of high fecal fat or poor absorption of glucose following a glucose tolerance test,[15] highly digestible liquid diets may be tried to supplement the daily diet (Table 10-2). However, further data is needed to verify the nutritional adequacy of these supplements, potential benefits, and side effects (e. g., diarrhea) to heart failure patients.

Dietary Sodium Restriction

One of the major dietary goals during chronic heart failure management is restriction of sodium intake. The degree of salt restriction depends on the stage and severity of heart failure. In the dog with early or mild failure, simple avoidance of treats and table food high in sodium may be adequate (Table 10-3). With recurrent or advanced chronic heart failure, moderate sodium restriction (13 mg/kg/day) may be needed. To accomplish this the daily ration must contain about 25 mg sodium per 100 g canned food or 90 mg per 100 g dry food.[5]

Most commercial dog foods contain excessive levels of sodium chloride (Table 10-4). Special prescription diets such as k/d, h/d (Hills Pet Products Inc, Topeka KS) are specially formulated to have low sodium content while meeting the overall nutritional needs of the cardiac patient. Do not assume that diets designed for geriatric dogs are low in sodium content.

Electrolyte disturbances are rare in dogs being fed restricted sodium diets.[10,23] Even when diuretics are administered, hyponatremia and hypokalemia are uncommon.[24] In animals with prolonged anorexia, especially cats treated with diuretics, hypokalemia frequently occurs. Cats with renal failure may also have increased urinary potassium excretion. Deleterious effects of hypokalemia are discussed elsewhere (chs. 4, 13, 14, and 15).

Home prepared diets may be employed. Recipes for dogs and cats are given (Table 10-5). Nutrient contents of human foods that may be used in basic recipes or as flavor enhancers are provided in Table 10-6. Foods to be avoided in basic recipes or for use in treats are listed in Table 10-3.

Anorexia and Dietary Habits

Dogs with heart failure are frequently older animals that have fixed dietary habits. Abruptly switching to a new diet is often unsuccessful. Guide-

Table 10-2 Liquid Diet Supplements

	Kcal/ml	g Protein/ml	mg Na/ml	Content of Supplement[a]
Ensure (Ross Lab)	1.06	0.04	0.84	Casein and soy protein, corn oil, and starch
Ensure Plus (Ross Lab)	1.50	0.05	1.1	Same as above but higher in protein and vitamins
Osmolite (Ross Lab)	1.06	0.04	0.55	Medium-chain triglycerides, corn, casein and soy protein, cornstarch
Compleat B (Doyle)	1.07	0.05	1.3	Beef puree, nonfat milk, corn oil, cereal and vegetable puree, orange juice
Meritene (Doyle)	0.96	0.06	0.88	Skim milk, casein, corn oil, corn syrup, sucrose
Precision HN (Doyle)	1.05	0.04	0.98	Egg white, medium-chain triglycerides, soybean oil, maltodextrin, sucrose
Sustacal (Mead Johnson)	1.01	0.06	0.93	Casein and soy protein, soy oil, sucrose, corn syrup
Vivonex (Norwich Eaton)	1.00	0.03	0.47	Free amino acids, safflower oil, glucose, oligosaccharides
High Nitrogen Vivonex (Norwich Eaton)	1.00	0.04	0.53	Free amino acids, safflower oil, glucose, oligosaccharides
Criticare HN (Mead Johnson)[b]	1.06	0.04	0.63	Casein, free amino acids, safflower oil, maltodextrin, cornstarch

[a] All contain vitamin and mineral supplements.
[b] Very palatable to cats.
(Ralston SL: Dietary management of chronic cardiac disease. p. 63. Proceedings of the Ninth Annual Kal Kan Symposium. Kal Kan Foods Inc, Vernon, CA, 1986, with permission.)

lines for changing diets are therefore suggested as follows[16]:

1. Switch the diet slowly over the course of 4 or 5 days, gradually replacing the old diet with the new.

2. Warm the new food to volatilize odors.
3. Add flavor enhancers in small amounts to the new food (Table 10-6).
4. Feed small amounts frequently.
5. If necessary, force feed through a nasogastric tube until the animal is nutritionally stabilized.

Table 10-3 Foods to Be Avoided in Heart Failure Diets

All preserved meats (e.g., corned beef, salami)
Canned fish (unless low-salt)
Beef kidney; liver
All cheese (unless low-salt)
Dried nonfat milk
Margarine or butter (unless low-salt)
Canned vegetables (unless low-salt)
All breads (unless low-salt)
Potato chips, pretzels, cornflakes
Dog "treats" (e.g., biscuits, rawhide)

(Modified from Ralston SL: Dietary Management of Cardiac Disease. p. 63. Proceedings of the Ninth Annual Kal Kan Symposium. Kal Kan Foods Inc, Vernon CA, with permission.)

OTHER CONDITIONS REQUIRING DIETARY MODIFICATION

Arterial Hypertension

In cases of arterial hypertension (diagnosed by blood pressure measurements) sodium intake should be reduced to 0.1 to 0.3 percent of the diet. Transition from high- to low-sodium diets should be gradual when moderate or advanced renal insufficiency exists. Salt restriction alone may permit adequate reduction in blood pressure with mild

Table 10-4 Sodium Content (mg/100 g Dry Matter) of Commercial Pet Foods

Dog Foods	Sodium (mg/100 g Dry Matter)	Cat Foods	Sodium (mg/100 g Dry Matter)
		Dry	
Cycle 2	740	Friskies Ocean Fish	877
Ken-L-Ration Biskit	600	Special Dinner Tuna &	
Gravy Train	563	Herring	615
Iams Chunks	540	Crave	600
Purina Dog Chow	508	Fish Ahoy	590
Gaines Meal	340	Kitten Chow	570
Average	550	Chef's Blend	535
		Iams	500
		Tamiami	485
		Cat Chow Original Blend	
		9-Lives Tuna	470
		Average	370
			561
		Semimoist	
Gainesburgers	950	9-Lives	737
Top Choice	812	Happy Cat	647
Prime	809	Tender Vittles	535
Average	857	Average	640
		Canned	
Mighty Dog	583	Purina 100 tuna	3,790★
Ken-L-Ration	1140	Fancy Feast Seafood	890
Friskies Dog Food	1036	Friskies Fish Flav	857
Kal Kan Chunks of Beef		Puss-N-Boots Fish	830
By-Products	894	Kal Kan Mealtime	790
Alpo Beef Chunks		9-Lives Tuna	730
Dinner	868	Friskies Buffet	
Average	904	Seafood Supper	690
		Bright Eyes	
		Seafood Supper	590
		Average (★excluded)	768
		Dietary prescription diets	
Canine *g/d*	300	Feline *c/d*	490
Canine *k/d*	230	Feline *k/d*	400
Canine *h/d*		Feline *h/d*	240
(canned)	90		
(dry)	55		

(Modified from Ross JN: Heart Failure. p. 11-30. In Lewis LN, Morris ML Jr (eds): Small Animal Clinical Nutrition. 3rd Ed. Mark Morris Associates, Topeka, KS, 1987, with permission.)

Table 10-5 Recipes for Homemade Diets for Dogs and Cats with Cardiac Disease

Highly Digestible Diet for Dogs	Low-Sodium Diet for Dogs	Restricted Mineral and Sodium Diet for Cats
½ cup farina cooked to make 2 cups	¼ lb lean ground beef or pork or chicken	1 lb regular ground beef or lamb or chicken cooked
1½ cups creamed cottage cheese (low salt)	2 cups cooked rice without salt	¼ lb liver
1 large egg, hard-cooked	1 tbsp vegetable oil	1 cup cooked rice without added salt
2 tbsp Brewer's yeast	2 tsp dicalcium phosphate	1 tsp vegetable oil
3 tbsp sugar		1 tsp calcium carbonate
1 tbsp vegetable oil		
1 tsp potassium chloride		
1 tsp dicalcium phosphate		
1 tsp calcium carbonate		
Balanced supplement that fulfills the canine minimum daily requirement for all vitamins and trace minerals.	Balanced supplement that fulfills the canine minimum daily requirement for all vitamins and trace minerals.	Balanced supplement which fulfills the feline minimum daily requirement for all vitamins and trace minerals.
Cook farina according to package directions, omitting salt. Cool. Add remaining ingredients to farina and mix well.	Braise meat, retaining fat. Add the remaining ingredients and mix.	Combine all ingredients.
Yield: 2.2 lb (1 kg)	Yield: 1 lb (0.5 kg)	Yield: 1¾ lb (0.8 kg)

Analysis		Analysis		Analysis	
Moisture %	75.8	Moisture %	68.5	Moisture %	64.0
Protein %	7.1	Protein %	6.3	Protein %	14.1
Fat %	3.7	Fat %	5.5	Fat %	13.8
Carbohydrate %	11.2	Carbohydrate %	17.7	Carbohydrate %	6.6
Fiber %	0.1	Sodium %[a]	.01	Ash %	1.5
Ash %	2.1	ME (Kcal)	660/lb	Calcium %	0.24
Calcium %	0.33			Phosphorus %	0.15
Phosphorus %	0.19			Magnesium %	0.014
Potassium %	0.36			Magnesium, mg/100 Kcal	8
ME (Kcal)	485/lb			Sodium %	0.06
Sodium %	0.16			ME (Kcal)	940/lb

[a] 50 mg sodium/100 g dry diet. ME, metabolizable energy as fed.
(Modified from Lewis LD, Morris ML Jr (eds): Small Animal Clinical Nutrition. 2nd Ed. p. A3-1. Mark Morris Associates, Topeka, KS, 1984.)

states of hypertension. However, additional drug therapy is required in more severe cases of systemic hypertension.[19]

Obesity and the Heart

Obesity may impose increased metabolic demands on the heart for oxygen with subsequent hemodynamic alterations. The syndrome of obesity is characterized by excessive accumulations of body fat due to imbalanced energy intake and utilization.

In some studies of obese human patients, oxygen consumption was increased and cardiac output elevated as a result of increased stroke volume. Elevated stroke volume was secondary to preload elevation due to blood volume expansion. Systemic vascular resistance was normal to low, facilitating increased cardiac output without systemic hypertension. Elevated left ventricular end-diastolic pressure (LVEDP) correlated with weight and was a consequence of increased preload. Pulmonary artery

Table 10-6 Nutrient Content of Human Foods that May be Used as Supplements or Substitutes in Basic Recipes[a]

Food	kcal	Protein (g)	Calcium (g)	Phosphorus (g)	Sodium (g)	Potassium (g)
Meats						
Chicken white meat	107	20	0.01	0.20	0.06	0.27
Pork, fresh cooked, lean and fat	391	24	0.01	0.27	0.06	0.28
Lean ground beef	179	21	0.01	0.19	0.06	0.24
Regular ground beef	268	18	0.01	0.16	0.06	0.22
Beef heart	108	17	0	0.18	0.09	0.23
Lamb, broiled or roasted	265	15	0.01	0.14	0.07	0.25
Eggs						
1 large (average = 50 g)	163	13	0.05	0.20	0.12	0.13
1 yolk (average = 17 g)	348	16	0.14	0.57	0.05	0.14
1 white (average = 33 g)	51	11	0.01	0.15	0.15	0.09
Dairy products						
Whole milk (1 cup = 244 g)	65	3.5	0.12	0.09	0.05	0.16
Skim milk (1 cup = 244 g)	59	3.6	0.12	0.10	0.06	0.18
Cottage cheese, creamed unsalted (1 cup = 225 g)	106	14	0.10	0.15	0.23	0.08
Yogurt, plain	64	5	0.15	0.12	0.05	0.19
Vegetables and fruits						
Avocado (California)	171	2	0.01	0.42	0.004	0.60
Banana	84	Trace	0.08	0.02	0.001	0.37
Carrots, raw, grated (1 cup = 110 g)	41	1	0.04	0.04	0.05	0.34
Corn, frozen (1 cup = 165 g)	79	3	0.003	0.07	0.001	0.18
Whole potato, boiled	77	2	0.007	0.05	0.006	0.40
Cereals[b]						
Corn grits, enriched (1 cup cooked = 245 g)	51	1	Trace	0.01	Trace	0.01
Farina (1 cup cooked = 245 g)	43	1	0.06	0.05	Trace	0.01
Oatmeal (1 cup cooked = 240 g)	54	2	0.01	0.05	Trace	0.07
Other grain products						
Macaroni, cooked 8–10 min (1 cup = 140 g)	110	3	0.01	0.05	Trace	0.06
Egg noodles, cooked (1 cup = 160 g)	125	4	0.01	0.06	Trace	0.04
Other						
Honey (1 tbsp = 21 g)	309	Trace	0.004	0.004	0.005	0.005
Butter, unsalted	721	Trace	0.03	0.02	0.01	0.02
Corn oil (1 tbsp = 14 g)	883	0	0	0	0	0
Molasses, blackstrap (1 tbsp = 20 g)	225	0	0.68	0.08	0.01	2.92

[a] All values are amounts per 100 g as fed.
[b] Cooked without added salt.
(Ralston SL: Dietary management of chronic cardiac disease. p. 63. Proceedings of the Ninth Annual Kal Kan Symposium. Kal Kan Foods Inc, Vernon, CA, 1986.)

and pulmonary capillary pressures were elevated secondary to increased LEVDP, as was right ventricular end-diastolic pressure and right atrial mean pressure. Left ventricular contractility was reduced despite increased ventricular filling pressures.[25]

Other investigators have suggested that similar changes were not due to impaired left ventricular performance but primarily to the hypervolemic state.[26] However, much evidence illustrates that hemodynamic changes are more than a physiologic adaptation to obesity and result from intrinsic myocardial changes that persist after weight reduction.[27,28]

In association with increased stroke vlume, left ventricular filling pressures and volume, and elevated left ventricular wall stress causes myocardial mass to increase. Secondary eccentric hypertrophy (wall thickening and chamber dilation) occurs.[29]

Arrhythmias have been associated with obesity and excessive weight loss. Obese humans with distinct eccentric left ventricular hypertrophy are prone to increased ventricular ectopy as compared with obese people without eccentric hypertrophy or with slender individuals.[30] Excessive weight loss, especially when achieved with high- protein, high-fat diets, has been associated with ventricular ectopy, ventricular fibrillation, and sudden death. The arrhythmias may be related to myocardial depletion of potassium or magnesium induced by lactic acidosis and natriuesis of fasting.[29] Weight loss in obese humans may be beneficial to the heart, however, by reducing ventricular sympathetic outflow, preload, afterload, and left ventricular hypertrophy.[31]

Obesity in dogs and cats can also adversely affect mechanical respiration, predisposing to obesity hypoventillation—the "pickwickian syndrome." This may be a contributing or complicating factor to cor pulmonale, a secondary form of right heart disease and failure.[32] Dietary management of the obese pet is necessary for successful management and has been summarized elsewhere.[33]

Taurine Deficiency

Taurine (2-aminoethanesulfonic acid) in mammals is derived from metabolism of sulfur amino acids (methionine and cysteine) through decarboxylation of cysteinesulfonic acid to hypotaurine, with subsequent oxidation to taurine.[34] In cats, however, taurine synthesis is minimal, and the amino acid is an essential nutrient.[35] Bile acids in the cat are conjugated almost exclusively with taurine. With dietary taurine depletion, bile acids are not conjugated to glycine as in other mammals. Instead, free bile acids are excreted.[36]

Taurine plays a prominent role as a neurotransmitter and neuromodulator in the central nervous system.[37,38] Degeneration of retinal photoreceptor cells is a clearly demonstrated result of taurine deficiency.[39] Taurine also plays a role in regulation of membrane excitability.[40] It is found widely distributed in the animal kingdom[41] but not in plants.

Recently, myocardial failure has been associated with plasma taurine depletion in cats fed commercial diets. Oral supplementation of taurine (250 to 500 mg/day) resulted in increased plasma taurine concentrations and normalization of left ventricular function. Most affected cats improved clinically (e.g., appetite) within 2 weeks of supplementation, and echocardiographically between 3 and 6 weeks, although a small subset died in the acute setting. Plasma taurine concentrations of affected cats was less than 20 nmoles/ml (normal = 31 to 147 nmoles/ml).[6] In humans, depressed myocardial taurine levels have been associated with congestive cardiomyopathy.[42] In other studies, elevation of myocardial taurine has been demonstrated in failing[43] and hypertrophied[44] hearts. Taurine supplementation in humans with congestive heart failure has resulted in reduced severity of clinical signs and symptoms.[45] These studies are prompting investigations into effects of taurine in the failing heart.

REFERENCES

1. Lewis LD, Morris ML Jr: Nutrition. p. 1-1. In Lewis LD, Morris ML Jr (eds): Small Animal Clinical Nutrition. 2nd Ed. Mark Morris Associates, Topeka, 1984

2. Buffington CA: Anorexia. p. 5-1. In Lewis LD, Morris ML (eds): Small Animal Clinical Nutrition. 2nd Ed. Mark Morris Associates, Topeka, 1984

3. Ettinger SJ, Suter PF: Low sodium diets and other drugs and methods indicated in cardiac therapy. p. 257. In Ettinger SJ, Suter PF (eds): Canine Cardiology. WB Saunders, Philadelphia, 1970

4. Smith TW, Braunwald E: The management of heart failure. p. 503. In Braunwald E (ed): Heart Disease. 2nd Ed. WB Saunders, Philadelphia, 1984

5. Ross JN Jr: Heart Failure. p. 11-1. In Lewis LD, Morris ML (eds): Small Animal Clinical Nutrition. 2nd Ed. Mark Morris Associates, Topeka, 1984

6. Pion PD, Kittleson MD, Rogers QR, et al: Myocardial failure in cats associated with low plasma taurine: A reversible cardiomyopathy. Science 237:697, 1987

7. Schlant RC, Sonnenblick EH: Pathophysiology of

heart failure. p. 319. In Hurst JW (ed): The Heart. Ed 6, Vol 2. McGraw-Hill, New York, 1986

8. Hosetetter TH, Pfeffer JM, Pfeffer MA, et al: Cardiorenal hemodynamics and sodium excretion in rats with myocardial infarction. Am J Physiol 245(Heart Circ Physiol 14):H98, 1983

9. Heymsfield SB, Smith J, Redd S, et al: Nutritional support in cardiac failure. Surg Clin North Am 61:635, 1981

10. Pensinger RR: Dietary control of sodium intake in spontaneous congestive heart failure in dogs. Vet Med Small Animal Clin 59:752, 1964

11. Thomas WP: Long-term therapy of chronic congestive heart failure in the dog and cat. p. 368. In Kirk RW (ed): Current Veterinary Therapy. Vol. VII. WB Saunders, Philadelphia, 1980

12. Pittman JG, Cohen P: The pathogenesis of cardiac cachexia. N Engl J Med 271:403, 1964

13. Blackburn GL, Gibbons GW, Bothe A, et al: Nutritional support in cardiac cachexia. J Thorac Cardiovasc Surg 73:480, 1977

14. Meguid MM, Collier MD, Howard LJ: Uncomplicated and stressed starvation. Surg Clin North Am 61:529, 1981

15. Sheffy BE: Nutrition and the immune response. J Am Vet Med Assoc 180:1073, 1982

16. Ralston SL: Dietary management of chronic cardiac disease. p. 63. In Proceedings of the Ninth Annual Kal Kan Symposium on Cardiology. Kal Kan Foods Inc, Vernon, CA, 1986

17. Dudrick SJ, Rhoades JE: Metabolism in surgical patients: Carbohydrates and fat utilization by oral and parenteral routes. p. 147. In Sabbiston DC Jr (ed): Davis-Christopher Textbook of Surgery. 12th Ed. Vol. 1. WB Saunders, Philadelphia, 1981

18. Malcolm R, Tozer TN: Clinical Pharmacokinetics: Concepts and Applications. Lea & Febiger, Philadelphia, 1980

19. Cowgill LD, Kallet AJ: Systemic hypertension. p. 360. In Kirk RW (ed): Current Veterinary Therapy. Vol. IX. WB Saunders, Philadelphia, 1986

20. Polzin DJ, Osborne CA: Update-conservative medical management of chronic renal failure. p. 1167. In Kirk RW (ed): Current Veterinary Therapy. Vol. IX. WB Saunders, Philadelphia, 1986

21. Polzin DJ, Osborne CA, Stevens JB, et al: Influences of modified protein diets on the nutritional status of dogs with induced chronic renal failure. Am J Vet Res 44:1694, 1983

22. Osborne CA, Polzin DJ: Conservative medical management of feline chronic polyuric renal failure. p. 1008. In Kirk RW (ed): Current Veterinary Therapy. Vol. VIII. WB Saunders, Philadelphia, 1983

23. Morris ML, Patton RL, Teeter SM: Low sodium diet in heart disease: How low is low? Vet Med Small Anim Clin 71:1225, 1976

24. Fox PR, Bond BR: Congestive Heart Failure in Dogs. Hoechst-Roussel Agri-Vet Co, Somerville, NJ, 1985

25. Divitiis O, Fazio S, Petitto M, et al: Obesity and cardiac function. Circulation 64:477, 1981

26. Kaltman AJ, Goldring RM: Role of circulatory congestion in the cardiorespiratory failure of obesity. Am J Med 60;645, 1976

27. Alexander JK, Peterson KL: Cardiovascular effects of weight reduction. Circulation 45:310, 1972

28. Backman L, Freyschuss V, Hallberg D, et al: Reversibility of cardiovascular changes in extreme obesity. Acta Med Scand 205:367, 1979

29. Messerli FH: Cardiopathy of obesity—a not-so-Victoria disease. N Engl J Med 314:378, 1986

30. Messerli FH, Ventura HO, Snyder DW: Eccentric left ventricular hypertrophy—a determinant of increased ventricular ectopy in obesity. J Am Coll Cardiol. abstract (in press)

31. MacMahon SW, Wilcken DEL, MacDonald GJ: The effect of weight reduction on left ventricular mass: a randomized controlled trial in young, overweight hypertensive patients. N Engl J Med 314:334, 1986

32. Fox PR: Cor pulmonale. p. 131. In Kirk RW (ed): Current Veterinary Therapy IX. W B Saunders Co, Philadelphia, 1986

33. Lewis LD, Morris ML Jr: Obesity. p.6-1. In Lewis LD, Morris ML (eds): Small Animal Clinical Nutrition. 3rd Ed. Mark Morris Associates, Topeka, 1987

34. Hayes KC: Taurine requirements in primates. Nutr Rev 43:65, 1985

35. Knopf K, Sturman JA, Armstrong MA, et al: Taurine: An essential nutrient for the cat. J Nutr 108:773, 1978

36. Rabin B, Nicolosi RJ, Hayes KC: Dietary influence on bile acid conjugation in the cat. J Nutr 106:1241, 1976

37. Davidson AN, Kaczmarek LK: Taurine—a possible neurotransmitter? Nature (London) 234:107, 1971

38. Oja SS, Lahdesmaki P: Is taurine an inhibitory neurotransmitter? Med Biol 52:138, 1974

39. Schmidt SY, Berson EL, Hayes KC: Retinal degeneration in cats fed casein. 1. Taurine deficiency. Invest Ophthalmol 15:47, 1976

40. Huxtable R, Bressler R: Effect of taurine on a muscle intracellular membrane. Biochem Biophys Acta 323:573, 1973

41. Jacobson JG, Smith LH: Biochemistry and physiology of taurine and taurine derivatives. Physiol Rev 48:424, 1968

42. Darsee JR, Heymsfield SB: Decreased myocardiol taurine levels and hypertaurinuria in a kindred with mitral-valve prolapse and congestive cardiomyopathy. N Engl J Med 304:129, 1981

43. Huxtable R, Bressler R: Taurine concentrations in congestive heart failure. Science 184:1187, 1974

44. Peterson MB, Mead RJ, Welty JD: Free amino acids in congestive heart failure. J Mol Cell Cardiol 5:139, 1973

45. Azuma J, Hasegawa H, Sawamura A, et al: Therapy of congestive heart failure with orally administered taurine. Clin Therap 5:398, 1983

11
Shock

Steve C. Haskins

Hypovolemic, septic, and cardiogenic shock has been the subject of several recent reviews.[1-4] Shock is characteristically a multisystemic disease that can be very difficult to treat. An improved understanding of hyopvolemia and its consequences has provided the basis for effective management of reversible hypovolemic shock. The widespread use of antibiotics and the intensive invasive management of the critically ill have saved many lives. It has also elevated our awareness of the incidence and complexities of septic shock, an event that claims a high mortality rate. There have been many modifications in the clinical approach and treatment modalities for shock. However, the therapeutic implications are diverse, and many are not well established at this time.

The early recognition of shock is crucial to successful clinical management. The purpose of this chapter is to review the common therapies that may be important in the management of hypovolemic, septic, and cardiogenic shock.

HYPOVOLEMIC SHOCK

An animal is hypovolemic when blood volume is diminished by whole blood loss or by extracellular fluid losses (third-space fluid accumulations, vom-

iting, diarrhea, or diuresis). The animal normally compensates for this hypovolemia by splenic and venous constriction to translocate blood from the venous capacitance vessels to the central arterial circulation, by arteriolar constriction to reduce diastolic runoff to help maintain diastolic blood pressure, and by an increase in heart rate to increase cardiac output. All these compensatory processes are an attempt to maintain mean arterial blood pressure so as to achieve adequate cerebral and coronary perfusion. If the initial blood loss is so severe or if these compensatory mechanisms are themselves compromised by disease such that adequate cerebral and coronary perfusion cannot be achieved, the animal will die of acute, severe, hypovolemic hypotension.

The compensatory arteriolar vasoconstriction, while temporarily supporting vital organ perfusion, does so at the expense of visceral and other peripheral organ perfusion. If the vasoconstriction is severe enough to interfere with the adequate delivery of oxygen and energy substrates to the tissues, or the removal of metabolites from the tissues, the animal is in hypovolemic shock. If blood volume is not restored by the endogenous redistribution of fluids from the interstitial to the intravascular fluid compartment, or, by the exogenous administration of fluids to the extent that the arterioles can dilate and reestablish visceral organ perfusion without causing excessive hypotension, the animal will succumb to the malperfusion of these peripheral tissues. In the face of hypoxia and the accumulation of multiple noxious metabolic products, the arterioles, after a time, lose their ability to remain constricted. The arterioles, unfortunately, dilate prior to the venules and blood begins to pool in the capillary beds of the tissues. The animal has passed from the normal compensatory, vasoconstrictive, ischemic, and reversible stage of hypovolemic shock to the decompensatory, vasodilative, congestive, pooling, and irreversible stage of shock. Essential blood volume now becomes trapped in the capillaries and sequestered in the surrounding tissues. Venous return, cardiac output, blood pressure, and vital organ perfusion decrease as the terminal event.

SEPTIC SHOCK

An animal is considered septic when its blood has become infected by bacteria, viruses, rickettsia, fungi, or protozoa. Bacterial infections are the most commonly recognized and may be gram-negative or positive, aerobic, or anaerobic. Many of these infections produce substances that are toxic to the host by a variety of mechanisms: (1) direct vasoactive activity or the release of vasoactive substances; (2) activation of coagulation, platelet, plasminogen, or prostaglandin cascades; (3) interfering with various phases of intermediary metabolism; or (4) inciting an inflammatory or immunologic response. When the infection is directly or indirectly affecting the animal to the extent that tissue energy production is compromised, septic shock has ensued.

Endotoxemia

Endotoxin is an extremely toxic and stable cell wall component of gram-negative bacteria that is released when the organism dies. The intact gastrointestinal (GI) mucosal barrier normally prevents the systemic absorption of naturally occurring enteric endotoxin. Gastrointestinal hypoxia or inflammation, however, predispose to free endotoxin absorption, without bacteremia.[5-8]

Endotoxin causes a marked increase in both cyclooxygenase and lipooxygenase metabolites of arachidonic acid.[9-10] Thromboxane A_2 and prostaglandins F_2 and E_2 (PGF_2 and PGE_2) are potent pulmonary vasoconstrictors and systemic vasodilators. Thromboxane is also a platelet aggregator. The leukotrienes are potent bronchoconstrictors that mediate an increased pulmonary microvascular permeability. Serotonin is increased following endotoxin administration and causes vasoconstriction and microvascular permeability.[11] Endotoxin causes direct and indirect complement-mediated cell damage,[12] and activates coagulation and platelet cascades.[13] Complement polypeptides increase vascular permeability, mast cell degranulation and histamine release (which induces a transient increase in microvascular permeability), vasoconstriction, and perivascular sequestration of neutrophils.[11] Neutrophils are heavily laden with superoxides and free radicals and proteolytic enzymes, which, when released, mediate extensive cellular destruction.[12,13]

Endotoxin is associated with a primary decrease in ventricular compliance and a depression of myocardial contractility and function.[14,15] The myocardial involvement is an early event in the endotoxic shock process. The precise cause is not known.

Endotoxin injection results in an initial sympathetic-mediated arteriolar constriction resulting in a decreased mesenteric, renal and muscle blood flow; venule dilation resulting in a decreased venous return; and hypotension resulting in a decreased cerebral and coronary blood flow.[16]

Bacterial Profiles of Systemic Sepsis

The heavy use of antibiotics associated with the development of resistant bacterial populations and the advances in invasive critical care technology are considered to be the cause for the increase in the incidence of gram-negative nosocomial infections in humans over the past 20 years.[17] Septicemia in humans is caused by gram-negative organisms approximately two-thirds of the time and by gram-positive organisms about one-third of the time.[18,19] Mixed infections occur 10 to 20 percent of the time. *Staphylococcus aureus* and streptococci are the most common gram-positive organisms, followed by pneumococci, *Haemophilus* and *Clostridia*.[18] *Esche-*

richia coli is the most common gram-negative organism followed by (in descending order) *Klebsiella pneumoniae, Pseudomonas* sp, *Enterobacter* sp, *Proteus* sp, *Bacteroides* sp, and *Serratia marcescens*.[17,18]

The distribution of bacteria causing septicemia in dogs is quite similar (Table 11-1); 30 to 70 percent being gram negative, 25 to 50 percent being gram positive, and 10 to 50 percent being mixed infections.[20,21] Anaerobic bacterial infections may be more common than is indicated in the above two studies.[22] *E. coli* was the most common organism (63 percent) in septicemic foals; 93 percent of the isolates were gram negative; 7 percent of the cultures were mixed.[23]

The therapeutic implications of identifiable patterns of bacterial infections is that an unknown infection in a random patient may be almost anything. Taking early cultures and sensitivities of known local infections is important because they guide an-

tibiotic choices if the patient becomes septicemic. Antibiotics must be broad spectrum to be effective when treating an unknown infection. Blood cultures should be submitted as soon as bacteremia is suspected and antibiotic selection changed if necessary when the results are available.

Origins of Systemic Sepsis

Bacteremia may originate from any infection that has diffuse exposure to blood such that large quantities of bacteria are able to invade the bloodstream within a relatively short period of time. In the dog[20,24] and the human,[17,19] the genitourinary tract (kidney, urinary bladder, prostate, uterus, and testicles) is the single most common cause of bacteremia. Gastrointestinal ischemia, inflammation or surgery, and pneumonia are the next most common sources. Pyothorax, peritonitis, hepatitis, oral in-

Table 11-1 Incidence of Bacterial Septicemia in Dogs

| | Hardie et al.[20] | | Hirsh et al.[21] |
Organism	Community Acquired (%)[a]	Hospital Acquired (%)[a]	(%)[a]
Gram-negative			
Escherichia coli	50	34	19
Klebsiella sp	12	14	7
Proteus sp	7	7	1
Pseudomonas sp	3	3	0
Salmonella sp	0	5	2
Enterobacter sp	0	2	1
Pasteurella sp	0	2	0
Total	72	67	30
Gram-positive			
Staphylococcus aureus	17	17	34
Streptococcus sp	9	10	11
Corynebacterium sp	0	2	4
Total	26	29	49
Anaerobes			
Bacteroides sp	0	0	1
Bacillus sp	0	0	4
Clostridium sp	2	0	4
Incidence of cultures with multiple organisms	24	54	10

[a] Expressed as a percentage of total isolates.

fections, and external wound or skin infections are common sources as well.

Early Recognition of Sepsis

Real proof of sepsis is based on a positive blood culture which, in itself, presents several major problems: (1) false-negative results occur up to 30 percent of the time.[17,19,20,24] Taking larger blood samples at repeated intervals minimizes the incidence of false negative results; (2) false-positive results (due to contaminants during the blood collection process) occur up to 25 percent of the time.[19] Careful antiseptic preparation of the skin puncture site and of the equipment used in the collection procedure minimizes the incidence of false positive results; (3) the 2- to 3-day lag period between the collection of the blood and the results of the culture and sensitivity make it an unrealistic prospective diagnostic aide. Sepsis is often advanced, and therapy should not be delayed until the results of the culture and sensitivity are available.

A presumptive diagnosis of sepsis should be made based on the recent past history of the patient and on the physical and laboratory findings. Therapy should commence as soon as the presumptive diagnosis is made. Blood should be taken for culture and sensitivity testing to verify efficacy of the antibiotic choice and to help identify probable appropriate antibiotics for future infections.

The recent past history of the patient should alert the clinician to patients at risk and is extremely helpful in making a presumptive diagnosis of sepsis. The history of a known infection, particularly of those systems previously identified as common sources of septicemia, in a patient exhibiting signs of septicemia is sufficient evidence to warrant a diagnosis of septicemia. In the absence of a known infection, the history of a procedure that could cause an infection would be sufficient (e.g., temporary or indwelling urinary catheter, an indwelling vascular catheter, surgery- particularly of those high-risk organ systems previously discussed, or a penetrating injury). Certain diseases or conditions predispose a patient to the acquisition of a systemic infection (e.g., diabetes mellitus, renal failure, hyperadrenocorticism, granulocytopenia, acute or chronic malnutrition,[25] and feline leukemia virus or other immunosuppressant diseases). Other thera-

pies predispose a patient to systemic infections (e.g., glucocorticosteroids or other immunosuppressant drugs, antibiotic therapy,[25,26] parenteral nutrition with lipids or protein hydrolysates).

A presenting clinical sign suggesting sepsis is a degree of mental obtundation more severe than that normally associated with the given stage of a disease process. Excessive depression in conjunction with an appropriate history should direct one to look specifically for septicemia.

For the purposes of this discussion, the physical signs and laboratory findings of septicemia are divided into two components: (1) septicemia, in which the animal is compensating for the infection in an appropriate manner, and (2) septic shock, in which the animal is being overwhelmed by the infection. These subdivisions are continuums of the same disease process and, although one may assume that there is a clear-cut difference between these syndromes, there is not. An individual patient will usually not manifest all the changes precisely as outlined or there may be overlaps and omittances of clinical signs. Although both syndromes are treated, similarly, there may be a different prognosis attendant to each disease process.

A suitable history, accompanied by two or more of the previously described physical and/or laboratory abnormalities in a patient that is becoming progressively more depressed, is sufficient to support a diagnosis of septicemia or septic shock. Either represents a serious imposition on patient homeostasis and treatment should commence immediately. The onset of the signs may be very slow and insidious or may be peracute and fatal over the course of just a few hours.

The physical signs associated with septicemia are depressed mentation and appetite, fever, and evidence of peripheral vasodilation (warmer than normal skin and appendages, dark red mucous membrane color or injected scleral vessels, less than 1-second capillary refill time, tachycardia, and tachypnea). The following hemodynamic changes are typical of a hyperdynamic state: tachycardia, increased cardiac output, decreased peripheral vascular resistance, decreased arterial blood pressure, increased pulmonary artery pressure and resistance, and decreased central venous pressure.[17,27,28] The hyperdynamic phase of the disease process may not occur if there is a large and rapid microorganism invasion of the bloodstream[27,29]; these patients may proceed directly to the hypodynamic phase of septic shock. Gastrointestinal signs may be observed.[3] A murmur may be evident if valvular endocarditis is a component of the disease process.

The laboratory findings of septicemia include leukocytosis with an increased percentage of immature polymorphonucleocytes, hyperglycemia, hypoalbuminemia, respiratory alkalosis, and increased serum alkaline phosphatase.[20] Vacuolated neutrophils, intraneutrophilic Döhle bodies, and hyperbilirubinemia are common in humans.[19]

The physical signs of septic shock are severe depression, anorexia, a subnormal temperature, tachycardia, tachypnea, peripheral vasoconstriction, and an increased core-to-toe web temperature.[30] The cardiovascular system generally is hypodynamic (e.g., decreased cardiac output, increased systemic and pulmonary resistance, pulmonary arterial pressure, and decreased systemic arterial and central venous pressures). Bloody diarrhea may be observed.[3] The laboratory findings may include a dramatic decrease in leucocyte count, hypoglycemia, respiratory alkalosis, metabolic acidosis, hemoconcentration, hypoalbuminemia, and marked increases in serum liver enzyme concentrations.[20,31]

Mortality Rate of Septic Shock and Septicemia

Mortality rates range between 6 and 33 percent in human gram-negative bacteremia when appropriate antibiotics are used, and between 30 and 53 percent when an inappropriate antibiotic is administered.[25,32] Twenty percent of bacteremic human patients enter shock when appropriate antibiotics are administered, and 50 percent enter shock when inappropriate antibiotics are used. The mortality rate in those patients developing septic shock varies between 40 and 80 percent[25,32] in the face of appropriate antibiotics and between 50 and 100 percent when inappropriate antibiotics are used.[25,32] The mortality rate from severe sepsis in dogs varies between 31 and 71 percent[20] and was reported to be 74 percent in septicemic neonatal foals.[23]

Mortality rate in septic shock varies directly with the fatality index of the underlying disease process.[18,25] The concurrence of uremia, congestive heart failure, diabetes, granulocytopenia, a hypodynamic cardiovascular system, the failure to develop a fever within the first 24 hours of the bacteremia, and preceding treatment with antibiotics, corticosteroids, and chemotherapeutic drugs increases the mortality of septic shock.[18,25]

Septicemia and septic shock can be aggressive diseases in terms of both their speed of onset and their high mortality rate. Clinicians must be alert to the possibility of these conditions, recognize early their clinical signs, and treat them aggressively when they develop.

TREATMENT OF SHOCK

Hypovolemic and particularly septic shock are systemic diseases. Appropriate therapy must therefore be multifaceted to be successful (Table 11-2). Fluid therapy remains the mainstay of shock therapy. Treatment of the infectious source, selection of appropriate antibiotics, and administration of glucocorticoids are also important. Hyperimmune serum is a new and exciting therapeutic modality which represents a major breakthrough in the treatment of gram-negative sepsis. Treatment of organ

Table 11-2 Treatment Considerations in Shock

Blood volume restoration
Blood pressure support
Remove or drain septic foci
Antibiotic treatment of sepsis
Glucocorticosteroids
Antiprostaglandins
Support of renal function
Correction of hypoglycemia
Correction of metabolic acidosis
Correction of coagulopathies
Antisera for gram-negative infections
    Lipopolysaccharide core antisera
    Multivalent oligosaccharide antisera
Support of pulmonary function
Protection of the gastrointestinal tract
Nutrition
Naloxone
Fibronectin
Granulocyte transfusion
Energy and energy substrates
Aprotinin

system dysfunction (e.g., hypotension, metabolic acidosis, hypoglycemia, coagulopathies, renal and pulmonary failure) is vital to the overall management of shock. In addition, many helper treatments have been shown to improve certain aspects of the shock process. These include nonsteroidal antiinflammatory drugs, energy substrate administration, fibronectin, naloxone, and aprotinin. Specific modalities of therapy and therapeutic strategies for treatment of hypovolemic and septic shock are listed subsequently. Cardiogenic shock is discussed at the end of this chapter and under myocardial diseases (Chs. 22 and 23).

Fluid Therapy

Restoration of an effective circulating blood volume is of primary importance in the management of hypovolemic and septic shock. The volume of fluid required often ranges between 40 to 90 ml/kg or more in dogs and about $\frac{1}{2}$ to $\frac{2}{3}$ of this volume in cats. The endpoint of fluid administration for a specific patient is determined by the alleviation of the peripheral vasoconstriction and the restoration of an acceptable pulse quality. Septic shock often requires surprisingly large volumes of fluid and objective measurements of the adequacy of blood volume restoration can be valuable: (1) the elevation of the central venous pressure to a high normal level (e.g., 5 to 10 cm H_2O), (2) elevation of pulmonary-capillary wedge pressure to a high normal level (e.g., 10 to 15 mmHg), or (3) the restoration of an acceptable arterial blood pressure (ABP) (e.g., greater than 60 mmHg mean; greater than 80 mmHg systolic). The restoration of hemodynamic balance may, however, occur in the face of inadequate restoration of organ perfusion.[33] Measures of organ function such as mucous membrane color, capillary refill time, toe-web temperature, urine output, and an improved mental status must be evaluated in addition to specific hemodynamic measurements.

Isotonic Sodium Replacement Fluids

The type of fluids to administer depends on the balance of blood constituent components. Generally, a clear crystalloid fluid containing a normal sodium concentration (130 to 154 mEq/L) with a bicarbonate-like anion (bicarbonate, lactate, acetate, or gluconate), such as lactated Ringer's, is the fluid of choice to start therapy. These fluids are economical and can be administered rapidly with minimal danger of inducing congestive heart failure, pulmonary edema or cerebral edema in animals without pre-existing complications of these organ systems.[34,35] If pulmonary edema does coexist with shock, fluid therapy must be monitored more carefully (e.g., central venous pressure measurement) and should be conservative to the extent that it restores acceptable (but not necessarily normal) cardiovascular function. If pulmonary edema is worsened in the process, it must also be treated in an appropriate manner.[36,37]

While subcutaneous, oral, or intraperitoneal fluid administration may be appropriate in states of simple dehydration, these routes are not direct enough for a life-threatening shock situation. Fluids must be administered intravenously.

Only about 20 to 30 percent of crystalloid fluids remain in the vascular fluid compartment 30 minutes after IV their administration.[38] The remainder readily diffuses across the endothelial membrane and is redistributed into the interstitial fluid compartment. The volume restoration achieved by crystalloid fluid administration may thus be fleeting. If hypotension or vasoconstriction recurs (fluid redistribution or continued bleeding may be the cause), further fluid administration, perhaps in the form of colloids or whole blood, is indicated.

Interstitial edema, due to the interstitial redistribution of fluids, may eventually interfere with pulmonary, cerebral, or GI function with aggressive fluid therapy programs. If this occurs, more specific colloid blood volume-expanding agents should be used. These agents are given subsequent to initial restoration of blood and interstitial volume with crystalloid fluids.

Excessive hemodilution is a common limitation to crystalloid fluid administration. Excessive hemodilution is defined as a packed cell volume below 20 percent, hemoglobin below 7 g/dl, and/or total protein below 3.5 g/dl or an albumin level below 1.5 g/dl. These values assume acute hemodilution (as opposed to chronic anemia, in which compensatory mechanisms can be called into force) in a patient with multisystem disease (with compensatory mechanisms that may be disabled). These guidelines will incorporate a margin of error that establishes at least a 99 percent confidence interval. The fact that many patients have survived more severe hemodilution cannot be extrapolated to critically ill patients. If the packed cell volume falls below 20 percent and further volume loading is indicated, the volume should be administered as whole blood. If the plasma protein levels alone fall below 3.5 g/dl and further volume loading is indicated, plasma or a plasma substitute should be administered.

The crystalloid fluid should contain a bicarbonate-like anion (bicarbonate, lactate, acetate, or gluconate) in order to prevent the dilutional acidosis induced by fluids without such anions (e.g., saline, Ringer's). If saline is used, the addition of 24 mEq/L of sodium bicarbonate will neutralize its acidifying tendency. In most instances, the lactate anion is quite satisfactory, even though hepatic metabolism is required in order for it to have an effect. Acetate and gluconate may be somewhat preferable to lactate, since these anions are metabolized by other tissues in addition to the liver.[39] Bicarbonate, has an immediate effect not requiring metabolism.

Other electrolytes such as sodium and potassium, unless known or suspected of being abnormal by virtue of pre-existing disease, receive little attention during this initial period of acute blood volume restoration. They can be dealt with in an appropriate manner once cardiovascular stabilization has been achieved.

Hypotonic fluids such as 5 percent dextrose in water and low sodium maintenance solutions should not be used for shock therapy. These are poor blood volume expanding agents and will cause excessive intracellular edema.

Hypertonic Saline

Hypertonic saline (2400 mOsm/L) has been shown to be an excellent extracellular and blood volume expanding crystalloid.[40–42] Following its administration, intracellular water is drawn into the extracellular compartment. Extracellular volume expansion far exceeds that from administration of similar volumes of isotonic crystalloid fluids.[40,41] The blood volume expanding effect is magnified and prolonged if the hypertonic saline is administered along with 6 percent dextran.[43]

In addition to the volume expanding effect, the infusion of hypertonic saline is associated with an increase in myocardial contractility, cardiac output, arterial blood pressure, tissue blood flow, and peripheral vasodilation, which may occur without an increase in vascular volume.[40,42,44] These effects may be transient[40,42] or sustained.[40,42,44] The mechanism for these effects is unknown but probably can be related to a cellular stabilizing effect, since hypertonic saline has been reported to normalize intracellular water and electrolyte balance and transmembrane potential in rats.[41]

Hypertonic saline may be especially efficacious in emergency situations in which a profound and quick volume effect is necessary and conventional fluids cannot be administered rapidly enough. The preadministration of hypertonic saline has been shown to magnify the subsequent response to isotonic fluids compared with controls.[42]

The intracellular fluid steal has not been associated with any recognized detrimental effects attributable to intracellular dehydration. Extracellular sodium concentration and osmolality rise only slightly due to the redistribution of intracellular fluids. Plasma potassium concentration[40] may be decreased, and it may be important to supplement potassium in hypokalemic patients.

Plasma

Plasma should be administered when the patient becomes excessively hypoproteinemic. The water-retaining capacity of albumin is 15 to 20 ml/g.[45,46] Plasma can serve as an amino acid source and can provide platelets (if fresh) and coagulation precursors (if fresh or fresh frozen).

Artificial Colloids

Dextran 70 is a high-molecular-weight polysaccharide with an average molecular weight of 70,000 (similar to that of albumin). It has a sustained water-retaining capacity of about 10 to 15 ml/g[47,48] (molecules smaller than MW 50,000 are rapidly excreted in the urine) and a half-life of about 24 hr.[49] The daily dose should not exceed 20 ml/kg, since high doses may be associated with hyperviscosity and a hemorrhagic diathesis. Rapid infusions may cause a thrombasthenia; therefore, infusion rates should not exceed 2 to 5 ml/kg/hr.

Dextran 40 (average MW 40,000) has a very short half-life (three hours) and is primarily used to decrease microvascular sludging, to improve tissue perfusion, and to provide transient volume restoration in the early phases of therapy.

Hetastarch (average MW 450,000) exhibits a duration of 12 to 48 hours[50] and could be used instead of dextran 70. However, at this writing it is considerably more expensive than dextran 70.

The artificial colloids are better blood volume expanders than crystalloid fluids alone.[44,49,51] They have a definite role in blood volume restoration therapy.

Whole Blood

Whole blood transfusions are indicated if the patient becomes excessively hemodiluted. Collected blood should be anticoagulated with heparin if it is to be immediately transfused, or with acid citrate dextrose (ACD) or citrate phosphate dextrose (CPD) if it is to be stored. Erythrocytes remain at least 70 percent viable for up to 3 weeks (ACD), or 4 weeks (CPD) when stored at 4°C.[52]

There are eight commonly identified canine erythrocytic antigens. Naturally occurring isoantibodies occur in about 15 percent of dogs.[53] Clinical transfusion reactions are unlikely except in autoimmune recipients. Although all erythrocytic antigens incite an antibody response, clinically significant transfusion reactions are only likely to occur following the second transfusion of dog erythrocyte antigen (DEA) 1.1 and DEA 1.2 and to a lesser extent, DEA 7. Potential donors should be typed (Bowling A, Bull R, personal communications) and negative for DEA 1.1 and 1.2 and perhaps DEA 7.

There are two recognized feline erythrocytic antigens.[54] Naturally occurring isoantibodies are uncommon in the cat as in the dog (about 5 percent of the population[54]) and therefore clinical transfusion reactions are unlikely with the first random transfusion. Severe transfusion reactions following repeated transfusions may be uncommon[55] but do occur.[56]

The necessity for crossmatching the blood of intended transfusions is not known. *In vitro* laboratory testing identifies mismatched combinations much more frequently than they are recognized clinically with random unmatched transfusions. Matches that are compatible *in vitro* are occasionally associated with clincal reactions. Theoretically, *in vitro* crossmatch testing will decrease the incidence of clinical and subclinical reactions and is therefore recommended if possible.

Autotransfusion of blood from a patient's body cavity directly back into the systemic circulation may be lifesaving in some emergency situations.[57] The blood may be collected via syringe or commercial collection system (Fenwal Labs [Div. Travenol] Deerfield, IL); should be anticoagulated if fresh; and should be filtered when administered.[58]

The rate of whole blood and plasma administration should be conservative so as to minimize the clinical manifestations of transfusion or histamine-mediated reactions to foreign protein. Infusion rates of 5 to 10 ml/kg/hr are usually satisfactory. However, rates up to 20 to 25 ml/kg/hr may be indicated in hypovolemic, hypotensive, and anemic patients.

Blood Pressure Support

The initial purpose of fluid therapy is to restore blood pressure and cerebral and coronary perfusion. Blood pressure can be easily monitored by external or internal methods.[59] Under some circumstances, effective fluid therapy cannot be achieved rapidly enough or, due to a component of heart failure, cannot be achieved at all without sympathomimetic support.

Blood or plasma should be administered until the hemoglobin, packed cell volume, and albumin or total protein have been elevated to an acceptable level. The necessary volume can be precalculated: [(blood volume × desired hemoglobin or protein concentration) − (blood volume × present hemoglobin or protein concentration) = grams of hemoglobin or protein to administer]. However, it is much simpler to realize that 10 and 40 ml/kg represent small and large transfusions, respectively, to administer a convenient dosage, and then remeasure packed cell volume or total protein.

α-Receptor agonists (norepinephrine, phenylephrine, or methoxamine) (Table 11-3) are indicated only in emergency situations when the patient is dying of hypotension, and when immediate pharmacologically induced vasoconstriction is the only

Table 11-3 Sympathomimetics

Drug (Receptor Activity)	Trade Name (Manufacturer)	Myocardial Chronotropy and Inotropy	Peripheral Vasomotor Tone	Dosage (IV)
Dopamine (dopa and ($\alpha++$; $\beta+++$)	Intropin (Arnar-Stone)	Increased	Variable	5–25 µg/kg/min (blood pressure support) 1–5 µg/kg/min (diuresis) (80–200 mg in 500 ml D_5W)
Dobutamine ($\alpha+$; $\beta+++$)	Dobutrex (Lilly)	Increased	Variable	2.5–40 µg/kg/min (100–400 mg in 500 ml D_5W)
Mephentermine ($\alpha+$, $\beta++$)	Wyamine (Wyeth)	Increased	Variable	0.1–0.75 mg/kg
Norepinephrine ($\alpha+++$; $\beta+$)	Levophed bitartrate (Winthrop-Breon)	Variable	Increased	1–10 µg/kg/min (1–4 mg in 500 ml D_5W)
Metaraminol ($\alpha+++$; $\beta+$)	Aramine (Merck Sharp and Dohme) Metaraminol bitartrate (Bristol; Invenex)	Variable	Increased	0.1–0.2 mg/kg
Methoxamine ($\alpha+++$; $\beta0$)	Vasoxyl (Burroughs Wellcome)	None	Increased	0.1–0.2 mg/kg
Phenylephrine ($\alpha+++$; $\beta0$)	Neo-Synephrine (Winthrop-Breon)	None	Increased	0.01–0.1 mg/kg
Ephedrine ($\alpha++$; $\beta+$)	(Vitarine)	Increased	Variable	0.05–0.2 mg/kg

means of restoring blood pressure in the time available. Continued use of these agents is contraindicated because they impair peripheral tissue perfusion severely, which may result in peripheral tissue failure.

Dopamine, dobutamine, and mephentermine (Table 11-3) provide good cardiotonic support with minimal peripheral vasoconstriction and are preferred for the support of blood pressure in the critically ill patient. Dopamine and dobutamine exhibit short durations of action and must be given by continuous intravenous infusion. Mephentermine can be administered intermittently, is least likely to cause ventricular arrhythmias and is the least potent of the three agents. Dopmine and dobutamine in-

fusions should be titrated to effect and monitored by arterial blood pressure (if available) or clinical signs.

Epinephrine could potentially be given during initial shock treatment but should not be continued because of its intense vasoconstrictor properties. Isoproterenol should not be used because of its intense vasodilator properties.

External compression devices have been shown to improve hemodynamics when applied to the hind legs and lower abdomen of a patient in shock. Although it was originally thought that the beneficial effects were attributable to the translocation of blood from these compressed areas to the central circulation, it is now believed that the beneficial effects are primarily due to increased peripheral vascular resistance.[60]

Removal or Drainage of the Septic Process

The source of infection should be removed (e.g., indwelling catheters, a pyometra) if feasible or drained and flushed thoroughly (e.g., pyothorax, peritonitis, cystitis, cellulitis). Patients must be hemodynamically stabilized as much as possible if general anesthesia is required.

Antibiotics

Appropriate antibiotic therapy is crucial in lowering the mortality rate from sepsis and septic shock.[25] The choice may be hindered by lack of available culture and sensitivity results at the initiation of therapy. A random infection may be gram negative, gram positive, aerobic, or anaerobic, in any combination. Prior cultures of known infections in the patient may be helpful if available. Direct smears of known infected sites may reveal the nature of the underlying infection and help guide initial antibiotic therapy. Previous cultures and sensitivities of similar infections also help guide antibiotic selection. If an animal becomes septicemic in the face of antibiotic prophylaxis, the invading organism is most assuredly resistant to the existing antibiotic and is likely to be resistant to many of the antibiotics commonly used in practice. The choice of antibiotic(s) when treating an unknown infection needs to be broad spectrum until specific *in vitro* sensitivity results become available.

Penicillins inhibit bacterial cell wall synthesis in actively growing organisms. Although there are several mechanisms of bacterial resistance to the penicillins, β-lactamase enzymatic inactivation is the most important.[61] *Staphylococcus* and the gram-negative enteric agents are β-lactamase producers and are therefore often resistant to β-lactamase-susceptible antibiotics (penicillin G, ampicillin, amoxicillin). Oxacillin, nafcillin, and cloxacillin have good gram-positive spectra; ticarcillin also has a reasonable gram-negative spectrum. Carbenicillin and the clavulanic acid-activated agents exhibit good broad-spectrum activity, including against *Pseudomonas*. Clavulanic acid is an irreversible β-lactamase

inhibitor that intensifies and broadens the anti-microbial effectiveness of the combined penicillin.[61] Streptococci, *Actinomyces*, *Actinobacillus*, *Pasteurella*, *Corynebacterium*, and all obligate anaerobes except *Bacteroides fragilis*, *Clostridium ranmosum*, and *Fusobacterium varium* are predictably sensitive to the penicillin antibiotics.[62]

Cephalosporin antimicrobial activity, like the penicillins, is dependent on the β-lactam ring to prevent cell wall synthesis. β-lactamase-producing bacteria are resistant to the effects of these antibiotics. First-generation (cephalothin, cephaloridine, cephapirin, cefazolin) and second-generation (cefamandole, cefoxitin) cephalosporins exhibit a predominantly gram-positive spectrum. They have intermediate effectiveness against common gram-negative enteric agents except *Klebsiella* and *Pseudomonas*,[63] as well as anaerobes.[22] Cephaloridine has the longest effective plasma activity in the dog with respect to its *in vitro* minimum inhibitory concentration (MIC) for all but *Pseudomonas*[63] but may be more nephrotoxic than other cephalosporins.[18] The other cephalosporins exhibit short durations of effective plasma activity. Second- and third-generation cephalosporins have a progressively greater gram-negative spectrum and β-lactamase resistance but at the expense of *S. aureus* activity.[63]

The aminoglycosides bind to bacterial ribosomes and inhibit protein synthesis. The new aminoglycosides (gentamicin, tobramycin, and amikacin) have a predominantly gram-negative spectrum, including *Klebsiella* and *Pseudomonas*, with a good effect against *S. aureus* and poor activity against streptococci, anaerobes, and fungi.[64] Streptomycin, neomycin, and kanamycin have become less effective in recent years and probably should not be relied on for treating unknown infections. Gentamicin-resistant gram-negative organisms are not rare,[65,66] particularly *Pseudomonas aeruginosa*. Polymyxin B, amikacin, and colistin are usually effective and tobramycin is often effective against these organisms.[66,67]

The aminoglycoside antibiotics are nephrotoxic (6 to 12 percent incidence in humans[18]), ototoxic, and vestibulotoxic. Their use is therefore not without potential disadvantages. Other potentially nephrotoxic agents should be minimized as much as possible. Carbenicillin or clavulanic acid-activated agents could, perhaps, be substituted for the aminoglycosides in patients with incipient renal failure.

Chloramphenicol is bacteriostatic with predominantly a gram-positive spectrum. It exhibits some gram-negative activity except against *E. coli*, *Pseudomonas*, *Klebsiella*, and *Enterobacter*.[68] Therefore, it is not of much use in the treatment of an unknown septicemia.

Erythromycin is a bacteriostatic antibiotic. It has a marginal gram-positive spectrum and displays no gram-negative activity.[68]

Trimethoprim-sulfadiazine is bacteriocidal. It displays only marginal activity against common gram-positive and -negative organisms and none against *Pseudomonas*[68] or anaerobes.[22]

The most common antibiotic resistance in one report[62] was to tetracycline, streptomycin, sulfonamides, kanamycin, neomycin, ampicillin, penicillin, and combinations thereof. Antibiotic selection(s) must be those most likely to be effective against the unknown infection. Combination therapies should widen the spectrum of activity and intensify the effectiveness by synergistic mechanisms of action. However, the efficacy of combination therapy over single bacteriocidal or bacteriostatic antibiotic therapy in known susceptible organisms or in the blind treatment of infections has not been proved.[25]

For initial therapy when antibiotic sensitivities are unknown, the following are recommended: an aminoglycoside (gentamicin, amikacin, or tobramycin) for the gram-negative organisms and staphylococci, and either a penicillin (especially carbenicillin or ticarcillin) or a cephalosporin for the anaerobes and streptococci.

A β-lactamase-resistant penicillin may be more effective than a susceptible one. Carbenicillin or clavulanic acid-activated amoxicillin or ticarcillin are effective broad-spectrum antibiotics when administered alone. Third-generation cephalosporins are expensive and have limited efficacy against staphylococci.

Anaerobes may be isolated from properly handled samples. They occur commonly in bite wounds, oropharyngeal abscesses, pleuropulmonary infections, and compound fractures.[22] Anaerobic infections are frequently associated with necrotic tissue, develop as a closed infection following a penetrating injury, and produce a very foul-smelling exudate.[22]

If an anaerobic infection is suspected and the patient's condition appears unresponsive to penicillin, either metronidazol, chloramphenicol, or clindamycin should be added to the treatment protocol.[68]

Although bactericidal antibiotics are almost exclusively used in the treatment of septic shock, their benefits should, perhaps, be re-evaluated. Bacteriostatic agents have been reported equally effective, on the average, as were bactericidal agents.[25] Cidal antibiotics were shown to increase endotoxin levels 8- to 9-fold and 10- to 2,000-fold (refs. 69 and 70, respectively) compared with controls. Static antibiotics were associated with a slight, slow increase in endotoxin levels which remained far below that of controls. It is apparent that significant amounts of endotoxin are released as a result of bactericidal antibiotic administration, and this may have important detrimental effects on the patient. A most interesting finding was that polymyxin B, a bactericidal agent, was associated with a significant decrease in endotoxin levels compared with control and the bacteristatic antibiotic.[69] This was attributed to the weak antiendotoxin effect of the antibiotic, a feature that this agent shares with colistin.[71]

Glucocorticosteroids

Pharmacologic doses of glucocorticosteroids have potential beneficial effects in all forms of shock, especially septic shock.[72–76] The mechanisms of their salutary effects are summarized in Table 11-4.

At pharmacologic doses, corticosteroids have been shown to improve tissue perfusion in many studies,[72–74,77,78] while failing to do so in others.[76,79] Although it is encouraging to see hemodynamic improvement following corticosteroid administration, it is not a prerequisite to their beneficial effects.[73,76,79]

Sequestration of leukocytes in the pericapillary tissues is thought to be a major cause of the development of relentlessly progressive pulmonary insufficiency in septic shock.[80] Corticosteroids decrease leukocyte margination, diapedesis, and perivascular leukocyte degeneration.[81–83]

Corticosteroids have recently been shown to reduce the absorption of endotoxins in experimental anterior mesenteric artery occlusion in cats.[8] The corticosteroids generally recommended for use in hypovolemic and septic shock are listed in Table 11-

Table 11-4 Beneficial Effects of Corticosteroids in Shock

Stabilizes cell and organelle membrane integrity
    Reduces leucocyte sequestration and degeneration
    Reduces platelet aggregation
    Reduces red cell sludging
    Reduces lyosomal degeneration
    Reduces capillary permeability
    Reduces intestinal autolytic lesions
    Reduces absorption of intestinal toxins

Improves cellular metabolism and gluconeogenesis
    Enhances gluconeogenesis
    Enhances lactate metabolism
    Increases ATP production
    Increases oxygen consumption

Improves capillary blood flow
    Decreases sludging
    Normalizes vasomotor tone and improves visceral
        organ perfusion
    Improves myocardial performance

Decreases production of myocardial depressant factor
    (but not its effect)

Inhibits complement-mediated granulocyte aggregation

Minimizes histologic organ damage

Reverses reticuloendothelial depression

Improves cerebral blood flow and preserves normal
    cerebral metabolic function

---

5. Evidence for efficacy of one drug over another is lacking at this time. Methylprednisolone sodium succinate has been shown to penetrate cells much faster than dexamethasone in one report.[84] However, several studies have failed to demonstrate greater antishock effects with either agent.[85-90] The antiendotoxin effects of dexamethasone paralleled the high plasma levels of the agent but not tissue levels.[91]

There appears to be no difference between the sodium succinate ester and sodium phosphate.[85,89,92] The sodium sulfate ester[91] and propylene glycol preparations[75] have been reported to be ineffective.

The optimal doses for hydrocortisone and methylprednisolone have been reported to be 300 and 30 mg/kg respectively.[93,94] No further improvement was noted when the doses were increased to 600 and 50 mg/kg respectively.[90,93,94] Similar effectiveness has been reported for dexamethasone at the optimal dose of 15 mg/kg.[90] No further improvement was noted when the dose was increased to 30 mg/kg.[90] Recommended shock dosages for the corticosteroids are listed in Table 11-5. It is generally recommended that hydrocortisone be repeated every 4 hours, prednisolone every 8 hours, and dexamethasone every 12 hours. The beneficial effects of corticosteroids are unique to massive bolus doses of these agents.[95]

The adverse effects of glucocorticoids listed in Table 11-6 are largely due to long-term use of supraphysiologic doses of these agents. Short-term use (less than 2 days) of massive doses is not associated with most of these effects. Short-term administration was associated with a transient inhibition of blood cortisol levels[95] and adenocorticotropic hormone (ACTH) responsiveness[96] but not adrenal atrophy. Short-term use decreases hydrogen ion and trypsin-induced GI epithelial damage during shock[97,98]; long-term administration is associated with GI hemorrhage, ulceration, and perforation.[99,100] Corticosteroids did not decrease phagocytosis *in vitro*.[84,101]

Cortiocosteroids have been shown to improve the shock state and to improve survival if administered prior to or immediately after the onset of shock. Whether corticosteroids improve overall long-term survival in clinical patients is still controversial.[102] This may be an unfair result to expect since many septic and otherwise shocky patients have lethal underlying diseases that would not be altered by steroids. Given that shock is a difficult disease to study, and in view of the vast array of potential short-term benefits from massive doses of corticosteroids, it seems advisable that they should be administered early in the therapeutic cascade.

Antiprostaglandins

It is clear that cyclo-oxygenase and lipoxygenase prostanoids (e.g., thromboxane, PGF_2, PGE_2, and the leukotrienes) are formed and released into the systemic circulation in increased quantities during septic shock in all species in which it has been studied. They cause marked hemodynamic changes. Their role as mediators of inflammation include pulmonary vasoconstriction, increased pulmonary cap-

Table 11-5 Available Corticosteroids for Shock Therapy

	Plasma Half-life[a] (min)	Biological Half-life[a] (hr)	Gluco-corticoid Potency[a]	Mineralo-corticoid Activity[a]	Equivalent Dose[a] (mg)	Approximate Physiologic Replacement Dose (mg/kg/day)	Pharmaco-logic Shock Dose (mg/kg)

Hydrocortisone
  Hydrocortisone sodium phosphate (Hydrocortisone phosphate; Merck Sharpe & Dohme)
  Hydrocortisone sodium succinate (A-hyroCort; Abbott) (Solu-Cortef; Upjohn)
	90–180	8–12	1	2	20	0.25–0.30	300

Prednisolone
  Prednisolone sodium phosphate (Hydeltrasol; Merck Sharpe & Dohme) (Cortisate-20; Burns-Biotec)
  Prednisolone sodium succinate (Solu-delta-cortef; Upjohn) (Prednisolone sodium succinate; Rugby)
	115–252	12–36	4	1	5	0.05–0.10	10–30

Methylprednisolone Methylprednisolone sodium succinate (Solu-medrol; Upjohn)	144–240	12–36	5	0	4	0.05–0.06	10–30
Dexamethasone Dexamethasone sodium phosphate (Azium SP; Schering) (Dalalone; O'Neal, Jones & Feldman) (Dexate-sp; Burns-Biotec) (Decadron phosphate; Organon)	200–300	36–72	25–30	0	0.75	0.01	6–15

[a] AMA Drug Evaluations, 5th ed. AMA, Chicago, 1983, p. 892.
Abbott, North Chicago, IL; Burns-Biotec, Omaha, NE; Beecham, Bristol, TN; Haver-lockhart, Shawnee, KS; Merck Sharpe & Dohme, West Point PA; Mayrand, Greensboro, NC; O'Neal, Jones & Feldman, Maryland Heights, MO; Organon, West Orange, NJ; Rugby, Rockville Centre, NY; Schering, Kenilworth, NJ; Tutag, Atlanta, GA; Upjohn, Kalamazoo, MI.

illary permeability, and systemic vasodilation. These changes can be detrimental to the patient.[103–107] Treatment with nonsteroidal antiprostaglandin anti-inflammatory drugs (Table 11-7) has been shown to normalize associated hemodynamic changes and improve survival in a wide variety of models and species.[104,107–114] Antiprostaglandin drugs do not affect the leukopenia, thrombocytopenia, pH and blood-gas changes, or the coagulopathies that occur during septic shock.[107,108,110] The effectiveness of these cyclo-oxygenase inhibitors is improved if they are administered along with fluids,[111] antibiotics,[110] and corticosteroids.[115] Indomethacin may be better than aspirin at ameliorating the hemodynamic response to sepsis.[107]

The antiprostaglandins have some serious deleterious effects. The most common appears to be GI ulceration and hemorrhage,[116–119] although GI lesions were not noted in dogs 7 days after administration of two doses of flunixin (1 mg/kg).[111] An-

Table 11-6 Adverse Effects
of Glucocorticosteroids

Immune suppression
Infection/septicemia
Adrenal suppression
Delayed wound healing
Pancreatitis (?)
Gastrointestinal mucosal necrosis
Diabetogenic (?)
Negative nitrogen balance
Hepatopathy

tiprostaglandins are not associated with renal dysfunction when given to normal dogs[120] but might be if there were a superimposed hemodynamic insult such as general anesthesia, hypotension, dehydration, or sepsis.[121-123] Continuous therapy with an antiprostaglandin may impair the inflammatory stage of wound repair but not the proliferative stage.[124]

It would appear that the cyclo-oxygenase inhibitors have important beneficial effects in septic shock. In spite of their potential adverse effects, serious consideration should be given to their administration.

Support of Renal Function

Renal failure is a common component of hypovolemic, endotoxic, and septic shock, as well as a potential consequence of some therapeutic measures

Table 11-7 Nonsteroidal Antiinflammatory
Drugs That Have Been Used in Shock in Dogs
and Cats

Drug	Dose
Aspirin	10 mg/kg
Indomethacin	10–20 mg/kg (repeated once at 2 hours)
Flunixin	1–2 mg/kg (repeated once at 2 hours)
Ibuprofen	5 mg/kg
Phenylbutazone	100 mg/kg
Aminopyrine	50 mg/kg (repeated 10 mg/kg hourly × 2)
Flufenamic acid	20 mg/kg (repeated 10 mg/kg hourly × 2)

(e.g., aminoglycoside and, to some extent, cephalosporin antibiotics; antiprostaglandins).[125] It is important to evaluate urine production as an indirect reflection of renal blood flow early in the course of shock therapy. If there is any doubt about urine production as determined by serial urinary bladder palpations, the bladder should be catheterized, even in septic shock patients.

The mainstay of renal blood flow support is fluid administration to restore blood volume and pressure. Once this is complete (as determined by central venous pressure or arterial blood pressure measurement, mucous membrane color and capillary refill time, and toe-web temperature), diuretic therapy should commence immediately.

Furosemide (5 mg/kg IV) promotes renal vasodilation and is a potent loop diuretic. If urine does not flow within 10 minutes, either one additional dose of furosemide should be administered or a different diuretic agent selected.

Mannitol or glucose (0.5 g/kg IV over a 20- to 30-minute period) osmotically increases blood volume and renal perfusion, and subsequently acts as an osmotic diuretic. If urine does not flow within 10 minutes following the end of the infusion, one should proceed to another agent, such as dopamine.

Dopamine (1 to 5 μg/kg/min) causes renal vasodilation via renal dopaminergic receptor stimulation, thereby improving renal blood flow and urine output. It is initiated at a low dose and increased (in 1-μg/kg/min increments at 10-minute intervals) until urine begins to flow or there is evidence of α-mediated peripheral vasoconstriction, which decreases renal blood flow. If dopamine is not effective, a combination of diuretics, dopamine, and fluid therapy may be used. The only further alternative is dialysis.

Correction of Hypoglycemia

Hypoglycemia is a common problem in septic shock[110,126] and can be severe when gluconeogenesis becomes compromised in the face of continued high glucose utilization.[127-129] Blood glucose concentration should be normalized by administering glucose as follows: an intravenous bolus of approximately 0.25 g/kg (0.5 ml of 50 percent dextrose) to restore normal blood glucose levels and a 5 to 10 percent glucose infusion (depending on the rate of fluid administration) to maintain the blood glucose at 80 to 180 mg/dl.

Correction of Metabolic Acidosis

Metabolic acidosis is a common complication of hyovolemic and septic shock.[110] Since the magnitude of its impact in shock is variable, it is helpful to measure the base deficit or bicarbonate deficit[130] and to calculate the amount of needed sodium bicarbonate as follows: base or bicarbonate deficit × body weight (kg) × 0.3. The 0.3 × kg figure is used as an approximation of extracellular fluid volume. In lieu of this absolute measurement, metabolic acidosis should be assumed to be present during shock. If the patient is moderately to severely affected, 3 to 5 mEq/kg, respectively, of sodium bicarbonate should be administered.

The adverse effects of bicarbonate, if administered too rapidly or in too great a quantity, include iatrogenic alkalosis, severe hypotension, vomiting, restlessness, paradoxical cerebrospinal fluid acidosis, cerebral edema, and hypercapnia. Therefore, no proportion of the calculated dose should be administered as a bolus. Rather, it should be administered over a period of 30 minutes. Bicarbonate administration increases the carbon dioxide production via carbonic acid equilibration. Animals that have no capacity to increase their minute ventilation due to their underlying disease process may become hypercapnic. These patients should receive positive pressure ventilation support or, perhaps, tromethamine (Abbott Laboratories, N. Chicago, IL), which alkalinizes the patient by binding hydrogen ion and consequently decreases blood carbon dioxide.[131] Since the metabolic derangement causing acidosis can be aggressive and the effects of the bicarbonate transient, the degee of metabolic acidosis should be requantitated 30 minutes after infusion of the bicarbonate.

Correction of Coagulopathies

Endothelial injury and tissue damage caused by hypoxia, endotoxins, exotoxins, and immune complexes expose collagen and release tissue thromboplastins into the systemic circulation. This activates the coagulation, (fibrinogenic) platelet, and plasmin (fibrinolytic) cascades. The coagulation and platelet cascades are also directly activated by endotoxin.[12,18] Plasmin degrades fibrin and fibrinogen; these degradation products inactivate fibrin monomers, platelets, and several coagulation factors, causing a hemorrhagic diathesis.[132]

If platelet and coagulation cascades predominate, a hypercoagulative state will be manifested. Small vessel thrombosis may cause microangiopathic hemolysis (histocytosis) and tissue ischemia. Postmortem fibrinolysis may negate histologic demonstration of these microinfarctions.[133] Intravascular coagulation almost always occurs in the face of poor capillary blood flow. The slower blood flows, the greater is its viscosity.[133] Hypercoagulability may also be potentiated by acidosis (less than 7.2 pH), high fibrinogen levels, increased platelet adhesiveness, and exogenous or endogenous catecholamines.[133]

If the anticoagulant plasmin cascade predominates, a hypocoagulative state will be manifested.[132] If the hypercoagulative state persists and coagulation precursors become depleted, a hypocoagulative state will develop.

The coagulation status of the patient can be evaluated by observing for evidence of abnormal clotting or bleeding from more than one site. This can be monitored by measuring prothrombin time, activated coagulation time, partial thromboplastin time, and thrombin time plus reptilase time[132] or by coagulation time in a nonanticoagulated test tube or capillary tube.[134–136] Platelet function can be evaluated by aggregometry or by counting numbers, by cuticle bleeding time (less than 5 min) and clot retraction time (less than 2 hours),[135] and by clinical manifestation of petechiae. Assessment of fibrin monomer and degradation products helps determine whether coagulation or fibrinolysis is activated (tests provide a false-negative result in 5 to 15 percent of human patients with activated coagulation/fibrinolysis[132]) but does not determine whether the patient is normo-, hyper-, or hypocoagulable or whether heparin or a plasma transfusion is indicated.

In all cases, effective treatment of the underlying disease process is the single most important therapeutic objective. The generous administration of fluids to enhance microcirculation and cause modest hemodilution, appropriate antimicrobial therapy, and drainage of infections are of paramount importance in this regard. If, after 4 hours of aggressive management, bleeding continues, the intravascular coagulopathy may require specific treatment.

Activated coagulation should be treated first with heparin in quantities sufficient to prolong the coagulation test being employed to 1.5 to 2 times normal. The effective dose of heparin is variable. One should start with 40 to 80 units/kg SC every 8 to 12 hours[132,137] and adjust the dose as necessary according to the coagulation test(s). A subcutaneous dose of 250 to 375 units/kg has been recommended for the cat.[136] Since heparin depends on antithrombin III for its anticoagulant effect, it may take 2 to 3 hours for a dose of heparin to take effect.[132] Heparin is inactive if the peripheral capillaries are acidotic or if the patient has a coagulase-induced coagulopathy.[133]

The activated platelet aggregation can be subdued by the administration of a nonsteroidal antiinflammatory agent or by dextran infusion. This may be important during heparin therapy, since heparin can potentiate platelet agglutination.[133] Aspirin may be the best thrombasthenic agent,[138] and should be administered at a dose of 25 mg/kg. It need not be repeated for 3 days.[139]

Hypocoagulative states may be due to inhibition of coagulation factors by fibrin or fibrinogen degradation products, or to a depletion of clotting factors. Factor or platelet deficiencies can be treated by administration of fresh plasma subsequent to heparin therapy. After heparin therapy has been instituted, persistent plasmin inactivation of coagulation factors may, as a last resort, be treated with an antifibrinolytic agent such as ethyl aminocaproic acid. The initial dose is 50 to 100 mg/kg IV followed by 30 mg/kg every 1 to 2 hours.[132] These two treatments should be administered only after effective heparin anticoagulation has been achieved to avoid iatrogenic thrombosis.

Lipopolysaccharide Core Antisera

Gram-positive sepsis may be managed effectively with appropriate antibiotics. However, with gram-negative infections, this is often difficult due to development of antibiotic resistance. The frequent occurrence and lethality of gram-negative septic shock make newly developed immunologic approaches treating these infections very important.

The oligosaccharide-specific side chains of cell walls are highly variable among different strains, species, and genera of gram-negative microorganisms. The development of antibodies to a particular gram-negative organism provides little cross-protection against another. By contrast, the core region and the biologically active lipid-A moiety of the outer cell wall membrane are relatively immunologically constant. Certain rough mutant strains of *Salmonella* and *E. coli* (J-5 strain) lack the O-specific side chains, which exposes the relatively homogeneous lipopolysaccharide core region. Although the core region is weakly immunogenic, core antiserum has been shown to provide protection against diverse populations of gram-negative organisms by neutralizing the biologically active lipopolysaccharide.[140–142] The core antibody exerts its protective effects primarily as a result of its antiendotoxin activity and not by enhancing opsonization or phagocytosis. Core antiserum is not yet commercially available. Although initial investigations are very promising, much more research needs to be done in this area before its clinical efficacy can be established.

Multivalent Oligosaccharide Antisera

If an animal were vaccinated with multiple strains and species of gram-negative bacteria, it would eventually produce a wide variety of O-specific antibodies. The serum could provide protection to a similar variety of clinical gram-negative infections.[143,144]

Antilipopolysaccharide serum serves not only as an antiendotoxin. It activates complement, which lyses the bacterial cell wall and opsonizes bacteria, facilitating neutrophil phagocytosis.[145]

Support of Pulmonary Function

As a result of autacoid (histamine, serotonin, bradykinin, cyclo-oxygenase, and lipoxygenase prostanoids) and direct endotoxin-induced endothelial damage, complement-mediated bacterial phagocytosis, perivascular neutrophil sequestration, and disintegration,[12,13,80] protein and fluids exude into the interstitium of the lung at a progressively increasing rate.[80,146,147] If the infiltrative process is sufficient to overload the ability of lymphatics to remove it, interstitial and eventually alveolar pulmonary edema develop. This sequence of events and the resulting hypoxemia is commonly referred to as *respiratory distress syndrome*. It is often delayed in onset, can be relentlessly self-progressive and ultimately fatal. The dog, rabbit, rat and mouse do not develop this pulmonary consequence of septic shock as readily as do the pig, sheep, cat, and human.[150]

Oxygen supplementation may suffice as an early supportive treatment. However, high-pressure positive-pressure ventilation is usually necessary.[148,149] The development of this diffuse infiltrative pulmonary process in dogs and cats has thus far been an ominous event, in our experience. Glucocorticosteroids have been shown to minimize the perivascular sequestration of neutrophils, to diminish their tendency to disintegrate once sequestered, and to help prevent the development of this respiratory distress syndrome if administered early in the disease process.[81–83]

Protection of the Gastrointestinal Tract

Gastrointestinal ulceration and hemorrhage in the dog and cat are not an uncommon consequence of hypovolemic, endotoxic, or septic shock. These pathologic changes could be attributed to the extreme hepatic venoconstriction (unique to the dog[151]), vasoconstrictive ischemia to intestinal mucosa, systemic hypotension-induced mucosal ischemia,[152] indirect actions via complement or prostaglandin activation, or direct cytotoxic effects.[153] The mucosal ischemia may exert cytotoxic effects directly by altering cellular metabolism or by impairing production of the protective mucous layer and gastric bicarbonate secretion. The latter exposes the GI tract to cytotoxic effects of gastric acid, bile, or pancreatic trypsin.[154,155]

The mainstay of GI protection is effective treatment of the underlying disease process (e.g., large volume fluid therapy to re-establish mucosal perfusion). Drugs such as cimetidine or ranitidine may be beneficial in that they decrease gastric acid secretion. Sucralfate may coat existing ulcers and prevent perforation. Aprotinin was reported not to decrease the incidence of hemorrhagic gastroenteritis in canine hypovolemic shock.[156]

Nutrition

Just as malnutrition predisposes to sepsis, proper nutrition is important in the prevention and treatment of sepsis.[157–159] Recent advances in parenteral and enteral nutrition have greatly improved this important aspect of critical patient care.[160,161]

Naloxone

β-Endorphin is elevated in septic and hypovolemic shock and has been shown to cause hypotension and pulmonary platelet trapping.[113] Naloxone administration (2 mg/kg/hr) has ameliorated the hypotension, hypoglycemia, acidosis, and pulmonary platelet trapping.[162–164] It has improved survival when administered alone[88] or with corticosteroids and antiprostaglandins.[88,115,165]

Fibronectin

Fibronectin is a circulating opsonizing glycoprotein that binds nonspecifically with microparticles to facilitate reticuloendothelial phagocytic activity.[166] Fibronectin is depleted in shock, trauma, or sepsis, resulting in reticuloendothelial depression. This can be reversed by fibronectin administration.[167]

Granulocyte Transfusion

Persistent leukopenia in septic patients is routinely associated with a high mortality rate.[18,32] It has led to several studies evaluating the efficacy of granulocyte transfusions in granulocytopenic septic patients.[18] The improvement in survival rates was dramatic, especially in those patients without spontaneous bone marrow recovery.[18] Granulocyte transfusion has been reported in the dog.[168,169]

Energy and Energy Substrates

On the assumption that irreversible shock is ultimately caused by a cellular energy deficit, adenosine monophosphate (ATP) or substrate infusion may help sustain cellular function and improve survival. Glucose and glucose-insulin-potassium have been reported to have beneficial effects in hypovolemic and septic shock.[170] Cyclic adenosine monophosphate (cAMP), Krebs cycle intermediates, and nicotinamide and adenosine administration have been reported to have some beneficial effects in septic but not in hemorrhagic shock.[170] ATP, particularly $ATP-MgCl_2$, has been reported to have beneficial effects in septic and hemorrhagic shock[170–174] However, not all reports are positive.[175] Further research needs to be done in this area before the efficacy of substrate and energy supplementation in the treatment of shock states can be established.

Aprotinin

Aprotinin (Bayvet, Division of Cutter Biological, Emeryville, CA) inhibits lysosomal proteolytic enzyme activity.[155] It was associated with a rapid regeneration of mitochondrial ATP[176] and improved myocardial function in hemorrhagic shock.[177] Topical aprotinin inhibits trypsin lysis of the ischemic gut[178] but was not found to be useful in preventing hemorrhagic gastroenteritis when administered parenterally in canine hemorrhagic shock.[156] Aprotinin may be useful in inhibiting neutrophil proteolytic pulmonary damage. Further clinical evaluation is necessary.

CARDIOGENIC SHOCK

Cardiogenic shock is defined as any abnormality that interferes with the forward outflow of blood from the heart to such an extent that adequate tissue perfusion is not achieved. Examples include acute or chronic heart failure, hypertrophic or congestive cardiomyopathy, arteriovenous shunts, outflow obstruction, excessive regurgitant fraction, thrombosis, pericardial fibrosis or tamponade, heartworm disease, or severe arrhythmias.

With inadequate capillary perfusion oxygen delivery to tissues becomes impaired. Removal of cellular metabolites is also important to maintain cellular viability. Accumulation of cellular metabolites may cause injury or death to the cells.

The patient may exhibit depression, weakness, syncope, and tachycardia with a weak, thready pulse. Reflex peripheral vasoconstriction is often apparent and arterial blood pressure is low. Central venous blood pressure and/or pulmonary capillary wedge pressure is high, depending on whether there is right or left heart failure, respectively, or both. Patients are generally tachypneic and hypocapneic in the absence of pulmonary edema, although pulmonary edema and hypoxemia may develop with left heart failure. Metabolic acidosis may also develop secondary to poor tissue perfusion. Arrhythmias of any description may be present.

Therapeutic Strategies

Therapy of cardiogenic shock is directed toward either (1) surgical correction of the underlying abnormality (e.g., stenotic or regurgitant valves, arteriovenous shunts, pericardial tamponade, pericardial fibrosis); or (2) administration of drugs that improve myocardial contractility in disorders of pump failure (e.g., dilated cardiomyopathy), reduce adreneric stimulation in disorders of diastolic dysfunction (hypertrophic cardiomyopathy), the administration of drugs or application of techniques that reduce afterload and/or preload, and control of serious arrhythmias.

An anticholinergic agent should be administered if the patient exhibits severe bradyarrhythmias which might further impair cardiovascular status. Temporary transvenous pacing may be required to increase cardiac output with complete atrioventricular block. Life threatening tachyarrhythmias may require appropriate antiarrhythmic therapy (e.g., drugs or electrical cardioversion).

Preload should be regulated in either left or right heart failure. If right-sided congestive heart failure is suspected, central venous pressure should be monitored. If left heart failure is suspected, pulmonary artery wedge pressure or diastolic pressure[179] should ideally be monitored in order to fine-tune preload reduction therapy. End-expiratory pressure or phlebotomy can be used to reduce excessive preload in acute life-threatening situations (e.g., fulminant pulmonary edema). Peripheral redistribution of central blood volume may also be accomplished by the careful administration of venodilators (Table 11-8). Care must be taken not to induce excessive hypotension. Reduction of extra-

Table 11-8 Vasodilating Agents

Drug Generic Name Brand Name (Source)	Mechanism of Action	Dose and Method of Administration (Onset, Peak, Duration)	Potential Adverse Effects
Morphine	Dilates primarily capacitance but also resistance vessels	0.05–0.2 mg/kg IM (10 min; 30–45 min; 2–4 hr)	CNS depression Respiratory depression Histamine-mediated hypotension (nausea, vomiting)
Acetylpromazine Acepromazine (Ayerst)	α-Receptor blockade	0.02–0.1 mg/kg IM (10 min; 30–45 min; 6–8 hr)	CNS depression
Hydralazine Apresoline (Ciba)	Direct arteriolar smooth muscle relaxant Little effect on venous capacitance vessels	0.2–0.5 mg/kg (10–20 min; 10–80 min; 2–8 hr)	With prolonged use: systemic lupus erythematosus Neuritis Blood dyscrasias
Diazoxide Hyperstat (Schering)	Direct arteriolar smooth muscle relaxant primarily on the resistance vessels	5 mg/kg rapidly IV (immed.; 5–10 min; 30 min to 10 hr)	Inhibits insulin release: hyperglycemia
Nitroprusside Nipride (Roche)	Direct arteriolar and venular smooth muscle relaxant	3 μg (0.5–10)/kg/min IV Dilute in D_5W, IV with continuous blood pressure monitoring (Immed; 1 min; 2 min)	Light sensitive; bottle must be covered with foil and kept for no longer than 4 hr Avoid in hepatic or renal failure Large doses may cause cyanide toxicity: Keep total dose below 1.5 mg/kg/2 hr. Treat with sodium nitrite (0.5–0.75 mg/kg slow IV) followed by sodium thiosulfate (0.2 g/kg slow IV) Thiocyanate accumulation (disorientation)

cellular fluid volume may be easily accomplished with potent diuretics such as furosemide. End-diastolic pressures should be maintained in the high-normal range to assure adequate filling pressures in the face of reduced myocardial compliance (common in many cardiomyopathic conditions). Pressures should not be allowed to increase above about 15 cm H_2O for central venous pressure or 18 mmHg for pulmonary capillary wedge pressure because of the danger of precipitating systemic or pulmonary edema, respectively.

Myocardial contractility may be stimulated (e.g., congestive cardiomyopathy) by the administration of catecholamine cardiotonic agents (dopamine, dobutamine, or mephentermine), digitalis glycosides, or the bipyridine derivatives amrinone and milrinone. Positive inotropes are not indicated for hypertrophic cardiomyopathy or other causes of cardiogenic shock in which contractility is normal.

Excess adrenergic stimulation is thought to underlie the development of hypertrophic cardiomyopathy and interruption of this influence has been shown to temporarily improve myocardial performance. Adrenergic blockers such as propranolol have been advocated for therapy.

Afterload reduction is not routinely recommended for cardiogenic shock because of the tendency to induce excessive hypotension. It may, perhaps, be indicated when compensatory vasoconstriction is believed to seriously impair tissue perfusion and venous cardiac return. Afterload reduction may be achieved by dopamine or dobutamine, amrinone, or furosemide,[180] or by the administration of specific arteriodilators (Table 11-8). Hypotension is a major complication of the use of arteriodilators in cardiogenic shock; since arterial blood pressure is often already low, dosages must therefore be conservative and the consequences of their administration monitored closely.

Intraaortic balloon counterpulsation has been demonstrated to improve cardiac output and myocardial oxygenation.[181-183] A balloon is inserted into the descending thoracic aorta via the femoral artery, phasically inflated at the time of aortic closure and deflated just prior to the next systole. The result is a reduction in the afterload against which the weak heart is required to pump, an increased mean arterial blood pressure, and cerebral and coronary perfusion.[184] Currently, this is largely a research technique.

REFERENCES

1. Kolata RJ, Burrows CF, Soma LR: Shock: pathophysiology and management. p. 32. In Kirk RW (ed): Current Veterinary Therapy. Vol. VII. WB Saunders, Philadelphia, 1980
2. Haskins SC: Shock. The Pathophysiology and Management of the Circulatory Collapse States. p. 2. In Kirk RW (ed): Current Veterinary Therapy. Vol. VIII. WB Saunders, Philadelphia, 1983
3. Hardie EM, Rawlings CA: Septic shock. Part I. Pathophysiology. Part II. Prevention, recognition, and treatment. Compend Cont Educ 5:369, 483, 1983
4. McAnulty JF: Septic shock in the dog: A review. J Am Anim Hosp Assoc 19:827, 1983
5. Papa M, Halperin Z, Rubinstein E, et al: The effect of ischemia of the dog's colon on transmural migration of bacteria and endotoxin. J Surg Res 35:264, 1983
6. Gathiram P, Gaffin SL, Wells MT, et al: Superior mesenteric artery occlusion shock in cats: Modification of the endotoxemia by antilipopolysaccharide antibodies (anti-LPS). Circ Shock 19:231, 1986
7. Gaffin SL, Grinbery Z, Abraham C, et al: Protection against hemorrhagic shock in the cat by human plasma containing endotoxin-specific antibodies. J Surg Res 31:18, 1981
8. Gaffin SL, Gathiram P, Wells MT: Effect of corticosteroid prophylaxis on lipopolysaccharide levels associated with intestinal ischemia in cats. Crit Care Med 14:889, 1986
9. Parratt JA: The role of arachidonic acid metabolites in endotoxin shock. I. Lipoxygenase products. p. 203. In Hinshaw LB (ed): Handbook of Endotoxin. Vol. 2. Pathophysiology of Endotoxin. Elsevier Science Publishers, New York, 1985
10. Flynn JT: The role of arachidonic acid metabolites in endotoxin shock. II. Involvement of prostanoids and thromboxanes. p. 237. In Hinshaw LB (ed): Handbook of Endotoxin. Vol 2: Pathophysiology of Endotoxin. Elsevier Science Publishers, New York, 1985
11. Morrison DC, Ulerutch RJ: The effect of bacterial endotoxins on host mediation systems. A review. Am J Pathol 93:526, 1978
12. Jacobs ER: Overview of mediators affecting pulmonary and systemic vascular changes in endotoxemia. p. 1. In Hinshaw LB (ed): Handbook of Endotoxin. Vol. 2. Pathophysiology of Endotoxin. Elsevier Science Publishers, New York, 1985
13. Fine DP: Role of complement in endotoxin shock. p. 129. In Hinshaw LB (ed): Handbook of Endotoxin. Vol. 2: Pathophysiology of Endotoxin. Elsevier Science Publishers, New York, 1985
14. Hinshaw LB: Cardiodepressant effects of endotoxin. p. 16. In: Hinshaw LB (ed): Handbook of Endotoxin. Vol. 2: Pathophysiology of Endotoxin. Elsevier Sciencce Publishers, New York, 1985
15. Archer LT, Benjamin BA, Beller-Todd BK, et al: Does LD_{100} E. coli shock cause myocardial failure? Circ Shock 9:7, 1982
16. Bond RF: Peripheral circulatory responses to endotoxin. p. 36. In Hinshaw LB (ed): Handbook of

Endotoxin. Vol. 2: Pathophysiology of Endotoxin. Elsevier Science Publishers, New York, 1985

17. Kreger BE, Craven DE, Carling PC, et al: Gram-negative bacteremia. III. Reassessment of etiology, epidemiology and ecology of 612 patients. Am J Med 68:332, 1980

18. Hruska JF, Hornick RB: Treatment of infection in septic shock. p. 482. In Cowley RA, Trump BF (eds): Pathophysiology of Shock, Anoxia, and Ischemia. Williams & Wilkins, Baltimore, 1982

19. Hamill RJ, Maki DG: Endotoxin shock in man caused by gram-negative bacilli. p. 55. In Proctor RA (ed): Handbook of Endotoxin. Vol. 4: Clinical Aspects of Endotoxin Shock. Elsevier Science Publishers, New York, 1986

20. Hardie EM, Rawlings CA, Calvert CA: Severe sepsis in selected small animal surgical patients. J Am Anim Hosp Assoc 22:33, 1986

21. Hirsh DC, Jang SS and Biberstein EL: Blood culture of the canine patient. J Am Vet Med Assoc 184:175, 1984

22. Dow SW, Jones RL, Adney WS: Anaerobic bacterial infections and response to treatment in dogs and cats: 36 cases (1983–1985). J Am Vet Med Assoc 189:930, 1986

23. Koterba AM, Brewer BD, Tarplee FA: Clinical and clinicopathological characteristics of the septicaemic neonatal foal: Review of 38 cases. Eq Vet J 16:376, 1984

24. Calvert CA, Greene CE, Hardie EM: Cardiovascular infections in dogs: Epizootiology, clinical manifestations and prognosis. J Am Vet Med Assoc 187:612, 1985

25. Kreger BE, Craven DE, McCabe WR: Gram-negative bacteremia. IV. Re-evaluation of clinical features and treatment in 612 patients. Am J Med 68:344, 1980

26. Glickman LT: Veterinary nosocomial (hospital-acquired) *Klebsiella* infections. J Am Vet Med Assoc 179:1389, 1981

27. Gahhos FN, Chiu RCJ, Bethune D, et al: Hemodynamic responses to sepsis: Hypodynamic versus hyperdynamic states. J Surg Res 31:475, 1981

28. Sugerman JH, Newsome HH, Greenfield LJ: Hemodynamics, oxygen consumption and serum catecholamine changes in progressive lethal peritonitis in the dog. Surg Gynecol Obstet 154:8, 1982

29. Hinshaw LB, Solomon LA, Holmes DD, et al: Comparison of canine response to *Escherichia coli* organisms and endotoxin. Surg Gynecol Obstet 127:981, 1968

30. Kolata RJ: The significance of changes in toe-web temperature in dogs in circulatory shock. Proc Gaines Vet Symp 28:21, 1978

31. Deysin M, Stein S: Albumin shifts across the extracellular space secondary to experimental sepsis. Surg Gynecol Obstet 151:617, 1980

32. Gudmundsson S, Craig WA: Role of antibiotics in endotoxin shock. p. 238. In Proctor RA (ed): Handbook of Endotoxin. Vol. 4: Clinical Aspects of Endotoxin Shock. Elsevier Science Publishers, New York, 1986

33. McNamara JJ, Suehiro GT, Suehiro A, et al: Resuscitation from hemorrhagic shock. J Trauma 23:552, 1983

34. Moss GS, Lowe RJ, Jelek J, et al: Colloid or crystalloid in the resuscitation of hemorrhagic shock: A controlled clinical trial. Surgery 89:434, 1981

35. Virgilio RW, Rice CL, Smith DE, et al: Crystalloid vs colloid resuscitation: Is one better? Surgery 85:129, 1979

36. Shires GT, Peitzman AB, Albert SA, et al: Response of extravascular lung water to intraoperative fluids. Ann Surg 197:515, 1983

37. Tranbaugh RF, Lewis FR: Mechanisms and etiologic factors of pulmonary edema, Surg Gynecol Obstet 158:193, 1984

38. Walser M, Selfin DW, Grollman A: Measurement of extracellular fluid with radiosulfate. J Clin Invest 31:669, 1952

39. Hartsfield SM, Thurmon JC, Corbin JE, et al: Effects of sodium acetate, bicarbonate and lactate on acid-base status in anaesthetized dogs. J Vet Pharmacol Therap 4:51, 1981

40. Nakayama SI, Sibley L, Gunther RA, et al: Small-volume resuscitation with hypertonic saline (2,400 mOsm/Liter) during hemorrhagic shock. Circ Shock 13:149, 1984

41. Nakayama SI, Kramer GC, Carlsen RC, Holcroft JW: Infusion of very hypertonic saline to bled rats: Membrane potentials and fluid shifts. J Surg Res 38:180, 1985

42. Kramer GC, Perron PR, Lindsey DC, et al: Small volume resuscitation with hypertonic saline dextran solution. Surgery 100:239, 1986

43. Smith GJ, Kramer GC, Perron P: A comparison of several hypertonic solutions for resuscitation of bled sheep. J Surg Res 39:517, 1985

44. Velasco IT, Pontieri V, Rocha-e-Silva M, et al: Hyperosmotic NaCl and severe hemorrhagic shock. Am J. Physiol 239:H664, 1980

45. Heyl JT, Gibson JG, Janeway CA: Studies on the plasma proteins. V. The effect of concentrated solutions of human and bovine serum albumin on blood volume after acute blood loss in man. J Clin Invest 22:763, 1943

46. Warren JV, Stead EA, Merrill JH, et al: Chemical,

clinical and immunological studies on the products of human plasma fractionation. IX. The treatment of shock with concentrated human serum albumin: A preliminary report. J Clin Invest 23:506, 1944

47. Hunt PS, Reeve TS: Arterial thrombus prevention and dissolution after low molecular weight dextran infusion in sheep. Med J Aust 54:539, 1967

48. Shoemaker WC, Monson DO: The effect of whole blood and plasma expanders on volume-flow relationships in critically ill patients. Surg Gynecol Obstet 137:453, 1973

49. Gruber VF: Blood Replacement. Springer-Verlag, New York, 1969

50. Hulse JD, Yacobi A: Hetastarch: An overview of the colloid and its metabolism. Drug Intell Clin Pharmacy 17:334, 1983

51. Allen D, Kvietyz PR, Granger DN: Crystalloids vs colloids: implications in fluid therapy of dogs with intestinal obstruction. Am J Vet Res 47:1751, 1986

52. Pichler ME and Turnwald GH: Blood transfusion in the dog and cat. Part I. Physiology, collection, storage and indications for whole blood therapy. Compend Cont Educ 7:64, 1985

53. Michel RL: Blood groups, typing and crossmatching of animal blood. Bull Am Soc Vet Clin Pathol 4:2, 1975

54. Auer L, Bell K: The AB blood group system in the domestic cat. Anim Blood Groups Biochem Genet 11:63, 1980

55. Marion RS, Smith JE: Survival of erythrocytes after autologous and allogenic transfusions in cats. J Am Vet Med Assoc 183:1437, 1983

56. Auer L, Bell K, Coates S: Blood transfusion reactions in the cat. J Am Vet Med Assoc 180:729, 1982

57. Crowe DT: Autotransfusion in the trauma patient. Vet Clin North Am 10:581, 1980

58. Turnwald GH: Blood transfusions in dogs and cats. Part II. Administration, adverse effects and component therapy. Compend Cont Educ 7:115, 1985

59. Haskins SC: Standards and techniques of equipment utilization. p. 60. In Sattler FP, Knowles RP, Whittick WG (eds): Veterinary Critical Care. Lea & Febiger, Philadelphia, 1981

60. Kaback KR, Sanders AB, Meeslin HW: MAST suit update. JAMA 252:2598, 1984

61. Wishart DF: Recent advances in antimicrobial drugs: The penicillins. J Am Vet Med Assoc 185:1106, 1984

62. Hirsh DC, Ruehl WW: A rational approach to the selection of an antimicrobial agent. J Am Vet Med Assoc 185:1058, 1984

63. Thomson RD, Quay JF, Webber JA: Cephalosporin group of antimicrobial drugs. J Am Vet Med Assoc 185:1109, 1984

64. Benitz AM: Future developments in the aminoglycoside group of antimicrobial drugs. J Am Vet Med Assoc 185:1118, 1984

65. Hennessey PW, Kohn FS, Bickford SM, et al: *In vitro* activity of gentamicin against bacteria isolated from domestic animals. Vet Med Small Anim Clin 66:1110, 1971

66. Roudebush P, Fales WH: Antibacterial susceptibility of gentamicin resistant organisms recovered from small companion animals. J Am Anim Hosp Assoc 18:649, 1982

67. Hirsh DC, Wiger N, Knox SJ: Susceptibility of clinical isolates of *Pseudomonas aeruginosa* to antimicrobial agents. J Vet Pharmacol Ther 2:275, 1979

68. Garvey MS, Aucoin DP: Therapeutic strategies involving antimicrobial treatment of disseminated bacterial infection in small animals. J Am Vet Med Assoc 185:1185, 1984

69. Goto H, Nakamura S: Liberation of endotoxin from *Escherichia coli* by addition of antibotics. Jpn J Exp Med 50:35, 1980

70. Shenep JL, Mogan KA: Kinetics of endotoxin release during antibiotic therapy for experimental gram-negative bacterial sepsis. J Infect Dis 150:380, 1984

71. Cooperstock MS: Inactivation of endotoxin by polymyxin B. Antimicrob Agents Chemother 6:422, 1974

72. Schumer W: Steroids in the treatment of clinical septic shock. Ann Surg 184:333, 1976

73. Shatney CH: The use of corticosteroids in the therapy of hemorrhagic shock. p. 465. In Cowley RA, Trump BR (eds): Pathophysiology of Shock, Anorexia, and Ischemia. Williams & Wilkins, Baltimore, 1982

74. Ferguson JL, Roesel OF, Bottoms GD: Dexamethasone treatment during hemorrhagic shock: Blood pressure, tissue perfusion and plasma enzymes. Am J Vet Res 39:817, 1978

75. White GL, White GS, Kosanke SD, et al: Therapeutic effects of predisolone sodium succinate vs dexamethasone in dogs subjected to E. coli septic shock. J Am Anim Hosp Assoc 18:639, 1982

76. Lefer AM, Martin J: Mechanism of the protective effect of corticosteroids in hemorrhagic shock. Am J Physiol 216:314, 1969.

77. Nagy S, Barankay T, Horpacsy G: Effect of corticosteroid treatment on renal blood flow in hemorrhagic shock. Eur Surg Res 2:333, 1970

78. Kusajima K, Wax SD, Webb WR: Effects of methylprednisolone on pulmonary microcirculation. Surg Gynecol Obstet 139:1, 1974

79. Repogle RL, Kundler H, Schottenfeld M: Hemo-

dynamic effects of dexamethasone in experimental hemorrhagic shock—Negative results. Ann Surg 174:126, 1971

80. Shasby DM, Hunninghake GW: Endotoxin-induced pulmonary leukostasis. p. 98. In Hinshaw LB (ed): Handbook of Endotoxin, Vol. 2: Pathophysiology of Endotoxin. Elsevier Science Publishing Co, New York, 1985

81. Jacobs HS, Moldow CF, Flynn PJ, et al: Therapeutic ramifications of the interaction of complement granulocytes and platelets in the production of acute lung injury. Ann NY Acad Sci 384:489, 1982

82. Hess ML, Manson NH: The paradox of steroid therapy: Inhibition of oxygen-free radicals. Circ Shock 10:1, 1983

83. Hammerschmidt DE, Flynn, PJ, Coppo PA, et al: Synergy among agents inhibiting granulocyte aggregation. Inflammation 6:169, 1982

84. Wilson JW: Cellular localization of ^{3}H-labeled corticosteroids by electron microscopic autoradiography after hemorrhagic shock. p. 275. In Glenn TM (ed): Steroids and Shock. University Park Press, Baltimore, 1974

85. Shatney CH, Lillehei RC: Serum complement levels in canine endotoxin shock: relation to survival and to corticosteroid therapy. Adv Shock Res 9:265, 1974

86. Ottosson J, Brandberg A, Erikson B, et al: Experimental septic shock—Effects of corticosteroids. Circ Shock 9:571, 1982

87. Sprung CL, Caralis PV, Marcial EH: The effects of high-dose corticosteroids in patients with septic shock. N Engl J Med 311:1137, 1984

88. Vargish T, Reynolds DG, Gurll NJ, et al: The interaction of corticosteroids and naloxone in canine hemorrhagic shock. J Surg Res 32:289, 1982

89. Erve PR, Earnest W, Schumer W: Antiendotoxic effect of water-soluble analogs of glucocorticoids. J Surg Res 18:567, 1975

90. Vargish T, Turner CS, Bond RF, et al: Dose-response relationships in steroid therapy for hemorrhagic shock. Am Surg 43:30, 1977

91. Imai T, Sakuraya N, Fujita T: Comparative study of antiendotoxic potency of dexamethasone based on its different ester types. Circ Shock 6:311, 1979

92. Hare LE, Yeh KC, Delzter CA, et al: Bioavailability of dexamethasone. II. Dexamethasone phosphate. Clin Pharmacol Ther 18:330, 1975

93. Altura BM, Altura BT: Peripheral vascular actions of glucocorticoids and their relationship to protection in circulatory shock. J Pharmacol Exp Ther 190:300, 1974

94. Altura BM: Glucocorticoid-induced protection in circulatory shock: Role of reticuloendothelial system function. Proc Soc Exp Biol Med 150:202, 1975

95. Toutain PL, Alvinerie M, Ruckebusch Y: Pharmacokinetics of dexamethasone and its effect on adrenal gland function in the dog. Am J Vet Res 44:212, 1983

96. Kemppainen RJ, Sartin JL: Effects of single intravenous doses of dexamethasone on baseline plasma cortisol concentrations and responses to synthetic ACTH in healthy dogs. Am J Vet Res 45:742, 1984

97. Haglund U, Abe T, Ahren C, et al: The intestinal mucosal lesions in shock. II. The relationship between the mucosal lesions and the cardiovascular derangement following regional shock. Eur Surg Res 8:448, 1976

98. Ritchie WP, Cherry KJ, Gibb A: Influence of methylprednisolone sodium succinate on bile-acid-induced acute gastric mucosal damage. Surgery 84:283, 1978

99. Toombs, JP, Caywood DD, Lipowitz AJ, et al: Colonic perforation following neurosurgical procedures and corticosteroid therapy in four dogs. J Am Vet Med Assoc 177:68, 1980

100. Sorjonen DC, Dillon AR, Powers RD, et al: Effects of dexamethasone and surgical hypotension on the stomach of dogs: Clinical, endoscopic, and pathologic evaluation. Am J Vet Res 44:1233, 1983

101. White GL, White GS: *In vitro* effects of prednisolone sodium succinate and *Escherichia coli* organisms on neutrophil survival, glucose utilization and *E. coli* clearance in canine blood. Am J Vet Res 43:1103, 1982

102. Kass EH: High-dose corticosteroids for septic shock. N Engl J Med 311:1178, 1984

103. Anderson FL, Jubiz W, Kralios AC, et al: Plasma prostaglandin levels during endotoxin shock in dogs. Circulation 45:II-124, 1972

104. Parratt JR, Sturgess RM: The effect of indomethacin in the cardiovascular and metabolic response to *E. coli* endotoxin in the cat. Br J Pharmacol 50:177, 1974

105. Fletcher JR, Ramwell PW, Herman CM: Prostaglandins and the hemodynamic course of endotoxin shock. J Surg Res 20:589, 1976

106. Ramwell PW, Fletcher JR, Flamenbaum WF: The arachidonic acid-prostaglandin system in endotoxemia. In Mattela MJ (ed): Proceedings of the Sixth International Congress on Pharmacology. Clin Pharmacol 5:175, 1975

107. Fletcher JR, Ramwell PW: Modification by aspirin and indomethacin of the haemodynamic and prostaglandin releasing effects of *E. coli* endotoxin in the dog. Br J Pharmacol 61:175, 1977

108. Fletcher JR, Ramwell PW: Indomethacin treatment following baboon endotoxin shock improves survival. Adv Shock Res 4:103, 1980

109. Fletcher JR: The role of prostaglandins in sepsis. Scand J Infect Dis 31 (suppl):55, 1982

110. Hardie EM, Kolata RJ, Rawlings CA: Canine septic peritonitis: Treatment with flunixin meglumine. Circ Shock 11:159, 1983

111. Hardie EM, Rawlings CA, Collins LG: Canine *Escherichia coli* peritonitis: Long-term survival with fluid, gentamicin sulfate and flunixin meglumine treatment. J Am Anim Hosp Assoc 21:691, 1985

112. Greenway CV, Murthy VS: Mesenteric vasoconstriction after endotoxin administration in cats pretreated with aspirin. Br J Pharmacol 43:59, 1971.

113. Almquist PM, Kuenzig M, Schwartz SI: Treatment of experimental canine endotoxin shock with ibuprofen: A cyclooxygenase inhibitor. Circ Shock 13:227, 1984

114. Jacobs ER, Soulsby ME, Bone RC: Ibuprofen in canine endotoxin shock. J Clin Invest 70:536, 1982

115. Almquist PM, Ekstrom B, Kuenzig M, et al: Increased survival of endotoxin-injected dogs treated with methylprednisolone, naloxone and ibuprofen. Circ Shock 14:129, 1984

116. Stewart THM, Hetenyl C, Rowse UH, et al: Ulcerative enterocolitis in dogs induced by drugs. J Pathol 131:363, 1980

117. Coles LS, Fries JF, Kraines RG, et al: From experiment to experience: Side effects of nonsteroidal anti-inflammatory drugs. Am J Vet Med 74:820, 1983

118. Romatowski J: Comparative therapeutics of canine and human rheumatoid arthritis. J Am Vet Med Assoc 185:558, 1984

119. Ewing GO: Indomethacin-associated gastrointestinal hemorrhage in a dog. J Am Vet Med Assoc 161:1665, 1972

120. Swain JA, Heyndrickx GR, Boettcher DH, et al: Prostaglandin control of renal circulation in the unanesthetized dog and baboon. Am J Physiol 229:826, 1975

121. Spyridakis LK, Bacia JJ, Barsanti JA, et al: Ibuprofen toxicosis in a dog. J Am Vet Med Assoc 188:918, 1986

122. Clive DM, Stoff JS: Renal syndromes associated with nonsteroidal anti-inflammatory drugs. N Engl J Med 310:563, 1984

123. Fink MP, MacVittie TJ, Casey LC: Effects of nonsteroidal anti-inflammatory drugs on renal function in septic dogs. J Surg Res 36:516, 1984

124. Donner GS, Ellison GW, Peyton LC: Effect of flunixin meglumine on surgical wound strength and healing in the rat. Am J Vet Res 47:2247, 1986

125. Barnes JL, McDowell EM: Pathology and pathophysiology of acute renal failure—A review. p. 324. In Cowley RA, Trump BF (eds): Pathophysiology of Shock, Anoxia, and Ischemia. Williams & Wilkins, Baltimore, 1982

126. Archer LT: Hypoglycemia in conscious dogs in live *Escherichia coli* speticemia. Circ Shock 3:93, 1976

127. Filkins JP, Cornell RP: Depression of hepatic gluconeogenesis and the hypoglycemia of endotoxin shock. Am J Physiol 227:778, 1974

128. Woolf LI, Groves AC, Duff JH: Amino acid metabolism in dogs with E. coli bacteremic shock. Surgery 85:212, 1979

130. Haskins SC: Blood gases and acid-base balance: Clinical interpretation and therapeutic implications. p. 201. In Kirk RW (ed): Current Veterinary Therapy. Vol. VIII. WB Saunders, Philadelphia, 1983

131. Wiklund L, Öquist L, Skoog G, et al: Clinical buffering of metabolic acidosis: Problems and a solution. Resuscitation 12:279, 1985

132. Bick RL: Disseminated intravascular coagulation and related syndromes: Etiology, pathophysiology, diagnosis and management. Am J Hematol 5:265, 1978

133. Hardaway RM: Pathology and pathophysiology of disseminated intravascular coagulation. p. 186. In Cowley RA, Trump BF (eds). Pathophysiology of Shock, Anoxia, and Ischemia. Williams & Wilkins, Baltimore, 1982

134. Byars TD, Ling GV, Ferris WA, et al: Activated coagulation time (ACT) of whole blood in normal dogs. Am J Vet Res 37:1359, 1976

135. Dodds WJ: Hemostasis and coagulation. p. 671. In Kaneko J (ed): Clinical Biochemistry of Domestic Animals. Academic Press, New York, 1980

136. Greene CE, Merriweather E: Activated partial thromboplastin time and activated coagulation time in monitoring heparnized cats. Am J Vet Res 43:1473, 1978

137. Ruehl W, Mills C, Feldman BF: Rational therapy in disseminated intravascular coagulation. J Am Vet Med Assoc 181:76, 1982

138. Gryglewski RJ, Korbut R, Ocetkiewicz A, et al: *In vivo* method for quantitation of anti-platelet potency of drugs. Naunyn Schmiedebergs Arch Pharmacol 302:25, 1978.

139. Greene CE: Effects of aspirin and propranolol on feline platelet aggregation. Am J Vet Res 46:1820, 1985

140. Pollack M, Huang AI, Prescott RK, et al: Enhanced survival in *Pseudomonas aeruginosa* septicemia associated with high levels of circulating antibody to *Escherichia coli* endotoxin core. J Clin Invest 72:1874, 1983

141. Ziegler EJ, McCutchan A, Fierer J, et al: Treatment of gram-negative bacteremia and shock with human antiserum to a mutant *Escherichia coli*. N Engl J Med 307:1225, 1982

142. Dunn DL, Mach PA, Condie RM: Anticore endotoxin F(ab')₂ equine immunoglobulin fragments protect against lethal effects of gram-negative bacterial sepsis. Surgery 96:440, 1984

143. Zanotti AM, Gaffin SL: Prophylaxis of superior mesenteric artery occlusion shock in rabbits by antilipopolysaccharide (Anti-LPS) antibodies. J Surg Res 38:113, 1985

144. Gaffin SL, Lachman E: The use of antilipopolysaccharide (anti-LPS) antibodies in the management of septic shock. S Afr Med J 65:158, 1984

145. Pudifin D, L'Hoste I, Duursma J, et al: Opsonization of gram-negative bacteria by antilipopolysaccharide antibodies. Lancet 1:1009, 1985

146. Rinaldo JE: Cellular mechanisms in adult respiratory distress syndrome, p. 396. In Snyder JV (ed): Oxygen Transport in the Critically Ill. Year Book Medical Publishers, Chicago, 1987

147. Sibbald WJ, Driedger AA: Pulmonary alveolarcapillary permeability in human septic respiratory distress syndrome. p. 372. In Cowley RA, Trump BF (ed): Pathophysiology of Shock, Anoxia, and Ischemia. Williams & Wilkins, Baltimore, 1982

148. Haskins SC: Physical therapeutics for respiratory disease. Semin Vet Med Surg 1:276, 1986

149. Snyder JV: The development of support ventilation: A critical summary. p. 283. In Snyder JV (ed): Oxygen Transport in the Critically Ill. Year Book Medical Publishers, Chicago, 1987

150. Crocker SH, Eddy DO, Obenauf RN: Bacteremia: Host-specific lung clearance and pulmonary failure. J Trauma 21:215, 1981

151. Archer LT: Pathologic manifestations of septic shock. p. 18. In Proctor RA (ed): Handbook of Endotoxin. Vol. 4. Elsevier Science Publishers, New York, 1986

152. Falk A, Myrvold HE, Sundgren O, et al: Mucosal lesions in the feline small intestine in septic shock. Circ Shock 9:27, 1982.

153. Livni N, Manny Y, Rabinovici N, et al: Effect of endotoxin on the dog kidney. Isr J Med Sci 13:339, 1977

154. Rees M, Bowen JC: Stress ulcers during live *Escherichia coli* sepsis. Ann Surg 195:646, 1982

155. Herlihy BL, Lefer Am: Selective inhibition of pancreatic proteases and prevention of toxic factors in shock. Circ Shock 1:51, 1974

156. Bottoms GD, Coppoc GL, Roesel OF, et al: Effect of the proteinase inhibitor aprotinin in the management of hemorrhagic shock in the dog. Am J Vet Res 39:1023, 1978

157. Mullen JL, Buzby GP, Matthews DC, et al: Reduction of operative morbidity and mortality by combined preoperative and postoperative nutritional support. Ann Surg 192:604, 1979

158. Sugerman HJ, Peyton JWR, Greenfield LJ: Gram-negative sepsis. Curr Probl Surg 180:408, 1981

159. Bistrian BR, Blackburn GL, Scrimshaw NS: Cellular immunity in semistarved states in hospitalized adults. Am J Clin Nutr 28:1148, 1975

160. Buffington CA: Anorexia. p. 5-1. In Lewis LD, Morris ML (eds): Small Animal Clinical Nutrition. 2nd Ed. Mark Morris Assoc. Topeka, 1984

161. Crowe DT: Tube feeding diets for nutritional support of the critically ill or injured patients. J Vet Emerg Crit Care Soc 1:8, 1985

162. Raymond RM, Harkima JM, Stoffs WV: Effects of naloxone therapy on hemodynamics and metabolism following a superlethal dosage of *Escherichia coli* endotoxin in dogs. Surg Gynecol Obstet 152:159, 1981

163. Almquist PW, Kuenzig M, Schwartz SI: The effect of naloxone and cyproheptadine on pulmonary platelet trapping, hypotension and platelet aggregability in traumatized dogs. J Trauma 23:405, 1983

164. Faden AI, Holaday JW: Experimental endotoxin shock: The pathophysiologic function of endorphins and treatment with opiate antagonists. J Infect Dis 142:229, 1980

165. Weissglas IS, Hinchey EJ, Chiu RCJ: Naloxone and methylprednisolone in the treatment of experimental septic shock. J Surg Res 33:131, 1982

166. Saba TM, Jaffe E: Plasma fibronectin (opsonic glycoprotein): Its synthesis by vascular endothelial cells and role in cardiopulmonary integrity after trauma as related to reticuloendothelial function. Am J Med 68:577, 1980

167. Scovell WA, Saba TM, Blumenstock FA, et al: Opsonic alpha 2 surface binding glycoprotein therapy during sepsis. Ann Surg 188:521, 1978

168. Bull RW: Granulocyte transfusions in the septic puppy. Vet Clin Pathol 9:48, 1980

169. Epstein RB, Zander AR: Granulocyte transfusions in leukopenic dogs. The granulocyte: Function and clinical utilization. Prog Clin Biol Res 13:227, 1977

170. Chaudry IH, Baue AE: The use of substrates and energy in the treatment of shock. Adv Shock Res 3:27, 1980

171. Chaudry IH, Baue AE: Overview of hemorrhagic shock. p. 189. In Cowley RA, Trump BF (eds): Pathophysiology of Shock, Anoxia and Ischemia. William & Wilkins, Baltimore, 1982

172. Chaudry IH, Sayeed MM, Baue AE: Effect of adenosine triphosphate-magnesium chloride administration in shock. Surgery 75:220, 1974

173. DiStazio J, Maley W, Thompson B, et al: Effects of ATP-MgCl$_2$ administration during hemorrhagic shock on cardiovascular function, metabolism and survival. Adv Shock Res 3:153, 1980

174. Hirasawa H, Oda S, Hayashi H, et al: Improved survival and reticuloendothelial function with intravenous ATP-MgCl$_2$ following hemorrhagic shock. Circ Shock 11:141, 1983

175. Peitzman AB, Shires GT, Illner H, et al: Effect of intravenous ATP-MgCl$_2$ on cellular function in liver and muscle in hemorrhagic shock. Curr Surg 38:300, 1981

176. Horpacsy G, Schnells G: Energy metabolism and lysosomal events in hemorrhagic shock after aprotinin treatment. Circ Shock 7:49, 1980

177. Davis D, Hilewitz H, Rogel S: Humoral factors in shock causing bradycardia and myocardial depression. Circ Shock 4:153, 1977

178. Bounous G: Mechanisms of intestinal lesion in shock. Gastroenterology 68:203, 1975

179. Sprung CL: The Pulmonary Artery Catheter. Methodology and Clinical Applications. University Park Press, Baltimore, 1983

180. Dikshit K, Vyden JK, Forrester JS, et al: Renal and extrarenal hemodynamic effects of furosemide in congestive heart failure after acute myocardial infarction. N Engl J Med 288:1087, 1973

181. Bardet J, Masquet C, Kahn C, et al: Clinical and hemodynamic results of intraaortic balloon counterpulsation and surgery for cardiogenic shock. Am Heart J 93:280, 1977

182. Kantrowitz A, Krakauer JS, Rosenbaum, et al: Phase-shift balloon pumping in medically refractory cardiogenic shock: Results in 27 patients. Arch Surg 99:739, 1969

183. Bregman D: Assessment of intra-aortic balloon counterpulsation in cardiogenic shock. Crit Care Med 3:90, 1975

184. Weber KT, Janicki JS: Intraaortic balloon counterpulsation: A review of physiological principles, clinical results, and device safety. Ann Thorac Surg 17:602, 1984

12

Hyperthyroidism and Other High Cardiac Output States

Betsy R. Bond

CARDIAC RESPONSE IN HYPERMETABOLIC AND HYPERKINETIC STATES

Cardiac output is the quantity of blood pumped by the heart through the systemic circulation per unit time. Transient increases in cardiac output may be normal physiologic responses to exercise or excitement. Prolonged increases in cardiac output, however, may be abnormal. Diseases that lower peripheral vascular resistance or increase tissue metabolism and oxygen demand, such as fever, thyrotoxicosis, or pregnancy, or that result in a hyperkinetic state, such as anemia, systemic arteriovenous (AV) fistula, may be causative.[1] Reductions in peripheral vascular resistance increase cardiac output by lowering afterload and reducing impedance to venous return, thereby increasing preload.[2,3] Resultant high-output heart failure is a condition in which cardiac output is markedly elevated before the development of heart failure and remains high afterward.[1]

Another factor contributing to high-output states is the venous pressure gradient—the pressure difference between small veins and the right atrium. This is the force that returns blood to the heart, determined primarily by the ratio of blood volume to capacitance in the systemic circulation. The larger the blood volume, the larger the venous pressure gradient. With increased venous return (i.e., preload), cardiac output increases, even in the face of normal cardiac function.

Compensatory mechanisms of cardiac dilation (in response to a larger blood volume), and hypertrophy may occur in association with increased demands imposed by a higher cardiac output.[1,2] Normally, the heart can tolerate changes resulting from these compensatory mechanisms. However, when abnormal metabolic conditions or hyperkinetic states are imposed on a heart with intrinsic myocardial dysfunction, congestive heart failure may occur if a combination of high-output states exists (e.g., anemia and AV fistula), or if the condition persists for a sufficient period of time. Cardiovascular adaptation to an abnormal workload depends on the state of myocardial function, the magnitude,

255

and rate of development of the extra systemic burden. The quicker the high-output state develops, the more likely it is that heart failure will ensue.[1]

The most common clinical condition leading to high-output heart failure is hyperthyroidism in cats (volume overload and impaired myocardial metabolism). Other causes in dogs and cats include anemia (volume overload and myocardial anoxia) and arteriovenous shunts (volume overload).

HYPERTHYROIDISM

Naturally occurring hyperthyroidism (thyrotoxicosis) is rare in the dog but is common in the older cat.[4-9] Feline hyperthyroidism results from overproduction of thyroxine (T_4) and triiodothyronine (T_3) by a benign functional adenoma (adenomatous hyperplasia) of one or both thyroid lobes. Thyroid carcinomas leading to hyperthyroidism are rare in the cat.[7-9]

A close relationship between thyroid hormones and the cardiovascular system has led to observations in human subjects that (1) hyperthyroidism may cause reversible cardiomyopathy in an otherwise healthy heart,[10,11] and (2) compensated heart failure may be decompensated by thyrotoxicosis.[2] Hyperthyroidism should therefore be considered an etiology in all middle aged to elderly cats (i.e., 7 years of age or older) with clinical evidence of cardiac disease.

Pathophysiology

Hyperthyroidism is a multisystemic disease that significantly affects energy metabolism and the cardiovascular system. It increases metabolic rate and oxygen consumption and decreases peripheral vascular resistance. Alterations in cardiovascular hemodynamics are secondary to (1) direct effects of thyroid hormone on the heart, and (2) adrenergic stimulation.[2,3,11-16]

Cardiac changes include marked increases in cardiac output, heart rate, ejection fraction, contractility, and pulse pressure. Myocardial oxygen consumption is elevated, and the increase in cardiac work in longstanding cases may augment cardiac hypertrophy or precipitate congestive heart failure.[2,3,13] The left ventricular ejection fraction is ele-

Table 12-1 Historical and Clinical Findings in 205 Cats with Hyperthyroidism

Clinical Finding	Percent of Cats
Weight loss	96
Polyphagia	77
Hyperactivity	68
Tachycardia	64
Polyuria/polydipsia	53
Cardiac murmur	54
Vomiting	49
Diarrhea	31
Increased fecal volume	28
Anorexia	28
Polypnea (panting)	28
Muscle weakness	22
Muscle tremor	14
Congestive heart failure	13
Dyspnea	13

(Peterson, ME: Feline hyperthyroidism. Vet Clin North Am 14:809, 1984.)

vated at rest but impaired during exercise.[16,17] The most important factors in the development of heart failure are the chronicity and rate of development of the thyrotoxic state and the presence and severity of underlying cardiac disease.[12,13]

History and Signalment

Feline hyperthyroidism is reported in cats ranging in age from 6 to 20 years. There is no breed or sex predilection.[7-9] The most common clinical signs include weight loss, polyphagia, hyperactivity, polyuria, polydipsia, vomiting, diarrhea, and increased fecal volume (Table 12-1). Approximately 10 percent of affected cats display a syndrome similar to apathetic hyperthyroidism in humans, in which the usual symptoms of hyperactivity are absent. This form of thyrotoxicosis is characterized by depression, weakness, anorexia, and occasionally congestive heart failure.[7-9,18] Since thyrotoxic cats do not necessarily display all these clinical signs, the absence of one or more should not exclude the diagnosis.[8]

Physical Examination

Cats with hyperthyroidism are generally thin or emaciated, with unkempt and matted hair coats. They may be hyperactive and difficult to handle, and may become dyspneic when excited.

Palpation of the neck may detect one or two enlarged thyroid lobes. This technique may be facilitated by extending the cat's head backward. The thumb and index finger should be gently passed over both sides of the trachea, starting proximally at the laryngeal area and moving distally toward the thoracic inlet. An enlarged thyroid gland may be felt to slip under the fingers. Occasionally, the thyroid gland descends into the thoracic inlet or thoracic cavity and is not easily palpated by this technique. Detection of the thyroid tumors must then be accomplished either by distally manipulating the thyroid lobe(s) proximally from the thoracic inlet, by evaluating serum thyroid hormone concentrations, or by radionuclide scanning.[8,9]

A systolic murmur and sinus tachycardia are auscultable in most thyrotoxic cats. A strong, bounding, rapid pulse and a prominent left apex precordial beat are generally present. Cats with associated congestive heart failure may exhibit dyspnea, muffled heart and lung sounds (due to pleural or pericardial effusion), an arrhythmia, or a gallop rhythm.[7-9,18]

Electrocardiography

The two most frequently observed electrocardiographic (ECG) abnormalities in feline hyperthyroidism are sinus tachycardia (heart rate $\geq$240 beats/min) and increased R-wave amplitude in lead II ($\geq$0.9 mV). Atrial and ventricular arrhythmias and intraventricular conduction disturbances are also commonly present[6,19,20] (Table 12-2). Direct action of thyroid hormones on the heart and the influence of catecholamines are responsible for many of the ECG disturbances. The ability of β-adrenergic blockers (e.g., propranolol) to decrease heart rate in the face of elevated thyroid hormone levels provides indirect evidence for the contribution of the sympathetic nervous system to these arrhythmias.[3,12,13] Tachycardia, increased R-wave amplitude, and many arrhythmias often resolve after successful therapy for hyperthyroidism has been administered[6,19] (Fig. 12-1).

Radiography

Thoracic radiographs commonly demonstrate cardiomegaly in thyrotoxic cats, especially of the left ventricle and left atrium.[7,18-20] Congestive heart failure, manifested as pulmonary edema, pleural effusion, or both, may be evident radiographically in 20 percent of affected cats. Therefore, a chest radiograph should be taken as part of the data base in hyperthyroid cats.[7] Many of these changes are partially or completely reversible after successful therapy (Fig. 12-2).

Echocardiography

Echocardiographic changes in feline hyperthyroidism (Table 12-3) parallel those found in humans. They include left ventricular dilation, left ventricular hypertrophy, and hypercontractility.[10,11,14-16,19-23] (Fig. 12-3). These may mimic primary myocardial disease (hypertrophic cardiomyopathy).[24] Many of these abnormalities resolve or revert toward normal after establishment of euthyroidism, especially the indices of contractility (Fig. 12-4). This indicates the reversible nature of many cardiac manifestations associated with hyperthyroidism.[11,14-16,19,21-23]

Table 12-2 Electrocardiographic Changes in 131 Cats With Hyperthyroidism

ECG Finding	No. of Cats	Percent of Cats
Tachycardia	87	66
Increased R-wave amplitude (lead II)	38	29
Prolonged QRS duration	23	18
Short Q-T interval	13	10
Atrial premature complexes	9	7
Left anterior fascicular block	8	6
Ventricular premature complexes	3	2
Right bundle branch block	2	2
First-degree atrioventricular block	2	2
Second-degree atrioventricular block with ventricular escape complexes	2	2
Atrial tachycardia	1	1
Ventricular tachycardia and bigeminy	1	1
Ventricular pre-excitation	1	1

(Peterson ME, Kintzer PP, Cavanagh PG, et al: Feline hyperthyroidism: Pretreatment clinical and laboratory evaluation of 131 cases. J Am Vet Med Assoc 183:103, 1983.)

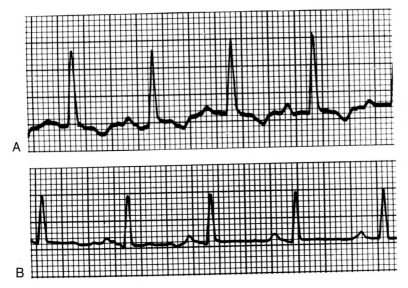

Fig. 12-1 Lead II electrocardiogram of a 9-year-old domestic shorthair cat with hyperthyroidism before (**A**) and 3 months after (**B**) thyroidectomy. (**A**) Left ventricular enlargement is indicated by tall R waves (1.35 mV) and widened QRS complexes (0.045 second). First-degree AV block is suggested by a P-R interval of 0.095 second. Heart rate is 200 beats/min. (**B**) R-wave amplitude, QRS width, and P-R interval have reverted to normal after thyroidectomy. Paper speed = 50 mm/sec; 1 cm = 1 mV.

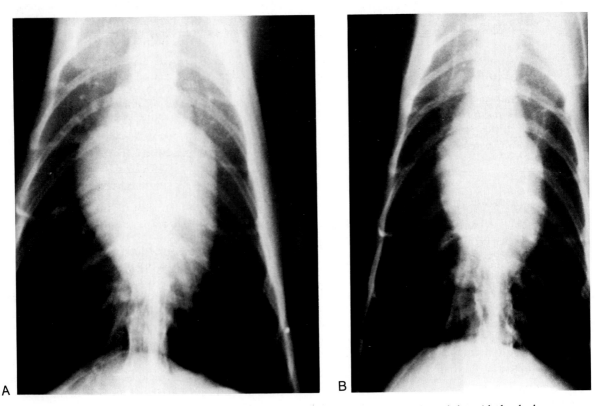

Fig. 12-2 Ventrodorsal radiographs of an adult domestic shorthair cat with a unilateral thyroid gland adenoma. (**A**) Pretreatment radiograph shows biatrial and left ventricular enlargement. (**B**) One month after thyroidectomy, these cardiac chambers are notably reduced in size.

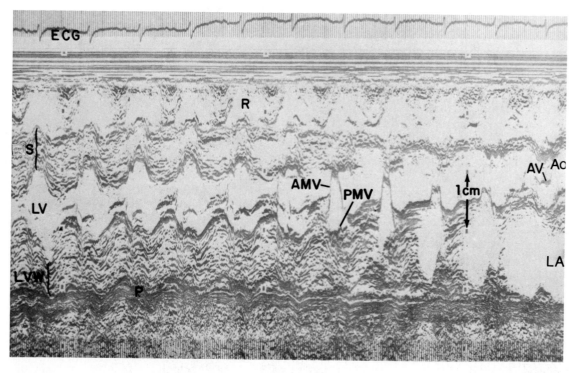

Fig. 12-3 M-mode echocardiogram of a 12-year-old domestic shorthair cat with untreated hyperthyroidism demonstrating a sweep from the cardiac apex (left) through the mitral valve region (center) to the aortic root–left atrial position (right). Hypertrophy of the interventricular septum (S) and left ventricular posterior wall (LVW), reduced left ventricular (LV) end-systolic dimension, and left atrial (LA) and right ventricular (R) enlargement are evident. Both ventricles contract hyperdynamically. ECG, electrocardiogram; AMV, anterior mitral valve leaflet; PMV, posterior mitral valve leaflet; AV, aortic valve; Ao, aorta; P, pericardium. Paper speed = 75 mm/sec.

Laboratory Findings

Mature leukocytosis, eosinopenia (stress response), and increased packed cell volume are commonly seen in affected cats. The most frequent biochemical abnormalities include elevations of serum alanine aminotransferase (ALT), aspartate aminotransferase (AST), alkaline phosphatase (SAP), and lactic dehydrogenase (LDH).[7–9] Histologic examination of the liver usually demonstrates only modest and nonspecific changes.[24] A small number of hyperthyroid cats develop mild to moderate hyperphosphatemia without evidence of renal insufficiency (Table 12-4). Baseline serum concentrations of T_4 and T_3 are elevated above normal range in most cats with hyperthyroidism. Not all cats with elevated serum T_4 concentrations, however, have elevated serum T_3 concentrations.[7,8]

Radionuclide Thyroid Imaging

Thyroid imaging (scanning) and thyroid radioiodine uptake are based on the principle that radionuclides are trapped and concentrated in the thyroid gland. The thyroid radioiodine uptake test uses isotopes of radioactive iodine (^{123}I, ^{131}I), which are taken up and stored in thyroid follicular cells such as stable iodine (^{127}I). Once within the cell, iodine is oxidized to iodide and incorporated into tyrosine groups of thyroglobulin, which help make up T_4 and T_3. The thyroid radioiodine uptake test directly

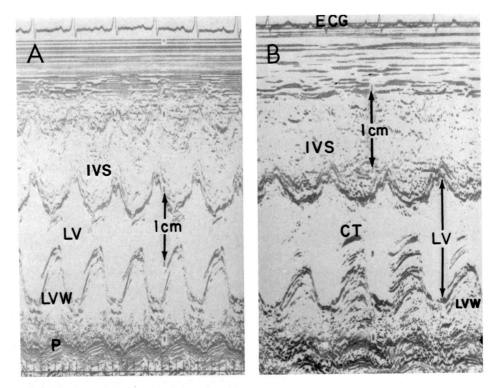

Fig. 12-4 M-mode echocardiograms at the left ventricular level just below the mitral valve from a 9-year-old domestic longhair cat before (**A**) and 5 months after (**B**) thyroidectomy for hyperthyroidism. (**A**) The left ventricle is hypercontractile, left-ventricular end-systolic dimension is reduced and hypertrophy of the interventricular septum (IVS) and left ventricular posterior wall (LVW) are evident. (**B**) Hyperdynamic contractility is reduced toward normal as evidenced by a diminished fractional shortening (compared to pretreatment). Left ventricular end-systolic dimension has normalized. There is less hypertrophy of the IVS and LVW. ECG, electrocardiogram; CT, chordae tendineae; LV, left ventricular chamber; P, pericardium. Paper speed = 75 mm/sec.

assesses thyroid gland function and is increased 24 hours after administration of the radioiodine in most cats with hyperthyroidism. This test is most useful in clinical determination of the radioactive iodine (^{131}I) dose for therapy of hyperthyroidism.[7,8,25]

Radionuclide thyroid scanning may be performed with isotopes of radioactive iodine (^{123}I or ^{131}I), but the agent most commonly used is pertechnetate ([99m]TcO$_4$). This is trapped and concentrated in the follicular cells such as iodine. Unlike ^{123}I and ^{131}I, however, [99m]TcO$_4$ is not bound to thyroglobulin or stored in the thyroid gland.[8] Although similar images are produced by radioiodine or [99m]TcO$_4$, the latter has advantages. First, the rapid uptake of [99m]TcO$_4$ permits the imaging procedure to begin 20 minutes after administration, as opposed to 4 and

24 hours for ^{123}I and ^{131}I, respectively. Second, higher doses of [99m]TcO$_4$ may be safely administered without delivering a high radiation dose, making for a more rapid scan. Finally, the quality of the [99m]TcO$_4$ thyroid scan may be superior to that of the radioiodine scan.[7,8,25]

Normal cats that are scanned display symmetric uniform distribution of radioactivity throughout both thyroid lobes. In hyperthyroid cats, thyroid imaging shows enlargement of both thyroid lobes in about 70 percent of affected cats. In the remaining 30 percent that have unilateral involvement, the normal contralateral lobe is completely suppressed and cannot be visualized on the scan. Therefore, thyroid scanning is useful in determining whether one or both thyroid lobes are involved (Fig. 12-5). Thyroid

Table 12-3 Echocardiographic Changes in 103 Cats With Untreated Hyperthyroidism

Echocardiographic Finding	Percent of Cats
Left atrial dilatation	67
Left ventricular dilation (end-diastole)	45
Left ventricular hypertrophy	
Interventricular septum	39
Left ventricular free wall	71
Increased contractile indices	
Shortening fraction	20
Velocity of circumferential fiber shortening	15

(Bond BR, Fox PR, Peterson ME: Unpublished data.)

imaging is also helpful in locating a thyroid lobe that has descended into the thoracic cavity, which cannot be palpated, and in detecting metastasis of functional thyroid adenocarcinoma.[7,8,25]

Treatment

Feline hyperthyroidism can be treated by three different methods: (1) chronic oral administration of an antithyroid drug, (2) surgical thyroidectomy of the affected lobe or lobes, and (3) radioactive iodine (^{131}I). There are advantages and disadvantages to each treatment modality, and several factors must be weighed in choosing the proper therapeutic strat-

Table 12-4 Laboratory Findings in 205 Cats with Hyperthyroidism

Test	Percentage of Cats Above Normal
Leukocyte count	42
Packed cell volume	47
RBC count	24
Hemoglobin concentration	16
Mean corpuscular volume	37
Serum alkaline phosphatase	72
Lactic dehydrogenase	64
Aspartate transaminase	61
Alanine transaminase	51
Total bilirubin	21
Blood urea nitrogen	28
Inorganic phosphorus	27

(Peterson ME: Feline hyperthyroidism. Vet Clin North Am 14:809, 1984.)

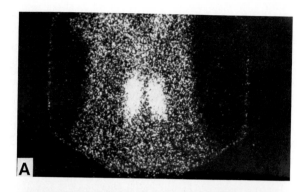

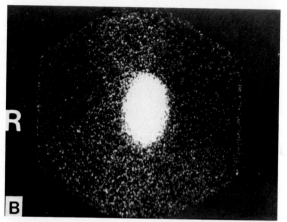

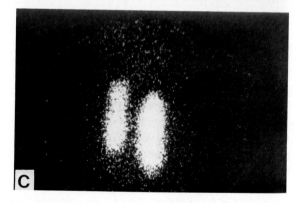

Fig. 12-5 Sodium pertechnetate thyroid scans of (**A**) clinically normal cat, (**B**) hyperthyroid cat with adenoma (adenomatous hyperplasia) of one thyroid lobe, and (**C**) hyperthyroid cat with bilateral thyroid gland adenomas. (**A**) Both thyroid lobes are symmetric in position and size with uniform distribution of radioactivity throughout the gland. (**B**) The adenomatous gland is greatly enlarged and descends toward the thoracic inlet; the uninvolved right lobe is not visualized. (**C**) Both lobes are enlarged and approximately similar in size and position. (Peterson ME, Kintzer PP, Cavanagh PG, et al: Feline hyperthyroidism: Pretreatment clinical and laboratory evaluation of 131 cases. J Am Vet Med Assoc 183:103, 1983.)

egy. Of major consideration is the presence of complicating cardiovascular disease (arrhythmias or congestive heart failure) or other major disorders (e.g., renal failure). The availability of an experienced surgeon, referral center for nuclear imaging and treatment, and the owner's desire to follow a certain therapeutic or economic course of therapy comprise practical considerations. Whatever form of therapy is chosen, the client must be informed that only thyroidectomy or radioactive iodine is curative.[8]

CHRONIC ORAL ANTITHYROID DRUG THERAPY

Two antithyroid drugs currently used to control feline hyperthyroidism are propylthiouracil (PTU)[26] and methimazole (MMI) (Tapazole, Eli Lilly, Indianapolis). These drugs lower serum T_4 and T_3 concentrations by inhibiting thyroid hormone synthesis. They do not destroy thyroid tissue. Therefore, relapse of the thyrotoxic condition will occur if the drug is discontinued or if owner compliance is poor. The initial daily oral dose of PTU is 50 mg tid; MMI is dosed at 5 mg tid. Serum T_4 concentrations should be assessed 2 to 3 weeks after initial administration, at which time most cats will be euthyroid. If serum thyroid concentrations are still elevated, daily dosages of PTU should be increased to 100 mg tid. Alternatively, MMI should be increased to 7.5 to 10 mg tid. Serum T_4 concentrations should be determined every 7 to 14 days thereafter and the dosages adjusted until euthyroidism is maintained. Serum T_4 concentrations should then be monitored monthly during chronic maintenance therapy to ensure stability of serum thyroid hormone levels.[9,27]

Some clients are unable to maintain an antithyroid drug dosage schedule of two or three daily doses. In such cases, the total daily dose of PTU or MMI may be given in a single daily administration. To be effective, these drugs must be given at least once daily, however, or the thyrotoxic condition will return.[8,9,26]

Adverse reactions to PTU or MMI constitute a major disadvantage to long-term oral antithyroid drug therapy. The most common clinical side effects are anorexia, lethargy, and vomiting; these symptoms occur more frequently with PTU than with

MMI. In most cats, these reactions are mild and resolve despite continued drug administration. If symptoms persist, the drug must be discontinued. Drug allergy (e.g., skin rash, facial swelling, and pruritus) may also occur in cats treated with PTU.[8,9,26,27]

Immune-mediated drug reactions represent potential serious side effects of PTU and MMI administration. The incidence of these reactions is about 8.5 percent with PTU[27] but less than 5 percent with MMI.[9] These include hemolytic anemia (often Coombs positive), thrombocytopenia, and granulocytopenia. Adverse clinical signs usually develop between the second and sixth weeks of therapy, but may occur at any time during treatment. Therefore, a complete blood count and platelet count should be monitored every 7 to 14 days for the first 6 weeks, and monthly thereafter. If anemia, granulocytopenia, or thrombocytopenia develops, the drug should be discontinued and appropriate supportive care instituted. Most clinical symptoms resolve within 2 weeks after the drug is withdrawn.[8,27]

Serum antinuclear antibodies (ANA) develop commonly in cats receiving MMI or PTU. The incidence increases as treatment duration lengthens. More than one-third of cats treated for more than 6 months with MMI develop ANA. However, despite this high incidence of MMI or PTU-related ANA, associated clinical signs of lupus is extremely rare.[9,27,28]

SURGERY (THYROIDECTOMY)

Surgical removal of affected thyroid lobe(s) is the treatment of choice for most cases of hyperthyroidism. It can be associated with significant morbidity and mortality.

Preoperative Considerations

Cats must be treated preoperatively with an antithyroid drug for at least 2 weeks, to minimize surgical risks and reduce complications associated with thyrotoxicosis.[8] Methimazole is the agent of choice because of its low incidence of adverse side effects.

If side effects develop and preclude antithyroid drug therapy, large oral or intravenous doses of stable iodine may be used to induce rapid lowering of thyroid hormone concentrations. Although iodine blocks T_4 and T_3 release from the thyroid gland, serum thyroid hormone concentrations may not normalize during this treatment, and the drug often loses its effect within a few weeks. Therefore, it should not be depended on for long-term therapy. Oral potassium iodide is dosed at 50 to 100 mg/day for 7 to 10 days prior to surgery.[8]

Propranolol, a β-adrenergic blocker, may be administered for 1 to 2 weeks preoperatively (2.5 to 5 mg bid to tid PO) to block many of the cardiovascular and neuromuscular effects of thyrotoxicosis and to control associated tachycardia, arrhythmias, and hyperexcitability. It should be used with caution, however, in cats with congestive heart fail-ure, since the negative inotropic effects of propranolol may depress cardiac function and worsen heart failure.[8,9] Propranolol does not reduce elevated serum thyroid hormone concentrations.

Operative Considerations

The surgical techniques for thyroidectomy have been described[9,29,30] (Fig. 12-6). Since most cats have bilateral functional thyroid adenomas, it is important to preserve parathyroid glands during bilateral thyroidectomy to avoid postoperative hypocalcemia. Even in unilateral thyroidectomy, care should be taken not to injure parathyroid glands.

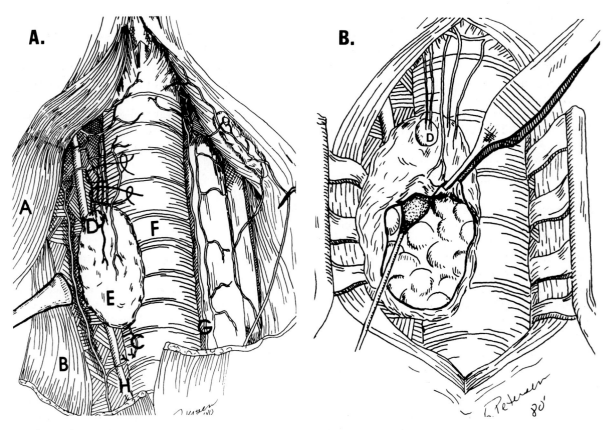

Fig. 12-6 (**A**) Unilateral thyroidectomy. The sternothyroideus and sternohyoideus muscles are retracted to reveal the thyroid mass. The cranial and caudal vessels are ligated and transected between the ligatures. A, sternohyoideus muscle; B, sternothyroideus muscle; C, caudal thyroid vein; D, external parathyroid gland; E, thyroid gland; F, trachea, G, recurrent laryngeal nerve; H, external carotid artery. (**B**) Bilateral thyroidectomy. The thyroid capsule has been incised. A cotton-tipped applicator facilitates blunt dissection of the thyroid parenchyma from the capsule. D, external parathyroid gland. (Black AP, Peterson ME: Thyroid biopsy and thyroidectomy. p. 388. In Bojrab MJ (ed): Current Techniques in Small Animal Surgery. 2nd Ed. Lea & Febiger, Philadelphia, 1983.)

Occasionally, a hyperfunctional thyroid lobe (adenomatous hyperplasia) may be only slightly enlarged and grossly mistaken for a normal thyroid lobe. In such cases, relapse of thyrotoxicosis will occur within 9 months, necessitating surgical removal of this lobe. Thus, preservation of parathyroid glands during hemithyroidectomy minimizes the risk of hypoparathyroidism if contralateral hemithyroidectomy later becomes necessary.[8,9]

Postoperative Complications

Many complications accompany thyroidectomy, including hypothyroidism, hypoparathyroidism, Horner's syndrome, and vocal cord paralysis. Hypocalcemia is the most serious side effect and may develop as a result of injury, devascularization, or inadvertent removal of the parathyroid glands. It is only a problem in cats that have had bilateral thyroid lobe removal. Clinical signs due to severe hypocalcemia will develop within 1 to 3 days after surgery. Therefore, serum calcium levels should be monitored daily for this period following bilateral thyroidectomy. Treatment is required only when low serum calcium concentrations (less than 6.5 mg/dl) are accompanied by signs of muscle tremor, tetany, or convulsions. Then, vitamin D therapy and calcium supplementation is instituted and continued for 2 to 3 months after surgery. At this time, an attempt should be made to reduce the dose of vitamin D and calcium gradually, monitoring serum calcium concentration at weekly intervals.[8,9,31]

Mild hypothyroidism occurs for 2 to 3 months following unilateral thyroidectomy, but serum thyroid hormone concentrations seldom fall low enough to require supplementation. If bilateral thyroidectomy has been performed, thyroxine (0.1 mg/day) should be administered 24 to 48 hours postoperatively. Occasionally, serum T_4 and T_3 concentrations return to normal several months after bilateral thyroidectomy, and T_4 administration may be discontinued.

Small remnants of thyroid tissue may remain attached to the thyroid capsule, and recurrent hyperthyroidism may develop. Therefore, serum T_4 concentrations should be monitored every 6 to 12 months in all hyperthyroid cats treated with surgical thyroidectomy.[8,9]

RADIOACTIVE IODINE

Radioactive iodine (^{131}I) is a simple, effective, safe method for treating feline hyperthyroidism. Its major drawback is the lack of available treatment centers and certain mandatory radiation safety restrictions and procedures that must be followed. Radioactive iodine is concentrated in the thyroid gland and selectively destroys hyperplastic or neoplastic thyroid tissue. After a single dose of ^{131}I, serum thyroid concentrations normalize within 2 weeks in most hyperthyroid cats. The two major adverse effects of therapy are persistent or recurrent hyperthyroidism because of inadequate ^{131}I therapy, and hypothyroidism from ^{131}I overdosage.[8,9,32]

Congestive Heart Failure and Hyperthyroidism

Most thyrotoxic cats develop reversible, secondary, hypertrophic cardiomyopathy.[18–20] Heart failure associated with hyperthyroidism may be manifested as pulmonary edema, pleural effusion, or both.[7] Prompt therapeutic return to euthyroidism may significantly reduce, if not eliminate, associated cardiovascular signs. Therefore, initial medical therapy is directed toward reversing the thyrotoxic state and reducing the effects of thyroid hormone on the cardiovascular system. Antithyroid drugs (PTU or MMI) are administered as previously described. Therapeutic thoracocentesis may be required if pleural effusion is severe. Diuretics should be administered to aid in the removal of edema or effusion (furosemide, 1 mg/kg bid to tid). Propranolol may be given if severe tachyarryhthmias are contributing to the heart failure state. Generally, it should not be used during the decompensated congestive heart failure state because its negative inotropic action may depress myocardial function. Oral maintenance dose is 2.5 mg (cats weighing less than 6 kg) or 5 mg (cats weighing more than 6 kg) bid to tid.[18] Once heart failure is controlled, definitive treatment of hyperthyroidism by surgical thyroidectomy or radioactive iodine therapy should be considered. Cats that are unable to undergo surgery or radiotherapy may be maintained indefinitely on antithyroid drugs, as long as there are no adverse effects.[8,9]

Digitalis (digoxin) has been used in severe right-sided heart failure or with atrial tachycardia, but its efficacy has not been proved. Hyperthyroid patients may be resistant to the effects of digitalis; its application is therefore in question.[33]

ANEMIA

In humans, a sustained increase in cardiac output occurs when the hematocrit falls below 25 percent, unless anemia is associated with a disease that produces an increase in viscosity (e.g., multiple myeloma). If anemia develops slowly, increased cardiac output results from tachycardia with little change in stroke volume. In chronic, severe anemia, heart rate may be normal or only minimally elevated. Cardiac output here is increased as a consequence of augmented stroke volume resulting from a reduction in blood viscosity and systemic arteriolar tone. Cardiac dilation and hypertrophy may be present.[1,34]

Unless a coexisting cardiac or hyperkinetic condition is present, anemia usually does not cause heart failure. If heart failure should occur, diuretics are advisable to help control extracardiac signs of effusion or pulmonary edema until the underlying cause of the anemia is corrected. Cardiac glycosides may be added if there is systolic (myocardial) failure. Vasodilators are probably of little help, as impedance to left ventricular emptying is already reduced.

ARTERIOVENOUS FISTULAS

Arteriovenous fistulas are abnormal communications between the arteries and veins that may be either congenital or acquired. Acquired causes are usually iatrogenic or traumatic,[35–37] but they may also result from infiltrative neoplasm or infection.[37] Patent ductus arteriosus (PDA) is the most common cause of congenital AV fistulas in dogs but is rare in the cat. Ventricular septal defects are centrally located AV fistulas representing the most frequent AV communication in felines. Uncommonly, congenital AV malformations are located peripherally.

Physical Examination

Physical examination findings in peripheral AV fistulas generally include dilation of involved arteries and veins with venous pulsation, a continuous focal vascular murmur, and a palpable thrill over the area of the fistula. Occlusion of the fistula often causes Branham's sign, an abrupt slowing of the heart rate. Hyperthermia may be noted over the fistula, and edema and ischemia may be present in distal tissues. There is a widened arterial pulse pressure (waterhammer pulse) due to a decrease in peripheral vascular resistance and rapid diastolic runoff into the venous circulation.[1,35–37]

Pathophysiology

The arteriovenous fistula acts as a bypass for normal blood flow. Initially, this reduces peripheral vascular resistance and decreases circulation to tissues served by the affected artery. With most peripheral shunts, flow to tissue distal to the shunt is maintained through collateral circulation, which develops by dilation of pre-existing unused arterioles. Therefore, venous hypertension and increased venous return to the heart occur. Hemodynamic responses include an increase in heart rate and peripheral vasoconstriction to restore arterial blood pressure. Neurohumoral, renal, and other fluid conservation mechanisms eventually expand blood volume. Left ventricular stroke volume is increased and cardiac output may be elevated as much as two to three times above normal. The magnitude of these changes depends primarily on the size of the fistula and original artery, and proximal arterial blood flow velocity.[35,37]

Chronic effects of AV fistulas are due to increased cardiac output resulting from increased venous return and decreased peripheral vascular resistance. These changes in blood volume and cardiac output expand the fistulous circuit, causing greater blood flow and volume. Congestive circulatory failure may ensue. Eventually, elevated venous pressure, pulmonary congestion, and edema can result. Mitral valvular insufficiency may occur secondarily. Myocardial failure secondary to volume overload may develop and contribute to congestive heart failure.[35]

Treatment

Surgical ligation or excision of the AV fistula is the treatment of choice, unless myocardial failure or pulmonary hypertension is present. Caution must be observed before surgically correcting fistulas.

Their repair may abruptly increase peripheral vascular resistance and increase myocardial stress. Diuretic administration may be necessary prior to surgical ligation.[1,35–37]

REFERENCES

1. Grossman W. Braunwald E: High-cardiac output states. p. 778. In Braunwald E (ed): Heart disease. 3rd Ed. WB Saunders, Philadelphia, 1988
2. de Groot WJ, Leonard JJ: Hyperthyroidism as a high cardiac output state. Am Heart J 79:265, 1970
3. Klein I, Levey GS: New perspectives on thyroid hormone, catecholamines, and the heart. Am J Med 76:167, 1984
4. McMillian FD, Sherding RG: Feline hyperthyroidism. Feline Pract 11:25, 1981
5. Holzworth J, Theran P, Carpenter JL, et al: Hyperthyroidism in the cat: Ten cases. J Am Vet Med Assoc 176:345, 1981
6. Peterson ME, Keene B, Ferguson DC, et al: Electrocardiographic findings in 45 cats with hyperthyroidism. J Am Vet Med Assoc 180:934, 1982
7. Peterson ME, Kintzer PP, Cavanagh PG, et al: Feline hyperthyroidism: Pretreatment clinical and laboratory evaluation of 131 cases. J Am Vet Med Assoc 183:103, 1983
8. Peterson ME: Feline hyperthyroidism. Vet Clin North Am 14:809, 1984
9. Peterson ME, Turrel JM: Feline hyperthyroidism. p. 1026. In Kirk RW (ed): Current Veterinary Therapy. Vol. IX. WB Saunders, Philadelphia, 1986
10. Cohen MV, Schulman IC, Spenillo A, et al: Effects of thyroid hormone on left ventricular function in patients treated for thyrotoxicosis. Am J Cardiol 48:33, 1981
11. Forfar JC, Muir AL, Sawers MB, et al: Abnormal left ventricular function in hyperthyroidism: Evidence for a possible reversible cardiomyopathy. N Engl J Med 307:1165, 1982
12. Forfar JC, Caldwell GC: Hyperthyroid heart disease. Clin Endocrinol Metab 14:491, 1985
13. Dillman WH: Thyroid hormones and the heart. Thyroid Today 6:1, 1983
14. Lewis BS, Ehrenfeld EN, Lewis N, et al: Echocardiographic left ventricular function in thyrotoxicosis. Am Heart J 97:460, 1979
15. Nixon JV, Anderson RJ, Mitchell LC: Alterations in left ventricular performance in patients treated effectively for thyrotoxicosis. Am J Med 67:268, 1979
16. Iskandrian AS, Rose L, Hakki AH, et al: Cardiac performance in thyrotoxicosis: Analysis of 10 untreated patients. Am J Cardiol 51:349, 1983
17. Shafer RB, Bianco JA: Assessment of cardiac reserve in patients with hyperthyroidism. Chest 78:269, 1980
18. Bond BR: Hyperthyroid heart disease in cats. p. 399. In Kirk RW (ed): Current Veterinary Therapy. Vol. IX. WB Saunders, Philadelphia, 1986
19. Moise NS, Dietze AE: Echocardiographic, electrocardiographic, and radiographic detection of cardiomegaly in hyperthyroid cats. Am J Vet Res 47:1487, 1986
20. Moise NS, Dietze AE, Mezza LE, et al: Echocardiography, electrocardiography, and radiography of cats with dilatation cardiomyopathy, hypertrophic cardiomyopathy, and hyperthyroidism. Am J Vet Res 47:1476, 1986
21. Bond BR, Fox PR, Peterson ME, et al: Echocardiographic characterization of feline thyrotoxic heart disease in the hyperthyroid and euthyroid state. (In press) J Am Vet Med Assoc, 1988
22. Levey GS: The heart and hyperthyroidism: Use of beta-adrenergic blocking drugs. Med Clin North Am 59:1193, 1975
23. Bond BR, Fox PR, Peterson ME: Echocardiographic evaluation of 45 cats with hyperthyroidism. J Ultrasound Med 2(suppl):184, 1983
24. Liu SK, Peterson ME, Fox PR: Hypertrophic cardiomyopathy and hyperthyroidism in the cat. J Am Vet Med Assoc 185:52, 1984
25. Peterson ME, Becker DV: Radionuclide imaging in 135 cats with hyperthyroidism. Vet Radiol 25:23, 1984
26. Peterson ME: Propylthiouracil in the treatment of feline hyperthyroidism. J Am Vet Med Assoc 179:485, 1981
27. Peterson ME, Hurvitz AI, Leib MS, et al: Propylthiouracil-associated anemia, thrombocytopenia, and antinuclear antibodies in cats with hyperthyroidism. J Am Vet Med Assoc 184:806, 1984
28. Aucoin DP, Peterson ME, Hurvitz AI, et al: Propylthiouracil-induced immune-mediated disease in cats. J Pharmacol Exp Ther 234:13, 1985
29. Birchard SJ, ME, Jacobson A: Surgical treatment of feline hyperthyroidism: Results of 85 cases. Am Anim Hosp Assoc 20:705, 1984
30. Black AP, Peterson ME: Thyroid biopsy and thyroidectomy. p. 388. In Bojrab MJ (ed): Current Techniques in Small Animal Surgery. 2nd Ed. Lea & Febiger, Philadelphia, 1983
31. Peterson ME: Treatment of canine and feline hypoparathyroidism. J Am Vet Med Assoc 181:1434, 1982

32. Turrel JM, Feldman EC, Hays M, et al: Radioactive iodine therapy in cats with hyperthyroidism. J Am Vet Med Assoc 184:554, 1984

33. Williams GH, Braunwald E: Endocrine and nutritional disorders and heart disease. p. 1725. In Braunwald E (ed): Heart Disease. 2nd Ed. WB Saunders, Philadelphia, 1984

34. Vatner SF, Higgins CB, Franklin D: Regional circulatory adjustments to moderate and severe chronic anemia in conscious dogs at rest and during exercise. Circ Res 30:731, 1972

35. Olivier NB: Pathophysiology of arteriovenous fistulae. p. 1051. In Slatter DH (ed): Textbook of Small Animal Surgery. WB Saunders, Philadelphia, 1985

36. Suter PF: Diseases of the peripheral vessels. p. 1062. In Ettinger SJ (ed): Textbook of Veterinary Internal Medicine. Vol. 1. 2nd Ed. WB Saunders, Philadelphia, 1983

37. Bouayad H, Feeney DA, Lipowitz AJ, et al: Peripheral acquired arteriovenous fistulas: A report of four cases and literature review. Am Anim Hosp Assoc 23:205, 1987

13

Cellular Mechanisms of Cardiac Arrhythmias

Kenneth H. Dangman
Penelope A. Boyden

The advent of microelectrode techniques during the late 1940s made possible the recording of transmembrane action potentials from single cardiac cells in isolated (*in vitro*) tissue preparations. This permitted exploration of electrophysiology and pharmacology of the regenerative responses responsible for these action potentials (Fig. 13-1). The cellular electrophysiology of normal and abnormal animal hearts has been studied intensely since the development of these techniques. Most microelectrode studies were designed primarily to provide insights into human cardiac physiology and pathophysiology. For the most part, however, these studies have been carried out in tissues from experimental animals with normal hearts or with experimentally induced pathology and/or arrhythmias. Clearly, these insights and conclusions are also of use to veterinary cardiologists. Understanding cellular mechanisms of cardiac arrhythmias should allow the practitioner to approach therapy on a more rational basis.

ELECTROPHYSIOLOGY OF THE NORMAL HEART

In order to understand how derangements of cellular electrophysiology can cause cardiac arrhythmias, it is first necessary to understand the normal electric function of cardiac tissues.

The clinically healthy heart usually remains in normal sinus rhythm. Normal sinus rhythm appears on the surface electrocardiogram as a sequence of three deflections (P, QRS, and T waves) (Fig. 13-2). The cardiac impulse of normal sinus rhythm begins in the pacemaker cells of the sinus, or sinoatrial (SA), node, where the transmembrane potential of the pacemaker cells gradually decreases during diastole, until threshold potential is attained. The specific pacemaker cell is not anatomically stable; changes in autonomic tone are thought to shift the pacemaker site within the node.

Diastolic depolarization in the sinus node begins from a maximum potential of about -60 mV and is thought to be produced by decay of a current i_K, which is an outward current carried by potassium ions. The upstroke of the sinus node action potential occurs when diastolic depolarization carries the membrane potential to the voltage threshold for the

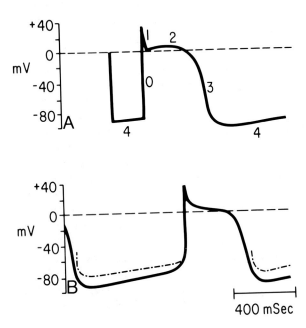

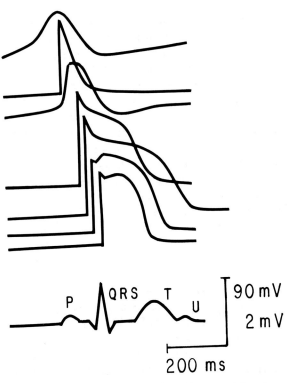

Fig. 13-2 Diagrammatic illustration of transmembrane action potentials in atrial and ventricular tissues during normal sinus rhythm. Traces, from top to bottom, show action potentials of sinus node cell, atrial myocardial fiber, AV node cell, His bundle fiber, distal Purkinje fiber, endocardial ventricular muscle cell, and epicardial ventricular muscle cell. Lowermost trace shows surface electrocardiogram (ECG). Note time and voltage calibration bars at lower right. Voltage calibration bar is 2 mV for ECG, 90 mV for action potentials.

Fig. 13-1 Diagrammatic representations of transmembrane action potentials. Heavy line shows output of microelectrode. Lighter dashed line (horizontal) shows zero or extracellular reference potential. Voltage level (in millivolts) shown along vertical axis. Note time bar at lower right. (**A**) Initially, voltage level is 0 when tip of the electrode is in extracellular fluid. As cell is impaled, voltage reading reflects intracellular potential. During diastole, the transmembrane potential is about −90 mV. When an action potential occurs, the polarization of the membrane reverses; transmembrane potential transiently spikes at +35 to +40 mV. This rapid upstroke is called phase 0. Repolarization occurs in three phases; phase 1 is the rapid repolarization phase that occurs 1 to 5 msec after the spike. Phase 2 is the slow repolarization that occurs during the action potential plateau. Phase 3 is the moderately rapid repolarization that occurs at the end of the plateau that carries the potential to diastolic levels (phase 4). (**B**) Spontaneously firing Purkinje fiber. Pacemaker activity in the heart occurs when phase 4 depolarization slowly carries membrane potential to the threshold voltage for inward current. Threshold voltage during diastole shown here as dashed line above the transmembrane potential. This pacemaker activity normally occurs in the SA node (see Fig. 13-2) and, if overdrive from the SA node is relieved, in subsidiary pacemaker tissues such as specialized atrial conduction tissue and ventricular Purkinje fibers (shown here).

onset of the slow inward current, which is largely carried by calcium ions. Sinus node depolarization, occurring as it does in a relatively small mass of tissue, is not reflected on the surface electrocardiogram (ECG).

After the sinus node pacemaker cell fires an action potential, the impulse conducts slowly throughout the node and then spreads to the adjacent cells of the atrial myocardium. The impulse then propagates from the perinodal atrial muscle fibers radially to the tissues of the right and left atria. This conduction may occur via specialized atrial conduction tracts. The transmembrane potentials of the atrial fibers have relatively high action potential amplitudes (100 to 110 mV) and maximum upstroke velocities (100 to 200 V/sec); thus, the impulse is conducted fairly quickly throughout these tissues. The wavefront of atrial depolarization produces the P wave of the electrocardiogram (Fig. 13-2).

The impulse is conducted from the atrial fibers into the atrioventricular (AV) node. The cells of the AV node are specialized to provide slow conduction; they are small and relatively poorly coupled electrically. The transmembrane action potentials of the nodal cells have low amplitudes and slow upstroke velocities and arise from relatively low diastolic potentials (about −60 mV). Thus, the wavefront of the cardiac impulse spreads slowly through this tissue. This slow conduction enables an appropriate interval (100 to 120 msec) to elapse between atrial and ventricular depolarization and contraction.

When the impulse emerges from the distal end of the AV node, it begins to invade the Purkinje fibers of the proximal His bundle. These Purkinje fibers have high diastolic potentials (about −90 mV), action potential amplitudes and maximum upstroke velocities. Once the impulse enters the His bundle, it can rapidly propagate via the more distal Purkinje fibers of the ventricular conduction system to the endocardial surfaces of the ventricles. The terminal subendocardial Purkinje fibers conduct the impulse to the subendocardial ventricular muscle. The conduction of the impulse in the AV node and the Purkinje fibers does not affect the surface ECG.

Conduction of the impulse in the ventricular myocardium, which progresses from the subendocardial layers to the subepicardial layers, is reflected in the QRS deflection. After the cardiac impulse is conducted to the outermost layers of the ventricular walls (the subepicardium), it is extinguished as the wavefront becomes surrounded with refractory or inexcitable tissues. The final event of the cardiac electric cycle is ventricular repolarization, which produces the T wave (see Fig. 13-2).

ELECTROPHYSIOLOGIC EFFECTS OF CARDIAC DAMAGE: GENERAL CONSIDERATIONS

Clinically significant arrhythmias seldom occur in the normal heart but are common in injured tissues. Indeed, it has long been recognized that the site and size of a zone of damage and the level of damage within that zone will affect the intensity and site of origin of the arrhythmias that occur.

Given that focal or diffuse injury to the myocardium can predispose to the development of arrhythmias, can we now identify any general changes in electrical activity that occur in the zones of damage that may underly this predisposition? To a limited extent, we can. Most acute experimental insults to *in vitro* myocardial tissues (including ischemia, anoxia, metabolic inhibition, stretch, and digitalis toxicity) and subacute or chronic injury to the in situ heart (experimentally produced myocardial infarction, naturally occurring congestive heart failure, and cardiomyopathies) will result in deterioration of the characteristic features of the myocardial action potential. That is, the diastolic potential of working myocardial cells and Purkinje fibers, typically −80 to −95 mV, will decrease. The maximum upstroke velocity, typically 100 to 800 V/sec in these cells, will decrease as well. Action potential plateaus of the ventricular fibers, which normally have durations of 0.2 to 0.5 seconds, can become markedly shortened. These effects, as explained below, can precipitate tachycardias or fibrillation in several ways.

Decreases in Diastolic Membrane Potential

It is now well established that the resting membrane potential (in ventricular or atrial muscle cells) or the maximum diastolic potential (in Purkinje fibers) will be shifted toward zero (i.e., become less negative) after focal damage by almost any agent. There are several possible causes for the decreases in diastolic potential that occur in these injured cells:

1. Decreased activity of the sarcolemmal sodium-potassium ATPase—the electrogenic sodium pump, which provides a net outward pump current as a result of the asymmetric transport of cations

2. Increased G_{Na} (inward sodium conductance)

3. Decreased G_K (outward potassium conductance)

All these changes would tend to result in an increase in net inward current and are likely to depolarize the cell. In addition, the decreased activity of the sodium pump may produce increased intracellular concentrations of sodium ion, decreased intracellular potassium ion concentrations, and increased potassium ion concentrations in the interstitial spaces of the myocardium. Such changes in concentration of potassium and sodium could also reduce the level of diastolic transmembrane potential by decreasing the magnitude of the electrochemical ionic gradients across the cell membrane.

A decrease in resting potential (in working myocardial fibers) or maximum diastolic potential (in Purkinje fibers) can exert several voltage-dependent changes in cellular electrophysiology. It can enhance ectopic impulse initiation by inducing either abnormal automaticity or triggered activity, or it can compromise conduction of the cardiac impulse and lead to conduction block and re-entrant excitation.

Decreases in the Amplitude and Rate of Rise of Phase 0

The major effect of decreases in diastolic potential on conduction is mediated through effects on phase 0 of the action potential (Fig. 13-3). In atrial or ventricular myocardial fibers (with takeoff potentials from about −60 mV to about −90 mV), conduction velocity is directly proportional to takeoff potential.

The amplitude and rate of phase 0 are important determinants of conduction velocity. In simple terms, action potentials with higher amplitudes and faster depolarization rates provide a better stimulus for induction of the regenerative response in downstream areas of membrane, which are in diastolic voltage ranges. Therefore, more distal membrane areas will be brought to threshold level more quickly by a robust action potential than by a depressed action potential. Thus, the robust impulse will be conducted more rapidly.

The amplitude and rate of phase 0 in turn are largely dependent on the intensity of the rapid inward sodium current. The inward sodium current is carried, according to the Hodgkin-Huxley formulation, through ion-selective channels in the cell membrane.[1] These channels are guarded by gates that impede ion fluxes; the opening and closing of these gates is both voltage and time dependent. It is believed that as the takeoff potential becomes less and less negative, more and more of the sodium

channels become inactivated (i.e., totally refractory to stimulation). Thus, as the takeoff potential is decreased from −90 to about −60 mV, the sodium current during phase 0 becomes less and less robust, the amplitude and rate of rise of the action potential is reduced, and the conduction velocity is decreased (Fig. 13-3).

We use the term *depressed fast responses* to describe action potentials occurring in partially depolarized atrial or ventricular myocardial cells or Purkinje fibers with take-off potentials between −75 and −60 mV. These action potentials may be important in the genesis of re-entrant arrhythmias. This is because the depressed fast responses will propagate more slowly than normal action potentials, facilitating re-entry. Also, if the impulse must traverse a zone of relatively inexcitable tissue, the depressed fast response, having an intrinsically lower stimulus efficacy than the normal responses, will be more likely to permit conduction blocks.

It has been shown that many of the class I antiarrhythmic drugs (e.g., lidocaine, procainamide, and bepridil) decrease upstroke and conduction velocity in cells with depressed fast responses in theraputic (low) concentrations, and that these concentrations do not affect normal action potentials.[2-4] This selective action could convert a zone of unidirectional conduction block to a zone of bidirectional block, and thus disrupt a re-entrant circuit. Therefore, local anesthetic effects on depressed fast responses may underly important antiarrhythmic actions of these drugs.

When the takeoff potential is reduced to a value less than −60 mV, the fast inward sodium channels are thought to be largely, if not entirely, inactivated. Yet action potentials still may occur in fibers with diastolic potentials of −55 to −35 mV. These action potentials, referred to as slow responses,[5] will be generated if sufficient slow inward current i_{si} can be elicited. The details are complicated, but it is thought that the slow inward current is carried exclusively by calcium ions.[6] The upstroke velocity of phase 0 of the slow-response action potentials is in the range of 1 to 5 V/sec; thus, they are conducted slowly (i.e., 0.02 to 0.05 m/sec). Obviously, the slow responses will provide less effective stimuli for regenerative responses than will normal or depressed fast responses. Therefore, slow-response-dependent action potentials are very likely to show

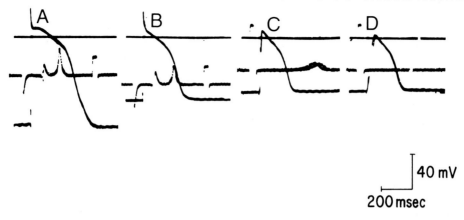

40 mV

200 msec

Fig.13-3 Effects of a decrease of resting membrane potential in a Purkinje fiber by elevation of extracellular potassium. Each panel shows a transmembrane action potential from a canine Purkinje fiber, the zero reference potential (horizontal line) for the action potential, and a differentiated signal obtained during the upstroke of the action potential. The horizontal placement of the differential trace is arbitrary. The peak of this differential recording is the maximal upstroke velocity of the action potential dV/dt_{max}. The differentiated trace also shows a square wave in each panel; this is a 200-V/sec calibration signal. Note that the gain on the differential amplifier is lower in the first two than in the second two panels. (**A**) Control action potential in Tyrode's solution (physiologic saline) containing 2.7 mM KC1; MDP is -92 mV, and dV/dt_{max} is 322 V/sec. (**B**) The KCl level is about 10 mM; the resting membrane potential is -66 mV, and the dV/dt_{max} is 200 V/sec. (**C**) Diastolic membrane potential is -58 mV, and the dV/dt_{max} shows two upstrokes of 20–26 V/sec. (**D**) The diastolic membrane potential is -55 mV, and the action potential became a slow response. No dV/dt_{max} could be determined; at rates under 5 V/sec, the deflection in the differential trace is too small to be measured. Shortly after this final photograph was taken, the membrane potential decreased slightly more, and no further action potentials were elicited.

variable conduction rates and unidirectional or bidirectional block. Partially depolarized myocardial tissues generating slow responses thus also provide the anatomic substrate for re-entrant arrhythmias.

Not all cardiac cells with resting potentials positive to -60 mV will support slow responses. The slow inward current is a weak current; if an appreciable outward (i.e., potassium) current is flowing, slow responses may not be elicited. If this is the case, enhancing the slow inward current may lead to slow-response action potentials. Phosphorylation of an internal site on one of the subunit proteins of the slow inward channel enhances i_{si}; a cyclic adenosine (cAMP)-dependent protein kinase catalyzes this phosphorylation. Therefore, catecholamines and phosphodiesterase inhibitors (caffeine, theophylline, and milrinone) can induce slow-response action potentials (Fig. 13-4). Therefore, it is possible that arrhythmias caused by β-adrenergic stimulation or increased sympathetic tone may be associated with slow-response action potentials. The specific mechanisms involved are described below.

It is likely that both slow-response and depressed fast-response action potentials can be found within or around the zone of pathology in most diseased hearts. This is because it is not probable that any type of cardiac damage, whether focal or diffuse, will produce an abrupt and totally uniform decrease in diastolic transmembrane potential throughout the affected area. Some cells may have takeoff potentials of -60 to -75 mV, partially inactivated fast sodium channels, and depressed fast responses. Other cells may have takeoff potentials of less than -60 mV and completely inactivated sodium channels. Some of these cells may support relatively robust slow-response action potentials and slow conduction, while other highly depolarized cells may show more tenuous slow responses with decremental conduction and block. Finally, some of the highly depolarized cells may have sufficiently strong outward (potassium) currents and weak inward (calcium) currents, such that they do not support any regenerative responses at all. Obviously, a zone of these highly depolarized fibers could produce a site of

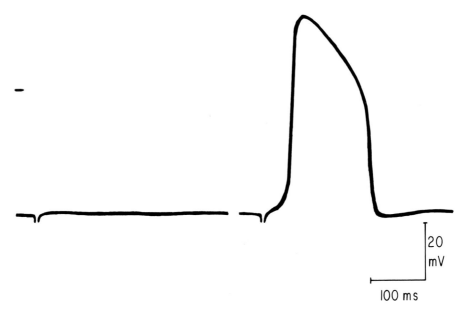

20
mV

100 ms

Fig. 13-4 Induction of slow-response action potential in canine ventricular muscle with milrinone. Resting potential − 40 mV. Left trace shows control. Right trace shows drug effect. This action, to increase the slow inward current, may help explain the positive inotropic effect of milrinone. (Modified from Canniff PC, Farah AE, Sperelakis N, Wahler GM: The effect of milrinone (Win 47203) on the in vitro electropharmacological properties of mammalian cardiac tissues. J Cardiovasc Pharmacol 7:813, 1985.)

either unidirectional or bidirectional conduction block.

Decreases in Action Potential Duration and Refractoriness

Many cardiac diseases result in changes in duration of action potential; either decreases or increases can occur. These changes in action potential duration can be important for arrhythmogenic mechanisms because recovery of excitability in normal atrial and ventricular myocardial cells accompanies repolarization (during phase 3 of the action potential). That is, excitability begins to recover after the cell has repolarized to about − 60 mV; the upstroke velocities of a premature action potential then increase more and more as the takeoff potential increases during the terminal portion of phase 3. Recovery of excitability is complete in normal myocardial cells or Purkinje fibers when maximum diastolic potential (or full diastolic potential) is achieved. Complete recovery of excitability occurs when the maximum rate of depolarization and action potential amplitude of a premature action po-

tential are essentially identical to those of the control action potentials elicited at the basic cycle length (Fig. 13-5). This rapid recovery of excitability is referred to as voltage-dependent refractoriness.

In cardiac tissues with takeoff potentials more positive than about − 70 mV, either depressed fast responses or slow-response action potentials will occur. In these tissues, refractoriness is a function of time as well as of voltage. That is, recovery of the amplitude and maximum rate of depolarization of a premature impulse extends well into phase 4 (Fig. 13-6). The different rates of recovery of excitability in normal and depressed segments of isolated canine Purkinje fibers are known to produce rate-dependent block[5] and are thought to underly re-entrant arrhythmias in canine ventricle.

SPECIFIC MECHANISMS FOR CARDIAC ARRHYTHMIAS

Much is known of the cellular mechanisms of arrhythmic activity in the mammalian heart. Arrhythmias can be caused by abnormalities of impulse ini-

Fig. 13-5 Example of voltage-dependent refractoriness. Record obtained in sheep Purkinje fiber preparation. Premature action potentials elicited at 14 different coupling intervals after primary beat; primary beat shown at the left. Early premature impulses occurring during phase 3 of the primary action potential produce only local responses. As fiber repolarizes, premature beats abruptly attain more normal amplitudes. At the beginning of phase 4, premature impulses have essentially normal amplitude (fourth premature upstroke from left). Amplitude and upstroke velocity do not increase further as the impulses are moved later and later into diastole. Note calibration bars at lower right. Vertical represents 20 mV, horizontal 100 msec.

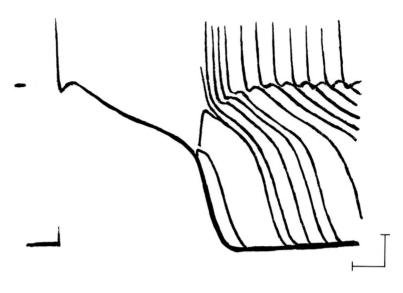

Fig. 13-6 Example of time-dependent refractoriness. Record in rabbit atrioventricular (AV) node preparation. Each trace shows superimposed electrograms or action potentials for primary beat and one of the six premature beats that were elicited at increasing coupling intervals. Upper trace shows atrial electrogram (AE), middle trace shows action potentials recorded from cell in the proximal region of the node (AN region). Lower trace (AH) shows record from distal region of the node. Note that the only premature impulse to propagate through the node is No. 6; premature impulse No. 5 produces only a subthreshold response, and Nos. 1 to 4 produce no effect at the distal node. In the AN cell, premature impulse No. 6 produces a normal action potential. Earlier impulses produce less and less response in the AN region, even though they arrive at the node after this region has fully repolarized. This is time dependent refractoriness. Note calibration bars at lower right; vertical bar is 25 mV, horizontal bar 50 msec. (Modified from Mendez C, Moe GK: Some characteristics of transmembrane potentials of AV nodal cells during propagation of premature beats. Circ Res 19:993, 1966.)

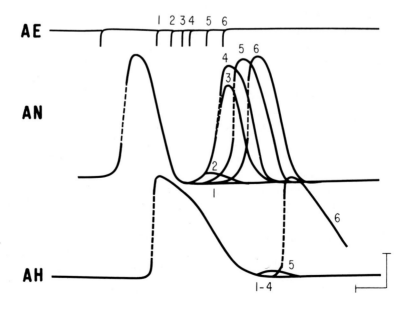

Table 13-1 Electrophysiologic Mechanisms
of Cardiac Arrhythmias

Arrhythmias caused by enhanced impulse initiation
  in ectopic foci:
    Automatic rhythms
      Normal automaticity
      Abnormal automaticity
    Triggered rhythms
      Early afterdepolarizations
      Delayed afterdepolarizations

Arrhythmias caused by abnormal impulse conduction
  Conduction blocks
  Re-entrant activation

Arrhythmias caused by simultaneous derangements
  of impulse initiation and impulse conduction

tiation, impulse conduction, or both.[7,8] Table 13-1
shows a simple classification system for these cellular mechanisms.

Arrhythmias Caused by Enhanced Impulse Initiation in Ectopic Foci

Ectopic arrhythmias caused by enhanced impulse initiation are generated by a specific cell (or small group of cells that are well coupled electrically) outside the sinus node. This cell or group of cells is referred to as the focus of the arrhythmia and are generally found at the center of the zone of earliest activation during the ectopic beats. The cells in the focus should display action potentials with a characteristic pacemaker configuration (Fig. 13-7). That is, they undergo rapid phase 4 depolarization that gradually leads to a regenerative response (the upstroke of the spontaneous action potential); a sharp inflection point at the foot of phase 0 will not occur. The presence of pacemaker fibers in a distinct ectopic focus distinguishes arrhythmias caused by enhanced impulse initiation from other arrhythmias, such as those caused by conduction block and/or re-entrant activation.[9] Two subtypes of arrhythmias caused by enhanced impulse initiation are recognized: automatic rhythms and triggered rhythms.[5]

AUTOMATIC RHYTHMS

Arrhythmias caused by automatic mechanisms occur when a subsidiary pacemaker site in the atria or ventricles becomes active and fires at a rate faster than that of the SA node. Automaticity is defined as spontaneous impulse generation occurring from a discrete pacemaker site, which (as opposed to triggering) does not depend on previous activation of that site for its initiation.[5] Automaticity can occur either as normal automaticity or as abnormal automaticity.

Normal automaticity occurs in the sinus node and in nonpathologic subsidiary pacemaker cells of the atria and atrioventricular junction. In ventricular tissues, normal automaticity only occurs in Purkinje fibers with high (approximately -90 mV) maximum diastolic potentials. Abnormal automaticity occurs in Purkinje fibers and working myocardial cells with markedly depolarized (approximately -55 mV) maximum diastolic potentials.

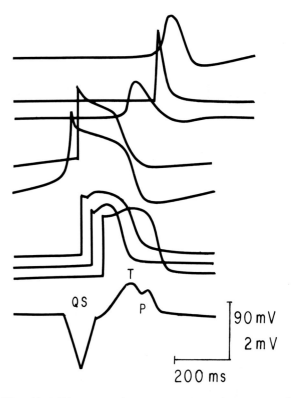

Fig. 13-7 Diagrammatic representation of sequence of depolarization during ventricular ectopic beat. Format as in Figure 13-2. Arrhythmia occurs because ectopic pacemaker in distal Purkinje fiber (fifth action potential from top) is firing rapidly. His bundle, AV node, atrial muscle, and sinoatrial (SA) node all are activated in retrograde direction, ventricular muscle activated in aberrant sequence. This results in a premature ventricular depolarization; note longer QRS duration with altered vectors, retrograde p wave in the ECG (bottom trace).

Normal Automaticity in Purkinje Fibers

Normal automaticity denotes spontaneous impulse initiation in canine, feline, and primate Purkinje fibers with normal maximum diastolic potentials (-80 to -95 mV) and occurs when overdrive from higher pacemakers is relieved (Fig. 13-8A). Normal automaticity also occurs in specialized atrial conduction fibers. The diastolic depolarization responsible for normal automaticity is generated by a net inward ionic current, which presumably reflects a balance of inward and outward currents.[10] While the detailed behavior of these currents is not entirely clear, at least four factors can contribute to the voltage time course of diastole in the normally automatic cardiac cell: (1) an inward current i_f, which is carried by Na^+ and K^+ ions, and which shows voltage and time dependence; (2) an outward current carried by potassium, which shows voltage dependence but is now thought not to have time dependence; (3) an outward current generated by activity of the electrogenic Na^+-K^+-ATPase (the sodium pump); and (4) the threshold voltage and onset char-acteristics of the fast inward (sodium) current that generates the upstroke of the action potential. Therefore, normal automaticity in Purkinje fibers is a complex phenomenon.

The electrophysiologic effects of antiarrhythmic drugs on normal automaticity may also be fairly complicated. Antiarrhythmic drugs can suppress normal automaticity directly at the cellular level by (1) decreasing the slope of diastolic depolarization, (2) increasing the threshold potential for the fast inward current, or (3) increasing the maximum diastolic potential, or (4) a combination of these effects. Antiarrhythmic drugs also can alter rate and rhythm of the heart indirectly, by interacting with autonomic nervous system reflexes or circulatory catecholamines.

Abnormal Automaticity

Abnormal automaticity is a form of impulse initiation that occurs in ectopic pacemakers with maximum diastolic potentials in the range of -60 to -40 mV (Fig. 13-9). It is thought to be an important

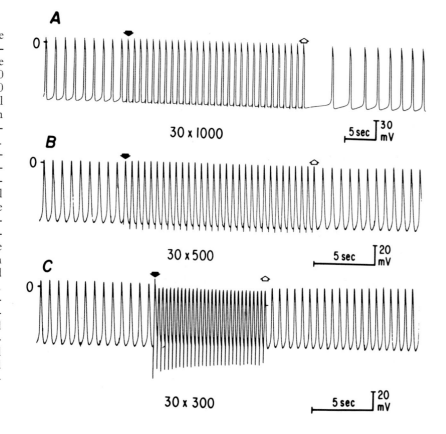

Fig. 13-8 Effects of overdrive stimulation on normal and abnormal automaticity in canine Purkinje fibers. (**A**) Effects of 30 beats at a cycle length of 1,000 msec (60 beats/min) on a normal preparation with maximum diastolic potential in the pacemaker region of about -90 mV. Postoverdrive suppression occurs after cessation of the stimulus train. (**B,C**) Effects of overdrive on fibers with abnormal automaticity. Neither overdrive hyperpolarization nor postoverdrive suppression of automaticity occurs. Note different time and voltage calibrations (shown below each panel) for (**B**) and (**C**) versus (**A**). (Dangman KH, Hoffman BF: Studies on overdrive stimulation of canine cardiac Purkinje fibers: Maximal diastolic potential as a determinant of the response. J Am Coll Cardiol 2:1183, 1983, Reprinted with permission from the American College of Cardiology.)

30 x 1000   5 sec   30 mV

30 x 500   5 sec   20 mV

30 x 300   5 sec   20 mV

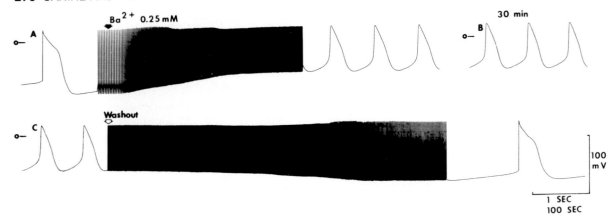

Fig. 13-9 Induction of abnormal automaticity in a normal canine Purkinje fiber by superfusion with Tyrode's solution containing barium chloride 0.25 mM. Exposure to barium (**A**) decreases maximum diastolic potential from about -90 mV to about -55 mV in 3 to 5 minutes. Rapid automaticity (abnormal automaticity) occurs. Abnormal automaticity is then sustained (**B**), until antiarrhythmic drugs are added or barium is washed out (**C**). This model of abnormal automaticity closely mimics naturally occurring forms in Purkinje fibers and myocardium damaged by ischemia or stretch. Traces obtained from a pen recorder with limited frequency response attenuates spikes. Note two different paper speeds; fast paper speed at beginning and end of (**A**) and (**C**) and throughout (**B**). Time and voltage calibrations at lower right. Zero reference potential at left of each panel. (Dangman KH, Miura DS. Electrophysiological effects of bethanidine sulfate on canine cardiac Purkinje fibers and ventricular muscle cells. J Cardiovasc Pharmacol 7:50, 1985.)

cause of atrial and ventricular arrhythmias.[11] Abnormal automatic activity can occur in the working myocardium of the atria or ventricles and in Purkinje fibers damaged by drug toxicity (i.e., digitalis), stretch, or ischemia. The balance of currents involved in the generation of abnormal automaticity may be more simple than those involved in normal automaticity, because abnormal automaticity occurs in a voltage range in which beat-to-beat activation and inactivation of the fast inward (sodium) current should be minimal. That is, because sodium influx during phase 0 is minimal in partially depolarized cells, the electrogenic sodium pump current will contribute minimally to diastolic voltage changes in pacemakers with abnormal automaticity. This may explain why abnormal automaticity, unlike normal automaticity, does not easily or frequently demonstrate postoverdrive suppression following a period of rapid stimulation (Fig. 13-8B,C). Diastolic depolarization in abnormal automaticity has been attributed to a time-dependent decrease of outward potassium current[6,12] or to the inward pacemaker current, i_f.[13] The upstroke of the action potentials in abnormal automaticity is carried by the slow in-

ward (calcium) current. The action potentials are characteristic of slow responses and can be abolished by slow inward current-blocking compounds, such as verapamil and nifedipine.[14]

The pharmacology of antiarrhythmic drug action on abnormal automaticity has become a major topic of interest only recently. As in the case of normal automaticity, it has been shown that antiarrhythmic drugs can slow or abolish abnormal automaticity directly by (1) decreasing the slope of diastolic depolarization, (2) increasing the threshold potential for the slow inward current, (3) increasing the maximum diastolic potential, or (4) some combination of the above. It is also possible that antiarrhythmic drugs might alter abnormal automaticity by indirect effects (i.e., occurring through interactions with the autonomic nervous system).

TRIGGERED ACTIVITY

Triggered activity is the second type of ectopic impulse generation that occurs from a discrete pacemaker site.[5] Triggered activity may be paroxysmal or continuous, but it occurs if and only if the pacemaker has previously been driven by an appropriate action potential or series of action potentials. That is, in contrast to automatic rhythms (which occur de novo), triggered rhythms only occur after an initiating beat that produce depolarizing afterpotentials. These afterpotentials are classified into two subgroups: early afterdepolarizations and delayed afterdepolarizations.

Early Afterdepolarizations

Early afterdepolarizations (EADs) occur during either phase 2 or 3 of the action potential. Triggered impulses occurring from maximum diastolic poten-

tials of -60 to -20 mV can be generated from these early afterdepolarizations. These triggered impulses may occur as coupled single beats or as salvoes of extra beats (Fig. 13-10). In Purkinje fibers, triggered beats from early afterdepolarizations can occur after exposure to high concentrations of antiarrhythmic drugs (e.g., quinidine, N-acetylprocainamide and cibenzoline); treatment with high concentrations of catecholamines, low oxygen tension, low pH (about 6.8); or myocardial infarction and exposure to toxic salts (e.g., barium chloride, cesium chloride), or organic toxins.[15–23]

In general, conditions that prolong action potential duration will tend to increase the amplitude of

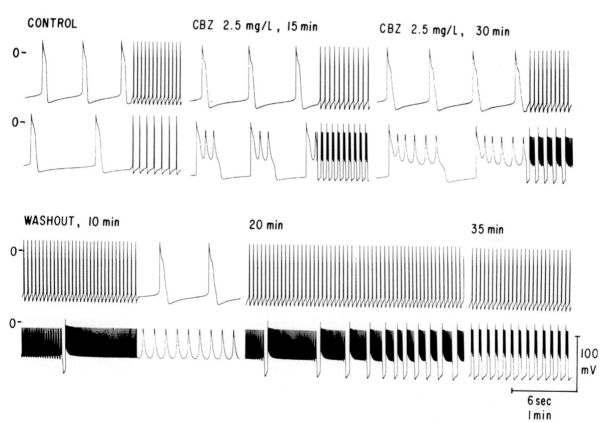

Fig. 13-10 Early afterdepolarizations in Purkinje fiber treated with cibenzoline. Records show one impalement (as upper and lower traces in each panel) from each of two separate Purkinje fiber preparations from one heart. Development of drug effects is shown in the upper two panels at center and right, and washout of drug effects shown in lower two panels. Times are as indicated. Note that early afterdepolarizations occur in impalement in lower trace, but not in upper. During washout, long salvoes of triggered impulses (resembling abnormal automaticity) occur. The duration of these salvoes gradually shortened as washout was continued. Format for time and voltage calibration as in Figure 13-10. (Dangman KH: Cardiac effects of cibenzoline. J Cardiovasc Pharmacol 6:300, 1984.)

early afterdepolarizations and consequently, the likelihood of triggering from the plateau level. Since the duration of action potentials decreases when the rate of stimulation is increased, early afterdepolarizations are generally abolished by rapid drive.[15] Indeed, early afterdepolarizations may be transiently suppressed if a single beat is imposed at a shortened cycle length.[15] Likewise, if a toxic drug or salt is present, early afterdepolarizations may emerge, if the dominant pacemaker rate is slowed.[15,20]

The ionic mechanisms of early afterdepolarizations are not entirely clear. It has been suggested that they occur when the sodium window current is increased[21] and repolarizing i_{K1} current is decreased during phase 3,[24] or if sodium-calcium exchange is increased.[25] The triggered impulses from EADs are abolished by most agents or conditions that shorten the duration of action potentials. Thus, increased extracellular potassium concentrations abolish EADs. Agents such as acetylcholine (ACh), lidocaine, and tetrodotoxin are also effective.[17,18,21,24]

Delayed Afterdepolarizations

The second electrophysiologic mechanism for triggered action potentials is the delayed afterdepolarization (DAD). DADs are afterdepolarizations occuring after full repolarization (Fig. 13-11). Triggered rhythms from DADs occur in isolated ventricular tissues following treatment with digitalis glycosides,[26-29] catecholamines,[30] and induction of myocardial infarction.[14,31] Atrial tissues have also been reported to support delayed afterdepolarizations and triggered activity following treatment with digitalis or catecholamines. Triggered activity from DADs can occur in coronary sinus tissues and mitral valve fibers.[32,33]

In Purkinje fiber preparations treated with catecholamines or toxic doses of a cardiac glycoside (e.g., ouabain 0.2 μM for 30 minutes), DADs can be easily elicited. The amplitude and coupling interval of these DADs is directly proportional to the rate and duration of the train of action potentials used to elicit them. The amplitude of delayed afterdepolarizations and the incidence of triggered activity can be decreased by a variety of agents, including acetylcholine, slow inward current-

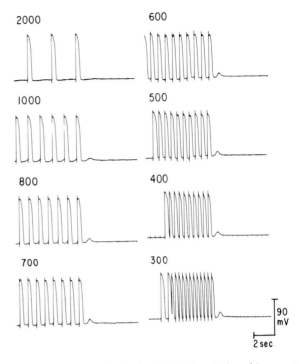

Fig. 13-11 Delayed afterdepolarizations induced in a goat Purkinje fiber by treatment with 1 μM isoproterenol. Each panel shows the effects of a stimulus train of 10 beats at cycle lengths of 2,000 and 400 msec. The train shown at 300 msec did not conduct 1:1 and so consists of a total of 14 beats. Note that as the cycle length is decreased, the amplitude of the delayed afterdepolarization increases, and the coupling interval decreases. Voltage and time calibrations shown at lower right. Maximum diastolic potential is approximately −94 mV throughout.

blocking compounds, local anesthetic drugs, and decreased calcium levels in the superfusate.

The ionic mechanisms of delayed afterdepolarizations are not clear.[6,10,34,35] It is agreed that DADs occur when intracellular calcium ion activity is increased. This engenders a novel transient inward current i_{TI} that may result from either (1) the opening of nonspecific ion channels that carry sodium and potassium fluxes i_{NaK}, or (2) inward currents created by electrogenic sodium-calcium ion exchange i_{NaCa}.

Arrhythmias Caused by Abnormal Impulse Conduction

Two types of arrhythmias can be caused by abnormalities of impulse conduction: bradycardias can result from conduction blocks, and tachycardias (or single or multiple premature depolarizations) can result from re-entrant activation.

CONDUCTION BLOCKS

A simple conduction block is most easily diagnosed from surface ECGs when failure of impulse propagation occurs at a critical point in the specialized conduction system. Such failures in conduction result in SA node exit block, second- or third-degree AV block, and bundle branch of hemibranch block. Small areas of block within the working atrial or ventricular myocardium probably do not give rise to clinically significant changes in cardiac activation patterns (unless the block leads to the production of re-entrant activity).

After a third-degree AV block, normal ventricular pacemakers usually will emerge to initiate a slow ventricular rhythm compatible with survival. In abnormal hearts, however, these pacemakers may not initiate a sufficiently rapid rhythm. This may lead to syncope or death. The appropriate therapy is often implantation of an electric pacemaker device.

RE-ENTRANT ACTIVATION

In normal sinus rhythm, the atria and ventricles are activated in a specific, efficient, and relatively constant pattern. Each normal cardiac impulse dies as the wavefront reaches the limits of the cardiac syncitium in the ventricular subepicardium. The myocardium is then activated again only after it is invaded by the next normal sinus impulse (see Fig. 13-2). If re-entrant activation occurs, the propagating impulse does not die out in the usual way; rather, it persists to re-excite the chambers of the heart after the end of the refractory period. Thus, re-entry can produce premature beats; either the atria or the ventricles can be involved in the re-entrant activity. In both canine and feline hearts, the refractory period of the atrium is approximately 150 msec, and the refractory period of the ventricular tissues is usually 200 to 500 msec. Therefore, an impulse capable of causing re-entry in hearts of these species must be sequestered in a zone of cardiac tissue for an appreciable time (so it can emerge and conduct at the end of the refractory period). In re-entry, the impulse does not remain stationary while awaiting the end

of the refractory period. The impulse must continue to conduct slowly through a pathway that is functionally or anatomically isolated from the rest of the myocardial syncitium. This isolated conduction pathway, which will generally be composed of a small percentage of the heart, must provide a route by which the impulse can return to the normal regions of the heart that have previously been excited. The pathway also must be sufficiently long to allow enough time for the impulse to continue to propagate until the end of the absolute refractory period.

The cardiac impulse propagates very quickly (1 to 5 m/sec) in normal atrial and ventricular myocardial fibers. This means that if re-entry were to occur in the normal myocardium, the length of the electrically isolated pathway needed for sequestration of the impulse would be very long. In the atrium, it would be at least 150 cm and in the ventricle it would be at least 200 to 500 cm. Electrically isolated pathways of this length are not likely to exist in the normal heart. In diseased hearts, however, conduction velocities can be slow. Therefore, the necessary pathway length for the isolated segment of a re-entrant circuit could be very short.[8]

In summary, the necessary conditions for development of re-entry are the occurrence of (1) unidirectional conduction block, and (2) slow conduction (relative to refractoriness of the surrounding cardiac cells). In the normal heart, the tissues most likely anatomic substrates for re-entry are those of the SA and AV nodes. This is because the nodal tissues have relatively poorly coupled cells, generate slow-response action potentials, and show time-dependent refractoriness. This may permit parallel conduction pathways with functional longitudinal dissociation to occur, and these parallel dissociated pathways may support re-entry.

In contrast to nodel tissues, the working atrial and ventricular myocardial tissues will support slow conduction and unidirectional conduction block only if significant pathology is present. Such re-entrant arrhythmias in the myocardium are generally considered of greater clinical significance than are the nodal arrhythmias. That is, life-threatening re-entrant arrhythmias are far more likely to occur in the diseased heart than in the normal heart. Two basic types of change in cellular electrophysiology of cardiac cells can predispose to the development of slow conduction and unidirectional conduction block: (1) decreases of maximum diastolic potential, and (2) increased dispersion of refractoriness.

Re-entry Dependent on Slow Conduction and Unidirectional Conduction Block in Partially Depolarized Tissues with Depressed Action Potentials

This type of re-entry can depend on an anatomic loop of tissue, composed of atrial, ventricular, or Purkinje fibers, with appropriate electrophysiologic characteristics. This is classic re-entry; descriptions of this type of re-entrant phenomena were reported by Mayer[36] in jellyfish mantle, by Mines[37,38] in AV rings of tortise ventricle, and by Schmitt and Erlanger[39] in ventricular preparations of turtle heart.

In the mammalian heart, the anatomy of the ventricular conduction system is such that after ischemic damage or stretch, pathways can occur that are functionally suitable for re-entry. The Purkinje system originates in the His bundle; it then divides into the left and right bundle branches. Each of these bundle brances then divides again and again, until the Purkinje system has fanned out over most of the endocardial surface of both ventricles. Each of the major bundles of Purkinje fibers is invested with a covering layer of connective tissue. This tends to keep it electrically isolated from the underlying ventricular muscle as well as from the other strands of Purkinje tissue running in parallel to it. In the His bundle and bundle branches, the strands of fibers usually anastomose quite freely. More peripherally, the terminal Purkinje arborize many times and contact endocardial ventricular muscle cells (Fig. 13-12). These ventricular muscle cells are connected syncytially. Therefore, junctional sites between Purkinje fibers and muscle can form anatomic loops. Normally, the cardiac impulse quickly propagates through all branches of the ventricular conduction system to the subendocardial ventricular muscle. Normal impulses are terminated in ventricular muscle when the advancing wavefronts collide and are surrounded by refractory tissue (Fig. 13-12).

Re-entry can occur in the distal Purkinje network if conduction velocity is decreased and unidirectional block occurs at a critical site (Fig. 13-13). Obviously, if there is a zone of damage that encompasses one or more of these Purkinje fiber-ventricular muscle loops, diastolic potential, action

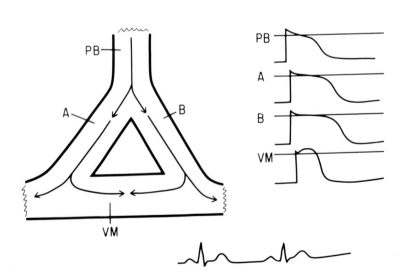

Fig. 13-12 Illustration of normal conduction of the cardiac impulse in the ventricular conduction system. Schmitt/Erlanger diagram[39] at left shows one of the bifurcations of the His-Purkinje system; PB denotes proximal bundle, A and B denote distal branches, and VM denotes ventricular muscle distal to branches. Action potential duration and refractory periods are longest in the gate regions of distal branches A and B. Impulse normally conducts down through the each branch and simultaneously activates endocardial ventricular muscle in contact with the ultimate transitional fibers of each branch. The wavefronts of activation then collide in the ventricular muscle zone and terminate. Action potentials at right from points indicated in drawing at left; action potentials diagrammatically indicate activation sequence in the ventricle, producing ECG of normal sinus rhythm, as shown below.

Fig. 13-13 Re-entry in the Schmitt/ Erlanger diagram.[39] Impulse propagates through proximal bundle (PB) and distal bundle A in the normal manner. Distal bundle B is damaged: antegrade impulse conducts slowly and decrementally through B (wavy line) and blocks in the damaged zone. The impulse conducts through the ventricle and re-enters the damaged zone from the distal margin. The impulse propagates back to the proximal bundle and re-enters the proximal bundle, where it continues to be conducted in the retrograde direction. This can give rise to a premature ventricular depolarization (displayed on ECG below). If every primary (sinus) impulse is followed by a premature depolarization, this can produce a bigeminal rhythm.

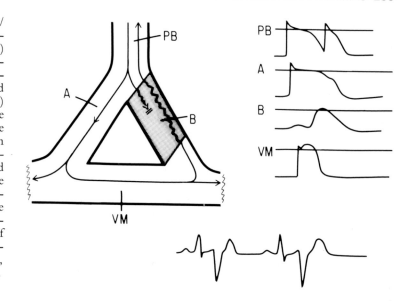

potential amplitude, and upstroke velocity may be reduced in the damaged fibers. Slow conduction and unidirectional block may occur. Since the intensity of insult in the damaged zone is rarely uniform, some areas within the loop will usually be more depressed than others. Unidirectional conduction block will usually occur in one of the areas of greatest depression. If, however, depression of the action potentials is too great, no conduction will be supported, and bidirectional conduction block will result. Under these circumstances, re-entry will not occur. Because the degree of depression is critical to the development of unidirectional conduction block, and this can vary from site to site in a zone of damage, re-entry is more likely to occur in a large zone of damage than a small one. Once a re-entrant circuit is established, it may lead to either single premature impulses or to multiple premature responses (tachycardia). Re-entrant tachycardias presumably resulting from continuous circling of the impulse around the loop are called circus movement tachycardias.

In some cases, the zone of damage may not have appropriate electrophysiologic characteristics (i.e., severely depressed enough action potentials) to precipitate re-entry at normal (sinus rhythm) cycle lengths. In these cases, re-entry may be provoked by premature impulses, which may originate from either supraventricular or ventricular foci. The pre-

mature impulses are more likely to precipitate re-entry because Purkinje fibers in a zone of damage will usually have a much longer refractory period than fibers in normal zones. If the depressed Purkinje fibers are activated prematurely, the premature impulse will be conducted more slowly, and have a greater tendency to block, than will an impulse elicited at the longer (normal) cycle length. In other words, premature impulses often can lead to re-entrant responses because at short cycle lengths there is a reduced safety factor for conduction in the myocardium.

Sites of re-entry over fixed anatomic pathways are not exclusively found in the peripheral Purkinje system. It is likely that similar re-entry loops could involve the His bundle and bundle branches, or the major proximal fascicles of the conduction system. In these cases, re-entry might occur as a result of bundle branch blocks or hemiblocks, respectively. Re-entry loops can also be formed in pathologic zones of working atrial or ventricular muscle. For example, atrial cardiomyopathy can produce areas of inexcitable tissue, which can create pathways for circus movement. Finally, the existence of an anatomically discrete loop is not an absolute requirement for the development of slow-conduction unidirectional conduction block and re-entry. Re-entry can occur in unbranched bundles of fibers or sheets of tissue if functional longitudinal dissociation occurs and is accompanied by slow conduction and unidirectional conduction block.

Re-entry Dependent on Dispersion of Refractoriness

Recently, it was demonstrated that re-entry can occur not only in depressed, depolarized tissues, but also in cardiac tissues in which the cells have normal diastolic potentials and rapid rates of depolarization. However, the same two basic electrophysiologic phenomena must be present to support re-entrant activation in these fully polarized tissues; that is, the preparation must still support unidirectional conduction block and slow conduction. While undamaged tissues probably will not exhibit slow conduction and unidirectional conduction block at normal sinus rates, both conduction abnormalities may occur during the propagation of premature impulses through relatively refractory cardiac tissues.

Re-entry occurring as a result of dispersion of refractoriness was described in isolated rabbit left atrium.[40–42] In this leading circle model, re-entry occurs in the absence of an anatomic obstacle (Fig. 13-14). The initiation of re-entrant activity is permitted when atrial fibers in close proximity to each other have different refractory periods. Re-entry can be initiated when a premature impulse fails to conduct through fibers with long refractory periods and conducts through fibers with shorter refractory periods. Eventually, the impulse returns to the initial site of unidirectional block in the retrograde direction after excitability recovers there. The impulse may then persist in a circus movement over an anatomically variable circuit with a perimeter of as little as 6 to 8 mm. The conduction velocity within the circuit is relatively slow because the impulses are propagating through partially refractory tissues. Impulses spread inward from the perimeter continuously, leading to a central zone of the re-entrant

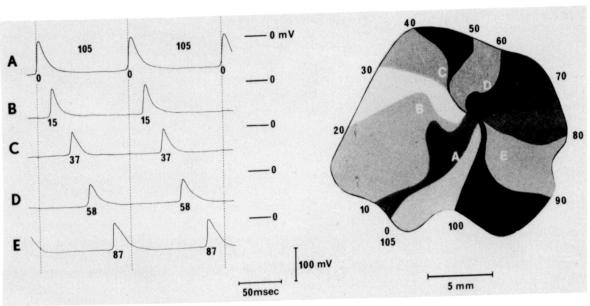

Fig. 13-14 Re-entrant activation in the rabbit left atrium, based on circus movement by the leading circle mechanism. The different shadings and numbers in the diagram at the right indicate the time in milliseconds during which the wavefront of activation passed that site in the preparation. Activation during one complete cycle occurs clockwise between time 0 and 105 msec. (**A**) Transmembrane action potentials recorded from five sites (labeled A through E) from the 6 o'clock position (**B**) during two beats of the tachycardia. Note time and voltage calibration bars center bottom, length scale right bottom. (Allessie MA, Bonke FIM, Schopman FJG: Circus movement in rabbit atrial tissue as a mechanism of tachycardia. III. The "leading circle" concept: A new model of circus movement in cardiac tissue without the involvement of an anatomic obstacle. Circ Res 41:9, 1977.)

circuit (i.e., is functionally inactive). The amplitudes of the action potentials and their maximum upstroke velocities decrease gradually from the periphery to the center of the circuit. Cells in the center of the re-entrant circuit produce only local responses rather than full action potentials dependent on regenerative responses. This is because they are continuously kept in a partially depolarized and refractory state by the circulation of the impulse about them. The length of the circuit and the circulation time of the loop are controlled by the conduction velocity and refractory period of the fibers composing it.

A second example of re-entry dependent on dispersion of refractoriness occurs in the AV node preparation. In AV node cells, the time needed for full recovery of excitability does not begin at the end of phase 3 but instead lasts well into phase 4. That is, these cells show time-dependent refractoriness rather than voltage-dependent refractoriness.[43] Re-entry can occur in this preparation because adjacent zones of the node are functionally different electrophysiologically. The recovery period can be different in the two zones of the node and, if these differences are significant enough, reentry can occur following a premature impulse. This is because, following a premature impulse, the differences in the refractory periods of the two populations of AV nodal cells functionally divide the node into two pathways. If conduction of the premature impulse through the node is slow enough, it may return to the atrium as a return extrasystole. If this return extrasystole propagates through the atrium at a time when the antegrade approaches to the node have recovered excitability, the impulse may again enter the AV node and conduct around the circuit. This can become a continuous process and may lead to paroxysmal supraventricular tachycardias with some degree of AV block.

Differences in refractoriness can also lead to reentry in the ventricle. Local differences in refractoriness can be accentuated by cardiac disease, producing a predisposition to re-entry. However, as in the examples cited in the atrium and the AV node, a premature impulse is needed to elicit re-entrant activity. An example of re-entrant activation of the ventricles dependent on differences in refractoriness would be the R-on-T phenomenon, in which ventricular fibrillation is elicited by premature impulses during the peak of the T wave.

Arrhythmias Caused by Simultaneous Derangements of Impulse Initiation and Impulse Conduction

It is probable that many of the arrhythmias occurring clinically are not caused by a single electrophysiologic mechanism but represent two or more mechanisms operating simultaneously. Perhaps the most simple example of these multifactorial arrhythmias is parasystole. Here, premature depolarizations in either the atria or the ventricles occur infrequently and are randomly distributed during diastole. Intervals between these ectopic impulses are whole-number multiples of one basic cycle length that is presumed to be the cycle length of an ectopic pacemaker. That is, parasystole is thought to reflect the activity of an independent ectopic pacemaker protected from sinus node overdrive by a complete entrance block, and the ectopic impulses are thought to reflect the escape of this ectopic impulse through a zone of variable exit block.

Another example of arrythmias caused by more than one mechanism occurring simultaneously is found in the multifocal ventricular arrhythmias in the digitalis intoxicated dog or cat. These arrhythmias may result from enhanced normal automaticity, delayed afterdepolarizations, and re-entrant activity.

Therefore, it is likely that arrhythmias encountered in veterinary practice often reflect multiple mechanisms. Many of these arrhythmias occur in digitalized animals or in animals with cardiomyopathic hypertrophy. Although identification of a specific electrophysiologic mechanism for these arrhythmias is a significant undertaking, it may prove more feasible in the near future.[9] The resultant information may help improve the effectiveness of pharmacologic therapy.

ACKNOWLEDGMENT

Original studies for and preparation of this chapter were supported entirely by a grant to KHD (HL-24354) from the National Heart and Lung and Blood

Institute, National Institutes of Health, U.S. Public Health Service.

REFERENCES

1. Noble D: The Initiation of the Heartbeat. Clarendon Press, Oxford, 1975
2. Allen JD, Brennan FJ, Wit AL: Actions of lidocaine on transmembrane potentials of subendocardial Purkinje fibers surviving in infarcted canine hearts. Circ Res 43:470, 1978
3. Dangman KH: Effects of bepridil on transmembrane action potentials recorded from canine cardiac Purkinje fibers and ventricular muscle cells; Insights into antiarrhythmic mechanisms. Naunyn-Schmied Arch Pharmacol 329:326, 1985
4. Dangman KH, Miura DS: Effects of therapeutic concentrations of procainamide on transmembrane action potentials of normal and infarct zone Purkinje fibers and ventricular muscle cells. J Cardiovasc Pharmacol (submitted, 1987)
5. Cranefield PF: The Conduction of the Cardiac Impulse: The Slow Response and Cardiac Arrhythmias. Futura Publications, Mount Kisco, NY, 1975
6. Noble D: The surprising heart: A review of recent progress in cardiac electrophysiology. J Physiol (Lond) 353:1, 1984
7. Hoffman BF, Rosen MR: Cellular mechanisms for cardiac arrhythmias. Circ Res 49:1, 1981
8. Wit AL, Cranefield PF: Reentrant excitation as a cause of cardiac arrhythmias. Am J Physiol 235:H1, 1978
9. Hoffman BF, Dangman KH: Demonstration of the mechanisms for arrhythmias in experimental animals. Ann NY Acad Sci 432:17, 1984
10. DiFrancesco D, Noble D: A model of cardiac electrical activity incorporating ionic pumps and concentration changes. Philos Trans Soc Lond B 307:353, 1985
11. LeMarec H, Dangman KH, Danilo P, Rosen MR: An evaluation of automaticity and triggered activity in the canine heart one to four days after myocardial infarction. Circulation 71:1224, 1985
12. Hiraoka M, Ikeda K, Sano T: The mechanism of Ba-induced automaticity in ventricular muscle fibers. J Mol Cell Cardiol 10(suppl I):35, 1978
13. Opie LH: The Heart. Physiology, Metabolism, Pharmacology and Therapy. Grune & Stratton, London, 1984
14. Dangman KH, Hoffman BF: Effects of nifedipine on electrical activity of cardiac cells. Am J Cardiol 46:1059, 1980
15. Dangman KH, Hoffman BF: *In vivo* and *in vitro* antiarrhythmic and arrhythmogenic effects of N-acetyl procainamide. J Pharmacol Exp Ther 217:851, 1981
16. Dangman KH: Cardiac effects of cibenzoline. J Cardiovasc Pharmacol 6:300, 1984
17. Roden DM, Hoffman BF: Action potential prolongation and induction of abnormal automaticity by low quinidine concentrations in canine Purkinje fibers. Relationship to potassium and cycle length. Circ Res 56:857, 1985
18. Coraboeuf E, Deroubaix E, Coulombe A: Acidosis induced abnormal repolarization and repeditive activity in isolated dog Purkinje fibers. J Physiol (Paris) 76:97, 1980
19. Hoffman BF, Cranefield PF: Electrophysiology of the heart. McGraw-Hill, New York, 1960
20. Brachmann J, Scherlag BJ, Rosenstraukh LV, Lazzara R: Bradycardia dependent triggered activity: Relevance to drug-induced multiform ventricular tachycardia. Circulation 68:846, 1983
21. Brown BS: Early afterdepolarizations induced by batrachytoxin: Possible involvement of sodium current. Fed Proc 42:581, 1983
22. Trautwein W: Membrane currents in cardiac fibers. Pharmacol Rev 15:277, 1963
23. Dangman KH, Hoffman BF: Effects of single premature stimuli on automatic and triggered rhythms in isolated canine Purkinje fibers. Circulation 71:813, 1985
24. Coraboeuf E: Role of ionic currents in the genesis of normal and abnormal automatisms in cardiac tissues. p. 1. In Antaloczy Z, Preda I (eds): Proceedings of the Eighth International Congress on Electrocardiology, 1981, Excerpta Medica, Amsterdam, 1982
25. Fischmeister R, Vassort G: The electrogenic Na-Ca exchange and cardiac electrical activity. I. Stimulation of Purkinje fibre action potential. J Physiol (Paris) 77:705, 1981
26. Rosen MR, Gelband H, Hoffman BF: Correlation between effects of ouabain on the canine electrocardiogram and transmembrane potentials of isolate Purkinje fibers. Circulation 47:65, 1973
27. Rosen MR, Gelband H, Merker C, Hoffman BF: Mechanisms of digitalis toxicity. Effects of ouabain on phase 4 of canine Purkinje fiber transmembrane potentials. Circulation 47:681, 1973
28. Ferrier GR, Moe GK: Effect of calcium on acetylstrophanthidin induced transient depolarization in canine Purkinje tissue. Circ Res 33:508, 1973
29. Karaguezian HS, Katzung BG: Voltage clamp studies of transient inward current and mechanical oscillations induced by ouabain in ferret papillary muscle. J Physiol (Lond) 327:255, 1982

30. Dangman KH, Danilo P, Hordof AJ, et al: Electrophysiologic characteristics of human ventricular and Purkinje fibers. Circulation 65:362, 1982
31. El Sherif N, Gough WB, Zeiler RH, Mehra R: Triggered ventricular rhythms in 1 day old myocardial infarction in the dog. Circ Res 52:566, 1983
32. Wit Al, Cranefield PF: Triggered and automatic activity in the canine coronary sinus. Circ Res 41:435, 1977
33. Wit AL, Cranefield PF: Triggered activity in cardiac muscle fibers of the simian mitral valve. Circ Res 38:85, 1976
34. Kass RS, Lederer WJ, Tsien RW, Weingart R: Role of calcium ions in transient inward current and aftercontractions induced by strophanthidin in cardiac Purkinje fibres. J Physiol (Lond) 281:187, 1978
35. Brown HF, Noble D, Noble SJ, Taupignon AI: Relationship between the transient inward current and slow inward currents in the sino-atrial node of the rabbit. J Physiol (Lond) 370:299, 1986
36. Mayer AG: Rhythmical Pulsation in scyphomedusae. Carnegie Inst Wash 47, 1906
37. Mines GR: On dynamic equilibrium in the heart. J Physiol (Lond) 46:350, 1913
38. Mines GR: On circulating excitations in heart muscles and their possible relation to tachycardia and fibrillation. Trans R Soc Can 8:43, 1914
39. Schmitt FO, Erlanger J: Directional differences in the conduction of the impulse through heart muscle and their possible relation to extrasystolic and fibrillary contractions. Am J Physiol 87:326, 1928–29
40. Allessie MA, Bonke FIM, Schopman FJG: Circus movement in rabbit atrial muscle as a mechanism of tachycardia. Circ Res 33:54, 1973
41. Allessie MA, Bonke FIM, Schopman FJG: Circus movement in rabbit atrial muscle as a mechanism of tachycardia. II. Role of nonuniform recovery of excitability in the occurrence of unidirectional block, as studied with multiple microelectrodes. Circ Res 39:168, 1976
42. Allessie MA, Bonke FIM, Schopman FJG: Circus movement in rabbit atrial tissue as a mechanism of tachycardia. III. The "leading circle" concept: A new model of circus movement in cardiac tissue without the involvement of an anatomical obstacle. Circ Res 41:9, 1977
43. Mendez C, Moe GK: Some characteristics of transmembrane potentials of AV nodal cells during propagation of premature beats. Circ Res 19:993, 1966

14

The Clinical Management of Cardiac Arrhythmias in the Dog and Cat

D. David Sisson

PATIENT EVALUATION: THE NEED FOR TREATMENT

An accurate electrocardiographic (ECG) interpretation is the essential, initial step toward the successful management of patients with cardiac arrhythmias. Certain arrhythmias are clearly life-threatening and require immediate therapy, regardless of the circumstances in which they occur. Other arrhythmias are observed so commonly in the general population that they are most certainly benign and can be safely ignored. However, the significance of most cardiac arrhythmias encountered in clinical practice is less certain. It is important to recognize that the need for therapy and the mode of therapy selected is determined as much by the unique circumstances of each patient as by the ECG features of the rhythm disorder. For example, infrequent unifocal premature ventricular beats are usually not treated in an otherwise healthy dog. This same rhythm disorder would be aggressively treated

when observed in a dog with severe subvalvular aortic stenosis and a history of syncope. Once a disorder of the heart rate or rhythm is detected, recorded, and classified, the emphasis of the clinical evaluation must shift to consideration of (1) the probable cause(s) of the arrhythmia, (2) the effects of the arrhythmia on the patient, and (3) the relative risk to the patient of the arrhythmia and the proposed therapeutic intervention.

Causes of Arrhythmias

The list of cardiac and extracardiac conditions associated with cardiac rate, rhythm, and conduction disturbances is long[1-33] (Tables 14-1 and 14-2). Admittedly, it may be difficult, if not impossible, to identify with certainty the etiology of an arrhythmia in some patients. Nonetheless, an attempt should always be made to identify any precipitating or aggravating causes of a cardiac arrhythmia. A detailed

Table 14-1 Common Cardiac Causes of Arrhythmia

Acquired Cardiac Disorders
    Myocarditis (all causes)
    Dilated cardiomyopathy
    Pericarditis
    Myocardial ischemia
    Trauma
    Arteriosclerosis
    Endocarditis
    Degenerative valvular disease
    Cardiac neoplasia
    Myocardial failure (all causes)
    Idiopathic fibrosis
    Hypertrophic cardiomyopathy

Congenital or Hereditary Defects
    Heart block (rare)
    AV bundle stenosis (Pugs)
    Preexcitation syndromes
    Sick sinus syndrome (?)
    Persistent atrial standstill
    Congenital anomalies such as:
        Subvalvular aortic stenosis
        Patent ductus arteriosis
        Pulmonic stenosis
        Tetralogy of Fallot

Table 14-2 Extracardiac Causes of Arrhythmia

Disorders of the Autonomic Nervous System
    Increased intracranial pressure
    Encephalitis
    CNS neoplasia
    Emotional stress
    Autonomic imbalance

Electrolyte and Acid-Base Disorders
    Hyperkalemia
    Hypokalemia
    Hypocalcemia and Hypercalcemia
    Hypomagnesemia

Disorders Causing Hypoxia
    Severe anemia
    Hypotension
    Shock (any cause)
    Thromboemboli
    Upper airway obstruction
    Pulmonary parenchymal diseases
    Ventilatory failure
    Pleural space diseases

Metabolic, Endocrine, Other Systemic Disorders
    Diabetes mellitus
    Hyperthyroidism
    Pheochromocytoma
    Sepsis
    Pancreatitis
    Gastric torsion
    Collagen-vascular diseases
    Coagulopathies
    Hyperviscosity syndromes

Mechanical Stimulation/Environmental Factors
    Cardiac catheterization
    IV catheters
    Pericardiocentesis
    Hyperthermia
    Thoracocentesis
    Rib fractures
    Surgical manipulation
    Hypothermia

Drugs
    Digitalis glycosides
    Sympathomimetics
    Diuretics
    Phosphodiesterase inhibitors
    Antiarrhythmic drugs
    Anesthetics (all)
    Xylazine
    Phenothiazines

history, thorough physical examination, and careful cardiovascular evaluation often will substantially simplify an otherwise directionless investigation of the almost limitless possibilities. Some of the more common potentially reversible causes of arrhythmias include disorders affecting the autonomic nervous system, endocrine diseases, metabolic disorders resulting in electrolyte or acid-base disturbances, hypoxia, heart failure, and a variety of systemic illnesses wherein the mechanism of arrhythmogenesis is ill defined (Table 14-3).

Identification of the underlying cause of an arrhythmia often produces gratifying results. Effective medical management of the heart failure state often resolves any associated rhythm disorders.[34] Restoration of normal serum potassium levels is all that is required to restore sinus rhythm in a number of different rhythm disturbances.[2,3,30,31,35] Prompt and vigorous treatment of any associated systemic disorder, such as profound anemia, sepsis, hyperthermia, pancreatitis, gastric torsion, or coagulopathy, may result in the spontaneous resolution of

Table 14-3 Systematic Approach to the Pet with Arrhythmia

History
    Age, breed, sex
    Previous medical/surgical disorders
    Current diseases
    Current drugs or medications
    Presenting clinical signs

Physical examination
    Complete general examination
    Cardiovascular evaluation
        Precordial palpation
        Auscultation (murmur, gallop rhythm, intensity of heart and lung sounds, heart rate-rhythm)
        Femoral pulse assessment
        Jugular venous pulse (cannon a waves)
        Response to vagomimetic maneuvers (carotid sinus massage, occular pressure)

Electrocardiography
    Assess rate, rhythm, electrocardiogram

Radiography
    Evidence of heart disease (cardiomegaly)
    Evidence of congestive heart failure (pleural, pericardial, or abdominal effusion, pulmonary edema)
    Nonselective angiocardiography
    Catheterization

Echocardiography
    Assess cardiac structure and function
    Evaluate cardiac shunts (bubble studies)

Clinical pathology (detect systemic/metabolic disorders)
    Hemogram
    Biochemical profile
    Electrolytes (serum potassium, sodium, chloride, calcium)
    Acid-base states (blood pH, PCO_2, bicarbonate)
    Serum T_3, T_4 levels
    Feline leukemia virus status (cats)
    Cytologic evaluation (effusions, masses)
    Heartworm serology

Hemodynamic assessment
    Capillary refill time, color
    Femoral arterial pulse pressure
    Relative state of depression
    Central venous pressure
    Urine output
    Arterial blood pressure

Assessment of pharmacologic therapy
    Clinical response to previous/current therapy
    Potential for abnormal drug metabolism and excretion (i.e., hepatic, renal failure)
    Previous/current adverse drug interactions or incompatabilities

(Fox PR, Kaplan P: Feline arrhythmias. p. 251. In Bonagura JD (ed): Contemporary Issues in Small Animal Practice. Vol. 7: Cardiology. Churchill Livingstone, New York, 1987.)

any associated arrhythmias.[3] In particular, any potentially arrhythmogenic drugs should be discontinued or reduced in dosage if toxicity is a possibility. Some of the more common offending agents include the digitalis glycosides, sympathomimetic drugs, anesthetics, aminophylline, thyroxine, and the antiarrhythmic agents themselves.[27-29,36-40]

Hemodynamic Effects of Arrhythmias

Therapy is almost always required when a rhythm disorder produces clinical signs in a patient as a result of an induced fall in cardiac output. Signs resulting from inadequate cardiac output include lethargy, exercise intolerance, weakness, ataxia, syncope, seizures, signs of systemic or pulmonary congestion, and sudden death. Patients suffering

from the latter are rarely presented for evaluation. By considering the hemodynamic consequences of an arrhythmia to the patient, the clinician can decide not only whether to treat but how urgent is the need for therapy. A careful history and physical examination is particularly important for the assessment of the hemodynamic consequences of a cardiac arrhythmia. The performance of the heart and, thus, the circulation are dependent primarily on (1) the ventricular rate, (2) the duration of the arrhythmia, (3) the site of origin of arrhythmia, (4) the presence of underlying cardiovascular disease, and (5) the presence of other disease processes that may adversely affect cardiac output or the perfusion requirements of the patient.[41]

The hemodynamic consequences of any rhythm disorder must be assessed in relationship to the physical condition of the patient being evaluated.[1,2,42–45] For example, the consequences of atrial fibrillation may be minimal in an otherwise healthy dog but are often catastrophic in a dog with advanced mitral regurgitation. Similarly, sinus bradycardia will have less impact in the healthy cat than in a cat with hyperthyroidism. In healthy dogs, cardiac output declines at heart rates greater than 180 beats/min as cardiac filling is impaired. Cardiac output also declines when the heart rate falls below 40 beats/min. When heart disease is present or when the demands on the heart are increased, less extreme changes in heart rate can result in clinical signs of low cardiac output. Circulatory function can often be adequately assessed by careful auscultation, palpation of arterial pulse rate and contour, evaluation of mucous membrane color, and examination for signs of pulmonary or systemic venous congestion. When these physical findings are equivocal in seriously ill patients, thoracic radiographs, central venous pressure monitoring, blood-gas determinations, and echocardiographic evaluation can be used to more accurately assess the hemodynamic effects of a rhythm disorder. This may require that the animal be referred.

Electrophysiologic Sequelae of Arrhythmias

Cardiac arrhythmias that are hemodynamically inconsequential are often treated in the absence of clinical signs because of the anticipated development of a more serious arrhythmia (Fig. 14-1). Frequent premature beats, pleomorphic (multifocal) premature ventricular beats, and premature beats encroaching upon the T wave (vulnerable period) of the preceding cardiac cycle are treated by most practicing cardiologists.[1,41,46] The initiation of prophylactic antiarrhythmic therapy implies that the examiner knows the likely future course of the observed arrhythmia in the patient being evaluated. To make this assessment, the clinician must consider the cause of the arrhythmia, the severity of underlying heart disease, the usual course of any concurrent systemic illnesses, and the natural history of the observed arrhythmia in the particular circumstances of the patient being evaluated. The propensity towards electric instability and sudden death has been documented in people with cardiomyopathy, in patients with subvalvular aortic stenosis, in dogs and cats with cardiomyopathy, in patients with digitalis intoxication, and in patients with congestive heart failure.[1,2,7,10,11,47–49]

In healthy animals, it is common practice to ignore infrequent unifocal premature ventricular beats that have a long coupling interval.[1,2,4] There is no convincing evidence that the suppression of premature ventricular contractions (PVCs) or even complex arrhythmias reduces the incidence of sudden death in healthy men.[50] Similar studies have not been performed in domestic animals. It is difficult to determine whether therapy is needed when ventricular arrhythmias are not causing hemodynamic changes but are observed in dogs suffering fom pancreatitis, gastric torsion, or other serious systemic diseases.[3,23–25,46] The efficacy of prophylactically administered antiarrhythmic therapy is controversial in humans and largely unstudied in domestic animals. Until well-designed studies are performed in the clinical setting, many therapeutic decisions must be guided by the experience and prejudices of the attending clinician.

PRINCIPLES OF THERAPY

Available Modes of Therapy

Once the decision to treat a patient with an arrhythmia is made, the mode of therapy must be selected. For a variety of reaons, electric cardioversion, surgical intervention, and pacemaker implantation have been rarely used in dogs and cats.[1] It must be emphasized that for many animals with symptomatic bradycardia there is no adequate substitute for an artificial cardiac pacemaker.[51,52] If survival of the patient with ventricular fibrillation is the goal, there is no adequate substitute for electric defibrillation.[53] Recognition and acceptance of the practical limitations of veterinary practice must temper the expectations of the clinician for success in the management of cardiac arrhythmias. The decision-making process in many instances is reduced to selection of the most appropriate drug(s). For example, only a few agents in clinical practice, such as parasympatholytic drugs (e.g., atropine, glycopyrrolate) and sympathomimetic drugs (e.g., iso-

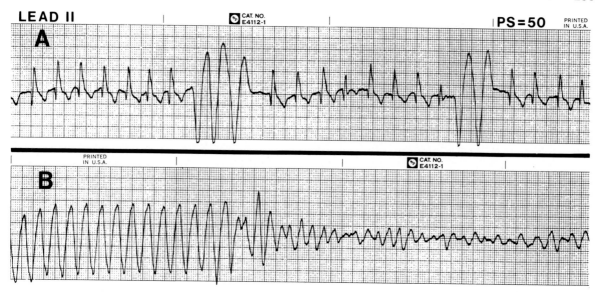

Fig. 14-1 Lead II recordings from a Doberman pinscher with atrial fibrillation and severe congestive heart failure due to dilated cardiomyopathy. Runs of ventricular premature complexes (**A**) precede the onset of life-threatening ventricular tachycardia and fibrillation (**B**) by less than 1 minute. PS = paper speed, 50 mm/sec.

proterenol, dopamine) can be used for the treatment of symptomatic bradycardia. By contrast, there is greater diversity in the drugs available for management of the pathologic tachycardias (Ch. 15).

Classification Schemes for Antiarrhythmic Drugs

Four to six categories of antiarrhythmic drugs have been devised by various investigators based on the electrophysiologic effects of these agents.[54–56] These classifications are useful to researchers trying to develop new antiarrhythmic drugs. They are also very useful guides for the selection of a drug based on its effectiveness for treating ventricular as opposed to supraventricular tachyarrhythmias. Agents that either lengthen atrioventricular (AV) nodal refractoriness, that depress slow-fiber conduction, or both, are used for the treatment of the supraventricular tachycardias and to slow the ventricular response to atrial flutter or fibrillation. These agents include propranolol, digitalis, and verapamil. Drugs such as quinidine or procainamide that lengthen atrial myocardial refractoriness are used to convert atrial fibrillation to normal sinus rhythm or to treat

refractory supraventricular tachycardias. Antiarrhythmic drugs that depress automaticity, inhibit fast-fiber conduction, and lengthen refractoriness of His-Purkinje fibers or ventricular muscle are selected to treat ventricular arrhythmias. Thus, lidocaine, procainamide, quinidine, propranolol, bretylium, phenytoin, or a number of investigational drugs are usually selected to treat or prevent ventricular tachycardia or fibrillation (Ch. 15).

There are significant limitations to the application of these classification schemes for the treatment of an individual patient. The surface ECG is unable to distinguish abnormal automaticity from after-depolarizations or from re-entry.[57] Thus, it is not possible to select an agent on the basis of a specific electrophysiologic mechanism of action. Furthermore, these classification schemes are based on the electrophysiologic effects of the drug in vitro in normal cardiac cells and do not always reflect the in vivo action of the drug in abnormal cells.[54–57] Nonetheless, these classifications are useful in avoiding adverse side effects engendered by combining like agents with additive toxicities. This is an important consideration when combination therapy is contemplated for a refractory arrhythmia.

Drug Selection

The selection of a particular antiarrhythmic drug is most appropriately made based on (1) clinical efficacy extrapolated from prior experience; (2) considerations of toxicity, (3) available routes of administration, and (4) the pharmacokinetic properties of the drugs as they affect dosing intervals.[41,57] Because studies of drug efficacy in animals with specific clinical disorders are limited, the choice of drug(s) in a particular setting must be based either on studies in experimental situations not resembling the actual circumstances of the patient or on studies of human patients with similar disorders. These considerations are discussed in more detail in those sections that describe the treatment of specific arrhythmias. It is important to emphasize that selection of a particular antiarrhythmic drug often requires consideration of its toxic effects or undesirable interactions with other drugs. Lidocaine is often used preferentially for life-threatening ventricular tachycardia not only because it is often effective and can be given intravenously, but also because it is relatively safe to administer in this circumstance. Intravenous quinidine would be inappropriate as an initial therapy because it often causes severe hypotension and would aggravate the condition of an already severely compromised patient.[58] Procainamide is often chosen over quinidine for the treatment of ventricular arrhythmias in digitalized patients. It is known that quinidine can increase serum and myocardial digoxin concentrations and precipitate digitalis toxicity.[59,60] If procainamide is not effective, quinidine can be used, but the dose of digoxin may have to be adjusted downward.

Knowledge of the available routes by which a drug may be administered is of great practical importance. In an emergency, the intravenous route is always preferred. If continuous intravenous infusion is not possible because of practical limitations, a drug must be selected that is available orally or by the intramuscular route. There are many instances when the oral route is unavailable (e.g., mandibular fractures, pancreatitis, gastric torsion, and in unconscious or obtunded patients). When long-term prophylactic therapy is indicated, the choice of drugs is greatly influenced by the required dosing interval. The realities of owner compliance usually dictate a dosing interval no more frequent than every 6 to 8 hours.

Therapeutic Goals

The goal(s) of each therapeutic intervention should be firmly established prior to beginning treatment. The expected result of treatment will vary with the arrhythmia, the individual circumstances of the patient, and the electrophysiologic effects of the drug administered. Digoxin may be administered to a dog with mitral regurgitation and frequent premature atrial beats in an effort to prevent the development of atrial tachycardia rather than to eliminate the premature beats. In the absence of underlying heart disease, the goal of quinidine therapy for atrial fibrillation is to restore and maintain sinus rhythm. In a dog or cat with cardiomyopathy, the goal for the treatment of atrial fibrillation is slowing of the ventricular response (rate) to the fibrillating atria. In these patients, digitalis is usually selected for initial therapy. Lidocaine is often administered to abolish ominous-appearing ventricular premature beats and to prevent ventricular tachycardia or fibrillation. Administration of bretylium to prevent ventricular tachycardia or fibrillation should not be expected to eliminate all premature beats. In cats with ventricular arrhythmias, the limited availability of effective drugs often mandates that the clinician accept a reduction in frequency rather than complete elimination of the arrhythmia. The importance of establishing a therapeutic goal must be emphasized whenever drug-resistant arrhythmias are encountered. The clinician must constantly assess and reassess the risk-benefit ratio of each intervention for every patient. Patient risk usually mounts progressively with each escalation of therapy, particularly when multiple agents are employed. These challenges to the intellect must be balanced by common sense and empathy for the patient. This is not to imply that aggressive therapy is never warranted nor is it meant to encourage surrender in the face of a difficult problem.

TREATMENT OF PATIENTS WITH BRADYARRHYTHMIAS

A rate-induced fall in cardiac output can result in clinical signs suggesting either cardiac or cerebral dysfunction. Transient and sporadic cerebral hypoperfusion is often manifested as episodic ataxia, weakness, syncope, or seizures. Recurrent episodes of prolonged cerebral anoxia may result in permanent brain damage and behavioral changes.[61] Chronic and persistent bradyarrhythmias are characterized by the development of exercise intolerance, lethargy, or overt heart failure.[62,63] Symptomatic bradycardia in dogs results most commonly from heart block or sinoatrial (SA) dysfunction (sick sinus syndrome or persistent atrial standstill).[15,64–66] Clinical signs are rarely observed in dogs with sinus bradycardia, particularly when the heart rate is in excess of 40 beats/min.

Sinus Bradycardia

The vast majority of dogs presented with sinus bradycardia are asymptomatic (for the arrhythmia) and do not require treatment. Vague signs of lethargy or depression accompanying the finding of sinus bradycardia usually reflect the presence of some other underlying disease and are not a result of low cardiac output. This fact can readily be demonstrated by performing an atropine challenge test. Following atropine administration, 0.02 to 0.05 mg/kg IM, SC, the heart rate almost always increases dramatically and the behavior of the affected dog remains unchanged. Electrocardiograms recorded following atropine administration often show initial accentuation of the bradycardia and first- or second-degree heart block. After 10 to 20 minutes, this centrally mediated increase in vagal tone disappears and sinus rhythm or sinus tachycardia develops. This pattern of response is normal and should not be interpreted as evidence of disease.[67]

In young, athletic, or sleeping dogs, sinus bradycardia is physiologic and is readily abolished by atropine or exercise. Sinus bradycardia from hypothermia, hypothyroidism, or hypokalemia is usually accompanied by historic or clinical findings that suggest the underlying problem. Affected dogs are best managed by correction of the underlying cause. Intracranial tumors, meningitis, increased intracranial pressure, mediastinal and cervical masses, obstructive jaundice, and a variety of other respiratory and abdominal disorders can increase vagal or reduce sympathetic tone resulting in an atropine- or catecholamine-responsive bradycardia.[41] Rarely is the resulting bradycardia severe enough to induce clinical signs in the absence of underlying heart disease.

Drug-induced bradycardias are more variably atropine responsive and may result in clinical signs if the heart rate is sufficiently slowed. β-blocking agents, calcium-channel blockers, anesthetics, morphine, phenothiazines, xylazine, digitalis, and the parasympathomimetic drugs may all induce a pronounced sinus bradycardia. Management is most logically instituted by (1) removing or hastening the elimination of the offending drug; (2) increasing the heart rate with atropine, isoproterenol or a temporary pacemaker; and (3) providing general supportive therapy for the patient in the form of intravenous fluid therapy as well as alleviation of hypothermia. Specific antidotes should be administered when available.

In cats sinus bradycardia may result from causes similar to the dog. Most commonly, severe systemic or metabolic disorders or cardiogenic shock associated with systolic dysfunction (feline dilated cardiomyopathy) are causative. At rates of 90 to 160 beats/min, the arrhythmia itself is usually benign (unless associated with shock or heart failure). The underlying condition must be identified and managed.[3,4]

Heart Block

Symptomatic heart block occurs most often as an idiopathic disorder of middle-aged or older dogs.[64–66] In most instances, myocardial and valvular function is normal, and the manifested signs are entirely due to the rhythm disturbance. Heart block in dogs may also result from bacterial endocarditis, infiltrative or hypertrophic cardiomyopathy, digitalis intoxication, and hyperkalemia.[68,69] Congenital complete heart block also occurs.[70] Complete heart block has been recorded in cats afflicted with hypertrophic cardiomyopathy.[71] First-degree and low-grade second-degree heart block in the dog most commonly result from increased vagal tone or the direct effects of drugs such as digitalis. In most instances, dogs with low-grade heart block do not require therapy and can be managed similarly to dogs with sinus bradycardia as described in the preceding section. Occasionally, high-grade second-degree or third-degree heart block occurs intermittently in dogs. This diagnosis must be confirmed by recording the ECG during the arrhythmic event. A 24-hour continuous ambulatory ECG recording greatly facilitates documentation of these uncommon arrhythmias.[72]

The only reliable method for the long-term management of symptomatic bradycardia due to heart block is the successful implantation of a permanent artificial cardiac pacemaker.[51,64–66] Vagolytic and adrenergic drugs cannot be relied on to restore and maintain a stable cardiac rhythm. Isoproterenol or dopamine can be used temporarily to increase the rate of discharge of the ventricular escape rhythm. This form of therapy is variably effective and is occasionally complicated by the development of rapid ventricular rhythms. Under no circumstances should antiarrhythmic drugs be administered to affected dogs prior to pacemaker implantation. Reduction of the rate of administration of isoproterenol or dopamine usually suffices for the control of these ventricular arrhythmias. Stabilization of patients with symptomatic heart block is best accomplished by pacemaker implantation. Fluid therapy and positive inotropic therapy are unnecessary, nor are they indicated in most patients with complete heart block. An increased heart rate best accomplishes the elimination of signs due to heart failure or hypotension in these circumstances (Fig. 14-2). The prognosis in dogs with idiopathic heart block is favorable and depends mainly on the skill of the team responsible for pacemaker implantation.[51, 64–66] In animals with endocarditis, infiltrative or hypertrophic cardiomyopathy, the prognosis is determined by the severity of the primary disease and is usually guarded to poor.

Sinus Node Dysfunction

The ECG findings in dogs with sinus node dysfunction (sick sinus syndrome) include sinus bradycardia, sinus arrest, or SA block together with failure of subsidiary (lower) pacemakers to form an adequate escape mechanism. Sinus node dysfunction has been described in female miniature schnauzers, dachshunds, and pugs.[15,73] Supraventricular tachyarrhythmias are observed in many affected dogs. The segregation of patients with sinus node dysfunction into those with (group 1) and those without (group 2) episodes of sinus or supraventricular tachycardia should not be made without

long-term ambulatory ECG recordings.[72,74] Many human patients as well as dogs categorized into group 1 based on a resting ECG show a high prevalence of supraventricular tachycardia when studied by continuous ECG monitoring. Most dogs that are symptomatic from sinus node dysfunction demonstrate episodic weakness or syncope. Sudden death is extremely uncommon.

The goals of therapy in dogs with sinus node dysfunction include maintenance of a stable heart rate and elimination of bradycardic and tachycardic episodes. Bradyarrhythmias in these patients are most reliably treated by permanent pacemaker implantation. Once the bradycardia is controlled by pacemaker implantation, any tachyarrhythmias can be managed by appropriate drug therapy. In most cases, digoxin or propranolol are used to prevent episodes of symptomatic paroxysmal supraventricular tachycardia. Both agents may aggravate sinus arrest and increase the frequency and severity of syncopal episodes when a pacemaker is not used. Most often, bradyarrhythmias in patients with sinus node dysfunction are poorly responsive to atropine or isoproterenol. The maintenance of stable blood levels of an orally administered vagolytic drug (isopropamide or propantheline bromide) or adrenergic drug (isoproterenol) is not a realistic goal over the life of the patient.[75] When pacemaker implantation cannot be accomplished, these methods can be resorted to and occasionally reduce the number of syncopal events to an acceptable level (as judged by the owner). Isoproterenol, atropine, and other vagolytic drugs should not be administered to dogs with supraventricular tachyarrhythmias, as they may markedly aggravate these arrhythmias. Asymptomatic dogs with an abnormal ECG are not treated. Because pacemaker implantation in the dog is often complicated by significant morbidity and mortality, it may be preferable to educate the owner rather than to treat mildly symptomatic patients (see Fig. 14-2).

Atrial Standstill

Persistent atrial standstill has been reported in English springer spaniels in association with a facioscapulohumeral type of muscular dystrophy.[76] Similar rhythm disturbances have been recorded in dogs with inflammatory or infiltrative diseases of the

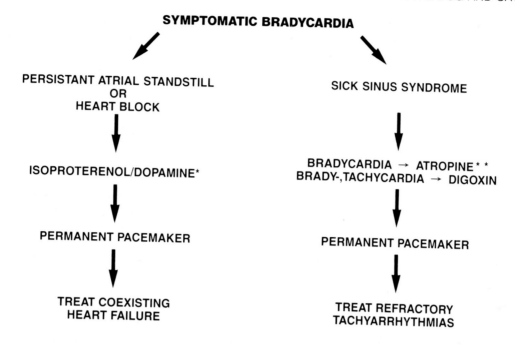

*Used only for temporary management by the intravenous route until pacing can be accomplished.
**Medical management not recommended for long-term therapy.

Fig. 14-2 Protocol for treating dogs and cats with symptomatic bradycardia. Successful long-term management relies heavily on the ability to implant an artificial pacemaker. In cats, management of underlying systemic or metabolic disorders or cardiomyopathy is usually required, as opposed to pacemaker implantation.

atrial myocardium.[77] In cats, persistent atrial standstill has been observed in association with dilated cardiomyopathy.[71] Once the diagnosis is made, therapy for persistent atrial standstill is similar to that described for complete heart block. An artificial pacemaker must be implanted to control the clinical signs. Evidence of myocardial failure is often present at the time of initial presentation or develops shortly after pacemaker implantation. This fact indicates that additional medical therapy may be required and that the long-term prognosis is uncertain in these patients.

More commonly encountered, however, is transient atrial standstill due to hyperkalemia resulting from lower urinary tract obstruction (especially in cats), renal failure or hypoadrenocorticism (Addison's disease).[3,30,35] Whenever the ECG features of this rhythm disorder are observed, hyperkalemia must be considered as a possibility and serum electrolyte levels determined. Therapy in such cases is

directed towards the immediate restoration of normal serum potassium levels and correction of the underlying disorder. When cardiac arrest appears imminent and additional time is required to lower serum potassium levels, calcium-containing solutions may be given intravenously to transiently antagonize the electrophysiologic effects of hyperkalemia.

TREATMENT OF PATIENTS WITH TACHYARRHYTHMIAS

Successful management of the pathologic tachycardias begins with characterization of the observed arrhythmia as ventricular or supraventricular. This differentiation is important because the classification and appropriate selection of antiarrhythmic drugs is based in large part on their ability to alter conduction, automaticity, or the effective refractory periods of specific cells found in the different regions of the heart. In the absence of cardiac hypertrophy or conduction disturbances, a normal QRS complex usually distinguishes a supraventricular from a ventricular arrhythmia. Occasionally, impulses from the atria are conducted aberrantly through the ventricles. This usually results from failure of recovery of a portion of the intraventricular conduction system. In most instances, the ECG characteristics of aberrantly conducted supraventricular beats resemble those of a right bundle branch block.[78] This is because the right bundle branch has the longest recovery time of the conduction system in most animals. Many other conduction patterns can occur, however. When ventricular arrhythmias originate high in the bundle of His, the resulting QRS complexes may have a normal configuration. These possibilities must always be considered, particularly, when a refractory arrhythmia is encountered.

When ventricular activation is abnormal and aberrancy is a consideration, other criteria for distinguishing ventricular from supraventricular rhythms should be sought. The relationship of P waves to QRS complexes often distinguishes supraventricular from ventricular arrhythmia. Ventricular tachycardias are often characterized by AV dissociation with the ventricular rate exceeding the atrial rate. The use of multiple leads and long tracings facilitates recognition of obscured P waves. When supraventricular tachycardias are sustained and characterized by aberrant conduction, vagal maneuvers may slow the rate sufficiently to permit recognition of P waves as they emerge from the T wave of the previous cycle. Identification of fusion or capture beats is important. Their presence indicates a diagnosis of a ventricular arrhythmia rather than aberrancy. When these methods fail, invasive electrodiagnostic evaluation, electric cardioversion, or response to medical therapy may satisfactorily supplement the ECG evaluation. Intravenous propranolol can be used as initial therapy safely in most patients wherein the ECG diagnosis is uncertain (Ch. 13).

Sinus Tachycardia

Sinus tachycardia is the expected physiologic response to exercise, pain, emotional stimuli, profound anemia, and inadequate tissue perfusion caused by hypovolemia or serious underlying heart disease. The diagnosis is usually straightforward and apparent from the patient's history and physical condition. Correction of the underlying problem by adequate fluid replacement, blood transfusions, or analgesics will usually eliminate the rapid heart rate and the need for therapy. Unless sinus tachycardia results in declining cardiac output or congestive signs, specific antiarrhythmic therapy is unnecessary. Propranolol has been advocated to slow the heart rate in cats with hyperthyroidism.[1–4,79] Most hyperthyroid cats can be rendered euthyroid in several days with propylthiouracil or methimazole. Definitive surgical therapy can be performed safely in most instances in 3 to 4 weeks, when the metabolic effects of the hyperthyroid state have abated. I do not recommend the routine use of propranolol in hyperthyroid cats. Although propranolol can be safely used in most affected cats, it can precipitate severe heart failure in cats with preexisting myocardial dysfunction.

In patients with signs of heart disease, sinus tachycardia resulting from increased sympathetic tone must occasionally be distinguished from a pathologic supraventricular tachycardia. The application of one or more vagal maneuvers, such as carotid sinus massage, ocular pressure, or provoking the diving reflex, often permits an accurate diagnosis in these circumstances. In dogs with sinus tachycardia, the heart rate usually slows gradually and transiently in response to vagal maneuvers. In contrast, when the rhythm is a reciprocating supraventricular tachycardia, vagal maneuvers often result in abrupt termination of the arrhythmia or transient heart block. When vagal maneuvers alone do not alter the heart rate, digoxin can be administered and the vagal maneuvers repeated, if necessary, to distinguish these arrhythmias. In addition, propranolol can be used to abolish the contribution of sympathetic tone or circulating catecholamines.

Supraventricular Tachycardias

The terminology of the supraventricular tachycardias is very confused in the literature. In this discussion, the term *supraventricular tachycardia* refers to any form of atrial or junctional tachycardia and excludes atrial flutter and atrial fibrillation. I prefer this usage because the surface electrocardiogram cannot reliably distinguish atrial from junctional foci.[41,52,80] Supraventricular tachycardias may occur with or without AV block and may be paroxysmal or sustained. The underlying mechanism of most supraventricular tachycardias is thought to be reentry, which may occur entirely within the SA node, in the atria, in the AV node, or may involve the combined participation of all these tissues.[80] In the presence of heart block, or when the arrhythmia is paroxysmal, supraventricular tachycardias are usually easily diagnosed. When supraventricular tachycardias are sustained, when the onset is unrecorded, and when QRS complexes are abnormal in form, the diagnosis is uncertain and is made accurately only if the possibility of aberrancy is considered. Supraventricular tachycardia may be observed in young patients with no other evidence of cardiac disease. In these circumstances, the possibility of pre-excitation via accessory AV pathways should be considered.

Short paroxysms of supraventricular tachycardia rarely produce signs in otherwise healthy animals. In these patients, therapy is not required unless there is a history of episodic weakness or collapse. Surprisingly, even sustained supraventricular tachycardias may be well tolerated in healthy animals, even when the heart rate exceeds 240 beats/min. However, the eventual development of heart failure is a well-documented sequela to sustained tachycardia indicating the absolute requirement for treatment in all patients with this arrhythmia.[81] In animals with structural heart disease, the hemodynamic consequences of these arrhythmias are serious and include profound hypotension and exacerbation of congestive heart failure. Sustained and paroxysmal supraventricular tachycardia often complicates those disorders wherein the atria are enlarged, such as mitral regurgitation in dogs and hypertrophic cardiomyopathy in cats.[1,2,4,32,33] Therapy is always indicated in these patients to abolish existing arrhythmia and to prevent future recurrences. Whenever supraventricular tachycardia occurs in a digitalized patient, the possibility of digitalis intoxication should be considered, particularly when AV block or AV dissociation is also present.

The goals of therapy in small animals with sustained supraventricular tachycardia include (1) slowing of excessively fast ventricular rates, (2) the restoration of sinus rhythm, (3) treatment of concurrently present heart disease, and (4) prevention of recurrence of the arrhythmia. Vagal maneuvers should be performed for initial management, as they may effect immediate restoration of sinus rhythm. If these efforts fail, pharmacologic agents are then given. The rationale of medical therapy is to prolong AV nodal refractoriness and to slow AV conduction by using drugs that have these electrophysiologic effects. Agents such as digoxin, propranolol, and verapamil may restore sinus rhythm by interrupting the reentry circuit or may simply slow the ventricular response by producing partial AV block. Vagal maneuvers should be tried following each pharmacologic intervention and before initiating additional drug therapy. If these efforts are unsuccessful, drugs that alter atrial myocardial refractoriness, such as quinidine or procainamide are given to dogs (but not cats). This approach also allows for the successful management of narrow QRS tachyarrhythmias that originate high in the bundle of His.

In the presence of heart failure or other evidence of hemodynamic instability, intravenous digoxin is indicated as the initial medicinal agent. If digitalization does not control the arrhythmia, intravenous propranolol is the usual alternative selected. Propranolol is administered cautiously and at low doses. It is repeated to effect, remaining cognizant of its negative inotropic effects, which can worsen congestive heart failure. Arrhythmias refractory to these therapies can often be terminated by intravenous verapamil, procainamide, quinidine, or, alternatively, by electric cardioversion. The relative merits of these latter therapies have not been critically evaluated in dogs or cats. Caution should be exercised with verapamil therapy, which can induce sinus arrest and high-grade heart block and with intravenous quinidine, which can evoke profound hypotension.[37,52] In asymptomatic patients, oral therapy is safer, and the same sequence of alternatives can be employed. Prophylactic therapy is usually necessary in affected animals. Digoxin is extremely well suited, by virtue of its required dosing interval, for chronic oral administration when long-term prophylaxis is desired.

In patients with atrial tachycardia and AV block or AV dissociation, digitalis is always withdrawn if intoxication is a possibility. All diuretics are also discontinued and serum potassium levels are evaluated. Hypokalemia is managed by cautious replacement therapy to avoid aggravation of existing heart block. Phenytoin or propranolol can be used to attempt control of excessive heart rates in canine patients (propranolol is used in cats). Paradoxically, supraventricular tachycardia with AV block is most effectively treated with digitalis in patients not already receiving this drug. If digoxin is ineffective, propranolol, quinidine, or procainamide can be judiciously added for dogs (only propranolol for cats). Digoxin should be avoided in patients with ventricular pre-excitation syndromes and widened QRS complexes. Aggravation of this tachyarrhythmia may result because digoxin often prolongs AV nodal refractoriness and shortens the refractory period of the accessory pathway providing favorable conditions for re-entry at very fast heart rates. The approach to small animal patients with supraventricular tachycardia is summarized in Figure 14-3.

Atrial Flutter and Atrial Fibrillation

Atrial flutter is an uncommon rhythm disorder in both dogs and cats.[1,2,4,71] The diagnosis of atrial flutter is straightforward when physiologic heart block permits recognition of characteristic saw-tooth-like flutter waves. The clinical associations and recommended therapy for this arrhythmia is identical to that of atrial fibrillation. At very rapid heart rates, atrial flutter resembles other supraventricular tachycardias. Fortunately, the therapeutic approach is similar for all these arrhythmias.

In contrast with atrial flutter, atrial fibrillation is one of the most common arrhythmias in the dog and is most often detected in dogs with the dilated form of cardiomyopathy or with advanced mitral regurgitation. Occasionally, atrial fibrillation is observed in dogs lacking other evidence of underlying heart disease. Atrial fibrillation has been observed in dogs following anesthesia and in dogs suffering from heatstroke, gastric dilation, or other serious trauma.[1,3,23,82,83] Atrial fibrillation also occurs in cats, albeit rarely. When it is recorded in this species, atrial fibrillation is frequently associated with hypertrophic cardiomyopathy.[1,2,4,33,71]

A logical goal of therapy for patients with atrial fibrillation is the restoration of sinus rhythm. Unfortunately, when the arrhythmia is chronic and when it is accompanied by underlying heart disease, conversion to sinus rhythm is difficult to achieve, whether by electric means or by quinidine administration.[1,83] Even when cardioversion succeeds, sinus rhythm cannot be maintained for a significant

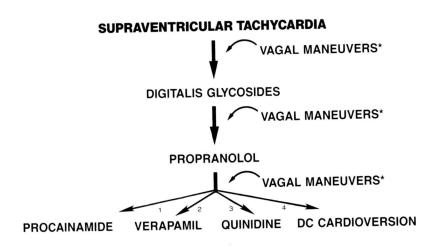

* Vagal maneuvers should be performed prior to each drug intervention.
1-4 Author's order of preference for the treatment of refractory arrhythmias.

Fig. 14-3 Protocol for treating sustained supraventricular tachycardia in dogs. This scheme can be modified for cats by omitting procainamide and quinidine. Reported clinical experience with verapamil and DC conversion is lacking.

period of time in these patients. For these reasons, efforts to restore sinus rhythm are confined to those dogs with little or no cardiac enlargement and adequate cardiac function. It is apparent that a thorough cardiovascular evaluation is mandatory in all dogs presenting with atrial fibrillation. Thoracic radiographs are necessary to detect signs of congestive heart failure and to evaluate heart size. Echocardiographic evaluation is particularly helpful for quantitative evaluation of cardiac function and atrial size. Most dogs with atrial fibrillation are large or giant breeds, and it is often difficult to know whether the arrhythmia is an early manifestation of developing myocardial disease or whether it represents a primary rhythm disturbance.

When atrial fibrillation is detected in a dog with a serious illness or in a dog recovering from recent trauma, no therapy is initially administered unless the ventricular rate is excessively fast (i.e., greater than 160 beats/min). Spontaneous reversion to sinus rhythm is a likely possibility if the heart is otherwise normal. If necessary, the ventricular rate can be slowed to acceptable levels with digoxin until the underlying illness or injury is resolved. If atrial fibrillation persists for more than 1 week, quinidine can be administered to encourage the conversion to sinus rhythm. Quinidine is also used to treat the occasional dog in which atrial fibrillation is detected as an incidental finding during routine physical examination. Aggressive follow-up and repeated recheck examination of these dogs is recommended because a significant number will probably develop signs of cardiomyopathy.

Most dogs with atrial fibrillation have obvious signs of advanced heart disease and heart failure. Digoxin is always indicated for the treatment of congestive heart failure in dogs with atrial fibrillation and a rapid heart rate. The primary goal of therapy with digoxin is a satisfactory reduction of the heart rate to about 120 to 160 beats/min. The precise heart rate attained is not as important as the improvement observed in the manifested clinical signs. If the dog is doing poorly and the heart rate remains elevated following digitalization, several options are available. First, adequate digitalization can be assessed either by evaluating serum digoxin levels or simply by modestly increasing the dose of digoxin. There is considerable individual variation in the serum level of digoxin tolerated by dogs; this

cannot be assessed without trial therapy. On the other hand, serum digoxin levels are useful in evaluating the possibility of marked underdosing. Other therapies designed to alleviate the heart failure state should be optimized as well. Alleviating pulmonary congestion and increasing cardiac output with diuretics, vasodilators, or angiotensin-converting enzyme inhibitors can reduce sympathetic tone and facilitate cardiac slowing.

When digitalization fails to slow the heart rate adequately, propranolol should be cautiously administered to accomplish this goal. Because of its negative inotropic effects, propranolol is initiated at low doses and the dose is gradually increased until a satisfactory response is attained (Chs. 8, 15, and 23). The value of other drugs, such as verapamil, in slowing the ventricular rate has not been adequately assessed in dogs with atrial fibrillation.[3,84] I do not recommend verapamil therapy until further studies have been reported. The approach to the treatment of dogs with atrial fibrillation is outlined in Figure 14-4.

Atrial fibrillation in cats relates directly to left atrial size.[32] Diseases of diastolic dysfunction (e.g., hypertrophic and restrictive cardiomyopathy) cause the greatest atrial enlargement.[2,4] Treatment is directed at the heart failure state and at slowing the ventricular rate. The latter is accomplished with either digitalis or propranolol, or both (Ch. 22).

Ventricular Premature Beats/ Ventricular Tachycardia

Ventricular arrhythmias are among the most common rhythm disturbances recorded in dogs and cats.[1-4] Premature beats and ventricular tachycardia are usually easily recognized on the ECG. Small animal patients with these arrhythmias can be categorized into four groups: group 1 patients are those that require immediate, intensive therapy due to impending ventricular fibrillation, circulatory collapse and death; group 2 patients are those that require prophylactic therapy to prevent a catastrophic arrhythmia; group 3 patients are those that require further monitoring prior to reclassification as group 2 or 4; and group 4 patients are those in which the arrhythmia can be safely ignored. The most formidable task in the management of ventricular arrhythmias is the evaluation and categorization of the

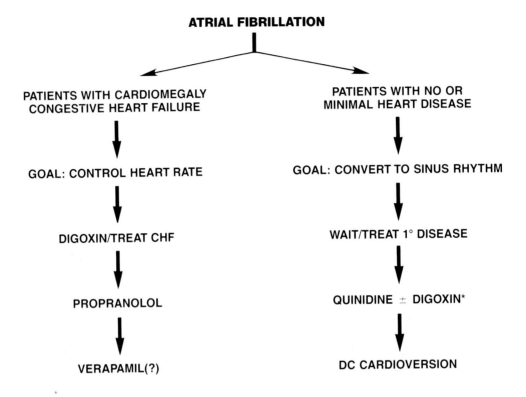

Fig. 14-4 Protocol for treating atrial fibrillation in dogs. Therapeutic strategies and goals are dependent on accurate cardiac structural and functional assessment (e.g., echocardiographic evaluation).

individual dog or cat with an arrhythmia. It must be appreciated that the identification of patients requiring therapy can never be made with 100 percent accuracy nor is the appropriate form of therapy obvious in all cases. As with other ECG disturbances, these judgments are best made by carefully evaluating each patient in order to determine the probable cause(s) of the arrhythmia, by accurately assessing the hemodynamic effects of the arrhythmia, and by making an informed judgement regarding the likelihood of progressive electric instability and sudden death.

Ventricular premature beats rarely cause significant hemodynamic impairment unless they are frequent. For this reason, the usual justification for the therapy of these arrhythmias is the prevention of a more serious arrhythmia. Ventricular premature beats are often classified on the basis of the following parameters:

1. Frequency—the number of premature beats per minute

2. Repetitiveness—singly occurring, bigeminal and trigeminal patterns, pairs and runs

3. Morphology—uniform (unifocal) or multiform (multifocal)

4. Coupling interval or proximity to the preceding beat—particularly in reference to the R-on-T phenomenon (i.e., the VPC occurs at the apex of the previous T wave)

Using these descriptors, certain warning arrhythmias have been defined that identify patients at risk of sudden death and in whom prophylactic therapy is indicated.[85,86] Thus, when the R-on-T phenomenon is observed, when more than 20 premature beats/min are recorded, when the premature complexes are multiform, or when pairs or runs of premature beats are observed, therapy is recommended.

It is noteworthy that these warning arrhythmias were originally identified in human patients with ischemic myocardial disease resulting from coronary insufficiency. With the possible exception of the R-on-T phenomenon, no clinical studies have been reported to confirm or repudiate the value of these criteria in species that rarely suffer from atherosclerosis. Other information may be of equal or greater value in making therapeutic decisions. These criteria are also borrowed from the experiences of cardiologists with human patients and include the following generalizations. Patients with premature ventricular beats should receive prophylactic therapy when (1) refractory heart failure is identified as a potential cause of the arrhythmia; (2) serious structural heart disease is identified, such as hypertrophic cardiomyopathy, dilated cardiomyopathy (particularly in boxers), advanced mitral regurgitation, and congenital defects, such as subvalvular aortic stenosis; (3) there is a history of unexplained weakness or collapse; and (4) an arrhythmia evidences progression to a more complex rhythm disorder and the primary disease of the patient is still evolving.[40,41,46,48,52]

Infrequent unifocal premature ventricular beats appear not to require treatment, particularly in healthy animals. In most instances, the arrhythmia is ignored or the patient is monitored as an outpatient for several weeks or months. If the rhythm disorder disappears or remains static, further evaluation is probably unnecessary. It is interesting that there is no convincing proof that the suppression of VPCs or even complex arrhythmias reduces the incidence of sudden death in healthy people.[50,87] It is not known whether the same holds true in dogs and cats. For this reason, the decision to treat, monitor, or ignore infrequent arrhythmias is often based on the whim of the attending clinician.

Ventricular tachycardia may be paroxysmal or sustained, have regular or irregular R-R intervals, be monomorphic, polymorphic, or pleomorphic in appearance, and may vary in rate from 60 to more than 200 beats/min. The management of ventricular tachycardia in dogs has also been modeled on therapeutic strategies devised in humans. Accelerated idioventricular rhythms are frequently observed in dogs that are acutely ill from some systemic disorder or that have been recently traumatized.[1,20,24–26] With this rhythm, uniform ventricular complexes occur at a rate of 60 to 140 beats/min, and the control of the cardiac rhythm is intermittently exchanged between the ventricular focus and the sinus node. This rhythm disorder rarely requires medical therapy, as it usually resolves spontaneously in 2 or 3 days. This is fortunate because this arrhythmia is difficult to suppress. Continuous ECG monitoring is prudent in affected dogs because a small percentage go on to develop more serious arrhythmias. Therapy is indicated when there is evidence of hemodynamic compromise of the patient, when serious underlying structural heart disease is present, or when this arrhythmia begins with a short coupling interval (R-on-T phenomenon).

Most other ventricular tachyarrhythmias are regarded as life threatening, and immediate therapy should be initiated. Life-threatening ventricular tachycardia is most appropriately managed by the administration of intravenous lidocaine. In the cat, lidocaine must be administered more slowly and in lower doses than in dogs.[1,2,71] Alternatively, electric cardioversion can be used, particularly in small animal patients that collapse from severe hemodynamic compromise. If lidocaine is ineffective, procainamide given intravenously is the best alternative for the treatment of dogs but it cannot be used in cats. Propranolol is the only other antiarrhythmic drug that can be safely administered intravenously to cats and is, therefore, the only practical alternative to lidocaine in this species. Propranolol is also used in dogs with arrhythmias refractory to both lidocaine and procainamide. Recently, bretylium has been accepted as the next line of defense, following lidocaine or procainamide therapy for ventricular tachycardia in human patients.[88,89] This agent is given intravenously over several minutes at a dose of 5 mg/kg and may be repeated at 15- to 30-minute intervals (dosages for humans). Bretylium does not always eliminate premature ventricular beats and in fact may transiently increase their frequency. It is very effective, however, for the prevention of ventricular fibrillation. Its value in dogs has not been critically evaluated. Quinidine can also be administered intravenously but it must be given very slowly. Quinidine often evokes profound hypotension and is usually a drug of last resort.

As these measures are being instituted, patient

evaluation must progress quickly and simultaneously. When profound hypotension is responsible for the initiation of the arrhythmia, vasoconstrictive therapies and fluid therapy may be life saving.[41] Acid-base and electrolyte disturbances must be restored to normal. If hypoxia initiated the event, the inciting cause must be identified and remedied. If digitalis toxicity is a likely cause, the slow infusion of potassium salts or phenytoin (in dogs) may effectively abort the arrhythmia. For refractory arrhythmias, striking the patient's chest (thump-version) may terminate ventricular tachycardia by mechanically inducing a premature systole that interrupts the re-entry circuit. Once the arrhythmia is successfully terminated, the emphasis of patient management is directed toward prevention of a recurrence. Antiarrhythmic therapy is usually continued by the intravenous route for several days and then switched to the oral or intramuscular route, depending on the individual requirements of the patient. The approach to patients with ventricular tachycardia is summarized in Figure 14-5.

Ventricular Flutter/Ventricular Fibrillation

Ventricular fibrillation is the terminal event in patients dying from a variety of causes, including many of the arrhythmias already discussed. Ventricular flutter resembles a sine wave in appearance while ventricular fibrillation is recognized by the presence of irregular undulations of the ECG tracing. There is no practical point to be made by distinguishing these arrhythmias from each other. The only reliable treatment for these arrhythmias is immediate electrical defibrillation.[41,53] If asystole or ventricular fibrillation suddenly develops, time should not be wasted recording an ECG or intubating the patient. When there is no heartbeat, an electric shock should immediately be administered.

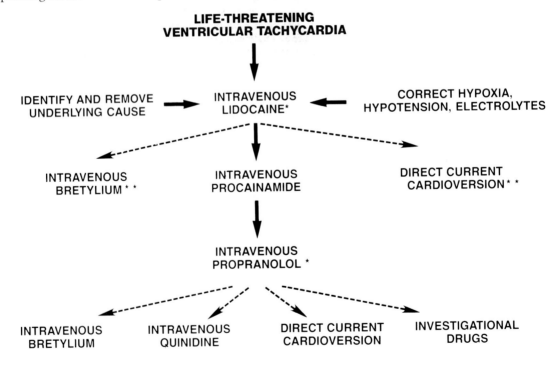

Fig. 14-5 Protocol for treating life-threatening ventricular tachycardia in dogs and cats. Immediate drug therapy combined with rapid identification and correction of precipitating or contributing causes are essential.

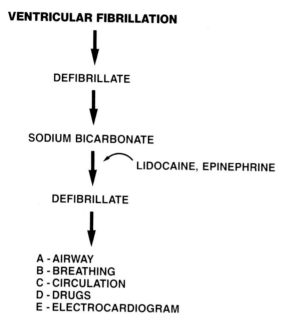

VENTRICULAR FIBRILLATION

↓

DEFIBRILLATE

↓

SODIUM BICARBONATE

↓ ⌒ LIDOCAINE, EPINEPHRINE

DEFIBRILLATE

↓

A - AIRWAY
B - BREATHING
C - CIRCULATION
D - DRUGS
E - ELECTROCARDIOGRAM

Fig. 14-6 Protocol for treating ventricular flutter or fibrillation in dogs and cats. Early electrical defibrillation, repeated if necessary, represents the best hope for successful resuscitation.

The ABCDE steps of resuscitation should not delay this intervention. The success of therapy is determined primarily by the interval of time between the onset of the arrhythmia and the administration of the electric shock.[90] If defibrillation is initially ineffective, sodium bicarbonate can be used to counteract the rapidly developing metabolic acidosis. Lidocaine and epinephrine can also be administered, but the most important therapy is the deliverance of another electric shock (Ch. 17).

The initial energy dose for ventricular defibrillation is 0.5 to 10 watt-sec/kg (W-sec/kg) when electrodes are applied externally to the chest wall.[91,92] The energy necessary for defibrillation is extremely variable; the most practical guidelines have been reported by Haskins[92] on the basis of patient weight:

<7 kg: 2 W-sec/kg

8–40 kg: 5 W-sec/kg

>40 kg: 5–10 W-sec/kg

Subsequent shocks should be delivered at twice the

initial dose. After successful defibrillation, immediate measures are taken to prevent a recurrence (Fig. 14-6). The cardiac rhythm must be monitored, the patient stabilized, and prophylactic antiarrhythmic therapy administered until the patient is out of danger.

REFERENCES

1. Tilley LP: Essentials of Canine and Feline Electrocardiography. 2nd Ed. Lea & Febiger, Philadelphia, 1985

2. Fox PR: Feline arrhythmias. p. 251. In Bonagura JD (ed): Contemporary Issues in Small Animal Practice. Vol. 7: Cardiology. Churchill Livingstone, New York, 1987

3. Fox PR: Cardiovascular disorders in systemic diseases. p. 265. In Tilley LP, Owens JM (eds): Manual of Small Animal Cardiology. Churchill Livingstone, New York, 1985

4. Fox PR: Feline myocardial diseases: A clinical approach. p. 57. In Proceedings of the Ninth Annual Kal Kan Symposium. Kal Kan Foods Inc, Vernon, CA, 1986

5. Bohn FK, Patterson DF, Pyle RL: Atrial fibrillation in dogs. Br Vet J 127:485, 1971

6. Lombard CW: Echocardiographic and clinical signs of canine dilated cardiomyopathy. J Small Anim Pract 25:59, 1984

7. Calvert CA, Chapman WL, Toal, RL: Congestive cardiomyopathy in Doberman Pinscher dogs. J Am Vet Med Assoc 181:598, 1982

8. Harpster N: Boxer cardiomyopathy. p. 329. In Kirk RW (ed): Current Veterinary Therapy. Vol. VIII. WB Saunders, Philadelphia, 1983

9. Bolton GR, Ettinger S: Paroxysmal atrial fibrillation in the dog. J Am Vet Med Assoc 158:64, 1971

10. Liu S-K, Maron BJ, Tilley LP: Canine hypertrophic cardiomyopathy. J Am Vet Med Assoc 174:708, 1979

11. Liu S-K, Tilley LP, Tashjian RJ: Lesions of the conduction system in the cat with cardiomyopathy. Recent Adv Stud Cardiac Struct Metab 10:681, 1975

12. Meierhenry EF, Liu S-K: Atrioventricular bundle degeneration associated with sudden death in the dog. J Am Vet Med Assoc 172:1418, 1978

13. James TN, Drake EH: Sudden death in Doberman Pinschers. Ann Intern Med 68:821, 1968

14. James TN, Robertson BT, Walso AL, et al: De subitaneis mortibus. XV. Hereditary stenosis of the His bundle in Pug dogs. Circulation 52:1152, 1975

15. Hamlin RL, Smetzer DL, Breznock EM: Sinoatrial syncope in Miniature Schnauzers. J Am Vet Med Assoc 161:1023, 1972

16. Muir WW: Electrocardiographic interpretation of thiobarbiturate-induced dysrhythmias in dogs. J Am Vet Med Assoc 170:1419, 1977

17. Buss DD, Hess RE, Webb AI, Spencer KR: Incidence of postanaesthetic arrhythmias in the dog. J Small Anim Pract 23:399, 1982

18. Zenoble RD, Hill BL: Hypothermia and associated cardiac arrhythmias in two dogs. J Am Vet Med Assoc 175:840, 1979

19. King JM, Roth L, Haschek M: Myocardial necrosis secondary to neural lesions in domestic animals. J Am Vet Med Assoc 180:144, 1982

20. Macintire DK, Synder TG III: Cardiac arrhythmias associated with multiple trauma in dogs. J Am Vet Med Assoc 184:541, 1984

21. King JM, Roth L, Haschek WM: Myocardial necrosis secondary to neural lesions in domestic animals. J Am Vet Med Assoc 180:144, 1982

22. D'Agrosa LS: Cardiac arrhythmias of sympathetic origin in the dog. Am J Physiol 233:H535, 1977

23. Muir WW: Gastric dilatation-volvulus in the dog, with emphasis on cardiac arrhythmias. J Am Vet Med Assoc 180:739, 1982

24. Muir WW, Bonagura JD: Treatment of cardiac arrhythmias in dogs with gastric distention-volvulus. J Am Vet Med Assoc 184:1366, 1984

25. Muir WW, Lipowitz AJ: Cardiac dysrhythmias associated with gastric dilatation-volvulus in the dog. J Am Vet Med Assoc 172:683, 1978

26. Muir WW, Weisbrode SE: Myocardial ischemia in dogs with gastric dilatation-volvulus. J Am Vet Med Assoc 181:363, 1982

27. Vassalle M, Greenspan K, Hoffman BK: An analysis of arrhythmias induced by ouabain in intact dogs. Circ Res 13:132, 1963

28. Wilmshurst PT, Webb-Preploe MM: Side effects of amrinone therapy. Br Heart J 49:447, 1983

29. Packer M: Vasodilator and inotropic therapy for severe chronic heart failure: Passion and skepticism. J Am Coll Cardiol 2:841, 1983

30. Schaer M: Hyperkalemia in cats with urethral obstruction: Electrocardiographic abnormalities and treatment. Vet Clin North Am 7:407, 1977

31. Watanabe Y: Antagonism and synergism of potassium and antiarrhythmic drugs. p. 68. In Bajusz (ed): Electrolytes and Cardiovascular Disease. S Karger, Basel, 1966

32. Boyden PA, Tilley LP, Liu S-K, et al: The effects of atrial dilatation on atrial cellular electrophysiology: Studies on cats with spontaneous cardiomyopathy. Circulation 56(suppl 3):II-48, 1977 (abst)

33. Boyden PA, Tilley LP, Pham TD: Effects of left atrial enlargement on atrial transmembrane potentials and structure in dogs with mitral valve fibrosis. Am J Cardiol 49:1896, 1982

34. Pitt B: Evaluation of the patient with congestive heart failure and ventricular arrhythmias. Am J Cardiol 57:19B, 1986

35. Willard MD, Schall WD, McCaw DE: Canine hypoadrenocorticism: Report of 37 cases and review of 39 previously reported cases. J Am Vet Med Assoc 180:59, 1982

36. Keene BW, Hamlin RL: Prophylaxis and treatment of digitalis-enhanced dysrhythmias with phenytoin in the dog. p. 118. In Proceedings of the American College of Veterinary Intern Medicine, Washington, DC, 1980 (abst)

37. Kawai C, Kanish T, Matsuyama E, Okazaki H: Comparative effects of three calcium antagonists, diltiazem, verapamil, and nifedipine on the sinoatrial and atrioventricular nodes. Experimental and clinical studies. Circulation 63:1035, 1981

38. Katz MJ, Zitnik RS: Direct current shock and lidocaine in the treatment of digitalis-induced ventricular tachycardia. Am J Cardiol 18:552, 1966

39. Musselman EE: Arrhythmogenic properties of thiamylal sodium in the dog. J Am Vet Med Assoc 168:145, 1976

40. Parmley WW, Chatterjee MB: Congestive heart failure and arrhythmias: An overview. Am J Cardiol 57:34B, 1986

41. Zipes DP: Arrhythmias. p. 167. In Andreoli KG, Fowkes VK, Zipes DP, Wallace AG (eds): Comprehensive Cardiac Care. CV Mosby, St Louis, 1983

42. Stewart HJ, Crawford JH, Hastings AB: The effect of tachycardia on the blood flow in dogs. I. The effect of rapid irregular rhythms as seen in auricular fibrillation. J Clin Invest 3:435, 1926

43. Yoran C, Yellin EL, Hori M, et al: Effects of heart rate on experimentally produced mitral regurgitation in dogs. Am J Cardiol 52:1345, 1983

44. Wichman J, Ertl G, Rudolph G, et al: Effect of experimentally induced atrial fibrillation on coronary circulation in dogs. Basic Res Cardiol 78:473, 1983

45. Sinno MZ, Gunnar RM: Hemodynamic consequences of cardiac dysrhythmias. Med Clin North Am 60:69, 1976

46. Vlay SC, Reid PR: Ventricular ectopy: Etiology, evaluation, and therapy. Am J Med 73:899, 1982

47. Pyle RL, Patterson DF, Chacko S: The genetics and pathology of discrete subaortic stenosis in the Newfoundland dog. Am Heart J 92:324, 1976

48. Francis GS: Development of arrhythmias in the patient with congestive heart failure: Pathophysiology, prevalence, and prognosis. Am J Cardiol 57:3B, 1986

49. Calvert CA: Dilated congestive cardiomyopathy in Doberman Pinschers. Compendium Cont Educ 8:417, 1986

50. Kennedy HL, Underhill SJ. Frequent or complex ventricular ectopy in apparently healthy subjects. A clinical study of 25 cases. Am J Cardiol 38:141, 1976

51. Fox PR, Matthiesen DT, Purse D, Brown NO: Ventral abdominal, transdiaphragmatic approach for implantation of cardiac pacemakers in the dog. J Am Vet Med Assoc 189:1303, 1986

52. Foster PR, Zipes DP: Pacing and cardiac arrhythmias. p. 605. In Mandel WJ (ed): Cardiac Arrhythmias—Their Mechanisms, Diagnosis, and Management. JB Lippincott, Philadelphia, 1980

53. Standards and guidelines for cardiopulmonary resuscitation (CPR) and emergency cardiac care (ECC). JAMA 244:453, 1980

54. Vaughan Williams EM: Classification of antiarrhythmic drugs. J Pharmacol Exp Ther 1:115, 1975

55. Bigger JT: Arrhythmias and antiarrhythmic drugs. Ann Intern Med 18:251, 1972

56. Gettes LS: On the classification of antiarrhythmic drugs. Mod Concepts Cardiovasc Dis 48:13, 1978

57. Zipes DP: Genesis of cardiac arrhythmias: Electrophysiological considerations. p. 581. In Braunwald E (ed): The Heart. WB Saunders, Philadelphia, 1988

58. Velebit V, Podrid P, Lown B, et al: Aggravation and provocation of ventricular arrhythmias by antiarrhythmic drugs. Circulation 65:886, 1982

59. Leahey EB Jr, Bigger JT Jr, Butler VP Jr, et al: Quindine-digoxin interaction: Time course and pharmacokinetics. Am J Cardiol 48:1141, 1981

60. Doering W: Digoxin-quinidine interaction. N Engl J Med 301:400, 1979

61. Meierhenry EF, Liu S-K: Atrioventricular bundle degeneration associated with sudden death in the dog. J Am Vet Med Assoc 172:1418, 1978

62. Lombard C, Tilley LP, Yoshioka M: Pacemaker implantation in the dog: Survey and literature review. J Am Anim Hosp Assoc 17:751, 1981

63. Bonagura JD, Helphrey ML, Muir WW: Complications associated with pacemaker implantation in the dog. J Am Vet Med Assoc 182:149, 1983

64. Lombard C, Tilley LP, Yoshioka M: Pacemaker implantation in the dog: Survey and literature review. J Am Anim Hosp Assoc 17:751, 1981

65. Bonagura JD, Helphrey ML, Muir WW: Complications associated with pacemaker implantation in the dog. J Am Vet Med Assoc 182:149, 1983

66. Sisson D: Permanent transvenous pacemaker implantation in the dog. In Proceedings of the Fourth Annual Veterinary Medical Forum 13:101, 1986

67. Averill KH, Lamb LE: Less commonly recognized actions of atropine on cardiac rhythm. Am J Med Sci 237:304, 1959

68. Robertson BT, Giles HD: Complete heart block associated with endocarditis in a dog. J Am Vet Med Assoc 161:180, 1972

69. Liu S-K, Maron BJ, Tilley LP: Canine hypertrophic cardiomyopathy. J Am Vet Med Assoc 174:708, 1979

70. Dear MG: Complete atrioventricular block in the dog: A possible congenital case. J Small Anim Pract 11:17, 1970

71. Tilley LP: Identification and therapy of cardiac arrhythmias in the cat. p. 41. In Proceedings of the Ninth Annual Kal Kan Symposium. Kal Kan Foods Inc, Vernon, CA, 1985

72. Woodfield JA, Thomas WP, Sisson DD: Diagnostic value of continuous ambulatory electrocardiography in detection of arrhythmia in dogs. Proceedings of the Fourth Annual Veterinary Medical Forum 14:55, 1986

73. Branch CE, Robertson BT, Becket SD, et al: An animal model of spontaneous syncope and sudden death. J Lab Clin Med 90:592, 1977

74. Crook BRM, Cashman PMM, Stott FD, et al: Tape monitoring of the electrocardiogram in ambulatory patients with sinoatrial disease. Br Heart J 35:1009, 1973

75. Marriott HJL, Myerburg RJ: Recognition and treatment of cardiac arrhythmias and conduction disturbances. p. 637. In Hurst JW (ed): The Heart. 4th Ed. McGraw-Hill, New York, 1978

76. Tilley LP, Liu S-K: Persistent atrial standstill in the dog and cat. p. 43. Scientific Proceedings of the American College of Veterinary Internal Medicine, New York, 1980 (abst)

77. Jeraj K, Ogburn PN, Edwards WD, et al: Atrial standstill, myocarditis and destruction of the cardiac conduction system: Clinicopathologic correlation in a dog. Am Heart J 99:185, 1980

78. Tilley LP: Aberrant ventricular conduction, a common ECG entity in the dog and cat. Proceedings of the Fourth Annual Veterinary Medical Forum 13:99, 1986

79. Birchard SJ, Peterson ME, Jacobson A: Surgical treatment of feline hyperthyroidism: Results of 85 cases. J Am Anim Hosp Assoc 20:705, 1984

80. Bigger JT, Goldreyer BN: The mechanism of supraventricular tachycardia. Circulation 42:673, 1970

81. Goldberger E: Supraventricular arrhythmias. p. 80. In Goldberg E (ed): The Treatment of Cardiac Emergencies. 3rd Ed. CV Mosby, St Louis, 1982

82. Bonagura JD, Ware WA: Atrial fibrillation in the dog: Clinical findings in 81 cases. J Am Anim Hosp Assoc 22:111, 1986

83. Ettinger SJ: Arrhythmias: Disturbances of the cardiac rate and rhythm. In Ettinger SJ, Suter PF (eds): Canine Cardiology. WB Saunders, Philadelphia, 1970

84. Johnson JT: Conversion of atrial fibrillation in two dogs using verapamil and supportive therapy. J Am Anim Hosp Assoc 21:429, 1985

85. Lown B, Wolf M: Approaches to sudden death from coronary heart disease. Circulation 44:130, 1971

86. Bigger JT, Wenger TL, Heisenbuttel RH: Limitations of the Lown grading system for the study of human ventricular arrhythmias. Am Heart J 93:727, 1977

87. Montague TJ, McPherson DD, Mackenzie BR, et al: Frequent ventricular ectopic activity without underlying cardiac disease: Analysis of 45 subjects. Am J Cardiol 52:980, 1983

88. Haynes RE, Tina CL, Copass MK, et al: Comparison of bretylium tosylate and lidocaine in the management of out-of-hospital ventricular fibrillation. A randomized clinical trial. Am J Cardiol 48:353, 1981

89. Bacaner M: Prophylaxis and therapy of ventricular fibrillation: Bretylium reviewed, lidocaine refuted. Int J Cardiol 4:133, 1983

90. Yakaitis RW, Every GA, Otto CW, et al: Influence of time and therapy on ventricular defibrillation in dogs. Crit Care Med 8:157, 1980

91. Geddes LA, Tacker WA, Rosborough JP et al: Electrical dose for ventricular defibrillation of large and small animals using precordial electrodes. J Clin Invest 53:310, 1974

92. Haskins SC: Cardiopulmonary resuscitation. Compendium. Cont Educ 4:170, 1982

15

Pharmacology and Pharmacokinetics of Antiarrhythmic Drugs

William W. Muir III
Richard A. Sams

The development and use of drugs to control heart rate and rhythm are firmly based on the knowledge that many cardiac arrhythmias result in deterioration of hemodynamics that could predispose to a fatal event.[1,2] The spectrum of drugs potentially useful as primary or secondary therapy for a cardiac arrhythmia often depends on the factors responsible for initiating the arrhythmia (Table 15-1). Cardiac arrhythmias induced by acid-base, electrolyte, and other local environmental disturbances (e.g., hypoxia, hypercarbia) are most appropriately treated by eliminating the cause. More specific and effective antiarrhythmic drug therapy, however, is indicated when the primary cause for the arrhythmia is irreversible (acquired or congenital heart disease) or cannot be eliminated within a relatively short period of time (e.g., ischemia, trauma, toxins). Ultimately, the proper choice of an antiarrhythmic drug should be founded on a thorough knowledge of the mechanisms responsible for the arrhythmia, the pharmacologic and pharmacodynamic properties of the

antiarrhythmic drug chosen, and the potential for drug toxicity and drug-drug interactions.

The cellular mechanisms and proposed hypotheses for the development and maintenance of cardiac arrhythmias (e.g., re-entry, automaticity, re-excitation) have been reviewed (Ch. 13). Unfortunately, the various hypotheses of arrhythmogenesis are not always easily applied to clinical situations, often making the choice for which antiarrhythmic drug or drugs to use empirical. Furthermore, the development of clinical arrhythmias is oftentimes multifactoral, making it difficult to assign specific antiarrhythmic drug therapy.[3] Categorization of antiarrhythmic drugs into various classes, however, has helped in highlighting their proposed mechanism(s) of action and in offering reasonable substitutes should adjunctive or alternative drug therapy be required.[4,5] This chapter describes the various classes of drugs used to treat cardiac arrhythmias, their pharmacology and pharmacokinetics, and indications for usage in dogs and cats.

Table 15-1 Common Clinical Causes
of Cardiac Arrhythmias

Central nervous system disease or trauma
Peripheral or reflex mediated alterations in neural tone
Infections (viral or bacterial)
Degenerative or fibrotic conditions
Congenital or acquired heart disease
Neurohumoral and endocrine influences
Acid-base and electrolyte disturbances
Hypoxia, hypercarbia, and temperature changes
Ischemia
Toxic substances and drugs

CLINICAL PHARMACOKINETICS

The pharmacologic effects of most drugs affecting the cardiovascular system are assumed to be a function of the drug concentration at various sites within the body. The concentration of a drug at these sites is a function of its rate and extent of absorption, distribution processes, metabolism, excretion, and protein binding. The development of safe and effective dosage regimens depends on the derivation of various pharmacokinetic parameters and knowledge of effective plasma concentrations of the drug. For example, the dose rate required to maintain an average or steady-state plasma drug concentration is obtained by the following equation:

Dose rate = total body clearance

$$\times \text{ average plasma drug concentration}$$

If the extent of bioavailability of a specific route of administration is known, the dose rate needs to be modified by dividing the right-hand side of the equation by the bioavailability. When the maximum and minimum plasma drug concentrations desired are known, the maximum time interval between doses can be calculated:

Time interval = $1.44 \times$ half-life

$$\times \ln \frac{\text{maximum plasma drug concentration}}{\text{minimum plasma drug concentration}}$$

where ln is the natural logarithm.

The time required to achieve steady-state plasma drug concentrations after initiating constant intravenous infusion or multiple dosing is approximately four half-lives of the drug. If it is necessary to achieve therapeutic drug concentrations more rapidly, a loading dose can be given at the time that the constant infusion or multiple dosing regimen is started. The loading dose is calculated:

Loading dose = desired plasma drug concentration

$$\times \text{ volume of distribution}$$

Early drug concentrations will be greater than desired if the drug is extensively distributed. Therefore, if the drug has a low therapeutic index, the loading dose should be divided or given slowly. Again, if bioavailability is incomplete, the appropriate correction can be made by dividing the right-hand side of the equation by the bioavailability.

Clearance is the most important term in defining the disposition of a drug. Individual organ clearances added together equal the total body clearance:

$$CL = CL_{\text{renal}} + CL_{\text{liver}} + CL_{\text{other}}$$

where CL represents clearance and subscripts indicate the organ involved. Other may represent lung, saliva, sweat, and additional sites of metabolism. If it is known, for example, that the drug is eliminated primarily by hepatic metabolism, the total body clearance approximates hepatic clearance.

Individual organ clearances can be expressed as follows:

$$CL = \text{organ blood flow} \times \text{extraction ratio}$$

The extraction ratio is an expression of the fraction of the drug molecules entering the organ that are removed by the organ. The extraction ratio ranges from zero for a noneliminating organ to unity for an organ that removes all drug molecules entering the organ. The maximum clearance of an organ can therefore equal the total blood flow to the organ.

The hepatic extraction ratio is approximated as follows:

$$E_{\text{hepatic}} = \frac{f_u \times CL_{\text{intrinsic}}}{Q_{\text{hepatic}} + f_u \times CL_{\text{intrinsic}}}$$

where f_u is the fraction of the drug unbound in blood, $CL_{\text{intrinsic}}$ is the intrinsic metabolic clearance, and Q_{hepatic} is the total hepatic blood flow rate. Hepatic clearance is therefore approximated by the following equation:

$$CL_{\text{hepatic}} = Q_{\text{hepatic}} \frac{f_\mu \times CL_{\text{intrinsic}}}{Q_{\text{hepatic}} + f_\mu \times CL_{\text{intrinsic}}}$$

If hepatic blood flow is much greater than the product of unbound fraction and intrinsic clearance, hepatic clearance reduces to the following equation:

$$CL_{hepatic} = fu \times CL_{intrinsic}$$

For drugs cleared in this manner, hepatic clearance is dependent on the unbound fraction and the intrinsic clearance but relatively independent of liver blood flow rate. Therefore, hepatic clearance of such low-extraction drugs will be influenced or affected by drug interactions and disease processes that affect protein binding of drugs and their intrinsic clearances. Intrinsic clearance, in turn, depends on the properties of hepatic microsomal enzymes which are subject to enzyme induction and enzyme inhibition.

In other cases in which the hepatic blood flow is less than the product of the unbound fraction and the intrinsic clearance, the hepatic clearance is approximated by the equation

$$CL_{hepatic} = Q_{hepatic}$$

Therefore, hepatic clearances of such "high-extraction" drugs will depend only on hepatic blood flow rates. The clearances of these drugs (e.g., propranolol and lidocaine) will not be significantly affected by alterations in plasma protein binding or intrinsic clearance.

The extent of oral bioavailability is determined not only by the fraction of the dose that is absorbed but also by the fraction of the absorbed dose that escapes hepatic metabolism. The latter fraction is readily estimated from the expression

$$F = 1 - E_{hepatic}$$

where F is the fraction of the absorbed dose escaping first-pass metabolism and $E_{hepatic}$ is the extraction ratio. First-pass metabolism of highly extracted drugs, such as lidocaine and propranolol, will be high, and the fraction escaping first-pass metabolism will be low. The converse is true for low-extraction drugs, such as phenytoin and tocainide.

CLASSIFICATION OF ANTIARRHYTHMIC DRUGS

Ultimately, the cause of all cardiac arrhythmias can be linked to the changes induced in the cellular membrane potential. Antiarrhythmic drugs have been classified into four groups on the basis of their electrophysiologic properties[5] (Table 15-2). It is hoped that this classification scheme will prove useful in the years to come.

Class 1 antiarrhythmic drugs are frequently referred to as membrane stabilizers and produce their principal electrophysiologic effects by depressing transmembrane sodium flux. Many of the drugs within this class also produce local anesthetic effects. The electrophysiologic alterations induced by the decrease in sodium flux are decreased automaticity, slowed conduction, prolonged refractoriness, and variable effects on action potential duration. Class 1 antiarrhythmic drugs have been subdivided into three groups (1A, 1B, 1C) on the basis of their ability to slow conduction velocity and alter action potential duration (Table 15-2). *Class 1A* drugs (which include quinidine, procainamide, and disopyramide) depress phase 0 of the action potential, depress conduction velocity, prolong action potential duration, and delay repolarization. Lidocaine, mexiletine, tocainide, and phenytoin are members of *class 1B*. They produce little to no effect on phase 0 of the action potential or conduction velocity in normal heart tissue, shorten action potential duration, and increase ventricular fibrillation threshold. *Class 1C* drugs (e.g., flecainide) cause marked depression of phase 0 of the action potential and conduction velocity but produce minimal effects on repolarization and refractoriness. The divergent electrophysiologic effects of the class 1 subgroups are characterized in Table 15-3.

Class 2 antiarrhythmic drugs produce antisympathetic or sympatholytic effects (Table 15-2). Although many antiarrhythmic drugs are noted for their effects on autonomic tone (Table 15-4), class 2 drugs include the β-adrenoceptor-blocking drugs and drugs with both α- and β-adrenoceptor antagonistic activity (e.g., lobetalol). This class of drugs produces their principal antiarrhythmic effects by inhibiting the stimulation of cardiac adrenergic receptors, particularly $β_1$-adrenoceptors. The role of $α_1$-adrenoceptor stimulation in producing cardiac arrhythmias was recently emphasized in acute ischemic and anesthetic (halothane, cyclopropane) feline and canine arrhythmia models.[6,7] These studies suggest that $α_1$-adrenoceptor stimulation may be important in spontaneously occurring arrhythmias and lends support to the clinical use of mixed α- and

Table 15-2 Classification and Electrophysiology of Antiarrhythmic Drugs

	Class 1A	Class 1B	Class 1C	Class 2	Class 3	Class 4
	Quinidine[a]	Lidocaine[a]	Flecainide[a]	Propranolol[a]	Amiodarone[a]	Verapamil[a]
	Procainamide	Tocainide	Encainide	Nadolol	Bretylium	Diltiazem
	Disopyramide	Mexiletine	Lorcainide[b]	Timolol	Bethanidine[b]	Nifedipine
	Acecainide[b]	Phenytoin	Propafenone[b]	Pindolol	Sotalol[b]	Gallopamil[b]
	Cibenzoline[b]	Aprindine[b]	Indecainide[b]	Atenolol	Clofilium[b]	Tiapamil[b]
	Pirmenol[b]	Ethmozine[b]		Metoprolol	Amiloride[b]	Nisoldipine[b]
	Ajmaline[b]			Acebutolol	N-acetylproca-	Nimodipine[b]
				Labetalol	inamide[b]	
				Sotalol[b]		
				Esmolol		

Effect of Drug on:

Normal automaticity	+	+/−	+	+	+	+
Abnormal automaticity	+	+	+	+/−	−	+
Triggered activity	−	−	−	+	−	+
Early and delayed after depolarizations	−/+	+	−	−	−	+
Re-entry	+	+	+	−	+	−
Fibrillation threshold	+/−	+	−	+/−	+	−

[a] First drug listed in each class is a prototypical drug.
[b] Investigational.
+, Effective; −, ineffective.

β-adrenoceptor-blocking drugs for known causes of arrhythmias. Clinically, the potentially beneficial effects of adrenoceptor-blocking drugs are dependent on the prevailing level of sympathetic tone. Larger drug dosages are required when sympathetic tone is high. Quinidine-like or membrane-stabilizing properties are frequently ascribed to many of

Table 15-3 Electrophysiologic Effects of Class I Antiarrhythmic Drugs

Electrophysiologic Characteristic	Class		
	Class 1A	Class 1B	Class 1C
Rate of rise of phase 0	↓	—	↓↓
Conduction velocity	↓	—	↓↓
Action potential duration	↑	↓	—

↓, decrease; ↑, prolong; —, little effect.

the β-adrenoceptor-blocking drugs, but they do not play a significant role in producing clinically relevant antiarrhythmic effects. Similarly, β_1 cardioselectivity, intrinsic sympathomimetic activity, and potency ratio do not appear to contribute to the antiarrhythmic effectiveness of this class of drugs.[8]

Compounds that prolong action potential duration and refractoriness without significantly depressing the rate of phase 0 or conduction velocity comprise *class 3* antiarrhythmic drugs (Table 15-2). Class 3 antiarrhythmic drugs are noted not only for their antiarrhythmic effects but for their purported ability to terminate and prevent ventricular fibrillation as well.[9] Clinical experience employing class 3 antiarrhythmic drugs (amiodarone, bretylium) as treatment for supraventricular or ventricular arrhythmias is limited in veterinary medicine and has not provided optimistic results.

Table 15-4 Sympathetic and Parasympathetic Effects of Antiarrhythmic Drugs

Drug	Sympathetic Effects	Parasympathetic Effects
Quinidine	α-Adrenoceptor blocker; β_1-stimulation?	Vagolytic
Procainamide	Ganglion blocking	
Disopyramide		Vagolytic
Lidocaine		
Phenytoin	Sympatholytic-CNS effect	
Tocainide		
Mexiletine		
Flecainide		Mild vagolytic
Propranolol	$\beta_{1,2}$-Adrenoceptor blocker	
Nadolol	$\beta_{1,2}$-Adrenoceptor blocker	
Timolol	$\beta_{1,2}$-Adrenoceptor blocker	
Pindolol	$\beta_{1,2}$-Adrenoceptor blocker and intrinsic sympathomimetic	
Atenolol	β_1-Adrenoceptor blocker	
Metoprolol	β_1-Adrenoceptor blocker	
Acebutolol	β_1-Adrenoceptor blocker	
Esmolol	β_1-Adrenoceptor blocker (moderately cardioselective)	
Labetalol	$\beta_{1,2}$-Adrenoceptor blocker, α_1-adrenoceptor blocker	
Bretylium	Initial norepinephrine release; late sympatholysis	
Verapamil	α-Adrenoceptor blocker; noncompetitive sympatholytic	
Digitalis	Sensitize baroreceptors; stimulate CNS; stimulate postganglionic sympathetic nerves; release norepinephrine from sympathetic nerve terminals	Increases vagal tone

Drugs that inhibit the entry of calcium ion into cells have collectively been termed calcium antagonists and comprise *class 4* antiarrhythmic drugs. These drugs do not themselves antagonize the effects of calcium ion but prevent its cellular influx (block the slow inward current) and are more appropriately termed calcium entry blockers. Calcium plays a pivotal role in regulating both the electric and mechanical activity of cardiac and vascular tissues.[10,11] Electrophysiologically, calcium is particularly important in maintaining normal automaticity and conduction within the sinoatrial (SA) and atrioventricular (AV) nodes. The potential therapeutic uses of calcium-entry blockers for the treatment of cardiovascular diseases in dogs and cats are listed in Table 15-5. Antiarrhythmic activity is one of the more prominent therapeutic effects of calcium entry blockers, although this action is not characteristic of all drugs in this group.[12] Only verapamil and diltiazem have emerged as clinically useful antiarrhythmic agents. Early clinical investigations studying the antiarrhythmic efficacy of calcium-entry blockers in dogs and cats have been discour-

aging. Additional research is required in order to more clearly define the appropriate criteria for the clinical use of class 4 antiarrhythmic drugs in dogs and cats.

Interestingly, *digitalis glycosides* (digitoxin, digoxin) are not placed into the antiarrhythmic scheme discussed above. The reason for this is un-

Table 15-5 Potential Clinical Uses of Calcium Entry-Blocking Drugs

Arrhythmias
    Paroxysmal supraventricular tachycardia
    Atrial fibrillation and flutter
    Atrioventricular nodal arrhythmias
    Premature ventricular depolarizations
    Ventricular tachycardia
Myocardial ischemia
Hypertropic cardiomyopathy
Pulmonary hypertension
Systemic hypertension
Chronic refractory heart failure?
Cardiopulmonary resuscitation?

certain. Although noted for their inotropic effects, digitalis glycosides produce indirect and direct antiarrhythmic effects.[13] Most of the antiarrhythmic actions of digitalis are due to increases in parasympathetic tone and, therefore, are supraventricular (Table 15-4). Digitalis glycosides increase vagal efferent activity and sensitize baroreceptors and ventricular receptors. The resultant increase in acetylcholine (ACh) release decreases sinus rate, depresses AV conduction velocity, prolongs AV refractoriness, enhances intra-atrial conduction, and depresses atrial specialized-fiber automaticity. Digitalis-induced increases in inotropy decrease cardiac size and increase myocardial perfusion, which may be partially responsible for improved intra-atrial conduction and the abolition of ventricular arrhythmias. Prolongation of the P-R interval, although inconsistent, is the most frequent ECG change observed during digitalis therapy. Digitalis derives its positive inotropic effects by producing dose-dependent inhibition of the Na^+, K^+-ATPase-dependent pump.[13] This action results in the accumulation of intracellular sodium that exchanges for extracellular calcium, thereby increasing intracellular calcium ion concentration. Increases in intracellular calcium ion result in a more forceful cardiac contraction but, if excessive, can predispose to the development of delayed afterdepolarizations and cardiac arrhythmias.

Toxic doses of digitalis cause depolarization and marked slowing of conduction in atrial and ventricular specialized fibers and the AV node. These actions predispose to a wide variety of conduction disturbances, including first-, second-, and potentially third-degree AV block, right or left bundle branch block, and re-enterant atrial or ventricular arrhythmias. The excessive accumulation of intracellular calcium ion can result in abnormalities in intracellular calcium kinetics resulting in oscillation of the resting membrane potential, delayed afterdepolarizations, and the development of automatic atrial and ventricular arrhythmias. More common toxic side effects include depression, restlessness, nausea, vomiting, anorexia, and diarrhea. Digitalis toxicity can usually be managed by decreasing or withdrawing digitalis therapy. Lidocaine and phenytoin are particularly effective in the dog for treating cardiac arrhythmias caused by digitalis toxicity. The simultaneous administration of furosemide, quinidine, verapamil, or amiodarone with digoxin can decrease the renal elimination of digoxin, increasing digoxin serum concentrations and predisposing to digitalis toxicity.[13] Hypokalemia decreases digoxin binding to skeletal muscle, increasing serum digoxin plasma concentrations and predisposing to digitalis toxicity.

Digitalis is indicated as antiarrhythmic therapy for nonsustained or sustained supraventricular tachycardia and atrial fibrillation. Therapeutic dosages of digitalis are frequently successful in abolishing arrhythmias that originate from or are dependent on the AV node. Digitalis usually produces a slowing of ventricular rate in patients with atrial fibrillation, during the early stages of heart failure. Infrequent premature ventricular depolarizations are occasionally abolished during digitalis therapy due to a a reduction in heart size and improved myocardial perfusion. Digitalis glycosides are contraindicated in patients with frequent premature ventricular depolarizations, ventricular tachycardia, or AV conduction disturbances and sick sinus syndrome. Extreme caution must be applied when considering their use in the treatment of patients with sinus bradycardia or supraventricular tachyarrhythmias caused by the presence of an accessory pathway.

PHARMACOLOGY OF ANTIARRHYTHMIC DRUGS

Quinidine

Quinidine is the prototypic class 1A antiarrhythmic drug. Like all class 1 antiarrhythmic drugs (Table 15-2), quinidine produces membrane-stabilizing effects derived from its inhibition of transmembrane sodium flux.[14,15] The decrease in transmembrane sodium flux results in a depression of conduction velocity and membrane responsiveness and decreases automaticity by depressing the slope of phase 4 depolarization. Prolongation of the action potential is a cellular electophysiologic effect shared by quinidine and other class 1A and 3 antiarrhythmic drugs (Table 15-2). This action combined with the ability of quinidine to depress conduction results in a marked prolongation of the effective refractory period in cardiac tissues. These direct cellular electrophysiologic effects are believed to be the primary mechanisms responsible for the antiarrhythmic efficacy of quinidine but are known to be extremely dependent on serum potassium concentrations.[15-17] Low serum potassium concentrations antagonize the depressant actions of quinidine, whereas high serum concentrations increase the ability of quinidine to depress conduction velocity, membrane responsiveness, and automaticity.

Clinically, the effects of quinidine are the result of direct cellular electrophysiologic actions and indirect actions mediated by competitive blockade of muscarinic cholinergic receptors (Table 15-4). The effect of quinidine on heart rate and rhythm is therefore dependent on the prevailing parasympathetic tone and the type of arrhythmia being treated (supraventricular versus ventricular). The parasympathetic nervous system innervates supraventricular tissues and proximal portions of the His-Purkinje system. The anticholinergic effects of quinidine predominate at low plasma concentrations and antagonize direct actions, increasing sinus node automaticity and AV conduction. Direct (depressant) electrophysiologic effects are produced when large doses of quinidine are used or accidental drug overdose occurs. At therapeutic concentrations, the direct and indirect electrophysiologic actions of quinidine combine to produce minimal to moderate increases in sinus rate, slight increases in QRS duration, and prolongation of the Q-T interval. The P-R interval usually remains unchanged due to the anticholinergic effects of quinidine and its purported ability to stimulate β-receptors within the AV node.[18] Acceleration of AV nodal conduction is an important consideration when treating patients with atrial fibrillation and flutter because of the potential to produce marked increases in ventricular rate. Clinically, digitalis has been used to slow AV conduction and prevent increases in ventricular rate in patients with supraventricular arrhythmias requiring quinidine therapy. Increasing plasma concentrations of quinidine generally lead to prolongation of the P-R interval and QRS duration. Increases in the QRS duration by more than 25 percent are usually indicative of quinidine toxicity.

Negative inotropism, vasodilation, and hypotension are produced by quinidine when administered at therapeutic dosages. These hemodynamic actions are not a problem in patients with normal cardiac function but must be considered during treatment of patients with compromised or compensated cardiac disorders. Quinidine produces vasodilation by blocking both α_1- and α_2-adrenoceptors.[19] The combination of the negative inotropic and vasodilatory effects of quinidine can produce marked decreases in arterial blood pressure, particularly following intravenous administration. Quinidine also has antimalarial, antipyretic, oxytocic, and skeletal muscle relaxant effects.[20]

Toxic quinidine concentrations produce a variety of deleterious cardiac effects that are extensions of its direct electrophysiologic and hemodynamic actions (Table 15-6). First-, second-, and third-degree AV block, intraventricular (i.e., bundle branch) block and ventricular tachycardia can be produced by quinidine. Ventricular arrhythmias are probably produced by marked depression of conduction of electrical impulses or increases in automaticity, possibly due to the ability of quinidine to induce early afterdepolarization. Direct depression of cardiac contractility and vasodilation cause decreased cardiac output, hypotension, and increased left ventricular end-diastolic pressure. Clinically, these changes are recognized by the development of lethargy, weakness, and pulmonary edema. Sodium bicarbonate, 1 mg/kg IV, can be used to partially reverse cardiotoxicity and hypotension. Metabolic alkalosis temporarily decreases serum potassium concentrations, thereby limiting the direct cellular effects of quinidine and increases quinidine binding to serum albumin. Protein-bound drugs are not believed to exert pharmacologic activity.

Quinidine has been reported to cause thrombocytopenia in humans.[20] Thrombocytopenia is believed to be caused by the interaction of a quinidine-evoked antibody with circulating platelets. Thrombocytopenia has not been documented during quinidine therapy in dogs and cats. Platelet counts in humans return to normal when quinidine therapy is discontinued. Nausea, vomiting, and diarrhea are the most frequently encountered adverse effect associated with oral quinidine therapy in dogs and cats. Unpublished clinical studies suggest that approximately 25 percent of all dogs treated with oral quinidine develop signs suggestive of gastrointestinal (GI) discomfort (Muir WW, Sams RA, unpublished data). The clinical incidence of GI side effects may be greater in cats.

Quinidine may precipitate the production of dig-

Table 15-6 Therapeutic Guidelines and Adverse Effects of Antiarrhythmic Drugs[a]

Drug	Tradename	Dose[a] and Route of Administration	Adverse Effects		
			Electrophysiologic	Hemodynamic	Other
Quinidine	Quinidine sulfate Quinidine gluconate Quinidine Dura-tabs	5–15 mg/kg qid PO 5–10 mg/kg IV slowly	Aggravation of arrhythmia, AV block; increased ventricular response in A fib	Mild negative inotrope, hypotension	Nausea, vomiting diarrhea, depression
Procainamide	Pronestyl Procan SR	5–15 mg/kg qid PO 5–10 mg/kg IV 20–50 μg/kg/min CRI[b]	Arrhythmia aggravation; AV block	Hypotension with IV use	Anorexia, nausea vomiting, lupus-like reaction
Disopyramide	Norpace	10–20 mg/kg q2h PO	Arrhythmia aggravation; AV block; increase in ventricular rate in A fib	Aggravates CHF; hypotension	
Lidocaine	Lidocaine	4 mg/kg IV 40–80 μg/kg/min IV CRI[b] (cats: 0.25–1 mg/kg IV over 5 min)	Arrhythmia aggravation Sinus bradycardia AV block	Minor	Drowsiness, ataxia, nystagmus, tremor vomiting, seizures
Tocainide	Tonocard	5–10 mg/kg tid PO	Same as lidocaine	Same as lidocaine	Same as lidocaine
Mexiletine		5–10 mg/kg bid-tid PO	Same as lidocaine	Same as lidocaine	Same as lidocaine
Phenytoin	Dilantin	30 mg/kg tid PO 10 mg/kg IV slowly	Minor	Minor	Depression, seizures
Flecainide	Tambocor	3–10 mg/kg tid PO	Arrhythmia aggravation; sinus bradycardia; AV block	Hypotension, decreased contractility	Depression, ataxia, nystagmus, vomiting leukopenia
Propranolol	Inderal	5–40 mg tid PO 0.1–0.3 mg/kg IV (cats: 0.2–1.0 mg/kg TID PO; 0.04–0.06 mg/kg IV slowly)	Bradycardia; AV block	Negative inotrope; hypotension	Depression, aggravation of pulmonary bronchoconstriction

Nadolol	Corgard	5–40 mg tid PO			
Timolol	Blocadren	0.5–5 mg tid PO			
Pindolol	Visken	1–3 mg tid PO	Bradycardia; AV block	Negative inotrope; hypotension	
Atenolol	Tenormin	0.5–1.0 mg/kg sid or bid PO			
Metoprolol	Lopressor	5–50 mg tid PO			
Amiodarone	Cordarone	10–20 mg/kg bid PO	Bradycardia; AV block	Negative inotrope; hypotension	Hypothyroidism, hyperthyroidism, pulmonary fibrosis, photosensitization, liver failure
Bretylium	Bretylol	5–10 mg/kg IV	Arrhythmia aggravation; tachycardia	Hypotension (late)	Nausea, vomiting
Verapamil	Calan Isoptin	1–5 mg/kg tid PO 0.25 mg/kg IV slowly	Bradycardia; AV block hypotension	Negative inotrope	Depression
Atropine Sulfate	Atropine	0.1–0.2 mg/kg sc IV	Tachycardia ventricular arrhythmies	Increased MVO_2 [c]	Depression, constipation
Glycopyrrolate	Robinul-V	0.05–0.01 mg/kg sc IV	Tachycardia	Increased MVO_2 [c]	Constipation

[a] All doses are for the dog, unless otherwise indicated.

[b] CRI, constant rate infusion; formula for CRI: Body weight (kg) × dose (µg/kg/min) × 0.36 = total dose in mg administered intravenously over 6 hours

[c] MVO_2, myocardial oxygen consumption.

italis toxicity in patients simultaneously administered quinidine and digoxin or in patients receiving chronic digoxin therapy to whom quinidine is administered to control cardiac arrhythmias. This drug-drug interaction is believed to be caused by a quinidine-induced decrease in the renal clearance of digoxin and the displacement of digoxin from skeletal muscle-binding sites.[21,22] The possibility of central nervous system (CNS)-induced toxicity with arrhythmia production due to an increased circulating plasma concentration of digoxin has also been suggested.[23] Digoxin-quinidine drug interaction can be avoided by reducing the dosage of digoxin prior to quinidine administration.

Quinidine is indicated for the treatment of supraventricular arrhythmias, including atrial premature depolarizations and AV junctional tachycardias in dogs and cats. Although effective in the treatment of ventricular premature depolarizations and tachycardia, the relatively high incidence of GI side effects mitigates against its routine use by this route. Quinidine is occasionally successful in converting atrial fibrillation of acute onset to normal sinus rhythm in the dog and can be used to depress conduction in the accessory pathway, thereby preventing repetitive ventricular tachycardia in patients with Wolff-Parkinson-White syndrome. Quinidine is contraindicated in patients with sinus bradycardia, sick sinus syndrome, frequent episodes of second-degree AV block, and during complete AV block. Quinidine-induced suppression of AV conduction and idioventricular pacemakers in a patient with a large number of blocked P waves or complete AV block could result in cardiac arrest. Quinidine should be administered cautiously to patients with heart failure or hyperkalemia, in order to avoid the precipitation of congestive symptoms.

Quinidine is a lipophilic weak base (pK$_a$ 4.0 and 8.6) that is rapidly and extensively distributed to peripheral tissues. It is extensively bound to plasma and tissue proteins and has a large volume of distribution[24] (Table 15-7).

Quinidine is eliminated by the kidneys and is metabolized by the liver; less than 40 percent of the dose is eliminated unchanged in the urine.[24,25] Since hepatic clearance (4.1 ml/min/kg) is less than hepatic blood flow, hepatic clearance is relatively insensitive to changes in hepatic blood flow but is sensitive to changes in binding and intrinsic clearance. For example, propranolol does not reduce quinidine clearance in spite of its reduction of hepatic blood flow.[26] The oral availability of quinidine is good and is not reduced by first-pass metabolism.

Quinidine competes for tissue-binding sites of some other drugs, most notably digoxin. Consequently, plasma digoxin concentrations rise during quinidine therapy due to displacement of digoxin from skeletal muscle and other tissue binding sites.[21,22] Furthermore, there is evidence that quinidine reduces the renal clearance of digoxin, although the precise mechanism is unknown.[21,22] Therefore, digoxin concentrations should be monitored during combined quinidine-digoxin therapy and the dosage of digoxin reduced, if necessary.

Procainamide

Procainamide is a class 1A antiarrhythmic drug with electrophysiologic properties similar to those of quinidine. Like quinidine, the electrophysiologic effects of procainamide are due both to direct and to indirect (anticholinergic) actions[14] (Table 15-4). Procainamide produces direct depression of automaticity in the SA node and atrial and ventricular specialized fibers. Atrial automatic tissues are more sensitive than are ventricular automatic tissues. The rate of phase 0 of the action potential is depressed by procainamide, resulting in a decrease in conduction velocity of electric impulses in all cardiac tissues. Procainamide depresses membrane responsiveness and excitability and prolongs action potential duration and refractoriness in atrial and ventricular specialized fibers and muscle.[20] The vagolytic effects of procainamide on supraventricular tissues (particularly the AV node) are less pronounced than those of quinidine. The direct depression of the AV node conduction velocity and the prolongation of refractoriness of procainamide are partially blunted by anticholinergic effects. Clinically, anticholinergic effects could be responsible for an increase in ventricular rate due to increased transmission of atrial impulses through the AV node. Therapeutic doses of procainamide, however, generally produce little or no effect on AV nodal conduction velocity or refractoriness in patients in normal sinus rhythm. The electrophysiologic effects of procainamide, like those of quinidine, are dependent on the extracellular potassium ion concentration. In-

Table 15-7 Pharmacokinetic Parameter Values for Various Antiarrhythmic Drugs in Healthy Dogs and Cats

Drug	CL_T (ml/min/kg)	CL_R (ml/min/kg)	V_d (L/kg)	$t_{1/2}$ (hr)	f (%)	F (%)	Reference
Dogs							
Quinidine	6.8	2.7	2.9	5.6	8.7	High	24,25
Procainamide	6.9–12.5	4.1–7.5	1.4–2.1	2.4	ND	85	[a]30,85
Disopyramide	25	3.8	3.0	1.2	20	70	31,35,36
Lidocaine	62	$<0.05 \times CL_T$	5.7	1.0	ND	Low	46–49
Phenytoin	4.0	$<0.05 \times CL_T$	1.2	3.3	65	40	53–56
Tocainide	4.2	1.3	1.7	4.7	ND	85	58
Mexiletine	ND	ND (variable)	>6.0	>4.0	ND	High	61,62
Amiodarone	21.1	ND	2.2	3.0	ND	Low	74
Propranolol	34–70	$<0.10 \times CL_T$	1.7–6.5	1.1	92–98.5	2–18	64,70–72
Bretylium	low	CL_T	low	9.1–10.5	ND	Low	78
Verapamil	62	0.3	4.5	0.8	ND	Low	83,84
Cats							
Quinidine	15.0	—	2.2	1.9		60	[b]
Lidocaine	—	—	—	0.75		Low	[b]
Phenytoin	30.0	—	—	>24.0		—	[b]
Propranolol	—	—	1.6	0.5		Low	[b]
Digoxin	—	—	—	33		880	[b]

CL_T, total body clearance; CL_R, renal clearance; V_d, volume of distribution; $t_{1/2}$, elimination half-life; f, protein binding; F, oral availability; ND, not determined.
[a] Davis LM: Personal communication.
[b] Sams RA, Muir WW: Unpublished data.

creases in extracellular potassium potentiate the depressant actions of procainamide.

Therapeutic dosages of procainamide produce ECG changes that are the result of the direct cellular electrophysiologic effects of the drug. Sinus rate remains unchanged or is minimally decreased. The P-R, QRS, and Q-T intervals are minimally prolonged. The magnitude of these changes is a reflection of the procainamide plasma concentration and can be used to monitor for toxic drug concentrations. A 25 percent increase in the QRS interval is an indication of procainamide toxicity.

Procainamide produces minimal cardiovascular depressant effects as compared with quinidine. Mild depression of cardiac contractility, as well as vasodilation and hypotension are produced when therapeutic dosages of procainamide are administered intravenously.[27] Intramuscular or oral administration of recommended dosages of procainamide produce insignificant changes in hemodynamics in dogs with normal myocardial function. Augmentation of

myocardial depression following procainamide administration to patients with heart failure is minimal, a function of dosage, and a function of the rate and route of administration.

Toxic dosages of procainamide produce hypotension and marked depression of AV conduction (Table 15-6). First-, second-, or third-degree AV block can occur. Depressed conduction in atrial and ventricular specialized fibers may initiate intraventricular block, precipitate tachyarrhythmias, or exacerbate existing arrhythmias. The precipitation of tachyarrhythmias by toxic dosages of procainamide or quinidine can result in syncope or lead to the sudden development of ventricular fibrillation.[20] Clinically, prolongation of the QRS and Q-T intervals (corrected for changes in heart rate) can be used as a therapeutic guide in order to avoid toxicity. Hypotension can be treated by administration of fluids, calcium-containing solutions, or catecholamines (e.g., dopamine, dobutamine). Patients receiving oral procainamide occasionally develop nausea, vomiting, and diarrhea. These GI effects are infrequent and generally subside when therapy is discontinued or reduced. A less frequent side effect of procainamide therapy, but an important clinical consideration, is the development of a systemic lupus erythematosus (SLE) syndrome and a neutropenia.[28] Depression, fever, and hepatomegaly are the more prevalent symptoms. The syndrome has only been observed in patients receiving large oral dosages of procainamide and disappears within a few days after reducing or discontinuing drug therapy. Procainamide is metabolized by the liver and excreted by the kidney. Renal excretion of procainamide is proportional to creatinine clearance. N-Acetylprocainamide, an active metabolite in humans, is not significant in dogs or cats (Muir WW, Sams RA, unpublished data). Drugs or diseases that interfere with liver metabolism or increase serum creatinine concentration should be expected to prolong procainamide elimination.

Procainamide, like quinidine, is indicated for the treatment of premature atrial and ventricular depolarizations, nonsustained and sustained atrial and ventricular tachycardias, and atrial fibrillation of recent onset.[20,29] Procainamide is not effective in converting chronic atrial flutter or fibrillation to sinus rhythm. Procainamide can be used to depress conduction of electric impulses across an accessory pathway, thereby reducing ventricular rate in animals with atrial flutter or fibrillation from Wolff-Parkinson-White syndrome. Clinically, procainamide enjoys a much greater popularity than quinidine because of the less frequent incidence of GI side effects. Procainamide should be used with extreme caution or avoided in patients with sinus bradycardia; sick sinus syndrome; first-, second-, or third-degree AV block; intraventricular conduction disturbances; and severely compromised hemodynamic function.

Procainamide is a lipophilic weak base (pK$_a$ 9.23) that is structurally related to procaine, but having greater stability to plasma esterases. Procainamide is rapidly and extensively distributed to extravascular tissues and, consequently, has a volume of distribution greater than total body water[30] (Table 15-7).

Total body clearance of procainamide in dogs is about 7 to 9 ml/min/kg at dosages of 8 to 26 mg/kg.[30] The relative contributions of renal and hepatic clearance to total clearance are unknown. N-Acetylprocainamide is a pharmacologically active metabolite that contributes to the pharmacologic effects in humans, but this metabolite is not found in significant concentrations in dogs or cats. If total clearance is due largely to hepatic metabolism, it would be expected that alterations in unbound fraction and liver enzyme activity would affect clearance and that alterations in liver blood flow would have little effect on clearance.

Plasma procainamide concentrations effective against ventricular arrhythmias produced by digitalis intoxication in dogs range from about 25 to 50µg/ml (Davis LE, personal communication). These concentrations are higher than in persons, perhaps due to the contribution of N-acetylprocainamide to the pharmacologic effect in man. These plasma concentrations can be attained with loading doses of 38.2 mg/kg followed by constant rate infusions of 16.3 mg/hr/kg. Plasma procainamide concentrations effective in controlling arrhythmias produced by coronary occlusion and digitalis intoxication in dogs have also been achieved after intravenous doses of 40 to 60 mg/kg.[30] Plasma procainamide concentrations required to abolish clinical arrhythmias are probably much lower than 25 to 50 µg/ml.

Disopyramide

Disopyramide is a class 1A antiarrhythmic drug with electrophysiologic and ECG properties similar to those of quinidine and procainamide.[14] Disopyramide has a long duration of action and produces few side effects in humans.[31] Unfortunately, these beneficial effects (i.e., long duration of action and fewer GI side effects) have not been observed in studies in dogs. Like quinidine and procainamide, disopyramide produces electrophysiologic effects in intact animals due to direct and indirect (i.e., anticholinergic) effects[32,33] (Table 15-4). Unlike quinidine and procainamide, however, the anticholinergic effects of disopyramide predominate at relatively low plasma concentrations. This results in increases in sinus rate and acceleration of AV conduction velocity when therapeutic dosages of disopyramide are administered. These observations dictate that disopyramide be used with caution in patients with atrial flutter or fibrillation in order to prevent excessive ventricular rates. The direct effects of disopyramide produce decreases in automaticity, conduction velocity, and increases in refractoriness. Large doses of disopyramide produce direct depression of AV conduction. These actions are dependent on the extracellular potassium concentration. Like quinidine and procainamide, disopyramide produces dose-dependent prolongation of the P-R, QRS, and Q-T intervals.

Therapeutic dosages of disopyramide produce significant decreases in myocardial contractility.[34] This effect is much more pronounced than quinidine and procainamide and leads to a reduction in cardiac output and an increase in left ventricular end diastolic pressure. Disopyramide therapy also produces vasoconstriction, resulting in an increase in peripheral vascular resistance. The mechanism for this latter effect is controversial but may lead to an increase in ventricular afterload and a further reduction in cardiac output. The deleterious cardiovascular effects of disopyramide are dose dependent and must be given serious consideration in patients with cardiac arrhythmias and heart failure.

The toxic manifestations associated with disopyramide therapy are primarily those caused by hypotension and myocardial depression, although electrophysiologic and ECG abnormalities similar to those produced by quinidine and procainamide can be expected (Table 15-6). Lethargy, weakness, and syncope may occur. Pulmonary congestion may develop or be exacerbated if dogs with compensated heart failure are treated with excessive doses of disopyramide. Anticholinergic actions may result in tachycardia. The incidence of severe adverse side effects with long-term disopyramide therapy in dogs and cats is unknown. Significant drug interactions involving disopyramide have not been reported.

Indications for disopyramide therapy are similar to those of quinidine and procainamide. Unifocal or multifocal, nonsustained or sustained, atrial or ventricular cardiac arrhythmias respond favorably to disopyramide therapy. Disopyramide can be used to treat atrial flutter or fibrillation of recent origin but could lead to excessively rapid ventricular rates prior to conversion to sinus rhythm. Disopyramide should be avoided in patients with chronic atrial fibrillation, compensated heart failure, sinus bradycardia, sick sinus syndrome, or pre-existing first-, second-, or third-degree AV block.

Disopyramide is a lipophilic weak base (pK$_a$ 8.36) that is rapidly and extensively distributed to extravascular tissues (Table 15-7). The binding of disopyramide to plasma α_1-acid glycoprotein is less extensive than in persons and consequently the volume of distribution is larger than in humans.[35]

Disopyramide is cleared by renal and hepatic mechanisms with approximately 20 percent of an intravenous dose eliminated unchanged in the urine. Hepatic metabolism is extensive and involves successive N-dealkylation of disopyramide.[35,36] Metabolites possess pharmacologic activity comparable to that of disopyramide and may contribute to its pharmacologic effects. Hepatic clearance is intermediate in magnitude between that of quinidine and propranolol.

Oral bioavailability is incomplete due to first-pass metabolism and averages about 40 percent. The half-life is somewhat larger after oral doses (2.4 hours) than after intravenous doses (1.1 hours).[35]

Disopyramide doses of 3 to 5 mg/kg IV slow the sinus rate in healthy dogs.[37] Maximum plasma concentrations after such doses are approximately 2 to 5 μg/ml. Owing to the rapid clearance and short half-life, disopyramide dosages need to be repeated frequently.

Lidocaine

Lidocaine, a local anesthetic, produces a variety of cellular electrophysiologic effects that are responsible for its class IB categorization.[14] Unlike class 1A antiarrhythmic drugs (i.e., quinidine, procainamide, disopyramide), therapeutic concentrations of lidocaine produce little effect on sinus rate, AV conduction velocity, and refractoriness. Lidocaine does not produce anticholinergic effects.[38] Lidocaine in low concentrations produces little to no depression of phase 4 depolarization in atrial and ventricular specialized fibers. Cardiac muscle membrane responsiveness, excitability, and conduction velocity are depressed to a lesser degree by lidocaine than by quinidine or procainamide and only at plasma concentrations of lidocaine in the high therapeutic or toxic range. In contrast to class 1A antiarrhythmic drugs, lidocaine shortens action potential duration in atrial and ventricular specialized fibers (Table 15-3), although the effective refractory period may be prolonged slightly.[20] Lidocaine is ineffective in significantly altering atrial refractoriness and conduction velocity which may be a partial explanation for its ineffectiveness in the treatment of supraventricular arrhythmias. The cellular electrophysiologic effects of lidocaine are dependent on the extracellular potassium concentration. Hyperkalemia intensifies the depressant action of lidocaine on cardiac membranes, resulting in the production of electrophysiologic effects more closely resembling those of quinidine. Clinically, the antiarrhythmic effects of lidocaine stem from its action on diseased or electrically abnormal cardiac tissues. Lidocaine causes marked suppression of automaticity and conduction velocity and prolongs refractoriness in hypoxic or damaged cardiac cells.[39] These effects are particularly evident in ventricular specialized (e.g., His-Purkinje) and muscle tissues. Lidocaine generally produces no change in P-R, QRS, or Q-T duration. The Q-T interval may decrease somewhat due to the ability of lidocaine to shorten action-potential duration. Occasionally, lidocaine produces sinus tachycardia. The mechanism for this latter effect is uncertain but may involve the CNS.

Therapeutic doses of lidocaine produce no change or minimal depression in cardiac contractility.[38] Intravenous bolus administrations or infusions of large dosages of lidocaine can produce transient and mild reductions in cardiac contractility and vasodilation that may result in transient decreases in cardiac output and arterial blood pressure. Slow bolus injections of therapeutic doses of lidocaine to dogs in heart failure produce no change in cardiac output, blood pressure, or heart rate.[40,41]

Central nervous system excitement is the most common toxic side effect associated with lidocaine administration to dogs and cats[42] (Table 15-6). Drowsiness and depression may occur when therapeutic concentrations of lidocaine are administered but are considered inconsequential. More frequently, agitation, disorientation, muscle twitching, nystagmus, and generalized tonic-clonic seizures are observed as the dose of lidocaine is increased. Convulsions are self-limiting and subside as the plasma lidocaine concentration decreases. Cats are seemingly more sensitive to the central nervous system side effects of lidocaine than dogs, emphasizing the need for caution during intravenous

bolus administration (Muir WW, Sams RA, unpublished data). Diazepam, 0.5 mg/kg, is effective in preventing lidocaine-induced seizures. Respiratory depression and arrest has been observed in unconscious dogs and cats recieving lidocaine to control arrhythmias due to traumatic myocarditis (Muir WW, Sams RA, unpublished data).

Lidocaine is rapidly metabolized by the liver. Consequently, hepatic metabolism of lidocaine is dependent upon liver blood flow.[43] Propranolol and cimetidine reduce hepatic blood flow. If administered concurrently with lidocaine, these drugs could decrease lidocaine elimination and predispose to lidocaine toxicity.[44,45]

Lidocaine is relatively ineffective in the treatment of supraventricular arrhythmias but is one of the most effective drugs currently available for the treatment of ventricular arrhythmias in dogs and cats. Unsustained and sustained premature ventricular depolarizations, unifocal and multifocal ventricular tachycardia, ventricular arrhythmias caused by halothane sensitization to catecholamines and digitalis toxicity respond favorably to lidocaine therapy. Lidocaine should be considered the drug of choice for the acute management of ventricular arrhythmias in patients with compensated or uncompensated heart failure. Lidocaine is potentially effective therapy for the treatment of atrial tachyarrhythmias and atrial flutter due to an accessory pathway but should be considered only if procainamide or quinidine has proven unsuccessful. Lidocaine should be administered cautiously to patients with sinus bradycardia, sick sinus syndrome, first- or second-degree AV block and is contraindicated in patients with third-degree AV block. The administration of lidocaine to a patient with complete heart block could abolish the idioventricular pacemaker resulting in cardiac arrest. Lidocaine should be used cautiously in compensated heart failure patients in order to prevent hypotension.

Lidocaine is a highly lipophilic weak base (pK$_a$ 7.85) that is rapidly and extensively distributed to extravascular tissues (Table 15-7). Consequently, it has a very large volume of distribution. Lidocaine is bound (44 to 71 percent) to plasma proteins, primarily α$_1$-acid glycoprotein.

The clearance of lidocaine is very high and is attributed primarily to hepatic metabolism, since only about 2 percent of an intravenous dose is recovered unchanged in the urine.[46,47] Major metabolites result from successive N-dealkylation and aromatic ring hydroxylation.[46] The N-dealkylated metabolites are pharmacologically active, possibly contributing to the antiarrhythmic and toxic effects of the drug. Hepatic clearance of lidocaine is perfusion rate-limited and varies with changes in hepatic blood flow. Propranolol decreases lidocaine clearance due to its reduction of hepatic blood flow.[48] Furthermore, patients in heart failure clear lidocaine more slowly than normal patients and require correspondingly lower dosages.

Although lidocaine is well absorbed following oral administration, nearly all of the dose is metabolized in the first pass through the liver.[46] High plasma concentrations of toxic metabolites after oral doses may be responsible for the emesis and other adverse signs noted. Therefore, lidocaine should not be given orally.

Therapeutic plasma lidocaine concentrations in persons range from 2 to 4 μg/ml with toxicity occurring at concentrations as low as 5 to 9 μg/ml. Concentrations in excess of 9 μg/ml in humans are frequently associated with toxicity. Tonic extension occurs in dogs at a mean lidocaine concentration of 8.2 μg/ml and ouabain-induced ventricular arrhythmias are abolished at a mean concentration of 6.2 μg/ml.[49] Concentrations required to abolish naturally occurring arrhythmias are probably much lower than this, perhaps 0.5 to 4.0 μg/ml.

Phenytoin

Phenytoin, an anticonvulsant, is classified as a class IB antiarrhythmic drug because its electrophysiologic effects on cardiac tissues, particularly ventricular specialized tissues, resemble those of lidocaine (Table 15-2). Phenytoin shortens action potential duration and increases the effective refractory period. Like lidocaine, phenytoin (when administered at therapeutic dosages) produces little to no effect on sinus rate, specialized tissue automaticity, conduction velocity and minimally increases refractoriness in normal heart tissues.[20] Phenytoin lacks anticholinergic properties but may increase AV conduction velocity due to its direct actions. The acceleration of atrioventricular conduction observed following phenytoin administration could cause an increase in ventricular rate in patients with atrial fibrillation. Dosages of phenytoin that produce plasma concentrations in the high therapeutic range cause depression of phase 0 of the action potential in atrial and ventricular muscle fibers and specialized tissues resulting in a decrease in conduction velocity of electrical impulses.[50] Phenytoin produces marked depression of automaticity and conduction velocity in damaged cardiac tissues.[39] This latter effect is believed to be responsible for phenytoin's antiarrhythmic efficacy in treating ventricular arrhythmias. Phenytoin produces no changes in the P-R and QRS intervals but may decrease the QT interval. Occasionally, the P-R interval decreases due to increases in AV conduction velocity.

Phenytoin produces minimal cardiovascular depression when administered at low infusion rates or orally.[20] Rapid intravenous administration can produce depression of myocardial contractility, vasodilation and hypotension. The majority of these effects are believed to be due to the water–propylene glycol mixture, in which phenytoin is solubilized. Slow intravenous or oral administration of phenytoin does not produce hemodynamic changes.

The oral administration of phenytoin is associated with few side effects other than CNS depression (Table 15-6). Rapid intravenous administration of phenytoin produces respiratory arrest, hypotension, and an exacerbation of cardiac arrhythmias. Most, if not all, of these adverse hemodynamic effects are attributed to the solvent which has a pH of 11 and contains 40 percent propylene glycol.[51] Bradycardia, atrioventricular block, cardiac arrest, and ventricular tachycardia are reported to occur following intravenous phenytoin administration. Central nervous manifestations of phenytoin toxicity include nystagmus, disorientation, and ataxia. Occasionally, anemia, pancytopenia and reticuloendothelial disorders are reported to occur in humans during chronic oral therapy.[52] These disorders regress when phenytoin therapy is discontinued.

Phenytoin is dependent on the liver and microsomal enzyme activity for its metabolism. Although specific drug interactions involving other cardiac drugs have not been emphasized, phenytoin, by stimulating microsomal enzymes, may enhance its own metabolism and that of other drugs dependent on the liver for elimination.

Phenytoin, like lidocaine, is effective in the treatment of ventricular arrhythmias. Clinical studies conducted to determine the efficacy of phenytoin in the treatment of naturally occurring supraventricular arrhythmias have been unanimously unsuccessful. Phenytoin is not effective in converting the acute onset of atrial flutter or fibrillation to sinus rhythm and may increase ventricular rate due to enhancement of AV conduction velocity. Digitalis-induced arrhythmias present a special situation for which phenytoin therapy is particularly effective.[52] Phenytoin will convert supraventricular and ventricular digitalis-induced arrhythmias to sinus rhythm. It is used clinically for this purpose in dogs. Contraindications for phenytoin therapy are similar to those of lidocaine. Phenytoin should be avoided in patients with sinus bradycardia, sick sinus syndrome, complete heart block and severe heart failure. The patient's current therapy should be closely scrutinized for drugs which may affect or be effected by the addition of phenytoin to the therapeutic regimen.

Phenytoin is a lipophilic weak acid (pK_a 8.3) that is structurally related to the barbiturates (Table 15-7). Phenytoin was previously known as diphenylhydantoin. The drug is rapidly and extensively distributed to extravascular tissues. Plasma-protein binding is not extensive and the volume of distribution is large.[53]

Phenytoin is cleared primarily by hepatic metabolism with only a small fraction of the dose eliminated unchanged in the urine.[54] Hepatic clearance in dogs (4.0 ml/min/kg) and in cats is much less than hepatic blood flow and is, therefore, relatively insensitive to changes in hepatic blood flow.[53] Hepatic clearance is subject to reduction due to inhibition of hepatic microsomal enzymes by chloramphenicol, pentobarbital, and other agents.[55] High doses of phenytoin are cleared more slowly than low doses, suggesting that phenytoin or a metabolite inhibits drug metabolism or that metabolism is saturable.[54]

The oral bioavailability of phenytoin in dogs is relatively poor. This is attributed to poor dissolution properties since first-pass metabolism is unimportant.[55,56]

The antiarrhythmic plasma concentration of phenytoin may be as high as 10 ug/ml in dogs. Oral phenytoin doses of 50 mg/kg/day to dogs produce peak plasma phenytoin concentrations ranging from about 2 to 7 μg/ml, which decline, to less than 1 μg/ml by 18 hours after the dose.[56] Peak and average plasma concentrations are only slightly higher after daily intramuscular doses of 50 mg/kg.[56] By contrast, cats became toxic after several daily oral doses of 10 mg/kg.[56]

Tocainide

Tocainide, an analog of lidocaine, is a Class 1B antiarrhythmic drug.[14] Tocainide is the product of the continuous search by the pharmaceutical industry to develop an orally active drug with electrophysiologic properties similar to those of lidocaine. Tocainide's electrophysiologic, antiarrhythmic, electrocardiographic, hemodynamic and toxic effects are identical to those of lidocaine.[57] Unlike lidocaine, however, tocainide's elimination is not significantly influenced by changes in liver blood flow thereby negating the potential influences of drugs like propranolol and cimetidine. Tocainide can be used as an alternative to lidocaine when oral therapy is feasible. Clinically tocainide is effective in the treatment of unifocal or multifocal premature ventricular depolarizations. Initial experience with tocainide as therapy for ventricular arrhythmias in dogs has been favorable although their has been a relatively high (40 percent) incidence of side effects (Muir WW, Sams RA, unpublished data). The most common side effects were nausea, vomiting, and anorexia (Table 15-6). Neurologic disturbances, including ataxia, disorientation, and twitching, have been observed in two dogs. Although clinical experience with tocainide in veterinary practice is limited, continued use will determine whether it will serve as an acceptable alternative to lidocaine.

Tocainide is a lipophilic weak base structurally related to lidocaine. Tocainide was synthesized in an effort to produce an antiarrhythmic agent with a lower clearance and greater oral availability than lidocaine (see Table 15-7). These objectives have been met with tocainide. The volume of distribution is greater than total body water but is substantially less than that of lidocaine. Total body clearance of tocainide is less than 10 percent of that of lidocaine and is attributed to both hepatic metabolism and renal excretion.[58] Approximately 30 percent of an intravenous dose is eliminated unchanged in the urine.[58] Hepatic clearance is approximately 2.9 ml/min/kg in healthy dogs[58] and is expected to be relatively insensitive to changes in hepatic blood flow.

Tocainide is well absorbed after oral administration and is not extensively metabolized on its first pass through the liver.[59] The half-life of tocainide is approximately 4.7 hours after intravenous doses and ranges from 8 to 12 hours after oral doses.[59]

Ectopic beats produced by occlusion of coronary arteries are suppressed at plasma tocainide concentrations of 15 to 30 μg/ml.[59] These concentrations can be achieved and maintained for about 5 hours after single oral doses of about 100 mg/kg.[59] However, doses required to abolish or reduce clinical arrhythmias are probably much lower than this.

Mexiletine

Mexiletine is a class 1B antiarrhythmic drug with electrophysiologic, antiarrhythmic, ECG, hemodynamic, and toxic effects similar to lidocaine and tocainide.[52] Like tocainide, mexiletine can be administered orally and possesses a relatively high degree of effectiveness. Studies in dogs with naturally occuring arrhythmias suggest that mexiletine should be effective in the treatment of unifocal and multifocal ventricular tachycardia.[60] Our observations in dogs administered mexiletine to treat ventricular tachycardia have produced only moderately encouraging results (Muir WW, Bonagura JD, unpublished results). Three of 10 dogs were converted to sinus rhythm, an additional four dogs demonstrated a decrease in the number of ventricular depolarizations, and three dogs did not respond. Three of 10 dogs vomited and became disoriented during therapy. Combining mexiletine with either β-adrenoceptor-blocking drugs or procainamide markedly increases antiarrhythmic efficacy and substantially reduces adverse side effects. Additional studies of naturally occuring arrhythmias in dogs and cats are required before mexiletine can be recommended. Mexiletine is rapidly absorbed from the GI tract. A basic drug with high lipid solubility, mexiletine is metabolized by the liver and is to a limited extent excreted unchanged by the kidney.[61] Renal excretion is dependent on urinary pH leading to large variation in the plasma elimination half-life. The elimination half-life of mexiletine varies from 4.5 to 7 hours in dogs being longer when the urine pH is alkaline.[62] Mexiletine is metabolized by hepatic mixed-funciton oxidases and, like lidocaine, metabolism is influenced by liver blood flow. Cimetidine

decreases the rate of mexiletine elimination. The volume of distribution of mexiletine is large due to its high lipid solubility. Therapeutic plasma concentrations range from 0.5 to 2 μg/ml.

Flecainide

Flecainide is a class 1C antiarrhythmic drug. Class 1C antiarrhythmic drugs (Tables 15-2 and 15-3) are noted for their ability to depress phase 0 of the action potential selectively, thereby producing a marked reduction in conduction velocity.[52,63] Therapeutic concentrations of flecainide produce relatively insignificant effects on sinus rate, atrioventricular conduction velocity, action potential duration or refractoriness. Conduction across accessory pathways is markedly depressed. Increased concentrations of flecainide produce direct dose-dependent depression of automaticity in the sinus node and atrial and ventricular specialized tissues. Dose-dependent prolongation of the QRS complex can be used as an index of flecainide effectiveness and toxicity. Intravenous flecainide administration produces direct depression of cardiac contractility and vasodilation, resulting in hypotension. These effects are evidenced after rapid intravenous administration and warrant consideration when flecainide is chosen to treat patients with cardiac arrhythmias and heart failure.

Toxic doses of flecainide produce bradycardia, intraventricular conduction disturbances, hypotension, and cardiac arrest. Aggravation of ventricular arrhythmias has been reported in humans. Nausea, vomiting, and anorexia have been observed in dogs (Muir WW, unpublished data).

Flecainide is potentially indicated as therapy for unifocal, premature, nonsustained or sustained ventricular arrhythmias in dogs. Initial experience using flecainide to treat nonsustained ventricular tachycardia in experimental dogs has not been encouraging.[63] Although 8 of 10 dogs were converted to sinus rhythm, 4 dogs developed bradycardia. One additional dog developed right bundle branch block and all 10 dogs demonstrated a transient period of hypotension which resolved within 10 to 20 minutes. Further experimental and clinical studies are required to determine the potential usefulness of flecainide in the treatment of ventricular arrhythmias in dogs. Flecainide and other class 1C antiarrhythmic drugs should be the treatment of choice for cardiac arrhythmias caused by an accessory pathway. Their relatively selective depression of conduction through accessory pathways make them ideal for this purpose. Flecainide is contraindicated in patients with sinus bradycardia, sick sinus syndrome, complete AV block, and intraventricular conduction disturbances. Initial investigations also caution against its use in multifocal ventricular tachycardia in patients with severe heart failure. Additional studies are needed to determine flecainide's antiarrhythmic efficacy and pharmacokinetics in dogs and cats.

Propranolol

Propranolol and all compounds that possess β-adrenoceptor blocking activity are grouped into class 2 antiarrhythmic drugs.[20] β-blocking drugs (Table 15-2) produce their beneficial effects upon heart rate and rhythm through indirect actions, specifically by inhibiting the effects of the adrenergic nervous system (Table 15-4) or exogenously administered adrenergic drugs (e.g., norepinephrine, epinephrine, isoproterenol, dopamine, and dobutamine).[64] Adrenergic stimulation of the heart increases sinus rate, enhances conduction velocity through the AV node, and decreases refractoriness. Automaticity in atrial and ventricular specialized fibers is enhanced by catecholamines. Differential decreases in ventricular muscle refractoriness produce an inhomogeneous pattern of repolarization which, in the setting of increased automaticity, can predispose to arrhythmias caused by re-entrant excitation. Propranolol and other β-adrenoceptor blocking drugs (see Table 15-2) slow sinus rate, depress conduction through the AV node and produce a more homogeneous pattern of repolarization. Increases in automaticity produced by increases in sympathetic tone are abolished. Dosages of propranolol that produce plasma concentrations in the high therapeutic range (>100 ng/ml) produce direct cellular electrophysiologic effects. These direct actions are characteristic of the class 1A antiarrhythmic drugs and have been referred to as quinidine-like effects.[52] The importance of quinidine-like effects during clinical therapy is controversial but unlikely to be significant. The electrocardiogram is minimally affected by propranolol, except for those changes induced by decreases in heart rate.

Propranolol and other β-adrenoceptor blocking drugs produce dose-dependent decreases in cardiac contractility and metabolic rate. Decreases in cardiac contractility and heart rate combine to produce decreases in stroke volume, cardiac output, arterial blood pressure, and myocardial oxygen consumption. These effects are particularly pronounced after intravenous administration and must be considered during oral therapy in patients with severe congestive heart failure or cardiomyopathy. Other important pharmacologic effects of propranolol are dependent on its nonselective β-adrenoceptor blocking activity (Table 15-8) and include decreases in renin release, bronchoconstriction, vasoconstriction and inhibition of insulin release.[65]

Toxic concentrations of propranolol produce bradycardia, cardiac failure, and hypotension (Table 15-6). Bronchospasm and hypoglycemia may occur. These particular effects can be prevented by the infusion of catecholamines (e.g., dopamine, dobutamine), which may precipitate cardiac rhythm disturbances. Central nervous system depression and disorientation may occur during therapy with propranolol and other highly lipophilic β-adrenoceptor blocking drugs. Propranolol therapy decreases liver blood flow, thereby decreasing the clearance of drugs dependent upon liver metabolism and liver blood flow for their elimination (e.g., lidocaine).[44] Propranolol markedly potentiates the depression of atrioventricular conduction produced by digitalis, calcium entry blocking drugs and class 1A antiarrhythmics. The simultaneous administration of propranolol and a calcium entry blocking drug (e.g., verapamil) can produce dramatic reductions in heart rate and cardiac contractility.

Propranolol is indicated as therapy for sinus tachycardia, supraventricular and ventricular arrhythmias, hypertrophic cardiomyopathy, hypertension, hyperthyroidism, and pheochromocytoma. Treatment of cardiac arrhythmias caused by accessory pathways is generally not successful. Therapy with propranolol is greatly influenced by the prevailing sympathetic tone and β-adrenoceptor numbers. Chronic stimulation of cardiac receptors by the adrenergic nervous system or catecholamines can result in a decrease in receptor numbers. The decrease in β-adrenoceptor numbers is termed down-regulation and is known to occur in patients with chronic congestive heart failure and cardio-

Table 15-8 Pharmacologic Properties of β-Adrenoceptor-Blocking Drugs

Drug	Relative β_1 Selectivity	Intrinsic Sympathomimetic Activity	Lipophilicity	Membrane-Stabilizing Activity
Propranolol	0	0	High	+
Nadolol	0	0	Low	0
Timolol	0	0	Low	0
Pindolol	0	+	Moderate	+
Metoprolol	+	0	Moderate	0
Atenolol	+	0	Low	0
Acebutolol	+	+ (weakly)	Low	+
Labetolol[c]	0	0	Low	0
Sotalol[a]	0	0	Low	0
Esmolol[b]	+	0	?	0

[a] Investigational.
[b] Short duration of action (10 to 20 minutes).
[c] Possesses α_1-adrenoceptor-blocking activity.
+, property exhibited; 0, property not exhibited.

myopathy. The administration of propranolol or any other β-adrenoceptor-blocking drug to a patient that has become dependent on adrenergic tone in order to maintain heart rate and cardiac contractility can be lethal. By contrast, receptor up-regulation may occur during chronic therapy with propranolol and other β-adrenoceptor-blocking drugs. Chronic therapy with propranolol, for example, may result in an increase in adrenergic receptor numbers or affinity resulting in severe cardiac arrythmias should therapy be suddenly discontinued.[65] Propranolol is contraindicated in patients with sinus bradycardia, AV block and severe congestive heart failure. Patients with chronic obstructive airway disease, undergoing anesthesia, or receiving calcium entry blocking drugs must be monitored closely if propranolol therapy is being considered.

Propranolol is a highly lipophilic weak base (pK$_a$ 9.45) which is highly bound to plasma α_1-acid glycoprotein and tissue proteins.[66] Consequently, propranolol is widely and extensively distributed to extravascular tissues and has a large volume of distribution (greater than total body water; Table 15-7).[67]

Propranolol is metabolized (primarily in the liver) to several oxidation products and their conjugates which are eliminated in the urine.[68,69] One of these oxidation products, 4-hydroxypropranolol, exhibits pharmacologic activity similar to that of pro-

pranolol and may contribute to its pharmacologic effect.[69]

Hepatic metabolism of propranolol is nonrestrictive (i.e., clearance is not affected by alterations in plasma protein binding or metabolic activity), perfusion-rate limited (i.e., clearance is affected by alterations in liver blood flow rate), and saturable. Consequently, the extraction ratio is high and dose dependent; only a small fraction of an oral dose escapes first-pass metabolism and reaches the systemic circulation.[70,71] Therefore, oral bioavailability is low but may increase with repeated doses as saturation of liver enzymes occurs. Likewise, oral availability increases with increasing doses.

The total body clearance of propranolol is very high, approaching or perhaps exceeding liver blood flow in dogs.[70,71] Alterations in liver blood flow due to physiologic variables (e.g., feeding), disease states (e.g., cardiac failure), or concomitant administration of drugs affecting cardiac output or liver blood flow would be expected to affect the clearance of propranolol. Feeding increases (52 percent) the clearance of intravenous propranolol; this is mostly due to an increase in hepatic blood flow, which remains elevated for 5 to 7 hours after feeding.[72] Propranolol decreases liver blood flow and decreases its own clearance as well as the clearance of other highly extracted drugs (e.g., lidocaine).[48]

The dose of propranolol required to suppress

catecholamine-induced arrhythmias is 0.1 to 1.0 mg/kg for intravenous dosing and 2 to 4 mg/kg for oral dosing. Doses may be given two to three times daily. Feeding does not affect the extent of oral absorption of propranolol but significantly delays the rate of absorption, shifting the time of peak plasma concentration from about 60 to 158 minutes.[72] Therapeutic plasma concentrations range from 40 to 85 ng/ml in human subjects and are probably near this range in dogs and cats.

Drugs other than propranolol that possess β-adrenoceptor blocking activity, are potentially useful in the treatment of cardiac arrhythmias in dogs and cats (Table 15-6). Metoprolol, atenolol, and acebutolol are *cardioselective* (β₁) adrenoceptor blocking drugs (Table 15-8) that offer specific advantages in patients with bronchospastic disorders or insulin-dependent diabetes mellitus.

Atenolol

Atenolol has been used successfully to reduce sinus rate, depress AV conduction, and eliminate premature ventricular depolarizations in dogs with naturally occurring heart disease. Atenolol has low lipohilicity and does not readily cross the blood-brain barrier, thereby decreasing the potential for CNS side effects. Once-daily dosing (0.2-0.5 mg/kg) is a practical advantage of atenolol therapy.

Pindolol

Pindolol is the only β-blocking drug that exhibits intrinsic sympathomimetic activity (Table 15-8). Although the practical significance of this observation is controversial, pindolol may prove useful in supporting a failing myocardium while inhibiting the potentially deleterious effects of a sudden increases in sympathetic tone. The potential benefit of pindolol as an alternative to propranolol in the treatment of dogs or cats with cardiac arrhythmias and bronchospastic disease remains to be determined. The dose is 0.25-0.5 mg/kg tid PO.

Labetolol

Labetolol is a unique nonselective β-adrenoceptor blocking drug that also possesses α₁-adrenoceptor blocking activity. α-Adrenoceptor stimulation is important in initiating cardiac arrhythmias during inhalation anesthesia with halothane and secondary to myocardial ischemia. Labetalol may prove to be more specific and effective than propranolol in the treatment of these latter causes for arrhythmias.

Amiodarone

Amiodarone is a class 3 antiarrhythmic drug initially introduced as a coronary artery dilator.[52] Like bretylium and other class 3 antiarrhythmic drugs, amiodarone is believed to produce its antiarrhythmic effects by causing marked prolongation of the action potential and effective refractory period in both atrial and ventricular tissues. Therapeutic doses of amiodarone decrease sinus rate and depress AV conduction velocity. The ECG from patients receiving amiodarone usually demonstrates a slowing of sinus rate, P-R and Q-T prolongation, and a flattening of the T wave. Initial clinical studies in dogs treated with oral amiodarone for refractory ventricular arrhythmias have not been encouraging. Cardiac contractility and arterial blood pressure are minimally depressed by therapeutic doses of amiodarone. Amiodarone decreases the renal excretion of digoxin.

Amiodarone is recommended as therapy for atrial and ventricular, unifocal or multifocal premature depolarizations.[73] Arrhythmias caused by an accessory pathway are particularly susceptible to treatment with amiodarone because of its ability to prolong refractoriness in specialized tissues. Amiodarone therapy in humans is associated with a significant number of side effects which include a gray or bluish discoloration of the skin, corneal microdeposits, alteration in thyroid function and rarely, pulmonary fibrosis.[52] Amiodarone-induced pulmonary fibrosis has resulted in death in humans. The extreme effectiveness of amiodarone in potentially lethal cardiac arrhythmias that are refractory to conventional antiarrhythmic therapy warrants its continued investigation in dogs with atrial and ventricular arrhythmias.

Amiodarone is a lipophilic weak base that has a large volume of distribution (2.22 L/kg).[74] At steady state, the concentration of amiodarone in the myocardium is almost ninety times its concentration in plasma reflecting the selective uptake of the drug in the heart. Furthermore, myocardial concentrations of the drug decrease much more slowly than plasma concentrations.

Amiodarone is cleared rapidly (CL_p = 21.0 + 7.0 ml/min/kg) by metabolism.[74] A major metabolite is N-desmethylamiodarone, which accumulates during chronic oral dosing. Serum digoxin concentrations increase when amiodarone is added to the therapeutic regimen. This could predispose to signs and symptoms of digitalis toxicity. The oral bioavailability is poor, probably due to extensive first-pass metabolism.

Bretylium

Bretylium is an antihypertensive drug which possesses Class 3 antiarrhythmic effects.[20] Other potentially useful drugs within this class that remain experimental include bethanidine, clofilium, N-acetylprocainamide, and sotalol (Table 15-2). Bretylium produces antiarrhythmic effects by both indirect and direct actions (Table 15-4). Bretylium therapy results in an initial release of catecholamines from adrenergic nerve terminals. This effect is transient and is followed by a prolonged period, during which norepinephrine release from postganglionic nerve terminals in inhibited. The direct actions of bretylium are limited to ventricular muscle and Purkinje tissues, in which it markedly prolongs action potential duration and the effective refractory period.[75] Bretylium increases the electric threshold necessary to induce ventricular fibrillation.[76] Clinically, the administration of bretylium in therapeutic dosages causes a transient increase in sinus and AV conduction velocity, presumably associated with the initial catecholamine release.[52] This is followed by a longer period during which heart rate and AV conduction are depressed. The ECG is not significantly changed by bretylium.

The intravenous administration of bretylium produces a biphasic hemodynamic response. Cardiac contractility, vascular tone and arterial blood pressure increase transiently (10 to 15 minutes) followed by a longer period during which heart rate and blood pressure are decreased. Cardiac contractility and cardiac output are not significantly affected during this second phase. Bretylium decreases pulmonary capillary wedge pressure by dilating venous capacitance vessels.

Toxicity associated with bretylium therapy is rare (Table 15-6). Hypotension is infrequent and, when it does occur, is easily treated with intravenous fluids. Ataxia, nausea, and vomiting may occur after rapid intravenous administration. No significant drug interactions have been reported in conjunction with bretylium therapy.

Bretylium has limited use as an antiarrhythmic drug in dogs and cats. It should not be used as a first-choice antiarrhythmic drug in the treatment of ventricular arrhythmias and is frequently unsuccessful when used in this manner. Bretylium is potentially indicated as therapy for life-threatening ventricular arrhythmias, including unifocal and multifocal ventricular tachycardia. Early studies in dogs and humans suggested that bretylium may be effective as a chemical defibrilling agent.[77] More recent investigations studying electrically induced ventricular fibrillation in experimental dogs suggest that bretylium will not restore sinus rhythm.[78] Poor results may be attributed in part to the fact that the onset of the antifibrillory effects of bretylium may be delayed for 4 to 6 hours following its administration. Clinically, if bretylium is to produce a beneficial effect, it should be administered early in the course of therapy and in conjunction with more conventional antiarrhythmic therapy. Bretylium should not be administered to extremely bradycardic or hypotensive patients.

Bretylium is a hydrophilic quaternary amine (i.e., it is ionized at all pH values). Its volume of distribution is lower than that of other drugs discussed in this chapter because of its greater polarity (Table 15-7).

The total clearance of bretylium is low and is attributed entirely to renal elimination.[78] Total clearance is diminished in those patients with renal dysfunction and the dose should be reduced accordingly. The limited volume of distribution and low clearance result in a comparatively long half-life of about 10.4 hours. Bretylium is well absorbed after intramuscular administration but is not absorbed after oral administration.

Antifibrillatory effects are related more closely to tissue drug concentration than to plasma drug concentration. Drug concentrations in plasma decline rapidly after intravenous dosing; tissue concentrations rise slowly, peaking at 1.5 to 6 hours.[78] Therefore, antifibrillatory effects are not seen immediately but are delayed for 3 to 6 hours after a single dose.

Intravenous doses of 2 to 6 mg/kg in dogs produce myocardial tissue concentrations which peak at 6 to 15 µg/ml in 3 to 6 hours. These concentrations increase ventricular fibrillation threshold 5- to 18-fold in dogs with or without myocardial ischemia.

Verapamil

Verapamil is a class 4 antiarrhythmic drug initially developed as a peripheral artery and coronary vasodilator.[20] Class 4 antiarrhythmic drugs derive their electrophysiologic and antiarrhythmic activity by producing dose dependent depression of transmembrane calcium flux through the slow channel.[79] This action has led to the terms slow-channel inhibitory drugs, calcium antagonists, and calcium-entry blockers (the last of which is preferred). Although a wide variety of compounds have been developed which inhibit calcium entry into cardiac cells, only verapamil and diltiazem demonstrate significant antiarrhythmic activity.[79] This action is believed to be due to their ability to depress the slow inward Ca^{2+} current and cause partial inhibition of the fast Na^+ current. Verapamil causes dose-dependent decreases in sinus rate and atrioventricular conduction velocity. Therapeutic dosages of verapamil fail to exert significant electrophysiologic effects on atrial or ventricular myocardium or specialized tissues. Verapamil decreases automaticity in ischemic or diseased atrial muscle. Dosages of verapamil that produce plasma concentrations in the high therapeutic range slow conduction in the His bundle. Verapamil produces prolongation of the P-R interval but otherwise does not induce significant alterations in the electrocardiogram.

Verapamil is a potent negative inotrope and vasodilator. Therapeutic dosages of verapamil cause decreases in cardiac contractility, vasodilation, and hypotension.[11] Large doses of verapamil can produce electromechanical uncoupling. These observations are particularly relevant to the treatment of patients with heart failure and must be considered whenever verapamil therapy is contemplated.

Toxic doses of verapamil produce sinus bradycardia, AV block, hypotension, and heart failure[10] (Table 15-6). These deleterious effects can be partially antagonized by the intravenous administration of calcium containing solutions or catecholamines. Verapamil decreases the renal clearance of digoxin resulting in increased serum digoxin concentrations.[80,81] The simultaneous administration of verapamil and β-adrenoceptor blocking drugs can lead to a sudden unexpected decrease in sinus rate or complete heart block.

Verapamil is recommended as therapy for supraventricular arrhythmias including sinus tachycardia, atrial premature depolarizations, paroxysmal atrial tachycardia, atrial flutter or fibrillation, and atrial tachyarrhythmias associated with an accessory pathway. Reciprocating supraventricular tachyarrhythmias originating from the atrioventricular node are responsive to verapamil therapy. Verapamil is particularly effective in slowing ventricular rate in patients with atrial fibrillation and has been used in conjunction with digoxin for this purpose. Verapamil is contraindicated in patients with sick sinus syndrome, AV conduction disturbances, and congestive heart failure. Arterial blood pressure should be monitored in patients receiving verapamil intravenously. Experience with verapamil in dogs and cats is limited, and initial clinical trials have been disappointing. A high incidence of cardiovascular side effects, including congestive symptoms, hypotension, and heart failure, are reported.[82] Additional clinical studies must be conducted before verapamil can be recommended as safe and effective therapy for the treatment of arrhythmias in dogs and cats.

Verapamil is a lipophilic weak base that is rapidly and extensively distributed to extravascular tissues (Table 15-7).

Total body clearance is very high due to extensive liver metabolism and possibly other routes of elimination.[83] Two metabolites resulting from successive N-demethylation are found in plasma after oral and intravenous dosing and may contribute to the pharmacologic effect.[83] The oral bioavailabilty of verapamil is low due to extensive first-pass metabolism.

There is a linear relationship between the logarithm of plasma verapamil concentrations and changes in AV conduction time, as estimated from the P-R interval of the surface ECG.[84] At a plasma concentration of 50 to 100 ng/ml, the P-R interval increases by about 50 msec. A dose of 30 mg of verapamil, given at a rate of 3 mg/min is well tolerated by 20-kg mongrel dogs. More rapid administration or higher doses leads to second-degree heart block and should be avoided.

INVESTIGATIONAL ANTIARRHYTHMIC DRUGS

A larger numer of antiarrhythmic drugs are currently being investigated in humans for potential clinical use (Table 15-2). Whether these drugs will provide beneficial antiarrhythmic benefits with minimal toxic side effects in dogs and cats remains to be determined.

REFERENCES

1. Resnekov L: Circulatory effects of cardiac dysrhythmias. Cardiovasc Clin 2:24, 1970
2. McIntosh HD, Morris JJ: The hemodynamic consequences of arrhythmias. Prog Cardiovasc Dis 8:330, 1966
3. Zipes DP: A consideration of antiarrhythmic therapy. (Editorial.) Circulation 72:949, 1985
4. Harrison DC: Antiarrhythmic drug classification: new science and practical applications. Am J Cardiol 56:185, 1985
5. Williams EMV: A classification of antiarrhythmic actions reassessed after a decade of new drugs. J Clin Pharmacol 24:129, 1984
6. Maze M, Smith CM: Identification of receptor mechanism mediating epinephrine-induced arrhythmias during halothane anesthesia in the dog. Anesthesiology 59:322, 1983
7. Penkoske PA, Sobel SE, Corr PB: Disparate electrophysiological alterations accompanying dysrhythmia due to coronary occlusion and reperfusion in the cat. Circulation 58:1023, 1978
8. Muir WW, Sams R: Clinical pharmacodynamics and pharmacokinetics of beta-adrenoceptor blocking drugs in veterinary medicine. Comp Cont Ed 6:156, 1984
9. Cardinal R, Sasyniuk BI: Electrophysiological effects of bretylium tosylate on subendocardial Purkinje fibers from infarcted canine hearts. J Pharmacol Expl Ther 204:159, 1978
10. Antman EM, Stone PH, Muller JE, Braunwald E: Calcium channel blocking agents in the treatment of cardiovascular disorders. Part 1. Basic and clinical electrophysiologic effects. Ann Intern Med 93:875, 1980
11. Stone PH, Antman EM, Muller JE, Braunwald E: Calcium channel blocking agents in the treatment of cardiovascular disorders. Part II. Hemodynamic effects and clinical applications. Ann Intern Med 93:886, 1980
12. Singh BN, Baky S, Nademanee K: Second-generation calcium antagonists: Search for greater selectivity and versatility. Am J Cardiol 55:214B, 1985
13. Hoffman BF, Bigger TJ: Digitalis and allied cardiac glycosides. p. 716. In Gilman AG, Goodman LS, Rall TW, Murad F (eds): The Pharmacological Basis of Therapeutics. 7th Ed. Macmillan, New York, 1985
14. Estes NAM, Garan H, McGovern B, Ruskin JN: Class I antiarrhythmic agents: Classification, electrophysiologic considerations, and clinical effects. p. 183. In Reiser HJ, Horowitz IN (eds): Mechanisms and Treatment of Cardiac Arrhythmias—Relevance of Basic Studies to Clinical Management. Urban and Schwarzenberg, Baltimore 1985
15. Nattel S, Bailey JC: Time course of the electrophysiological effects of quinidine on canine cardiac Purkinje fibers: Concentration dependence and comparison with lidocaine and disopyramide. J Pharmacol Exp Ther 225:176, 1983
16. Materson BJ, Caralis PV: Risk of cardiac arrhythmias in relation to potassium imbalance. J Cardiovasc Pharmacol 6:S493, 1984
17. McGovern B: Hypokalemia and cardiac arrhythmias. (Editorial views.) Anesthesiology 63:127, 1985
18. Chassaing C, Duchene-Marullaz P, Paire M: Mechanism of action of quinidine on heart rate in the dog. J Pharmacol Exp Ther 222:688, 1982
19. Schmid PG, Nelson LD, Mark AL, et al: Inhibition of adrenergic vasoconstriction by quinidine. J Pharmacol Exp Ther 188:124, 1974
20. Bigger JT, Hoffman BF: Antiarrhythmic drugs. p. 748. In Gilman AG, Goodman LS, Rall TW, Morod F (eds): The Pharmacological Basis of Therapeutics. 7th Ed. Macmillan, New York, 1985
21. Leahey EB, Bigger JT, Butler VP Jr: Quinidine-digoxin interaction. Time course and pharmacokinetics. Am J Cardiol 48:1141, 1981
22. Warner NJ, Leahey EB Jr, Hougen JJ, et al: Tissue digoxin concentrations during the quinidine-digoxin interaction. Am J Cardiol 51:1717, 1983
23. Lathers CM, Roberts J: Are the sympathetic neural effects of digoxin and quinidine involved in their action of cardiac rhythm. J Cardiovasc Pharm 7:350, 1985
24. Neff CA, Davis LE, Baggot JD: A comparative study of the pharmacokinetics of quinidine. Am J Vet Res 33:1521, 1972
25. Hiatt E, Quinn G: The distribution of quinine, quin-

idine, cinchonine, and cinchonidine in fluids and tissues of dogs. J Pharmacol Exp Ther 83:101, 1985

26. Mayersohn M, Perrier D, Fenster P, Marcus FI: Steady-state plasma concentrations of quinidine and propranolol. Clin Pharmacol Ther 97:678, 1979

27. Badke FR, Walsh RA, Crawford MH, et al: Hemodynamic effects of N-acetylprocainamide compared with procainamide in conscious dogs. Circulation 6:1142, 1981

28. Ellroot AG, Murata GH, Riedinger MS, et al: Severe neutropenia associated with sustained-release procainamide. Ann Intern Med 100:197, 1984

29. Wu D, Denes P, Bauernfiend, R, et al: Effects of procainamide on atrioventricular nodal re-entrant paroxysmal tachycardia. Circulation 57:1171, 1978

30. Bagwell EE, Walle, Drayer DE, et al: Correlation of the electrophysiological and antiarrhythmic properties of the N-acetyl metabolite of procainamide with plasma and tissue concentrations in the dog. J Pharmacol Exp Ther 197:38, 1976

31. Ranney RE, Dean RR, Karim A, Radzialowski FM: Disopyramide phosphate: pharmacokinetic and pharmacologic relationships of a new antiarrhythmic agent. Arch Int Pharmacodyn 191:162, 1971

32. Kus T, Sasyniuk B: Electrophysiological actions of disopyramide phosphate on canine ventricular muscle and Purkinje fibers. Circ Res 37:844, 1975

33. Heel RC, Brogden RN, Speight TM, Avery GS: Disopyramide: a review of its pharmacological properties and therapeutic use in treating cardiac arrhythmias. Drugs 15:331, 1978

34. Walsh RA, Horwitz LD: Adverse hemodynamic effects of intravenous disopyramide compared with quinidine in conscious dogs. Circulation 60:1053, 1979

35. Karim A, Cook C, Novotney RL, Zagarella J and Campion J: Pharmacokinetics and steady-state myocardial uptake of disopyramide in the dog. Drug Metab Dispos 6:338, 1978

36. Cook CS, Karim A and Sollman P: Stereoselectivity in the metabolism of disopyramide enantiomers in rat and dog. Drug Metab Dispos 10:116, 1982

37. Yeh BK, Sung P, Scherlag BJ: Effects of disopyramide on electrophysiological and mechanical properties of the heart. J Pharm Sci 62:1924, 1973

38. Harrison DC, Alderman EL: The pharmacology and clinical use of lidocaine as an antiarrhythmic drug. Modern Treatm 9:139, 1972

39. Hondeghem LM, Grant AO, Jensen RA: Antiarrhythmic drug action: selective depression of hypoxic cardiac cells. Am Heart J 87:602, 1974

40. Mason DT, DeMaria AN, Amsterdam EA, et al: Antiarrhythmic agents I: mechanisms of action and clinical pharmacology. Drugs 5:261, 1973

41. Mason DT, DeMaria AN, Amsterdam EA, et al: Antiarrhythmic agents II: therapeutic considerations. Drugs 5:292, 1973

42. Ikeda M, Dohi T, Tsujimoto A: Inhibition of gamma-aminobutyric acid release from synaptosomes by local anesthetics. Am Soc Anesth 38:495, 1983

43. Feely J, Wade D, McAllister CB, et al: Effect of hypotension on liver blood flow and lidocaine disposition. N Engl J Med 307:866, 1982

44. Branch RA, Shand DG, Wilkinson GR, Nies AS: The reduction of lidocaine clearance by dl-propranolol. N Engl J Med 303:373, 1980

45. Lineberger AS, Sprague DH, Battaglini JW: Sinus arrest associated with cimetidine. Anesth Analg 64:554, 1985

46. Keenhagan JB, Boyes RN: The tissue distribution, metabolism, and excretion of lidocaine in rats, guinea pigs, dogs and man. J Pharmacol Exp Ther 180:454, 1972

47. Wilcke JR, Davis LE, Neff-Davis CA, Koritz GD: Pharmacokinetics of lidocaine and its active metabolites in dogs. J Vet Pharmacol Ther 6:49, 1983

48. Branch RA, Shand DG, Wilkinson GR, Nies AS: The reduction of lidocaine clearance by dl-propranolol: An example of hemodynamic drug interaction. J Pharmacol Exp Ther 184:515, 1973

49. Wilcke JR, Davis LE, Neff-Davis CA: Determination of lidocaine concentrations producing therapeutic and toxic effects in dogs. J Vet Pharmacol Ther 6:105, 1983

50. Rosen MR, Hoffman BF: Mechanisms of action of antiarrhythmic drugs. Circ Res 32:1, 1973

51. Louisa S, Kutt H, McDowell F: The cardiocirculatory changes caused by intravenous dilantin and its solvent. Am Heart J 74:523, 1967

52. Lucchesi BR, Patterson ES: Antiarrhythmic drugs. p. 329. In Antonaccio MJ (ed): Cardiovascular Pharmacology. 2nd Ed. Raven Press, New York, 1984

53. Sanders JE, Yeary RA, Powers JD, deWet P: Relationship between serum and brain concentrations of phenytoin in the dog. Am J Vet Res 40:473, 1979

54. Dayton PG, Cucinell SA, Weiss M, Perel JM: Dose-dependence of drug plasma level decline in dogs. J Pharmacol Exp Ther 158:305, 1967

55. Sanders JE, Yeary RA: Serum concentrations of orally administered diphenylhydantoin in dogs. J Am Vet Med Assoc 172:153, 1978

56. Roye B, Serrans EE, Hammer RH, Wilder BJ: Plasma kinetics of diphenylhydantoin in dogs and cats. Am J Vet Res 34:947, 1973

57. Anderson JL: Mason JW, Winkle RA, et al: Clinical electrophysiologic effects of tocainide. Circulation 57:685, 1978

58. Berlin-Wahlen A, Barcus JC, Keenhagen JB, et al: Elimination of N-(2-aminoacyl)-2,6-xylidines after intravenous infusion in dogs. Acta Pharm Suec 14:417, 1977

59. Coltart DJ, Berndt TB, Kernoff R, Harrison DC: Antiarrhythmic and circulatory effects of Astra W36095—A new lidocaine-like agent. Am J Cardiol 34:35, 1974

60. Campbell NPS, Kelly JG, Adgey AAJ, Shanks RG: The clinical pharmacology of mexiletine. Br J Clin Pharmacol 6:103, 1978

61. Prescott LF, Pottage A, Clements JA: Absorption, distribution and elimination of mexiletine. Postgrad Med J 53:50, 1977

62. Beckett AH, Chidomere EC: The distribution and excretion of mexiletine in man. Postgrad Med J 53:60, 1977

63. Dobmeyer D, Muir WW, Schaal SF: Antiarrhythmic effects of flecainide against canine ventricular arrhythmias induced by two-stage coronary ligation and halothane-epinephrine. J Cardiovasc Pharmacol 7:238, 1985

64. Muir WW, Sams RA: Clinical pharmacodynamics and pharmacokinetics of Beta-adrenoceptor blocking drugs in veterinary medicine. Comp Cont Ed 156:156, 1984

65. Shiroff RA, Mathis J, Zellis R, et al: Propranolol rebound: a retrospective study. Am J Cardiol 41:778, 1978

66. Evans GH, Nies AS, Shand DG: The disposition of propranolol. III. Decreased half-life and volume of distribution as a result of plasma binding in man, monkey, dog and rat. J Pharmacol Exp Ther 186:114, 1973

67. Vu VT, Abramson FP: The pathways of propranolol metabolism in dog and rat liver 10,000 g supernatant fractions. Drug Metab Dispos 8:300, 1980

68. Walle T, Oatis JE, Walle UK, Knapp DR: New ring hydroxylated metabolites of propranolol. Drug Metab Dispos 10:122, 1982

69. Fitzgerald JD, O'Donnell SR: Pharmacology of 4-hydroxypropranolol, a metabolite of propranolol. Br J Pharmacol 43:222, 1971

70. Orme CF, Orme ML, Buranapong P, Macelean D, Breckenridge AM and Dollery CT: Contribution of the liver to the overall elimination of propranolol. J Pharmacokinet Biopharm 4:17, 1976

71. Kates RE, Keene BW, Hamlin RL: Pharmacokinetics of propranolol in the dog. J Vet Pharmacol Ther 2:21, 1979

72. Bai SA, Walle UK, Walle T: Influence of food on the intravenous and oral doses kinetics of propranolol in the dog. J Pharmacokinet Biopharm 13:229, 1985

73. Swan JH, Chisholm AW: Control of recurrent supraventricular tachycardia with amiodarone hydrochloride. Can Med Assoc J 114:43, 1976

74. Latini R, Connolly SJ, Kates RE: Myocardial disposition of amiodarone in the dog. J Pharmacol Ex Ther 224:603, 1983

75. Bigger JT Jr, Jaffe CC: The effect of bretylium tosylate on the electrophysiologic properties of ventricular muscle and Purkinje fibers. Am J Cardiol 27:82, 1971

76. Sanna G, Arcidiacono R: Chemical ventricular defibrillation of the human heart with bretylium tosylate. Am J Cardiol 32:982, 1973

77. Breznock EM, Kagan K, Hibser NK: Effects of bretylium tosylate on the in vivo fibrillating canine ventricle. Am J Vet Res 38:89, 1977

78. Anderson JL, Patterson E, Conlon M, et al: Kinetics of antifibrillatory effects of bretylium: Correlation with myocardial drug concentrations. Am J Cardiol 46:583, 1980

79. Katz AM: Basic cellular mechanisms of action in the calcium-channel blockers. Am J Cardiol 55:2B, 1985

80. Klein HO, Kaplialinsky, E: Verapamil and digoxin: Their respective effects on atrial fibrillation and their interaction. Am J Cardiol 50:894, 1982

81. Kuhlman, J: Effects of verapamil, diltiazem, and nifedipine on plasma levels and renal excretion of digitoxin. Clin Pharmacol Ther 38:667, 1985

82. Newman RK, Bishop VS, Peterson DF, et al: Effect of verapamil on left ventricular performance in conscious dogs. J Pharmacol Exp Ther 201:723, 1977

83. McIlhenny HM: Metabolism of [^{14}C] verapamil. J Med Chem 14:1178, 1971

84. McAllister RG Jr, Bourne DWA, Dittert LW: The pharmacology of verapamil. I. Elimination kinetics in dogs and correlation of plasma levels with effect on the electrocardiogram. J Pharmacol Exp Ther 202:38, 1977

85. Papich MG, Davis LE, Davis CA, et al: Pharmacokinetics of procainamide hydrochloride in dogs. Am J Vet Res 47:2351, 1986

16

Cardiovascular Syncope

Robert H. Lusk, Jr.
Stephen J. Ettinger

Syncope is the complete loss of consciousness due to deprivation of oxygen or glucose-energy substrates that transiently impairs cerebral metabolism. In contrast to other organs, the metabolism of the brain is entirely dependent on oxygen perfusion. Limited storage of high-energy phosphates in the brain makes its energy supply dependent on the oxidation of glucose extracted from blood. Cessation of cerebral blood flow for as little as 10 seconds leads to a loss of consciousness.[1]

Syncope must be considered a symptom complex rather than a primary disease. The differential diagnosis of cardiovascular syncope is extensive (Tables 16-1 and 16-2). Noncardiovascular disorders may cause similar signs and must be included in the differential diagnosis (e.g., neurogenic seizures, narcolepsy, catalepsy, episodic weakness, hypoglycemia, acute hemorrhage, and diseases associated with reduced alertness).[2] Syncope is almost always a reversible clinical state but can occasionally result in sudden death.[3]

In dogs and cats, a syncopal event may begin with generalized muscle weakness, which leads to ataxia. It can progress to collapse and loss of consciousness. The animal may initially become motionless with relaxed skeletal muscles. This relaxed state is often followed by uncoordinated muscle movements giving the impression of seizurelike activity. Loss of muscle sphincter control may initiate involuntary urination and/or defecation. The patient often cries out during the episode. This is related to a release of central nervous system activity. Syncope, seizures, and episodic weakness are often difficult to distinguish from each other.[2-5]

CAUSES OF SYNCOPE

Cardiovascular syncope can be classified into two major categories (Table 16-1). One group includes animals with a normal heart but with peripheral vascular and/or neurogenic dysfunction. These abnormalities are difficult to recognize clinically. The other group includes primary cardiac dysfunction with normal peripheral vascular and nervous systems. These disorders represent most of the causes of clinically recognizable syncope.[2-5]

Peripheral Vascular or Neurologic Dysfunction (Normal Heart)

Vasovagal and vasodepressor syncope can occur in healthy patients. In dogs and cats it is associated with marked excitement. Respiration rate usually

TABLE 16-1 Causes of Cardiovascular and
Cardiopulmonary Syncope

Peripheral vascular or neurologic dysfunction with normal heart
    Vasovagal
    Postural hypotension
    Hyperventilation
    Carotid sinus hypersensitivity
    Glossopharyngeal neuralgia
    Deglutition
Cardiovascular dysfunction
    Intracardiac obstruction to blood flow
        Aortic stenosis
        Pulmonic stenosis
        Ball thrombus
        Hypertrophic obstructive cardiomyopathy
    Extracardiac obstruction to blood flow
        Cardiac tamponade
        Constrictive pericarditis
        Dirofilariasis
    Arrhythmias
        Tachycardias
        Bradycardias
        Bradycardia-tachycardia (sick sinus) syndrome
        Atrioventricular block (high-grade second degree, third degree)
    Cardiopulmonary dysfunction
        Cough (tussive) syncope
        Right-to-left shunts (congenital heart disease)
        Pulmonary hypertension
        Pulmonary emboli
    Myocardial infarction

(Modified from Ettinger SJ: Weakness and syncope. p. 83. In Ettinger SJ (ed): Textbook of Veterinary Internal Medicine. Diseases of the Dog and Cat. 2nd Ed. Vol. 1. WB Saunders, Philadelphia, 1983.)

increases and the animal appears weak and confused. Hemodynamically there is peripheral arterial vasodilation and venoconstriction. The cardiac output fails to rise despite a decrease in peripheral vascular resistance and venoconstriction. Concomitant increased vagal activity produces bradycardia. This associated bradycardia in humans can be blocked with atropine, but the fainting episode still occurs. Therefore, the decreased heart rate is not the sole cause. Humans with postural hypotension develop a fall in blood pressure when rising from a supine position.

When evaluating an animal for postural hypoten-sion the following clinical causes should be considered: drug therapy (β-adrenergic blockers, vasodilators, antihypertensives and tranquilizers), intravascular volume depletion (diuretics, vomiting, diarrhea), diabetes mellitus, and Addison's disease (hypoadrenocorticism).[1-4]

The hyperventilation syndrome is associated with anxious or hyperexcitable pets. Resultant overaeration of alveoli and a relative decrease in alveolar and arterial PCO_2 may result. Decreased PCO_2 may cause progressive cerebral arterial vasoconstriction and peripheral vasodilation. This leads to a progressive decrease in cerebral perfusion.[1]

Carotid sinus hypersensitivity may cause changes in vasomotor tone and heart rate. Afferent impulses from baroreceptors activates the vagal center and inhibitory neurons of the vasomotor center. Vagal traffic to the heart increases while sympathetic outflow to the heart and vessels decrease. Vasodilation, decreased blood pressure, bradycardia, reduced cardiac output, and syncope may result. This syndrome can occur in conjunction with neoplasia, inflammatory processes of the neck, or tight collars.[6]

Glossopharyngeal neuralgia and deglutination syncope have been reported in humans. In the former, pain from the middle ear, soft palate or pharynx may be transmitted afferently via the vagal and glossopharyngeal nerves centrally. Reflex hypotension and syncope can result. In the latter, syncope has been initiated by swallowing, usually in association with exophageal tumors, diverticulum or spasm.

Cardiovascular Dysfunction

Cardiac disorders represent most of the clinically recognizable causes of syncope. They have in common a transient but marked reduction in cardiac output due to obstruction to blood flow, arrhythmias, or cardiopulmonary dysfunction (Tables 16-1 and 16-2).

Obstruction to blood flow can cause cardiac output to become relatively fixed. During exercise, systemic vascular resistance normally decreases, in part due to metabolite induced vasodilation. If cardiac output is restricted by a disease such as aortic stenosis, hypotension and syncope can result. Ball thrombi in cats with cardiomyopathy can reduce preload by decreasing ventricular filling. Arrhyth-

Table 16-2 Syncopal-Associated Disease

Type of Syncope	Pathophysiology			Physiologic Event
1. Obstruction to Cerebral Blood Flow	Arteriosclerosis Thrombosis Embolus Neoplasia Trauma			Cerebrovascular accident Transient ischemic attack Tussive syncope Hyperventilation
2. Cardiogenic	Heart Rate Rhythm	↓ Heart rate		Heart block Tachycardia bradycardia syndrome Vasodepressor syncope Carotid sinus hypersensitivity
		↑ Heart rate		Supraventricular tachycardia Ventricular tachycardia
	Obstruction			Asymmetric hypertrophy (IHSS) Myxoma Pulmonary hypertension Ischemic heart disease Heartworm disease
3. Blood pressure	↓ Cardiac output	↓ Heart rate		Cardiogenic
		↓ Stroke volume	Contractility	Cardiogenic
			↓ Filling → ↓ Volume	Blood loss Adrenal insufficiency Tussive syncope
			↓ Venomotor tone	Postural hypotension vasodilator drugs Hyperventilation
	↓ Peripheral resistance	Vascular		
		↓ Sympathetic stimulation		Micturition syncope Adrenergic-blocking drugs Postural hypotension Vasodepressor syncope Carotid sinus hypersensitivity
4. Blood constituency	↓ O_2			Cardiopulmonary
	↓ Glucose			Reactive or fasting hypoglycemia

(Ettinger SJ: Weakness and syncope, p. 84. In Ettinger SJ (ed): Textbook of Veterinary Internal Medicine, Diseases of the Dog and Cat. 2nd Ed. Vol. 1. WB Saunders, Philadelphia, 1983.)

mias may accompany these disorders and contribute to syncope.[2]

Cardiac tamponade or constrictive pericarditis impede diastolic filling. This increases intraventricular end-diastolic pressure, reduces ventricular end-diastolic volume and decreases cardiac output. Compensatory sinus tachycardia, increased peripheral vascular resistance, increased systemic and pulmonary venous pressure may eventually become inadequate.[7] Syncope can result, especially when the animal is stressed or excited.

Syncope accompanying hypertrophic cardiomyopathy (HCM) is common in dogs but rare in cats.[8,9] The obstructive form of HCM may be due to a dynamic movement of the anterior mitral valve leaflet toward the ventricular septum during systole. A sudden reduction in left ventricular filling or arrhythmia may also contribute to syncope.[10]

Arrhythmias may significantly reduce cardiac output. Ventricular filling may be diminished by rapid heart rates (e.g., ventricular or supraventricular tachycardias) or lack of atrial contraction (e.g., atrial fibrillation or atrial standstill, especially in the setting of organic heart disease). Decreased cardiac output can result from severe bradycardia (e.g., complete atrioventricular block) or prolonged asystole (e.g., sick sinus syndrome). Deleterious effects of the arrhythmias on coronary perfusion and myocardial function may also be contributory.[1]

Cough or tussive syncope is very common in older, small breed dogs with murmurs of mitral insufficiency. These pets have a high incidence of acquired chronic AV valve disease, collapsing trachea, and chronic obstructive pulmonary disease.[2,4] The mechanisms of syncope may include several factors such as an acute reduction in cardiac output, peripheral dilation following the cough, markedly increased cerebrospinal fluid pressure with secondary intracranial capillary and venous compression, increased cerebral vascular resistance due to hypocapnia of coughing, and a "concussive effect" caused by a sudden, increased intracranial pressure transmitted from the thorax and abdomen via the cerebrospinal fluid.[11,12]

Approach to the Syncopal Patient

Cardiac syncope must be differentiated from a variety of other disease processes. The clinician must completely review the patient history, which, along with the physical examination, is the most important factor in reaching a correct diagnosis. The frequency, clinical characteristics of the animal before and after the syncopal episode, and relative occurrence of syncopal events must be ascertained. The client should be questioned as to circumstances which may relate to syncope (e.g., exertion, coughing, hot environment). A complete medication history must always be obtained.

A complete and thorough physical examination must be conducted. It should include a detailed neurologic and cardiovascular evaluation. Careful attention must be paid to auscultation of the heart, palpation of the pulses, capillary refill time and mucous membrane color assessment.

Most syncopal diseases can be diagnosed from the history and physical examination. To elucidate the more difficult cases, a systematic clinical data base must be generated. This should include a blood panel with hemogram and complete biochemical profile. A 10-lead ECG is mandatory to detect arrhythmias, infer acid–base and electrolyte abnormalities and suggest ventricular or atrial enlargement. If the cause of syncope remains unknown the workup may be expanded to include a 24-hour ambulatory ECG.[13–16] Cardiac catheterization may be performed but echocardiography is preferred due to increased information yield and greatly reduced patient risk. When blood pressure monitoring becomes more widely available, postural pressure measurements may yield valuable information in a small subset of patients.

The treatment of syncope depends on accurate identification and characterization of the underlying or inciting disorder. Specific breed associations with common causes of syncope are listed[15] (Table 16-3). Appropriate medical and surgical management is discussed elsewhere (Chps. 8, 14, 15, 29, 30).

TABLE 16-3 Specific Breed Associations with Common Causes of Syncope

Breed	Common Causes of Syncope
Boxer	Ventricular arrhythmias, cardiomyopathy, vasodepressor syncope (?)
Brachycephalic breeds	Upper airway obstructive syndromes
Dachshund	Sick sinus syndrome
Doberman pinscher	Ventricular arrhythmias, dilated cardiomyopathy, His-bundle disease
English springer spaniel	Atrial muscular dystrophy (silent atrium)
German shepherd	Ventricular arrhythmias, dilated cardiomyopathy, pericardial disease, hemangiosarcoma; AV nodal disease
Miniature schnauzer	Sick sinus syndrome (especially females)
Pug	His-bundle stenosis

(Keene BW: Differential diagnosis of syncope. p. 220. Proceedings of the Fifth Annual Veterinary Medicine Forum. Am Coll Vet Intern Med, 1987.)

ACKNOWLEDGMENT

Dr. Robert H. Lusk, Jr. was supported by the Berkeley Veterinary Research Foundation, Inc.

REFERENCES

1. Sobel BE, Roberts R: Hypotension and syncope. p. 952. In Braunwald E (ed): Heart Disease. A Textbook of Cardiovascular Medicine. Vol. 1. 2nd Ed. WB Saunders, Philadelphia, 1984
2. Ettinger SJ: Weakness and Syncope. p. 34. In Ettinger SJ (ed): Diseases of the Dog and Cat. 2nd Ed. Vol. 1. WB Saunders, Philadelphia, 1983
3. Beckett SD, Branch CE, Robertson BT: Syncopal attacks and sudden death in dogs: Mechanisms and etiologies. J Am Anim Hosp Assoc 14:378, 1978
4. Ettinger SJ, Suter PF: Canine Cardiology. WB Saunders, Philadelphia, 1970
5. Kudenchuk PJ, McAnulty JM: Syncope: Evaluation and treatment. Mod Conc Cardiov Dis 54: 1985
6. Boudoulas H, Lewis RP: Cardiac syncope: Diagnosis, mechanism, and management. p. 521. In Hurst JW (ed): The Heart. 6th Ed. McGraw-Hill, New York, 1986
7. Silber EN, Katz LN: Heart Disease. Macmillan, New York, 1975
8. Liu SK, Tilley LP, Maron BJ: Canine hypertrophic cardiomyopathy. J Am Vet Med Assoc 174:708, 1979
9. Fox PR: Feline myocardial diseases. p. 337. In Kirk RW (ed): Current Veterinary Therapy. Vol. VIII. WB Saunders, Philadelphia, 1983
10. Wenger NK, Goodwin JF, Roberts WC: Cardiomyopathy and myocardial involvement in systemic diseases. p. 1181, In Hurst JW (ed): The Heart. 6th Ed. McGraw-Hill, New York, 1986
11. McIntosh HD, Estes EH, Warren JV: The Mechanisms of Cough Syncope. Am Heart J 52:70, 1956
12. Shepherd JT, Vanhoutte PM: The Human Cardiovascular System. Facts and Concepts. Raven Press, New York, 1979
13. Bauer T, Saal AK: Special diagnostic techniques for the evaluation of cardiac disease. p. 87. In Tilley LP, Owens JM (eds): Manual of Small Animal Cardiology. Churchill Livingstone, New York, 1985
14. Tilley LP: Essentials of Canine and Feline Cardiology. 2nd Ed. Lea & Febiger, Philadelphia, 1985
15. Keene BW: Differential diagnosis of syncope. p. 220. Proc Fifth Annu Vet Med Forum, Am Coll Vet Intern Med, 1987
16. Woodfield JA: A diagnostic approach to syncope: The Holter monitor. p. 732, Proc Fifth Annu Vet Med Forum, Am Coll Vet Intern Med, 1987

17

Cardiopulmonary Resuscitation

A. Thomas Evans

When cardiac arrest occurs, effective artificial circulation must be re-established within a few minutes or irreversible brain damage may result. Artificial circulation can be supported by external cardiac compression or by massaging the heart directly through a thoracotomy incision. The decision to initiate cardiopulmonary resuscitation (CPR) is based on the fundamental assumption that the brain may still be viable even though the heart has stopped.

One of the first attempts at improving circulation was external cardiac compression using cats in 1878.[1] External cardiac massage produced blood pressures of 60 to 100 mmHg in a study reported in 1934.[2] It was soon appreciated that dogs could withstand up to 8 minutes of ventricular fibrillation if external cardiac compression was applied.[3] Closed chest cardiac massage was later popularized by Kouwenhoven and co-workers in 1960.[4]

The modern history of CPR underwent an initial period of serendipitous discovery, followed by periods of skepticism, complacency, and, finally, acceptance.[5,6] Modern, effective methods of CPR are now addressing a new area of concern—resuscitation and protection of the brain. With increasing success at restarting the heart, researchers are now focusing on injury, which may occur during reperfusion of the ischemic-anoxic brain.[7]

Changing concepts of traditional CPR techniques and brain pathophysiology are incorporating new therapeutic strategies. A thorough understanding of pathophysiologic mechanisms, cellular biology, and biochemistry may help in formulating more effective treatment protocols.

PATHOPHYSIOLOGY OF CARDIAC ARREST

The popular maxim quoting 4 to 6 minutes as the length of cardiac arrest time before brain damage occurs probably arose from early canine studies.[8,9] It is actually possible for the central nervous system (CNS) to withstand anoxia for longer intervals, perhaps up to 60 minutes, without irreversible injury under certain investigational conditions.[10,11] However, the brain behaves differently during actual CPR and its postresuscitation period. Those experimental neuronal survival times cannot be duplicated under clinical conditions.

Four phenomena have been suggested to account for the shorter neuronal viability during CPR: (1) a progressive postresuscitation hypoperfusion that commences soon after reperfusion and continues for as long as 18 hours[12-14]; (2) hydrolysis of membrane phospholipids with continued arachidonic acid production[15]; (3) reperfusion injury due to cell membrane lipid peroxidation[16]; and (4) neuronal calcium overloading.[17,18]

MECHANISMS OF INJURY

Postresuscitation Hypoperfusion

The concept of the no-reflow phenomenon describes lack of cerebral perfusion following brain ischemia.[12] It is a syndrome of progressive hypoperfusion in the postischemic brain unrelated to microthrombi and not totally explainable by increases in intracranial pressure.[13,19-21] More likely, progressive small vessel resistance in certain regions of the brain reduces cortical blood flow to as low as 5 percent of normal.[19] Accumulation of arachidonic acid or its by-products as described below may be contributory.

Production of Free Fatty Acids

Free fatty acids (FFAs) and their metabolites damage brain structure and function by disrupting cell membranes.[18] During cerebral anoxia, or even with incomplete ischemia, tissue arachidonic acid accumulates because of reduced catabolic enzyme activity. Arachidonic acid may lead to the production of prostaglandins, thromboxanes, and leukotrienes, causing neuronal damage.

Metabolism of arachidonic acid has several clinically significant consequences in the development of cerebral injury. Arachidonic acid synthesis is inhibited during ischemia but augmented during hypoperfusion. Via the enzyme cyclooxygenase, arachidonic acid is transformed into the intermediate prostaglandin G_2 (PGG_2), which is then converted to PGH_2. Reactive oxygen free radicals are generated as a by-product but are normally scavenged and prevented from accumulating in brain tissue.[16,18] Conversion of PGH_2 to PGI_2 is facilitated by prostacyclin synthetase, which can be inhibited during brain ischemia-anoxia by fatty acid hydroperioxides.[18] PGI_2 causes vasodilation and inhibition of platelet aggregation.[7] Thus, these potential beneficial effects may be reduced during brain ischemia.

Thromboxanes are synthesized from cyclic endoperoxides.[7] Thromboxane A_2 promotes platelet aggregation and vasoconstriction. Ischemia may shift the balance of prostacyclin-thromboxane A_2 production in favor of the latter, increasing the potential for vasoconstriction and tissue hypoperfusion.

A third group of compounds, the leukotrienes, are also synthesized from arachidonic acid.[18] They have a stimulatory effect on smooth muscle and change the permeability of cell membranes. These actions are detrimental to the brain and may contribute to hypoperfusion and loss of ionic gradients across cell membranes.

Free Radical Production

Free radicals may be produced in concert with ischemia during the reperfusion stage of cardiac arrest due to the abundance of reducing equivalents (e.g., nicotinamide adenine dinucleotide, xanthine oxidase, nicotinamide adenine dinucleotide phosphate, cytochrome P-450 reductase). Biochemical systems that normally keep superoxide ions in check (e.g., superoxide dismutase, catalase) are overwhelmed by the sudden increase in superoxide ions and their injurious by-products, such as hydroxyl radicals.

Sites of resultant cellular injury involve double bonds of polyunsaturated fatty acid side chains in membrane lipids. These double bonds are rearranged by oxygen-based free radicals in lipid peroxidation reactions. This results in changes in membrane fluidity and permeability.[22] Free radical production has been detected in dog myocardium, cat intestine, and transplanted kidney.[23] These changes could potentially lead to accelerated lipid peroxidation following cerebral reperfusion.

Almost any cellular molecule can be a target of free radical reactions.[24] Terminal SH groups in proteins containing the amino acid cystine or methionine can be cross-linked, and aromatic amino acids can be oxidized. Affected enzymes would probably become nonfunctional. Na^+-K^+-ATPase can be inhibited by membrane lipid peroxidation, which would slow or prevent recovery of the intracellular environment.

Lipid peroxidation reaction rates are fastest when lipids are arranged in a monolayer.[25] Organelle and cellular membranes are obvious targets for free radical attacks because they present a large number of highly unsaturated fatty acids in a monolayer arrangement. These reactions shorten fatty acid chains, contribute to other peroxidation by-products, and increase cell membrane viscosity.

Free iron is a catalyst for initiation of lipid peroxidation.[26] Iron is present in the brain as part of the ferritin molecule, in transport proteins (transferrin), in hemoglobin, and in myoglobin. Reducing agents necessary to make iron available as a catalyst are more plentiful during brain ischemia and reperfusion.[27]

Hydroxyl radicals form during lipid peroxidation. Free iron catalyzes this reaction, resulting in damage to cellular proteins and lipids. The resultant cellular destruction may contribute to patient degeneration late in cardiac arrest. Recognition of free radicals has stimulated interest in protecting the brain during the reperfusion phase of cardiac arrest with drugs to ameliorate free-radical-induced cellular injury.[28] Experimental use of an iron chelator (deferoxamine) to bind free iron has improved the outcome of cardiac resuscitation in rats.[28] Lipid peroxidation following reperfusion was experimentally reduced in dogs given deferoxamine.[29] Thus, a new type of treatment to minimize reperfusion brain injury may be available in the future.

Other Mechanisms of Brain Injury

Altered calcium homeostasis during brain ischemia-anoxia may be related to brain injury during cardiac arrest. Normally, intracellular calcium is maintained 10^{-4} times below the extracellular concentration by energy-dependent ionic pumps.[30] A shift of calcium into intracellular locales and subsequent loss of membrane ionic gradients may contribute to calcium overloading. This loss of calcium homeostasis may partially explain postischemic hypoperfusion, arachidonic acid accumulation, free radical formation, and postischemic mitrochondrial injury. Loss of plasma membrane integrity may result in a nonfunctioning cell.[31]

Energy failure is a concept that has been used to explain ischemic-anoxic brain injury. It is usually defined in terms of phosphocreatine, adenosine triphosphate, adenosine diphosphate, and adenosine monophosphate concentrations that are depleted in the ischemic brain. However, there are shortcomings in this theory. In certain other CNS disturbances, such as status epilepticus and hypoglycemia, the degree of neuronal damage does not correlate with the fall in cerebral energy state.[18,32]

MANAGEMENT OF CARDIAC ARREST

When you prepare for an emergency, the emergency ceases to exist. Cardiac arrest is an abrupt cessation of cardiac output, with subsequent loss of effective tissue perfusion. There are several causes:

1. *Ventricular fibrillation*: chaotic, uncoordinated, ineffective ventricular motions accompanied by an electrocardiogram (ECG) without discernible P-QRS-T complexes
2. *Ventricular asystole*: cessation of ventricular electrical activity accompanied by a flat ECG
3. *Electromechanical dissociation*: recognizable ECG QRS complexes, feeble ventricular contractions with absence of significant blood pressure and arterial pulses.

Cardiovascular collapse (extreme bradycardia or tachycardia, hypotension, advanced shock) and prolonged respiratory arrest (i.e., due to airway obstruction, suffocation, severe respiratory disease, drugs, anesthetic agents) can also lead to cardiac arrest. The focus of therapeutic intervention may vary depending on the inciting cause.

Effective cardiopulmonary resuscitation necessitates coordinated team participation, which necessitates preplanned guidelines and a rehearsed division of effort. An appropriately maintained "crash cart" should be organized in advance with drug doses posted or, if shelf life allows, previously drawn up. All equipment must be in good functional order.

CLINICAL RECOGNITION

Clinical signs of impending or actual cardiac arrest are striking and should prompt immediate initiation of CPR. Animals may be observed gasping for air or unconscious, without ventilatory attempts. Mucous membranes will be pale or cyanotic, and femoral pulses and audible heart beats will be absent. Pupils may be dilated, and the eyes seem to be staring into space. Hemorrhage from surgical sites is diminished and appendage tone is absent. Autonomic release of bowel and bladder muscle control may result in defecation or urination.

Lack of a femoral arterial pulse or palpable heartbeat does not necessarily indicate cardiac arrest. Arterial pulses are difficult to palpate externally when systolic pressure is less than 50 mmHg. ECG monitoring is therefore essential.

CARDIOPULMONARY RESUSCITATION

Application of artificial ventilation and restoration of circulation through manual cardiac compression should be initiated until a stable cardiovascular status is achieved or CPR is abandoned. The objectives of CPR are listed in Table 17-1.

Airway

Establishment or confirmation of a patent airway is the initial concern when beginning CPR. Endotracheal intubation, or rarely tracheostomy, should

Table 17-1 Objectives of Cardiopulmonary Resuscitation

Airway
    Establish and maintain an open airway
    Endotracheal Intubation

Breathing
    Intermittent positive-pressure ventilation

Circulation
    External cardiac compression
        Especially in animals weighing less than 10 kg
    Internal cardiac compression
        Large dogs or after 2 minutes of external compression

Drugs (see Table 17-2)

ECG monitoring
    Defibrillation; cardiac drug therapy

Follow-up support and monitoring
    Cardiopulmonary and CNS function
    Data base

be performed as the first step. In one clinical trial, all survivors of cardiac arrest had endotracheal tubes in place prior to the arrest.[33]

Breathing

Effective ventilation plays a major role in managing acidemia of cardiac arrest. Artificial ventilation should use 100 percent oxygen if possible. Intermittent positive pressure may be applied to the endotracheal tube using a mouth-to-tube technique, to the reservoir bag on an anesthetic machine or non-rebreathing circuit, or to a self-inflating resuscitation bag. A rate of 7 to 9 breaths/min is recommended. The delivered inspiratory volume should approximate a normal chest excursion. Ventilation need not be stopped to accommodate cardiac massage.

Circulation

Two clinical methods to reinstitute stroke volume and circulation artificially are commonly used. One is external cardiac compression. Blood flow is generated by increasing intrathoracic pressure by externally compressing the chest. The other is direct cardiac massage through a thoracotomy incision.

EXTERNAL CARDIAC COMPRESSION

External cardiac compression (closed-chest CPR) may be attempted initially during the first 2 minutes of cardiac arrest. The resultant hemodynamic effects are probably due to changes in intrathoracic pressure generated by this technique.[34] Manual thoracic compression should be appled directly over the heart for one-third of the cycle at a minimal rate of 60 cycles/min. Vital organ perfusion pressures and blood flow in dogs have been shown to be more dependent on duration and magnitude of compression than on rates. Moreover, high repetition chest compression may be tiring to perform for prolonged periods of time and rates of 150/min are not more efficacious than 60/min.[34]

Other maneuvers to increase intrathoracic pressure during closed chest CPR have been suggested. Abdominal binding may increase intraabdominal pressure to prevent paroxysmal diaphragmatic motion during chest compression.[35,36] Interposed abdominal compression during CPR has been shown to increase cerebral perfusion, but the degree of improvement may not be sufficient to protect the brain.[37,38]

Successful thoracic compression with simultaneous positive-pressure ventilation should improve mucous membrane color, produce a palpable femoral arterial pulse, and reduce pupillary size. If the desired effects are not achieved, the CPR technique should be modified to use more or less compressive force, a longer compression phase, and a slightly different site for thoracic compression or to increase intravenous fluid administration to promote venous return.[39]

DIRECT CARDIAC COMPRESSION

In dogs weighing more than 10 kg, closed-chest CPR may not produce adequate cerebral perfusion to prevent severe neurologic injury.[40–43] Therefore, it should not be used longer than 2 minutes before the decision is made to begin open-chest CPR (Fig. 17-1).

Internal cardiac massage should be initiated when external cardiac compression is not likely to be effective or if the thorax is already opened or severely traumatized. Direct heart visualization is also advantageous in helping detect pericardial tamponade, inadequate ventricular filling between compressions, and ventricular fibrillation.[39]

An emergency thoractomy is performed at the left fifth or sixth intercostal space. The hair may be clipped but time should not be spent to prepare the skin aseptically. Care should be taken when making the incision to avoid cutting the lungs, the intercostal arteries along the caudal rib edges, or the internal thoracic artery lateral to the sternum. The pericardial sac need not be opened to massage the heart unless pericardial tamponade occurs due to blood or transudate accumulation. The pericardium should not be closed following successful resuscitation.

The heart may be massaged directly using enough force to produce ventricular emptying. Adequate ventricular filling should be allowed before the next compression.

After successful CPR, care must be taken to prepare the skin edges aseptically. Thoracic lavage should be performed and a broad-spectrum systemic antibiotic used. A chest drain may be required to evacuate the thorax and re-establish negative pressure.

DRUG THERAPY

Epinephrine is the most effective drug for stimulating the heart and increasing coronary and cerebral blood flow during CPR. It is a potent positive chronotrope and inotrope. The α-adrenergic agonistic effects of epinephrine cause peripheral vasoconstriction, which may strongly contribute to its beneficial action in cardiac arrest.[44–46] Peripheral vasoconstriction may increase peripheral vascular resistance and diastolic blood pressure, improve venous return to the heart, and raise filling pressures. Cardiovascular responses to epinephrine include increased heart rate, contractility, automaticity, systemic vascular resistance, arterial blood pressure, and myocardial oxygen requirement.

Other α-adrenergic agonists may be as effective as epinephrine in restarting the arrested heart. They include *phenylephrine, metaraminol,* and *methoxamine*.[39,47–48] Isoproterenol (β-adrenergic agonist) and phenothiazines (α-adrenergic receptor blockers) should not be used during the acute phase of CPR[39] (Table 17-2).

The most effective catecholamine for use in CPR may vary from patient to patient. Comparison of epinephrine, *dopamine* and *dobutamine* in a dog asphyxial and fibrillatory arrest model showed that dobutamine was not effective in the initial treatment of cardiac arrest. Dopamine was equivalent to epinephrine, however, in the percentage of successful treatments.[48] Epinephrine or dopamine may induce ventricular fibrillation but are not contraindicated when myocardial stimulation is necessary. Catecholamine-induced arrhythmias may be exacerbated by hypoxia, acidosis, halothane anesthesia, and myocardial trauma. Avoidance of these agents in similar settings is recommended when cardiac stimulation is not necessary. Bradycardia may be responsive to atropine or isoproterenol and vascular volume expansion. Postresuscitation hypotension may be corrected with dobutamine, dopamine, or mephentermine as a result of their positive inotropic and blood pressure-maintaining qualities.[39]

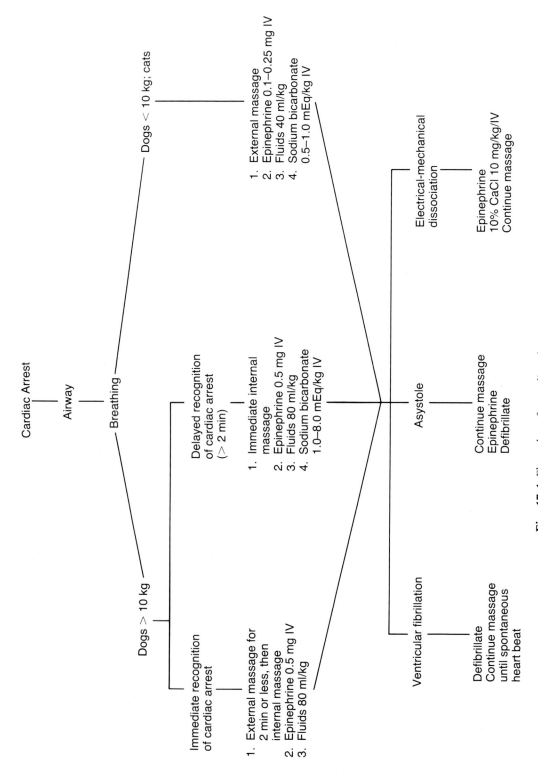

Fig. 17-1 Flow chart for cardiopulmonary resuscitation.

Calcium chloride has often been generically recommended for the initial treatment of cardiac arrest. Recent evidence has questioned its effectiveness, and it may not improve the outcome of CPR. [49-51] Moreover, brain injury from ischemic anoxia is thought to be mediated by a loss of calcium homeostasis.[37,52,53] Therefore, the administration of calcium to an intracellular environment in which the concentration of calcium is excessive may be contraindicated. Additional liabilities of calcium administration include sinus tachycardia, ventricular arrhythmias, cell membrane hyperstabilization (inhibiting depolarization), and myocardial tetany.[39,49,51]

There are several specific indications for calcium administration. One is electromechanical dissociation, in which the heart is still weakly beating and brain ischemia has presumably not yet developed. Secondarily, since calcium antagonizes the effect of hyperkalemia on excitable cells, it may be useful when arrest or near-arrest is caused by hyperkalemia due to hypoadrenocorticism, urethral obstruction, or acute renal failure. In addition, calcium administration should be considered if arrest is induced by calcium antagonists (e.g., verapamil).

Acidosis accompanies ventilatory and circulatory arrest. Metabolic acidosis results from generation of lactic acid during hypoxia-induced anerobic metabolism. Respiratory acidosis occurs from hypercarbia due to carbon dioxide retention in ventilatory failure.[54] Acidosis may depress diastolic depolarization and suppress spontaneous activity.[55] It may also depress the electric threshold required to cause ventricular fibrillation, decrease myocardial contractility, increase pulmonary vascular resistance, and diminish the response to catecholamines.[56-60]

Prompt and efficient artificial ventilation aids in oxygenation and carbon dioxide excretion and is a major factor in managing the acidemia of cardiac arrest. An important contributor to refractory acidosis is persistent ventilatory insufficiency.[61]

Sodium bicarbonate is given for the management of metabolic acidosis. Its administration results in a buffer reaction. Elevation of blood pH occurs by combination of bicarbonate (HCO_3^-) ions with hydrogen (H^+) ions:

$$HCO_3^- + H^+ \rightleftharpoons H_2CO_3 \rightleftharpoons CO_2 + H_2O$$

Thus, carbon dioxide is generated. However, when adequate artificial alveolar ventilation is provided during CPR, it is eliminated through the lungs, thereby raising blood pH.[54]

How much sodium bicarbonate to give when treating cardiac arrest is difficult to estimate. For example, cardiac arrest that is treated immediately may not require bicarbonate therapy. Adequate ventilation may permit managment of acidosis in patients who are not previously acidotic.[62] However, a 10- to 15-minute period of cardiac arrest prior to effective initiation of CPR requires a large dose of bicarbonate. By contrast, 3 minutes of fibrillatory arrest followed by 18 minutes of external CPR with standard artificial ventilation may result in an alkalemia from respiratory alkalosis. Only after 18 minutes of CPR does the blood pH become less than 7.40.[63]

In general, small doses of sodium bicarbonate (0.5 to 1.0 mEq/kg) may be beneficial during external CPR when combined with artificial ventilation to maintain blood pH. If internal CPR techniques are used, a larger dose may be necessary (e.g., 1.0 to 8.0 mEq/kg).[64] Close attention to adequate alveolar ventilation is necessary to ensure that generated carbon dioxide is eliminated.

Excessive sodium bicarbonate administration may be problematic. Resultant metabolic alkalosis may cause leftward displacement of the oxyhemoglobin dissociation curve and depress oxygen release to tissues. Alkalemia may acutely lower the concentration of serum potassium by inducing an intracellular shift. Cerebrospinal fluid acidosis can result if CO_2 is generated and rapidly diffuses across the blood-brain barrier. Catecholamines may be inactivated. Calcium salts may precipitate in preparations containing bicarbonate.[54]

Effective circulating blood volume and venous return require fluid volume replacement for successful resuscitation. After several minutes of CPR without fluid replacement, cardiac stroke volume may decline, and organ perfusion becomes compromised. Diffusion of adenine into interstitial fluid may contribute to blood volume reduction during cardiac arrest by dilating arterioles and reducing peripheral vascular resistance.[65]

Fluid administration for *vascular volume expansion* should initially employ a rate used for shock treatment (80 ml/kg in the dog, 40 ml/kg in the cat), depending on the patient's needs. Lactated Ringer's

Table 17-2 Drugs Used during and after Cardiac Resuscitation

Drug (Receptor Activity)	Trade Name (Manufacturer)	Myocardial Chronotropy and Inotropy	Peripheral Vasomotor Tone	Major Indication	Dosage (IV)
Sympathomimetic drugs					
Catecholamines					
Epinephrine (α + + +; β + + +)	Adrenalin (Parke-Davis)	Increased	Increased	Cardiac arrest	0.25–0.5 mg (2.5–5 ml 1:10,000 solution) for average-sized dog (15 kg); cat: 0.1–0.25 mg
Norepinephrine (α + + +; β +)	Levophed bitartrate (Breon)	Variable	Increased	Vasoconstriction	0.01–0.1 mg for average-sized dog
Dopamine (dopa and β + + +; α + +)	Intropin (Arnar-Stone)	Increased	Variable	Increase visceral perfusion; Blood pressure support	50–200 mg in 500 ml D_5W—dog; 2–10 mg in 250 ml D_5W—cat (to effect; start 2.5μg/kg/min)
Isoproterenol (α 0; β + + +)	Isuprel (Winthrop)	Increased	Decreased	Cardiac stimulation	0.2–0.5 mg in 250 ml D_5W (to effect; start 0.01 μg/kg/min)
Dobutamine (α +; β + + +)	Dobutrex (Lilly)	Increased	Variable	Blood pressure support	100–400 mg in 500 ml D_5W—dog; 4 to 20 mg in 250 ml D_5W—cat (to effect; start 5 μg/kg/min)
Noncatecholamines					
Mephentermine (α +; β + +)	Wyamine (Wyeth)	Increased	Variable	Blood pressure support	0.1–0.5 mg/kg—dog
Metaraminol (α + + +; β +)	Aramine (Merck, Sharp & Dohme) Metaraminol bitartrate (Bristol, Invenex)	Variable	Increased	Vasoconstriction	0.1–0.2 mg/kg—dog
Methoxamine (α + + +; β 0)	Vasoxyl (Burroughs Wellcome)	None	Increased	Vasoconstriction	0.1–0.2 mg/kg—dog
Phenylephrine (α + + +; β 0)	Neo-Synephrine (Winthrop)	None	Increased	Vasoconstriction	0.01–0.1 mg/kg—dog

Other therapeutic agents

Agent	(Manufacturer)	Effect	Purpose	Dosage
Calcium	(Bristol; Invenex; Vitarine)	Variable	Increase cardiac output; Electrical-mechanical dissociation	10% CaCl 1.5 to 2.0 mg/dog; 0.05–0.01 ml/kg—cat; 10% CaGluc 6 to 8 ml for average-sized dog
Sodium bicarbonate			To prevent the severe acidosis associated with extremely poor tissue perfusion	0.5 to 1.0 mEq/kg bolus if closed CPR (small dogs; cats); 1.0 to 8.0 mEq/kg bolus if open CPR and if several minutes of anoxia (large dogs)
Sodium-containing replacement solutions	(Abbott; Cutter; McGraw)		To fill the increasing capacity of the vascular compartment and generate a suitable venous return	40 ml/kg (dog); 20 ml/kg (cat) of lactated Ringer's or equivalent solution very rapidly, then slow drip
Atropine	Atropine sulfate (Bristol)	Increased (Chronotropy)	To minimize parasympathetic influences on the heart	0.01 to 0.02 mg/kg
Lidocaine HCl	Xylocaine (Abbott; Astra; Bristol; Invenex)		To stabilize excitable cell membranes and depress ectopic ventricular pacemaker activity (class II)	1 to 2 mg/kg bolus; repeat to 8 mg/kg (max.). Mix 1 to 2 mg/ml D_5W; administer 10 to 50 μg/kg/min (to effect)—dog; cat: 0.25–1.0 mg/kg over 5 min.
Procainamide	Pronestyl (Squibb)	Increased; Decreased	To stabilize excitable cell membranes and depress ectopic ventricular pacemaker activity (class I)	1 to 5 mg/kg; 10 to 50 μg/kg/min (to effect)—dog
Propranolol HCl	Inderal (Ayerst)	Decreased	Beta-receptor blocking agent	0.05 to 0.3 mg/kg—dog; cat: 0.25 mg in 1 ml saline, give 0.2 ml boluses to effect
Mannitol	(Travenol; Merck, Sharp & Dohme)		Osmotic reduction in perivascular cellular and interstitial edema and diuresis	0.5 to 1 gm/kg

(Modified from Haskins SC: Cardiopulmonary resuscitation. p. 377. In Kirk RW (ed): Current Veterinary Therapy. Vol. VIII. WB Saunders, Philadelphia, 1983. Reprinted with permission from WB Saunders Co.)

or equivalent solution is recommended. After normalization of heart rate and rhythm, the infusion rate can be reduced as required to maintain cardiac output and organ perfusion. Excessive fluid volume or infusion rate may cause acute pulmonary edema and resuscitation failure. By contrast, deterioration of cardiovascular parameters may require further fluid administration. This can be accomplished with another loading dose of crystalloid sodium replacement fluids, colloid blood volume expanders, hypertonic salt solutions, or whole blood.[66]

Colloid blood expanders are particulate fluids whose large molecular size prevents rapid leakage across vascular membranes. Dextran 40 parenteral solution, a high-molecular-weight polysaccharide, has been used to maintain fluid volume without overloading the vascular compartment. It is hypertonic and initially attracts water into the vascular space, increasing plasma volume and decreasing blood viscosity. It also acts as a free radical scavenger. Dosage is 2.0 g/kg, and administration over several hours is required to prevent vascular overload.

Alternatively, a hypertonic solution may be formulated with 8 g NaCl added to 1 L of lactated Ringer's solution. This may be slowly infused over a 12-hour period as required to maintain arterial pressure without requiring a large infusion volume. If arterial pressures can be maintained without excessive fluid replacement, the hypertonic salt solution is not required.

Whole blood administrations may be indicated in the anemic, hypovolemic patient. The concentration of hemoglobin should be maintained above 6.0 g/dl (PCV > 18 to 20 percent).[39]

Other therapeutic agents are administered during cardiac arrest to correct problems if they occur (Table 17-2). For example, frequent ventricular premature complexes are treated with lidocaine. Hypotension continuing after adequate fluid therapy can be treated with drugs that cause peripheral arterial vasoconstriction. Dopamine has been effective during the postresuscitation period to maintain blood pressure and correct oliguria. However, one canine study has documented dopamine-induced cerebral vasoconstriction.[67] After resuscitation, dogs normally undergo a period of hypertension. It would therfore be unusual for dopamine to be re-

quired to maintain arterial blood pressure for long periods of time.

TERMINATION OF CPR

The CPR effort should continue as long as brain viability seems possible. Most successful recoveries are accomplished within 10 to 15 minutes.[33] With good brain perfusion during resuscitation, success may occur up to 30 to 40 minutes after cardiac arrest. The decision to discontinue CPR is based on cardiovascular unresponsiveness or brain death after appropriate techniques and therapeutic modalities have been adequately performed.

POSTRESUSCITATION MANAGEMENT

Although the initial goal of CPR is to re-establish a state of spontaneous heartbeat and effective circulation, maintenance of cerebral circulation and oxygenation comprises the primary concern during postresuscitation support.

In the responsive animal that is breathing spontaneously, the clinician should continue ECG monitoring and start or maintain intravenous infusion with lactated Ringer's solution. Lidocaine should be administered if ventricular arrhythmias occur, using a bolus or constant-rate infusion technique. Atropine may be useful in small doses if severe sinus bradycardia occurs. The hemodynamic status should be assessed by checking mucous membrane color and refill time, arterial pulse (i.e., strength, quality, and rate), and urine output. The heart rate and lungs should be auscultated and a thoracic and/or abdominal radiograph evaluated. A hemogram, urine analysis, and biochemical profile should be analyzed.

Other patients may require more intensive care. They may have required more prolonged external chest compression (resulting in internal injuries) or may have received multidrug therapy; they may display decreased responsiveness, require continued intubation (spontaneous breathing absent or present), or display unstable ECG activity or systemic blood pressure. Ventilatory support and ECG monitoring must be continued. Factors precipitating or contributing to cardiac arrest should be evaluated and corrected (e.g., including hypoxia, acidosis or alkalosis, sepsis, hypovolemia, electrolyte imbalances, drug intoxication, severe hypothermia or hyperthermia, uremia, anemia, anesthesia, and neurologic injury).

Treatment of the brain after cardiac arrest is the most important aspect of CPR once a stable cardiac rhythm is established. Various protective measures and agents have been reported to help minimize postresuscitation neurologic injury. Iron chelators, calcium antagonists, barbiturates, free radical scavengers, and antiprostaglandins have displayed some effectiveness in ameliorating neurologic deficits. Pathophysiology of ischemic-anoxic neurologic injury is complex and will ultimately require a therapeutic strategy that addresses the multifactorial nature of this injury.

DEFIBRILLATION (ELECTRIC COUNTERSHOCK)

Ventricular fibrillation may occur as a terminal manifestation of many extracardiac diseases. It must be converted immediately to ventricular asystole if cardiopulmonary support and stimulation is to be successful. A high-energy electric charge of short duration is introduced to the myocardium between two paddles through the chest wall (external defibrillation) or applied to the heart (internal defibrillation). The charge depolarizes the entire heart, permitting re-establishment of a normal rhythm. Both AC and DC current defibrillation is used, but the latter is recommended.[39]

Considerable patient variation exists regarding the amount of energy required for successful defibrillation. In general, small energies should first be used with repeated countershocks delivered at progressively increased energy-level settings.[39,68] External defibrillation should be dosed at an energy (watt-seconds) of 2/kg (<7 kg body wt), 5/kg (8 to 40 kg wt) and 5 to 10/kg (>40 kg body wt); internal defibrillation can use 0.2 to 0.4 watt-sec/kg.[69] Prolonged periods of ventricular fibrillation may require increased defibrillation energies and result in a lower rate of successful defibrillation.

Meticulous attention to the principles of resuscitation will increase the success rate of electric de-fibrillation. Adequate support therapy includes proper oxygenation and ventilation, control of acid-base status, and enhancement of fibrillation coarseness with epinephrine.

Excessive electric current can cause morphologic cardiac lesions.[70] Resultant myocardial injury may promote ECG abnormalities.[71]

REFERENCES

1. Boehm R: V. Arbeiten aus dem pharmakologischen Institute der universitat Donpat: 13, Ueber Widerbelebung nach Vergiftungen und Asphyxie. Arch Exp Pathol Pharmakol 8:68, 1978
2. Tournade A, Rocchisani L, Mely G: Etude expérimentale des effêts circulatoires qu'entraînent la respiration artificielle et la compression saccadée du thorax chez le chien. Compt Rend Soc Biol 117:1123, 1934
3. Gurvich HL, Uniev GS: Restoration of heart rhythm during fibrillation by condenser discharge. Am Rev Soviet Med 4:252, 1947
4. Kouwenhoven WB, Jude JR, Kickerbocker GG: Closed chest cardiac massage. JAMA 173:1064, 1960
5. Criley JM, Niemann JT, Rosborough JP: Cardiopulmonary resuscitation research 1960–1984: Discoveries and advances. Ann Emerg Med 13:756, 1984
6. Weale FE, Rothwell-Jackson RL: The efficiency of cardiac massage. Lancet 1:990, 1962
7. White BC, Winegar DC, Jackson RE, et al: Cerebral cortical perfusion during and following resuscitation from cardiac arrest in the dog. Am J Emerg Med 2:128, 1983
8. Heymans C: Survival and revival of nervous tissues after arrest of circulation. Physiol Rev 30:325, 1950
9. Weinberger LM, Gibbon MH, Gibbon JH: Temporary arrest of circulation to the central nervous system. I Physiologic effects. Arch Neurol Psychol 43:615, 1940
10. Ames A III: Earliest irreversible changes during ischemia. Am J Emerg Med 1:139, 1983
11. Hossman KA: Neuronal survival and revival during and after cerebral ischemia. Am J Emerg Med 1:191, 1983
12. Ames A III, Wright RL, Kowada M, Thurston JM, Majno G: Cerebral ischemia. II. The no-reflow phenomenon. Am J Pathol 52:437, 1968
13. Rehncrona , Abdul-Rahman A, Siesjo BK: Local cerebral blood flow in the post ischemic period. Acta Neurol Scand 60(suppl):294, 1979
14. White BC, Winegar CP, Henderson O, et al: Pro-

longed hypoperfusion in the cerebral cortex following cardiac arrest and resuscitation in dogs. Ann Emerg Med 12:414, 1983

15. Nemoto DM, Shiu GK, Nemmer JP, et al: Free fatty acid accumulation in the pathogenesis and therapy of ischemic-anoxic brain injury. Am J Emerg Med 1:175, 1983

16. Demopolous HB, Flamm ES, Pictronigro DD, Seligman ML: The free radical pathology and the microcirculation in the major central nervous system disorders. Acta Physiol Scand 492(suppl):91, 1980

17. Vykocil F, Kritz M, Bures J: Potassium selective microelectrodes used for measuring the extra-cellular brain K^+ during spreading depression and anoxic depolarization in rats. Brain Res 39:255, 1972

18. Siesjo BK: Cell damage in the brain: A speculative synthesis. J Cereb Blood Flow Metab 1:155, 1981

19. Gadzinski DS, White BC, Hoehner PJ: Canine cerebral cortical blood flow and vascular resistance post cardiac arrest. Ann Emerg Med 11:58, 1982

20. Chaiang J, Kowada M, Ames A III, et al: Cerebral ischemia. III. Vascular changes. Am J Pathol 52:455, 1968

21. Drewes LR, Gilboe DD, Betz AL: Metabolic alterations in brain during anoxic-anoxia and subsequent recovery. Arch Neurol 29:385, 1973

22. Halliwell B, Gutteridge J: Oxygen toxicity, oxygen radicals, transition metals, and disease. Biochem J 219:1, 1984

23. McCord JM: Oxygen-derived free radicals in postischemic tissue injury. N Engl J Med 312:159, 1985

24. Freeman BA, Crapo JD: Free radicals and tissue injury. Lab Invest 47:412, 1982

25. Mead JF: Free radical mechanisms of lipid damage and consequences for cellular membranes. p. 51. In Prior WA (ed): Free Radicals in Biology and Medicine. Vol. 1. Academic Press, New York, 1983

26. Aust SD, Morehouse LA, Thomas CE: Role of metals in oxygen radical reactions. J Free Radicals Biol Med 1:3, 1985

27. Rehncrona S: Brain acidosis. Ann Emerg Med 14:770, 1985

28. Babbs CB: Role of iron ions in the genesis of reperfusion injury following successful cardiopulmonary resuscitation: Preliminary data and a biochemical hypothesis. Ann Emerg Med 14:777, 1985

29. Komara JS, Nayini NR, Bialek H, et al: Brain iron delocalization and malondialdehyde production following cardiac arrest (abstract). Ann Emerg Med 14:507, 1985

30. Katz AM, Reuter H: Cellular calcium and cardiac cell death. Am J Cardiol 44:188, 1979

31. Mead JF: Free radical mechanisms of lipid damage and consequences for cellular membranes. p. 51. In Pryor WA (ed): Free Radicals in Biology. Academic Press, New York, 1976

32. Agardh CE, Kalimo H, Olsson Y, Siesjo BJ: Hypoglycemic brain injury: Metabolic and structural findings in the rat cerebellar cortex during profound insulin-produced hypoglycemia and in the recovery period following glucose administration. J Cereb Blood Flow Metab 1:85, 1981

33. Gilroy BA, Dunlop BJ, Shapiro HM: Outcome from cardiopulmonary resuscitation in cats: Laboratory and clinical experience. J Am Anim Hosp Assoc 23:133, 1987

34. Halpern HR, Tsitlik JE, Guerei AD, et al: Determinants of blood flow to vital organs during cardiopulmonary resuscitation in dogs. Circulation 73:539, 1986.

35. Rudikoff MT, Maughan WL, Effron M, et al: Mechanisms of blood flow during cardiopulmonary resuscitation. Circulation 61:345, 1980

36. Bircher N, Safar P, Stewart R: A comparison of standard, MAST-augmented and open-chest CPR in dogs. A preliminary investigation. Crit Care Med 8:147, 1980

37. White BC, Hildebrandt JF, Evans AT, et al: Prolonged cardiac arrest and resuscitation in dogs: Brain mitrochondrial function with different artificial perfusion methods. Ann Emerg Med 14:383, 1985

38. Koehler RC, Chandra N, Guerci AD, et al: Augmentation of cerebral perfusion by simultaneous chest compression and lung inflation with abdominal binding after cardiac arrest in dogs. Circulation 67:266, 1983

39. Haskins SC: Cardiopulmonary resuscitation. p. 377. In Kirk RW (ed): Current Veterinary Therapy. Vol. VIII. WB Saunders, Philadelphia, 1983

40. Jackson RE, Joyce K, Danosi SF, et al: Blood flow in the cerebral cortex during cardiac resuscitation in dogs. Ann Emerg Med 13:657, 1984

41. Sanders AB, Kern KB, Ewy GA, et al: Improved resuscitation from cardiac arrest with open-chest massage. Ann Emerg Med 13:676, 1984

42. Safar P: Recent Advances in cardiopulmonary-cerebral resuscitation: A review. Ann Emerg Med 13:856, 1984

43. White BW, Aust SD, Arfors KE, Aronson LD: Brain injury by ischemic anoxia: Hypothesis extension—A tale of two ions? Ann Emerg Med 13:862, 1984

44. Redding JS, Pearson JW: Resuscitation from asphyxia. JAMA 182:283, 1962

45. Yakatis RW, Otto CW, Blitt CD: Relative importance of alpha and beta adrenergic receptors during resuscitation. Crit Care Med 7:293, 1979

46. Otto CW, Yakaitis RW, Blitt CD: Mechanism of action of epinephrine in resuscitation form asphyxial arrest. Crit Care Med 9:364, 1981

47. Hopkins JA, Shouemaker WC, Greenfield S: Treatment of surgical emergencies with and without an algorithm. Arch Surg 115:745, 1980

48. Otto CW, Yakaitis RW, Redding JS, Blitt CD: Comparison of dopamine, dobutamine, and epinephrine in CPR. Crit Care Med 9:358, 1981

49. Hughes WG, Ruedy JR: Should calcium be used in cardiac arrest? Am J Med 81:285, 1986

50. Stueven HA, Thompson BM, Aprahamian C, Tonsfeldt DJ: Calcium chloride: Reassessment of use in asystole. Ann Emerg Med 13:820, 1984

51. Stempien A, Katz AM, Messineo FC: Calcium in cardiac arrest. Ann Intern Med 105:603, 1986

52. Fiskum G: Involvement of mitochondria in ischemic cell injury and in regulation of intracellular calcium. Am J Emerg Med 2:147, 1983

53. Borgers M, Thone F, Van Reempts J, Verheyen F: The role of calcium in cellular dysfunction. Am J Emerg Med 2:154, 1983

54. White RD: Cardiovascular pharmacology: Part 1. p. VII-1. In McIntyre KM, Lewis AJ (eds): Textbook of Advanced Cardiac Life Support. American Heart Association, Dallas, 1981

55. Hecht HH, Hutter OF: Action of pH on cardiac Purkinje fibers. Fed Proc 23:157, 1964 (abst)

56. Mitchell JH, Wildenthal K, Johnson RL: The effects of acid-base disturbances on cardiovascular and pulmonary function. Kidney Int 1:375, 1972

57. Cingolani HE, Faulkner LS, Mattiazzi AR, et al: Depression of human myocardial contractility with "respiratory" and "metabolic" acidosis. Surgery 77:427, 1975

58. Sinaha R, Tinker MA, Hizon R, Gerst PH: Metabolic acidosis and lung mechanics in dogs. Ann Rev Respir Dis 106:881, 1972

59. Kerber RE, Sarnat W: Factors influencing the success of ventricular defibrillation in man. Circulation 60:226, 1979

60. Houle DB, Weil MH, Brown EB, Campbell GS: Influence of respiratory acidosis on ECG and pressor responses to epinephrine, norepinephrine, and metaraminol. Proc Soc Exp Biol Med 94:561, 1957

61. Filmore SJ, Shapiro M, Killip J: Serial blood gas studies during cardiopulmonary resuscitation. Ann Intern Med 72:465, 1970

62. Bishop RL, Weinsfeldt ML: Sodium bicarbonate administration during cardiac arrest. JAMA 235:506, 1976

63. Sanders AP, Ewy GA, Taft TV: Resuscitation and arterial blood gas abnormalities during prolonged cardiopulmonary resuscitation. Ann Emerg Med 13:676, 1984

64. Krause GS, Joyce KM, Nayini NR, et al: Cardiac arrest and resuscitation: Brain iron delocalization during reperfusion. Ann Emerg Med 14:1037, 1985

65. Berne RM, Rubio R, Dobson JG, Curnish RR: Adenosine and adenine nucleotides as possbile mediators of cardiac and skeletal muscle blood flow regulation. Circ Res 28/29(suppl I):115, 1971

66. Jelenko C III, Williams JB, Wheeler BA, et al: Studies in shock and resuscitation, I: use of a hypertonic, albumin-containing, fluid demand regimen (HALFD) in resuscitation. Crit Care Med 7:157, 1979

67. Toda N: Reactivity in human cerebral artery: Species variation. Fed Proc 44:326, 1985

68. Resnekov L: High energy electrical current in the management of cardiac dysrhythmias. p. 589. In Mandel WJ (ed): Cardiac Arrhythmias. JB Lippincott, Philadelphia, 1980

69. Geddes LA, Tacker WA, Rosborough JP, et al: Electrical dose for ventricular defibrillation of large and small animals using precordial electrodes. J Clin Invest 53:310, 1974

70. Tedeschi CG, White CW Jr: A morphologic study of canine hearts subjected to fibrillation and manual compression. Circulation 9:916, 1954

71. Resenkov L, McDonald L: Appraisal of electroconversion in treatment of cardiac dysrhythmias. Br Heart J 30:786, 1968

DISEASES OF THE CARDIOVASCULAR SYSTEM

18

Congenital Heart Disease in Dogs

N. Bari Olivier

DEFINITION AND ETIOLOGY

Congenital heart defects are technically defined as morphologic heart disorders that are present at birth. However, the term is commonly used to include a greater spectrum of cardiovascular disorders, including those of major blood vessels.

The etiology of congenital heart disease is complex and incompletely understood. Selected lesions, such as aortic stenosis, pulmonic stenosis, patent ductus arteriosus (PDA), and conotruncal abnormalities, have a well-documented genetic (hereditary) basis in specific breeds.[1,2] Other factors, such as environmental influences, may also be contributory. Alternatively, both genetic and environmental influences may be causative. According to this theory, three risk factors are identified: (1) a genetic potential for the lesion, (2) exposure to an environmental trigger during a vulnerable period of cardiac development, and (3) a genetically determined susceptibility to the environmental trigger. The relative role of each risk factor varies for each animal. For example, the genetic potential for the lesion may be so strong that a defect occurs regardless of environmental influences. Similarly, environmental effects alone could be sufficient to cause a defect.

However, the greatest risk stems from the interaction of all three risk factors.

CLINICAL SIGNS

Dramatic changes occur in the postnatal period in cardiovascular and pulmonary anatomy and physiology (Ch. 1). Congenital defects may present only mild physiologic disturbances in utero but become life-threatening immediately after birth. Both the congenital defect and physiologic environment may change. Because congenital heart disease is a dynamic process, the morbidity is subject to change as well.

Complex or severe lesions are often fatal during the first few hours or days after birth and, therefore, rarely recognized. The early mortality associated with such lesions undoubtedly influences the reported incidence of congenital heart defects. In less severely affected animals, clinical signs associated with congenital heart disease are usually apparent by the first few months after birth. Exceptions include disorders with minimal morphologic or hemodynamic alterations. Recognition or suspicion of congenital heart disease often occurs during initial preventive medical care when a cardiac murmur, abnormal arterial or venous pulses, cyanosis, or poor growth are detected. In some cases, signs of heart failure such as coughing, respiratory difficulty, or excercise intolerance are noticed by the owner who then seeks medical advice.

Early recognition of congenital heart disease may confer a better prognosis. The tendency for progression of the primary disease or development of irreversible sequela (e.g., obstructive pulmonary vascular disease) emphasizes the importance of early diagnosis and treatment if necessary.

Most clinical signs associated with congenital heart disease relate to congestive heart failure or poor tissue oxygen delivery. They are nonspecific and include respiratory difficulty, exercise intolerance, general unthriftiness, posterior paresis, generalized weakness, depression, syncope, or seizures. Some clinical signs of congenital heart disease originate from organ systems other than the heart. For example, vascular ring disorders may be associated with esophageal entrapment with regurgitation as the dominant sign. Other congenital heart defects may represent only one component of a more complex generalized embryologic disorder.

The presence of abnormal cardiovascular signs in a history, physical examination, or data base, including radiographs and electrocardiogram (ECG), cannot automatically be attributed to congenital heart disease. Acquired heart lesions can be sustained at a young age (inflammation or infection) and produce signs similar to congenital heart defects. More definitive diagnostic tests may be required to verify and define the presence of a congenital cardiac anomaly.

Most congenital cardiovascular anomalies produce an audible *murmur*, the most common clinical finding. Careful and systematic auscultation therefore represents one of the most effective screening techniques for detecting congenital heart disease. Murmurs unaccompanied by anatomic abnormalities of the heart ("innocent murmurs") occur but are uncommon. Thus, all murmurs in dogs should be considered potentially pathologic until proved otherwise by a diagnostic workup. To provide the most diagnostic information, murmurs should be characterized as to their timing, intensity, character (e.g., crescendo, plateau, harsh, musical), and location (point of maximal intensity and radiation).

Algorithms for classifying congenital defects based on the presence and type of murmur are particularly helpful in initiating a list of differential diagnoses.[3]

In addition to cardiac murmurs, characterization of *heart sounds* can provide important diagnostic information. For example, the second heart sound (S_2) has two components that normally occur in rapid succession. The first component (A_2) is normally associated with aortic valve closure and the second (P_2) with pulmonic valve closure. The interval between these two components is short in most normal dogs, and a distinction often cannot be made between the two sounds. The A_2 to P_2 interval is only slightly prolonged during normal inspiration and usually can not be detected during auscultation. However, abnormal prolongation of the A_2 to P_2 interval may cause audible splitting of S_2. This can be associated with large left-to-right shunts, obstructions to right ventricular outflow, or delayed right ventricular contraction due to right bundle branch block associated with congenital defects. Splitting of S_2 can also be due to prematurity of the A_2 component, as occurs in some cases of mitral regurgitation or with a ventricular septal defect. In addition to splitting, the intensity of S_2 may also provide important clues. Muffled or absent aortic or pulmonic components are common with stenosis or incompetence of the respective valve. Increased intensity of the second sound is sometimes associated with pulmonary or systemic hypertension.

Gallop rhythms are the occurrence of three or four heart sounds in a cardiac cycle. They can result from a variety of heart-sound combinations. Gallop rhythms produced by audible third or fourth heart sounds (S_3 and S_4, respectively) are pathologic in dogs and cats. They may indicate increased, early atrioventricular (AV) flow (S_3 gallop) or high end-diastolic ventricular pressure with a vigorous atrial systole (S_4 gallop).

Cyanosis is a blue discoloration of mucous membranes and other areas in which dense capillary networks lie near the surface. In a young dog, it is highly suggestive of a right-to-left cardiac shunt and is a key differentiating sign in differentiating specific defects. Congenital heart disease causes cyanosis primarily due to arterial hypoxemia (central cyanosis) rather than due to low blood flow or biochemical causes. The presence of cyanosis depends on the absolute amount of reduced hemoglobin rather than the percentage of oxygen saturation. Five grams or more of reduced hemoglobin per 100 ml blood is considered the threshold for the detection of cyanosis.[4] Thus, for any degree of arterial hypoxemia, the tendency and severity of cyanosis is related to the amount of hemoglobin in the blood. This explains why cyanosis is rarely detected in anemic dogs regardless of the arterial oxygen tension and why cyanosis is more common and severe in polycythemic subjects. Because cyanosis is a subjective assessment and dependent on several factors, direct measurement of arterial oxygen tension or hemoglobin saturation may be required in equivocal cases.

Two features common to almost all cyanotic congenital heart defects are a defect in the partitions of the heart or great vessels and an obstruction to pulmonary blood flow. This favors right-to-left shunting with ejection of unsaturated venous blood into the systemic circulation.

Polycythemia is often present in cyanotic animals and represents an adaptive response to chronic arterial hypoxemia. Mild to moderate polycythemia is generally considered a desirable physiologic response. By contrast, severe polycythemia (hematocrits >65 percent) can be harmful. Severe polycythemia increases the viscosity of blood and resistance to blood flow, which may place an additional burden on a compromised heart. In addition, sluggish blood flow can impair tissue oxygenation and promote intravascular thrombogenesis.

Evaluating *arterial* and *venous pulses* can also offer valuable diagnostic information. Pulse strength (determined by the pulse pressure and vascular compliance) as well as pulse character (rate of rise and fall of the pulse) should be assessed visually and by palpation. For example, a hypokinetic arterial pulse may be associated with aortic stenosis or low cardiac output while jugular venous distention or pulsations are indicative of right-sided heart disorders.

In addition to a thorough history and complete physical examination, the minimum data base for an animal with a suspected congenital heart defect includes an ECG (at least six leads) and high-quality dorsoventral and lateral thoracic radiographs.

The ECG is essential for evaluating the cardiac rhythm. Although it is somewhat insensitive for an assessment of cardiomegaly, it sometimes displays evidence of atrial or ventricular enlargement and usually illustrates ventricular dominance. It can also be used as one of several criteria to estimate the severity of certain defects such as ventricular outflow obstructions. As an example, if the ECG indicates severe right ventricular enlargement in a dog with a pulmonic stenosis murmur, a significant obstruction can be suspected and the need for further diagnostic evaluation and possibly surgical corrections anticipated.

Thoracic radiographs are indispensible in the evaluation of congenital heart disease. An evaluation of the size of the cardiac silhouette and intrathoracic blood vessels can be made. They are particularly important in assessing pulmonary vascularity and cardiac chamber enlargement patterns. Nonselective and selective contrast radiographs are also useful in quantifying the severity of some lesions and in identifying some of the complex congenital heart defects.

Additional diagnostic tests to complement the data base include arterial and venous blood gases, echocardiography (including Doppler ultrasonic examinations), selective cardiac catheterization, and occasionally lung biopsies to assess pulmonary vascular histology. Two-dimensional echocardiography and Doppler examinations offer the opportunity for repeated assessment of a patient with congenital heart disease without the risks and expense of cardiac catheterization or other invasive techniques.

When an ultrasonic examination is not conclusive, nonselective angiography or cardiac catheterization may be needed. Nonselective angiography is relatively safe and easy to perform but provides limited information. Right-sided and some left-sided lesions (e.g., pulmonic stenosis, aortic stenosis) or right-to-left shunts can often be detected in cats and small dogs. Left-to-right shunts, however, are generally poorly illustrated nonselectively. Selective cardiac catheterization has been the gold standard for an accurate appraisal of most congenital heart defects. Pressure measurements, flow determinations (cardiac output), oximetry, and selective angiographic studies may be performed. Some types of diagnostic information, such as vascular resistance calculations, can only be made using data from a cardiac catheterization. The obvious drawback is its invasive nature, expense, and the risks of anesthesia and catheterization procedure.

IDENTIFYING THE LESION

Recognizing the existence of heart disease is only the first step in the diagnositic process. Information provided by the minimum data base may suggest the physiologic nature of the disorder (e.g., intracardiac shunt, ventricular outflow obstruction). However, a more precise characterization of the lesion and its physiologic consequences is usually needed, particularly if surgical therapy is anticipated.

Interpretation of data requires evaluating essential diagnostic questions in a systematic approach[5] (Table 18-1). These questions promote classification of the defect according to key differentiating physiologic features. Not all questions are relevent in all cases, but the first two should be considered obligatory. The presence of cyanosis or, more objectively, arterial hypoxemia (question 1) can be determined by physical examination (and arterial blood-gas analysis if available). An assessment of pulmonary blood flow (question 2) can be made from examination of the radiographic size of the pulmonary vessels. The third and fourth questions often require multiple sources of information including, in some cases, echocardiography or cardiac catheterization. The dominant ventricle (normally the left ventricle) may be indicated by ECG changes in the QRS pattern or by ventricular asymmetry using radiographic or echocardiographic evaluation. Determining whether pulmonary hypertension exists (question 5) requires invasive direct pressure measurements obtained during cardiac catheterization. Implicit in question 5 is appraisal of pulmonary vascular resistance which requires measurements of pulmonary blood flow. Referral for catheterization is necessary for these assessments.

On the basis of these answers, a list of differential diagnoses can be formulated from which a specific diagnosis can be made[5] (Table 18-2). Some of the defects are listed in more than one category, indicating the variable expression of these congenital diseases.

SPECIFIC CONGENITAL DEFECTS

Patent Ductus Arteriosus

Patent ductus arteriosus, the most common congenital heart defect in dogs, results from a failure of the ductus to close after birth. Functional ductal closure (contraction) normally occurs within the first 72 hours after birth, and anatomic closure is complete within the first few weeks. PDA is usually an isolated defect but can be associated with a variety of additional anomalies, the most common being persistence of the left cranial vena cava. PDA is more commonly seen in pure-breed dogs, with a distinct predilection for females. Specific breeds with increased risk for defective ductal closure include miniature poodles, keeshonds, cocker spaniels, German shepherds, Pomeranians, collies, and Shetland sheepdogs. A genetic basis for defective closure has been documented in poodles.[6] In these poodles, the defect appears to be influenced by many genes, each acting additively with a genetic threshold for patency (complete phenotypic expression). Dogs with genotypes just below this threshold may still transmit the defect to offspring and often have incomplete phenotypic expressions, such as a ductal diverticulum.

NATURAL HISTORY

The natural history depends on the size of the ductus and the pulmonary vascular resistance. Most commonly, a large ductus exists with pulmonary vascular resistance that is considerably less than the systemic circulation. A large left to right shunt results. Signs of left-sided congestive heart failure are

Table 18-1 Key Diagnostic Questions for Evaluating Congenital Heart Disease

1. Is the patient cyanotic (or hypoxemic)?
2. Is pulmonary arterial blood flow increased or decreased?
3. Does the malformation(s) originate in the left or right heart (or both)?
4. Which is the dominant (i.e., dilated or hypertrophied) ventricle?
5. Is pulmonary hypertension present?

Table 18-2 Classification of Congenital Heart Disease According to Their Physiologic Features

Acyanotic without a shunt

Malformation originating in the left heart
    Aortic stenosis
    Interrupted aortic arch
    Aortic coarctation
    Aortic regurgitation
    Congenital mitral regurgitation
    Congenital mitral stenosis
    Primary endocardial fibroelastosis
Malformation originating in the right heart
    Pulmonic stenosis
    Congenital pulmonic regurgitation
    Tricuspid dysplasia (Ebstein's anomaly and other forms)

Acyanotic with a shunt

Shunt at atrial level
    Isolated ASD
    Incomplete endocardial cushion defect
    ASD with mild PS
    Anomalous pulmonary venous connections
Shunt at ventricular level
    Isolated VSD
    Incomplete endocardial cushion defect
    VSD with mild PS
    VSD with aortic regurgitation
    Right ventricular origin of both great vessels with a subcrystal VSD and low pulmonary vascular resistance
Shunt at great vessel level
    PDA
    Aorticopulmonary window
    Truncus arteriosus with low pulmonary vascular resistance
Shunt at multiple levels
    Complete endocardial cushion defect
    VSD with PDA
    VSD with ASD

Cyanosis

Increased pulmonary blood flow
    Complete transposition of the great arteries
    Truncus arteriosus
    Common atrium
    Tetralogy of Fallot with a PDA
    Right ventricular origin of both great vessels
Normal or decreased pulmonary blood flow
    Dominant left ventricle
        Tricuspid atresia
        Tricuspid dysplasia with ASD
    Dominant right ventricle
        Normal or low pulmonary artery pressure
            Pulmonary stenosis or atresia with a VSD (tetralogy of Fallot and others)
            Pulmonic stenosis with R-L ASD
            Complete transposition of the great arteries with severe pulmonic stenosis
            Right ventricular origin of both great vessels with pulmonic stenosis
            Truncus arteriosus with hypoplasia of the pulmonary arteries
        Increased pulmonary artery pressure
            Any of several defects with obstructive pulmonary vascular disease increasing pulmonary vascular resistance (ASD, VSD, PDA or aorticopulmonary window, truncus arteriosus, right ventricular origin of both great vessels)

(Data from refs. 13, 14, 37, 44–47, 52, and 53.)
ASD, atrial septal defect; VSD, ventricular septal defect; PDA, patent ductus arteriosus; PS, pulmonic stenosis; R-L, right to left shunting

noted in more than 25 percent of affected dogs.[7,8] Mitral regurgitation is a frequently recognized complication. It is usually a sequela to left heart dilation and stretching of the mitral valve apparatus. Severely dilated hearts may also develop arrhythmias, particularly atrial fibrillation and premature ventricular contractions.

Untreated dogs face a mortality of 60 to 70 percent during the first few years of life.[7] Mitral regurgitation and arrhythmias significantly increase the risk of death. Dogs surviving the initial 6 to 12 months may develop obstructive pulmonary vascular disease secondary to the shunt-related increase in pulmonary blood flow.[9–11] The increased pulmonary vascular resistance can lead to severe pulmonary hypertension, reversal of the shunt flow and occasionally, right heart failure.

Two major types of atypical manifestation may be detected. Rarely, older affected animals display minimal clinical signs. They represent a minority of dogs and may have a small, perhaps partially closed ductus arteriosus. Although they tend to be more vulnerable to other cardiopulmonary insults, these dogs can have a near-normal life expectancy. Another unusual manifestation of a PDA is severe pulmonary hypertension that persists after birth because high pulmonary vascular resistance persists from the *in utero* circulation. Bidirectional or reverse shunting through the ductus is common in these dogs. They may actually live normal lives for several months or even years. However, signs of respiratory difficulty, weakness, posterior paresis, syncope, or signs of arterial thromboembolism usually become evident by 2 to 3 years of age. Survival beyond 5 to 7 years in these cases is unusual.

PATHOPHYSIOLOGY AND HEMODYNAMICS

An increase in central blood volume occurs in response to the large left-to-right shunt through most PDAs. Typically, aortic pressure exceeds pulmonary artery pressure throughout the cardiac cycle. Nevertheless, systolic and mean pulmonary arterial pressures are usually mildly to moderately elevated due to the high pulmonary artery flow and direct communication with the high aortic pressure. Right heart filling pressures are usually normal. By contrast, left heart filling pressure and pulmonary venous pressure are elevated due to the volume overload. Although not commonly measured, effective cardiac output is probably normal at rest and with mild activity in most dogs. Systolic arterial pressure is usually elevated (sometimes dramatically) due to the increased stroke volume. Diastolic arterial pressure is low because of the diastolic shunting through the pulmonary circulation. The result is a very wide arterial pulse pressure. Development of mitral regurgitation exacerbates left heart volume overload and increases pulmonary venous pressures even further.

Increased pulmonary artery flow at higher pressures tends to elicit pulmonary vascular changes.[12]

Medial hypertrophy and intimal proliferation develop and gradually progress to fibrosis and vessel obliteration. Increased pulmonary vascular resistance and pressure can result. These changes are progressive and, although initially reversible, may reach a nonreversible stage. Pulmonary vascular resistance and pressure can increase sufficiently to create right-to-left shunting through the ductus. The volume overload of the pulmonary circulation and left heart are then relieved but at the expense of a pressure overload of the right heart and pulmonary arteries and a right-to-left shunt.

DIAGNOSIS

Most dogs with a PDA have normal growth and are alert at rest. The most prominent physical finding is a continuous murmur at the left cardiac base (see Figs. 3-2 and 3-5). The diastolic component of the murmur can be very localized, although the systolic component tends to radiate extensively. A murmur of mitral regurgitation often can be ausculted at the left apex. A prominent left apical heart impulse can usually be palpated. Lung sounds are often increased in intensity and rales and other signs of pulmonary congestion or edema may be noted in advanced cases. The arterial pulses are strong, with a rapid diastolic decline (waterhammer pulse). Cyanosis and jugular distention or pulsations are absent in uncomplicated cases. As pulmonary vascular resistance increases, the murmur becomes attenuated, beginning with the diastolic component. With bidirectional or reverse-shunting PDAs, the left basilar murmur is faint or absent, and a loud S_2 may be heard. A right-to-left shunting PDA may cause arterial hypoxemia and cyanosis, depending on the magnitude of the shunt. Cyanosis is classically differential, affecting the caudal mucous membranes only. However, it can be generalized if aortic blood flow is turbulent and retrograde flow of unsaturated blood occurs to the brachycephalic arteries.

In early uncomplicated cases, the ECG is generally unremarkable. Increased QRS amplitude, prolongation of the P and QRS waves, ST slurring or depression, and large T waves are common ECG finding with advanced disease, indicating left heart enlargement (Fig. 18-1). Arrhythmias such as sinus tachycardia, atrial fibrillation, and premature ven-

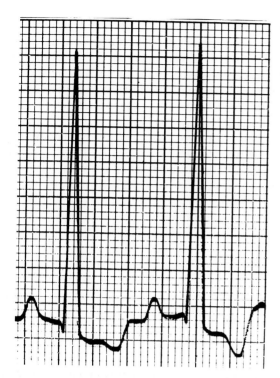

Fig. 18-1 Lead II electrocardiogram (ECG) from a collie with left-to-right shunting patent ductus arteriosus and left-sided heart failure. R waves are tall (3.7 mV) and P waves are wide (0.05 sec) indicating left ventricular and left atrial enlargement, respectively. 1 cm = 1 mV. Paper speed = 50 mm/sec. (Courtesy of Dr. Philip Fox.)

tricular contractions are occasionally noted. With reverse shunting (i.e., right-to-left) PDAs, ECG changes suggestive of right ventricular enlargement (Ch. 4) are usually present.

With a left-to-right shunting PDA, thoracic radiographs typically illustrate severe cardiomegaly, especially of the left heart. Enlargement of pulmonary arteries and veins is indicative of increased pulmonary flow. The radiographic triad of ascending aortic dilation, main pulmonary artery enlargement, and left atrial enlargement in the dorsoventral view is fairly specific for a PDA (Fig. 18-2). Radiographic evidence of pulmonary congestion and edema is frequently seen in advanced cases.

An aorticopulmonary septal defect[13] can exhibit clinical and radiographic signs similar to those of a PDA, with the exception that it lacks dilation of the ascending and proximal descending aorta. This distinction may be difficult to appreciate from an anal-

ysis of plain radiographs. Truncus arteriosus[14] is another lesion that could be confused with a PDA, although the former usually exhibits generalized cyanosis and abnormal radiographic orientation of the great vessel(s).

The diagnostic features of a right-to-left shunting PDA differ from those of a left-to-right PDA. Murmurs are usually absent with a right-to-left shunt. The radiographs may have features of left and right heart enlargement if the increased pulmonary vascular resistance was acquired. An aneurysmal dilation of the descending aorta in the area of the ductus arteriosus is often observed in the dorsoventral radiograph. The peripheral lung fields may appear hypovascular. A cyanotic patient (especially differen-

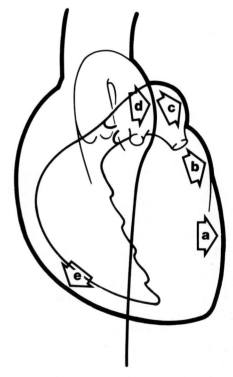

Fig. 18-2 Schematic dorsoventral view of the heart with changes due to volume overload caused by a patent ductus arteriosus (PDA). Characteristic radiographic signs in this view include a convex left ventricular border (a), left atrial enlargement with prominence of the left auricular appendage (b), enlarged pulmonary trunk (c), and bulging of the aortic arch (d). Pulmonary arteries and veins may be enlarged. If pulmonary hypertension develops, right ventricular enlargement may occur (e). (Courtesy of Dr. Peter Lord.)

tial cyanosis) without a murmur and with ECG and radiographic evidence of right ventricular enlargement is highly suggestive of a right-to-left PDA but could also be confused with Eisenmenger's complex.

Ancillary diagnostic tests that may be required are ultrasonography (including Doppler echocardiography) and cardiac catheterization. The ductus arteriosus is difficult to visualize directly with echocardiography. It is occasionally imaged as an echolucent communication between the aorta and main pulmonary artery on a short-axis sweep of the heart. Left atrial dilation with a dilated hyperdynamic left ventricle typifies most left-to-right PDAs. A dilated aorta with prominent systolic motion may also be imaged (see Fig. 6-35). A continuous flow disturbance (turbulence) and high-velocity retrograde flow toward the pulmonic valve can be detected if a pulsed Doppler sampling gate is placed in the proximal pulmonary artery. Doppler echocardiography can also document retrograde flow into the left atrium, if mitral regurgitation is present. Reverse PDAs are difficult to detect echocardiographically, unless the ductus is visualized and retrograde ductal flow is detected by Doppler. Echocardiography can be useful, however, to eliminate or document other differential diagnoses, such as atrial or ventricular septal defects.

Cardiac catheterization is rarely required for diagnosis unless radiographic, ECG, or echocardiographic evidence of right ventricular enlargement is noted in a left-to-right shunting ductus, or if a right-to-left shunting ductus is suspected but unconfirmed. In these cases, cardiac catheterization will permit the measurement of pulmonary artery pressure and flow and calculation of pulmonary vascular resistance. This will help distinguish pulmonary hypertension secondary to high ductal flow from pulmonary hypertension from high resistance (yet not high enough for right-to-left shunting). Cardiac catheterization or angiocardiography will also definitively illustrate the ductus angiographically (Fig. 18-3), help detect the direction of shunting (Fig. 18-4), and provide hemodynamic information (Fig. 18-5).

TREATMENT

Early surgical ligation is the treatment of choice for a left-to-right shunting PDA. If congestive heart failure is present, preoperative stabilization is needed (e.g., cage rest, diuretics, supplemental ox-

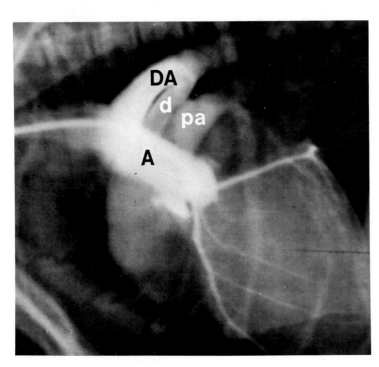

Fig. 18-3 Lateral left ventriculogram from a dog with left-to-right shunting patent ductus arteriosus. A large ductus (d) is visualized connecting the descending aorta (DA) with the pulmonary artery (pa). A, aorta. (Courtesy of Dr. Bruce W. Keene.)

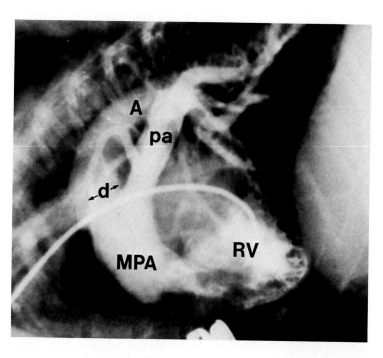

Fig. 18-4 Lateral view of a selective angiocardiogram from a 9-month-old female cocker spaniel with a reverse (i.e., right-to-left shunting) PDA. This right ventricular phase demonstrates simultaneous opacification of the main pulmonary artery (MPA) and descending aorta (A). A PDA (d) is visible. Pulmonary arteries (pa) are tortuous and blunted peripherally, suggesting pulmonary hypertension. RV, right ventricle. (Courtesy of Dr. Philip Fox.)

ygen or vasodilators) prior to anesthesia and surgery. Positive inotropic therapy is generally not indicated, since left ventricular performance is usually adequate. Digitalis, however, can be useful to control complicating supraventricular tachyarrhythmias.

Reductions in left heart size and resolution of mitral regurgitation can usually be expected if surgical correction is successful before 1 year of age (Ch. 28). Surgical ligation is also recommended for high-resistance pulmonary hypertensive PDAs that are still shunting left to right, although resolution of the pulmonary hypertension is often incomplete. Surgery is not generally recommended for right-to-left shunting PDAs. Although successful ductal closure can be associated with a decline in pulmonary artery pressure, a detrimental postoperative increase in pulmonary artery pressure is more common in these cases.

Pulmonic Stenosis

Pulmonic stenosis is a common congenital defect in dogs, occurring approximately once in every 1,000 live births. Three types of pulmonic stenosis are recognized, including supravalvular stenosis (rare) and valvular and subvalvular forms. In dogs,

a combination of valvular and subvalvular stenosis frequently occurs. Lesions causing pulmonic stenosis may be morphologically similar. For example, subvalvular stenosis may result from a discrete fibrous ring or tunnel or from muscular infundibular hypertrophy.

Pulmonic stenosis is usually an isolated defect, but it can potentially occur with many other congenital disorders or as a component of complex anomalies such as tetralogy of Fallot. Breeds with increased risk include the English bulldog, beagles, Chihuahuas, samoyeds and cocker spaniels.

NATURAL HISTORY

Most dogs with pulmonary stenosis have mild to moderate pressure gradients across the pulmonic valve and are asymptomatic.[15,16] Dogs with severe pulmonic stenosis, however, may exhibit progressive exercise intolerance, syncope, or right heart failure. Moderate to severe pulmonic stenosis can be a progressive disorder due to infundibular muscular hypertrophy or fibrosis and secondary right ventricular outflow obstruction. Dogs with severe obstructions typically begin to have symptoms of low-output heart failure and even congestive right

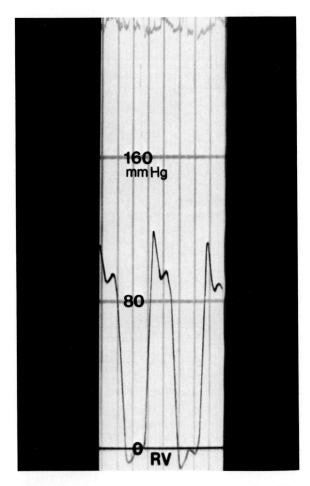

Fig. 18-5 Right ventricular pressure tracing from a dog with a right-to-left shunting PDA. Systolic right ventricular pressure (approximately 120 mmHg) is greatly elevated. (Courtesy of Dr. Philip Fox.)

heart failure between their first and third years of life. They rarely survive beyond 4 years if untreated.

PATHOPHYSIOLOGY AND HEMODYNAMICS

In order to sustain stroke volume in the face of an outflow obstruction, the right ventricle must generate a higher systolic pressure than normal. The pressure gradient across the stenosis is related to the magnitude and rate of blood flow through the stenotic valve divided by the cross-sectional area of the stenosis. The magnitude of decrease in right ventricular outflow tract cross-sectional area is also an index of severity and is not influenced by changes in blood flow or flow rate. From a pathophysiologic viewpoint, the right ventricular systolic pressure is as important as the size of the obstruction. Obstruction size, gradients, and systolic ventricular pressures are all interrelated.

Increased systolic ventricular pressure increases systolic myocardial wall stress and right ventricular external work, which are major determinants of myocardial oxygen consumption. Concentric hypertrophy develops to provide a greater mass of muscle with which to generate these increased pressures and also (by increasing wall thickness), to reduce right ventricular wall stress (law of Laplace). To an extent, hypertrophy is a beneficial compensatory response. However, marked hypertrophy places an increased demand on right ventricular blood flow and can actually exacerbate right ventricular obstruction by encroaching on an already narrowed ventricular outflow tract. Obstruction to ventricular flow is a systolic phenomenon; therefore, diastolic right heart filling pressures are usually normal or only sightly increased. Increased filling pressure may occur if myocardial compliance is reduced due to extensive hypertrophy or ischemia or if volume overload becomes a complicating factor due to pulmonary regurgitation, tricuspid regurgitation, or a compensatory response to reduced cardiac output.

A number of complications can result from severe pulmonic stenosis. High right ventricular systolic pressures can retard right ventricular myocardial perfusion. The resultant myocardial ischemia and fibrosis may initiate arrhythmias or depress ventricular performance. The high-velocity flow beyond a subvalvular stenosis can also damage the pulmonic valve leading to pulmonic regurgitation and right ventricular volume overload.

DIAGNOSIS

A systolic murmur is characteristically heard over the left heart base, which is usually harsh, crescendo, or crescendo-decrescendo and fairly localized to the lower second or third intercostal space (see Figs. 3-2 and 3-3). The second heart sound may be split (see Fig. 3-3), although this is usually difficult to detect because the P_2 component is reduced in intensity or obscured by the heart murmur. A prominent right ventricular apex beat may be detected. Jugular distention and pulsations are present in about one-third of cases. Arterial pulses feel normal unless low-output failure develops.

The ECG may be normal with mild pulmonic stenosis or display right ventricular enlargement with a right axis shift when the stenosis and pressure gradient is significant. Right ventricular enlargement on the ECG (see Fig. 4-15) suggests the need for additional diagnostics (i.e., cardiac catheterization) and possibly surgical repair.

Analysis of the thoracic radiographs reveals right ventricular enlargement and varying degrees of poststenotic dilatation of the main pulmonary artery (Fig. 18-6). Peripheral pulmonary arteries and veins are normal or small. Right atrial enlargement may be noted on the dorsoventral view in severe cases.

Echocardiography can identify the compensatory right ventricular hypertrophy and thereby provide an approximate assessment of the severity of obstruction. In addition, poststenotic dilatation of the pulmonary artery can be directly imaged with two-dimensional echocardiography (see Fig. 6-35, frame 3; Fig. 18-7, frames 2 and 3). Thickened and poorly moving pulmonary valve leaflets may be visualized in valvular pulmonic stenosis although the latter may also occur due to low cardiac output from other causes. Ventricular septal motion is often paradoxic due to right ventricular pressure overload. Doppler echocardiography is an important noninvasive method of detecting the turbulent blood flow associated with both pulmonic and aortic stenosis.[17] Pulsed-Doppler techniques provide the added advantage of delineating regional flow velocities within the heart and proximal great vessels. Pressure gradients across a stenotic lesion can be estimated if

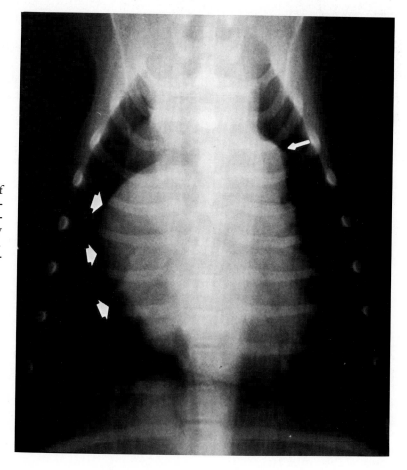

Fig. 18-6 Dorsoventral radiograph of a dog with pulmonic stenosis. Poststenotic dilatation of the main pulmonary artery is evident at approximately the 2 o'clock position (thin arrow). Right ventricular enlargement is outlined by the three thick arrows.

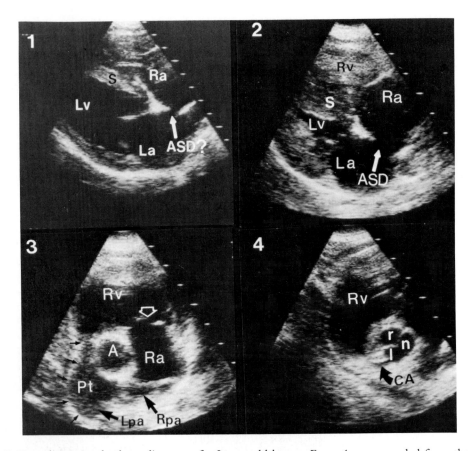

Fig. 18-7 Two-dimensional echocardiogram of a 2-year-old boxer. *Frame 1* was recorded from the right intercostal position and shows a long-axis view of the heart. While a patent foramen ovale is suggested by the septal dropout (arrow), a thin membrane spanning the apparent defect cannot be excluded. Note that there is tapering of the atrial septum in the region of the suspected defect instead of the T sign (i.e., an effect caused by echo-beam width artifact in which the edge of a septal defect is elongated and delineated, as opposed to just dropping out). This makes diagnosis of an ASD less likely. Additional imaging planes and contrast echocardiography may be helpful in making the correct diagnosis. *Frame 2* is a similar view recorded from a different boxer with a large ostium secundum defect. The right atrium is dilated; right ventricular dilation and hypertrophy is present because of concurrent pulmonic stenosis. In *frame 3* the dilated pulmonic trunk (poststenotic dilatation) is outlined (small black arrows) in this short-axis view. In *frame 4*, the aortic leaflets are labeled and the left coronary artery (CA) is seen. A contrast echocardiogram demonstrated a right to left shunt in this dog (see Fig. 6-32). Lv, left ventricle; Ra, right atrium, S, interventricular septum; La, left atrium; ASD, atrial septal defect; Rv, right ventricle; A, aorta; Pt, main pulmonary trunk; Lpa, left pulmonary artery; Rpa, right aortic cusp; l, left aortic cusp; n, noncoronary cusp; r, right coronary cusp; open arrow, tricuspid valve. (Courtesy of Dr. N. Sydney Moise.)

the velocity of blood flow beyond the obstruction can be measured with these techniques.

A diagnosis of pulmonic stenosis must take into consideration other congenital heart defects. The left basilar ejection-type murmur is similar to that of aortic stenosis. These lesions are usually differentiated by demonstrating ECG and radiographic evidence of right ventricular enlargement, which is absent in uncomplicated aortic stenosis. Atrial septal defects with a large left-to-right shunt can have a murmur of relative pulmonic stenosis and radiographic evidence of right heart enlargement but usually also exhibit radiographic signs of pulmonary overcirculation which is not present with pulmonic stenosis.

Cardiac catheterization or echocardiography is indicated to verify the diagnosis and to assess the location and severity of the obstruction. Right ventricular angiography illustrates the lesion and poststenotic dilation of the pulmonary artery (Fig. 18-8). The ratio between main pulmonary artery width and valve annulus obtained from right ventricular angiography may be useful in identifying pulmonic stenosis and distinguishing this from other congenital malformations.[15] Typical hemodynamic findings include an increased right ventricular systolic pressure with at least a 15 mmHg pressure differential between the right ventricle and pulmonary artery (Fig. 18-9).

TREATMENT

Other than the medical control of arrhythmias, the treatment of pulmonic stenosis is surgical. Surgery is generally indicated if the pressure gradient exceeds 80 mmHg, if severe right ventricular hypertrophy exists, or if the patient is symptomatic. Young dogs with gradients of 40 to 80 mmHg should be followed closely because of the risk of developing secondary infundibular hypertrophy or fibrosis. Serial physical and ECG examinations are indicated with follow-up radiographs, echocardiograms, and possibly cardiac catheterization if progression is suspected. Asymptomatic dogs with mild gradients do not require any therapy and can be expected to perform well as pets.

The use of negative inotropic drugs such as β-adrenergic blockers has been suggested for muscular subvalvular stenosis to reduce contractility and the resulting dynamic obstruction. The effectiveness of this form of therapy, however, has not been determined in dogs.

Aortic Stenosis

Obstruction to blood flowing from the left ventricle into the aorta is a common congenital heart defect in dogs, occurring slightly less frequently

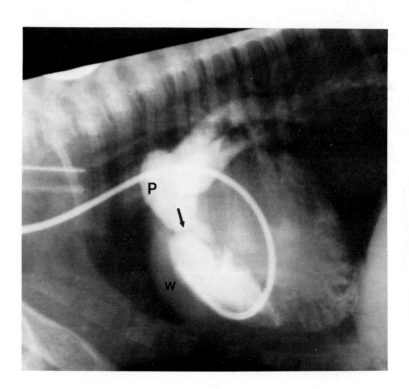

Fig. 18-8 Selective right ventriculogram of a dog with valvular pulmonic stenosis. The leaflets of the pulmonic valve are thickened and dysplastic (arrow). Note marked poststenotic dilation of the main pulmonary artery (P) and marked hypertrophy of the right ventricular cranioventral wall (W).

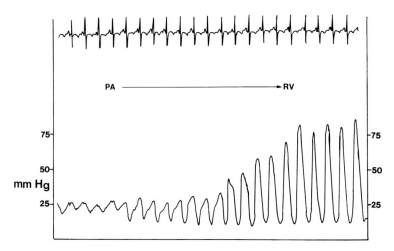

Fig. 18-9 Pressure tracing recorded from the main pulmonary artery (PA) and right ventricle (RV) of a dog with pulmonic stenosis. As the catheter is withdrawn from the PA (approximately 28 mmHg) into the RV (approximately 85 mmHg), a systolic pressure gradient of 55 to 60 mmHg occurs. An electrocardiogram (ECG) is recorded above the pressure tracing.

than pulmonic stenosis. The stenotic lesion can be supravalvular, valvular, or subvalvular in location. Supravalvular stenosis is a rare naturally occurring congenital lesion but can be induced experimentally by vitamin D supplementation in pregnant bitches.[18] Subvalvular aortic stenosis is the most common form, accounting for approximately 90 percent of all cases. Valvular lesions are the second most common form of aortic stenosis in dogs.

Breeds with an increased risk for aortic stenosis include Newfoundlands, boxers, German shepherds, golden retrievers, and German shorthair retrievers. The defect has also been recognized in smaller breeds such as terriers. A genetic basis has been identified in Newfoundland dogs by an incompletely understood mechanism that resembles an autosomal-dominant form of transmission.[2] Although aortic stenosis is usually an isolated defect, it sometimes occurs with mild aortic regurgitation, concurrent pulmonic stenosis, or mitral regurgitation. Association with other defects occurs sporadically.

In subvalvular aortic stenosis, the anatomic (phenotypic) expression may not occur for several weeks after birth.[2] The mildest lesions are fibrous nodules in the subvalvular region of the left ventricular outflow tract. Progression of these lesions can occur to form a distinct ridge, band, or collar of obstructive fibrous tissue just below the valve. In severe cases, the fibrous tissue can be extensive, involving the mitral valve leaflets.

NATURAL HISTORY

The occurrence of clinical signs is related to the severity of left ventricular obstruction. Dogs with mild stenosis (resting gradients <30 mmHg) generally remain asymptomatic and have a normal life expectancy. Moderate stenosis (30 to 70 mmHg gradients) is associated with variable signs and symptoms, including exercise intolerance and syncopal episodes. These signs are more common in dogs, with severe gradients exceeding 70 mmHg. The severity and frequency of signs tend to increase with time in dogs with moderate to severe stenosis and are potentiated by exercise or excitement. Severely affected dogs are susceptible to unexpected death, which probably results from a lethal arrhythmia. Coexisting aortic or mitral regurgitation increases the severity of symptoms and are significant additive risk factors of early mortality.

PATHOPHYSIOLOGY AND HEMODYNAMICS

The pathophysiology of aortic stenosis is similar to pulmonic stenosis and relates to a ventricular pressure overload. Higher systolic pressures must be generated to maintain an adequate stroke volume. Compensatory left ventricular hypertrophy develops and is quantitatively related to the severity of obstruction. Mild to moderate obstructive lesions may remain rather stable once a dog is mature. By contrast, dogs with severe stenosis can experience progression of the obstructive lesion due to hypertrophy of the left ventricular outflow tract.

Demand for left ventricular myocardial blood flow is increased with aortic stenosis due to increases in systolic myocardial wall stress, external ventricular work, and muscle mass associated with the defect. As a result, the left ventricular myocardium, particularly the subendocardial region, is susceptible to ischemia and associated risk of myocardial depression and arrhythmia generation.

The pathophysiology of aortic stenosis is due to both the reduced capacity to increase cardiac output and to ischemic myocardial damage. Increases in cardiac output are accomplished by increasing heart rate and to a lesser degree, stroke volume; the former increases myocardial oxygen requirements and imposes greater demands on myocardial blood flow, while the latter requires generation of higher ventricular systolic pressure. When the physiologic limits for myocardial blood flow and systolic pressure generation are attained, cardiac output reaches its peak, which may be insufficient to sustain physical efforts such as exercise. If ventricular pressure rises high enough, left ventricular receptors can be stimulated that induce reflex vasodilation and bradycardia.[19,20] Weakness or syncope may result. Myocardial ischemia can predispose to arrhythmias, depress contractility, and decrease left ventricular diastolic compliance.

The hemodynamics of aortic stenosis are predictably dependent on the severity of obstruction. Mild anatomic forms of the lesion usually do not exhibit a pressure gradient despite the presence of a faint (often inconsistent) murmur.[2] More commonly, however, are gradients over 20 mmHg. Left ventricular filling pressures are normal or only slightly elevated unless mitral or aortic regurgitation is present or the left ventricle is stiff due to excessive hypertrophy. Cardiac output is normal at rest in all but the most severely affected animals. The ability to increase cardiac output in response to exercise is attenuated. Metabolic vasodilation of skeletal muscle vasculature is also attenutated and contributes to muscular weakness and exercise intolerance.[21,22] The obstruction to flow may prolong left ventricular ejection resulting in a slow rate of aortic pressure rise and a reduction in peak aortic pressure.

DIAGNOSIS

The most striking physical feature of a physiologically significant left ventricular obstruction is a systolic, crescendo, or crescendo-decrescendo murmur heard best at the left cardiac base over the third to fourth intercostal space (see Figs. 3-2 and 3-5). The murmur may have a high-pitched musical tone and may radiate extensively, particularly to the right thoracic inlet and cranially along the carotid arteries. A prominent, sometimes sustained, left apical impulse may be palpated on dogs with significant obstruction. Palpation and characterization of the arterial pulse may help differentiate aortic stenosis from pulmonic stenosis which can have a similar-sounding murmur. Dogs with significant aortic stenosis tend to have a slow-rising and attenuated arterial pulse, whereas dogs with pulmonic stenosis usually have a normal arterial pulse.

The ECG of dogs with mild stenosis (gradients <30 mmHg) is usually normal. More severe stenosis is often associated with tall prolonged (widened) QRS complexes indicative of left ventricular enlargement. Depression of the S-T segment or a tall T wave is evident in some advanced cases and may represent myocardial ischemia. Ischemia can also lead to conduction defects that may manifest as abrupt notches in the QRS complex. Arrhythmias, including premature ventricular contractions, ventricular tachycardia or atrial fibrillation are also occasionally identified and may be elicited by exercise.

Radiographically, left ventricular enlargement is variable, but poststenotic dilation of the proximal aorta is frequently observed. Left ventricular enlargement is usually more evident on the dorsoventral view and appears as an elongation of the left ventricular silhouette (Fig. 18-10). The pulmonary vasculature is normal unless mitral regurgitation is also present and leads to left atrial and pulmonary venous enlargement.

Physiologically significant forms of subvalvular aortic stenosis are relatively easy to identify echocardiographically, using either M-mode or two-dimensional formats. Variable thickening of the ventricular septum and left ventricular free wall (see Fig. 6-34) and an echo-dense ridge, band or tunnel in the left ventricular outflow tract can usually be seen (Fig. 18-11). Left ventricular fractional short-

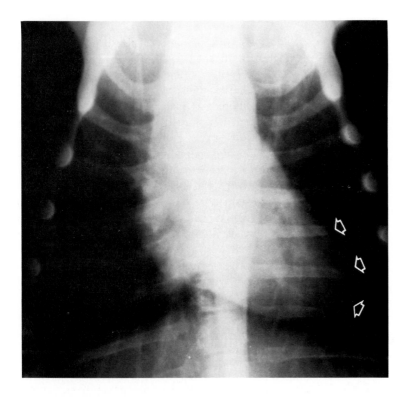

Fig. 18-10 Dorsoventral radiograph of a young dog with subvalvular aortic stenosis. Left ventricular enlargement is evident as an elongated left ventricular silhouette (arrows).

ening is usually normal or increased. If the stenosis involves the aortic valve, it may appear thickened and exhibit a diminished systolic range of motion. The poststenotic dilatation of the ascending aorta can also be visualized (see Fig. 6-34). Partial closure of the aortic valve in mid-systole may be seen with severe subvalvular stenosis. Excessive systolic fluttering of the aortic valve and systolic cranial (anterior) motion of the mitral valve (see Fig. 6-33) are also associated findings. Doppler studies illustrate the turbulent flow beyond the stenosis and demonstrate delayed peak aortic flow velocity. Esti-

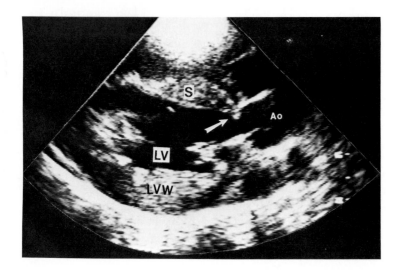

Fig. 18-11 Two-dimensional echocardiogram (long-axis view) of a dog with subaortic stenosis. There is severe hypertrophy of the interventricular septum (S) and left ventricular posterior wall (LVW). A ridge of fibrous tissue (arrow) is present in the left ventricular outflow tract. LV, left ventricular chamber; Ao, aorta.

mations of the pressure gradient across the stenosis can be made noninvasively using pulsed or continuous wave Doppler. Higher gradients are associated with higher poststenotic blood velocity and turbulence. Aortic regurgitation, if present, can often be demonstrated as retrograde blood flow below the aortic valve during early diastole with this technique.

Cardiac catheterization currently provides the most reliable and accurate hemodynamic information. Dogs with mild anatomic lesions and very low-intensity murmurs usually do not have pressure gradients across the stenotic region.[2] More severely affected animals commonly have gradients of 20 to 100 mmHg (Fig. 18-12). The effects of anesthesia on stroke volume and myocardial contractility can sometimes result in misleadingly low-pressure measurements and must be considered when assessing catheterization data. Oximetry values are normal. Selective angiography will illustrate left ventricular hypertrophy, an obstructive (stenotic) lesion, and poststenotic aortic dilation (Fig. 18-13). A contrast injection just above the aortic valve is usually made to check for aortic regurgitation.

THERAPY

The mortality associated with surgical repair of subvalvular stenosis in dogs is relatively high (e.g., approximately 25 percent).[23,24] For this reason, surgical therapy is generally reserved for dogs with prominent signs, marked left ventricular hypertrophy, or ECG evidence of myocardial ischemia or arrhythmias. Asymptomatic dogs with pressure gradients greater than 80 mmHg should also be considered for surgery because of the risks for secondary myocardial injury and unexpected death. β-Adrenergic blockers have been recommended to prevent arrhythmias and early mortality in patients with aortic stenosis without myocardial failure. The efficacy of this treatment in dogs is unknown. Additional antiarrhythmic agents may be needed if arrhythmias already exist. Other forms of medical therapy, such as positive inotropes and vasodilators, are generally contraindicated.

Ventricular Septal Defects

Defects in the ventricular septum are relatively common in dogs, accounting for approximately 5

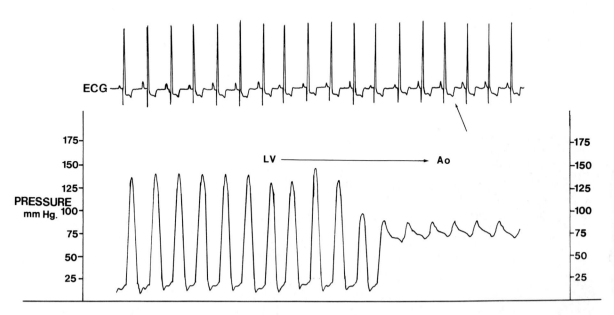

Fig. 18-12 Pressure tracing recorded from the aorta (Ao) and left ventricle (LV) in a dog with subvalvular aortic stenosis. Left ventricular systolic pressure is elevated (approximately 140 mmHg). As the catheter is withdrawn from the left ventricle (LV) to the aorta (Ao), a systolic pressure gradient (approximately 50 mmHg) occurs. The electrocardiogram (ECG) displays S-T segment depression (arrow), which may suggest myocardial ischemia.

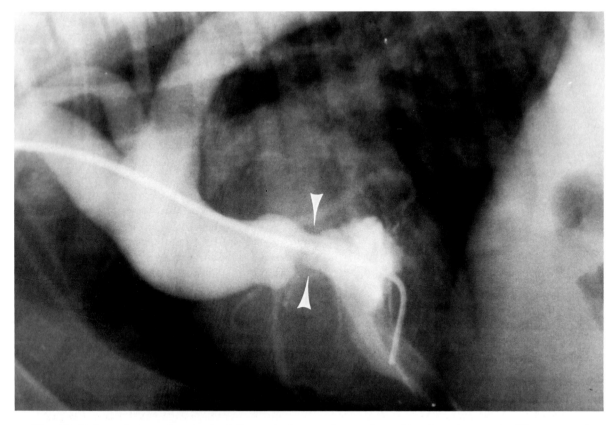

Fig. 18-13 Lateral view of a selective left ventriculogram from a dog with subaortic stenosis. The narrowed eccentric left ventricular outflow tract (between arrow heads) is due to a subvalvular fibrous ring. Poststenotic dilation of the ascending aorta is evident.

to 10 percent of all congenital heart defects or about 1 per 2,000 live births.[25] Most VSDs create a communication between the two ventricles. Left ventricular to right atrial communications are also possible with defects of the endocardial cushion type.[26] Most isolated VSDs in dogs occur in the membranous region of the septum beneath the cranial (anterior) aspect of the tricuspid septal leaflet. Septal defects also can occur below the pulmonic valve (supracristal defects) but only rarely in the muscular region of the septum.

As with most congenital heart defects, the etiology of VSDs is incompletely understood. A genetic cause is suspected and has been demonstrated as a polygenic trait in the spectrum of conotruncal defects of keeshonds.[1] Other breeds thought to have an increased risk include English bulldogs.[27] VSDs may occur as isolated abnormalities but are also components of complex anomalies, such as tetralogy of Fallot, double outlet right ventricle, and truncus arteriosus.

NATURAL HISTORY

The history of VSD depends on the severity of the defect and ranges from a complete lack of signs with small defects to congestive heart failure and death with large defects. Many dogs have small defects with mild left-to-right shunts. These dogs remain asymptomatic and may even experience spontaneous closure of the defect.[28] By contrast, symptomatic dogs commonly exhibit respiratory signs from congestive heart failure and exercise intolerance during the first 18 months of life.[29] Clinical signs may remain relatively stable or progress to include syncope, seizures, and cyanosis within a few years. This is associated with reversal of the shunt direction following the development of obstructive pulmonary vascular disease. Increased susceptibility to respiratory infections is another potential complication for all dogs with a VSD and occurs in about 50 percent of cases.[29]

Untreated symptomatic dogs can be expected to have a significantly shorter life span and commonly die within months of the diagnosis. This is particularly true for cyanotic patients with a right-to-left shunt.

PATHOPHYSIOLOGY AND HEMODYNAMICS

The location of the VSD has a minor influence on the pathophysiology with two exceptions. Membranous and supracristal defects can be associated with secondary aortic regurgitation due to defective structural support of the aortic valve or flow distortion of the valves (Venturi effect). Defects in the muscular septum are also somewhat unique in that they may decrease in size during systole and thus limit shunt flow. The importance of defect location, however, is much less than defect size and status of pulmonary vascular resistance.

Small defects provide significant restriction to systolic shunting and induce little hemodynamic change. These restrictive VSDs are characterized by a large systolic pressure gradient between the two ventricles. Systolic pressures in the right ventricle and pulmonary artery are only slightly increased in these cases. Larger defects may still be somewhat restrictive but allow a considerable shunt flow if pulmonary vascular resistance is low. In these cases, variable systolic hypertension occurs in the right ventricle and pulmonary artery. Pulmonary vascular resistance, or specifically the difference between pulmonary and systemic vascular resistance, becomes more important in determining shunt flow as the size of the defect increases. In the extreme case where the ventricular septum is functionally absent, the ratio of pulmonary to systemic flow is determined entirely by the respective differences in vascular resistance. Equilibration of aortic and pulmonary artery systolic pressures may result.

Increased pulmonary flow at high systolic pressures may cause secondary obstructive pulmonary vascular disease and subsequent increases in both systolic and diastolic pulmonary artery pressure.[30–32] These vascular changes tend to be progressive and may lead to right heart pressures that exceed those in the left. This reverses the shunt direction from left to right to right to left and is called *Eisenmenger's physiology* or *syndrome*. Right-to-left shunting resulting from acquired infundibular stenosis of the right ventricle (acquired or pseudo-tetralogy of Fallot) is an uncommon sequela of a VSD in dogs.

The normal direction of left-to-right shunt flow through a VSD produces a volume overload of the pulmonary circulation and left heart. As a result, left heart filling pressures are increased in proportion to the magnitude of the shunt. The combination of increased pulmonary flow with increases in pulmonary arterial and venous pressures promotes pulmonary edema. Aortic regurgitation, if present, can exacerbate the increased left ventricular end-diastolic pressure and volume. Because shunting occurs predominantly during systole, the right ventricle is usually spared from dilation and increased filling pressure unless the defect is extremely large.

DIAGNOSIS

The classic murmur of a VSD is harsh and holosystolic with the point of maximal intensity at the right cranial sternal border (see Figs. 3-2, 3-4, and 3-5), although murmurs and heart sounds associated with VSDs can be quite variable. The murmur may be present only during early systole if the defect is small and partially closes during contraction or if the defect is large and accompanied by pulmonary hypertension. The more common holosystolic murmur of a fixed, small to moderately-sized VSD can be either plateau, crescendo, or crescendo-decrescendo in character. Occasionally, a left basilar murmur due to relative pulmonic stenosis can be heard due to large flow rates through the fixed cross-sectional area of the right ventricular outflow tract. This is particularly true of supracristal defects in which the shunt is functionally from left ventricle to pulmonary artery.[32] The second heart sound is often split (see Fig. 3-3) with retention of respiratory influences, although this may be obscured by the murmur. A loud second heart sound can sometimes be heard in dogs with pulmonary hypertension. Murmurs are typically absent in cyanotic patients with a right-to-left shunt.

Arterial pulses are variable, being normal with small defects, brisk with large moderately shunting defects, and depressed with very large shunts that cause congestive heart failure. Jugular pulses are absent unless severe pulmonary hypertension and right ventricular failure are present.

Dogs with high pulmonary vascular resistance and Eisenmenger's syndrome usually exhibit generalized cyanosis that is accentuated with exercise. Varying degrees of polycythemia are usually present in these cases.

Normal ECGs are expected for dogs with small defects. Evidence of left atrial and ventricular enlargement may be seen with large left to right shunts. Evidence of right heart enlargement is absent unless obstructive pulmonary vascular disease and severe pulmonary hypertension develop. A variety of arrhythmias can be associated with VSDs ranging from AV nodal or intraventricular conduction defects to supraventricular and ventricular tachyarrhythmias. Conduction defects such as right bundle branch block may be more common with membranous VSDs because of their proximity to the normal conduction pathways.

Hemodynamically significant VSDs usually have radiographic signs of left heart enlargement with increased pulmonary vascularity, although considerable variation exists. The radiographic signs are similar to those of a left-to-right PDA except that the degree of left heart enlargement and pulmonary overcirculation is generally less with a VSD, and the aortic dilation common with a PDA is absent with a VSD. Reverse-shunting VSDs exhibit variable radiographic findings. Right ventricular or biventricular enlargement is usually evident. Pulmonary vascular markings range from small or normal to large and tortuous.

Echocardiographically, dilation of the left heart and pulmonary artery can usually be detected if the left-to-right shunt is significant. Defects larger than 1 cm often can be directly visualized as an echolucency in the ventricular septum just below the aortic valve (Fig. 18-14). Additional findings occasionally include altered septal motion due to conduction defects and diastolic fluttering of the aortic and/or mitral valve if secondary aortic regurgitation develops. Fractional shortening of the left ventricular wall is usually exaggerated unless myocardial failure develops or a right-to-left shunt develops. Right-to-left shunting can be visualized with contrast echocardiography using a venous injection of echocontrast material. Noninvasive identification of left-to-right shunting, however, requires pulsed Doppler ultrasonic techniques. Pulsed Doppler signals from the right side of a left-to-right shunting restrictive VSD illustrate high blood velocities and varying degrees of turbulence.

The clinical appearance of a VSD can be similar to several other congenital defects. Supracristal defects, for example, can produce murmurs similar to

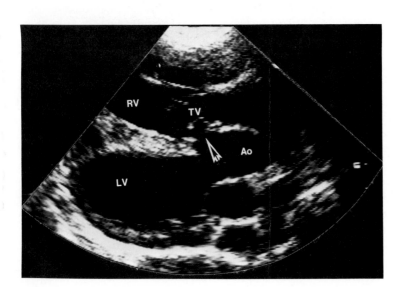

Fig. 18-14 Two-dimensional echocardiogram (long-axis view) of a dog with membranous ventricular septal defect. It is visualized as an echolucency (arrow) just below the tricuspid valve (TV) and aorta (Ao). LV, left ventricle; RV, right ventricle.

pulmonic stenosis. It may be differentiated from pulmonic stenosis by lack of right ventricular enlargement on radiographs or the electrocardiogram and by radiographic evidence of pulmonary overcirculation. By contrast, reverse-shunting VSDs are physiologically similar to those of tetralogy of Fallot, but the former does not usually have an associated pulmonic stenosis murmur. If the diagnosis is in question, however, a cardiac catheterization is indicated for confirmation, to determine shunt severity and the potential for successful repair. Angiocardiographic visualization of the defect (Fig. 18-15) may be important if surgical correction is considered. Oximetry permits calculation of relative blood flows (Q) in the pulmonary (Q_p) and systemic (Q_s) circulations. Measurements of pulmonary flow may also be important to calculate pul-

monary vascular resistance. Systolic pulmonary hypertension can be associated with left-to-right shunting VSDs without increased pulmonary vascular resistance in nonrestrictive VSDs. This underscores the value of calculating resistance from flow and pressure data obtained during the cardiac catheterization.

TREATMENT

Not all dogs with a VSD require therapy. Asymptomatic patients with small shunts ($Q_p : Q_s$ Ratio <2) usually perform well as pets without the need for surgical therapy. These dogs may occasionally experience respiratory signs due to congestion, which can be treated with diuretics and/or arterial vasodilators. Dogs with $Q_p : Q_s$ ratios of >2.5 are

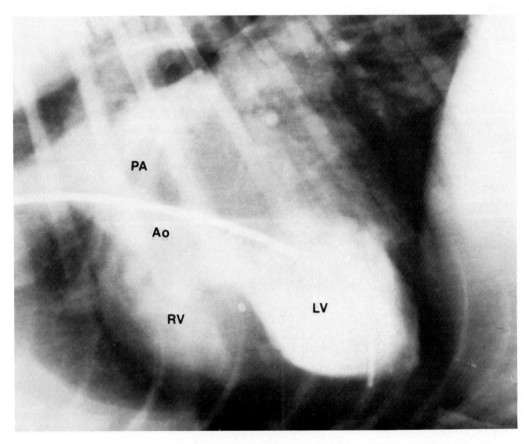

Fig. 18-15 Right lateral view of a selective left ventriculogram in a dog with a left-to-right shunting ventricular septal defect. Injection was made in the left ventricle (LV). Contrast medium appears in the right ventricle (RV). Both the aorta (Ao) and the pulmonary artery (PA) are therefore opacified.

at risk of developing obstructive pulmonary vascular disease and should be considered surgical candidates, regardless of clinical signs. Primary anatomic repair of the VSD or pulmonary artery banding to reduce pulmonary overcirculation constitute surgical options for such patients. Successful primary repair is physiologically superior to pulmonary artery banding but requires open-heart surgery and is associated with greater risk and expense. Pulmonary artery banding offers a reliable and relatively easy way to reduce shunt flow in mature dogs that have normal or only slight increased pulmonary vascular resistance.

Dogs with small left-to-right shunts with high pulmonary vascular resistance (greater than two times normal or greater than 50 percent of systemic resistance) pose a greater therapeutic problem. Banding the pulmonary artery could reverse the shunt flow and is therefore not generally recommended. Primary anatomic closure is the only treatment likely to be effective in these cases but does not guarantee an end to the progression of obstructive pulmonary vascular disease.

Dogs wtih bidirectional or reverse shunting through a VSD are generally not considered surgical candidates. Vasodilators such as hydralazine, captopril, and prazosin have been suggested as potential medical therapies for right-to-left shunting patients as a means to reduce pulmonary vascular resistance. Unfortunately, these drugs produce inconsistent effects on the pulmonary vasculature and often preferentially dilate systemic vessels, increasing the right-to-left shunt. The management of these shunts should include exercise restriction and, in cyanotic patients, periodic phlebotomy to maintain the hematocrit below 60 percent. Low-dose aspirin therapy is also recommended to reduce the risk of arterial thromboembolism.

Atrial Septal Defects

Atrial septal defects (ASDs) are anatomically distinguished from other interatrial communications such as a patent foramen ovale by partial or complete absence of normal septal tissue (see Fig. 1-3). Three major types of ASDs occur, but all are relatively uncommon in dogs. A sinus venosus ASD occurs high in the atrial septum near the junction of the pulmonary vein and left atrium.[33] Ostium secundum defects are located in the middle of the septum, bounded dorsally and ventrally by atrial septal tissue. An ostium primum defect occurs low in the atrial septum, with ventricular septum or AV valves forming its ventral border. It is considered an incomplete form of an endocardial cushion defect.[34,35]

Atrial septal defects may be isolated lesions or may occur in conjunction with a variety of other defects, including pulmonic stenosis and tricuspid dysplasia. A genetic basis is suspected in most cases with Old English sheepdogs, samoyeds, and boxers considered to be at increased risk.[23]

NATURAL HISTORY

Most dogs with an isolated ASD are asymptomatic. By contrast, signs associated with large ASDs include exercise intolerance, syncope, and respiratory manifestations of congestive heart failure before 1 year of age. Asymptomatic dogs may become symptomatic if other hemodynamic stresses are superimposed, such as tricuspid regurgitation. Dogs with ASDs also seem to be more susceptible to pulmonary problems, including lower respiratory tract infections. Unlike a VSD or PDA, atrial septal defects are rarely associated with obstructive pulmonary vascular disease.

Asymptomatic dogs usually have a normal lifespan. Mild signs do not usually progress and are also compatible with a relatively normal life span. Such dogs frequently experience temporary exacerbation of clinical signs. By contrast, severely affected dogs may develop signs of congestive heart failure or frequent syncopal episodes and rarely survive beyond 4 years without treatment.

PATHOPHYSIOLOGY AND HEMODYNAMICS

The net shunt through an ASD is usually left to right. Instantaneous flow may be quite variable, changing slightly with respiration or heart rhythm and even temporarily shunting right to left.

The magnitude of the net shunt is dependent on the size of the defect, the relative cross-sectional area of the two AV valves, and the relative diastolic compliance of the two ventricles. Volume overloading of the right atrium, right ventricle, and pulmonary vessels occurs and forms the basis for the hemodynamic alterations and clinical signs. The volume overload results in increased end-diastolic pressure in the right heart. Marked right ventricular dilation can distort the tricuspid valve apparatus, leading to tricuspid regurgitation. This places an additional volume load on the right atrium. In these cases, right atrial pressure may actually exceed left atrial pressure, causing reversal of the shunt.

Right ventricular systolic performance is usually normal or even enhanced despite the increase in work imposed by the volume overload. Systolic pressures in the right ventricle and pulmonary artery are usually normal or only slightly increased.

The pathophysiology of an ASD can be considerably different if other lesions exist. For example, with pulmonic stenosis, right ventricular compliance may be reduced and right atrial pressure elevated with the result being either a small left-to-right shunt or a right-to-left shunt.

DIAGNOSIS

Small defects rarely produce clinical signs. There is no murmur associated with the atrial shunt flow due to the low velocity of blood flow. Larger shunts may produce physical signs in the form of wide and fixed splitting of S_2 with a loud P_2 component (see Fig. 3-3). Large shunts may also be associated with a relative pulmonic stenosis murmur due to high flow across this valve. Arterial pulses are usually normal. Jugular distention and pulsations can sometimes be identified in dogs with large defects or if right ventricular failure has developed. Auscultation of the lung fields may reveal accentuated bronchovesicular sounds, crackles, wheezes, or rales, if pulmonary congestion develops secondary to increased pulmonic blood flow.

The ECG is relatively insensitive to the hemodynamic changes induced by most ASDs. Occasionally, right ventricular enlargement patterns will be evident if the shunt flow is large.

Thoracic radiographs are often normal with small defects. Large defects with considerable shunt flow can more than double the $Q_p : Q_s$ ratio. This may cause right heart enlargement and dilation of pulmonary arteries and veins. The left atrium is usually normal in size although varying degrees of enlargement may occur.

Echocardiography (Figs. 18-7 and 18-16; see also

Fig. 6-32) provides the opportunity to visualize the ASD directly from several imaging planes. Pseudo-ASD images (echolucency or dropout in the midseptal region) are common artifacts in normal dogs. Careful interpretation of atrial septal images is therefore required when considering an atrial septal defect. Detection of shunt flow is possible by means of contrast echocardiography or pulsed Doppler techniques. Intravenous contrast echo studies are best suited for demonstrating right-to-left shunts (see Fig. 6-32). Occasionally, left-to-right shunts can be visualized due to the dilutional effect of the shunt on the contrast media as the media enters the right atrium. Alternatively, a left-to-right shunt can sometimes be transiently reversed in an anesthetized animal by sustained positive pressure inflation of the lungs (similar to a Valsalva maneuver). Pulsed Doppler examinations can demonstrate the left-to-right shunt flow as a low-velocity signal beginning late in ventricular systole and continuing through diastole. A brief right-to-left flow signal can sometimes be recognized during isovolumetric ventricular contraction.

Cardiac catheterization is the most reliable method of diagnosing an ASD. The defect may occasionally be crossed with a catheter introduced from the right atrium, permitting a selective left atrial injection to demonstrate the shunt. Alternatively, a pulmonary artery contrast injection can demonstrate the left-to-right shunt as the left atrium is highlighted.

An assessment of the defect size and location is important if surgical correction is anticipated. Oximetry data reveal an increase in oxygen saturation at the atrial level and also permits calculation of the pulmonary to systemic flow ratio ($Q_p : Q_s$). This ratio is calculated from regional oxygen saturation values as follows:

$$Q_p : Q_s - (Sat_{ao} - Sat_{cvc})/(Sat_{ao} - Sat_{pa})$$

where ao is aorta, cvc is cranial vena cava, and pa is pulmonary artery. Ratios greater than 2 are generally considered hemodynamically significant. Pulmonary artery pressure may be normal or increased, depending on the magnitude of the shunt and the pulmonary vascular resistance. If pulmonary artery pressures are increased, cardiac output measurements should be conducted to permit calculation of pulmonary vascular resistance.

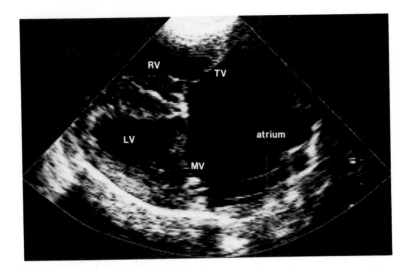

Fig. 18-16 Two-dimensional echocardiogram from a dog, four-chamber view, illustrating complete absence of the interatrial septum. Normally, atrial septal tissue would extend in a plane similar to the ventricular septum, partitioning a left and right atrial chamber. LV, left ventricle; RV, right ventricle; MV, mitral valve; TV, tricuspid valve.

THERAPY AND PROGNOSIS

Most dogs with an ASD do not require therapy and are often undiagnosed because of a lack of clinical signs. These dogs can be expected to have normal lifespans. Dogs that experience mild or intermittent signs of congestive heart failure can often be successfully managed medically using low-sodium diets and diuretic therapy.

Surgical closure of an ASD is not routinely conducted because of the risks and expense of open heart surgery. However, surgical closure should be considered for any dog with severe or progressive signs, with large defects with a $Q_p:Q_s$ greater than 2.5, and if pulmonary vascular resistance is elevated. Surgical closure can also be beneficial in dogs with right-to-left shunts. Palliative surgical procedures such as pulmonary artery banding are not usually recommended because shunt direction could be reversed if right ventricular diastolic compliance decreases.

Tetralogy of Fallot

In 1888, Etienne-Louis Fallot published a description of a congenital heart malformation characterized by a large VSD, pulmonary stenosis, right ventricular hypertrophy, and a dextropositioned aorta overiding the ventricular septum. Despite the distinct anatomic description, this tetralogy can be sim-plified to two physiologically important variables—a large VSD and varying degrees of pulmonary stenosis. The right ventricular hypertrophy is merely a compensatory change and the degree of aortic malpositioning is highly variable and insignificant from a hemodynamic point of view. Although Fallot's tetrad remains distinct anatomically, its clinical designation generally includes any large VSD accompanied by hemodynamically significant pulmonic stenosis, irrespective of aortic position or fibrous continuity between the semilunar and AV valves.

Combinations of a VSD and pulmonic stenosis have been recognized in a variety of breeds, including poodles, schnauzers, keeshonds, and terriers. In the keeshond, the defect is genetically transmitted as a spectrum of disorders called conotruncal defects.[1] These include isolated VSDs, pulmonic stenosis, tetralogy and tetralogy-like defects, and persistent truncus arteriosus. The mode of inheritance appears to be a polygenic trait similar to a PDA. Matings between affected dogs or matings of affected dogs to normal first-degree relatives gave results that resembled simple dominant inheritance. However, outcrosses to unrelated normal dogs without a history of congenital defects resulted in a proportion of affected offspring much lower than expected for a single dominant gene hypothesis.[1]

Ventricular septal defect-pulmonic stenosis combinations can also be complicated by other defects, such as PDA or an atrial septal defect. Maldevelopment of the peripheral pulmonary arteries is also frequently observed. A right aortic arch may be present in some cases.

NATURAL HISTORY

Dogs with VSD-pulmonic stenosis generally fall into one of two clinical categories: asymptomatic dogs with a murmur, or dogs with exertional respiratory difficulty, cyanosis, and other signs.[36] Approximately 80 percent of affected dogs become symptomatic during the first year of life.[25] Asymptomatic dogs include those with mild to moderate pulmonic stenosis, while symptomatic dogs usually have severe pulmonic stenosis and a bidirectional or right-to-left shunt through the VSD. The separation of these two groups of dogs is somewhat simplified, since the clinical manifestations of the disease encompasses a wide range. For example, dogs with a large VSD and minimal pulmonic stenosis show physiologic effects similar to those from an isolated VSD, and may be asymptomatic (so-called "pink tetralogy") or develop congestive heart failure due to a large left-to-right shunt.

Additional signs occasionally observed in symptomatic dogs include stunted growth, severe exercise intolerance, syncope, or seizures.[37] Signs of arterial thromboembolism may occur, particularly if secondary polycythemia develops.

Tetralogy-like defects tend to progress with time. Progression of the disease occurs for a number of reasons, the most common being hypertrophy of the infundibular region which exacerbates obstruction to pulmonary flow. Other complications include a reduction in collateral pulmonary blood flow and tricuspid or aortic regurgitation. Thus, even asymptomatic dogs are at risk of developing serious complications. The life expectancy for untreated symptomatic dogs is significantly reduced, with death occurring by 2 years of age. Occasionally, mildly symptomatic dogs will survive well into adult life. Right heart failure is an uncommon but potential sequela in dogs surviving the first few years of life. It is more likely to occur if pulmonary or tricuspid regurgitation superimposes a volume load on the right ventricle.

PATHOPHYSIOLOGY AND HEMODYNAMICS

The physiologic consequences of tetralogy-like defects primarily depend on three factors: the size of the VSD, the degree of pulmonic stenosis, and (less importantly) the systemic vascular resistance. At one end of the spectrum, with a large VSD and minimal pulmonic stenosis, a left-to-right shunt occurs. A volume overload is imposed on the pulmonary circulation and left heart similar to that caused by an isolated nonrestrictive VSD. The spectrum of manifestations of tetralogy can be appreciated by considering progressive increases in the obstruction to pulmonary flow. As the stenosis increases, the left-to-right shunt decreases. At the point where resistance to flow into the pulmonary artery exceeds systemic vascular resistance, a right-to-left shunt develops. Thus, the direction of shunt flow is determined by the relative resistances of the pulmonary and systemic circulation, not the degree of aortic dextroposition.

In some cases, infundibular muscular hypertrophy contributes to the pulmonic stenosis, especially during muscular contraction. In these cases, the direction of shunt may vary, tending toward right to left during excitement, exertion, or with any other cause for increased cardiac output or myocardial contractility.

Patients with severe pulmonic stenosis and a right-to-left shunt usually have reduced pulmonary blood flow that may be supplemented primarily by bronchial artery collaterals. The development and severity of systemic desaturation depend on both the magnitude of right-to-left shunt and the pulmonary blood flow. For example, if extensive collateral circulation can maintain pulmonary flow at near-normal levels, cyanosis may not develop despite a significant right-to-left shunt.

Right ventricular systolic pressure is invariably increased. This is not necessarily a manifestation of the pulmonic stenosis since a nonrestrictive VSD can also lead to high systolic pressures. The peak right ventricular pressure rarely exceeds systolic aortic pressure unless obstruction to pulmonary flow is severe and the VSD is small and restrictive. Right ventricular end-diastolic pressures range from normal to increased, although overt right heart failure is uncommon. The pulmonary artery pressure is classically reduced in cyanotic patients due to decreased flow, although normal or even high pressures are sometimes present if concurrent defects in the peripheral pulmonary vasculature exist. Left heart volumes and filling pressure are reduced in cyanotic patients.

DIAGNOSIS

Major findings from the physical examination are the murmur, cyanosis (if the pulmonic stenosis is severe), and often stunted growth. A holosystolic right sternal border murmur can be heard in addition to the systolic left basilar pulmonic stenosis murmur if the stenosis is mild. However, the pulmonic stenosis murmur predominates in most cases. The character of this murmur can provide clues about the severity of obstuction. Loud murmurs persisting throughout systole are associated with less severe forms of obstruction, and a left-to-right shunt. The murmur becomes softer and shorter as the severity of pulmonic stenosis increases due to preferential shunting into the aorta (see Figs. 3-2 through 3-5). A continuous murmur is rarely heard. If present, it is indicative of severe pulmonic stenosis or atresia and extensive systemic collateralization through bronchial arteries or a PDA. Arterial pulses are usually normal and jugular pulsations are typi-

cally absent. A prominent cardiac apex impulse can often be palpated on the right precordium. Polycythemia is often present in cyanotic patients.

The ECG of dogs with VSD-PS varies according to the degree of pulmonic stenosis. Occasionally, it may be normal or show evidence of left heart enlargement if a large left-to-right shunt is present. Typically, severe pulmonic obstruction is present and associated with right ventricular dominance in the form of a severe right axis shift and right ventricular enlargement pattern (see Fig. 4-15). A supraventricular tachycardia may be present at rest, which can increase dramatically in response to exertion.

The radiographic appearance of a tetralogy is variable. The classic findings include a normal or slightly enlarged cardiac silhouette with right ventricular enlargement. Pulmonary vessels are clearly visible but smaller than normal. The main pulmonary artery varies in size. It may be small with pulmonary valve atresia or with severe infundibular stenosis. Alternatively, a poststenotic dilation may be observed secondary to valvular pulmonic stenosis. The left atrium may be small if pulmonary flow is reduced. Occasionally, a right aortic arch can be identified radiographically.

Echocardiography may assist the diagnosis (Figs. 18-17 and 18-18; see also Figs. 6-31 and 6-35). Right ventricular hypertrophy, a small left atrium, pul-

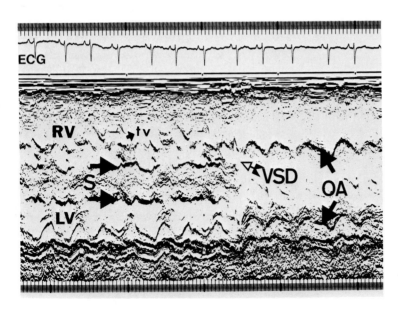

Fig. 18-17 M-mode echocardiographic sweep from the cardiac apex to base in a keeshond puppy with tetralogy of Fallot. Overriding of the aorta (OA) is readily apparent as a dropout of echoes between the interventricular septum (S) and aorta. This is due to the ventricular septal defect (VSD) (open arrow). Right ventricular enlargement, interventricular septal hypertrophy, and decreased left ventricular chamber dimension are present. RV, right ventricular chamber; LV, left ventricular chamber; tv, tricuspid valve; ECG, electrocardiogram. (Courtesy of Dr. N. Sydney Moise.)

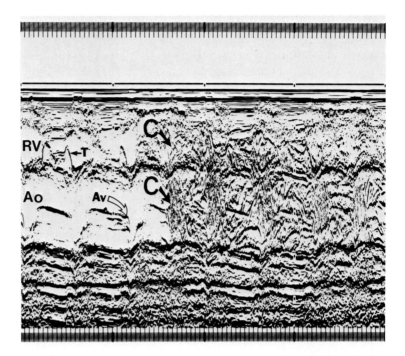

Fig. 18-18 Nonselective contrast M-mode echocardiogram of the keeshond puppy in Figure 17-17. Microbubbles injected into the cephalic vein cause contrast echoes (C) to appear in the right ventricle (RV) and, almost simultaneously, in the aorta (Ao), demonstrating a right-to-left intracardiac shunt. T, tricuspid valve; Av, aortic valve. (Courtesy of Dr. N. Sydney Moise.)

monic stenosis, a VSD, and dextropositioned aorta may be imaged. Right-to-left shunts across the VSD may be demonstrated with contrast echocardiography. These findings may help distinguish tetralogy from *Eisenmenger's syndrome* (any communication between systemic and pulmonary circulations producing pulmonary vascular disease and secondary right-to-left shunting) and *Eisenmenger's complex* (VSD, pulmonary vascular disease, and right-to-left shunting of blood).

Despite the aid of echocardiography, tetralogy-like defects can be difficult to confirm noninvasively. Clinically, they may be indistinguishable from other lesions, such as truncus arteriosus, double outlet right ventricle, and Eisenmenger's disorders.[37] A complete cardiac catheterization is usually needed to confirm the lesion, assess the hemodynamics, and evaluate the pulmonary stenosis and peripheral pulmonary vessels. Common catheterization findings include angiographic and hemodynamic demonstration of pulmonic stenosis and angiographic or oximetry evidence of the VSD. If a true tetralogy of Fallot exists, the aorta can often be catheterized from the right ventricle. An injection of contrast media above the aortic valve permits an

assessment of systemic collaterals to the pulmonary circulation. Measurement of pulmonary artery pressure is important in older dogs to distinguish tetralogy-like lesions from cases with a VSD and acquired infundibular stenosis ("acquired tetralogy of Fallot"), the latter being a nonsurgical disease. If the pulmonary stenosis is severe, however, pulmonary arterial catheterization is difficult and possibly dangerous. In these cases, a right ventricular contrast injection demonstrates both the stenosis and usually the right-to-left shunting VSD (Fig. 18-19).

TREATMENT

Dogs with minimal pulmonic stenosis (gradient <30 mmHg) and a left-to-right shunt can usually be managed conservatively, similar to management of an isolated VSD. The potential for progression of pulmonary stenosis or obstructive pulmonary vascular disease must be considered. If the stenosis is severe, more aggressive therapies should be considered, including primary surgical repair of the VSD and pulmonary stenosis, surgical creation of systemic-pulmonary shunts, and β-adrenergic blocker therapy. Primary surgical repair would be

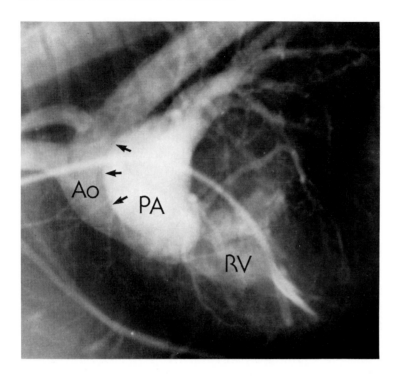

Fig. 18-19 Lateral view of a selective right ventriculogram in a 5-month-old, female terrier. Contrast material is injected into the right ventricle (RV). The aorta (Ao) and pulmonary artery (PA) opacify simultaneously, suggesting a right-to-left shunting ventricular septal defect (VSD) with an overriding aorta. The main pulmonary artery displays a poststenotic dilation (arrows). Severe right ventricular hypertrophy is present. These changes are compatible with tetralogy of Fallot. (Courtesy of Dr. Philip Fox.)

the ideal choice were it not for the mortality and expense associated with open-heart surgery. Creation of a shunt between a systemic artery and pulmonary artery is a palliative procedure that increases pulmonary blood flow. It is primarily indicated for cyanotic patients suffering from hypoxic symptoms that are not candidates for primary repair (Ch. 28). β-Adrenergic blockers can be used if surgical therapy is not feasible or as an adjunctive form of therapy before and after surgical palliation.[38] The desired effects of β-adrenergic blockade are to reduce myocardial contractility (primarily for dynamic infundibular stenosis), increase systemic vascular resistance, reduce heart rate, and alter the oxyhemoglobin dissociation in favor of oxygen unloading.[39]

Another aspect of treatment is the control of polycythemia. Hematocrits greater than 60 percent are associated with a significant increase in blood viscosity. This increases the risk of thromboembolic disease and can adversely affect cerebral perfusion. Maintaining hematocrits below 60 percent by periodic phlebotomy reduces these risks, yet still permits an increase in the oxygen carrying capacity of the blood. Low-dose aspirin therapy is also rec-

ommended in patients with a right-to-left shunt to reduce the risk of thromboembolism.

Atrioventricular Valve Malformations

Malformations of either one or both AV valves are occasionally recognized as congenital defects in dogs.[40–43] These malformations can be of several forms. All are associated with some degree of abnormal valve function and cause either regurgitation or stenosis, or both. Mitral and tricuspid regurgitation are the most common manifestations, depending on which of the two AV valves are involved. Affected valves have thickened or redundant leaflets, abnormal chordae tendineae or papillary muscles, or attachments (see Fig. 32-1). Other valvular malformations occur as components of congenital heart disease complexes such as cleft mitral valves associated with endocardial cushion defects.

Malformations of AV valves have not been recognized with enough frequency to identify specific breeds with increased risk or to verify a genetic cause. AV valve malformations are occasionally associated with other defects, such as ASDs.

NATURAL HISTORY

Malformations of AV valves are frequently associated with signs of congestive heart failure at an early age. Signs include exercise intolerance coughing, dyspnea, ascites, and peripheral edema, depending on which valve is involved. Arrhythmias are common and may contribute to episodic weakness or syncope. Clinical signs are usually progressive, especially if myocardial failure develops secondarily. Dogs with congenital valvular regurgitation rarely survive beyond 4 years of age. Similar mortality can be expected for stenotic valves unless surgical correction is performed.

PATHOPHYSIOLOGY AND HEMODYNAMICS

The major physiologic result for either AV valvular regurgitation or stenosis is increased atrial volume and pressure. High pressures are responsible for causing pulmonary congestion and edema. A reduced capacity to increase cardiac output may occur. A significant volume overload is also delivered to the ventricle associated with the valvular regurgitation.

Supraventricular arrhythmias may develop in response to severe atrial dilation. As the ventricular rate increases, less time is available for complete diastolic filling, particularly if the valve is stenotic. A decrease in stroke volume and cardiac output may result. Cardiac performance can be further embarrassed if myocardial function is depressed. Reduction in contractility is occasionally associated with AV valve malformations, especially regurgitant forms. It is not clear whether this is a primary manifestation of the congenital defect or whether it develops secondary to chronic ventricular volume loading.

DIAGNOSIS

A presumptive diagnosis of congenital AV valvular regurgitation can usually be made in a young dog from a holosystolic apical murmur (see Figs. 3-2 and 3-4). Jugular pulsations are common with severe tricuspid malformations. The ECG will usually portray an enlargement pattern for the involved atria and ventricle if the valve is predominantly regurgitant. Supraventricular tachyarrhythmias or ventricular conduction disturbances such as bundle branch blocks may also be noted. Plain thoracic radiographs also depict enlargement of the involved chambers. Occasionally, the atrial dilation may be so severe that recognition of the individual cardiac chamber regions becomes difficult. Venous congestion, pulmonary edema, and pericardial, thoracic, or abdominal effusions may be evident with severe lesions.

Malformed stenotic valves are characterized by a low-intensity diastolic murmur with radiographic evidence of atrial (but not ventricular) enlargement. Radiographic signs of venous engorgement and edema are similar to those of regurgitant valves.

Echocardiography may show changes due to volume overload and chamber enlargement, may be helpful in identifying valvular stenosis, and assessing myocardial performance. If a diagnosis is still in doubt, cardiac catheterization may be needed (Fig. 18-20). This is particularly true for stenotic valves, which could be confused with some forms of restrictive myocardial disease. Demonstration of a diastolic pressure gradient across the valve would confirm a suspicion of stenosis. Manipulating a catheter across such a valve is often difficult, however.

TREATMENT

Dogs with regurgitant valves are generally treated medically. Low-sodium diets, diuretics, and venodilators may relieve some of the signs of congestive heart failure. Arterial vasodilators may actually reduce the severity of the regurgitation and shift the balance of total ventricular stroke volume more toward the arterial circulation. Positive inotropic drugs may be helpful if depressed myocardial performance is identified echocardiographically. Although clinical improvement may be noted following these therapies, progression of the disease can, and usually does, continue to occur.

Some dogs with stenotic valves can also be managed effectively with medical therapy. Judicious use of low-sodium diets, diuretics, and venodilators may reduce the signs of congestion, although always at the risk of reducing cardiac output. Surgery

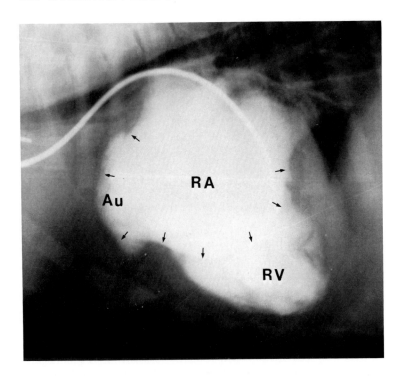

Fig. 18-20 Lateral view of a right ventriculogram in a 3-month-old male Old English sheepdog with tricuspid valve dysplasia. Contrast material is injected into the right ventricle (RV). The right atrium (RA) is opacified due to tricuspid regurgitation. The RV is dilated. The RA and right auricular appendages are profoundly enlarged (arrows). Au, right auricle. (Courtesy of Dr. Philip Fox.)

is another potential therapeutic option. Partial valvulotomy can relieve the obstruction to the point where clinical signs are resolved or significantly reduced. However, the benefits of surgical correction must be considered with the expense and risks of intracardiac surgery and at the risk of surgically creating severe, potentially fatal valvular regurgitation.

Vascular Ring Anomalies

Malposition of the great vessels is a relatively common congenital cardiovascular disorder in dogs, accounting for approximately 7 percent of all cases.[25,44-48] Multiple types of abnormal vascular orientation occur, including a right aortic arch, double aortic arch, right ductus (ligamentum) arteriosus, and aberrant origin of a subclavian artery (see Fig. 1-4). More than 90 percent of vascular ring disorders are due to a right aortic arch and a left ductus (ligamentum) arteriosus.

Vascular rings are frequently associated with a left cranial vena cava and occasionally a patent ductus arteriosus. Breeds with increased risk include German shepherds and Irish setters. A genetic cause is

suspected, although the mode of inheritance is unclear.

NATURAL HISTORY

Most dogs with a vascular ring disorder are symptomatic. Stunted growth and esophageal regurgitation are prominent signs occurring shortly after weaning during the first 6 months of life. Signs of aspiration pneumonia may also occur. Dogs with a double aortic arch may also exhibit signs of tracheal entrapment, such as respiratory stridor, wheezing, coughing, or cyanosis.[46,47] Dogs with vascular slings caused by an aberrant subclavian artery may be asymptomatic.

Clinical signs may be slowly progressive due to generalized debilitation and progression of the esophageal dilation. Untreated symptomatic dogs are usually unthrifty and have a shorter life expectancy.

PATHOPHYSIOLOGY

Abnormal orientation of a great vessel results in a discordant spatial relationship to the heart and other great vessels.[44,47] A constricting ring or sling of cardiovascular structures can result, entrapping the esophagus and occasionally the trachea. Cardiovascular hemodynamics are usually normal with clinical signs related entirely to organ entrapment.

The vascular ring created by a right aortic arch is bounded dorsally and to the right by the aortic arch, to the left by the ligamentum arteriosum and main pulmonary artery, and ventrally by the base of the heart (see Fig. 19-13). A similar ring is formed by a left aortic arch and a right ligamentum arteriosum. The confluence of the right and left sides of a double aortic arch form a ring that is completed centrally by the base of the heart. Both the esophagus and the trachea are entrapped in these cases. Incomplete rings or vascular slings are formed when the right subclavian artery originates from a left aortic arch or when the left subclavian originates from a right aortic arch. In either case, the subclavian artery passes obliquely over the esophagus, forming a partial esophageal obstruction.

Regurgitation is the result of food retention in the dilated portion of the esophagus proximal to the obstruction. The cause of esophageal dilation, however, is not known. Both mechanical effects of food retention and esophageal motility disorders have been suggested. The latter mechanism is supported by the frequent observation of weak peristalsis of the dilated region of the esophagus. A reduction in the number of myenteric nerve cells in the wall of the dilated esophagus has been demonstrated in dogs with a right aortic arch.[47] This could result in altered motility due to abnormal intrinsic esophageal innervation. The occasional occurrence of poststenotic esophageal dilation[48] also suggests the possibility of a generalized esophageal motility disorder. It is not clear whether these motility abnormalities are a primary defect or occur secondary to esophageal obstruction and dilation.

DIAGNOSIS

A presumptive diagnosis of a vascular ring disorder is usually based on the history of frequent regurgitation beginning shortly after weaning. The physical examination findings are often normal, although affected dogs are usually underweight. If distended with food or gas, the dilated cervical esophagus can occasionally be palpated near the tho-

racic inlet. Fever and signs of respiratory disease may be evident if aspiration pneumonia exists.

Thoracic radiographs usually suggest the diagnosis. Ventral displacement of the cranial thoracic trachea and a widened mediastinum are frequently observed on plain films. Displacement of the descending aortic silhouette to the right is occasionally observed. Radiographic signs of aspiration pneumonia may also be evident. An esophagram confirms the diagnosis in most cases by illustrating the esophageal stricture over the base of the heart and esophageal dilation (usually limited to the prestenotic region, although poststenotic dilation is occasionally observed).

TREATMENT

Surgical separation of the constricting vascular ring is usually the preferred treatment. Adjunctive therapy often includes dietary management in the form of frequent, small, liquid, or semiliquid meals fed from an elevated position. The success of therapy, however, can be quite variable. Residual signs such as occasional regurgitation commonly occur.[45]

REFERENCES

1. Patterson DF: Genetic aspects of cardiovascular development in dogs. p. 1. In Van Praagh R (ed): Etiology and Morphogenesis of Congenital Heart Disease. Futura, Mount Kisco, NY, 1980

2. Patterson DF: Two hereditary forms of ventricular outflow obstruction in the dog. p. 43. In Nora JJ (ed): Congenital Heart Disease—Causes and Processes. Futura, Mount Kisco, NY, 1984

3. Thomas WP: Congenital Heart Disease. p. 301. In Kirk RW (ed): Current Veterinary Therapy. Vol. VIII. WB Saunders, Philadelphia, 1983

4. Guntheroth WG: Congenital malformations of the heart. p. 446. In Rushmer RF (ed): Cardiovascular Dynamics. 4th Ed. WB Saunders, Philadelphia, 1976

5. Perloff JK: Formulation of the problem. p. 1. In Perloff JK (ed): The Clinical Recognition of Congenital Heart Disease. 2nd Ed. WB Saunders, Philadelphia, 1978

6. Patterson DF, Pyle RL, Buchanan JW, et al: Hereditary patent ductus arteriosus and its sequela in the dog. Circ Res 29:1, 1971

7. Eyster GE, Eyster JT, Cords GB, Johnston J: Patent

ductus arteriosus in the dog: characteristics of occurrence and results of surgery on one hundred consecutive cases. J Am Vet Med Assoc 168:435, 1976

8. Wolfe DA: Patent ductus arteriosus in dogs: A surgical review and simplified technique. J Am Anim Hosp Assoc 15:323, 1979

9. Buchanan JW, Patterson DF, Pyle RL: Plexiform lesions in young dogs with hereditary patent ductus arteriosus and pulmonary hypertension. Circulation 50(suppl III): 1974 (abst 192)

10. Zook BC: Some spontaneous cardiovascular lesions in dogs and cats. Adv Cardiol 13:148, 1974

11. Legendre AM, Appleford MD, Eyster GE, Dade AW: Secondary polycythemia and seizures due to right-to-left shunting patent ductus arteriosus in a dog. J Am Vet Med Assoc 164:1198, 1974

12. Esterly JA, Glagore S, Ferguson DJ: Morphogenesis of intimal obliterative hyperplasia of small arteries in experimental pulmonary hypertension. Am J Pathol 52:325, 1968

13. Eyster GE, Dalley JB, Chaffee A, et al: Aorticopulmonary septal defect in a dog. J Am Vet Med Assoc 167:1094, 1975

14. Chen HC, Bussiom P: Persistent truncus arteriosus in a dog. Vet Pathol 9:379, 1972

15. Fingland RB, Bonagura JD, Myer CW: Pulmonic stenosis in the dog: 29 cases. J Am Vet Med Assoc 189:218, 1986

16. McCaw D, Aronson E: Congenital cardiac disease in dogs. Mod Vet Pract 65:509, 1984

17. Requarth JA, Goldberg SJ, Vasko SD, Allen HD: In vitro verification of doppler prediction of transvalve pressure gradient and orifice area in stenosis. Am J Cardiol 53:1369, 1984

18. Friedman WF, Roberts WC: Vitamin D and the supravalvular aortic stenosis syndrome. Circulation 34:77, 1966

19. Mark AL, Abboud FM, Schmidt PG, Heistad DD: Reflex vascular responses to left ventricular outflow obstruction and activation of ventricular baroreceptors in dogs. J Clin Invest 52:1147, 1973

20. Mark AL, Kioschos JM, Abboud FM: Abnormal vascular responses to exercise in patients with aortic stenosis. J Clin Invest 52:1138, 1973

21. Zelis RD, Mason DT, Braunwald E: A comparison of the effects of vasodilator stimuli on peripheral resistance vessels in normal subjects and in patients with congestive heart failure. J Clin Invest 47:960, 1968

22. Zelis RD, Mason DT, Braunwald E: Partition of blood flow to the cutaneous and muscular beds of the forearm at rest and during leg exercise in normal subjects and in patients with heart failure. Circ Res 24:799, 1969

23. Eyster GE, DeYoung B: Cardiac disorders. p. 1069. In Slatter D (ed): Textbook of Small Animal Surgery. WB Saunders, Philadelphia, 1985

24. Breznock EM, Whiting V, Pendrays D: Valved apico-aortic conduit for relief of left ventricular hypertension caused by discrete subaortic stenosis in dogs. J Am Vet Med Assoc 182:51, 1983

25. Patterson DF: Canine congenital heart disease: Epidemiology and etiological hypothesis. J Small Anim Pract 12:263, 1971

26. Clark DR, Anderson JG, Paterson C: Imperforate cardiac septal defect in a dog. J Am Vet Med Assoc 156:1020, 1970

27. Mulvihill JJ, Priester WA: Congenital heart disease in dogs: Epidemiologic similarities to man. Teratology 7:73, 1973

28. Breznock EM: Spontaneous closure of ventricular septal defects in the dog. J Am Vet Med Assoc 157:1343, 1970

29. Eyster GE, Whipple RD, Anderson LK, et al: Pulmonary artery banding for ventricular septal defects in dogs and cats. J Am Vet Med Assoc 170:434, 1977

30. Feldman EC, Nimmo-Wilkie JS, Pharr J: Eisenmenger's syndrome in the dog: Case reports. J Am Anim Hosp Assoc 17:477, 1981

31. Turk JR, Miller JB, Sande RD: Plexogenic pulmonary arteriopathy in a dog with ventricular septal defect and pulmonary hypertension. J Am Anim Hosp Assoc 18:608, 1982

32. Okubo S, Nakai M, Tomino T: Relevance of location of defect and pulmonary vascular resistance to the intracardiac pattern of left-to-right shunt flow in dogs with experimental ventricular septal defects. Circulation 73:775, 1986

33. Jeraj K, Ogburn PH: Atrial septal defect (sinus venosus type) in a dog. J Am Vet Med Assoc 177:342, 1980

34. Troy GC, Turnwald GH: Atrial fibrillation and abnormal ventricular conduction presented as right bundle branch block in a dog with an atrial septum primum defect. J Am Anim Hosp Assoc 15:417, 1979

35. Hamlin RL, Smith CR, Smelzer DL: Ostium secundum type interatrial defects in the dog. J Am Vet Med Assoc 143:149, 1963

36. Clark DR, Ross JN, Hamlin RL, Smith CR: Tetralogy of Fallot in the dog. J Am Vet Med Assoc 152:462, 1968

37. Pyle RL: Congenital heart disease. p. 933. In Ettinger SJ (ed): Textbook of Veterinary Internal Medicine. 2nd Ed. WB Saunders, Philadelphia, 1983

38. Eyster GE, Anderson LK, Sawyer DC, et al: Beta-adrenergic blockade for management of tetralogy of

Fallot in a dog. J Am Vet Med Assoc 169:637, 1976

39. Garson A, Gillette P, McNamara D: Propranolol: the preferred palliation for tetralogy of Fallot. Am J Cardiol 47:1098, 1981

40. Liu S, Tilley LP: Malformations of the canine mitral valve complex. J Am Vet Med Assoc 167:465, 1975

41. Liu S, Tilley LP: Dysplasia of the tricuspid valve in the dog and cat. J Am Vet Med Assoc 169:623, 1976

42. Lord PF, Wood A, Liu S, Tilley LP: Left ventricular angiocardiography in congenital mitral valve insufficiency of the dog. J Am Vet Med Assoc 166:1069, 1975

43. Eyster GE, Anderson L, Evans AT: Ebstein's anomaly: A report of 3 cases in the dog. J Am Vet Med Assoc 170:709, 1977

44. van den Ingh T, van der Linde-Sipman JS: Vascular rings in the dog. J Am Vet Med Assoc 164:939, 1974

45. Shires PK, Liu W: Persistent right aortic arch in dogs: a long term follow-up after surgical correction. J Am Anim Hosp Assoc 17:773, 1981

46. Martin DG, Ferguson EW: Double aortic arch in a dog. J Am Vet Med Assoc 183:697, 1983

47. Ellison G: Vascular Ring anomalies in the dog and cat. Comp Cont Educ 2:693, 1980

48. Clifford DH: Effect of persistent aortic arch on the ganglial cells of the canine esophagus. J Am Vet Med Assoc 158:1401, 1971

19

Congenital Feline Heart Disease

Philip R. Fox

INCIDENCE

It is important to identify congenital cardiovascular malformations so that early pharmacologic therapy, surgical correction, or palliation can be instituted, and an accurate prognosis formed. Since cardiomyopathies can affect cats as young as 5 months of age, myocardial disorders represent the principal differential diagnosis for congenital heart diseases. Congenital lesions may be lethal within the first few days or months of life. By contrast, many congenital defects do not impose serious hemodynamic burdens, and affected cats may survive into adulthood or old age.

Feline congenital cardiovascular anomalies have received less attention than their canine counterparts. Reported necropsy incidences include 28 per 1,000 autopsies (2.8 percent) at the Angell Memorial Hospital over a 22-year period[1] and 19 per 1,000 autopsies (1.9 percent) at the Animal Medical Center during a 14-year interval.[2] When this prevalence is combined with that of acquired heart disease (cardiomyopathies), which ranges from 8.5[2] to 15[3–8] percent, congenital cardiovascular disorders represent approximately one-ninth to one-fourth of feline cardiovascular disorders. The relative frequency of the more common feline congenital cardiovascular defects is listed (Table 19-1).

ETIOLOGY

The factors causing feline congenital heart disease are unknown. Familial patterns have been reported for several breeds. Siamese cats have been associated with aortic stenosis (AS),[9] patent ductus arteriosus (PDA),[9] atrioventricular (AV) valve malformation,[10] endocardial fibroelastosis,[1,9,11–13] and persistent atrial standstill with atrial fibrosis.[13,14] Domestic shorthair cats have been associated with ventricular septal defects (VSD) and AV malformations. Genetic transmission has been demonstrated only for endocardial fibroelastosis in the Burmese breed.[15–17] An inherited metabolic disease caused by α-L-iduronidase deficiency (mucopolysaccharidosis I) has been associated with mitral valve thickening and mitral insufficiency in a family of domestic shorthair cats.[18]

A male sex predisposition has been recorded for various cardiac anomalies, including AV valve mal-

Table 19-1 Relative Incidence of the Most Common Feline Congenital Cardiovascular Anomalies

Cardiovascular Anomaly	Percentage of Reported Cases
Atrioventricular valve malformations (mitral valve complex malformation, tricuspid valve complex dysplasia)	17
Ventricular septal defect (VSD)	15
Endocardial fibroelastosis	11
Patent ductus arteriosus (PDA)	11
Vascular anomalies (persistent right aortic arch, venous anomalies)	8
Aortic stenosis (AS)	6
Tetralogy of Fallot (TF)	6
Atrial septal defect (ASD)	4
Common atrioventricular canal	4
Pulmonic stenosis (PS)	3

Data from Refs. 1 and 2.

formation (5:1), aortic stenosis (3:0), endocardial fibroelastosis (9:5), and tricuspid dysplasia (6:1).[1,19] Sex-linked inheritance has not been demonstrated.

CLINICAL FINDINGS

The age at which clinical signs occur depends more on the severity of the lesion and associated hemodynamic impairment than on the specific type of lesion. Seriously affected cats may die during the postnatal period or by 6 to 12 months of age. On the other hand, less severely affected cats, especially those with malformations of the AV valves, may reach adulthood and old age.[1,2,4,19-23] Key diagnostic questions aid in the evaluation of congenital cardiovascular disorders (see Tables 18-1 and 18-2).

The history may include an account of neonatal littermate mortality. Retarded or stunted growth, exercise intolerance, and dyspnea after exertion may be characteristic of severely affected individuals. Vascular ring anomalies may cause regurgitation. Because clinical signs are generally related to congestive heart failure, reported abnormalities may include dyspnea, abdominal distention, and a pounding heartbeat. Coughing is not a feature, even when pulmonary edema is severe. Many cats are asymptomatic, and cardiac anomalies are first detected during routine examination or at the time of initial vaccinations or elective neutering. Although males are more commonly affected, this provides little useful information, since cardiomyopathies have also been reported to show male predominance in some studies. There is no consistent breed predilection.

Physical examination must be thorough and meticulous to capture information critical for diagnosis.[1,4,20-24] Cyanosis should be looked for in the resting and mildly stressed condition and can provide useful information (Table 19-2). Jugular venous distention and pulsation may develop with right-sided heart failure or with lesions affecting the right heart (e.g., tricuspid dysplasia; right-to-left shunting ASD, VSD, PDA; tetralogy of Fallot). Arterial pulse character may be difficult to assess, but in some cats, certain abnormalities may be detectable. A left-to-right shunting PDA causes a widened pulse pressure caused by diastolic runoff of blood from the aorta into the pulmonary artery. A brisk, bounding B-B shot or waterhammer pulse results. Aortic stenosis with a significant gradient may cause a hypokinetic pulse with delayed upstroke, although diminished pulse amplitude may result from congestive heart failure of any cause. Thoracic pre-

Table 19-2 Differential Diagnoses for Cyanosis caused by Congenital Heart Disease

Symmetric cyanosis (cranial and caudal mucous membranes equally affected)
  Respiratory failure (e.g., congestive heart failure)
  Right to left shunt
    Atrial septal defect
    Ventricular septal defect
    Communication at root of great vessels

Differential cyanosis (caudal mucous membrane cyanosis greater than cranial membranes)
  Right-to-left shunting
  Patent ductus arteriosus

Peripheral cyanosis (cyanotic foot pads, nail beds)
  Arterial thromboembolism
  Vegetative embolization
  Shock

cordial palpation may indicate the point of maximal heart murmur intensity, disclose thrills (abnormal vibrations accompanying grade ⅚ or louder murmurs), indicate the relative strength and location of the precordial (apex) beat, and detect arrhythmias. Auscultation provides invaluable information for disease characterization. Most congenital heart diseases produce systolic murmurs. Murmur location (e.g., cardiac base versus apex) and character (e.g., ejection or crescendo-decrescendo versus regurgitant or plateau) are usually of greater diagnostic value than timing (unless the murmur is continuous). Classic auscultatory characteristics of the common cardiac anomalies are listed in Table 19-3. Variations are common, multiple defects may be present, and occasionally, serious heart defects may occur in absence of a murmur. Lung sounds may be silent if pleural effusion is present or may reveal rales due to pulmonary edema. Occasionally, a gallop rhythm may be auscultated.

The ECG is an indispensible part of the data base. It is less reliable in cats than in dogs for indicating cardiac chamber enlargement caused by volume overloads; often the ECG is normal. Arrhythmias are uncommon. Because the most common heart defects (AV valve malformations, VSD) cause the fewest ECG alterations, a normal ECG does not indicate lack of congenital heart disease or offer a better prognosis. Nevertheless, left ventricular enlargement (e.g., R wave in lead II taller than 0.9 mV or wider than 0.04 seconds) may be detected with severe defects (e.g., PDA). By contrast, anomalies causing pressure overloads often result in ECG abnormalities. This is especially true for pulmonic stenosis, tetralogy of Fallot, and right-to-left shunting PDA (i.e., right-axis deviation; deep S waves in leads I, II, III, aVF, CV$_6$LU, CV$_5$LL); and aortic stenosis (tall R waves). Occasionally, right bundle branch block occurs with a large ventricular or atrial septal defect.

Thoracic radiographs complement physical examination and ECG findings. They provide important information regarding the affected cardiac chambers (e.g., atrial or ventricular enlargement) or great vessels (e.g., poststenotic dilatation). These changes result from anatomic and hemodynamic effects of the cardiovascular defect. The extent of cardiac enlargement may indicate stage or severity of the disease. Evaluation of pulmonary vasculature may suggest vascular hypertension, various circulatory patterns, and shunts.[24,25] Radiographic changes are detailed in Chapters 5 and 18.

Nonselective angiocardiography provides invaluable information about cardiovascular structure. This technique is practical for most clinical settings and it helps differentiate many congenital from acquired myocardial diseases. Certain congenital anomalies, such as PDA, PS, tetralogy of Fallot, and

Table 19-3 Characterization of Cardiac Murmurs Associated with Congenital Heart Defects

Anomaly (Congenital Cardiac Defect)	Heart Murmur Characteristics		
	Timing	Location	Quality
Aortic stenosis (AS)	Systolic	L. 3 ICS	Ejection
Pulmonic stenosis (PS)	Systolic	L. 2-3 ICS	Ejection
Tetralogy of Fallot	Systolic	L. 2-3 ICS; R. sternal border (occas.)	Ejection
Ventricular septal defect (VSD)	Systolic	R. sternal border; L. 5-6 ICS	Regurgitant
Atrial septal defect (ASD) (endocardial cushion defect)	Systolic	L. 2-3 ICS; L. 5-6 ICS	Regurgitant/Ejection
Mitral valve complex malformation	Systolic	L. 5-6 ICS	Regurgitant
Tricuspid valve dysplasia	Systolic	R. 4-5 ICS	Regurgitant
Patent ductus arteriosus (PDA)	Continuous	2-3 ICS	Machinery

ICS, intercostal space; L. 2-3 ICS; left cardiac base; 4-6 ICS, cardiac apex.

AS, are easily recognized. Diagnosis of other lesions, such as VSD, AV valve malformations and vascular ring anomalies, may be aided when nonselective angiocardiography is combined with other elements of the data base.[25–27] Cardiac catheterization provides more definitive information but increases morbidity and mortality.

Echocardiography has greatly facilitated recognition and assessment of congenital anomalies. Direct visualization of atrial and ventricular septal defects, subaortic stenosis, and AV valve malformations may be made. The cardiac response to such defects (i.e., cardiac chamber hypertrophy, dilatation, or poststenotic dilatation of great vessels) may be detected. Right-to-left shunts (ASD, VSD, PDA) may be documented using contrast echocardiographic techniques.[28–30] Pulsed and continuous-wave Doppler echocardiography have the potential benefit of identifying regurgitant flows and may be useful in the future to estimate ventricular pressures and pressure gradients.

ABNORMAL PHYSIOLOGY

Congenital cardiovascular defects may influence functional and structural circulatory development. Postnatal morphologic changes usually reflect the response of the heart and vessels to the congenital anomaly. Anatomic and physiologic cardiovascular changes may continue from prenatal through adult life. While some lesions may functionally resolve (e.g., ventricular septal defect), other cardiocircuulatory lesions may impose progressive pressure or volume overloads on affected cardiac chambers.

Some congenital diseases may cause physiologic abnormalities despite normal anatomy. For example, electrophysiologic pathways for ventricular pre-excitation or cardiac conduction system disruptions may be undetectable at birth but manifest later in life.

Fetal and transitional circulations have been discussed (Ch. 1). The detailed accounts of pathophysiologic and hemodynamic consequences of specific congenital anomalies are discussed under congenital canine diseases (Ch. 18).

SPECIFIC CARDIOVASCULAR DEFECTS

Patent Ductus Arteriosus

The clinical incidence of PDA is 0.2 in 1,000[36] to 0.07 in 1,000[2]; it comprised 6.5 to 9.5 percent of autopsy congenital feline heart defects.[1,2] In humans[31] and dogs[32] PDA is an inherited trait, but in cats, only familial tendencies have been reported.[9,33] There may be a slightly higher incidence in the Siamese breed. A female preponderance was found in five of eight unrelated cats,[34–37] but predisposition to females has not been proved. Clinical signs may occur from 1 month to 5 years of age and include either right- or left-sided congestive heart failure, or both. PDA has been recorded in association with other congenital heart defects, including atrial and ventricular septal defects and tricuspid dysplasia.[1,2,37,38]

The classic physical examination finding in a left-to-right shunting PDA is a continuous (machinery) murmur that is loudest over the left cardiac base. It is accentuated during late systole and early diastole. The latter is due to diastolic shunting of blood from aorta to pulmonary artery. Variation in location may occur, and the murmur may be diffusely present over the left precordium. This is especially true if secondary mitral regurgitation or multiple congenital anomalies are present. A palpable precordial thrill is usually present over the point of maximal murmur intensity. Femoral arterial pulses are hyperkinetic (water hammer), associated with the large left ventricular stroke volume and diastolic pressure runoff through the patent ductus.

The ECG usually displays evidence of left ventricular enlargement (R wave in lead II taller than 0.9 mV or wider than 0.04 second) (Fig. 19-1A) Left atrial enlargement may be suggested by P waves in lead II wider than 0.04 second. Occasionally, the ECG is normal.

Radiography and echocardiography demonstrate left atrial and ventricular enlargement due to increased venous blood return to these chambers. In the DV or VD radiographic view, left ventricular enlargement is particularly evident as a long heart; dilatation of the descending aorta and main pulmonary artery due to blood turbulence in the ductus region may also be present (see Fig. 18-2). Non-

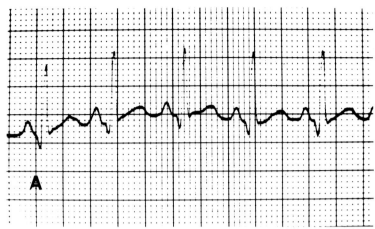

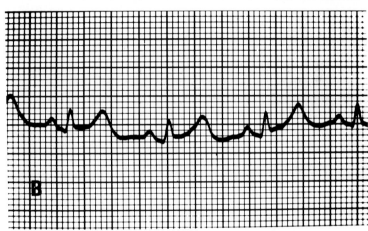

Fig. 19-1 Lead II electrocardiograms from a 4-month-old female domestic short-hair cat. (**A**) Electrocardiogram before surgery for a patent ductus arteriosus. Left ventricular enlargement is suggested by the tall R wave (1.2 mV) and widened QRS complex (0.05 second). (**B**) Six months postoperatively, these changes have resolved. 1 cm-1 mV. Paper speed = 55 mm/sec.

selective angiocardiography displays left atrial and ventricular enlargement and outlines the PDA (Figs. 19-2 and 19-3). Pulmonary overcirculation is evident radiographically. Two-dimensional echocardiography may identify the ductus, but generally this is difficult.

Rarely, pulmonary hypertension occurs, causing right-to-left shunting through the ductus. Clinical signs in these cases include cyanosis (predominantly of the caudal mucous membranes), weakness, syncope, loss of diastolic murmur, maintenance of the systolic murmur, loud or split second heart sound (S$_2$), and dyspnea. The ECG may suggest right ventricular enlargement (right axis shift) and right atrial enlargement (P waves in lead II greater than 0.2 mV). Radiographs show right heart enlargement and tortuous pulmonary arteries. Main pulmonary artery and descending aortic bulges may persist in the DV view. With two-dimensional echocardi-

ography, diagnosis of reverse-shunting PDA can be made by injecting microbubble-laden saline into a peripheral vein and observing microbubbles in the descending aorta or across the ductus. Right ventricular hypertrophy will also be present. Bidirectional shunting has been reported[35] and observed by the author. Catheterization reveals high right ventricular and pulmonary artery pressures.

Surgical correction of left-to-right shunting PDA has been described utilizing left lateral thoracotomy at the fourth,[36] fifth,[35] and sixth[20,34] intercostal spaces. Selection of the optimal surgical site may be facilitated by nonselective angiocardiography to indicate the interspace that provides greatest exposure. Postoperatively, reduction of cardiac size and normalization of the electrocardiogram and pulmonary circulation usually occurs (Fig. 19-1B).

Surgery may be harmful when pulmonary artery pressure exceeds aortic pressure (i.e., right to left

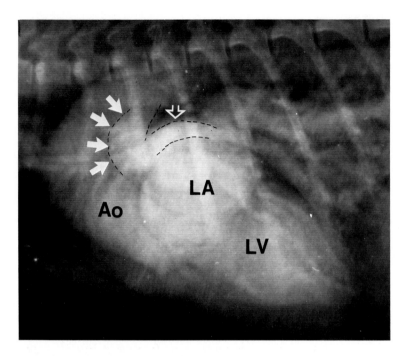

Fig. 19-2 Nonselective preoperative angiocardiogram from the same cat in Figure 19-1. Note dilation of the left atrium (LA) and left ventricle (LV); the lungs are overcirculated due to the extra volume of blood shunted from the aorta to the pulmonary artery. The patent ductus arteriosus is visible (closed arrows) between the descending aorta and pulmonary artery (open arrow). Ao, aorta.

shunts). Ductus ligation may cause right-sided heart failure in these cases by eliminating the right-to-left conduit.

Ventricular Septal Defect

The VSD usually occurs high in the membranous ventricular septum below the aortic valve, covered by the septal tricuspid valve leaflet (i.e., subaortic and infracrystal).[1,2,4,20] Occasionally, VSD may occur elsewhere in the muscular septum. It is often associated with other cardiac anomalies.[1,2,37–40] Examples include a large suboartic VSD as part of tetralogy of Fallot or high membranous VSD and low atrial septal defect creating a common atrioventricular canal (endocardial cushion defect). One-third of isolated VSDs have been associated with tricuspid valve dysplasia.[2]

Typically, the VSD permits left-to-right shunting from the left ventricle to the right ventricular outflow tract. This causes pulmonary overcirculation, increases venous return to the left atrium and ventricle, imposes a volume overload on the left heart, and results in dilatation and hypertrophy. Occasionally, large defects cause equalization of ventricular pressures, right ventricular hypertrophy, and

right-to-left shunting (Eisenmenger's physiology). Bidirectional shunting is fairly common.

Clinical signs are variable. They may occur in kittens during the first few days or weeks of life, become significant by 1 year of age, or cause only a murmur and cardiomegaly through adulthood.[2,4] Characteristically, a loud, harsh, holosystolic murmur is present at the right cranial sternal border (fourth or fifth intercostal space) and often at the left apex (Table 19-3). Mitral and tricuspid valve murmurs occur with endocardial cushion defects. The ECG is usually normal but may display left atrial, biatrial, or left ventricular enlargement. Right bundle branch block may occasionally occur.

Radiographic signs are usually unremarkable with small defects. Large defects may result in left atrial and ventricular enlargement, pulmonary overcirculation, and variable right ventricular enlargement. Nonselective angiocardiography may on occasion allow identification of contrast shunting from the left ventricle to right ventricular outflow tract (Fig. 19-4).

Two-dimensional echocardiography may provide visualization of the VSD and display left atrial and ventricular dilatation. Contrast echocardiographic studies may disclose right-to-left or bidi-

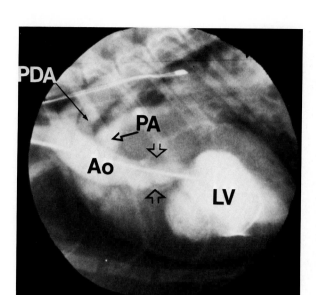

Fig. 19-3 Selective left ventricular catheterization of a young cat. A patent ductus arteriosus (PDA) is visible between the aorta (Ao) and pulmonary artery (PA). A subvalvular aorta stenosis is also visualized between the open arrows. The left ventricle (LV) is severely hypertrophied due to the fixed outflow obstruction caused by the aortic stenosis. (Courtesy of Dr. John D. Bonagura.)

rectional shunting. Doppler echocardiography may identify the shunt and indicate the blood flow pathway.

Catherization may make it possible to identify the lesion and assess the degree of shunting. Noninvasive procedures (i.e., echocardiography), however, are safer.

Therapy is individualized depending on the type of heart failure (left or right sided) and severity. Furosemide is used to control edema or effusions. Digoxin is added if severe right-sided failure occurs. Small VSDs are usually well tolerated. Spontaneous closure has been observed.[1] For hemodynamically significant lesions, pulmonary artery banding may be performed palliatively to increase right ventricular systolic pressure and reduce the degree of left-to-right shunting.[41,42] Open-heart surgical correction has been rarely attempted.[40]

Atrial Septal Defect

An ASD may complicate other anomalies,[37,38] but an isolated ASD is uncommon.[1,2,20] A lesion in the lowermost portion of the interatrial septum is known as a primum atrial septal defect. When located high in the atrial septum, it is termed a secundum defect. An ASD usually permits blood to shunt from the left to right atrium. This imposes a volume overload on the right atrium, right ventricle, and pulmonary arteries. Right-sided heart failure may result.

Clinical signs are variable, and a small ASD may go undetected. A soft systolic ejection murmur representing a relative pulmonic stenosis may be heard in the pulmonic valve region (left base). This may be caused by a large stroke volume ejected across the pulmonic valve. Theoretically, a soft diastolic murmur due to increased blood volume crossing the tricuspid valve, and a split S_2 caused by asynchronous aortic and pulmonic valve closure may occur. If pulmonary hypertension or pulmonic stenosis is present, cyanosis may be observed. A low (primum) ASD may interrupt the conduction system, and the ECG may display right bundle branch block. Often, the ECG is unremarkable. Radiography and echocardiography may identify right atrial and ventricular enlargement caused by volume overloading. With echocardiography, ventricular septal motion may be paradoxic due to right ventricular diastolic overloading. In the short-axis view, diastolic flattening of the interventricular septum results from diastolic right ventricular pressure overload but normal left ventricular circular geometry returns during systole. Right-to-left or bidirectional shunting may be detected using contrast echocardiography or Doppler echocardiography. A low (primum) ASD may be associated with altered mitral valve morphology, creating mitral insufficiency.

Therapy for heart failure includes diuretics and positive inotropes. Pulmonary artery banding may be considered for palliative treatment of large defects to reduce left-to-right shunting.[21]

Persistent Common AV Canal (Endocardial Cushion Defect)

When a low ASD (ostium primum) occurs with a high membranous VSD at the coronary sinus level, a single conduit (common AV canal) between all four heart chambers is formed.[1,2,4,20,39,43,44] It is usually associated with malformation of the AV valves.[20,39,44] Severe volume overload of all chambers may result from left-to-right shunting and AV

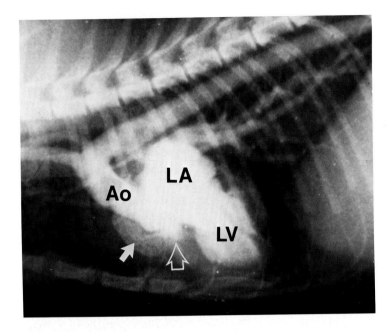

Fig. 19-4 Nonselective angiocardiogram (left ventricular phase) from a 7-month-old female domestic shorthair cat with a high ventricular septal defect. Contrast can be seen shunting from the left ventricle (LV) across the upper ventricular septum (open arrow), appearing in the right ventricular outflow tract, and opacifying the pulmonary artery (solid arrow). The defect was verified by echocardiography. LA, left atrium; Ao, aorta.

valvular insufficiency. If pulmonary hypertension develops from increased pulmonary blood flow, right-to-left shunting and cyanosis results.

Severely affected cats may have murmurs compatible with mitral and tricuspid insufficiency and relative pulmonic stenosis. The ECG may suggest cardiac chamber enlargement patterns or conduction defects, especially right bundle branch block. Radiography and echocardiography may reveal massive generalized cardiomegaly. The defect may be suggested during selective angiocardiography when dye injected into the region of the common AV canal outlines all chambers simultaneously.[20] Alternatively, the defect may be imaged noninvasively using echocardiography (Fig. 19-5).

Affected cats may die postpartum. Others display stunted growth, with death occurring by 6 to 10 months of age.[2,20] Therapy for heart failure employs diuretics and digoxin. Prognosis is usually grave.

Atrioventricular Valve Malformation and Dysplasia

Anomalies of the mitral and tricuspid valves constitute the most common feline congenital heart defect. They are characterized by long, thick, or hypoplastic valve leaflets, which are sometimes adhered to the septum; aberrant, short, fused, or absent chordae tendineae; papillary muscle hypoplasia, hypertrophy, fusion, malplacement (usually upwardly positioned); abnormal insertion between papillary muscles and AV valves; and secondary atrial and ventricular dilation.[2,20,45] Tricuspid dysplasia is often associated with a VSD or mitral valve complex malformation.[2,37,38] Acquired myocardial diseases (cardiomyopathies) often coexist with congenital AV valve complex lesions.

Clinical signs are variable and depend on the severity of the lesions. Most commonly, cats are mildly affected. They may remain compensated for life and have a heart murmur associated with affected valves (i.e., mitral or tricuspid insufficiency). Severe lesions cause volume overload of associated cardiac chambers. Left- or right-sided heart failure, or both, and death may occur as early as 6 months of age. The ECG may display atrial or ventricular enlargement patterns or may be normal. Radiography may show generalized or specific (e.g., left atrial and ventricular) cardiac chamber enlargement.

Echocardiography may display atrial and ventricular dilatation and abnormal valve leaflets and chordal attachments (Figs. 19-6 and 19-7). Accentuated fractional shortening may sometimes be observed. Upward malposition of left ventricular pap-

Fig. 19-5 Two-dimensional echocardiogram from a young cat with an endocardial cushion defect. The anomaly is formed by a low atrial septal defect (ostium primum) and high membranous VSD. This causes a single opening (common atrioventricular canal) between all four heart chambers. LA, left ventricle; LV, left ventricle; RA, right atrium; RV, right ventricle. (Courtesy of Dr. John D. Bonagura.)

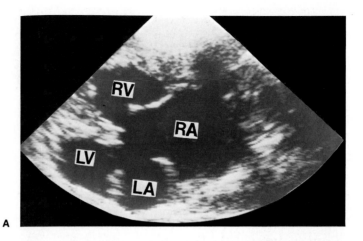

A

Fig. 19-6 Two-dimensional echocardiographic short-axis view at the mitral valve level recorded from the right intercostal position from an adult cat with tricuspid valve dysplasia. An abnormally elongated tricuspid valve (tv) is present within a severely enlarged right ventricle. This finding is compatible with Ebstein's anomaly, a congenital defect of the tricuspid valve. S, interventricular septum; MV, mitral valve.

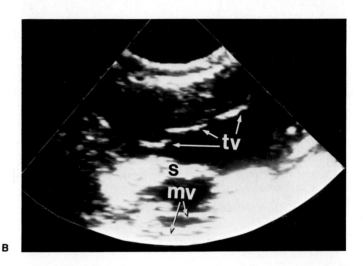

B

Fig. 19-7 Two-dimensional echocardiogram, long-axis view recorded at the right intercostal position from a 12-year-old female domestic short-hair cat with mitral valve malformation. The papillary muscle (P) is upwardly displaced (i.e., toward the mitral valve orifice). It attaches directly to the anterior mitral valve leaflet (between large arrows), which is shortened and malformed. Chordae tendineae at this attachment are short and indistinct. The left atrium (LA) is enlarged secondary to resultant mitral regurgitation. S, interventricular septum; Ao, aorta; LV, left ventricle; RV, right ventricle; W, left ventriculaar posterior wall.

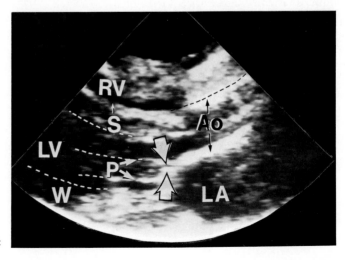

C

illary muscles suggests malformation of the mitral valve complex and can be best visualized in the two-dimensional long-axis view (Fig. 19-7). Abnormal AV valve leaflets, chordae tendineae, and paradoxic ventricular septal motion may be observed.

If congestive heart failure develops, standard therapies are applied. Vasodilators (e.g., captopril, 3.12 to 6.25 mg PO BID to TID), furosemide, and digoxin have been beneficial in some cases of congestive heart failure.

Aortic Stenosis

Fixed obstruction to left ventricular outflow may be supravalvular,[39,46] valvular,[1,2] or subvalvular[39] in location. A fibrous stenotic ring may be present just above (supravalvular) or below (subvalvular) the aortic valve. In the former, the aortic valve is also malformed.[39,46] Wide morphologic variation in stenosis severity is not a feature of AS in cats, as it is in dogs.[44]

Reduction in left ventricular outflow causes elevated pressures and compensatory hypertrophy. Increased blood flow velocity through the stenotic ring causes turbulence. This results in a loud left or right basilar systolic ejection murmur (radiating rightward and cranially), poststenotic dilatation of the ascending aorta and aortic arch, and, potentially, a palpable thrill at the point of maximal murmur intensity. Femoral arterial pulses may be weak (hypokinetic). Exertional syncope may occur.

Clinical findings may be present by 4 to 6 months of age and include stunted growth, exertional syncope, or exercise intolerance. Occasionally, affected cats are asymptomatic, and the murmur is detected during routine examination for vaccination. The ECG may be normal or show left ventricular enlargement (R wave in lead II taller than 0.9 mV), left-axis deviation, left anterior fascicular block, tall T waves or ST segment deviation (compatible with ischemia or hypoxia), or ventricular arrhythmias. Radiography shows severe enlargement of the left ventricle, poststenotic dilation of the ascending aorta, and sometimes left atrial enlargement. Echocardiography may demonstrate left ventricular hypertrophy and poststenotic aortic dilatation. Catheterization may reveal increased left ventricular pressures and systolic pressure gradients across the ventricular outflow tract. Angiocardiography (se-

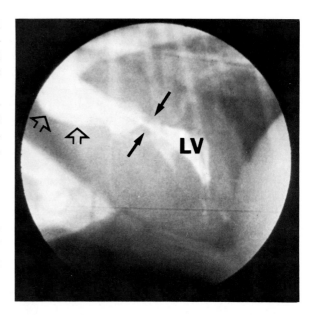

Fig. 19-8 Selective left ventriculogram in a young cat with subaortic stenosis. The stenosis appears as a fibrous ring below the aortic valve (between closed arrows). Poststenotic dilatation of the ascending aorta is evident (open arrows). The left ventricular cavity (LV) is very small due to compensatory concentric left ventricular hypertrophy. (Courtesy of Dr. John D. Bonagura.)

lective or nonselective) illustrates left ventricular hypertrophy, the obstructive aortic lesion, and poststenotic aortic dilatation (Figs. 19-3 and 19-8).

Therapy is unrewarding. Congestive heart failure is treated with furosemide. β-Adrenergic blockers (propranolol, 2.5 to 5 mg BID) may be given to reduce myocardial oxygen demand, resulting from ventricular hypertrophy or for ventricular arrhythmias. Most affected cats develop severe left-sided heart failure or sudden death before 1 year of age. One cat was observed by the author to survive almost 2 years.

Pulmonic Stenosis

Isolated PS is rare.[1,2,39,47,48] More commonly, pulmonic stenosis accompanies other heart defects. It comprises one of the four essential components of tetralogy of Fallot,[1,2,4,20,21,48-56] has been reported with an aorticopulmonary septal defect[57] and tricuspid stenosis with right ventricular hypoplasia.[58]

Stenotic lesions may be supraventricular, valvular, or subvalvular. The rarity of isolated lesions precludes generalizations regarding sites of stenosis. Right ventricular outflow obstruction causes pressure overload on the right ventricle.

Clinical signs include stunted growth, a loud ejection murmur heard best at the left base that may radiate to the right base, a murmur of tricuspid insufficiency, prominent jugular venous pulse, syncope, and right-sided congestive heart failure. The ECG may show a right ventricular enlargement pattern and right-axis deviation in the frontal plane. Thoracic radiographs display marked right ventricular enlargement and prominent main pulmonary artery. Lung fields may be normal or undercirculated. Echocardiography indicates right ventricular hypertrophy. Ventricular septal geometry is abnormal on the short-axis two-dimensional echocardiogram, remaining flat during systole and diastole. This is in contrast to changes described for right ventricular overload (e.g., ASD). The tricuspid valve may be easier to image than normal due to right ventricular enlargement. Catheterization may reveal elevated right ventricular systolic and end-diastolic pressure. Angiocardiography illustrates right ventricular hypertrophy, the stenotic lesion, and poststenotic dilation of the main pulmonary trunk (Fig. 19-9). Tricuspid regurgitation may be present.

Too few cases have been followed to describe a typical natural history. Successful palliative surgery (e.g., valvulotomy, or patch-graft technique) is theoretically possible but has not been reported.

Tetralogy of Fallot

The four principal components of this tetralogy are (1) subaortic (high membranous) VSD, (2) right ventricular outflow obstruction, (3) overriding or dextropositioned aorta, and (4) right ventricular hypertrophy. The most common cause of obstruction to right ventricular outflow in cats is marked hypertrophy of the crista supraventricularis and infundibular portion of the right ventricular free wall.[2,49–53] Elevation of right ventricular pressure causes right-to-left shunting. Unoxygenated blood passes through the VSD into the left ventricle and into the aorta overriding the septal defect. This causes symmetric cyanosis and hypoxemia. Right ventricular hypertrophy occurs secondary to right ventricular pressure overload.

Clinical signs include shunting, weight loss, cyanosis, and episodes of dyspnea or collapse exacerbated by exercise or excitement.[1,2,49–56] Some cats become incapacitated from systemic hypoxia by 5 or 6 months of age. A systolic heart murmur over the pulmonic and often tricuspid valve areas may be accompanied by a thrill at the left basilar region. The hematocrit and packed cell volume are usually elevated and often exceed 70 percent.[50,51,53,54] Congestion of retinal vessels with venous tortuosity and retinal detachment may result from hyperviscosity.[51]

The ECG is variable. Right-axis deviation and right ventricular enlargement patterns are usually present.[20,49,55,56] However, normal[51,54] and leftward[49] mean electric axis orientations in the frontal plane have been recorded.

Radiography displays moderate to severe right ventricular enlargement (Fig. 19-10). Pulmonary arteries appear normal or small due to shunting of blood away from them. Nonselective angiocardiography can demonstrate simultaneous opacification of the aorta and pulmonary artery following injection of dye into the right ventricle (Fig. 19-11). Cardiac catheterization will record elevated right ventricular systolic pressures (115 to 260 mmHg).[49,52]

Echocardiography may reveal right ventricular hypertrophy, VSD, dextropositioned aorta, and small pulmonary arteries. Echocardiographic contrast studies using microbubble-laden saline demonstrate right-to-left shunting across the VSD.

Most reported cats with tetralogy of Fallot have been euthanized due to incapacitating dyspnea, hypoxia, and cyanosis. Congestive heart failure is infrequent. Occasionally, animals survive into adulthood. Cats affected at the ages of $2\frac{1}{2}$ years[54] and 5 years[53] have been reported.

Medical therapy has included oral β-adrenergic blockade with propranolol[20,53] (5 mg BID) and repeated phlebotomies (10 ml/kg/day) in which the withdrawn blood volume is replaced by an electrolyte solution.[51] The action of propranolol may involve depression of myocardial contractility,[59] increased peripheral vascular resistance,[60] and increased tissue oxygen availability by shifting the hemoglobin-oxygen dissociation curve.[61] Beneficial

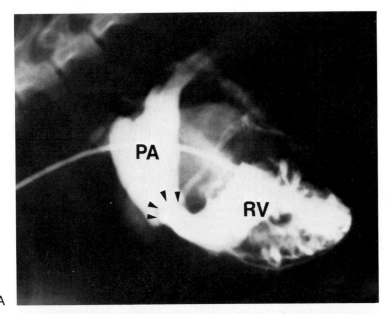

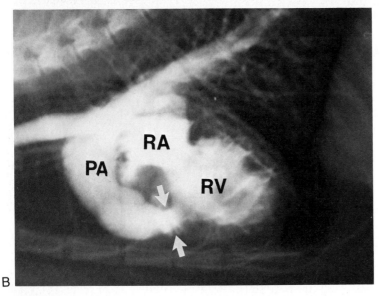

Fig. 19-9 Angiocardiograms of two young cats with pulmonic stenosis (PS). (**A**) Selective right ventriculogram displaying valvular PS. The fibrotic pulmonic valve forms a caplike semilunar crescent (arrowheads). Severe poststenotic dilatation of the pulmonary artery (PA) is noted. (**B**) Nonselective angiocardiogram illustrating subvalvular pulmonic stenosis (arrows) due to hypertrophy of the crista supraventricularis and infundibular portion of the right ventricular free wall. Poststenotic dilatation of the PA is evident. RA, right atrium; RV, right ventricle.

effects have been reported in a dog affected with tetralogy of Fallot.[62]

Surgical palliation may be attempted using procedures to redirect underoxygenated blood from systemic to poorly perfused pulmonary circulation. These techniques include the Blalock-Taussig procedure to anastomose the left subclavian to the right pulmonary artery[63] or Pott's procedure to anastomose the aorta to the right pulmonary artery.[64] Attempts at direct anastomosis of the right auricular appendage and main pulmonary artery to return systemic venous blood directly to the underperfused lungs,[56] and Pott's technique,[50] have been reported. Clinical application of procedures based on the Blalock-Taussig shunt were reported with postoperative follow-up of 44 days[50] and 10 months.[56]

Primary Endocardial Fibroelastosis

Congenital endocardial fibroelastosis has been documented as an inherited anomaly in Burmese cats[16,17,65] and has been observed in the Siamese

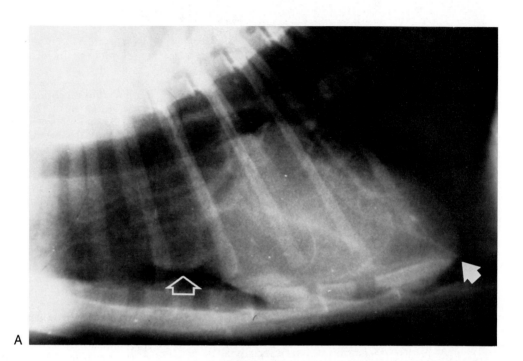

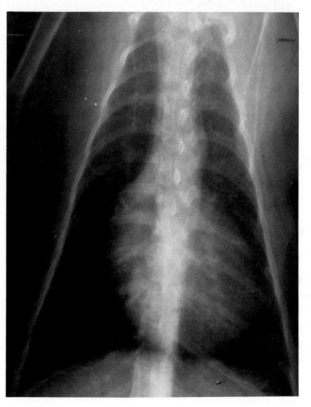

Fig. 19-10 Thoracic radiographs of a 6-month-old female domestic short-hair cat with tetralogy of Fallot and severe right ventricular enlargement. (**A**) In the lateral view, sternal contact is greatly increased causing the cardiac apex to be elevated (closed arrow). Displacement of the ascending aorta causes a protrusion of the aortic arch (open arrow). Right auricular enlargement or poststenotic dilatation of the pulmonary artery can cause the same effect. (**B**) In the dorsoventral view, the right ventricle is rounded and globular. Lung fields in both views are lucent.

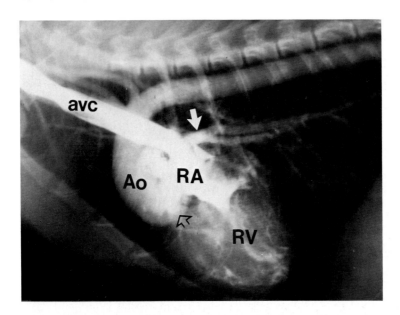

Fig. 19-11 Nonselective angiocardiogram of the same cat described in Figure 19-10. Radiograph was exposed immediately after injection of contrast into the jugular vein. The aorta (Ao) and pulmonary artery (white arrow) opacify simultaneously. This is because blood shunts right-to-left through the high VSD into the dextropositioned (overriding) aorta. Pulmonary artery branches are much smaller than normal due to undercirculation caused by the pulmonic stenosis (open arrow). The right ventricle (RV) is hypertrophied and enlarged. The irregular structure adjacent to the right atrium (RA) and overlying the ascending aorta is the right auricle. avc, anterior vena cava.

breed.[2,9,33] It is characterized by diffuse mural endocardial thickening by collagenous and elastic tissue. Severe cardiac dilatation occurs, especially of the left atrium and ventricle.

Clinical signs can develop between 3 weeks and 6 months of age,[1,2] including dyspnea, cyanosis, and sudden death. Auscultation may reveal gallop rhythms, tachycardia, mitral insufficiency, heart murmurs, or dull heart and lung sounds due to hydrothorax. The ECG may show left ventricular enlargement (tall R waves in lead II), T-wave changes, or conduction disturbances. Radiography shows generalized cardiomegaly, especially left sided. Extracardiac signs of pleural, pericardial, and occasionally abdominal effusion may be present.[1] Endocardial edema and lymphatic dilatation may occur in early stages, suggesting a possible association between lymphatic obstruction and EFE.[65] The disease course is usually short and fatal.

Endocardial fibroelastosis may occur secondary to other acquired or congenital cardiovascular diseases or lesions.[2,66] Gross and microscopic changes often are not specific. Thus, it is often difficult to make a definitive diagnosis of endocardial fibroelastosis and, for all practical purposes, primary and secondary forms are clinically indistinguishable.

Vascular Ring Anomalies

Congenital malformations of the great vessels and associated structures occur infrequently. Persistent right aortic arch is the predominant feline vascular ring anomaly.[67-75] It results when the aorta develops from the right fourth embryonic arch instead of its left counterpart. Because the left ductus arteriosus (forming the ligamentum arteriosum) persists between the main pulmonary artery and anomalous right aorta, the esophagus passing through the ring is constricted. The ring is formed by the aorta on the right, the ligamentum arteriosum and pulmonary trunk on the left and heart base below (Fig. 19-12).

Clinical signs may appear after weaning, when solid diets are introduced. Because of esophageal constriction, regurgitation of undigested food is the primary client complaint. Radiography shows localized esophageal dilation cranial to the heart on lateral survey radiographs. Diagnosis is confirmed with an esophagram (Fig. 19-13) in which a saccular contrast-filled cranial esophagus narrows abruptly at the fourth intercostal space dorsal to the heart.[25] Angiocardiography is indicated if additional cardiovascular anomalies such as PDA or persistent left cranial vena cava are suspected.[75]

Treatment involves surgical separation of the

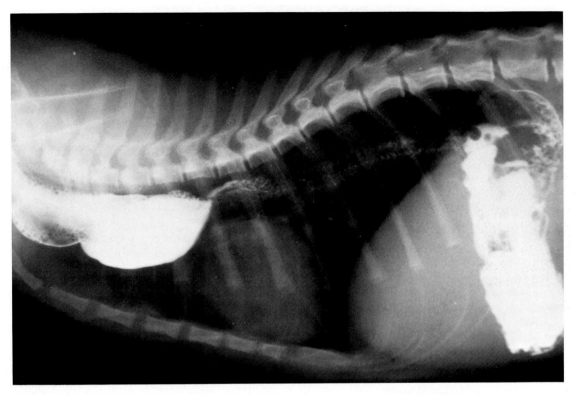

Fig. 19-12 Right lateral esophagram of a 16-week-old male domestic short-hair cat with a persistent right aortic arch. This vascular anomaly causes esophageal constriction cranial to the heart base and precardiac esophageal dilation. The distal esophagus from the heart base to the diaphragmatic hiatus is unaffected.

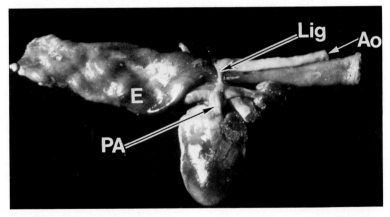

Fig. 19-13 Left lateral view of a persistent right aortic arch and vascular ring anomaly from a kitten. A constricting ring is formed around the esophagus. This results from the ligamentum arteriosum (Lig) (formerly ductus arteriosus) situated dorsally and to the left connecting the main pulmonary artery (PA) (to the left and ventrally) to the descending aorta (Ao) (dorsally and to the right). The latter was derived anomalously from the right fourth aortic arch. The heart base is ventral to the esophagus. Precardiac dilation of the esophagus (E) results. (Courtesy of Dr. John D. Bonagura.)

constricting ring by transecting the ligamentum arteriosum.[71–74] Esophageal dilation usually persists, although in some cases clinical signs are abolished postoperatively.

Other vascular anomalies have been rarely reported in conjunction with esophageal obstruction. These include double aortic arch,[33] retroesophageal right subclavian artery,[1] and a complex anomaly formed by the left aortic arch, right ligamentum arteriosum, and a segment of right dorsal aorta.[76]

Vascular congenital defects that do not cause esophageal obstruction may occur. Reported cases include double outlet right ventricle,[1,2,77,78] transposition of the great arteries,[79] persistent truncus arteriosus,[2] aortic-caudal vena caval fistula,[80] intrahepatic arteriovenous fistula,[81] and venous anomalies. The latter include persistent left vena cava,[53,82] duplication of the caudal vena cava,[1,2] common pulmonary vein stenosis,[1] and portosystemic shunts.[1,83–87]

Excessive Left Ventricular Moderator Bands

A morphologically distinct pattern of abnormal left ventricular moderator band networks and congestive heart failure has been described.[88] There is extreme variation of gross cardiac structural changes (e.g., left ventricular hypertrophy or dilation) and density of moderator band networks (Ch. 23 and 32). Since these aberrant bands have been identified in 1-day-old kittens, they appear to represent a congenital cardiac anomaly. Their association or impact on myocardial diseases, however, is unclear.

Other Anomalies

A number of rare feline congenital cardiovascular defects have been reported. These include tricuspid stenosis and right ventricular hypoplasia, right atrial wall hypoplasia, patent foramen ovale,[2] congenital right ventricular myocardial hypoplasia (Uhl's anomaly),[89] cor triatriatum,[90] partial or complete pericardial agenesis,[91] and persistent atrial standstill with atrial fibrosis.[13,14]

REFERENCES

1. Harpster NK: The cardiovascular system. p. 820. In Holzworth J (ed): Diseases of the cat. Vol. I. WB Saunders, Philadelphia, 1987
2. Liu SK: Pathology of feline heart diseases. Vet Clin North Am 7:323, 1977
3. Bond BR, Fox PR: Advances in feline cardiomyopathy. Vet Clin North Am 4:1021, 1984
4. Fox PR, Tilley LP, Liu SK: The cardiovascular system. p. 249. In Pratt PW (ed): Feline Medicine. American Veterinary Publications, Santa Barbara, CA, 1983
5. Fox PR: Feline myocardial diseases—A clinical approach. p. 57. Proceedings of the Ninth Annual Kal Kan Symposium, Vernon, California, 1986
6. Fox PR: Feline heart disease. p. 65. Scientific Proceedings of the American Animal Hospital Association, 1986
7. Fox PR: Feline cardiomyopathy. p. 157. In Bonagura JD (ed): Contemporary Issues in Small Animal Practice. Vol. 7: Cardiology. Churchill Livingstone, New York, 1987
8. Fox PR: Myocardial disorders. In Ettinger SJ (ed): Textbook of Veterinary Internal Medicine. 3rd Ed. WB Saunders, Philadelphia, 1989
9. Severin GA: Congenital and acquired heart diseases. J Am Vet Med Assoc 151:1733, 1967
10. Wilkinson GT: Dyspnea in the cat. I. Etiology (familial defect of tricuspid valve in Siamese). J Small Anim Pract 8:543, 1967
11. Noden DM: Normal development and congenital birth defects in the cat. p. 1248. In Kirk RW (ed): Current Veterinary Therapy. Vol. IX. WB Saunders, Philadelphia, 1986
12. Zook BC: Some spontaneous cardiovascular lesions in dogs and cats. Adv Cardiol 13:148, 1974
13. Patterson DF: Hereditary defects of the cardiovascular system in the dog and cat. Proceedings of the Fourth Annual American College of Veterinary Internal Medicine Forum. Vol 11. p. 9, 1986
14. Tilley LP, Liu SK: Persistent atrial standstill in the dog and cat. Proc Am Coll Vet Intern Med :43, 1983 (abst)
15. Paasch LH, Zook BC: The pathogenesis of endocardial fibroelastosis in Burmese cats. Lab Invest 42:197, 1980
16. Zook BC, Paasch LH, Chandra RS, et al: The comparative pathology of primary endocardial fibroelastosis in Burmese cats. Virchows Arch Pathol Anat 390:211, 1981
17. Zook BC, Paasch LH: Endocardial fibroelastosis in Burmese cats. Am J Pathol 106:435, 1982

18. Haskins ME, Jezyk PF, Desnick RJ, et al: Alpha-L-iduronidase deficiency in a cat: A model of mucopolysaccharidosis. I. Pediatr Res 13:1294, 1979

19. Liu SK, Tilley LP: Dysplasia of the tricuspid valve in the dog and cat. J Am Vet Med Assoc 169:623, 1976

20. Bolton GR, Liu SK: Congenital heart diseases of the cat. Vet Clin North Am 7:341, 1977

21. Bonagura JD: Congenital heart disease. p. 1. In Bonagura JD (ed.): Cardiology. Contemporary Issues in Small Animal Practice. Vol. 7: Cardiology. Churchill Livingstone, New York, 1987

22. Edwards NJ, Tilley LP: Congenital heart defects. p. 155. In Bojrab MJ (ed): Pathophysiology in Small Animal Surgery. Lea & Febiger, Philadelphia, 1971

23. Fox, PR: Feline congenital heart disease. Proceedings of the Fifth Annual Medical Forum of the American College of Veterinary Internal Medicine, 1987

24. Thomas WP: Congenital heart disease. p. 301. In Kirk RW (ed): Current Veterinary Therapy. Vol. VIII. WB Saunders, Philadelphia, 1983

25. Suter PF: Thoracic Radiography. A Text Atlas of Thoracic Diseases of the Dog and Cat. Peter F. Suter, Wettswil, Switzerland, 1984

26. Owens JM, Twedt DC: Nonselective angiocardiography in the cat. Vet Clin North Am 7:309, 1977

27. Fox PR, Bond BR: Nonselective and selective angiocardiography. Vet Clin North Am 13:259, 1983

28. Pipers FS, Hamlin RL: Clinical use of echocardiography in the domestic cat. J Am Vet Med Assoc 176:57, 1980

29. Bonagura JD: M-mode echocardiography: Basic principles. Vet Clin North Am 13:299, 1983

30. Bonagura JD, Pipers FS: Diagnosis of cardiac lesions by contrast echocardiography. J Am Vet Med Assoc 183:396, 1983

31. Lamy M, de Greuchy J, Schweisguth O: Genetic and nongenetic factors in the etiology of congenital heart disease: Study of 118 cases. Am J Hum Genet 9:17, 1957

32. Patterson DT, Pyle RL, Buchanan JW, et al: Hereditary patent ductus arteriosus and its sequellae in the dog. Circ Res 29:1, 1971

33. Van der Linde-Sipman JS, Van den Ingh TS, Koeman JP: Congenital heart abnormalities in the cat: A description of sixteen cases. Zentralbl Vet A 20:419, 1973

34. Cohen JS, Tilley LP, Liu SK, et al: Patent ductus arteriosus in five cats. J Am Anim Hosp Assoc 11:95, 1975

35. Jeraj KJ, Ogburn P, Lord PF, et al: Patent ductus arteriosus with pulmonary hypertension in a cat. J Am Vet Med Assoc 172:1432, 1978

36. Jones CL, Buchanan JW: Patent ductus arteriosus: Anatomy and surgery in a cat. J Am Vet Med Assoc 179:364, 1981

37. Dear MG: An unusual combination of congenital cardiac anomalies in a cat. J Small Anim Pract 11:37, 1970

38. Perkins RL: Multiple congenital cardiovascular anomalies in a kitten. J Am Vet Med Assoc 160:1430, 1972

39. Liu SK: Pathology of feline heart disease. p. 341. In Kirk RW (ed): Current Veterinary Therapy. Vol. V. WB Saunders, Philadelphia, 1974

40. Weirich WF, Blevins WE: Ventricular septal defect repair. Vet Surg 7:2, 1978

41. Eyster GE, Whipple RD, Anderson LK, et al: Pulmonary artery banding for ventricular septal defect in dogs and cats. J Am Vet Med Assoc 170:434, 1977

42. Mann PGH, Stock JE, Sheridan JP: Pulmonary-artery binding in the cat. A case report (ventricular septal defect). J Small Anim Pract 12:45, 1971

43. Liu SK, Ettinger S: Persistent common atrioventricular canal in two cats. J Am Vet Med Assoc 153:556, 1968

44. Bonagura JD: Congenital heart disease. In Ettinger SJ (ed): Textbook of Veterinary Internal Medicine. 3rd Ed. WB Saunders, Philadelphia, 1989

45. Liu SK, Tilley LP: Dysplasia of the tricuspid valve in the dog and cat. J Am Vet Med Assoc 169:623, 1976

46. Liu SK: Supravalvular aortic stenosis with deformity of the aortic valve in a cat (also endocardial fibrosis). J Am Vet Med Assoc 152:55, 1968

47. Hawe RS: Pulmonic stenosis in a cat. J Am Anim Hosp Assoc 17:777, 1981

48. Tashjian RJ, Das KM, Palich WE, et al: Studies on cardiovascular disease in the cat. Ann NY Aca Sci 127:581, 1965

49. Bolton GR, Ettinger SJ, Liu SK: Tetralogy of Fallot in three cats. J Am Vet Med Assoc 164:1117, 1974

50. Bush M, Pieroni DR, Goodman DG, et al: Tetralogy of Fallot in a cat. J Am Vet Med Assoc 161:1679, 1972

51. Lombard CW, Twitchell MJ: Tetralogy of Fallot, peristent left cranial vena cava and retinal detachment in a cat. J Am Anim Hosp Assoc 14:624, 1978

52. Eyster GE, Weber W, McQuilllan W: Tetralogy of Fallot in a cat. J Am Vet Med Assoc 171:280, 1977

53. Hawe RS, Witter WR, Wilson JB: Tetralogy of Fallot in a five-year old cat. J Anim Hosp Assoc 15:329, 1979

54. Van Heerden, Lourens DC: Tetralogy of Fallot in a two-and-one-half year old cat. J Am Anim Hosp Assoc 17:129, 1981

55. Kirby D, Gillick A: Polycythemia and tetralogy of Fallot in a cat. Can Vet J 15:114, 1974

56. Miller CW, Holmberg DL, Bowden V, et al: Microsurgical management of tetralogy of Fallot in a cat. J Am Vet Med Assoc 186:708, 1985

57. Will JW: Subvalvular pulmonary stenosis and aorticopulmonary septal defect in the cat. J Am Vet Med Assoc 154:913, 1969

58. Lord PF, Liu SK, Carmichael JA: Congenital tricuspid stenosis with right ventricular hypoplasia in the cat. J Am Vet Med Assoc 153:300, 1968

59. Naylor WG, Chipperfield D, Lowe TE: The negative inotropic affect of beta-receptor blocking drugs on human heart muscle. Cardiovasc Res 3:30, 1969

60. Honey M, Chamberlain DA, Howard J: The effect of beta-sympathetic blockade on arterial oxygen saturation in Fallot's tetralogy. Circulation 30:501, 1964

61. Oski FA, Miller LD, Delivoria-Papadopoulos M, et al: Oxygen affinity in red cells: Changes induced in vivo by propranolol. Science 175:1372, 1972

62. Eyster GE, Anderson LK, Sawyer DC, et al: Beta adrenergic blockade for management of tetralogy of Fallot in a dog. J Am Vet Med Assoc 169:637, 1976

63. Blalock A, Taussig HB: The surgical treatment of malformation of the heart in which there is pulmonary stenosis and pulmonary atresia. JAMA 12:189, 1945

64. Pott's WJ, Smith S, Bibson S: Anastomosis of the aorta to a pulmonary artery: Certain types in congenital heart disease. JAMA 132:627, 1946

65. Paasch LH, Zook BC: The pathogenesis of endocardial fibroelastosis in Burmese cats. Lab Invest 42:197, 1980

66. Van Vleet JF, Ferrans VJ: Myocardial diseases of animals. Am J Pathol 124:1, 1986

67. Jessop L: Persistent right aortic arch in the cat causing esophageal stenosis. Vet Rec 72:91, 1960

68. Hathaway JE: Persistent right aortic arch in a cat. J Am Vet Med Assoc 147:255, 1965

69. Evans I, Keahs WH: Persistent right aortic arch in a cat. Vet Med Small Anim Clin 66:1090, 1971

70. Core SH, Dominy WR: Persistent right aortic arch in a cat. Vet Med Small Anim Clin 74:822, 1979

71. Reed JH, Bonasch H: The surgical correction of persistent right aortic arch in a cat. J Am Vet Med Assoc 140:142, 1962

72. Uhrich SJ: Report of a persistent right aortic arch and its surgical correction in a cat. J Small Anim Pract 4:337, 1963

73. Lawther WA: Diagnosis and surgical correction of persistent right aortic arch and eosophageal achalasia in the dog and cat. Aust Vet J 46:326, 1970

74. Ellison GE: Vascular ring anomalies in the dog and cat. Comp Cont Ed 2:693, 1980

75. Wheaton LG, Blevins WE, Weirich WE: Persistent right aortic arch associated with other vascular anomalies in two cats. J Am Vet Med Assoc 184:848, 1984

76. Van der Linde-Sipman JS: Vascular ring caused by a left aortic arch, right ligamentum arteriosum and part of the right dorsal aorta in a cat. Zentralbl Vet A 28:569, 1981

77. Northway RB: Use of an aortic homograft for surgical correction of a double outlet right ventricle in a kitten. Vet Med Small Anim Clin 74:191, 1979

78. Jeraj K, Ogburn PN, Jessen CA, et al: Double outlet right ventricle in a cat. J Am Vet Med Assoc 173:1356, 1978

79. Straw RC, Aronson EF, McCaw DL: Transposition of the great arteries in a cat. J Am Vet Med Assoc 187:634, 1985

80. Bolton GR, Edwards NJ, Hoffer RE: Arteriovenous fistula of the aorta and caudal vena cava causing congestive heart failure in a cat. J Am Anim Hosp Assoc 12:463, 1976

81. Legendre AM, Krahwinkel DJ, Carrig CB, et al: Ascites associated with intrahepatic arteriovenous fistula in a cat. J Am Vet Med Assoc 168:589, 1976

82. Zeiner FN: Two cases of coronary venous drainage by a persistent left superior vena cava in a cat. Anat Rec 129:275, 1957

83. Vulgamott JC, Turnwald GH, King GK, et al: Congenital portocaval anomalies in the cat: Two case reports. J Anim Hosp Assoc 16:915, 1981

84. Rothuizen J, Van de Ingh TS, Voorhout G, et al: Congenital portosystemic shunts in sixteen dogs and cats. J Small Anim Pract 23:67, 1982

85. Birchard SJ: Surgical management of portosystemic shunts in dogs and cat. Comp Cont Ed 6:795, 1984

86. Scavelli TD, Hornbuckle WE, Roth L, et al: Portosystemic shunts in cats: Seven cases (1976–1984). J Am Vet Med Assoc 189:317, 1986

87. Martin RA, Freeman LE: Shunt identification and surgical management of portosystemic shunts. Semin Vet Med Surg 2:302, 1987

88. Liu SK, Fox PR, Tilley LP: Excessive moderator bands in the left ventricle of 21 cats. J Am Vet Med Assoc 180:1215, 1982

89. Atwell RB: Uhl's anomaly in a cat associated with severe right-sided cardiac decompensation. J Small Anim Pract 21:121, 1980

90. Gordon B, Trautvetter E, Patterson DF: Pulmonary congestion associated with cor triatriatum in a cat. J Am Vet Med Assoc 180:75, 1982

91. Walker EL Jr, Zessman JE: A case of an incomplete pericardial cavity in the cat. Anat Rec 113:459, 1952

20

Chronic Valvular Disease in the Dog

Bruce W. Keene

Chronic valvular disease (CVD) is the most common heart disease of dogs, affecting a large percentage of the geriatric canine population and causing disability and death in many of those afflicted. CVD is a degenerative disorder that may infrequently affect cats. However, the disease is of major clinical significance only in the dog. Other causes of valvular disease or insufficiency (e.g., congenital lesions, papillary muscle dysfunction, annular dilation secondary to dilated cardiomyopathy, traumatic valve disruption) are described elsewhere.

Epidemiologic studies have estimated the overall incidence of CVD in the canine population to be from 17 to 40 percent, depending on the diagnostic criteria and methods employed. In one investigation, it was found that 58 percent of dogs aged 9 years and older had pathologic evidence of severe CVD.[1] As this study was based on pathologic findings at necropsy, it is unlikely that all animals with lesions were suffering from the clinical effects (i.e., heart failure) of the disease. Despite this disclaimer, it is clear from both the veterinary literature and clinical practice that CVD is a common disease in dogs, especially if one considers the geriatric population. In general, small breeds are affected much more commonly than large, and males are affected

approximately 1.5 times more frequently than are females. The lesions of CVD occur most often in the atrioventricular (AV) valves, with involvement of the mitral valve alone present in approximately 60 percent of the cases in one series.[2] Involvement of both the mitral and tricuspid valve is seen in approximately one-half as many cases as have mitral disease alone. Isolated tricuspid valve disease is infrequently identified. Chronic acquired degenerative lesions of the aortic and/or pulmonic valves are rarely seen in dogs.

ETIOLOGY AND PATHOLOGY

Although the disease has been recognized clinically for many years and numerous descriptive and correlative pathologic studies have been performed, the etiology of CVD remains unknown. The relatively recent recognition of the mitral valve prolapse syndrome in man has generated renewed interest in CVD in the dog, as the histopathologic descriptions of the valvular lesions are quite similar. In the dog, the valvular lesions of CVD are termed *endocardiosis*. Other terms that have been used for this condition recently (in light of the findings in humans) include

409

mucoid valvular degeneration and *myxomatous transformation of the AV valves.* Grossly, when compared with the normal age-matched mitral valve apparatus, endocardiosis results in shrunken, nodular, distorted AV valves and chordae tendineae (Fig. 20-1). Gross lesions are graded based on the severity of the changes present. Lesions vary from a few small discrete nodules at the commissure of the valve to large coalescing plaquelike deformities that cause shortening, thickening, and rolling of the leaflets, with weakening and nodularity of the chordae. In advanced stages, degeneration of the chordae tendineae may progress to rupture, with catastrophic consequences for the patient. Pathologic changes often develop in the left atrium (e.g., dilation, jet lesions, tears, endocardial fibrosis) secondary to the

volume overload imposed by the incompetent valve.

While the cause of endocardiosis is unknown, some progress has been made in understanding the cellular and molecular changes underlying the characteristic gross valvular lesions. More precise characterization of these changes may shed light on the etiology. This could eventually offer a more effective primary therapeutic approach directed at the valve itself. Currently, pharmacologic management is directed at the hemodynamic consequences resulting from advanced valvular disease.

The histologic basis for endocardiosis is the proliferation of loose tissue in the spongiosa layer of the valve, accompanied by deposition of increased extracellular matrix containing what was formerly

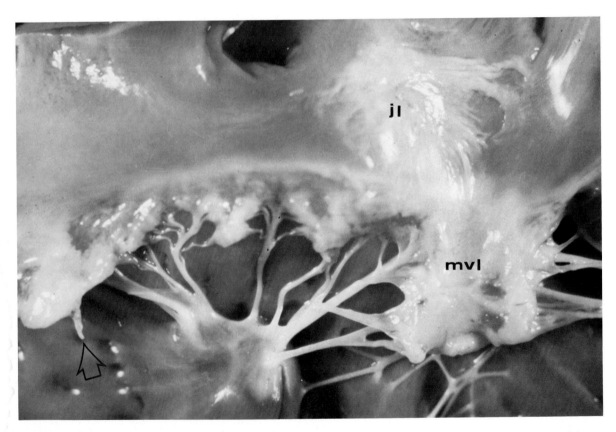

Fig. 20-1 Mitral valve apparatus affected by severe endocardiosis. Note the thickening and nodularity of the mitral valve leaflets (mvl), the jet lesion in the left atrium above the valve (jl), and a ruptured chorda tendinea (arrow). (Photo courtesy of Dr. Richard Dubielzig.)

known as acid mucopolysaccharide.[3] Rapid strides in molecular and cell biology over the past decade have resulted in a better understanding of the structure and some of the functions of the extracellular matrix. Glycosaminoglycans (GAGs), formerly known as mucopolysaccharides, play a major role in determining the composition and physical properties of the extracellular matrix. They are hydrophilic molecules with a high negative charge. GAGs have been divided into seven groups distinguished by their sugar residues as well as by the type of linkage between the sugars and the number and location of sulfate groups. These structural features determine in part the flexibility, stiffness, water content, and other physical properties of the molecules. GAG chains can form hydrated gels and occupy large amounts of space by adopting extended random-coil conformations, which have a very large volume-to-mass ratio.[4] Such a configurational change or deposition of such a material in a valve leaflet could result in the swelling and loose connective tissue changes typical of endocardiosis.

Collagen is the major protein of the extracellular matrix. Collagens are a family of characteristic fibrous proteins that have in common a stiff core of three polypeptide chains intertwined to form a regular helix (the α-chain). At least five distinct types of collagen have been identified based on their molecular formulae, tissue distribution, and distinctive chemical and physical properties.[5] Considering the gross and histopathologic nature of endocardiosis, it is reasonable to speculate that the nodular thickening and proliferation in the spongiosa, combined with the structural weakening of the valve and chordae tissue, are related to defective or degenerative alteration in either the valve collagen or GAG, or both.

In humans, disorders of collagen synthesis, content, or organization (dyscollagenosis) are thought to be the initiating event in the myxomatous changes of mitral valve prolapse.[6] An absence of type III and AB collagens was implicated in one case report.[7] These types of defects have also been reported in human patients with mitral valve prolapse in conjunction with other known connective tissue disorders, such as Ehlers-Danlos syndrome and Marfan's syndrome.[8] This indirect evidence, occurring as it does in a species (humans) in whom

the histopathologic lesions are so similar to those of the dog, supplies fertile ground for speculation. The breed and sex predilection of chronic valvular heart disease could also support a theory of genetic predisposition to the development of a connective tissue disorder. Indeed, the breeds that are primarily afflicted with CVD are often the same ones that are predisposed to intervertebral disc disease, anterior cruciate ligament rupture, and other disorders that could possibly be explained by an extracellular matrix defect. Definitive studies will need to be performed in the dog, however, before real progress can be made.

PATHOPHYSIOLOGY

The basic physiologic abnormality in CVD is mechanical, consisting of improper coaptation of the mitral leaflets during left ventricular systole. The severity of the hemodynamic burden imposed will depend primarily on the size of the regurgitant orifice and the aortic impedance to the ejection of blood. How well the lesion is tolerated by the patient depends on these factors, as well as on the rate at which regurgitation develops, the capacity of the left atrium to dilate (compliance), and the general health of the myocardium and patient.

Chronic mitral regurgitation imposes a volume overload on both the left ventricle and left atrium. The compensatory response of the heart includes dilation of those chambers to accommodate the increased volume accompanied by myocardial hypertrophy, in an attempt to maintain ventricular function and normalize wall stress. This response is known as eccentric hypertrophy.[9] In chronic mitral regurgitation, the compliance (change in volume for a given change in pressure) of the left heart chambers also increases, allowing them to accommodate a larger volume of blood for any given level of end-diastolic pressure.[10] These compensatory mechanisms serve to maintain forward stroke volume in the face of even large regurgitant volumes and also protect the patient from developing signs of congestive heart failure by allowing large volumes of blood to enter the left atrium at relatively low pressures. In many cases of endocardiosis, patients with the typical murmur may remain compensated and asymptomatic for years.

These compensatory mechanisms do have limits, however, and eventually either forward output falls or left atrial pressure rises (or both) in response to a progressive hemodynamic burden. Signs of heart failure ensue. In some cases, the left atrium may enlarge to such a degree that the left mainstem bronchus is compressed, resulting in clinical signs (e.g., cough), even before the onset of markedly elevated left atrial pressure and subsequent pulmonary edema. Often, there is a gradual progression of clinical signs, beginning with mild exertional dyspnea or cough, and ending with intractable biventricular heart failure.

Three major physiologic complications may interrupt the normally slow progression of chronic mitral regurgitation and hasten the demise of the patient. First, cardiac arrhythmias may arise in the dilated and overworked atrium or ventricle. Supraventricular tachyarrhythmias (e.g., atrial premature complexes, paroxysmal atrial tachycardia, atrial fibrillation) may reduce the time available for ventricular filling, increase myocardial oxygen demand, abolish effective atrial contraction (and thus precipitate elevation of left atrial pressure) and exacerbate pulmonary edema. Ventricular arrhythmias, while not as common, may also compromise cardiac output and put the patient at risk for sudden death due to ventricular fibrillation. Second, a markedly dilated and hypertrophied left atrium may eventually reach its elastic limit and tear, resulting in cardiac tamponade and cardiovascular collapse. Third, major chordae tendineae may succumb to disease and/or hemodynamic stress and rupture, abruptly increasing the regurgitant volume, raising left atrial pressure, and precipitating or worsening pulmonary edema.

The development of actual myocardial failure as a result of chronic volume overload is difficult to document. The most sensitive parameter of muscle function, contractility (an intrinsic property of the muscle defined as the speed of fiber shortening at zero load), is impossible to measure directly in the intact animal. Furthermore, most of the clinically useful noninvasive ejection phase indicies of contractility are rendered inaccurate by the low-pressure popoff valve created by mitral regurgitation. Although still controversial, recent evidence obtained using an echocardiographic end-systolic volume index in dogs with congestive heart failure secondary to chronic valvular heart disease suggests that most canine patients have normal or only mildly depressed myocardial function.[11] This finding conflicts with indirect conclusions drawn from earlier pathologic studies, which showed that focal areas of myocardial necrosis, fibrosis, and intramural coronary arteriosclerosis and infarction were common in animals with clinical signs of chronic valvular heart disease.[12] The investigators assumed based on this pathological evidence that the myocardial lesions were an important contributing factor in the pathogenesis of heart failure in these dogs. Because of the previously mentioned problems in estimating myocardial function in dogs with mitral regurgitation and the serious questions involved in extrapolating pathologic data into physiologic findings, this controversy is not likely to be settled in the very near future. Correlative pathophysiologic studies, possibly incorporating endomyocardial biopsy (currently being used to answer this question in humans) may be necessary to answer whether myocardial failure plays a significant role in the pathogenesis of CVD. It is hoped that validation of a physiologic technique to quantitate myocardial function in dogs with mitral regurgitation will be forthcoming as well. Only then can the corollary question, Is positive inotropic support indicated in the management of CVD?, be satisfactorily addressed.

It is important to remember that although tricuspid regurgitation is not as common as mitral valve disease, this lesion coexists with mitral insufficiency in a significant number of animals. Tricuspid regurgitation may result in right-sided heart failure with attendant jugular venous pulsations (large v waves), ascites, and pleural effusion. Even in the absence of significant tricuspid regurgitation, right ventricular failure may develop as a result of chronic stress on the right ventricle caused by the increased work of filling the left side of the heart.

CLINICAL DIAGNOSIS AND ASSESSMENT

The diagnosis of CVD is often first made on routine physical examination conducted for an unrelated complaint in absence of clinical signs of disease. Early in the evolution of chronic mitral or tricuspid regurgitation, the compensatory mechanisms discussed above protect the patient from clinical manifestations of the disease. Subclinical disease (New York Heart Association class I) may be present for many years without causing any sign of heart failure. Cardiac auscultation is thus the key to early diagnosis of mitral or tricuspid insufficiency.

Dogs with symptomatic CVD are generally presented because of complaints related to dyspnea, tiring, restlessness, cough, syncope, or ascites. All these complaints in the symptomatic CVD patient are usually accompanied by weight loss. The signalment (e.g., middle-aged to older small-breed male) may also raise the clinician's index of suspicion for CVD. It is important to remember, however, that small coughing dogs—even those with typical murmurs of CVD—may be coughing due to causes unrelated to valvular insufficiency or heart failure. The cough reflex is elicited mainly via irritant receptors, which are much more plentiful in large airways (e.g., stimulated by bronchitis, tracheal collapse) than in alveoli or bronchioles. Even life-threatening pulmonary edema usually results in dyspnea and tachypnea without severe coughing until late in its progression. The differential diagnostic challenge of CVD is frequently not whether the disease is present, but whether or not the CVD is responsible for the patient's clinical signs (Table 20-1). This question can only be answered reliably in most cases after completion of the physical examination and evaluation of thoracic radiographs, electrocardiogram (ECG), and clinical laboratory tests.

Auscultation

The classic murmur of mitral insufficiency is holosystolic or plateau shaped and heard best at the left fifth intercostal space (the cardiac apex). There it is transmitted through the solid structures of the heart to the chest wall. Because the regurgitant jet may radiate dorsally, cranially, or even caudally, the murmur may also be heard well (sometimes even louder) toward the left base. Mild regurgitation may cause a more decrescendo murmur of shorter duration. Therefore, any systolic murmur or mid-systolic click in a middle-aged or older dog should raise the suspicion of CVD. It is important to emphasize

Table 20-1 Diagnostic Implications of Common Historical and Physical Findings[a]

Finding	Diagnostic Implications
Obesity	With few exceptions, respiratory disease: Heart failure usually causes dramatic weight loss and is therefore seen rarely in obese canine patients.
Pronounced sinus arrhythmia	Primary respiratory disease: Pronounced sinus arrhythmia is usually lost due to high sympathetic tone in heart failure.
"Honking" cough without dyspnea or exercise intolerance	Respiratory disease: Pulmonary edema may cause coughing, but honking cough with preservation of exercise ability is usually due to large airway compression/irritation (e.g., collapsed trachea).
Small breed male	Heart disease: Males are more often affected by a ratio of about 1.5:1 (a weak criterion for differentiation).
Loud cardiac murmur	No consistent correlation exists between murmur intensity (loudness) and hemodynamic severity of valvular regurgitation.
Crackles (e.g., rales)	Nonspecific finding occurring in pulmonary edema, bronchitis, pneumonia, and pulmonary fibrosis. Chest radiographs are necessary to differentiate the cause of crackles accurately.

[a] Differentiation of cough due to pulmonary edema caused by chronic mitral insufficiency from primary respiratory diseases.

that the intensity (loudness) of the murmur of mitral or tricuspid regurgitation does not correlate with its hemodynamic significance.[13] While the auscultatory features may range from a soft, squishing holosystolic murmur to a loud, musical whoop heard without the aid of a stethoscope, the clinician must rely on the supporting clinical and radiographic data base to determine the hemodynamic significance of the insufficiency.

Documentation of tricuspid insufficiency may be difficult, since it usually coexists with mitral insufficiency, and the murmur of mitral insufficiency frequently radiates to the tricuspid area. A precordial thrill on the right hemithorax, abnormal jugular venous pulsations (*v* waves), and marked differences in the pitch or character of the murmurs on the left and right sides of the chest are all signs that support the diagnosis of tricuspid insufficiency. Presence of a third or fourth heart sound (gallop rhythm) may signal abnormal ventricular stiffness and impending failure, and should prompt a thorough investigation even in a previously asymptomatic patient. Likewise, the discovery of an arrhythmia (e.g., premature or dropped beats) during auscultation should prompt completion of a cardiac data base, including an ECG.

Auscultation of the lungs is also an essential part of assessing the patient with CVD. In the asymptomatic animal with a typical murmur of mitral valvular insufficiency, the lung sounds are expected to be normal. The presence of crackles (rales) should be investigated radiographically in all patients, remembering that they are a nonspecific finding that may attend pulmonary fibrosis, pneumonia, bronchitis, or edema.[14]

Radiography

Although the diagnosis of CVD is generally made during cardiac auscultation, high-quality, inspiratory, lateral, and dorsoventral (or ventrodorsal) chest radiographs are an important adjunct for assessing the hemodynamic consequences of CVD and associated clinical signs (Chap 5). Radiographic findings in CVD vary widely, depending on the duration and severity of valvular insufficiency. In symptomatic patients, significant dilation of the left atrium and ventricle is typically evident (see Figs. 5-3 through 5-5). The rare exception occurs with severe acute mitral regurgitation, as accompanies rupture of a primary chordae tendineae before extensive valvular endocardiosis has developed. In this instance, the compliance of the left atrium and ventricle has not been given the opportunity to increase gradually in adaptation to a slowly imposed volume load. Thus, cardiomegaly may be minimal in the face of florid regurgitation and severe radiographic

evidence of left heart failure (e.g., pulmonary edema).

The extent and severity of extracardiac signs of heart failure are often variable. Pulmonary venous congestion and edema are often present in symptomatic CVD patients and are the radiographic correlates of left heart failure. Occasionally, the left atrium will be unusually compliant, and massive left atrial enlargement may exist without evidence of pulmonary edema. On radiographs, the expanding left atrium can often be seen to compress the left mainstem bronchus, identifying a major cause of cough in CVD patients. Other common radiographic findings are right heart enlargement, the result of tricuspid insufficiency, pulmonary venous hypertension, or concurrent chronic pulmonary disease associated with cor pulmonale. Pleural effusion, ascites, hepatomegaly, and distention of the caudal vena cava are all potential changes associated with right ventricular failure in CVD patients.

Electrocardiography

Electrocardiography is a useful and necessary tool in the assessment and management of CVD. However, there are no pathognomonic ECG signs of either the disease or the syndrome of heart failure resulting from the disease. Left atrial enlargement usually results in widening (>0.04 sec in small breeds) and notching of the P waves (P-mitrale). Left ventricular enlargement frequently causes augmentation of the R-wave voltage in lead II or aVF (>2.5 mV in small breeds). Widening of the QRS complex beyond 0.065 sec accompanied by notching of the R-wave descent may be associated with myocardial disease. If the patient is examined early in the course of the disease and at regular intervals thereafter, the gradual evolution of these signs may be informative.

Most symptomatic patients at presentation will exhibit sinus tachycardia or normal sinus rhythm, reflecting increased sympathetic tone associated with heart failure. Therefore, documentation of marked sinus arrhythmia in a coughing patient suspected of having heart failure secondary to CVD should prompt reconsideration of the cause of the patient's signs. Occasionally, patients with concurrent heart failure and severe primary pulmonary disease (e.g., chronic bronchitis, obstructive lung disease, tracheal collapse) will maintain excessive vagal tone and sinus arrhythmia, but this situation is relatively rare. Supraventricular premature complexes are commonly seen in advanced cases, probably representing a manifestation of atrial stress and distention. Serious supraventricular rhythm disturbances (those that are hemodynamically significant), such as paroxysmal supraventricular tachycardia, atrial tachycardia, atrial flutter, and atrial fibrillation, may pose a significant problem in managing CVD in some patients. Ventricular dilation, hypoxia, and stress predispose these patients to ventricular premature complexes as well, and a few patients may require specific antiarrhythmic therapy for symptomatic ventricular tachyarrhythmias.

Echocardiography

Ultrasonic examination of the heart (echocardiography) has been of limited usefulness in the management of CVD. Although the valvular lesions of advanced CVD are often identifiable as smooth thickenings of the mitral leaflets, and the exact extent of left atrial and ventricular enlargement can be documented (see Figs. 6-37 through 6-39), neither the one-dimensional (ice-pick) view of the M-mode nor even the two-dimensional echocardiogram permits reliable assessment of mitral or tricuspid valve coaptation. Because the diagnosis of CVD is generally based on the presence of a murmur of mitral insufficiency in conjunction with the history, clinical presentation, and radiographic findings, echocardiography is rarely needed. One major exception to this occurs in breeds such as the cocker spaniel, which are commonly subject to both CVD and dilated cardiomyopathy. Dilated cardiomyopathy with associated mitral regurgitation resulting from papillary muscle dysfunction, annular dilation, or ventricular dyssynergy can be difficult to differentiate from primary CVD in these patients. Echocardiographic examination usually permits a definitive diagnosis to be made based on ventricular function indices (e.g., normal or hyperdynamic wall motion in most cases of CVD versus severely hypodynamic in dilated cardiomyopathy). Separation of these patients is of significant practical importance since both prognosis and therapy generally differ greatly between the two diseases.

While echocardiography has proved useful in sep-arating patients with primary mitral regurgitation from those with primary dilated cardiomyopathy, it is less sensitive in identifying more subtle differences in ventricular function in the presence of valvular insufficiency.[15] The reason is that the accuracy of most echocardiographic derived indices of ventricular function depends (in part) on the conditions under which ventricular ejection takes place. In the presence of mitral regurgitation, the ventricle also ejects blood backwards into the relatively low-pressure left atrium. This requires less work for the amount of myocardial fiber shortening accomplished. In the presence of significant mitral insufficiency, the ventricle will appear hyperdynamic if it is healthy, since it is contracting against a reduced load. For the same reason, it may appear to contract normally even if serious myocardial disease is present.[16] Without knowing the exact extent of the regurgitation, it becomes impossible using conventional echocardiographic imaging, to know to what extent the echo-derived indices of ventricular function are being affected by CVD.

To address this problem, a human classification system was devised for surgical mitral valve replacement. It is based on the echocardiographically calculated end-systolic volume index to preoperatively differentiate human patients with normal myocardial function (and thus, a good postoperative prognosis) from those with mild, moderate, or severe myocardial dysfunction.[17] This has been applied to dogs with CVD in an attempt to better quantitate the extent of myocardial dysfunction in these patients.[18] While there are potential limitations in techniques that extrapolate measurements across species, this study represents the best functional data currently available in veterinary medicine. On the basis of these data, it has been suggested that myocardial failure is not a major contributor to heart failure in most dogs with CVD.[18] Once validated in the dog, the end-systolic volume index, or some related echocardiographic parameter will certainly find a place in the assessment, staging, and therapeutic management of CVD.

THERAPY

Ideally, therapy of CVD would be directed at improving the function of the defective valve, either through surgical repair or replacement. Surgical management is not economically and technically practical in veterinary medicine. The management of CVD is therefore concerned with ameliorating the clinical signs of heart failure, keeping the pet as comfortable and fit as possible until the disease progresses to the point where optimal pharmacologic manipulation of preload, afterload, heart rate, rhythm, and contractility no longer result in adequate hemodynamic compensation. Considering the pathophysiology of CVD in dogs, this therapy must be directed primarily toward (1) reducing the venous pressures to alleviate edema and effusions; (2) maintaining adequate cardiac output to prevent signs of weakness, lethargy, and azotemia; and (3) reducing the cardiac workload and regurgitant fraction, if possible, to forestall problems associated with severe chamber enlargement and increased myocardial oxygen demand. Complications resulting from therapy (e.g., arrhythmias, drug intoxications) must also be managed.[19,20]

Therapy for CVD is instituted in stages, based on the nature and severity of the patient's clinical signs. Cage rest and a stress-free environment are important to reduce the cardiac workload.

In general, preload reduction may be accomplished by drugs or interventions that reduce blood volume or increase venous capacitance. Sodium restricted diets, diuretics, and venodilators are all effective in controlling the clinical signs of CVD related to elevations in venous pressures. Deciding which of these interventions to use in a particular patient at a given time involves consideration of a variety of factors. These include the severity of clinical signs, expected level of owner compliance, and personal experience with these agents.

As a rule, mild to moderate salt restriction can be accomplished with minimal difficulty in most canine patients (Ch. 10). Dogs with heart failure have a reduced capacity to excrete sodium loads, resulting in an increased blood volume. Restriction of salt (but not water) intake by eliminating salty treats, gradual dietary salt reduction by mixing a commercial low-sodium diet with the normal ration, or preparation of a homemade salt-restricted diet can help minimize renal fluid retention. Strict salt restriction (e.g., limiting total sodium intake to 12 mg/kg/day) is much more difficult to accomplish and may be unnecessary if diuretics are used.

Diuretics (e.g., furosemide) are generally well tolerated and quite effective when dietary salt restriction either fails to control signs of venous congestion or is impractical. If they are used overzealously, however, dehydration, reduced cardiac output, hypokalemia, and azotemia are potential complications.

Venodilators (e.g., nitroglycerin) and drugs that have both arterial and venous dilating properties (e.g., prazosin, captopril) may be effective in controlling signs of venous congestion. They need to be used with appropriate caution and knowledge of potential side effects (e.g., hypotension, tachycardia, decreased cardiac output). Pending more definitive clinical and pharmacodynamic information in the dog, venodilating drugs are generally used after the patient has become refractory to conventional doses of diuretics or instead of diuretics for the occasional patient that cannot tolerate diuretic therapy. Morphine may reduce anxiety in severely dyspneic (class IV) CVD patients, and is also useful as an emergency venodilator.

Cardiac output can be difficult to maintain and evaluate in the symptomatic CVD patient. All therapy to reduce venous congestion has the potential to reduce cardiac output, necessitating a relatively cautious, monitored therapeutic approach. Cardiac output can be assessed via pulmonary artery catheterization and direct measurement by an indicator dilution technique. While this is feasible in some institutional settings, it is expensive and invasive and uses technology that is not generally available in most private practices. Clinical indicators of cardiac output (e.g., muscle strength, activity level, serum creatinine concentration, capillary refill time, and venous PO_2) are more widely available. They must be used conscientiously and in combination to assess patient response to therapy or the need for additional treatment.

Drugs with arterial vasodilating properties may improve cardiac output in CVD, while reducing regurgitant fraction and myocardial workload. These drugs include hydralazine, a direct-acting arterial dilator, as well as nitroprusside, prazosin, and captopril, which dilate both arteries and veins through a variety of mechanisms (Ch. 8). Hydralazine has been shown to be of clinical and hemodynamic benefit in patients with CVD.[21,22] In general, it is recommended that the dosage of hydralazine be titrated in the hospital in order to find an appropriate dose (i.e., one that provides improvement of cardiac output and reduction of regurgitant fraction without excessive hypotension and tachycardia). Titration is most accurately performed by monitoring the arterial blood pressure and/or venous PO_2. However, hydralazine is still useful in the absence of these technical capabilities by using parameters of clinical response (e.g., resolution of cough, pulmonary edema, and increased activity level) as the endpoint of titration. Dosage adjustment over a few days may be required in this fashion. Captopril and prazosin also seem to be clinically useful in managing CVD in some patients. Controlled clinical studies are now under way to evaluate further the hemodynamic effects of several vasodilators in the dog.

Controlling serious tachyarrhythmias will improve cardiac output and reduce cardiac workload and possibly the amount of mitral or tricuspid regurgitation. Since cardiac muscle failure does not appear to be a significant contributor to most cases of heart failure caused by CVD, the use of positive inotropes (e.g., digitalis, dobutamine, dopamine) is not indicated unless there is evidence of myocardial failure. Digitalis is reserved for treating patients with persistent supraventricular tachyarrhythmias, right ventricular failure, or advanced heart failure refractory to diuretics and vasodilators. The use of digitalis and other positive inotropes in heart failure secondary to CVD is still a controversial topic. The views expressed here are based on the currently available veterinary literature and on my own clinical experience and should not be construed as dogma.

Therapy for CVD must be individually tailored for the patient, owner, and practitioner. In asymptomatic stages of the disease (class I), client education, reassurance, and support are all that are necessary. Digitalis, diuretics, or even rigid salt restriction are not indicated or justifiable at this stage. In symptomatic patients (class III or IV), every effort should be made to define the source of clinical signs accurately (e.g., radiographic evidence of pulmonary edema versus lack of edema but cough due to left atrial compression of the left mainstem bronchus). Treatment should then be based on these findings. For example, the patient with bronchial compression requires agents to reduce atrial size (such as hydralazine) to decrease regurgitant fraction, and furosemide to reduce blood volume. Ther-

apy can be adjusted over several days. In contrast, the patient with severe pulmonary edema and dyspnea at rest (class IV) presents as a medical emergency. Acquisition of parts of the data base (e.g., radiography) may need to be temporarily postponed in these critical patients. Morphine, furosemide, cage rest, 40 percent oxygen supplementation, and a bronchodilator may be lifesaving when the primary problem is pulmonary edema resulting from elevated capillary hydrostatic pressure (Ch. 9). Arterial vasodilation, thoracocentesis, or antiarrhythmic therapy may also be indicated based on information obtained from the data base.

Provided significant drug interactions are avoided, and the owner is willing and able to comply with the treatment regimen, CVD patients are often better managed with a combination of moderately dosed drugs that affect more than one hemodynamic parameter than with maximal (and potentially toxic) doses of any single agent. The clinician must remember, however, that overly complex, poorly explained, or inadequately labeled medications are a major cause of client noncompliance and subsequent therapeutic failure. It is critical that the client understand at the outset that therapy for heart failure is individualized and that drugs and dosages may need to be changed based on the pet's response. Clients must clearly understand that these adjustments do not necessarily signal therapeutic failure. However, they must be gently made to realize that failure is indeed inevitable. Detailed information regarding drug dosages and preparations used in the management of heart failure, pulmonary edema, and arrhythmias can be found in chapters 8, 9, 14, 15.

REFERENCES

1. Whitney, JC: Observations on the effect of age on the severity of heart valve lesions in the dog. J Small Anim Pract 15:511, 1974
2. Buchanan, JW: Chronic valvular disease (endocardiosis) in dogs. Adv Vet Sci Comp Med 21:75, 1977
3. Whitney, JC: Cardiovascular pathology. J Small Anim Pract 8:459, 1967
4. Chakrabarti B, Park JW: Glycosaminoglycans: Structure and interaction. CRC Crit Rev Biochem 8:225, 1980

5. Hay ED: Extracellular matrix. J Cell Biol 91:205s, 1981

6. King BD, Clark MA, Baba N, et al: "Myxomatous" mitral valves: Collagen dissolution as the primary defect. Circulation 66:288, 1982

7. Hammer D, Leir CV, Baba N, et al: Altered collagen composition in a prolapsing mitral valve with ruptured chordae tendineae. Am J Med 67:863, 1979

8. Brandt KD, Summer RD, Ryan TJ, et al: Herniation of mitral leaflets in the Ehlers-Danlos syndrome. Am J Cardiol 36:524, 1975

9. Brown OR, DeMots H, Kloster FE, et al: Aortic root dilatation and mitral valve prolapse in the Marfan's syndrome. Circulation 52:651, 1975

10. Braunwald E: Valvular heart disease. p. 1023. In Braunwald E (ed): Heart Disease. A Textbook of Cardiovascular Medicine. WB Saunders, Philadelphia, 1988

11. Kittleson MD, Eyster GE, Knowlen GG, et al: Myocardial function in small dogs with chronic mitral regurgitation and severe congestive heart failure. J Am Vet Med Assoc 4:455, 1984

12. Detweiler DK, Patterson DF: The prevalence and types of cardiovascular disease in dogs. Ann NY Acad Sci 127:481, 1965

13. Shillingford JP: The estimation of severity of mitral incompetence. Prog Cardiovasc Dis 5:252, 1962

14. Forgacs P: The functional basis of pulmonary sounds. Chest 73:339, 1978

15. McDonald IG: Echocardiographic assessment of left ventricular function in mitral valve disease. Circulation 59:1218, 1979

16. Urschel CW, Covell JW, Sonnenblick EH et al: Myocardial mechanics in aortic and mitral valvular regurgitation: The concept of instantaneous impedance as a determinant of the performance of the intact heart. J Clin Invest 47:867, 1968

17. Borow KM, Green LH, Mann T, et al: End-systolic volume as a predictor of postoperative left ventricular performance in volume overload from valvular regurgitation. Am J Med 68:655, 1980

18. Kittleson MD, Eyster GE, Knowlen GG, et al: Myocardial function in small dogs with chronic mitral regurgitation and severe congestive heart failure. J Am Vet Med Assoc 184:455, 1984

19. Bonagura JD, Hamlin RL: Treatment of heart disease: An overview. p. 319. In Kirk RW (ed): Current Veterinary Therapy. Vol. IX. WB Saunders, Philadelphia, 1986

20. Sisson D: Acquired valvular heart disease in dogs and cats. p. 59. In Bonagura JD (ed): Contemporary Issues in Small Animal Practice. Vol. 7: Cardiology, Churchill Livingstone, New York, 1987

21. Hamlin RL, Kittleson MD: Clinical experience with hydralazine for treatment of otherwise intractable cough in dogs with apparent left-side heart failure. J Am Vet Med Assoc 180:1327, 1982

22. Kittleson MD, Eyster GE, Olivier NB, Anderson LK: Oral hydralazine therapy for chronic mitral regurgitation in the dog. J Am Vet Med Assoc 182:1205, 1983

21

Endocarditis and Bacteremia

Clay A. Calvert

Bacteremia is defined as the presence of bacteria in the circulating blood. Under certain circumstances, bacteremia may lead to sequestration of bacteria and colony formation in special sites or structures of the body. In dogs, the heart valves are commonly identified sites of bacterial sequestration resulting in bacterial endocarditis. Bacterial endocarditis occurs in cats but is rare.

The incidence of bacteremia and bacterial endocarditis in dogs and cats in unknown. This is largely due to the fact that blood cultures are not usually a component of the minimum data base of patients exhibiting clinical signs and having laboratory evidence consistent with bacteremia. Particularly in cats, the procurement of multiple blood samples of relatively large volumes for bacterial culture is often impractical. Nonetheless, blood cultures should be procured, especially in dogs weighing more than 10 kg, when bacteremia is suspected.

EPIZOOTIOLOGY

Bacteremia develops as a normal but transient phenomenon whenever bacteria-laden mucosal surfaces such as the nasopharynx and the gastrointestinal (GI), and genital mucosa have been traumatized.[1-4] The presence of circulating antibody titers to normal microflora support the concept of transient asymptomatic bacteremia.[5] Pathologic bacteremia occurs when the bloodstream is seeded via venous and lymphatic drainage sites of infection anywhere in the body.[1-4] Fluid accumulation, high tissue pressure, surgical or physical manipulation of abscesses, areas of cellulitis, or other infected tissues favor lymphatic and venous spread of bacteria to the systemic circulation.[6,7] Bacteria entering the bloodstream are usually rapidly removed by circulating and fixed macrophages of the mononuclear-phagocyte system of the liver, spleen, and bone marrow and by neutrophils in capillaries, especially in the lungs.[8]

The clinical signs associated with bacteremia may be peracute, acute, subacute, or chronic. Peracute bacteremia is associated with clinical signs that develop and fulminate over a period of several hours. It is usually the result of gram-negative infections, usually by *Escherichia coli* or *Salmonella* spp., wherein endotoxemia occurs producing severe clinical and hemodynamic abnormalities. Peracute gram-negative sepsis is most often the result of intestinal mucosal barrier interruption by gram-negative pathogen overgrowth, intestinal obstruction, traumatic intestinal perforation, intestinal surgery, or prolonged surgical procedures involving the liver or urogenital tract.[9] Acute bacteremia develops over a period of several days. It is most often the result of gram-negative infections, but may result from *Staphylococcus aureus* infection.[9] Subacute bacteremia develops and persists for several weeks or longer and is usually the result of gram-positive infections.[9]

Chronic bacteremia is a sequela of acute or subacute bacteremia that has often not been previously recognized. It is always associated with a focus of persistent infection. Chronic bacteremia may result from microorganisms of low pathogenicity (e.g., *Brucella canis*) or from sequestration of bacterial colonies on heart valves, bone, or sites of abscessation in the liver, spleen, kidneys, or muscles. Chronic bacteremia may be of indeterminable duration and is usually the result of gram-positive infections, especially with inappropriate antibiotic therapy. The clinical signs are subtle or vague and many laboratory and clinical findings commonly seen with acute bacteremias are absent or less pronounced.[6,9,10] Bacterial endocarditis associated with chronic bacteremia may be diagnosed only after the clinical signs of left-sided congestive heart failure develop. In many such cases, a history can be elicited of undiagnosed fever and gastrointestinal signs having occurred 6 weeks to 3 months earlier.

The prevalence of bacterial endocarditis has been reported to be from 0.6 to 6.6 percent.[11–16] Although particular breed predilections have not been consistently reported, German shepherds may be predisposed.[14,17] In general, large male dogs have been reported to be more frequently affected.[13,14,17]

The incidence of bacteremia among a hospital population was approximately 1 percent of the internal medicine case load and 0.3 percent of the general hospital accessions.[18] Of 165 bacteremic dogs identified among 663 (25 percent) dogs, blood cultures were procured because of suspected sepsis. Of 165 bacteremic dogs, 77 (46 percent) had bacteremia alone, 45 (27 percent) had bacterial endocarditis and 43 (27 percent) had discospondylitis. The mean and median ages of dogs with bacteremia were 5.3 and 5.0 years, respectively (range, less than 1 to 11 years), which was similar to that of dogs with bacterial endocarditis (4.9 and 4.5 years; range, 2 to 13 years). Although there were equal numbers of male and female dogs affected with bacteremia alone, there was almost a 2:1 male-to-female ratio of dogs with bacterial endocarditis.[18]

The predisposition of large, male dogs to bacterial endocarditis has been observed.[17,19] The prostate gland would be a logical source of infection that could account for a male predisposition. Although chronic or subacute bacterial prostatitis is identified in some bacteremic dogs, a causal relationship is difficult to prove. Nonetheless, the prostate gland should be suspected as a source of infection in large, male, middle-aged, or older dogs with suspected bacteremia. Bacteriuria is commonly associated with bacteremia and bacterial endocarditis but may be related to either a cause or an effect.[9]

In the face of bacteremia, a predisposing cause and/or a source of infection should be sought. The administration of corticosteroids has been associated with bacteremia and bacterial endocarditis.[9,17,18] In some instances, these drugs have been administered for the treatment of apparently unrelated problems. When prescribed at high dosages or for protracted periods, bacteremia may develop. The only clinical signs of bacteremia may be fever, vomiting, and diarrhea. The indiscriminant use of fixed-dose antibiotic-steroid combination drugs or repositol corticosteroids is discouraged. Of 96 dogs with bacteremia alone or bacterial endocarditis (excluding peracute infections), abscesses, cellulitis, fistulas, and infected wounds (12 percent) were the most common predisposing conditions. Upper urinary tract infections (7 percent), surgery (7 percent), neoplasia (6 percent), prostatic infections (5 percent), oral infections (5 percent), and pyodermas (2 percent) were the other most often identified problems that may have predisposed dogs to bacteremia.[17] Most organisms isolated from these dogs were gram positive (i.e., primarily coagulase positive *Staphylococcus aureus*). A causal affect between oral or prostatic infections and bacteremia is probably underestimated.

PATHOGENESIS

A number of different bacteria have been associated with bacteremia and bacterial endocarditis in dogs, most often *S. aureus*, *E. coli,* and β-hemolytic streptococci.[9,11,13,14,17–24] Most bacteria identified in bacteremic dogs are aerobes. The incidence of anaerobic bacteremia is unknown.

Infections involving the skin, subcutis, bone, urogenital tract, lung, prostate gland, oral cavity, liver, intestine, and perianal tissues have all been incriminated as sources of bacteremia.[8,9,13,14,16,21] Bacteremia has been associated with routine dental prophylaxis in dogs,[25–27] but the incidence of pathologic bacteremia or bacterial endocarditis resulting from these procedures is probably very low.

It has been assumed that prior heart valve damage is an important predisposing factor for valvular bacterial endocarditis. Experimentally, it is difficult to induce bacterial endocarditis of heart valves in dogs unless their valves have been physically or chemically damaged, or unless clumped or highly virulent bacteria are used.[28] However, the prevalence of valvular bacterial endocarditis in dogs with congenital heart defects is low.[17] Most dogs with confirmed valvular bacterial endocarditis have no history of valvular disease or congenital heart defects.[17,19,24] The role of early subclinical mitral valvular endocardiosis (fibrosis, polysaccharidosis)[29,30] as a factor predisposing to bacterial endocarditis is unknown. The most common congenital heart defect associated with valvular bacterial endocarditis in dogs is subaortic stenosis.[17,31,32] The aortic valve cusps may be damaged by blood flow turbulence created by the subvalvular obstruction, thereby predisposing to bacterial infection.

Endogenous, stress-related, fibrin-platelet heart valve vegetations have been produced in experimental animals and observed in humans with a number of diseases.[33] Bacterial infection of these lesions is common.[34] These sterile vegetations have been hypothesized to result from endogenous stress injury and to be important in some instances of bacterial endocarditis.[35,36] Various stress conditions have been shhown to predispose laboratory animals to bacterial endocarditis by causing interstitial edema or other structural changes in heart valves.[37,38] Stress or endothelial injury leading to collagen exposure has been shown to result in platelet aggregation.[39] Subsequent bacteremia may result in colonization of the platelet-fibrin thrombus. The pathogenesis of subacute bacterial endocarditis in humans has been reported to involve these platelet-fibrin thrombi.[40] In addition, it is believed that prior valvular damage and a high titer of agglutinating antibody against the infective bacteria is required.[28,40–47] Certain virulent bacteria may not require prior heart valve damage or formation of a sterile platelet-fibrin thrombus.[28,48,49]

Certain bacteria have a greater ability to adhere to normal canine heart valves.[50] Adherence tendencies may depend on the ability of bacteria to produce dextran, which is important in the adherence properties of bacteria such as S. aureus and Pseudomonas.[39,51] Streptococci and staphylococci can adhere to normal heart valves and are two of the three bacteria most often involved in canine bacteremia and bacterial endocarditis.[9,17,18] Proteases produced by S. aureus and β-hemolytic streptococci are capable of damaging endothelia that could result in a platelet-fibrin thrombus and subsequent bacterial colonization.[52]

The pathophysiologic manifestations of gram-negative bacteremia tend to be more fulminant and severe than those of gram-positive bacteremia, primarily because of the effects that circulating endotoxin have on the complement, kallikrein, fibrinolytic, and coagulation pathways. Regardless of the specific offending gram-negative bacteria, the associated clinical manifestations are identical.[8] Bacteremia may be associated with clinical signs due to exotoxins or endotoxins. Endogenous pyrogen release is initiated by bacteremia, resulting in fever. The continual or intermittent shedding of bacteria into the bloodstream, hypersensitivity to bacteria, and septic embolization of organs, especially the kidneys, are associated with most extracardiac manifestations of bacteremia and bacterial endocarditis.

Purulent inflammation or abscess formation is common in organs that receive their vascular supply via an end-arteriole network with little anastomosis. Secondary embolic abscesses, splenomegaly, and hematuria are more often associated with bacterial endocarditis than with bacteremia alone.[8] Metastatic infection can result in life-threatening complications. Virtually all dogs with bacterial endocarditis of the left heart experience multiple continuous embolization and renal infarction, which may lead to renal failure. Renal failure was present in 6 of 61 dogs (10 percent) with bacterial endocarditis at the time of diagnosis.[17] Septic embolization of the spleen occurs in most dogs with bacterial endocarditis, but clinically apparent complications are uncommon.[17] Occasionally, splenic abscessation causes unresponsive fever with progressive leukocytosis.

Increased serum alkaline phosphatase (SAP) activity, hypoalbuminemia, and hypoglycemia are often associated with bacteremia.[9,18] Elevated SAP activity is statistically more common with gram-negative infections, particularly *E. coli*.[9,18] Circulating endotoxin has been reported to affect hepatic excretory mechanisms and may contribute to intrahepatic cholestasis.[53]

Hypoalbuminemia is a common manifestation of most types of bacteremia. Subacute and chronic bacteremia may result in transcapillary leakage due to immune-mediated or embolic vasculitis. Certain bacterial toxins, including proteases produced by *S. aureus* and β-hemolytic streptococci, are known to produce endothelial damage that may lead to leakage of plasma.[52] Canine endotoxemia is associated with increased vascular permeability, which permits albumin to leak into the extravascular compartment.[54] Sepsis is also associated with reduced hepatic synthesis of albumin.[54] Approximately one-half of bacteremic dogs examined for hepatic function in one study had increased sulfobromphthalein retention, suggesting reduced hepatic function.[9]

Hypoglycemia may occur in bacteremic patients, usually in association with increased SAP activity and/or hypoalbuminemia. In these patients, hypoglycemia may result from increased utilization by leukocytes.[55] However, incubation of normal blood with bacteria alone has not been shown to cause a significant decrease in blood glucose.[56] Hypoglycemia has been associated with marked leukocytosis from noninfectious causes.[57] In bacteremic patients, hypoglycemia may also result from the effects of bacteria or bacterial toxins on the intermediary metabolism of glucose.

Subacute and chronic bacteremia can result in antigenic stimulation of the immune system. Circulating immunoglobulin increases as a protective response, but hypersensitivity reactions can occur. Circulating immune complexes may be deposited in many tissues, leading to polyarthritis, myositis, vasculitis, and glomerulonephritis. Antinuclear antibody, lupus erythematosus, and Coombs' test results may be positive in dogs with subacute and chronic bacteremia.[17] Circulating autoantibodies have been detected in dogs with bacterial endocarditis and polyarthritis.[58]

Table 21-1 Selected Necropsy Findings in 44 Dogs with Bacterial Endocarditis

Gross Necropsy Findings	Dogs Affected	
	No.	%
Distribution of heart valve lesions		
Mitral	30	71
Aortic	16	34
Aortic only	10	23
Mitral and aortic	6	14
Pulmonic	1	2
Tricuspid	6	14
Tricuspid only	4	9
Systemic embolization and infarcts		
Kidney	35	80
Spleen	35	80
Kidney and spleen	20	45
Left ventricle	19	43
Lungs	9	20
Brain	2	4.5
Iliac artery	1	2.2
Congenital heart defects	4	9
Endocardiosis	6	13.6
Glomerulonephritis	7	16

(Calvert CA: Valvular bacterial endocarditis in the dog. J Am Vet Med Assoc 180:1080, 1982.)

Valve damage and dysfunction, microembolization of the myocardium, and cardiac rhythm disturbances are the principal cardiac consequences of bacteremia and bacterial endocarditis. The mitral (see Fig. 32-8) and aortic valves are most often affected.[17,19] The distribution of gross lesions in one large study is listed in Table 21-1.

Vegetations of the aortic or mitral valve lead to valvular regurgitation (insufficiency), which causes volume overload of the heart. Left-sided congestive heart failure may occur. In the author's experience, aortic valve insufficiency in association with bacterial endocarditis always leads to intractable left-sided congestive heart failure if the patient survives the consequences of bacteremia. Heart failure usually develops from 4 to 12 weeks after the onset of clinical signs associated with bacteremia. Mitral insufficiency alone seldom results in heart failure within the first year after the diagnosis. Gradual,

Table 21-2 Clinical Findings in Dogs with Bacteremia and Bacterial Endocarditis

Clinical Findings	Bacteremia (N = 77) No.	%	Bacterial Endocarditis (N = 45) No.	%
Fever (>39.4°C)	58	75	32	70
Sinus tachycardia	25	32	9	41
Vomiting	13	17	16	35
Lameness	15	19	15	34
Shifting	5	6	8	18
Cardiac murmur	5	6	33	74
Systolic	5	6	33	74
Diastolic	0	0	6	13
Ventricular arrhythmia	4	5	12	27
Renal failure	1	1	5	11
Heart failure	0	0	7	16
Myopathy	3	4	2	4
Sudden death	0	0	4	8

N, total number of dogs.

CLINICAL MANIFESTATIONS

The clinical signs associated with bacteremia alone and bacterial endocarditis are similar (Table 21-2). The incidence of lameness, sinus tachycardia, heart murmurs, cardiac rhythm disturbances, embolic complications, and immune-mediated phenomena is greater with bacterial endocarditis (Table 21-3).[9,17,18] Gram-negative sepsis usually manifests peracute clinical signs. Bacterial endocarditis, however, tends to be acute or subacute, often due to a gram-positive microorganism. Frequently, this subacute disease is manifested by low-grade or episodic fever (although body temperature is sometimes normal), mild leukocytosis with either a mild left shift and monocytosis or without a left shift, low normal or slightly low serum albumin concentration, occasionally increased serum alkaline phosphatase activity, and, occasionally, hypoglycemia. Chronic bacterial endocarditis results from a failure to clinically recognize the acute or subacute stage of the disease.

Dogs with bacteremia often display some combination of fever, lethargy, anorexia, and GI disturbances at the time of initial bacteremia. Following the initial clinical signs, dogs with bacterial endocarditis variably manifest fever, lameness, myalgia, lethargy, and anorexia. Dogs with subacute or chronic bacterial endocarditis may exhibit signs of left-sided congestive heart failure, especially if the aortic valve has been damaged. Acute cardi-

progressive left atrial and left ventricular enlargement occurs, but the incidence and time course of heart failure in such cases are unknown.

Multiple small septic emboli affect the myocardium of bacterial endocarditis patients. Rarely, multiple myocardial abscesses develop.[17,31,32] Usually, arrhythmias are the primary consequences of myocardial embolization.[17] Although both ventricular and supraventricular tachyarrhythmias occur, the former are most common.[17,18] In one report, 4 of 77 dogs (5 percent) with bacteremia alone had ventricular tachyarrhythmias (usually unifocal ventricular extrasystoles) compared with an incidence of 12 of 45 dogs (27 percent) with bacterial endocarditis (Table 21-2).[18] The incidence of arrhythmias is certainly underestimated because of the brief recording period of routine electrocardiography. Major coronary artery occlusion and myocardial infarction have been reported[59,60] but are unusual in dogs with bacterial endocarditis.[17]

Aortic valvular endocarditis may lead to a dissecting valve ring abscess with infection of the septum or of a major component of the atrioventricular (AV) conduction system.[61] AV heart blocks have been reported in dogs[32,62] but are uncommon. In a series of 61 dogs with bacterial endocarditis, only 1 dog experienced complete block.[17]

Table 21-3 Incidence of Selected Clinical Abnormalities in 61 Dogs with Bacterial Endocarditis

Clinical Abnormalities	Dogs with Abnormality No.	%
Fever	51	83
Leukocytosis	50	82
Heart murmur	46	74
Lameness	21	34
Fever + leukocytosis + heart murmur	27	44
Fever + leukocytosis + murmur + lameness	11	18

(Calvert CA: Valvular bacterial endocarditis in the dog. J Am Vet Med Assoc 180:1080, 1982.)

ogenic pulmonary edema occurring in breeds not normally affected by mitral valve endocardiosis or cardiomyopathy is often the result of bacterial endocarditis. In such cases, there is usually no history of a pre-existing heart murmur, or a heart murmur may be absent at the time of presentation. Acute, severe, refractory pulmonary edema in large-breed dogs may be due to bacterial endocarditis of the aortic valve. In the Doberman pinscher, acute pulmonary edema is usually the result of dilated cardiomyopathy, which can be easily confirmed by echocardiography. Decompensated dilated cardiomyopathy in other large and giant breeds is usually manifest as bilateral congestive heart failure.

A history of predisposing factors may be elicited for many dogs with bacteremia.[16–18] They include immunosuppressive drug therapy (including cancer chemotherapy), intravenous catheters, surgery, abscesses, cellulitis, infected wounds, pyoderma, urinary tract infection (especially prostatitis), ulcerative gingivitis, or stomatitis.[9,17,18,20]

Physical examination findings of patients with bacteremia and bacterial endocarditis vary with the stage of disease and associated sequela. Early in the course of bacterial endocarditis a heart murmur may be absent.[17,61–64] In some dogs, lameness or po-

lyarthritis may be the dominant clinical sign. However, lameness is an inconsistent finding in dogs with bacterial endocarditis, and a classic shifting-leg lameness is seen in few dogs.[17] In some, heart failure or renal failure may distract the clinician's attention from an infectious disease. In one study, fever was detected in 42 of 61 dogs (70 percent) at some time during the course of illness.[17]

Systolic heart murmurs were detected in 45 of 61 dogs (74 percent) in one study.[17] The murmur was of recent onset or latent in 41 percent of these animals. In my experience, the systolic murmur of rapidly changing character, described in association with endocarditis in human beings, is less common in dogs. The presence of a systolic murmur whose intensity increases over a short period of time or evidence of a diastolic murmur (Fig. 21-1) is an ominous sign. A diastolic murmur is almost always due to aortic valve regurgitation and is strongly suggestive of vegetative endocarditis.[17,65]

The arterial pulse of dogs with bacterial endocarditis is often unremarkable. A hyperkinetic pulse may result from increased stroke volume due to mitral insufficiency. In the presence of aortic valve regurgitation the stroke volume is increased, but the regurgitant fraction causes the pulse pressure to de-

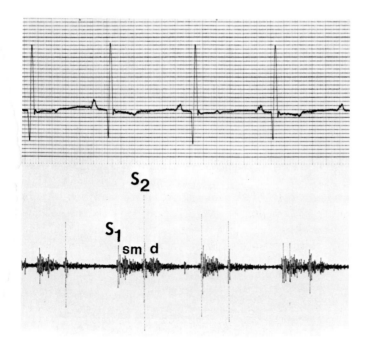

Fig. 21-1 Phonocardiogram (200 to 500 Hz) from a dog with bacterial endocarditis involving the mitral and aortic valves. A simultaneous electrocardiogram was recorded to facilitate timing of phonocardiographic events. A systolic murmur (sm) is seen between the first heart sound (S_1) and second heart sound (S_2). An early diastolic murmur (d) follows S_2.

crease quickly after systole, producing a "water-hammer" pulse.

Although cardiac rhythm disturbances commonly occur in association with bacterial endocarditis, they are usually single ectopic beats or short paroxysms of tachycardia. These are easily overlooked or not detected during physical examination (Table 21-2).

The presence of lameness, joint pain, muscle pain, and stiffness may suggest either immune-mediated disease or septic embolization of various tissues. Lumbar or abdominal pain on palpation may suggest renal or splenic inflammation secondary to septic embolization, infarction, or abscess formation.

Occasionally, erosion of an artery occurs following septic embolization, and hemorrhage occurs. Thrombophlebitis may also produce pain and edema of an extremity. Vasculitis is commonly associated with bacteremia and although petechial and ecchymoses of the mucous membranes or retina are possible,[66] such findings in spontaneous cases are uncommon.[9,17,18]

CLINICAL PATHOLOGY

The leukograms of dogs with bacteremia alone and bacterial endocarditis are similar. A neutrophilic leukocytosis with an appropriate left shift and monocytosis is present in most dogs with bacteremia and in virtually all dogs with bacterial endocarditis at some point during the course of disease. Leukopenia and an inappropriate left shift are more common with bacteremia alone, usually in association with peracute and acute gram-negative infections. Leukopenia and inappropriate left shifts are less often associated with bacterial endocarditis because of a lower incidence of gram-negative bacteremia and a general tendency for a subacute time course. Monocytosis is the most common consistent leukogram abnormality[9,17,18] and is usually present even in chronic low-grade infections. A profound leukocytosis and left shift are often absent in chronic bacterial endocarditis. Prior antibiotic therapy may also result in white blood cell (WBC) counts less than 20,000/mm³. In one study, 11 of 59 dogs (19%) with bacterial endocarditis did not have a detected leukocytosis.[17] A mature neutrophilia and monocytosis associated with leukocytoses of variable degrees, occasionally as high as 50,000/mm³, is consistent with chronic bacterial endocarditis. The absence of fever and leukocytosis were recorded in fewer than 10 percent of affected dogs.[17]

A normocytic normochromic anemia is commonly seen with subacute or chronic bacterial endocarditis and is usually nonregenerative. Thirty-five of 59 dogs (60 percent) with bacterial endocarditis had packed cell volumes less than 37 percent at the time of diagnosis.[17] A regenerative anemia is occasionally encountered and is probably the result of erythrocyte destruction from physical forces associated with vegetative lesions or blood flow turbulence. Two of nine dogs (22 percent) with regenerative anemias in which Coombs' tests were performed were positive.[17]

Serum chemistry abnormalities are commonly recorded in dogs with bacteremia and bacterial endocarditis. Of 95 dogs tested, hypoalbuminemia (less than 2.5 mg/dl), a twofold or greater elevation of serum alkaline phosphatase (SAP), and hypoglycemia (less than 70 mg/dl) were detected in 48 (51 percent), 46 (48 percent), and 23 (24 percent) dogs, respectively.[18] Increased SAP activity was associated with both gram-positive and gram-negative infections but was statistically more likely with the latter.[18] Hypoglycemia seldom occurred in the absence of increased SAP activity and/or hypoalbuminemia.

Proteinuria, occult hematuria, and pyuria may occur in association with bacteremia. Proteinuria and occult hematuria may be more common with bacterial endocarditis, in which renal infarction, glomerulonephritis, and pyelonephritis are common sequelae. Pyelonephritis may be either a cause or effect of bacterial endocarditis.

THORACIC RADIOGRAPHY

Thoracic radiographs are usually of little value in the diagnosis of bacteremia and bacterial endocarditis. Left-sided congestive heart failure (e.g., left atrial enlargement, pulmonary edema, and distention of the cranial lobar veins) may be evident at the time of physical examination (Fig. 21-2). However, most dogs do not have radiographically obvious cardiomegaly at the time of diagnosis. Dogs with chronic bacterial endocarditis may develop left atrial

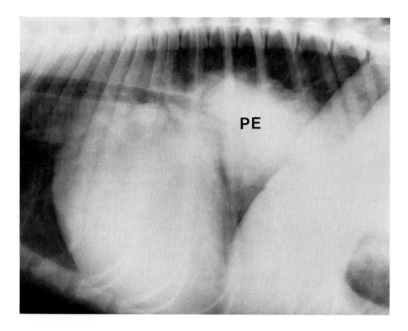

Fig. 21-2 Left lateral thoracic radiograph of a 5-year-old male boxer with bacterial endocarditis and vegetative lesions involving the aortic valve. There is a marked increase in pulmonary density at the perihilar region with air bronchograms suggesting an alveolar pattern. The left atrium is slightly enlarged. This infiltrate is compatible with pulmonary edema (PE).

enlargement. The long-term prognosis in such cases is unknown.

Bacterial endocarditis of the tricuspid or pulmonic valves, although uncommon, produces multiple embolization of the pulmonary arterial system. Focal areas of mixed interstital and alveolar lung disease are usually present and consistent with septic embolization and pneumonia.

ELECTROCARDIOGRAPHY

The electrocardiograms (ECGs) of dogs with bacterial endocarditis are frequently abnormal.[17,21,62] Ventricular tachyarrhythmias represent the most common arrhythmias. In most cases, they are not life-threatening, although exceptions are noted. AV blocks, supraventricular arrhythmias, evidence of chamber enlargement, and ST segment changes are seen occasionally.[32,60] The frequency of cardiac arrhythmias is probably underestimated because of the limited duration of clinical heart rhythm monitoring.

ECHOCARDIOGRAPHY

The echocardiogram is important in the diagnosis of bacterial endocarditis and in monitoring cardiac function in surviving dogs.[19] Echocardiography makes possible the presumptive diagnosis of valvular endocarditis in the absence of positive blood cultures and diastolic heart murmurs. Vegetations of 3- to 4-mm thickness can be detected. Those on the aortic valve are relatively easy to detect (Fig. 21-3; see also Fig. 6-43) as opposed to mitral valve apparatus vegetations (Fig. 21-4) with M-mode echocardiography. Two-dimensional ultrasonography is a more accurate technique for detecting vegetative lesions (see Fig. 6-44). Diastolic fluttering of the anterior mitral valve leaflet and vibration of the interventricular septum often occur from aortic valve regurgitation due to aortic valve vegetative lesions. This can be detected by M-mode echocardiography (Fig. 21-5).

OTHER DIAGNOSTIC TESTS

In my experience, dogs with bacterial endocarditis have elevated erythrocyte sedimentation rates. A normal sedimentation rate may be an important negative finding when the diagnosis of bacterial endocarditis is considered. A normal sedimentation rate weighs heavily against the diagnosis in human beings.[16,17,67]

Tests of immune-mediated disease are occasionally positive in dogs with bacterial endocarditis.[17]

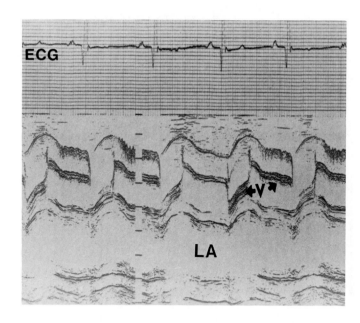

Fig. 21-3 M-mode echocardiogram at the aortic valve level from a 4-year-old German short-hair pointer with bacterial endocarditis. Vegetative lesions (arrows) are visible as increased echoes on the aortic valve leaflets in systole and diastole. LA, left atrium; ECG, electrocardiogram; V, vegetative lesions.

Although one-half to one-third of affected human beings have a significant rheumatoid factor titer,[68] none of six affected dogs tested was positive.[17] The presence of phagocytic reticuloendothelial cells in a peripheral blood smear and teichoic acid antibodies have, on occasion, lent support to the diagnosis of bacterial endocarditis in human beings whose blood culture results were negative.[68]

Recently, radionuclide techniques have been applied to the diagnosis of bacterial endocarditis. Gallium-67 citrate will concentrate in portions of the myocardium and endocardium involved in an infective process, although false-positive and -negative test results occur.[67,69]

Intraleukocyte bacteria may be demonstrated in buffy coat smears of venous blood in approximately 50 percent of human beings with bacterial endocarditis, some of whom had negative blood culture results.[70,71] Smears have been positive in patients with bacteremia or bacterial endocarditis that had received antimicrobial therapy. A simple method of performing leukocyte smears has been described.[70] One drop of unanticoagulated venous blood is placed on a clean glass coverslip and incubated in a moist Petri dish for 25 minutes at 37°C. The clot on the coverslip is gently washed off with normal (0.9 percent) saline, and the coverslip with attached leukocytes is immersed in fixative (methanol or glu-teraldahyde) prior to Giemsa staining and microscopic examination.

MICROBIOLOGY

Although a number of different bacteria have been isolated from bacteremic dogs, the most often incriminated agents are S. aureus, E. coli, and β-hemolytic streptococci.[9,11,13,14,17,18,22,23] Although anaerobic bacteria have been isolated from dogs with bacterial endocarditis,[32] their incidence is unknown. Bacteremia caused by S. aureus may be the most common identified type.

S. aureus bacteremia tends to produce an acute or subacute syndrome. Peracute bacteremia usually develops from gram-negative infections. E. coli is the most commonly isolated gram-negative bacterium in bacteremic patients.[9,18] Gram-positive bacteremia tends to develop in association with cutaneous wounds and infections, some urinary tract infections, catheter induced infections, and some instances of stomatitis or periodontal disease. Gram-negative bacteremia is usually associated with intestinal and abdominal disorders, abdominal surgery, perianal disease and surgery, and some cases of intravenous or urinary catheter-induced infec-

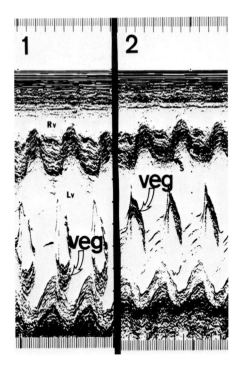

Fig. 21-4 M-mode echocardiograms at the mitral valve level from a mature Saint Bernard with bacterial endocarditis. Vegetative lesions (veg) are visible as an abnormal mass of echoes on the posterior mitral valve (*frame 1*) and anterior mitral valve (*frame 2*) leaflets. RV, right ventricle; LV, left ventricle; S, septum. (Courtesy of Dr. N. Sydney Moise.)

tions. Only 1 to 50 organisms may be present per milliliter of bacteremic blood sample.[71]

Bacteremia originating from extravascular sites is often transient or intermittent, so blood cultures performed at inappropriate times may be negative. Because bacteremia often precedes the development of a fever spike by 1 hour or more, it is difficult, in some cases, to determine the best time for culture sample procurement.[72] Bacteremia associated with endocarditis is qualitatively continuous but quantitatively variable.[62] Many blood samples may be drawn without obtaining positive cultures.[73,74] In humans, a standard sampling protocol is three blood samples drawn within 24 to 48 hours.[75,76] Positive cultures were obtained in 88 percent of affected dogs with endocarditis when more than one sample was drawn.[17]

False-positive results of blood cultures due to contamination by skin microflora usually involve such organisms as *Corynebacterium, Bacillus,* and some streptococci. *S. epidermidis* should be considered as a contaminant unless multiple cultures from other sites contain the organism as well.

False-negative blood culture results may be obtained when the patient has received prior antibiotic therapy. Culture of specimens from such patients in hypertonic medium increases the recovery of infecting organisms by preventing destruction of the cell wall-deficient bacteria that result from antimicrobial therapy.[77] Sucrose added to the medium helps to inactivate residual antimicrobial activity of the blood.[72] Antibiotic influences may be neutralized prior to culture by collecting blood in commercially available bottles (ARD, Marion Scientific, Kansas City, MO) that contain antimicrobial compounds. Other common causes of negative blood cultures are right-side or chronic bacterial endocarditis, uremia, failure to culture for anaerobic bacteria, and nonbacterial etiology.[74]

The skin over the venipuncture site should be shaved and prepared by alternately wiping the skin with 70 to 90 percent alcohol and scrubbing with an inorganic iodine soap. This sequence should be repeated three or more times. Ungloved hands should not touch the site during the collection procedure. Multiple samples should be taken within a 24-hour period from different sites. A minimum of 10 ml blood should be taken for each sample. If anaerobic cultures are sought, 20 ml blood should be drawn and the volume divided equally. Negative pressure should not be applied to the syringe as the needle is withdrawn through the skin. Alternatively, the syringe may be detached from the needle prior to withdrawal. To avoid contamination, a new needle is placed in the syringe prior to injection of the blood sample into the culture bottle. The culture bottle stopper should be disinfected prior to injection. Care should be taken to avoid the entry of room air into vacuum culture bottles. Clotted and citrated blood are inappropriate for culture because the fibrin clot decreases the frequency of microbe isolation.

DIAGNOSIS

The definitive antemortem diagnosis of bacterial endocarditis requires

1. Clinical signs and laboratory data consistent with the diagnosis

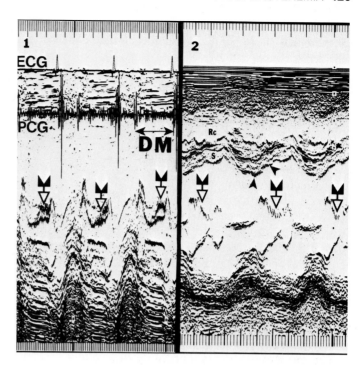

Fig. 21-5 M-mode echocardiograms at the mitral valve level displaying several characteristics of bacterial endocarditis. Frame 1 is an echophonocardiogram from an adult boxer. Diastolic fluttering of the mitral valve leaflets are illustrated (arrows). This is caused by a diastolic regurgitant jet of blood from the aortic valve made incompetent by vegetative lesions. A diastolic murmur (DM) is evident on the phonocardiogram (PCG). Frame 2 is an Echocardiogram from a 5-month-old English bulldog with congenital aortic insufficiency. Diastolic fluttering of the mitral valve (open arrows) and interventricular septum (arrowheads) is noted. RC, right ventricular chamber; S, interventricular septum; ECG, electrocardiogram. (Courtesy of Dr. N. Sydney Moise.)

2. A cardiac murmur of recent onset
3. Positive blood culture results

The presence of echocardiographic abnormalities indicative of bacterial endocarditis is very useful, especially in subacute and chronic cases, in the absence of a heart murmur, when the recent onset of a murmur is in doubt, and when blood culture results are negative. Particularly in the absence of a heart murmur with negative blood culture results, the clinical signs associated with bacteremia and bacterial endocarditis may be difficult to distinguish from those of immune mediated diseases.

Concomitant disorders such as heart failure, renal failure, neoplasia, abscesses, cellulitis, indwelling catheters, and infected wounds often are present in bacteremic dogs. Fever, lethargy, GI signs, myalgia, lameness, and hematologic abnormalities occurring in dogs affected by predisposing factors should alert the clinician to the possibility of bacteremia. Hypoalbuminemia, especially when associated with increased serum alkaline phosphatase activity and hypoglycemia, is strongly indicative of bacteremia.[9] Neoplasia, heart failure, and renal failure may distract the clinician from considering an infectious process. In one study, 14 of 59 cases (24 percent) contained ample information for the di-agnosis but bacterial endocarditis was not suspected.[17]

THERAPY

The important principles of the treatment of bacteremia and bacterial endocarditis are as follows:

1. Obtain blood cultures and perform bacterial antibiotic sensitivity tests.
2. Identify and treat sources of infection.
3. Identify concomitant problems, such as heart failure, renal failure, hypoglycemia, and hypoalbuminemia.
4. Employ bactericidal antibiotics.
5. Ensure high serum antibiotic levels (using high dosages).
6. Employ antibiotics that penetrate fibrin.
7. Ensure prolonged antibiotic therapy duration.
8. Repeat blood cultures following antibiotic therapy.

Despite the primary concern with the infective agent, concomitant predisposing disorders should not be overlooked. Urinary and intravenous catheters should be removed when sepsis is suspected, and potential sites of infection should be drained, debrided, or otherwise treated.

In the critically ill patient, antibiotic therapy should be started prior to the return of blood culture results.[79] Although this approach has inherent shortcomings such as selection for microbial resistance, critically ill patients with presumed infections should still be treated as soon as possible. Subsequent therapeutic adjustments may be made on the basis of culture results.

Bactericidal antibiotics are the drugs of choice in the treatment of bacteremia and bacterial endocarditis. Several antibiotics are usually given in sequence for a total of 6 to 8 weeks for the treatment of bacterial endocarditis. Bacteriostatic antibiotics, if used at all, should conclude rather than initiate the sequence.

On the basis of predisposing infections or other factors, time course of infection, known patterns of associated bacteria, and their antimicrobial sensitivity patterns, the antibiotics most likely to be effective can be predicted. This knowledge is important when blood culture results are negative and in critically ill patients prior to blood culture results. Most strains of *S. aureus* are sensitive, *in vitro*, to cephalosporins, aminoglycosides, erythromycin, and chloramphenicol. However, most are resistant to penicillin, ampicillin, and trimethoprim. Most isolates of *E. coli* are sensitive to gentamicin and cephalothin but resistant to ampicillin and chloramphenicol. β-hemolytic streptococci are usually sensitive to penicillin, ampicillin, cephalosporins, and chloramphenicol but are usually resistant to erythromycin, aminoglycosides, and trimethoprim. *Pseudomonas* spp are usually resistant to most practical, cost-allowable antibiotics except gentamicin and amikacin. Because *Pseudomonas* spp are recognizable early in their *in vitro* colony growth, when suspected, antibiotic sensitivity should be tested against third generation cephalosporins, carbenicillin, and amikacin. *Pseudomonas* spp are often sensitive to polymyxin B and colistimethate, but the use of these antibiotics is associated with significant problems.

In general, cephalothin, gentamicin, and chloramphenicol are most effective in vitro, for gram-positive bacteria while gentamicin and cephalothin are most effective against gram-negative agents. Thus, a combination of gentamicin with penicillin, ampicillin, or a cephalosporin is the logical choice for treatment of life-threatening bacteremia in the absence of laboratory identification of an organism or its antibiotic sensitivity. Subsequently, appropriate adjustments in therapy may be possible based on antibiogram results.

The incidence of anaerobic bacteremia in dogs is unknown and the antibiotic sensitivity patterns of these microbes are different from those of aerobes. Anaerobic infections should be suspected in the presence of periodontal disease, deep abscesses, granulomas, peritonitis, osteomyelitis, septic arthritis, and septic pleural effusions.[25–27,80–83] In general, most isolates of anaerobic bacteria are sensitive in vitro, to penicillin, ampicillin, cephalosporins, clindamycin, chloramphenicol, or metronidazole. Trimethoprim-sulfadiazine or trimethoprim-sulfamethoxasole is effective against gram-negative anaerobes.

In order to ensure adequate serum antibiotic concentrations, higher than normal dosages of antimicrobial drugs are indicated. Therapy should be initiated by the intravenous route and continued for 5 to 10 days, if feasible. Sodium or potassium penicillin may be given at a dosage of 20,000 to 40,000 units/kg every 4 to 6 hours, depending on the urgency. Ampicillin or cephalothin may be given at a dosage of 20 to 40 mg/kg every 6 hours. Gentamicin is usually administered at a dosage of 2 mg/kg every 8 hours and may be given for 5 to 14 days. Close attention must be paid to renal function when drugs are administered at higher than normal dosages and when gentamicin is employed in this manner.

Parenteral treatment should be continued for 14 to 21 days but this is not always practical. Subcutaneous administration of ampicillin, cephalothin and gentamicin may be substituted for the IV route when necessary or after 5 to 10 days of IV treatment. Ideally, oral antibiotic therapy should be instituted only after there is clinical and leukogram evidence of improvement.

Gram-negative bacteremia is more difficult to control when it accompanies neutropenia, hypogammaglobulinemia, diabetes mellitus, or renal failure, all of which generally predispose patients to this type of infection. Combination antibiotic therapy is often employed for gram-negative infections because they are associated with more acute progression and high mortality. Although clinical evidence supports the use of carbenicillin or ticarcillin with aminoglycosides for *Pseudomonas* and *Proteus*, these drugs must be given separately because of known *in vitro* incompatibilities. Amikacin, unlike tobramycin and gentamicin, is not inactivated *in vitro* by penicillins.[84–86] Continuous IV infusion of aminoglycosides has been recommended,[87] although associated increased nephrotoxicity has been reported.[1]

Patients with gram-negative bactermia must be closely monitored. Although clinical and hematologic evidence of improvement often occurs initially, relapse is common. Acquired antimicrobial resistance may develop rapidly. Clinical signs of resurging bacteremia include deterioration of mucous membrane color, increasing capillary refill time, increasing toe-web-to-rectal temperature differential, decreasing blood pressure, and increasing heart rate. Detection of these signs of early deterioration indicate a need for intensified therapy including adjustments of antibiotic treatment. Amikacin, tobramycin, or a third-generation cephalosporin may stem the tide of bacteremia.

PROGNOSIS

Several factors influence the natural course of bacteremic disorders including adequacy of therapy, severity of bacteremia, source of infection, delay before treatment, concomitant disorders, and the age of the patient. The prognosis is better when abscesses, cellulitis, skin, and wound infections are the source of bacteremia but is worse when gram-negative bacteria are involved because of the potentially fatal complications associated with endotoxemia. The mortality of 19 bacteremic dogs with hypoalbuminemia and elevation of serum alkaline phosphatase activity and 17 dogs with these abnormalities plus hypoglycemia were significantly higher (77 percent and 65 percent, respectively) than that of 31 dogs (13 percent) without these abnormalities. Abnormalities of serum albumin concentration or serum alkaline phosphatase activity alone did not correlate with an increased mortality rate.[9]

All dogs having aortic valve endocarditis in one study died.[9] Although many survived the initial complications of bacteremia, aortic valvular insufficiency resulted in intractable left-sided congestive heart failure in most dogs within 4- to 6 weeks. One

dog survived for 6 months. The appearance of a latent diastolic murmur or the increasing intensity of a systolic murmur is an ominous sign.

Bacterial endocarditis affecting only the mitral valve is associated with a better prognosis. Seven out of 15 dogs (47 percent) for example with no evidence of aortic valve involvement in one study survived.[17] Recent improvements in survival is attributable to an increased awareness or index of suspicion of bacterial endocarditis, rapid diagnosis, and aggressive appropriate therapy.

Late relapse and death occur in some dogs, usually when bacteriostatic antibiotics are chosen for treatment. The premature termination of antibiotic therapy may also result in relapse and death in bacteremic dogs, particularly when associated with bacterial endocarditis.

Renal failure has developed in a number of dogs one to several years after having survived bacterial endocarditis. Apparently, septic embolization and infarction of the kidneys during bacteremia are the causes of renal failure.

The indiscriminate use of corticosteroids, even with antibiotics as prophylaxis, is detrimental to bacteremic patients. Prophylactic antibiotic treatment is usually ineffective unless the type of bacteria and its antibiotic sensitivity are known. Bacterial resistance to frequently used antibiotics, such as ampicillin, is common. Thus, effective prophylactic antibiotic therapy usually requires the use of combinations of antibiotics, often including an aminoglycoside. Even then, the tendency to select for resistance bacteria is increased. Another common cause of corticosteroid administration to bacteremic dogs is the similarity in clinical manifestations of bacteremic and immune-mediated diseases. The survival rate of 17 dogs with bacterial endocarditis given corticosteroids was only 12 percent compared with an overall survival rate of 20 percent in 45 dogs that did not receive corticosteroids and a survival rate of 40 percent in a third group of 20 dogs wherein rapid diagnosis and optimum therapy were provided.[17]

REFERENCES

1. Everett ED, Hirschmann JV: Transient bacteremia and endocarditis prophylaxis. Medicine (Baltimore) 56:61, 1977

2. Reith AF, Squier TL: Blood cultures of apparently healthy persons. J Infect Dis 51:336, 1932

3. Orloff MJ, Peskin GW, Ellis HL: A bacteriologic study of human portal blood. Implications regarding hepatic ischemia in man. Ann Surg 148:738, 1958

4. Reith AF: Bacteria in the muscular tissues and blood of apparently normal animals. J Bacteriol 12:367, 1926

5. Loesche WJ: Indigenous human microflora and bacteremia. p. 40. In Kaplan EL, Taranta AV (eds): Infective Endocarditis. American Heart Association Symposium, Dallas, Texas, 1977

6. Bennett IL, Beeson PB: Bacteremia: A consideration of some experimental and clinical aspects. Yale J Biol Med 25:241, 1954

7. Kornegay JN, Barber DL: Discospondylitis in dogs. J Am Vet Med Assoc 177:337, 1980

8. Petersdorf RG: Disorders caused by biologic agents. p. 725. In Wintrobe MM, Thorn GW, Adams R, et al (eds): Principles of Internal Medicine. McGraw-Hill, New York, 1974

9. Calvert CA, Greene CE, Hardie EM: Cardiovascular infections in dogs: epizootiology, clinical manifestations, and prognosis. J Am Vet Med Assoc 187:612, 1985

10. Okall CC, Elliott SD: Bacteremia and oral sepsis. Lancet 2:869, 1935

11. Schornagel H: Endocarditis. Tijdschr Diergeneesk 63:57, 1936

12. Winquist G: Topagrafisk och etiologisk samman-stallning au de fibrinosa och ulcerosa endokarditerna hos en de av vora husdjur. Skand Vet Tieskr 35:575, 1945

13. Shouse CL, Meier H: Acute vegetative endocarditis in the dog and cat. J Am Vet Med Assoc 129:278, 1956

14. Lundh T: Fibrinous endocarditis in dogs. Acta Vet Scand 5:17, 1964

15. Jones TC, Zook BC: Aging changes in the vascular system of animals. Ann NY Acad Sci 127:671, 1975

16. Detweiler DK, Patterson DF, Huber K, et al: The prevalence of spontaneously occurring cardiovascular disease in dogs. Am J Public Health 51:228, 1961

17. Calvert CA: Valvular bacterial endocarditis in the dog. J Am Vet Med Assoc 180:1080, 1982

18. Calvert CA, Greene CE: Bacteremia in dogs: Diagnosis, treatment, and prognosis. Comp Cont Educ 8:179, 1986

19. Lombard CW, Buergelt CD: Vegetative bacterial endocarditis in dogs: Echocardiographic diagnosis and clinical signs. J Small Anim Pract 24:325, 1983

20. Hardie E, Rawlings CA, Calvert CA: Severe sepsis in selected small animal surgery patients. J Am Anim Hosp Assoc 22:33, 1986

21. Murdoch DB, Baker JR: Bacterial endocarditis in the dog. J Small Anim Pract 18:687, 1977

22. Luginbuhl H, Detweiler DK: Cardiovascular lesions in dogs. Ann NY Acad Sci 127:517, 1965

23. Kirchhoff Von H, Amtsberg G, Bisping W, et al: Untersuchungen zur Atiologie und Pathogenese der Endokardiose und Endokarditis des Hunds. Dtsch Tiererztl Wochenschr 80:428, 1973

24. Drazner FH: Bacterial endocarditis in the dog. Comp Cont Educ 1:918, 1979

25. Black AP, Crichlaw RT, Saunders JR: Bacteremia during ultrasonic teeth cleaning and extraction in the dog. J Am Anim Hosp Assoc 16:611, 1980

26. Fontine WT, Sims S, Donavan ML: Bacterial contamination associated with dental procedures in dogs. J Am Anim Hosp Assoc 5:150, 1969

27. Silver JG, Martin L, McBride BC: Recovery and clearance rates of oral microorganisms following experimental bacteremias in the dog. Arch Oral Biol 20:675, 1979

28. Blahd M, Frank I, Saphir O: Experimental endocarditis in dogs. Arch Pathol 27:424, 1939

29. Detweiller DK, Patterson DF: The prevalence and types of cardiovascular diseases in dogs. Ann NY Acad Sci 127:481, 1965

30. Buchanan JW: Chronic valvular disease in dogs. Adv Vet Sci Comp Med 21:75, 1977

31. Muna WFT, Ferrans VS, Pierce JE, et al: Discrete subaortic stenosis in Newfoundland dogs: Association of infective endocarditis. Am J Cardiol 41:746, 1978

32. Bonagura JD: Bacterial endocarditis. p. 1052. In Ettinger SJ (ed): Textbook of Veterinary Internal Medicine. WB Saunders, Philadelphia, 1983

33. Treedman L, Valone J: Experimental infective endocarditis. Prog Cardiovasc Dis 22:169, 1979

34. Durack DT, Beeson PB, Petersdorf RG: Experimental endocarditis. III. Production and progress of the disease in rabbits. Br J Exp Pathol 54:142, 1973

35. Lillehei CW, Bobb JRR, Visscher MB: Occurrence of endocarditis with valvular deformities in dogs with arteriovenous fistulae. Proc Soc Exp Biol Med 75:9, 1950

36. Angrist A, Oka M, Nakas R: Interstitial oedema in valvular endocarditis. Ann NY Acad Sci 156:480, 1969

37. Highman B, Altland PD: Effect of exposure and acclimatization to cold on susceptibility of rats to bacterial endocarditis. Proc Soc Exp Biol Med 110:663, 1962

38. Miller AJ, Pick R, Kline IK, et al: The susceptibility of dogs with chronic impairment of cardiac lymph flow to staphylococcal valvular endocarditis. Circulation 30:417, 1964

39. Gutschik E, Christensen N: Experimental endocarditis in rabbits. Acta Pathol Microbiol Scand 86B:215, 1978

40. Weinstein L: Infective endocarditis. p. 1136. In Braunwald E (ed): Heart Disease: A Textbook of Cardiovascular Medicine. WB Saunders, Philadelphia, 1984

41. Rowlands DT, Vakelzadeh J, Sherwood BF, et al: Experimental bacterial endocarditis in the opossum. Am J Pathol 58:295, 1970

42. Vakelzadeh J, Rowlands DT, Sherwood BF, et al: Experimental bacterial endocarditis in the opossum. J Infect Dis 122:89, 1970

43. Jartner BS, Helmboldt CI: Streptococcal bacterial endocarditis in chickens. Vet Pathol 8:54, 1971

44. Musher DM, Richie Y: Bacterial clearance and endocarditis in American opposums. Infect Immun 9:1126, 1974

45. Carrizosa J, Tanphaichitra D, Levison ME: Experimental *Bacteroides fragilis* endocarditis in rabbits. Infect Immun 15:871, 1977

46. Santoro J, Levison ME: Rat model of experimental endocarditis. Infect Immunol 17:913, 1978

47. Jones JET: Bacterial endocarditis in the pig with special reference to streptococcal endocarditis. J Comp Pathol 90:11, 1980

48. Dick GF, Schwartz WB: Experimental endocarditis in dogs. Arch Pathol 42:159, 1946

49. Jones JET: The experimental production of endocarditis in the pig. J Pathol 99:307, 1969

50. Gould K, Ramirez-Rhonda CH, Holmes RK, et al: Adherence of bacteria to heart valves in vitro. J Clin Invest 56:1364, 1975

51. Ramirez-Rhonda CH: Adherence of *Streptococcus mutans* to normal and damaged canine aortic valves. Clin Res 25:382A, 1977

52. Straus DC: Protease produced by *Streptococcus sanguis* associated with sub-acute bacterial endocarditis. J Infect Immun 38:1037, 1982

53. Utili R, Abernathy CO, Zimmerman HJ: Cholestatic effects of *Escherichia coli* endotoxin on the isolated perfused rat liver. Gastroenterology 70:248, 1976

54. Deysine M, Stein S: Albumin shifts across the extracellular space secondary to experimental infection. Surg Gynecol Obstet 141:617, 1980

55. Hinshaw LB, Archer LT, Beller BK, et al: Glucose utilization and the role of blood in endotoxin shock. Am J Physiol 233:71, 1979

56. Miller SI, Wallace RJ, Musher DM, et al: Hypoglycemia as a manifestation of sepsis. Am J Med 68:649, 1980

57. Goodenow TJ, Malarkey WB: Leukocytosis and artifactural hypoglycemia. J Am Vet Med Assoc 237:1961, 1977

58. Bennett D, Gilbertson MM, Grennan D: Bacterial endocarditis with polyarthritis in 2 dogs associated with circulating autoantibodies. J Small Anim Pract 19:185, 1978

59. Nielsen SW, Nielsen LB: Coronary embolism in valvular bacterial endocarditis in the dog. J Am Vet Med Assoc 125:376, 1954

60. Fregin GF, Luginbuhl H, Guarda F: Myocardial infarction in a dog with bacterial endocarditis. J Am Vet Med Assoc 160:956, 1972

61. Lerner PI, Weinstein L: Infective endocarditis in the antibiotic era. N Engl J Med 274:199, 1966

62. Pelletier LL, Petersdorf RG: Infective endocarditis. Medicine (Baltimore) 56:287, 1977

63. Kaye D: Changes in the spectrum, diagnosis, and management of bacterial and fungal endocarditis. Med Clin North Am 57:941, 1953

64. Weinstein L, Rubin RH: Infective endocarditis. Prog Cardiovasc Dis 16:239, 1973

65. Fisher FW: Heart disease in the dog. J Small Anim Pract 13:553, 1972

66. Walker WF, Hamburger M: A study of experimental staphylococcal endocarditis in dogs. J Lab Clin Med 53:931, 1959

67. Gregoratos G, Karliner JS: Infective endocarditis. Med Clin North Am 63:173, 1979

68. Gleckman R: Culture negative bacterial endocarditis. Am Heart J 94:125, 1977

69. Wiseman J, Rouleau J, Rigo P, et al: Gallium-67 imaging for the technique of bacterial endocarditis. Radiology 110:135, 1976

70. Powers DL, Mandell GL: Intraleukocyte bacteria in endocarditis patients. JAMA 227:312, 1974

71. Studer JP, Glauser MP, Schapira M: Value of examining buffy coats for intragranulocytic micro-organisms in patients with fever. Br Med J 1:85, 1979

72. Washington JA: Blood cultures: principles and techniques. Mayo Clin Proc 50:91, 1975

73. Beeson PB, Brammon ES, Warren JV: Observations on the sites of renewal of bacteria from the blood in patients with bacterial endocarditis. J Exp Med 8:9, 1945

74. Griffith GC, Levinson DC: Subacute bacterial endocarditis. Calif Med 71:403, 1949

75. Cannady PB, Sanford JP: Negative blood cultures in infective endocarditis. South Med J 69:1420, 1976

76. Washington JA: Blood cultures, principles, and techniques. Mayo Clin Proc 50:91, 1945

77. Agarwal AK: Culture-negative infective endocarditis. Postgrad Med J 72:123, 1982

78. Sokolow M, McIlroy MB: Clinical Cardiology. Lange Medical, Los Altos, CA, 1979

79. Schimpff S, Satterlee W, Young VM, et al: Therapy

with carbenacillin and gentamicin in febrile cancer patients. N Engl J Med 284:1061, 1971

80. Berg JN, Falls WH: Canine and feline anaerobic infections. Scope 21:2, 1977

81. Hirsch DC, Bilberstein EL, Jang SS: Obligate anaerobes in veterinary practice. J Am Vet Med Assoc 176:326, 1979

82. Walker RD, Richardon DC, Bryant MJ, et al: Anaerobic bacteria associated with osteomyelitis in domestic animals. J Am Vet Med Assoc 192:814, 1983

83. Caywood DD, Wallace LJ, Broden TD: Osteomyelitis in the dog: A review of 67 cases. J Am Vet Med Assoc 172:943, 1978

84. McLaughlin JE, Reeves DS: Clinical laboratory evidence for inactivation of gentamicin by carbenicillin. Lancet 1:261, 1971

85. Noone P, Pattison JR: Therapeutic implications of interactions of gentamicin and penicillin. Lancet 2:575, 1971

86. Holt HA, Broughall JM, McCarthy M, et al: Interaction between aminoglycoside antibiotics and carbenicillin or ticarcillin. Infection 4:107, 1976

87. Feld R, Valdivieso M, Bodey GP, et al: Antimicrobial activity in serum and urine as a therapeutic guide in bacterial infections. J Infect Dis 129:187, 1974

88. Bodey GP, Rodriguez V, Valdivieso M, et al: Amikacin treatment of infections in patients with malignant disease. J Infect Dis 134(suppl):5421, 1976

22

Feline Myocardial Disease

Philip R. Fox

Cardiomyopathies are structural or functional abnormalities of the myocardium. The term *primary cardiomyopathy* denotes myocardial disorders that exclude diseases resulting from ischemic, hypertensive, vascular, pulmonary parenchymal, acquired valvular, congenital, or other cardiovascular derangements.[1-3]

Classification schemes have been proposed using physiologic, pathologic, or clinical features, although no single method defines all variables completely (Table 22-1). The folllowing features have been used to characterize myocardial disease: (1) primary or idiopathic (describes the heart muscle as the sole source of disease whose etiology is unknown) and secondary (relates the myocardial disorder to identifiable systemic or metabolic disease); (2) etiology (e.g., carnitine or taurine deficiency cardiomyopathy); (3) pathology (e.g., infiltrative cardiomyopathy); (4) clinical presentation (e.g., congestive cardiomyopathy); (5) myocardial structure (e.g., hypertrophic or dilated cardiomyopathy), and (6) myocardial function (e.g., systolic or diastolic failure).[1-35] Strict categorization is not always possible, and intergrade and merging forms are common (Table 22-2). Progressive changes in cardiac chamber structure and function may occur,

and categories may overlap. Current concepts favor classifications of intergrading cardiac performance (e.g., systolic or diastolic dysfunction) with heart chamber morphology.[1,2,11-14,18,19,24,25,27-34] This has been facilitated through the growing availability of echocardiography.

INCIDENCE

Cardiomyopathies represent the majority of feline cardiovascular diseases. A necropsy survey of 4,933 feline autopsies reported an 8.5 percent incidence of primary myocardial disease versus a 1.9 percent occurrence of congenital heart defects.[8] The clinical incidence has been estimated at 12 to 15 percent when secondary cardiomyopathies are taken into consideration.[16]

DIAGNOSTIC APPROACH

Historically, diagnosis and treatment have been based on structural classification inferred from history, physical examination, electrocardiography (ECG), and plain-film radiography. While this data

Table 22-1 Classification of Feline Myocardial Diseases

Primary (idiopathic) cardiomyopathies
    Hypertrophic
    Dilated (congestive)
    Restrictive
    Intermediate of intergrade

Secondary cardiomyopathies
    Metabolic
        Endocrine
            Thyrotoxicosis
            Acromegaly
            Uremia[a]
        Nutritional
            Taurine deficiency
            Selenium/vitamin E deficiency[a]
            Obesity
    Infiltrative
        Neoplasia
        Glycogen storage diseases[a]
        Mucopolysaccharidosis[a]
        Leukemia
    Fibroplastic
        Endomyocardial fibrosis
        Endocardial fibroelastosis
    Hypersensitivity[a]
    Physical agents
        Hyperpyrexia
        Hypothermia
    Toxic
        Doxorubicin
        Catecholamines
        Lead
        Ethanol
    Inflammatory
        Infectious
            Viral[a]
            Bacterial
            Protozoal
            Fungal
            Algal
        Noninfectious collagen diseases[a]
    Genetic
        Hypertrophic cardiomyopathy[a]
        Dilated cardiomyopathy[a]
        Endocardial fibroelastosis
    Miscellaneous
        Ischemia
        Muscular dystrophy[a]
        Conduction system disorders
        Excessive left ventricular moderator bands[b]

[a] Suspected but not proved.
[b] Association and contribution to myocardial diseases unclear.

Table 22-2 Necropsy Classification: 452 Cats with Myocardial Disease[a] (10/81–4/84), The Animal Medical Center

Morphologic Classification	No. of Cats	Percentage of Total
Dilated cardiomyopathy	109	24
Hypertrophic cardiomyopathy	144	32
Restrictive cardiomyopathy	19	4
Intermediate or intergrade cardiomyopathy	180	40

[a] Includes primary and secondary cardiomyopathies.

base is often suitable for diagnosing heart disease in dogs (especially canine dilated cardiomyopathy), it is insufficient for accurate classification of feline myocardial disorders. Nonselective angiocardiography may provide additional information about cardiac chamber morphology and suggest abnormal hemodynamic states (e.g., prolonged circulation time).[27–29] However, these findings are often inaccurate in all but classic forms of cardiomyopathy. Moreover, sedation and radiographic contrast agents are associated with significant morbidity and mortality in decompensated patients or when arrhythmias are present. Echocardiography provides a rapid noninvasive technique for assessing cardiac structure and function and is the preferred diagnostic modality when available.[31–34]

Heart failure should be clinically approached as a syndrome resulting from systolic or diastolic dysfunction associated with morphologic cardiac changes. Congestive signs and related hemodynamic abnormalities can then be appropriately treated while potential etiologic factors are investigated with laboratory and other diagnostic procedures.

PRIMARY CARDIOMYOPATHIES

Heart Failure Due to Systolic Dysfunction

Systolic dysfunction, or myocardial or pump failure, results when the ventricles fail to generate normal contractile force. Classically, all four cardiac chambers are greatly dilated, cardiac output is severely reduced, end-systolic and end-diastolic ventricular volumes are increased, and myocardial wall tension is elevated.[1,2] Congestive heart failure results from both depressed contractility and failure (or overcompensation) of neuroendocrine, hepatorenal, and peripheral vascular compensatory mechanisms. Systolic dysfunction varies from mild to severe and is coupled with heterogenous structural variations. Prognosis is not directly related to indices of contractility.

Dilated (Congestive) Cardiomyopathy

Etiology

Dilated cardiomyopathy (DCM) in classic form results in profound cardiac dilatation, severely reduced contractility, and cardiogenic shock. A wide variation in degree of systolic impairment and structural change occurs, however. The reported incidence of DCM varies from approximately 17 to 20 percent of necropsies[8,26] to about 40 percent in clinical studies.[18] This may be attributable to dissimilar criteria for classification, changes in causative factors (e.g., nutrition), or regional population differences.

The etiology of primary (idiopathic) DCM is unknown. It may represent the end-stage result of myocardial injury caused by various metabolic, toxic, or infectious agents.[1,2,21,35] Taurine deficiency has recently been associated with DCM and reversible myocardial failure in cats.[21] Myocardial toxins including anthracyclines (especially doxorubicin)[3,36,37] and cyclophosphamide[38] have induced DCM in humans and animals. Microvascular hyperreactivity with myocytolysis, reactive hypertrophy and progressive systolic dysfunction has been demonstrated in the Syrian hamster.[39] Familial transmission in humans is considered rare.[1,2,40] Metabolic deficiencies have been demonstrated in human familial DCM, including carnitine deficiency.[41,42] Carnitine-linked defects of myocardial metabolism have been demonstrated in association with canine DCM.[43] Infective (viral) and immunologic factors have been implicated in some cases of DCM based on myocardial nuclear changes, high viral antibody titers in some affected people, circulating immune complexes in cases of human myocarditis-associated DCM, and immuunoregulatory defects.[44–46] Selenium deficiency has been associated with DCM in man (Keshan's disease)[47,48] and animals,[3,49] although it has not been proven to be the sole cause of myocardial disease.

PATHOPHYSIOLOGY

Depressed ventricular contractile performance (i.e., systolic or pump dysfunction) is the predominant function abnormality.[1,2] Cardiac chamber dilation may be present prior to clinical signs if stroke volume is maintained by compensatory mechanisms (e.g., sympathetic, renal, and hormonal responses; increased end-diastolic fiber length). Sinus tachycardia may contribute to maintain cardiac output in canine DCM, but this finding is uncommon in affected cats. Elevated ventricular end-diastolic pressures may result from reduced systolic emptying and increased end-systolic residual volume. Alterations in left ventricular relaxation and diastolic compliance coexist with impaired contractile function and contribute to elevated filling pressures.[50,51] Ventricular dilatation causes geometric distortion of the atrioventricular (AV) valve apparatus, leading to mitral regurgitation.[3,6,12,18,20,24,25] This further reduces forward stroke volume and contributes to left atrial dilatation. The latter predisposes to atrial arrhythmias, especially atrial fibrillation.[52,53] Sudden arrhythmias often herald acute cardiac decompensation, although the ECG may be normal in some cases. With atrial fibrillation or other tachyarrhythmias, resultant loss of atrial systole and reduced time for diastolic filling decreases cardiac output. Inadequate forward flow produces clinical signs of low output failure (Table 22-3) as muscles and organs become poorly perfused. Decreased renal perfusion stimulates the renin-angiotensin-aldosterone system, which increases cardiac preload and afterload. Enhanced sympathetic activity also increases preload and peripheral vascular resistance. The latter further reduces cardiac output.[1,2] Ventricular hypertrophy may occur as a compensatory mechanism to reduce wall tension and pressure according to the law of Laplace.[54] Congestion, effusions, and signs of low cardiac output ultimately develop. Cardiogenic shock may result.

PATHOLOGY

Necropsy reveals a globular heart with severe dilation of all four cardiac chambers (see Fig. 32-11). Heart weights are significantly greater than normal. Ventricular walls become abnormally thin, although various degrees of compensatory hypertrophy may be present. Papillary muscles and trabeculae are atrophied. Focal endocardial fibrosis may be present. AV valve circumference is usually enlarged but valve leaflets are normal. Cardiac muscle cells may display various degrees of degeneration ranging from coagulation, granulation, and sarcoplasmic vacuolization to myocytolysis.[3,9,11-14,18,19,25,26,55]

CLINICAL FINDINGS

Signalment suggests young to middle-aged cats. Ages range from 5 months to 16 years, with a mean of about $7\frac{1}{2}$ years.[9,18] All breeds are affected; Siamese, Abyssinian, and Burmese breeds display a particularly high incidence. Reports of sex predisposition vary from male dominance[9] or slight female dominance,[16] to relatively equal distribution.[24,25]

Presenting clinical signs are usually vague. They include anorexia, dyspnea, lethargy, or emesis for 1 to 3 days duration. Paresis of a front or rear leg results from acute embolization. Syncope is rare.[18,19,24,25]

Physical examination reveals lethargy, depression, and dehydration (usually 5 to 8 percent). Hypothermia is usually present or is recorded shortly after admission. Auscultation may detect a gallop rhythm (usually S_3) and a left and/or right apical systolic heart murmur. Lung sounds may reveal crackles due to pulmonary edema. Alternatively or in addition, heart and lung sounds may be muffled if significant pericardial or pleural effusion is present. The left cardiac apex beat (precordial impulse) and femoral arterial pulse are weak. Hydroperitoneum and hepatomegaly can occur if right-sided heart failure is present (Table 22-3 above).

Electrocardiography displays normal sinus rhythm in about one-half of affected cats, while bradycardia is recorded in less than one-fourth. The reported incidence of left ventricular enlargement (R wave in lead II greater than 0.9 mV or QRS complex

Table 22-3 Clinical Features of Heart Failure Due to Systolic (Myocardial or Pump) Failure

Forward heart failure (i.e., decreased cardiac output, reduced tissue perfusion)
    Dyspnea (subacute or chronic)
    Lethargy
    Depression
    Weakness
    Reduced cardiac apex beat
    Muffled or soft heart sounds
    Hypokinetic femoral pulses
    Hypothermia

Backward heart failure (i.e., elevated venous pressures behind the failing ventricles)
    Dyspnea
    Muffled heart/lung sounds (effusions)
    Hepatomegaly
    Hydroperitoneum
    Peripheral edema (rare)

Other Findings
    Cardiomegaly
    S_3 gallop rhythm
    Vomiting
    Murmur (mitral/tricuspid insufficiency)
    Various arrhythmias

Examples
    Idiopathic dilated cardiomyopathy
    Taurine deficiency myocardial failure
    Doxorubicin cardiotoxicity

duration greater than 0.04 seconds) is 25 to 39 percent.[18,25] Ventricular premature complexes have been recorded in almost one-half of affected cats in one study[18] but less commonly by other investigators.[6,12,25] Various other arrhythmias are occasionally detected.

Radiographs classically display generalized severe cardiomegaly, which is often silhouetted by pleural effusion (Fig. 22-1). Pulmonary venous congestion or mild pulmonary edema may be present concurrently but is often obscured. A characteristic round, globoid ventricular apex may be evident in the ventrodorsal view. A dilated caudal vena cava, hepatomegaly, and hydroperitoneum may be present[6,7,11-14,16,18-20,24,25,29,30] (Table 22-4).

Nonselective angiocardiography may display moderate left atrial enlargement, severe left and right ventricular dilation, atrophic papillary mus-

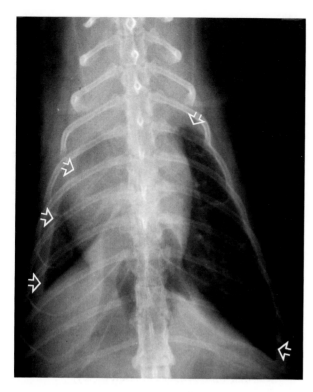

Fig. 22-1 Dorsoventral thoracic radiograph of an 8-year-old male domestic short-hair cat with dilated cardiomyopathy and right-sided congestive heart failure. Pleural effusion is present, causing the lung lobes to retract (arrows) and silhouetting the cranial heart. Severe generalized cardiomegaly is evident.

cles, reduced aortic diameter, and slow circulation time[11–14,18,19] (Table 22-4; Fig. 22-2). Hazards associated with angiocardiography are due to tranquilizer-related arrhythmias and adverse reactions to contrast medium.[28] Thus, it should not be performed in severely decompensated animals.

Echocardiography provides rapid, safe, and accurate noninvasive evaluation of cardiac function as well as structure (Fig. 22-3). Diagnostic features include greatly enlarged ventricular end-diastolic and end-systolic dimensions; significantly depressed indices of left ventricular contractility (e.g., decreased left ventricular ejection time, prolonged pre-ejection period, decreased fractional shortening, and prolonged velocity of circumferential fiber shortening; aortic root, interventricular septal, and left ventricular free wall hypokinesis); moderate left atrial and severe right ventricular dilation.[12,16,18,19,24,25,31–34]

Left ventricular free wall and interventricular septal thickness may be reduced or appear normal if compensatory hypertrophy has occurred.

Clinical laboratory abnormalities are common.[11–13,24,25] Most cats are azotemic (e.g., blood urea nitrogen, 35 to 60 mg/dl; normal = 20 to 30 mg/dl) resulting from reduced cardiac output, decreased water consumption, anorexia, and fluid sequestration (effusions). Low plasma taurine levels (less than 20 nM/ml) occur in cats fed taurine-deficient diets.[21] Mild hyperglycemia may be present. With thromboembolic disease, coagulopathies are common. Disseminated intravascular coagulation may occur in association with consumptive coagulopathy, liver-mediated coagulopathy, or from effects of thromboembolism. In addition, elevation in serum lactic acid dehydrogenase, creatinine phosphokinase, alanine aminotransferase (SGPT), and aspartate aminotransferase (SGOT) are recorded during thromboembolism.[56,57]

Differential diagnosis includes other causes of congestive heart failure. Congenital cardiac anomalies must be considered, especially lesions causing volume overload (e.g., ventricular septal defect, AV valve dysplasia, common AV canal). Pericardiodiaphragmatic hernia and pericardial diseases may cause generalized severe cardiomegaly. Acquired valvular disease, endocarditis, and heart-base tumors are rare. All causes of pleural effusion must be evaluated. These include feline infectious peritonitis, chylothorax, pyrothorax, neoplasia, and other systemic or metabolic disorders. Thyrotoxicosis and hypertrophic or restrictive cardiomyopathy may also cause right-sided heart failure. Since cardiogenic shock may dominate the clinical presentation diseases inducing a shocklike state must be considered.

Treatment of Heart Failure Due to Systolic (Pumping) Dysfunction

The overall goals for therapy of disorders resulting from systolic failure (e.g., dilated cardiomyopathy) are listed (in Table 22-5).[1,2,11–14,18,19,21,22–25,36,41,43,58–68] Treatment may be divided into immediate and maintenance therapeutic strategies. Drug doses are listed (in Table 22-6).

Table 22-4 Nonselective Angiocardiographic Features
of Myocardial Diseases

Structural Characteristic	Type of Cardiomyopathy		
	Dilated	Hypertrophic[a]	Restrictive
Left ventricle			
Shape	Globular	Slitlike	Irregular (intracavitary fibrosis)
Dilation	↑ ↑ ↑	0	0 or ↑
Hypertrophy	0	↑ ↑ ↑	↑ ↑ or ↑ ↑ ↑
Papillary muscles	Thin	Hypertrophied	Hypertrophied
Systolic volume	↑ ↑	↓ or ↓ ↓	N or ↓
Diastolic volume	↑ ↑ ↑	N or ↓	N or ↓
Left atrium			
Size	↑	↑ ↑ or ↑ ↑ ↑	↑ ↑ or ↑ ↑ ↑
Mitral regurgitation	↑	↑ or ↑ ↑	↑ ↑ or ↑ ↑ ↑
Right ventricle			
Size	↑ ↑ ↑	N to ↑ ↑	N to ↑ ↑
Congestive heart failure			
Left sided	↑	↑ ↑ ↑	↑ ↑
Right sided	↑ ↑ ↑	↑ (↑ ↑ ↑ late)	↑ (↑ ↑ ↑ late)
Circulation time	↓ ↓ ↓	N or ↑	N, ↓, ↑

[a] Cannot easily differentiate from left ventricular hypertrophy caused by thyrotoxicosis.
N, normal; 0, absent; ↑, mild; ↑ ↑, moderate, ↑ ↑ ↑, severe.

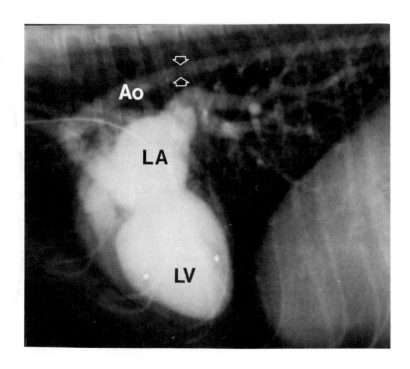

Fig. 22-2 Nonselective angiocardiogram of a young adult domestic short-hair cat with dilated cardiomyopathy. The left atrium (LA) is moderately enlarged and the left ventricle (LV) is severely dilated. Papillary muscles are thin and atrophic (asterisks). The aorta (Ao) is thin and poorly opacified (arrows) suggesting reduced contractility and diminished forward stroke volume. There is residual contrast material in the pulmonary artery.

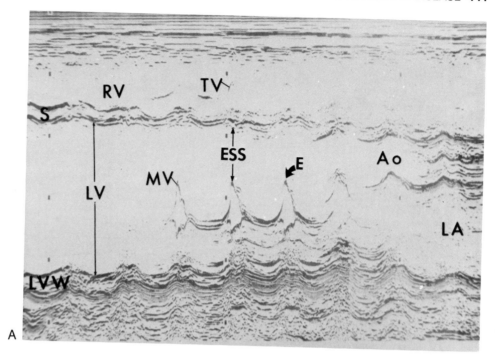

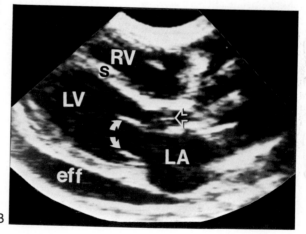

Fig. 22-3 (**A**) M-mode echocardiogram from a 3-year-old female domestic short-hair cat with dilated cardiomyopathy recorded from the right intercostal position. From left to right, the transducer is rotated from the left ventricular apex to the aortic root/left atrial position. The left and right ventricles (LV, RV) are severely dilated. Interventricular septal (S) and left ventricular posterior wall (LVW) motion is hypokinetic, indicating reduced myocardial contractility. The E point (E) of the anterior mitral valve (MV) is widely separated from the septum indicating LV dilation. The left atrium (LA) is severely enlarged. TV, tricuspid valve; Ao, aortic root; ESS, E-point septal separation. (**B**) Two-dimensional echocardiogram (long-axis view) recorded from the right intercostal position from a 4-year-old male Siamese cat with dilated cardiomyopathy. The left ventricle (LV), right ventricle (RV), and left atrium (LA) are severely dilated. Pericardial effusion (eff) is present. Closed curved arrows, mitral valves; open arrow, aortic valve. (**A** modified from Bond BR, Fox PR: Advances in feline cardiomyopathy. Vet Clin North Am 14:1021, 1984.)

Table 22-5 Therapeutic Strategies for Treating Systolic (Myocardial) Failure (e.g., Dilated Cardiomyopathy)

Optimize ventricular performance
  Pharmacologic intervention of
    Preload (ventricular filling pressure)
    Afterload (resistance to ventricular emptying
    Contractility
    Heart rate and rhythm
Eliminate congestive signs (edema, effusion)
  Diuretics
  Vasodilators
Correct contributing factors
  Treat etiologic causes
    Taurine deficiency
  Manage precipitating diseases
    Severe anemia
    Thyrotoxicosis
Administer special therapies
  Aspirin (if thromboembolism)
  Fluid administration (shock, dehydration)
  Mechanical fluid removal
    Thoracocentesis
    Pericardiocentesis
  External (environmental) heat supplementation
Avoid cardiosuppressive or toxic agents
  Withhold negative inotropes
    β-Adrenergic blockers (e.g., propranolol)
    Calcium-channel blockers (e.g., verapamil)
  Avoid cardiotoxic therapies
    Chemotherapy (e.g., doxorubicin)
Modify (individualize) therapy
  Correct dietary imbalances
  Reduce or eliminate cardiac drugs, where possible

IMMEDIATE THERAPY

Mechanical fluid removal (thoracocentesis) to reduce the physical restraint on lung expansion should be initiated when auscultation reveals muffled heart and lung sounds associated with dyspnea; 100 to 300 ml of pleural effusion may be removed acutely without untoward effects. A mild pneumothorax may result if the needle punctures a lung, but this rarely poses a clinical problem. I prefer a 19- to 21-gauge 1.9-cm-long butterfly needle (Medi-Wing, Sherwood Medical). Further diagnostic tests (e.g., ECG, radiographs) may then be done more safely.

Diuretics are administered as a next step to reduce edema or effusion by inhibiting renal tubular reabsorbtion of sodium or its accompanying anions.[66]

Furosemide, a potent loop diuretic, is most commonly selected (Lasix, Hoechst). Cats are highly sensitive to its effects; the initial dose is 1.1 mg/kg IV or IM bid. Diuresis may occur within 30 minutes. For cats previously receiving oral maintenance furosemide, this dose is sometimes increased to 2.2 mg/kg bid to tid. Overzealous administration, however, may severely reduce ventricular filling (preload), cause azotemia and electrolyte abnormalities, reduce cardiac output, and prolong renal clearance of certain drugs (e.g., digoxin).[11–14,16,18,19,24,25,66,67] Homeostatic factors (e.g., aldosterone, antidiuretic hormone) may eventually diminish diuretic action.[67]

Positive inotropic agents are administered to stimulate the depressed myocardium based on the presumption of adequate myocardial or contractile reserve.[61–65] Classically, digoxin (Lanoxin, Burroughs Wellcome) has been used. Intravenous digitalization has been advocated in severely affected cats employing a total calculated dose of 0.005 mg/kg lean body weight. One-half the dose is injected, followed 1 hour later by one-fourth of the total calculated dose. The last one-fourth of the dose is repeated but may be omitted if ECG evidence of digitalis toxicity (e.g., progressive bradycardia, development of AV block or other arrhythmia) occurs.[11–14,24,25]

Synthetic sympathomimetic amines possess greater inotropic activity than digoxin and provide a finer control for acute management of cardiogenic shock. Dopamine (Intropin, American Critical Care), a norepinephrine precursor, directly stimulates cardiac β₁-adrenergic receptors as well as causing release of myocardial stores of norepinephrine.[70] The latter mechanism may limit its efficacy if such stores are depleted.[71] At lower doses, it stimulates renal dopaminergic receptors promoting renal cortical blood flow and diuresis. At high doses, it stimulates α₁-adrenergic receptors, resulting in increased systemic arterial and venous pressures.[72,73] This vasoconstrictor activity is undesirable, as it increases impedance to ventricular ejection. Tachycardia, arrhythmias, and increased myocardial oxygen demand are other potential adverse effects. Recommended dose is 2 to 5 μg/kg/min administered by constant-rate infusion.

Dobutamine (Dobutrex, Lilly) exerts its positive inotropic effects through stimulation of myocardial

Table 22-6 Drugs Used in the Treatment of Feline Myocardial Diseases

Drug	Use	Feline
Positive inotropes	Increase myocardial contractility	
Digoxin (lanoxin, Burroughs Wellcome)	Life-threatening supraventricular arrhythmias	Rapid IV:0.005 mg/kg IV divided (half initially, then $\frac{1}{4}$ of total calculated dose at $\frac{1}{2}$ to 1 hr. intervals)
	Maintenance inotropic support	Maintenance (oral): 1.9–3.2 kg–0.031 mg (i.e., $\frac{1}{4}$ of 0.125 mg tab) q 48–72 hr; 3.3–6.0 kg–0.031 mg q 24–48 hr; 6.0 kg–0.031 mg sid to bid
Dobutamine (Dobutrex, Lilly)	Short-term inotropic support	2–10 μg/kg/min IV CRI
Dopamine (Intropin, American Critical Care)	Same	2–5 μg/kg/min IV CRI
Diuretics	Reduce congestion, effusions	
Furosemide (Lasix, Hoechst)		1.1–4.4 mg/kg IV, IM, PO, sid to tid
Hydrochlorthiazide-spironolactone (Aldactazide, Searle)		2.2–4.4 mg/kg PO bid
Hydrochlorthiazide (Hydrodiuril, Merk)		2 to 4 mg/kg PO bid

α- and β-adrenergic receptors.[64,74,75] It has little effect on heart rate or blood pressure, when administered at doses of 5 to 10 μg/kg/min, exerts a lesser effect on the sinoatrial (SA) node (and therefore heart rate) than on myocardial tissue and does not stimulate renal dopaminergic receptors.[58,64,76] Attenuation of hemodynamic effects have been reported in man requiring upward dose titration.[77] However, improved exercise performance and functional classification have resulted from short-term dobutamine administration.[78,79]

A common adverse side effect of dobutamine administration in cats is seizures.[12,24,25] These are typically focal facial seizures, but occasionally become generalized. Seizures have been observed at infusion rates as low as 5 μg/kg/min. They stop as soon as the dobutamine infusion is discontinued, and often do not reoccur when the dose is reduced by 50 percent. If seizures continue at the reduced dosage, dopamine may be substituted for dobutamine.

A new class of potent inotropic drugs has emerged whose action involves inhibition of cardiac phosphodiesterase F-III. These nonadrenergic, nonglycoside inotropes also possess mild to moderate arteriolar dilating properties.[65] Amrinone (Inocor, Sterling) has been used in dogs (1 to 3 mg/kg IV bolus followed by a constant rate infusion of 10 to 100 μg/kg/min) for short-term inotropic support. The dose in cats may be similar, but pharmacokinetics have not been reported. Milrinone, a derivative of amrinone, has been studied experimentally but is not yet commercially available. It has been shown to improve left ventricular contractile force in cats when infused at 1 μg/kg/min. An oral dose of 0.5 to 1.0 mg/kg bid has proved effective in dogs, but similar studies have not been completed in cats.[80]

The use of β-adrenergic blocking drugs in human dilated cardiomyopathy has been controversial. They are intended to protect against increased sympathetic tone accompanying heart failure.[81,82] However, lack of improvement has been reported,[83] as well as clinical deterioration associated with withdrawal of the β-blocking therapy.[84] At present, propranolol is administered to cats to slow the ventricular rate when supraventricular tachyarrhythmias are unresponsive to digoxin or for management of ventricular arrhythmias.[11-14,18, 24,25] The use of β-adrenergic blockers in situations in which heart rate and rhythm are controlled is speculative and potentially deleterious.

Judicious fluid therapy is beneficial to combat the effects of shock and circulatory failure. Intravenous fluid supplementation helps prevent severe reduction in preload (and cardiac output) and reduces vascular volume contraction caused by diuretics, anorexia and shock. A mixture of 0.45 percent NaCl (or half-strength lactated Ringer's solution) with 2.5 percent dextrose in water (D_5W) is given at a submaintenance dose of 20 to 35 ml/kg/day slowly IV, in two or three divided doses. Potassium chloride must often be supplemented (e.g., 5 to 7 mEq for each 250 ml fluids). Serum electrolytes should be monitored. The infusion rate and dose varies with each patient and must be balanced to optimize cardiac output without exacerbating pulmonary edema or effusions.[11,12,24,25] Central venous pressure (CVP) monitoring may provide a helpful guide to gauge infusion rate. Increases in CVP exceeding 2.5 cm H_2O within 30 minutes may indicate hypervolemia.[85] In such situations, the fluid infusion rate should be reduced by 50 percent, or infusion temporarily discontinued. If pulmonary edema develops, prompt discontinuation of fluids should be followed by an IV bolus of furosemide (1.1 mg/kg). Subcutaneous fluid administration may then be substituted for the IV route.

Vasodilators are theoretically useful to reduce resistance to left ventricular ejection and thereby improve cardiac performance. They should not be given if hypotension or cardiogenic shock is present unless blood pressure can be maintained with other agents (e.g., dopamine). Their place in the therapeutic strategy of this disease has not yet been clearly defined and efficacy is still undetermined. Nevertheless, several agents have been advocated on the basis of subjective clinical experience. Two percent nitroglycerin ointment (Nitro-Bid, Marion) has profound venodilating effects, and some action on arteriolar beds. It has significant action on cutaneous and skeletal muscle beds with lesser activity in visceral organs.[86] However, the venodilating action may actually reduce cardiac output in heart failure

states in which ventricular filling pressures are not elevated.[87] Hydralazine, an arteriolar dilator, has been used (0.5 to 0.8 mg/kg bid) with subjective improvement in a small number of cats.[19] Captopril (Capoten, Squibb), an angiotensin enzyme converting inhibitor, is a balanced vasodilator that acts on both arterial and venous beds. Its efficacy in treating heart failure has been documented in humans[88,89] and dogs.[90] In cats, captopril has been dosed at 3.12 to 6.25 mg PO bid to tid. Anorexia and hypotension (manifested as weakness and lethargy) are the most common side effects.[12,24,25]

Since hypothermia is common during the decompensated state, external environmental heating is an important adjunct to therapy. This is easily accomplished using a heat lamp placed at an appropriate distance to avoid thermal burns. Supplemental environmental heating should be continued until a compensated state is achieved.

Dramatic improvements have been reported after oral taurine supplementation in cases in which myocardial failure is associated with taurine deficiency.[21] Therefore, this amino acid is supplemented immediately (500 mg PO bid) whenever dilated cardiomyopathy is suspected. Clinical improvement may take 1 to 2 weeks to be apparent. Thus, the immediate therapy described above is necessary to stabilize the patient pending potential response to taurine administration.

MAINTENANCE THERAPY

If cardiogenic shock can be reversed and the heart failure state compensated, oral drug maintenance may be instituted. Drug-related toxicity, dehydration, decreased cardiac output (e.g., overzealous preload reduction) and prerenal azotemia constitute common problems during the first 3 to 7 days of therapy.

Furosemide is given at 1.1 to 2.2 mg/kg sid to bid. Higher doses (2.2 to 4.4 mg/kg bid to tid) may be required to manage recurrent heart failure or in refractory cases.[11-14,24,25] A combination of hydrochlorthiazide and spironolactone (Aldactazide, Searle) has also been used (2.2 to 4.4 mg/kg) for chronic maintenance,[18,19] although the thiazide may be ineffective in the presence of renal dysfunction.[91] Since prerenal azotemia is common in affected cats, furosemide is often preferred. Diuretic dosage must be specifically tailored to individual needs, and administration should be temporarily discontinued if anorexia, azotemia, or dehydration occur.

Digoxin may be given in pill or elixir form. Although higher plasma levels and more accurate dosing can be achieved with the elixir,[92,93] it is less palatable to cats. The 0.125-mg tablet is readily tolerated, but its small size inhibits accurately dividing it into less than one-fourth of a tablet (0.031 mg).[11,12] Males may develop higher serum levels than females of the same body weight, and food administered in conjunction with digoxin may decrease drug absorption.[92,93] The biologic half-life of digoxin in healthy cats given a single IV injection is 33.3 ± 9.5 hours. The mean half-life after chronic oral administration of elixir (0.05 mg/kg bid) was 79 hours (range, 33 to 202 hours),[94] indicating that digoxin elimination is capacity limited in the cat.

Digoxin toxicity is a greater clinical problem than is underdigitalization. Anorexia and depression are early signs of toxicity.[11–14,16,24,25] Vomiting accompanies more severe intoxication. Clinical illness in normal cats given toxic doses may last up to 96 hours.[92,93] In cardiomyopathic cats with reduced cardiac output and renal insufficiency, digoxin toxicity may persist up to seven days.[12,24,25] Toxic plasma concentrations in healthy cats ranged from 2.4 to 2.9 ng/ml,[94] but some cardiomyopathic cats display clinical signs of toxicity at half this level (Fox PR, unpublished data). Concurrent therapy with digoxin tablets (0.01 mg/kg PO q48h), aspirin (80 mg/kg Q48H), furosemide (2 mg/kg PO bid), and commercial low-salt diet (h/d, Hills) predisposed normal cats to digoxin toxicity. The precise mechanism of altered digoxin kinetics was not identified.[95] The most striking ECG evidence of digoxin toxicosis in one study was ST segment elevation, and PQ interval prolongation may be noted at nontoxic concentrations.[94] The maintenance dose is highly individualized and may vary with disease progression. Based on a calculated dose of 0.005 to 0.01 mg/kg lean body weight and normal renal function, the following guidelines are suggested: for cats weighing 1.9 to 3.2 kg, one-fourth of a 0.125-mg digoxin tablet every 2 to 3 days; for cats weighing 3.3 to 6.0 kg, one-fourth of a tablet daily or every other day; and for cats weighing more than 6.0 kg, one-fourth tablet daily (occasionally, bid)[11–12,24,25]

Vasodilator drugs have been used for maintenance therapy in compensated cats unable to tolerate digoxin or where a significant component of mitral insufficiency is suspected. Captopril dosed at 3.12 to 6.25 mg (one-eighth to one-fourth of a 25-mg tablet) bid to tid may be tolerated in this setting for long periods.[11,12]

Dietary modifications should include elimination of diets with low taurine formulations. Oral taurine supplementation should continue if concern exists about dietary deficiency or when plasma taurine is less than 20 nM/ml.[21] Prescription diets for sodium restriction (h/d, Hills) may be tried or home preparation formulas used.

Prognosis during the period of initial management (cardiogenic shock) is generally guarded to poor, but is improving as a result of advances in diagnostic recognition (especially by echocardiography), refinements in therapeutic protocols, and identification of myocardial failure associated with taurine deficiency. Mortality is highest during the first 5 to 7 days. If extracardiac signs of edema or effusions can be controlled, hydration maintained, and taurine supplemented, many cats resume eating and prognosis improves. Thromboembolic disease is a grave complication. Cardiogenic shock confers a poor prognosis although some will respond to aggressive therapy. Survival exceeding 4 years has occasionally been observed.[11,12] Taurine supplementation may improve the outcome in taurine-deficient cats, and clinical signs may improve within 2 to 3 weeks of this therapy. Echocardiographic changes (e.g., left ventricular end-diastolic and end-systolic dimensions, fractional shortening) begin to improve in approximately 3 weeks.[21] In some individuals, systolic function may improve dramatically, and maintenance cardiac drugs may be discontinued. The incidence of taurine deficiency dilated cardiomyopathy is the focus of current investigations.

Heart Failure Due to Diastolic Dysfunction

Ventricular hypertrophy or fibrosis may result from various primary or secondary myocardial disorders[3–20,23–26] that decrease left ventricular compliance (i.e., increase myocardial stiffness) and impede diastolic filling. Systolic (pumping) function is usually adequate. Clinical signs result from diastolic dysfunction caused by impaired ventricular relaxation, myofibrillar architectural disarray, abnormal ventricular cavity shape, endomyocardial fibrosis, or ventricular cavity distortion.[1–3,96,97]

Left ventricular hypertrophy is an important compensatory response to chronic left ventricular pressure or volume overload.[98] It may be observed with various systemic, metabolic, or infiltrative diseases, or in athletic individuals, or it may be idiopathic. Hypertrophy may represent an appropriate, adaptive response or be associated with depressed cardiac function and structural changes.[1–3,12,15,17, 18,25] The clinical significance of left ventricular hypertrophy and its therapeutic and prognostic implications depend on accurate characterization of causative factors and their correction, where possible. Echocardiography is the most accurate noninvasive method to detect hypertrophy. All potential identifiable causes of left ventricular hypertrophy (e.g., thyrotoxicosis, renovascular hypertension, pressure overload) should be investigated. Angiographic or echocardiographic evidence of left ventricular hypertrophy does not therefore automatically equate with a diagnosis of idiopathic hypertrophic cardiomyopathy.

Hypertrophic Cardiomyopathy

ETIOLOGY

Hypertrophic cardiomyopathy (HCM) is a common feline myocardial disorder with a heterogeneous morphologic expression. The etiology is unknown. Human studies have demonstrated familial transmission with an autosomal-dominant mode of inheritance as well as nonfamilial varieties.[99–101] Other possible etiologies include enhanced myocardial responsiveness to circulating catecholamines or excessive catecholamine production,[102] abnormal compensatory hypertrophy resulting from myocardial ischemia or fibrosis,[101,103] and a primary collagen abnormality with secondary ventricular hypertrophy.[104] It may be possible that HCM is not a single disease but represents a group of etiologically different disorders.[101]

PATHOPHYSIOLOGY

Although it is morphologically heterogeneous, HCM characteristically represents increased muscle mass due to a hypertrophied nondilated left ventri-

cle. The principal pathophysiologic consequence is elevated left ventricular end-diastolic pressure in the face of a normal or reduced end-diastolic volume.[1,2,6,101] Global left ventricular diastolic function is adversely affected through several interrelated abnormalities.[101,105–107] A decrease in early rapid diastolic filling results from reduced ventricular distensibility (i.e., compliance) and prolonged (or incomplete) relaxation.[105,106] Increased muscle stiffness may be caused by fibrosis or myocardial cell disorganization,[108] while ventricular chamber stiffness results from increased muscle stiffness and muscle mass (hypertrophy).[101] Mitral regurgitation develops from distortional changes in the mitral valve apparatus (resulting from ventricular hypertrophy) or from interference with normal mitral valve closure due to anterior motion of the mitral valve during mid-systole.[101,109] The left atrium dilates in response to increased end-diastolic pressures, and pulmonary venous pressures eventually become elevated.

Left ventricular function is hyperdynamic.[110] Ventricular ejection may be nearly completed during the first third of the systolic ejection period.[108,111] The development of an intraventricular pressure gradient (i.e., a dynamic subaortic obstruction to left ventricular outflow) has received much attention in human HCM,[101] and has been demonstrated in the cat[6] and dog.[112] Affected individuals may exhibit anterior motion of the mitral valve leaflet across the outflow tract to the ventricular septum during early systole. This may cause mechanical impedence to left ventricular ejection, increase systolic intraventricular pressures, myocardial wall stress, and oxygen demand.[101] The clinical incidence and role of dynamic subaortic pressure gradients in dogs and cats, however, is unknown.

PATHOLOGY

The principal pathologic feature of primary (idiopathic) HCM is abnormal left ventricular hypertrophy and increased ventricular muscle mass in absence of a causative systemic or cardiac disease. A number of nonspecific but predictable characteristics may be present:

1. Left ventricular hypertrophy is a hallmark and may vary in pattern and extent in humans[102] and

animals.[3,6,8,9,55,112–117] In dogs, disproportionate thickening of the ventricular septum (asymmetric septal hypertrophy) is the rule.[112,114–116] In cats, about two-thirds to three-fourths of affected animals have symmetric left ventricular hypertrophy.[116,117]

2. Ventricular septal disorganization (greater than 5 percent of the tissue section) has been reported in 27 percent of affected cats. This occurred only in those with asymmetric septal hypertrophy.[116,117]

3. Fibrous connective tissue may be present focally or diffusely in the endocardium,[8,55,115–117] conduction system,[117] or myocardium.[8,55]

4. Narrowed small intramural coronary arteries are recognized histologically[55,101] and may be components of the hypertrophied ventricle.

5. Heart weight/body weight ratio is increased.[116]

6. Decompensated animals may display evidence of left and/or right-sided congestive heart failure, although the former is more common in cats.[11,12,55,114–117]

7. Thromboembolic disease frequently accompanies cardiac decompensation in felines but not canines.[12]

CLINICAL FINDINGS

There is a wide age range of affected cats (5 months to 17 years),[7,15,116,117] with a mean age of 4.8[19] to 7 years.[116] Domestic short-hair cats are most frequently reported followed by the domestic longhair. The Persian breed may be predisposed.[6,9] This disease is rare in the Siamese, Burmese, and Abyssinian breeds which are instead predisposed to dilated cardiomyopathy. Males are more commonly affected and represent 23 to 87 percent of reported studies.[6,8,18,55,116,117]

The predominant clinical sign is acute dyspnea associated with pulmonary edema or biventricular failure (Table 22-7). Anorexia and vomiting may precede clinical signs by 1 or 2 days. Paresis of a front leg or posterior paralysis may result from thromboembolic disease. Sudden death may occur.[7,11,12,18,19,24,25]

Auscultation may disclose a diastolic gallop rhythm, usually the fourth heart sound (S_4), rales, soft systolic murmur (I to II/VI) over the mitral and/

Table 22-7 Clinical Features of Heart Failure Due to Diastolic Dysfunction (Decreased Ventricular Compliance)

Forward cardiac output usually adequate

Backward heart failure (i.e., elevated venous pressures behind failing ventricle)
  Dyspnea (acute)
  Tachypnea
  Pulmonary rales/rhonchi
  Normal heart sounds (unless effusions)
  Normal or accentuated cardiac apex beat
  Normal femoral pulses
  Hypothermia

Other findings
  Cardiomegaly
  S_4 gallop rhythm
  Murmur (mitral/tricuspid insufficiency)
  Left anterior fascicular block
  Various arrhythmias
  Vomiting

Examples
  Hypertrophic cardiomyopathy
  Restrictive cardiomyopathy

or tricuspid valve areas and arrhythmias. Heart and lung sounds will be muffled if significant pleural or pericardial effusion is present. The left precordial apex beat is usually palpably normal or hyperdynamic. Paresis and absence of femoral arterial pulses accompany distal aortic thromboembolism.[7,11–14,18,19,24,25]

Electrocardiographic abnormalities have been recorded in 35 to 70 percent of affected cats.[6,19] The most commonly reported findings are conduction disturbances of which only left anterior fascicular block is most consistent. The latter is rare in other forms of primary myocardial diseases. Left ventricular enlargement patterns (QRS greater than 0.04 second; R_{II} greater than 0.9 mV) are present in some cats but are not diagnostic for HCM. Arrhythmias occcur in one-fourth to one-half of affected cats with ventricular premature complexes predominating.

Plain-film radiography may show mild to moderate left ventricular enlargement with moderate to severe left atrial enlargement (Table 22-4). The latter is particularly obvious on the dorsoventral view. Pulmonary venous congestion, interstitial and/or alveolar pulmonary densities (suggesting pulmonary edema), and occasionally slight pleural effusion occur most commonly. Pulmonary edema in cats may be patchy and focal (Fig. 22-4) rather than located in the perihilar region as with dogs. Severe diffuse edema is rarely seen with systolic failure (i.e., dilated cardiomyopathy) but is common with diastolic dysfunction (i.e., hypertrophic or restrictive cardiomyopathies). With chronic or advanced HCM, cardiomegaly may be generalized and accompany extracardiac signs of severe biventricular failure (e.g., pleural, pericardial or abdominal effusion, hepatosplenomegaly, pulmonary edema).[11–14,16,18,19,24,25]

Nonselective angiocardiography discloses left ventricular free wall hypertrophy, severe reduction of the left ventricular chamber (often slitlike in appearance) and extremely hypertrophied papillary muscles (Table 22-4; Fig. 22-5). The left atrium is moderately to severely dilated. Pulmonary veins may be tortuous due to elevated left ventricular end-diastolic pressure. Circulatory transit time may be normal or accelerated. Ball thrombi may occasionally be present in the left atrium or ventricle.[11–14,16,24,25,27–29]

Echocardiography is the most sensitive technique for evaluation of left ventricular hypertrophy (Fig. 22-6) and noninvasively allows assessment of myocardial function. Hypertrophy of the ventricular septum and left ventricular free wall, decreased left ventricular internal dimensions, normal to elevated fractional shortening, and right ventricular dilation (late in the disease course of some cases) may be evident. Left atrial enlargement is often marked. Pericardial or pleural effusion or left heart ball thrombi may be imaged. Occasionally, systolic anterior motion of the mitral valve and partial systolic closure of the aortic valve may be noted.[16,18,19,24,25,31–34]

Differential diagnosis must include all causes of

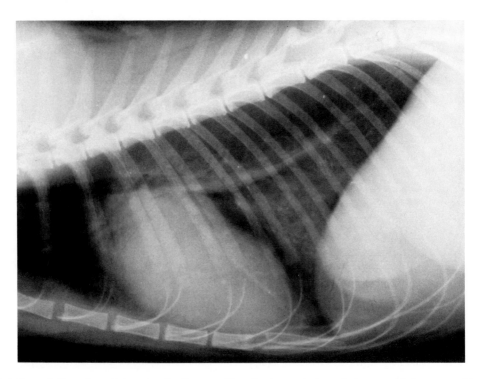

Fig. 22-4 Lateral thoracic radiograph of a 5-year-old male domestic long-hair cat with hypertrophic cardiomyopathy and left-sided congestive heart failure. There is a focal interstitial and alveolar pulmonary pattern caudal to the heart compatible with pulmonary edema. This infiltrate cleared after furosemide administration. Severe left ventricular enlargement is evident.

Fig. 22-5 Nonselective angiocardiogram of a 6-year-old male domestic short-hair cat with hypertrophic cardiomyopathy. The left atrium (LA) is extremely dilated. The left ventricular cavity is greatly narrowed due to hypertrophy of the myocardium and papillary muscles. There is residual contrast medium in the right ventricular outflow tract and pulmonary artery (asterisk). Ao, aorta; pv, pulmonary veins; LV, left ventricular cavity. (Modified from Fox PR: Feline cardiomyopathy. p. 157. In Bonagura JD (ed): Cardiology. Contemporary Issues in Small Animal Practice, Vol. 7. Churchill Livingstone, New York, 1987.)

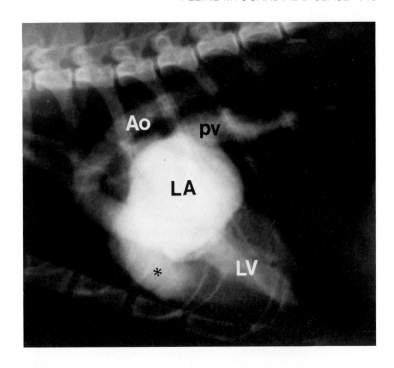

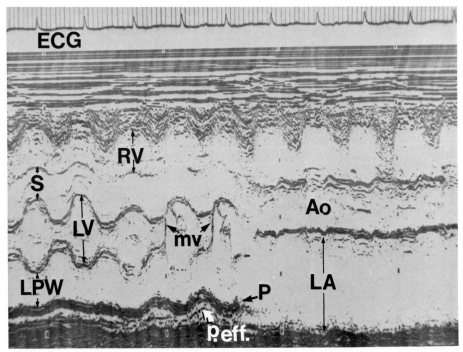

Fig. 22-6 M-mode echocardiogram of a 4-year-old male domestic short-hair cat with hypertrophic cardiomyopathy recorded at the right intercostal position. The transducer is rotated from left ventricular (LV) apex (left) to the aortic root (Ao) and left atrium (LA) at the base (right). The left ventricular posterior wall (LPW) and interventricular septum (S) are hypertrophied. The left atrium is severly dilated, and enlarged. A mild pericardial effusion (p. eff.) is evident. P, pericardium; mv, mitral valve; ECG, electrocardiogram.

left ventricular hypertrophy.[17] Congenital aortic stenosis, thyrotoxicosis,[15] restrictive and infiltrative cardiomyopathy,[8,12,24] and systemic hypertension[119] should be considered. Since right-sided congestive heart failure may be present, congenital and acquired heart diseases as well as extra-cardiac causes of effusions must be evaluated. Severe pericardial effusion may occasionally accompany HCM. Pericardial diseases and feline infectious peritonitis constitute other sources of pericardial effusion.[18,120]

Restrictive Cardiomyopathy

Restrictive cardiomyopathy occurs when diastolic ventricular volume and stretch (i.e., compliance) is impaired by endocardial, subendocardial, or myocardial fibrosis or infiltrative disease. It is characterized by elevated ventricular filling pressures with normal or near normal systolic function.[1,2,121-123] Hemodynamically, it resembles restrictive pericarditis. Limitation of ventricular filling reduces preload and ultimately, cardiac output. In cases of extensive endomyocardial fibrosis, the left ventricular chamber may become obliterated.

Confusion regarding terminology may occur, since some literature has designated restrictive cardiomyopathy under the terminology of intermediate cardiomyopathy.[18,19] Mild, diffuse, or focal fibrosis may accompany all forms of myocardial diseases but fibrosis does not constitute the predominant morphologic abnormality in most disorders,[8] nor does it significantly impair diastolic function. The term intermediate cardiomyopathy is better reserved for morphologic disorders characterized by ventricular dilatation with or without hypertrophy, often with mild to moderate reduction in systolic function.[12,24,25]

Restrictive cardiomyopathy is the least common of the feline primary (idiopathic) myocardial disorders. Primary RCM is not reported in the dog. Endocardial fibrosis without eosinophilia is the predominant form of primary feline RCM. Secondary causes are rare and result from infiltrative, neoplastic, or infectious disorders.[3,8,9,12-14,16,24,25,124] The etiology of the primary disease is unknown.

Reported ages vary from 8 months to 19 years.[8,9,18,19,124] There is no particular breed predisposition. A male predominance was reported at one institution,[8,9,124] and an approximately equal sex distribution at another.[18,19]

Clinical signs are quite variable and include left-sided failure (pulmonary edema), right-sided failure (pleural, pericardial, or abdominal effusion) or bi-ventricular heart failure. A high incidence of thromboembolic disease accompanies this disorder. Anorexia and vomiting may be present for a short but variable period of time. Clinical signs usually develop or worsen acutely.[8,9,12,18,19,24,25,124]

Physical examination findings usually include dyspnea, paresis (from thromboembolism), and hypothermia. Auscultatory abnormalities include muffled heart and lung sounds (from pleural effusions), rales (from pulmonary edema), gallop heart rhythms, systolic murmurs of mild to moderate intensity at the left and/or right cardiac apex, and irregularities in heart rate and rhythm. Femoral arterial pulse deficits and occasionally hepatomegaly or ascites may be palpated.[9,12,18,19,24,25]

Electrocardiographic abnormalities have been recorded in 31[9] to 70[19] percent of affected cats. Left atrial and ventricular enlargement patterns are common. Ventricular and supraventricular arrhythmias are frequently recorded.

Plain radiography usually displays an interstitial and alveolar pattern associated with pulmonary edema or moderate to severe pleural effusion. A globoid cardiac silhouette occasionally results from pericardial effusion. If pericardial or pleural effusion is absent or minimal, dramatic left atrial enlargement may be evident. This is typified on the lateral view by a large left atrial bulge elevating the trachea over the heart base and on the dorsoventral view by pronounced left auricular enlargement. The left ventricle may be enlarged in both radiographic projections. Pulmonary veins are often prominent and tortuous. Hepatomegaly and mild to moderate ascites may be present.[12,18,19,24,25,124]

Nonselective angiocardiography has provided the most sensitive means of clinical diagnosis, although it is associated with slight morbidity and mortality. Characteristic changes include left ventricular hypertrophy with an irregular, often obliterated, left ventricular cavity, severe left atrial enlargement, and tortuous pulmonary veins (Table 22-4; Fig. 22-7). Left atrial or ventricular thrombi may be present.[9,11-14,16,19,24,25,28]

Catheterization has demonstrated mitral regurgitation, left ventricular filling defects, and mor-

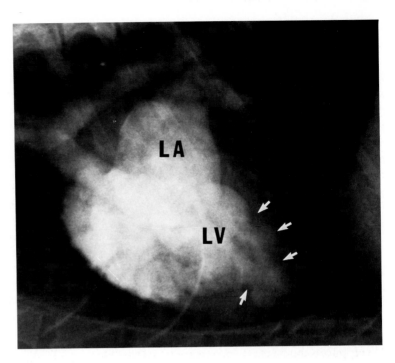

Fig. 22-7 Nonselective angiocardiogram of a 9-year-old female domestic short-hair cat. The left atrium (LA) is severely dilated. The left ventricle (LV) is hypertrophied and irregular, especially at the apex and caudal wall (arrows) and displays many filling defects. At necropsy there was extensive endocardial fibrosis compatible with restrictive cardiomyopathy. (Fox PR: Feline cardiomyopathy, p 170. In Bonagura JD (ed): Contemp Issues Small Anim Pract. Vol 7. Churchill Livingstone, New York, 1987)

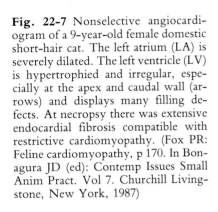

phologic mid-left ventricular stenosis. Intraventricular pressure gradients correlating with these structural alterations have been demonstrated.[9,20]

Echocardiography may demonstrate hypertrophy of the left ventricular septum and free wall, severe left atrial enlargement, normal to mildly depressed indices of left ventricular performance (i.e., fractional shortening, velocity of circumferential fiber shortening), and occasionally abnormal or depressed motion of the ventricular septum or left ventricular free wall. The left ventricular internal dimensions are usually reduced. With M-mode echocardiography, a sweep from the apex to mitral valve position often discloses an irregular ventricular chamber filled with extraneous echoes. These are associated with extensive fibrosis and occasionally cavity obliteration. Two-dimensional echocardiography confers the ability to better visualize loss of normal left ventricular chamber symmetry and permits visualization of distorted fused papillary muscles. Increased endocardial echogenicity has been observed. Right ventricular dilation is often evident.

Gross pathologic findings include a heart weight to body weight ratio greater than normal due to increased left ventricular mass (hypertrophy). Extreme left atrial and auricular enlargement is common. Hypertrophy of the left ventricle with pronounced diffuse endocardial thickening and myocardial fibrosis is the pathologic hallmark. Fibrous adhesions between the papillary muscles and myocardium, distortion and fusion of chordae tendineae, and mitral valve leaflets may be seen. Aortic or cardiac chamber thromboemboli may occur.[3,8,9,12,124]

Differential diagnosis must include all forms of heart disease that result in ventricular hypertrophy and congestive heart failure. Since left ventricular hypertrophy is a dominant feature of RCM and older cats are often affected by this disease, thyrotoxicosis and systemic hypertension must be considered. Secondary causes of increased endomyocardial echogenicity and left ventricular chamber obliteration must include neoplastic and infectious diseases. Constrictive pericarditis may clinically resemble RCM.

Treatment of Heart Failure Associated with Diastolic Dysfunction

Hypertrophic and restrictive cardiomyopathy may progress along several pathophysiologic pathways: (1) diastolic dysfunction, (most common); (2)

dynamic subaortic obstruction (uncommon); (3) myocardial fibrosis and ishemia; and (4) a burnout phase resulting in end-stage depression of ventricular contractility. Clinical signs may therefore result from one or more of these factors. Therapy for heart failure resulting from hypertrophic or restrictive cardiomyopathy should ideally employ strategies tailored toward the underlying predominant abnormality and individualized on the basis of clinical signs and echocardiographic findings[1,2,59,101,121] (Table 22-8)

Hypertrophic Cardiomyopathy

Therapeutic strategies have been modified for cats from human protocols.[1,2,11–14,16,18,19,24,25,59,101,121] Responses are variable, and therapy must be individualized. Diuretics and β-adrenergic blockade have long been the cornerstone of medical therapy (Tables 22-6 and 22-8).

Diuretics are initially administered (furosemide 1.1 mg/kg IV or IM bid to tid) to reduce left ven-

Table 22-8 Therapeutic Strategies for Treating Heart Failure Due to Diastolic Dysfunction (Hypertrophic Cardiomyopathy)

Eliminate congestive signs (pulmonary edema, effusions)
    Diuretics
    Mechanical fluid removal

Reduce diastolic dysfunction
    Improve ventricular compliance
    Decrease contractility, increase, ventricular filling
    β-Adrenergic blockade (e.g., propranolol)

Manage arrhythmias
    Supraventricular
        Digoxin; propranolol
    Ventricular
        Propranolol; lidocaine

Avoid drugs or conditions predisposing to dynamic left ventricular outflow obstruction
    Positive inotropes (e.g., digoxin)
    Arteriolar dilators (e.g., captopril, hydralazine)
    Severe preload reduction (overdiuresis)
Administer special therapies
    Aspirin (if thromboembolism)

tricular end-diastolic, mean left atrial, and pulmonary capillary pressures. After 24 to 36 hours, dosing may be decreased to sid or bid and changed from parenteral to oral. Pulmonary edema is usually very responsive to this potent loop diuretic agent. Thereafter, furosemide is gradually reduced to the lowest effective dose. Some cats remain stable on 1.1 mg/kg given every other day. Alternatively, maintenance therapy with a hydrochlorthiazide-spironolactone combination drug (Aldactazide, Searle) may be used (2.2 mg/kg/day).[18,19]

With disease progression, left-sided heart failure may worsen and right-sided heart failure develop. This requires upward dose titration of furosemide (2.2 to 4.4 mg/kg tid). Refractory right-sided heart failure may respond to the addition of a second diuretic agent acting at a different site in the nephron (e.g., hydrochlorothiazide, 1 to 2 mg/kg PO bid). While furosemide rarely causes electrolyte imbalance, combination diuretic therapy must be monitored closely for azotemia, hyponatremia, or hypokalemia.[12,24,25]

In cases of severe fulminating pulmonary edema, the initial furosemide dose may be increased to 2.2 mg/kg IV or IM bid or tid. Supplemental oxygen therapy (40 to 60 percent oxygen-enriched inspired gas) in these cases may be beneficial to improve pulmonary gas exchange by increasing the driving force for oxygen diffusion into alveolar capillaries. Preload reduction can be enhanced with 2 percent nitroglycerin ointment ($\frac{1}{8}$ to $\frac{1}{4}$ inch applied cutaneously to the ear pinna every 4 to 6 hours for 24 to 36 hours).[11–14,24,25]

β-Adrenergic blockade with propranolol has been the mainstay of medical human treatment. It inhibits sympathetic cardiac stimulation and diminishes myocardial oxygen requirements by reducing heart rate, left ventricular contractility and systolic myocardial wall stress.[125–127] Left ventricular diastolic compliance may improve indirectly through reduction of heart rate or myocardial ischemia.[121,128] While similar beneficial effects have not been proved with feline HCM, propranolol is still advocated for these reasons. Oral dose is 2.5 mg bid to tid in cats weighing less than 6 kg and 5 mg bid to tid in cats weighing more than 6 kg. Propranolol is usually administered 24 to 36 hours after diuretic therapy is initiated, unless sinus tachycardia or ventricular arrhythmias are present. In the latter case, it is coadministered with diuretics. The questions of whether prophylactic therapy for asymptomatic patients is warranted has not been answered.

Calcium-channel blockers, especially verapamil, have been shown to be effective in management of human HCM. Multiple factors contribute to their clinical effectiveness, including reduction in heart rate, blood pressure, a mild negative inotropic effect (reducing myocardial oxygen consumption),[129] and improvement of rapid diastolic ventricular filling.[130] Unfortunately, clinical trials with this drug are lacking in cats. Until further research is completed, verapamil cannot be recommended.

Certain drugs have been considered harmful in human hypertrophic cardiomyopathy based on their propensity to increase dynamic left ventricular outflow obstruction. They include drugs that increase contractility (digitalis), lower arterial pressure, or decrease ventricular volume (overdiuresis, vasodilators).[1,2,101,121] Occasionally, however, use of these drugs may be considered. Severe right-sided heart failure unresponsive to diuretics and dietary sodium restriction may require digitalis, as may supraventricular tachycardias. Vasodilators (e.g., captopril have also been used for refractory right-sided failure. Untoward effects have not been clinically observed by the author with these drugs in stated situations.

Prognosis is guarded to good, depending on disease progression, concomitant arrhythmias, and development of thromboembolic disease. Atrial fibrillation or severe, refractory right-sided congestive heart failure confers a poor prognosis. Thromboemboli may be associated with acute decompensation. If the heart failure state can be successfully managed, distal aortic embolism and associated signs may resolve. Repeated embolic episodes, however, usually follow. Sudden death may occur, but survival exceeding 6 years has been observed.

Restrictive Cardiomyopathy

Treatment involves managing pulmonary edema; pleural, pericardial, or abdominal effusions; and arrhythmias. Therapeutic strategies are similar to those listed for hypertrophic cardiomyopathy and are most successful with uncomplicated left-sided failure. Success may be short-lived due to throm-

boembolic disease, exacerbation of heart failure, or malignant arrhythmias.

HEART FAILURE ASSOCIATED WITH MYOCARDIAL DISEASES OF UNSPECIFIED OR MIXED MYOCARDIAL DYSFUNCTION

Intergrade or Intermediate Cardiomyopathies

Myocardial diseases may be progressive or regressive. During their natural course they may exhibit various structural alterations (e.g., dilation and hypertrophy) within one or both functional categories of systolic or diastolic dysfunction. The cardiomyopathic process may not be clearly definable from history, physical examination, or radiographic or angiocardiographic findings. Variable states of compensation and heart failure may develop over time.[12,24,25] Intergrade or intermediate cardiomyopathies are common. Thus, frequent diagnostic reevaluations, especially with echocardiography, are often required for accurate and timely characterization of the disease state. Serum taurine levels should be checked in cats displaying systolic (pumping) failure. Diets should be appropriately modified or taurine supplemented.

EXCESSIVE LEFT VENTRICULAR MODERATOR BANDS AND HEART FAILURE

A pathologic syndrome has been reported in which distinct changes in cardiac structure with abnormal moderator bands have been associated with heart failure. These changes relate to abnormal moderator band networks bridging the left ventricular septum, free wall, or papillary muscles.[10-12] The heart weight to body weight ratios in these cats are lower than in other forms of primary cardiomyopathy (Chs. 19 and 32).

Abnormal, diffuse moderator band networks have been identified in these cats with congestive heart failure and myocardial structural changes.[10] Since they have been identified in kittens as young as 1 day of age, in some cases at least, aberrant moderator bands may represent a form of congenital heart disease. In other cases, individuals up to 13 years old have been identified with abnormal moderator band networks, cardiac dilation, or hypertrophy and congestive heart failure.

Clinical findings are quite variable and include anorexia, dyspnea, hypothermia, left- and/or right-sided congestive heart failure, gallop rhythms, systolic heart murmurs, thromboembolic disease, and arrhythmias. ECG changes in 21 reported cases included right bundle branch block in six cats, left anterior fascicular block in four cats, first- and third-degree AV block in three cats, and sinus bradycardia in four cats. Cardiomegaly was a consistent radiographic finding. Cardiac catheterization in two cats demonstrated normal systolic but elevated left ventricular end-diastolic pressure (30 to 40 mmHg). Necropsies reveal a tendency for left ventricular hypertrophy in younger cats (mean age, 4 years) or dilation in older cats (mean age, 8.7 years). Microscopic myocardial changes were similar to those recorded with dilated and hypertrophic forms of cardiomyopathy.[10]

Diagnosis is often difficult due to heterogeneous nature of clinical and structural abnormalities. Nonselective angiocardiography has been insensitive for identifying moderator band networks. Recently, M-mode and two-dimensional echocardiography have facilitated moderator band recognition and provides valuable information about cardiac structure and function. Moderator bands may be imaged in the left ventricular cavity and traversing the ventricular septum and free wall[12,24,25] (Fig. 22-8).

Differential diagnoses include aortic or mitral valve vegetations, flail aortic or mitral valves, pedunculated thrombi, and tumors.[131,132] Other forms of primary or secondary myocardial disease may mimic the heart failure state associated with this abnormality.

Treatment of Heart Failure Associated with Intermediate Cardiomyopathy

Therapy is individualized on the basis of predominant pathophysiologic manifestations and clinical findings (Tables 22-3 through 22-5 above). Furosemide is administered (1.1 to 2.2 mg/kg IV or IM) to aleviate extracardiac manifestations of congestive failure (pulmonary edema, effusions). Digoxin is

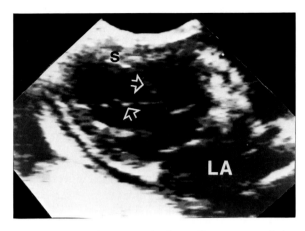

Fig. 22-8 Two-dimensional echocardiogram recorded at the right intercostal position from a young domestic short-hair cat (long-axis view). An aberrant network of moderator bands traverses the interventricular septum (S) and left ventricular posterior wall (arrows). The left atrium (LA) is enlarged and mild pericardial effusion is present.

added (as described under feline DCM) if severe right-sided heart failure or supraventricular tachyarrhythmias are present. Lidocaine (0.25 to 1.0 mg/kg IV over 5 minutes) or propranolol (2.5 to 5 mg PO bid to tid) is administered for serious ventricular arrhythmias (frequent or multifocal ventricular premature complexes or ventricular tachycardia). Oral taurine supplementation and dietary change is necessary in taurine deficient cats. Other contributory factors (e.g., hyperthyroidism) must be detected and corrected.

THROMBOEMBOLIC DISEASE ASSOCIATED WITH CARDIOMYOPATHY

Thromboembolism is a frequent complication associated with feline myocardial disorders.[3–14,16,18–20,24,25,29,55–57,133] Thrombosis is clot formation within a cardiac chamber or vessel lumen. Embolization occurs when a clot or other foreign material lodges within a vessel. At necropsy thromboembolism has been reported in up to 48 percent of myopathic cats (e.g., 48 percent in HCM,[4–6] 29 percent in RCM,[8] 25 percent in DCM,[5,6] and 14 percent with excessive left ventricular moderator bands[10]).

The overall clinical incidence of feline thromboembolism, however, is less than indicated by autopsy data.

Distal aortic (saddle) embolization occurs in more than 90 percent of cats affected with thromboembolic disease. The brachial artery may sometimes be occluded, and mural thrombi are occasionally present in the left atrium or ventricle.[8] Various other organs may become embolized.

PATHOPHYSIOLOGY

Pathogenesis of thrombosis involves one or more of three essential conditions[134-136]: (1) local vessel or tissue injury, (2) circulatory stasis, and (3) altered blood coagulability. Because these factors are variably present in cardiomyopathic cats, thromboembolic disease is a consistent complication.

Pathologic changes involving atrial and ventricular endothelial surfaces may present reactive surfaces to circulating blood. This may trigger a thrombotic process by inducing platelet adhesion and aggregation with subsequent activation of the intrinsic clotting cascade. Endocardial thickening may occur with all myocardiopathies and is most common with the restrictive and hypertrophic forms.[8] These lesions may be patchy, focal, or diffuse and are composed of hyaline, fibrous, and granulation tissue with collagenous fibers.

Blood flow may be altered in myopathic hearts. Left atrial and auricular enlargement results from mitral regurgitation or elevated end-diastolic pressure. Regional circulatory stasis may result. Intracavitary stasis may follow functional or anatomic mid-ventricular stenosis (especially in the apical region)[20] or may accompany chronic heart failure.[136] Abnormal left ventricular moderator bands may contribute to altered circulation.[11]

Hypercoagulable states commonly accompany thromboembolic disease in cardiomyopathic cats. Disseminated intravascular coagulation associated with consumptive coagulopathy, liver-mediated coagulopathy, or thromboembolism was present in more than 75 percent of affected cats in one study.[56] In addition, feline platelets are very reactive and responsive to serotonin-induced aggregation.[137] Serotonin is a vasoactive amine released from platelets during the platelet release reaction and is present in high concentration in feline platelets.[138]

Collateral circulation plays a critical role in clinical thromboembolic disease. For example, experimental distal aortic ligation does not duplicate the clinical syndrome caused by a saddle embolus. However, experimentally induced aortic thromboembolism simulates the naturally occurring syndrome.[139,140] This underscores the importance of vasoactive substances (e.g., serotonin) released by the clot and their effects on collateral circulation.[141] Chemicals such as thromboxane A_2 also cause vasoconstriction.[142] Its synthesis can be reduced by antiprostaglandin drugs such as aspirin.[143]

Ischemic neuromyopathy is a predictable consequence of arterial occlusion and in particular, of clot associated inhibition of collateral circulation.[144] Ischemia abolishes rapid axoplasmic neuronal flow causing conduction failure, which becomes irreversible after 5 or 6 hours. Distal aortic (saddle) embolization causes peripheral nerve lesions starting at the mid thigh region. The majority of nerve fibers display Wallerian-type degeneration while some exhibit damage to the myelin sheath only. Clinically, duration of initial ischemia is sufficient to cause loss of peripheral nerve function and induce pathological neuromuscular changes. Focal necrosis, myophagia, and architectural changes may be evident histologically.[144] Distal limbs below the stifle are most severely injured. Cranial tibial muscles are more effected than gastrocnemius muscles, inhibiting hock flexion more than extention. Hip flexion and extension is maintained. The result is a dragging motion of the hind legs. Distal limb sensation is severely affected.[56]

CLINICAL MANIFESTATIONS

Clinical signs are attributable to congestive heart failure (e.g., dyspnea) or effects of specific organs or arteries embolized (e.g., azotemia from renal infarction) (Table 22-9). Most cats present with a lateralizing posterior paresis due to saddle embolus at the distal aortic trifurcation. Anterior tibial and gastrocnemius muscles are often firm or become hard by 12 to 18 hours after embolization due to ischemic myopathy. Occasionally, a single brachial artery is embolized, causing monoparesis. Renal, mesenteric, or pulmonary embolization may cause death. Intermittent claudication is occasionally the only clinical complaint.[56]

Table 22-9 Clinical Findings Associated
with Thromboembolism

Acute pain
Vocalization

Acute paresis
Lateralizing posterior paresis
Monoparesis
Intermittent claudication

Pallor–affected footpads

Pulselessness—affected limbs

Hypothermic distal limb extremities

Firm gastrocnemius and cranial tibial muscles

Cyanotic vascular nail beds

Congestive heart failure
Dyspnea
Tachypnea
Weakness
Anorexia
Cardiomegaly
Pulmonary edema
Effusions
Murmur/gallop rhythm
Arrhythmias

Laboratory abnormalities
Prerenal azotemia
Elevated alanine aminotransferase
Elevated aspartate aminotransferase
Elevated lactate dehydrogenase
Elevated creatine phosphokinase
Hyperglycemia
Lymphopenia
Disseminated intravascular coagulation

DIAGNOSTIC EVALUATION

If thromboembolism is suspected based on history and clinical signs a minimum data base should be generated. This includes thoracic radiographs, an ECG, a biochemical profile, and feline leukemia virus test.

Approximately one-half of affected cats have heart murmurs or gallop rhythms. Common ECG abnormalities include supraventricular arrhythmias, cardiac chamber enlargement (especially left atrium and ventricle), and left anterior fascicular block. Most affected cats appear clinically dehydrated. This is usually reflected by mild prerenal azotemia.

Serum concentrations of alanine aminotransferase (SGPT) and aspartate aminotransferase (SGOT) are elevated by about 12 hours and peak by 36 hours postembolization, indicating hepatic and skeletal muscle inflammation and necrosis. Lactate dehydrogenase (LDH) and creatine phosphokinase (CPK) enzymes are greatly increased shortly after embolization indicating widespread cellular injury. They may remain elevated for weeks. Hyperglycemia, mature leukocytosis, and lymphopenia may be present.[56]

Thoracic radiographs typically display cardiac chamber enlargement. Most affected cats have associated extracardiac signs of congestive heart failure (e.g., pulmonary edema, pleural effusion).

Echocardiography provides rapid, noninvasive assessment of cardiac structure and function and detects intracardiac thrombi when present. It facilitates early accurate characterization of the cardiomyopathic disorder and assists in formulating appropriate therapy and prognosis.

Nonselective angiocardiography in the stabilized patient aids diagnosis if echocardiography is not available. It provides additional information by determining the anatomic extent of thromboembolism and assessing collateral flow (Fig. 22-9).

Differential diagnoses for acute posterior paresis should include trauma, intervertebral disc extrusion, spinal lymphosarcoma, and fibrocartilagenous infarction. However, physical examination findings coupled with the presence of a gallop rhythm, arrhythmia, or radiographic evidence of heart failure are often diagnostic.

TREATMENT

Therapy is directed toward managing the heart failure state as previously discussed. Propranolol should be avoided, as it has no demonstrated antithrombotic effects[145] and may enhance peripheral vasoconstriction through β-adrenergic receptor blockade.

Surgical embolectomy is contraindicated. This is because affected cats are a high surgical risk due to decompensated heart failure, hypothermia, disseminated intravascular coagulation, and arrhythmias.[11–14,24,25,56,57,146] In addition, significant ischemic neuromyopathy has usually occurred in most instances preoperatively. It is not surprising

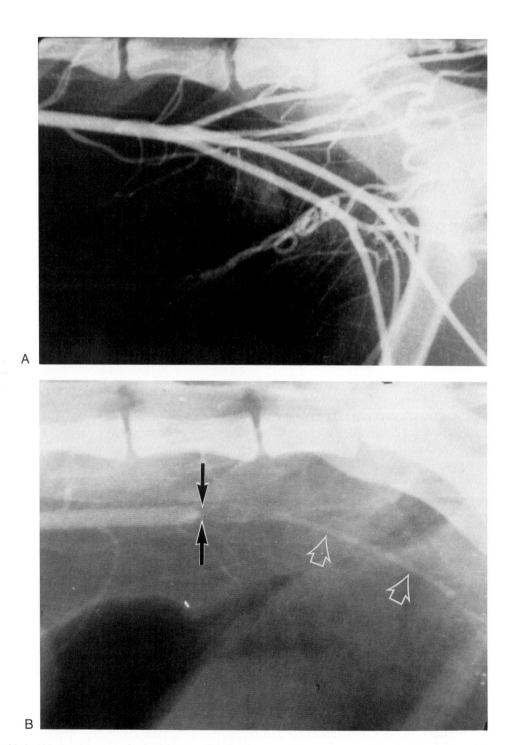

Fig. 22-9 (A) Angiogram of a healthy cat illustrating normal vascular anatomy in the region of the aortic trifurcation. **(B)** Distal aortic saddle embolus (closed arrow). There is a small column of contrast dye distal to the block (open arrows) indicating partial recanalization.

that results of embolectomy have been poor. Embolectomy catheters have also proved ineffectual.[18]

Various medical treatments have been used for acute and chronic management of thromboembolic disease,[134,147] although most are empirical. Arteriolar dilation with acetylpromazine maleate and hydralazine has been proposed to improve collateral circulation.[18] However, vasodilation may not be uniform. With hydralazine; for example, splanchnic, coronary, cerebral, and renal blood flow is increased,[147] but flow to muscle beds is not dramatically altered.[148,149] Moreover, it has not been demonstrated that hydralazine or acetylpromazine alter platelet-induced reduction of collateral flow caused by vasoactive substances such as serotonin.

Thrombolytic agents have been widely used in man but are only recently being investigated in cats. Streptokinase administered in a model of experimentally induced feline aortic thromboembolism failed to produce significant improvement as measured by venous angiograms or thermal circulatory indices.[150] Some agents (e.g., streptokinase, urokinase) act by generating the nonspecific proteolytic enzyme plasmin through conversion of the proenzyme plasminogen. This causes a generalized lytic state with the incipient hazard of bleeding complications.[151] More ideal thrombolytic agents such as tissue plasminogen activator have higher specificity.[152] It has been administered to a small number of cats with spontaneous distal aortic thromboembolism with variable results.[154] Currently, this drug is prohibitively expensive.

Anticoagulants have no effect on established thrombi. Their use has been based on the premise that by retarding clotting factor synthesis or accelerating their inactivation, thrombosis from activated blood clotting pathways can be prevented.

Heparin acts by binding to antithrombin III, enhancing its ability to neutralize activated factors XII, XI, X, IX, and thrombin.[153] This prevents activation of the coagulation process. It is administered as an initial IV dose of 1,000 USP units, followed 3 hours later by 50 USP units/kg SC. The latter is repeated at 6- to 8-hour intervals.[18] The dose is then adjusted to prolong clotting time 2 or 2.5 times the pretreatment baseline index value. Bleeding is a major complication and clotting profiles must be evaluated.

Warfarin has been proposed for chronic oral maintenance in cats surviving an embolic episode.[18] This coumadin drug impairs hepatic vitamin K metabolism, a vitamin necessary for synthesis of procoagulants (factors II or prothrombin, VII, IX, and X).[155] The initial dosage (0.5 to 1.0 mg/day) is adjusted to prolong the prothrombin time to twice the normal value.[18] Beneficial results have not been clinically documented.

Anti-platelet aggregating drugs are theoretically beneficial during and after a thromboembolic episode to prevent further embolic events. Aspirin induces a functional defect in platelets by inactivation, through acetylation, of cyclo-oxygenase, an enzyme critical in thromboxane A_2 synthesis.[156,157] The latter is an arachidonic acid derivative that induces platelet activation. This occurs mainly through platelet adenosine diphosphate release, the common pathway in platelet aggregation.[135] Vasoconstriction results from released platelet thromboxane A_2 and serotonin.

Aspirin dosed at 1.25 mg per cat (about 25 mg/kg) effectively inhibits platelet function for 3 to 5 days.[145,158] Collateral circulation has been demonstrated to improve in aspirin treated cats with experimentally induced aortic thrombosis.[143] Recommended dose is one-fourth of a 5-grain tablet every second to third day.[11,12,143,145,158]

Much concern exists regarding potential inhibition of prostacyclin synthesis by aspirin.[159] Prostacyclin, the major cyclo-oxygenase product in vascular endothelium, causes vascular vasodilation[160] and inhibition of platelet aggregation.[161] The optimal aspirin dose that will inhibit thromboxane A_2 production but that will spare vascular endothelial prostacyclin synthesis has not yet been established for cats.

With successful management of the heart failure state, motor ability may begin to return within 10 to 14 days. By 3 weeks, significant motor function (i.e., hock extension and flexion) has often returned, typically better in one leg than in the other.[12,24,25,56] Recovery may be due to remyelination of nerves injured by ischemia. Ischemic myopathy affects the cranial tibial muscles more severely than others, which seems to correlate with later clinical return of hock flexional ability. Motor function may be completely normal by 4 to 6 weeks, although a conscious proprioceptive deficit or conformational abnormality (e.g., extreme hock flexion) may persist in one leg. Complete reinervation of damaged nerves may require more time.

PROGNOSIS

Short-term prognosis depends on the nature and responsiveness of the underlying myocardial disorder and heart failure state. Most affected cats experience additional thromboembolic episodes although post embolization survival of 4 years has been observed.

Secondary Cardiomyopathies

Secondary cardiomyopathy designates myocardial structural or functional alterations resulting from known systemic or metabolic abnormalities (Table 22-1 above). Overlap may occur between functional and structural categories. For example, neoplastic or fungal myocardial infiltration may cause secondary restrictive cardiomyopathy and diastolic dysfunction; doxorubicin toxicity and feline taurine deficiency may result in systolic dysfunction and dilated cardiomyopathy.[1–3,10–21,24,25, 42–49,124,162–165] As offending stimuli or etiologies are identified, the primary (idiopathic) cardiomyopathies will eventually be classified as secondary myocardial disorders. This should enable a more rational and effective approach toward prevention, treatment, or potentially cure.

Many noninfectious agents may directly or indirectly damage the myocardium. Injury may be acute or chronic, transient or permanent, dose or rate limited. Inflammation (myocarditis) may or may not be present. Stimuli for myocardial injury may involve drugs, chemicals, toxins, physical agents, nutritional disorders, and a variety of systemic and metabolic diseases.[1–3,17]

Hyperthyroidism is a polysystemic disorder resulting from excessive levels of the thyroid hormones thyroxine (T_4) and triiodothyronine (T_3). It is one of the most common feline endocrine disorders[162–180] with a reported incidence at one institution of approximately 1 of every 300 cats.[165] Alteration in cardiovascular hemodynamics are secondary to direct effects of thyroid hormone on the heart and increased adrenergic stimulation.[166–169] A hyperkinetic state may result with ensuing high output heart failure.[162,166–173] This condition is discussed in Chapter 12.

Cardiotoxicity may result from certain chemotherapeutic protocols or from chemical and physical agents. Arrhythmias (ventricular, supraventricular, and conduction abnormalities), dilated cardiomyopathy and congestive heart failure is reported in dogs receiving cumulative doses ranging from greater than 240 mg/m^2 to 150 mg/m^2 or less.[181,182] Cats appear more resistant to cardiotoxic effects of doxorubicin than do dogs. A chronic cumulative dose of 100 to 125 mg/m^2 did not result in cardiotoxicity when studied in 30 cats,[183] and arrhythmias were recorded in only 1 of 14 cats receiving up to 180 mg/m^2.[184] In another feline study three cats receiving higher doses (265 to 320 mg/m^2) displayed histologic cardiac lesions but no clinical signs of heart failure.[185]

Other agents may cause myocardial injury including hydrocarbons, mercury, arsenic, and selenium deficiency. Physical agents such as heat stroke and hypothermia, blunt or penetrating trauma, electric shock, or hypersensitivity reactions may be injurious as well.[1–3]

Secondary cardiac neoplasms greatly outnumber primary heart tumors in the cat[186,187] (Patnaik AK, personal communication, 1987). The heart is the most common site of hemangiosarcoma metastasis, but primary right atrial origin is rare.[186]

Lymphosarcoma occasionally infiltrates the myocardium. Approximately 10 to 15 percent of feline lymphosarcoma cases have histologic evidence of myocardial infiltration with neoplastic or atypical lymphocytes. This percentage increases to about 20 percent when cases of leukemia with lymphoma are considered (Patnaik AK, personal communication, 1987).

Myocarditis represents inflammation of myocytes, interstitium, or vascular structures. Clinical expression is variable ranging from asymptomatic focal inflammation to generalized myocarditis with fatal arrhythmias and congestive heart failure. Myocarditis of suspected viral origin was recorded in 25 cats.[124] Twenty-one had an acute clinical course composed of dyspnea, depression, and leukocytosis for 1 to 2 days prior to death. Subendocardial petechiae or diffuse hemorrhage, endoymocardial infiltration with lymphocytes and plasma cells, and myocytolysis were common findings. Other cats with chronic endomyocarditis and restrictive cardiomyopathy died of congestive heart failure. Severe, diffuse endocardial fibrosis was the prominant feature; endomyocardial fibrosis and arteriosclerosis was marked in advanced cases. Diagnosis of myocarditis is usually ellusive. Therapy is supportive. Congestive heart failure or arrhythmias are treated in standard fashion.

Toxoplasma gondii can occasionally cause myocarditis as part of a polysystemic process or in immunosuppressed animals. Immune suppression from drugs or disease (e.g., feline leukemia virus) may cause encysted bradyzoites to excyst rapidly, proliferate, and exacerbate myocarditis.[188] Neonatal toxoplasmosis and myocarditis (multifocal necrosis with tachyzoites) has been reported in kittens aged 18 and 32 days.[189] Death was probably due to pneumonia. In a group of 20 cats with toxoplasmosis, histologic lesions were found in 12 but were only severe in one cat. Cysts and bradyzoites were rare in these lesions and clinical signs of heart disease were usually absent.[18] Thus, *Toxoplasma* induced myocarditis is apparently overshadowed in most cases by its more dominant systemic effects.

Bacterial myocarditis can result from sepsis, bacterial endocarditis or pericarditis. Abscessation, valvular vegetation, or focal suppurative myocarditis may result. Fever and arrhythmias provide clinical suspicion. Echocardiography provides an accurate imaging technique for valvular vegetations[190] and can occasionally detect myocardial abscesses. Vegetative endocarditis is rare in cats and the mitral valve is most commonly involved.[8,18,190,191]

Miscellaneous myocardiopathies have been reported. Persistent atrial standstill associated with a fascioscapulohumeral-like skeletal muscular dystrophy occurs in dogs and with dilated cardiomyopathy in cats (especially Siamese).[192] Enlarged paper-thin atria are usually present. Myocardial fibrosis and focal myocarditis and necrosis are sometimes evident.

Two subclasses of genetic mucopolysaccharidosis (MPS), diseases resulting from defects in glycosaminoglycan metabolism, have been reported from cats—MPS I (Hurler's syndrome) in domestic short-haired cats[193] and MPS VI (Maroteaux-Lamy syndrome) in Siamese cats.[194] Cardiac involvement has not been significant in these cases, although it has been important in their human counterparts.[195]

Conduction system lesions in cats with cardiomyopathy may occur. They include AV nodal degeneration and fibrosis bundle branch infiltration and degeneration.[8,196]

REFERENCES

1. Wenger NK, Goodwin JF, Roberts WC: Cardiomyopathy and myocardial involvement in systemic disease. p. 1181. In Hurst JW (ed): The Heart. McGraw-Hill, New York, 1986
2. Wynne JW, Braunwald E: The cardiomyopathies and myocarditides. p. 1410. In Braunwald E (ed): Heart Disease. 3rd Ed. WB Saunders, Philadelphia, 1988
3. Van Vleet JF, Ferrans V: Myocardial diseases of animals. Am J Pathol 124:98, 1986
4. Tilley LP, Liu SK: Cardiomyopathy and thromboembolism in the cat. Fel Pract 5:32, 1975
5. Liu SK, Tilley LP, Lord PF: Feline cardiomyopathy. Recent Adv Stud Card Struct Metab 10:627, 1975
6. Tilley LP, Liu SK, Gilbertson SR, et al: Primary myocardial disease in the cat: A model for human cardiomyopathy. Am J Pathol 87:493, 1977
7. Harpster N: Feline cardiomyopathy. Vet Clin North Am 7:355, 1977
8. Liu SK: Pathology of feline heart diseases. Vet Clin North Am 7:323, 1977
9. Liu SK, Tilley LP: Animal models of primary myocardial diseases. Yale J Biol Med 53:191, 1980
10. Liu SK, Fox PR, Tilley LP: Excessive moderator bands in the left ventricle of 21 cats. J Am Vet Med Assoc 180:1215, 1982
11. Fox PR: Feline myocardial diseases. p. 337. In Kirk RW (ed): Current Veterinary Therapy. Vol. VIII. WB Saunders, Philadelphia, 1983
12. Fox PR: Myocardial diseases. In Ettinger SJ (ed): Textbook of Veterinary Internal Medicine. 3rd Ed. WB Saunders, Philadelphia, 1989
13. Fox PR, Tilley LP, Liu SK: The cardiovascular system. p 249. In Pratt PW (ed): Feline Medicine. American Veterinary Publications, Santa Barbara, CA, 1983
14. Tilley LP, Liu SK, Fox PR: Myocardial disease. p 1029. In Ettinger SJ (ed): Textbook of Veterinary Internal Medicine. 2nd Ed. Vol I. WB Saunders, Philadelphia, 1983
15. Liu SK, Peterson ME, Fox PR: Hypertrophic cardiomyopathy and hyperthyroidism in the cat. J Am Vet Med Assoc 185:52, 1984
16. Bond BR, Fox PR: Advances in feline cardiomyopathy. Vet Clin North Am 14:1021, 1984

17. Fox PR: Cardiovascular disorders in systemic diseases. p. 265. In Tilley LP, Owens JM (eds): Manual of Small Animal Cardiology. Churchill Livingstone, New York, 1985

18. Harpster NK: The cardiovascular system. p. 820. In Holzworth J (ed): Diseases of the Cat. Vol I. WB Saunders, Philadelphia, 1986

19. Harpster NK: Feline myocardial diseases. p. 380. In Kirk RW (ed): Current Veterinary Therapy. Vol. IX. WB Saunders, Philadelphia, 1986

20. Lord PF, Wood A, Tilley LP, et al: Radiographic and hemodynamic evaluation of cardiomyopathy and thromboembolism in the cat. J Am Vet Med Assoc 164:154, 1974

21. Pion PD, Kittleson MD, Rogers Q, et al: Myocardial failure in cats associated with low plasma taurine: A reversible cardiomyopathy. Science 237:764, 1987

22. Report of the WHO/ISFC task force on the definition and classification of cardiomyopathies. Br Heart J 44:672, 1980

23. Goodwin JF: Congestive and hypertrophic cardiomyopathies. A decade of study. Lancet 1:731, 1970

24. Fox PR: Feline myocardial diseases—A clinical approach. p. 57. Presented at the Proceedings of the Ninth Annual Kal Kan Symposium, Vernon, Calif, 1986

25. Fox PR: Feline cardiomyopathy. p. 157. In Bonagura JD (ed): Contemporary Issues in Small Animal Practice. Vol. 7: Cardiology. Churchill Livingstone, New York, 1987

26. Liu SK: Pathology of feline heart disease. p. 341. In Kirk RW (ed): Current Veterinary Therapy. Vol. V. WB Saunders, Philadelphia, 1974

27. Owens JM, Twedt DC: Nonselective angiocardiography in the cat. Vet Clin North Am 7:309, 1977

28. Fox PR, Bond BR: Nonselective and selective angiocardiography. Vet Clin North Am 13:259, 1983

29. Suter PF: Thoracic Radiography. A Text Atlas of Thoracic Diseases of the Dog and Cat. Peter F. Suter, Wettswil, Switzerland, 1984

30. Suter PF: The radiographic diagnosis of canine and feline heart disease. Comp Cont Ed 3:441, 1981

31. Pipers FS, Hamlin RL: Clinical use of echocardiography in the domestic cat. J Am Vet Med Assoc 176:57, 1980

32. Bonagura JD: M-mode echocardiography: Basic principles. Vet Clin North Am 13:299, 1983

33. Soderberg SF, Boon JA, Wingfield WA, et al: Echocardiography as a diagnostic aid for feline cardiomyopathy. Vet Radiol 24:66, 1983

34. Bonagura JD, Herring DS: Echocardiography: Acquired heart disease. Vet Clin North Am 15:1209, 1985

35. Adelman AG, Wigle ED, Felderhof CH, et al: Current concepts of primary cardiomyopathy. Cardiovasc Med 2:495, 1977

36. Greene HL, Reich SD, Dalen JE: How to minimize doxorubicin toxicity. J Cardiovasc Med 7:306, 1982

37. Ferrans VJ: Overview of cardiac pathology in relation to anthracycline cardiotoxicity. Cancer Treatm Rep 62:955, 1978

38. Gottdiener JS, Appelbaum FR, Ferrans VJ, et al: Cardiotoxicity associated with high dose cyclophosphamide therapy. Arch Intern Med 141;758, 1981

39. Factor SM, Minase T, Cho S, et al; Microvascular spasm in the cardiomyopathic Syrian hamster: A preventative cause of focal myocardial necrosis. Circulation 66:342, 1982

40. Berko B, Swift M: X-linked dilated cardiomyopathy. N Engl J Med 316:1186, 1987

41. Waber LJ, Valle D, Neill C, et al: Carnitine deficiency presenting as familial cardiomyopathy: A treatable defect in carnitine transport. J Pediatr 101:700, 1982

42. Rebouche CJ, Engel AG: Carnitine metabolism and deficiency syndromes. Mayo Clin Proc 58:533, 1983

43. Keene BW, Panciera DL, Regitz V, et al: Carnitine-linked defects of myocardial metabolism in canine dilated cardiomyopathy. Proceedings of the Fourth Annual Veterinary Medicine Forum. Vol II. 14:54, 1986 (abst)

44. Dec GW, Palacios IF, Fallon JT, et al: Active myocarditis in the spectrum of acute dilated cardiomyopathies. N Engl J Med 312:885, 1985

45. Maisch B, Deeg P, Liebau G, et al: Diagnostic relevance of humoral and cytotoxic immune reactions in primary and secondary dilated cardiomyopathy. Am J Cardiol 52:1072, 1983

46. Unverferth DV: The etiology of idiopathic dilated cardiomyopathy. p. 213. In Unverferth DV (ed): Dilated Cardiomyopathy. Futura, Mount Kisco, NY, 1985

47. Editorial: Selenium in the heart of China. Lancet 2:889, 1979

48. Johnson RA, Baker SS, Fallon JT, et al: An occidental case of cardiomyopathy and selenium deficiency. N Engl J Med 304:1210, 1981

49. Hsu FS, Du SJ: Cardiac diseases in swine. In Roberts HR, Dodds WJ (eds): p. 134. Pig Model for Biomedical Research. Pig Research Institute, Taiwan, Republic of China, 1982

50. Grossman W, McLaurin LP, Rolett EL: Alterations

in left ventricular relaxation and diastolic compliance in congestive cardiomyopathy. Cardiovasc Res 13:514, 1979

51. Lord PF: Left ventricular diastolic stiffness in dogs with congestive cardiomyopathy and volume overload. Am J Vet Res 37:953, 1976

52. Boyden PA, Tilley LP, Pham TD, et al: Effects of left atrial enlargement on atrial transmembrane potentials and structure in dogs with mitral valve fibrosis. Am J Cardiol 49:1896, 1982

53. Boyden PA, Tilley LP, Albala A, et al: Mechanisms for atrial arrhythmias associated with cardiomyopathy: a study of feline hearts with primary myocardial disease. Circulation 69:1036, 1984

54. Benjamin IJ, Schuster EH, Bulkey BH: Cardiac hypertrophy in idiopathic dilated congestive cardiomyopathy: A clinicopathologic study. Circulation 64:422, 1981

55. Van Vleet J, Ferrans VJ, Weirich WE: Pathologic alterations in hypertrophic and congestive cardiomyopathy of cats. Am J Vet Res 41:2037, 1980

56. Fox PR: Feline thromboembolism associated with cardiomyopathy. Presented at the Proceedings of the Fifth Annual Veterinary Medicine Forum, American College of Veterinary Internal Medicine, p. 714, 1987

57. Fox PR, Dodds WJ: Coagulopathies observed with spontaneous aortic thromboembolism in cardiomyopathic cats. Proc Am Coll Vet Intern Med :83, 1982 (abstr)

58. Maskin CS, Le Jemtel MD, Sonnenblick EH: Inotropic drugs for treatment of the failing heart. Cardiovasc Clin 14:1, 1984

59. Goodwin JF: The frontiers of cardiomyopathy. Br Heart J 48:1, 1982

60. Spodick DH: Effective management of congestive cardiomyopathy. Arch Intern Med 142:689, 1982

61. Sonnenblick EH: Force-velocity relations in mammalian heart muscle. Am J Physiol 202:931, 1962

62. Dyke SE, Urschel CW, Sonnenblick EH, et al: Detection of latent function in acutely ischemic myocardium in dogs: Comparison of pharmacologic inotropic stimulation and post extrasystolic potentiation (PESP). Circ Res 36:490, 1975

63. Spann JF Jr, Covell JW, Eckberg DL, et al: Contractile performance of the hypertrophied and chronically failing cat ventricle. Am J Physiol 223:1150, 1972

64. Colucci WS, Wright RF, Braunwald E: New positive inotropic agents in the treatment of congestive heart failure. Mechanisms of action and recent clinical developments (First of two parts) N Engl J Med 314:290, 1986

65. Colucci WS, Wright RF, Braunwald E: New positive inotropic agents in the treatment of congestive heart failure. Mechanisms of action and recent clinical developments (Second of two parts) N Engl J Med 314:349, 1986

66. Opie LH, Kaplan NM: Diuretic therapy. p. 111. In Opie LH (ed): Drugs for the Heart. Grune & Stratton, Orlando FL, 1987

67. Brest AN: Clinical pharmacology of diuretic drugs. Cardiovasc Clin 14:31, 1984

68. Cohn JN: Vasodilator therapy for heart failure: The influence of impedance on left ventricular performance. Circulation 48:5, 1973

69. Hirota Y, Shimizu G, Kaku K, et al: Mechanisms of compensation and decompensation in dilated cardiomyopathy. Am J Cardiol 54:1033, 1984

70. Goldberg LI: Cardiovascular and renal actions of dopamine: Potential clinical implications. Pharmacol Rev 24:1, 1972

71. Chidsey CA, Sonnenblick EH, Morrow AG, et al: Catecholamine excretion and cardiac stores of norepinephrine in congestive heart failure. Am J Med 39:442, 1965

72. Beregovich J, Bianchi C, Rubler S, et al: Dose-related hemodynamic and renal effects of dopamine in congestive heart failure. Am Heart J 87:550, 1974

73. Goldberg LI: Dopamine-clinical uses of endogenous catecholamine. N Engl J Med 291:707, 1984

74. Kenakin TP: An in vitro quantitative analysis of the alpha adrenoceptor partial agonist activity of dobutamine and its relevance to inotropic selectivity. J Pharmacol Exp Ther 216:210, 1981

75. Ruffolo RR Jr, Spradlin TA, Pollock GD, et al: Alpha and beta adrenergic effects of the stereoisomers of dobutamine. J Pharmacol Exp Ther 219:447, 1981

76. Kittleson MD: Dobutamine. J Am Vet Med Assoc 177:642, 1980

77. Unverferth DV, Blanford M, Kates RE, et al: Tolerance to dobutamine after a 72 hour continuous infusion. Am J Med 69:262, 1980

78. Unverferth DV, Magorien RD, Altshuld R, et al: The hemodynamic and metabolic advantages gained by a three-day infusion of dobutamine in patients with congestive cardiomyopathy. Am Heart J 106:29, 1983

79. Liang C, Sherman LG, Wellington K, et al: Sustained improvement of cardiac function in patients with congestive heart failure after short-term infusion of dobutamine. Circulation 69:113, 1984

80. Knowlen GD: Positive inotropic drugs in heart failure. p. 323. In Kirk RW (ed): Current Veterinary Therapy. Vol. IX. WB Saunders, Philadelphia, 1986

81. Swedberg K, Hjalmarson A, Waagstein F, et al: Beneficial effects of long-term beta-blockade in congestive cardiomyopathy. Br Heart J 44:117, 1980

82. Waagstein F, Hjalmarson A, Swedberg K, et al: Beta-blockers in dilated cardiomyopathies: They work. Eur Heart J 4(suppl A):173, 1983

83. Ikram H, Fitzpatrick MA: Beta blockade for dilated cardiomyopathy: The evidence against therapeutic benefit. Eur Heart J 4(suppl A):179, 1983

84. Swedberg K, Hjalmarson A, Waagstein F, et al: Adverse effects of beta-blockade withdrawal in patients with congestive cardiomyopathy. Br Heart J 44:134, 1980

85. Booth HW Jr, Clark DR, Merton DA: Cardiovascular effects of rapid infusion of crystalloid in the hypovolemic cat. J Small Anim Pract 26:477, 1985

86. Vatner SF, Pagani M, Rutherford JD, et al: Effects of nitroglycerin on cardiac function and regional blood flow distribution in conscious dogs. Am J Physiol 234:H-244, 1978

87. Smith TW, Braunwald E: The management of heart failure. p. 503. In Braunwald E (ed): Heart Disease. WB Saunders, Philadelphia, 1984

88. Captopril Multicenter Study Group: A placebo trial of captopril in refractory chronic congestive heart failure. J Am Coll Cardiol 2:755, 1983

89. Levine E, Franciosa JA, Cohn JN: Acute and long-term response to an oral converting enzyme inhibitor, captopril, in congestive heart failure. Circulation. 62:35, 1980

90. Knowlen GG, Kittleson MD, Nachreiner RF, et al: Comparison of plasma aldosterone concentration among clinical status groups of dogs with chronic heart failure. J Am Vet Med Assoc 183:991, 1983

91. Frazier HS, Yager H: Drug therapy: The clinical use of diuretics. N Engl J Med 288:246, 1973

92. Erichsen DF, Harris SG, Upson DW: Therapeutic and toxic plasma concentrations of digoxin in the cat. Am J Vet Res 41:2049, 1980

93. Erichsen DF, Harris SG, Upson DW: Plasma levels of digoxin in the cat: some clinical applications. Am Anim Hosp Assoc 14:734, 1978

94. Bolton GR, Powell AA: Plasma kinetics of digoxin in the cat. Am J Vet Res 43:1994, 1982

95. Snyder PS, Atkins CE, Keene BW: The effect of aspirin, furosemide and commercial low salt diet on digoxin kinetics in normal cats. p. 922. Presented at the Proceedings of the Fifth Annual Veterinary Medicine Forum, American College of Veterinary Internal Medicine, 1987 (abst 66)

96. Braunwald E, Lambrew CT, Morrow AG et al: Idiopathic hypertrophic subaortic stenosis. Arc 29/30 (suppl 4):1, 1964

97. Sanderson JE, Gibson DG, Brown DJ et al: Left ventricular filling in hypertrophic cardiomyopathy: An angiographic study. Br Heart J 39:661, 1977

98. Panidis IP, Kotter MN, Facc JF, et al: Development and regression of left ventricular hypertrophy. J Am Coll Cardiol 3:1309, 1984

99. Ciro E, Nichols PF III, Maron BJ: Heterogeneous morphologic expression of genetically transmitted hypertrophic cardiomyopathy. Circulation 67:1227, 1983

100. Maron BJ, Mulvihill JJ: The genetics of hypertrophic cardiomyopathy. Ann Intern Med 105:610, 1986

101. Maron BJ, Bonow RO, Cannon RO, et al: Hypertrophic cardiomyopathy. Interrelations of clinical manifestations, pathophysiology and therapy (First of two parts). N Engl J Med 316:780, 1987

102. Perloff JK: Pathogenesis of hypertrophic cardiomyopathy: Hypothesis and speculation. Am Heart J 101:219, 1981

103. Goodwin JF: Prospects and predictions for the cardiomyopathies. Circulation 50:210, 1974

104. James TN, Marshall TK: De subitaneis mortibus XII. Asymmetrical hypertrophy of the heart. Circulation 51:1149, 1975

105. Stewart S, Mason DT, Braunwald E: Impaired rate of left ventricular filling in idiopathic subaortic stenosis and valvular aortic stenosis. Circulation 37:8, 1968

106. Gaasch WH, Levine HJ, Quinones MA, et al: Left ventricular compliance: mechanisms and clinical implications. Am J Cardiol 38:645, 1976

107. Hanrath P, Mathey DG, Siegert R, et al: Left ventricular relaxation and filling pattern in different forms of left ventricular hypertrophy: An echocardiographic study. Am J Cardiol 45:15, 1980

108. St. Johns, Lie JT, Anderson KR, et al: Histopathological specificity of hypertrophic obstructive cardiomyopathy; myocardial fibre disarray and myocardial fibrosis. Br Heart J 44:433, 1980

109. Wigle ED, Sasson Z, Henderson MA, et al: Hypertrophic cardiomyopathy: The importance of the site and the extent of hypertrophy. A review. Prog Cardiovasc Dis 28:1, 1985

110. Pouleur H, Rousseau MF, van Eyll C, et al: Force-velocity-length relations in hypertrophic cardiomyopathy: evidence of normal or depressed myocardial contractility. Am J Cardiol 52:813, 1983

111. Grose R, Strain J, Spindola-Franco H: Angiographic and hemodynamic correlations in hypertrophic cardiomyopathy with intracavitary systolic pressure gradients. Am J Cardiol 58:1085, 1986

112. Thomas WP, Mathewson JW, Suter PF, et al: Hy-

pertrophic obstructive cardiomyopathy in a dog: Clinical, hemodynamic, angiographic and pathologic studies. J Am Anim Hosp Assoc 20:253, 1984

113. Swindle MM, Huber AC, Kan JS, et al: Mitral valve prolapse and hypertrophic cardiomyopathy in a pup. J Am Vet Med Assoc 184:1515, 1984

114. Liu SK, Maron BJ, Tilley LP: Hypertrophic cardiomyopathy in the dog. Am J Pathol 94:497, 1979

115. Liu SK, Maron BJ, Tilley LP: Canine hypertrophic cardiomyopathy. J Am Vet Med Assoc 174:708, 1979

116. Maron BJ, Liu SK, Tilley LP: Spontaneously occurring hypertrophic cardiomyopathy in dogs and cats: A potential animal model of a human disease. p. 73. In Kaltenbach M, Epstein SE (eds): Hypertrophic Cardiomyopathy. Springer-Verlag, Berlin, 1982

117. Liu SK, Maron BJ, Tilley LP: Feline hypertrophic cardiomyopathy: Gross anatomic and quantitative histologic features. Am J Pathol 102:388, 1981

118. Maron BJ, Wolfson JK, Epstein SE, et al: Intramural ("small vessel") coronary artery disease in hypertrophic cardiomyopathy. J Am Coll Cardiol 8:545, 1986

119. Cowgill LD, Kallet AJ: Systemic hypertension. p. 360. In Kirk RW (ed): Current Veterinary Therapy. Vol. IX, WB Saunders, Philadelphia, 1986

120. Rush JE, Keene BW, Fox PR: Retrospective study of pericardial disease in cats. p. 922. Presented at the Proceedings of the Fifth Annual Veterinary Medicine Forum, American College of Veterinary Internal Medicine, 1987 (abst 67)

121. Maron BJ, Bonow RO, Cannon RO, et al: Hypertrophic cardiomyopathy. Interrelations of clinical manifestations, pathophysiology, and therapy (second of two parts). N Engl J Med 316:844, 1987

122. Benotti JR, Grossman W, Cohn PF: Clinical profile of restrictive cardiomyopathy. Circulation 61:1206, 1980

123. Chew CYC, Ziady GM, Raphael MJ, et al: Primary restrictive cardiomyopathy: Non-tropical endomyocardial fibrosis and hypereosinophilic heart disease. Br Heart J 39:399, 1977

124. Liu SK: Myocarditis and cardiomyopathy in the dog and cat. Heart Vessels 1(suppl 1):122, 1985

125. Cohen LS, Braunwald E. Amelioration of angina pectoris in idiopathic hypertrophic subaortic stenosis with beta-adrenergic subaortic stenosis with beta-adrenergic blockade. Circulation 35:847, 1967

126. Thompson DS, Nagvi N, Juul SM, et al: Effects of propranolol on myocardial oxygen consumption, substrate extraction and haemodynamics in hypertrophic obstructive cardiomyopathy. Br Heart J 44:488, 1980

127. Flamm MD, Harrison DC, Hancock EW: Muscular subaortic stenosis: Prevention of outflow obstruction with propranolol. Circulation 38:846, 1968

128. Hess OM, Grimm J, Krayenbuehl HP: Diastolic function in hypertrophic cardiomyopathy: effects of propranolol and verapamil on diastolic stiffness. Eur Heart J 4(suppl F):47, 1983

129. Rosing DR, Idanpaan-Heikkila U, Maron BJ, et al: Use of calcium-channel blocking drugs in hypertrophic cardiomyopathy. Am J Cardiol 55(suppl 185-B) 1985

130. Bonow RO, Dilsizian V, Rosing DR, et al: Verapamil-induced improvement in left ventricular diastolic filling and increased exercise tolerance in patients with hypertrophic cardiomyopathy: Short and long-term effects. Circulation 72:853, 1985

131. Choo MH, Chia BL, Wu DC, et al: Anomaous chordae tendineae: A source of echocardiographic confusion. Angiology 33:756, 1982

132. Feigenbaum H: Echocardiography. 4th Ed. Lea & Febiger, Philadelphia 1986

133. Flanders J: Feline aortic thromboembolism. Comp Cont Educ 8:473, 1986

134. Furster V, Chesebro JH: Antithrombotic therapy: Role of platelet-inhibitor drugs. I. Current Concepts of thrombogenesis: Role of platelets (first of three parts). Mayo Clin Proc 56:102, 1981

135. Hirsch J: Hypercoagulability. Semin Hematol 14:409, 1977

136. Edwards WD: Aneurysms and mural thrombi of the left ventricle. Mayo Clin Proc 56:129, 1981

137. Weiser MG, Kociba GJ: Platelet concentration and platelet volume distribution in healthy cats. Am J Vet Res 45:518, 1984

138. Dodds WJ: Platelet function in animals: Species specificities. p. 45. In de Gaetano G, Garattini S (eds): Platelets: A Multidisciplinary Approach. Raven Press, New York, 1978

139. Imhoff RK: Production of aortic occlusion resembling acute aortic embolism syndrome in cats. Nature (Lond) 192:979, 1961

140. Schaub RG, Meyers KM, Sande RD, et al: Inhibition of feline collateral vessel development following experimental thrombolic occlusion. Circ Res 39:736, 1976

141. Schaub RG, Meyers KM, Sande RD: Serotonin as a factor in depression of collateral blood flow following experimental arterial thrombosis. J Lab Clin Med 90:645, 1977

142. Grygleski RJ: Prostaglandins, platelets and atherosclerosis. CRC Crit Rev Biochem 7:291, 1980

143. Schaub RG, Gates KA, Roberts RE: Effect of aspirin on collateral blood flow after experimental thrombosis of the feline aorta. Am J Vet Res 43:1647, 1982

144. Griffiths IR, Duncan ID: Ischaemic neuromyopathy in cats. Vet Rec 104:518, 1979

145. Allen DG, Johnstone IB, Crane S: Effects of aspirin and propranolol alone and in combination on hemostatic determinants in the healthy cat. Am J Vet Res 46:660, 1985

146. Buchanan JW, Baker GJ, Hill JD: Aortic embolism in cats: Prevalence, surgical treatment and electrocardiography. Vet Rec 79:496, 1966

147. Schneeweiss A: Drug Therapy in Cardiovascular Diseases. Lea & Febiger, Philadelphia, 1986

148. Freis ED: Changing attitudes to hypertension. Ann Intern Med 78:141, 1973

149. Oblad B: A study of the mechanism of the hemodynamic effects of hydralazine in man. Acta Pharmacol Toxicol 20(suppl 1):1, 1963

150. Killingsworth CR, Eyster GE, Adams T, et al: Streptokinase treatment of cats with experimentally induced aortic thrombosis. Am J Vet Res 47:1351, 1986

151. Kaplan AP, Castellino FJ, Collen D, et al: Molecular mechanisms of fibrinolysis in man. Thromb Haemost 39:263, 1978

152. Sherry S: Tissue plasminogen activator (t-PA). N Engl J Med 313:1014, 1985

153. Rosenberg RD, Lam L: Correlation between structure and function of heparin. Proc Natl Acad Sci USA 76:1218, 1979

154. Pion PD, Kittleson MD, Peterson S, et al: Thrombolysis of aortic thromboemboli in cats using tissue plasminogen activator: Clinical data. p. 925. Presented at the Proceedings of the Fifth Annual Veterinary Medicine Forum, American College of Veterinary Internal Medicine, 1987 (abstr 72)

155. Bell RW: Metabolism of Vitamin K and prothrombin synthesis: Anticoagulants and the vitamin K-epoxide cycle. Fed Proc 37:2599, 1978

156. Roth GJ, Stanford N, Majerus PW: Acetylation of prostaglandin synthesis by aspirin. Proc Natl Acad Sci USA 72:3073, 1975

157. Hamberg M, Svensson J, Samuelsson B: Thromboxanes: A new group of biologically active compounds derived from prostaglandin endoperoxides. Proc Natl Acad Sci USA 72:299, 1975

158. Greene CE: Aspirin and feline platelet aggregation. J Am Vet Med Assoc 188:1820, 1985

159. Preston FE, Whipps, Jackson CA, et al: Inhibition of prostacyclin and platelet thromboxane A_2 after low dose aspirin. N Engl J Med 304:76, 1981

160. Moncada S, Gryglewski R, Bunting S, et al: An enzyme isolated from arteries transforms prostaglandin endoperoxides to an unstable substance that inhibits platelet aggregation. Nature (Lond) 263:663, 1976

161. Armstrong JM, Lattimer N, Moncada S, et al: Comparison of the vasopressor effects of prostacyclin and 6-oxoprostaglandin F_1-alpha with those of prostaglandin E_2 in rats and rabbits. Br J Pharmacol 62:125, 1978

162. Peterson ME, Kintzer PP, Cavanaugh PG, et al: Feline hyperthyroidism: pretreatment clinical and laboratory evaluation of 131 cases. J Am Vet Med Assoc 183:103, 1983

163. Hoenig M, Goldschmidt HM, Ferguson DC, et al: Toxic nodular goiter in the cat. J Small Anim Pract 23:1, 1982

164. Peterson ME: Feline hyperthyroidism. Vet Clin North Am 14:809, 1984

165. Peterson ME, Turrel JM: Feline hyperthyroidism. p. 1026. In Kirk RW (ed): Current Veterinary Therapy. Vol. I. WB Saunders, Philadelphia, 1986

166. Ingbar SH, Woeber KA: The thyroid gland. p. 117. In Williams RH (ed): Textbook of Endocrinology. 6th Ed. WB Sauunders, Philadelphia, 1981

167. Klein I, Levey GS: New perspectives on thyroid hormone, catecholamines, and the heart. Am J Med 76:167, 1984

168. Forfar JC, Caldwall GC: Hyperthyroid heart disease. Clin Endocrinol Metab 14:491, 1985

169. Grossman W, Braunwald E: High cardiac output states. p. 807. In Braunwald E (ed): Heart Disease. 2nd Ed. WB Saunders, Philadelphia, 1984

170. Bond BR: Hyperthyroid heart disease in cats. p. 399. In Kirk RW (ed): Current Veterinary Therapy. Vol. IX. WB Saunders, Philadelphia, 1986

171. Bond BR: Hyperthyroidism and other high cardiac output states. In Fox PR (ed): Canine and Feline Cardiology. Churchill Livingstone, New York, 1988

172. Jacobs G, Hutson C, Dougherty J, et al: Congestive heart failure associated with hyperthyroidism in cats. J Am Vet Med Assoc 188:52, 1986

173. Moise NS, Dietze A, Mezza E, et al: Echocardiography, electrocardiography, and radiography of cats with dilatation cardiomyopathy, hypertrophic cardiomyopathy and hyperthyroidism. Am J Vet Res 47:1476, 1986

174. Moise NS, Dietze AE: Echocardiographic, electrocardiographic, and radiographic detection of cardiomegaly in hyperthyroid cats. Am J Res 47:1487, 1986

175. Peterson ME, Keene BW, Ferguson DC, et al: Electrocardiographic findings in 45 cats with hyperthyroidism. J Am Vet Med Assoc 180:934, 1982

176. Bond BR, Fox PR, Peterson ME, et al: Echocardiographic findings in 103 cats with hyperthyroidism. J Am Vet Med Assoc (in press), 1988

177. Bond BR, Fox PR, Peterson ME: Echocardiographic evaluation of 45 cats with hyperthyroidism. J Ultrasound Med 2(suppl):184, 1983

178. Peterson ME, Hurvitz AI, Leib MS, et al: Propylthiouracil-associated hemolytic anemia, thrombocytopenia and antinuclear antibodies in cats with hyperthyroidism. J Am Vet Med Assoc 184:806, 1984

179. Birchard SJ, Peterson ME, Jacobson A: Surgical treatment of feline hyperthyroidism: results of 85 cases. J Am Anim Hosp Assoc 20:705, 1984

180. Meric SM, Hawkins EC, Washabau RJ, et al: Serum thyroxine concentrations after radioactive iodine therapy in cats with hyperthyroidism. J Am Vet Med Assoc 188:1038, 1986

181. Van Vleet JF, Ferrans VJ, Weirich WE: Cardiac disease induced by chronic adriamycin administration in dogs and an evaluation of vitamin E and selenium as cardioprotectants. Am J Pathol 99:13, 1980

182. Loar AS, Susaneck SJ: Doxorubicin-induced cardiotoxicity in five dogs. Semin Vet Med Surg 1:68, 1986

183. Mauldin N, Matus R, Patnaik A, et al: A prospective study of efficacy and toxicity of doxorubicin and cyclophosphamide used in treatment of selected malignant tumors in 30 cats. J Vet Int Med 2 (in press), 1988

184. Jeglum KA, de Guzman E, Young KM: Chemotherapy of advanced mammary adenocarcinoma in 14 cats. J Am Vet Med Assoc 187:157, 1985

185. Cotter SM, Kamki PJ, Simon M: Renal disease in five tumor-bearing cats treated with adriamycin. J Am Anim Hosp Assoc 21:405, 1985

186. Tilley LP, Bond B, Patnaik A, et al: Cardiovascular tumors in the cat. J Am Anim Hosp Assoc 17:1009, 1981

187. Patnaik AK, Liu SK: Angiosarcomas in cats. J Small Anim Pract 18:191, 1977

188. Jacobson RH: Toxoplasmosis—Feline infections and their zoonotic potential. p. 1307. In Kirk RW (ed): Current Veterinary Therapy. Vol. VII. WB Saunders, Philadelphia, 1980

189. Dubey JP, Johnstone I: Fatal neonatal toxoplasmosis in cats. J Am Anim Hosp Assoc 18:461, 1982

190. Yamaguchi RA, Pipers FS, Gamble DA: Echocardiographic evaluation of a cat with bacterial vegetative endocarditis. J Am Vet Med Assoc 183:118, 1983

191. Shousse CL, Meier H: Acute vegetative endocarditis in the dog and cat. J Am Vet Med Assoc 129:278, 1956

192. Tilley LP, Liu SK: Persistent atrial standstill in the dog and cat. Proc Am Coll Vet Intern Med 43, (abstr), 1983

193. Haskins ME, Jezyk PF, Desnick RJ: Mucopolysaccharidosis in a domestic short-haired cat: A disease distinct from that seen in the Siamese cat. J Am Vet Med Assoc 175:384, 1979

194. Haskins ME, Aguirre GD, Jezyk PF, et al: The pathology of feline arylsulfatase B deficient mucopolysaccharidosis. Am J Pathol 101:657, 1980

195. Renteria VG, Ferrans VJ, Roberts WC: The heart in the Hurler syndrome: Gross, histologic and ultrastructural observations in five necropsy cases. Am J Cardiol 38:487, 1976

196. Liu SK, Tilley LP, Tashjian RJ: Lesions of the conduction system in the cat with cardiomyopathy. Recent Adv Stud Card Struct Metab 10:681, 1975

23

Canine Myocardial Disease

Philip R. Fox

INCIDENCE

Cardiomyopathy refers to diseases of myocardial structure or function exclusive of disorders caused by valvular disease, congenital heart defects, and pulmonary parenchymal or vascular disturbances. Classification schemes may be based on anatomic, functional, and pathophysiologic features and are presented in Chapter 22. Causes and classifications of canine myocardial diseases are listed in Table 23-1.[1-15]

Canine myocardial diseases comprise a smaller percentage of total cardiovascular disorders in dogs than cats. Specific clinical or necropsy incidence has not been reported, although dilated cardiomyopathy is relatively common. There is less functional and structural heterogeneity in canine than feline cardiomyopathies. However, several breeds display marked variation with respect to pathophysiologic changes and clinical presentation.[8-13] These differences are most notable among "giant breeds," the Doberman pinscher, boxer, and English cocker spaniel breeds.[6-26]

DIAGNOSTIC STRATEGIES

The diagnosis of dilated cardiomyopathy has been based historically on structural classification in-ferred from history, physical examination, electrocardiography (ECG), and plain-film radiography.[8-14,27-30] In addition, echocardiography provides a rapid, accurate, noninvasive technique for assessing cardiac structure and function.[31-33] As a result, invasive studies are rarely required for diagnosis. Endomyocardial biopsy has been used to document biochemical and inflammatory myocardial abnormalities,[34-36] although this procedure is currently considered experimental.

When combined with the above data base, heart failure may be clinically approached as a syndrome of systolic or diastolic dysfunction associated with morphologic cardiac changes. Treatment is directed toward relieving congestive signs and correcting related hemodynamic abnormalities and arrhythmias.

PRIMARY (IDIOPATHIC) CARDIOMYOPATHIES

Heart Failure Due to Systolic Dysfunction

Systolic (i.e., myocardial or pump) failure occurs when the ventricle is unable to generate enough contractile force. Examples include primary (idiopathic) dilated cardiomyopathy or secondary dilated car-

Table 23-1 Causes of Canine Myocardial Disease

Primary (idiopathic) cardiomyopathies	Secondary cardiomyopathies (*continued*)
Hypertrophic	Toxins
Dilated (congestive)	Doxorubicin
Restrictive[a]	Cobalt
Intermediate or intergrade	Catecholamines
	Lead
Secondary cardiomyopathies	Ethanol
Metabolic	Inflammatory
Endocrine	Infectious
Thyrotoxicosis	Viral
Pheochromocytoma	Bacterial
Hyperadrenocorticism (Cushing's disease)	Protozoal
Uremia[a]	Fungal
Hypothyroidism[a]	Algal
Carnitine deficiency	Rickettsial
Nutritional[a]	Noninfectious
Selenium/vitamin E deficiency	Collagen diseases[a]
Obesity	
	Genetic
Infiltrative	Hypertrophic cardiomyopathy[a]
Neoplasia	Dilated cardiomyoatphy[a]
Glycogen storage diseases[a]	Endocardial fibroelastosis (?)
Fibroplastic	Miscellaneous
Endomyocardial fibrosis	Ischemia
Endocardial fibroelastosis	Muscular dystrophy
	Conduction system disorders
Hypersensitity	
Physical agents	
Hyperpyrexia	
Hypothermia	

[a] Suspected but not proven.

diomyopathy resulting from toxins (e.g., doxorubicin), infection (e.g., canine parvovirus), or inflammation (e.g., physical agents).[2,3,7–14] In the classic form, all four cardiac chambers are severely dilated (Table 23-2). There is reduced cardiac output and index; increased end-systolic and end-diastolic ventricular volume; increased end-diastolic, atrial, pulmonary wedge, and central venous pressure, and excessive wall tension. Congestive heart failure results from depressed contractility and failure (or overcompensation) of neuroendocrine, hepatorenal, and peripheral vascular compensation mechanisms. The degree or extent of systolic dysfunction may vary depending on the etiology and stage of disease, and can range from mild to severe contractile impairment.

Dilated (Congestive) Cardiomyopathy

ETIOLOGY

The etiology of primary (idiopathic) dilated (congestive) cardiomyopathy is unknown. It may represent the end-stage result of myocardial injury caused by various metabolic, toxic, or infectious agents.[1–3] Myocardial toxins, including anthracyclines (especially doxorubicin)[7,37,38] and cyclophos-

Table 23-2 Breed-Related Features of Canine Idiopathic Dilated Cardiomyopathy[a]

Clinical Features	Large/Giant Breeds (Classic Form)	Doberman Pinscher	Boxer	English Cocker Spaniel
Age	6 mo–14 yr (4–6-yr avg)	2.5–14.5 yr (6.5-yr avg)	6 mo–15 yr (8-yr avg)	10 mo–9 yr (5–6-yr avg)
Sex	Predominantly male	Predominantly male	Approximately equal	Approx. equal; male predisposition in one study
Electrocardiography	Atrial fibrillation common; LVE; Ventricular ectopia	Sinus, LVE, or LBBB pattern; ventricular arrhythmias common; atrial fibrillation in 20%	Ventricular arrhythmias common (LBBB pattern)	RII, aVF > 3.0 mV (early changes); deep Q waves leads II, aVF; APCs common in one study
Radiography	Generalized cardiomegaly; biventricular heart failure	LAE; acute severe pulmonary edema; pleural effusion mild, uncommon	N or cardiomegaly	Generalized cardiomegaly; pulmonary edema
Echocardiography	Ventricular dilation; reduced contractility (FS)	Ventricular dilation, reduced contractility (FS); B shoulder inconsistent; asymptomatic cases—excessive EPSS most sensitive (LV dimensions may be almost N; Ao wall excursion N before onset of CHF	N to ventricular dilation; contractility N to depressed	LV dilation (usually); one-fourth with N contractility (FS)
Other		Cardiogenic shock common during CHF	Clinical categories: I: asymptomatic with arrhythmias II: syncope with arrhythmias III: CHF with arrhythmias Arrhythmias often refractory	Chronic AV valvular disease (endocardiosis) common; long asymptomatic period common (usually with ECG evidence of LVE)
Prognosis	6-mo survival, 25–40%; some survive more than 24 months	Grave; most die within 6–8 weeks	Category I: 2 years II: 1–2 years III: <6 mo; sudden death possible	Guarded

[a] Much overlap occurs between findings and breed characteristics should not be considered pathognomonic. (Data from refs. 6, 8, 13, 16, 18, 20, 26, 58.)
APCs, atrial premature complexes; AV, atrioventricular; CHF, congestive heart failure; ECG, electrocardiogram; EPSS, mitral valve E-point (interventricular) septal separation; FS, fractional shortening; LAE, left atrial enlargement; LBBB, left bundle branch block (i.e., QRS > 0.07 seconds, upright lead II, aVF); LVE, left ventricular enlargement; N, normal, Ao, aorta.

phamide,[39] have caused dilated cardiomyopathy in humans and animals. Microvascular hyperreactivity with myocytolysis, reactive hypertrophy, and progressive systolic dysfunction has been demonstrated in the Syrian hamster.[40] Familial transmission in humans is rare.[2,3,41] Metabolic deficiencies have been demonstrated in human familial dilated cardiomyopathy, including carnitine deficiency.[42,43] Carnitine-linked defects of myocardial metabolism have been demonstrated in association with canine dilated cardiomyopathy.[34] Infective (viral) and immunologic factors have been implicated in some cases of human dilated cardiomyopathy based on myocardial nuclear changes, high viral antibody titers, circulating immune complexes, and immunoregulatory defects.[44–46] Selenium deficiency has been associated with dilated cardiomyopathy in humans (Keshan's disease)[47,48] and animals,[7,49] although it has not been proved to be the sole cause of myocardial disease. Taurine deficiency has recently been implicated as a cause of reversible myocardial failure in felines.[50]

PATHOPHYSIOLOGY

The principal functional defect is depressed ventricular contractile performance.[1–3] Cardiac chamber dilation may be present before the appearance of clinical signs, if stroke volume is maintained by compensatory mechanisms. Sinus tachycardia may help maintain cardiac output transiently. Ventricular end-diastolic pressures may be elevated by reduced systolic emptying and increased end-systolic residual volume, which represent additional compensatory mechanisms that temporarily maintain cardiac output. Alterations in left ventricular relaxation and diastolic compliance coexist with impaired contractile function and contribute to elevated filling pressures.[51,52] Ventricular dilation causes geometric atrioventricular (AV) valve apparatus distortion, resulting in mitral regurgitation.[7,8,11,53] This further reduces forward stroke volume and contributes to left atrial dilation. Atrial enlargement predisposes to atrial arrhythmias, especially atrial fibrillation.[54,55] The resultant loss of atrial contribution and reduced time for diastolic filling decreases cardiac output. Inadequate forward flow produces clinical signs of low-output failure as muscles and organs become poorly perfused (Table 22-3). Decreased renal perfusion stimulates the renin-angiotensin-aldosterone system, increasing preload and afterload. Enhanced sympathetic activity contributes to increased preload and peripheral vascular resistance, further reducing cardiac output.[2,3] Ventricular hypertrophy may occur as a compensatory mechanism to reduce wall tension and pressure, according to the law of Laplace.[56] Congestive signs ultimately develop.

PATHOLOGY

Necropsy shows a globular-shaped heart with severe dilation of all cardiac chambers. Ventricular walls become abnormally thin, although various degrees of compensatory hypertrophy may be present. Papillary muscles and trabeculae are atrophied. Focal endocardial fibrosis may be present. Valve leaflets are normal, but AV valve circumference is usually enlarged. Histologic changes include various degrees of myocardial cellular degeneration, ranging from coagulation, granulation, and sarcoplasmic vacuolization to myocytolysis.[2,3,6,7,10–13,20]

GENERAL CLINICAL FINDINGS

Affected animals are usually young (6 months to 14 years, mean:4 to 6 years), predominantly male, and of large and giant breeds. Clinical signs often occur acutely and include dyspnea, coughing, syncope, exercise intolerance, or abdominal distention. In other animals, signs occur over 3 to 7 days and include partial anorexia, weight loss (often pronounced), and mild to moderate lethargy.

Physical examination demonstrates abnormalities consistent with low cardiac output (weakness), left-sided heart failure (dyspnea due to pulmonary edema), or right-sided heart failure (i.e., muffled heart and lung sounds due to effusions). Biventricular failure may sometimes be present. The decompensated dog is typically weak, displays prolonged capillary refill time, and has pale mucous membranes and hypokinetic femoral arterial pulses. Jugular venous distention or pulsations, abdominal distention (ascites), and hepatosplenomegaly may be detected. Auscultation often indicates a left or right apical murmur of mild to moderate intensity due to

Table 23-3 Clinical Signs and Electrocardiographic Findings in Boxer Cardiomyopathy

Clinical Findings	Harpster (N = 63)[a]		Fox (N = 103)[b]	
	N	%	N	%
Age (years, mean)	1–15(8.2)		0.5–15(8.0)	
Male	36	57.8	53	51.4
Female	27	42.2	50	48.5
Syncope	22	34.3	36	34.9
Cough	15	23.4	26	25.2
Dyspnea	8	12.4	13	12.6
Weight loss	7	10.9	12	11.6
Electrocardiographic findings				
Sinus rhythms				
Normal sinus rhythm	20	31.7	7	6.8
Sinus arrhythmia	NR		32	31.1
Sinus tachycardia	11	17.5	15	14.6
Atrial arrhythmias				
Supraventricular premature complexes	7	11.1	6	5.8
Paroxysmal atrial tachycardia	4	6.3	1	0.9
Atrial fibrillation	7	11.1	2	1.9
Ventricular arrhythmias				
Ventricular premature complexes				
Rare/occasional	23	36.5	15	14.6
Frequent	22	34.9	14	13.6
Ventricular tachycardia	27	42.9	12	11.6
Other findings				
QRS interval >0.07 seconds	9	14.3	9	8.7
RII >3.0 mV	7	11.1	3	2.9

NR, not reported.
[a] Data from Harpster.[26]
[b] Data from Fox.[57]

AV valvular insufficiency. A rapid irregular heart rate and a third heart sound (S_3) gallop rhythm may be present. Muffled heart and lung sounds may be due to diminished contractility or the dampening effects of pericardial and pleural effusion. Increased bronchovesicular sounds and inspiratory crackles may be evident. Weight loss may be obvious, resulting in accentuated ribs and dorsal spinous vertebral processes.[6–13,15–26]

Electrocardiography usually suggests left heart enlargement, conduction abnormalities, or tachyarrhythmias.[6,8–13,15–19,21–28] The most common arrhythmia is atrial fibrillation, a rapid totally irregular supraventricular tachycardia without P waves (Fig. 23-1; see also Fig. 4-39). It is usually detected during initial physical examination or develops dur-

ing the early stages of treatment. Less frequently, paroxysmal atrial tachycardia (see Fig. 4-37) or sinus tachycardia (often with atrial premature complexes) is recorded. Sinus rhythm is seen consistently only with dilated cardiomyopathy in Doberman pinschers and English cocker spaniels. Ventricular arrhythmias (see Figs. 4-42, 4-43, and 14-1) may be present or coexist with supraventricular rhythm disorders as singles, pairs, or triplets of ventricular premature complexes. Occasionally, paroxysmal or sustained ventricular tachycardia is recorded. Left ventricular enlargement is often present (R wave in lead II taller than 3.0 mV or QRS duration wider than 0.065 second with ST-T segment slurring). With severe pericardial or pleural effusion, R waves may be small (less than 1.0 mV). Left atrial enlarge-

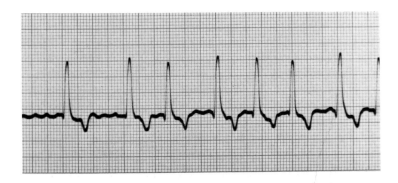

Fig. 23-1 Lead II electrocardiogram from a 5-year-old male Great Dane with dilated cardiomyopathy and atrial fibrillation. The rhythm is rapid and totally irregular. P waves are absent. 1 mV = 0.5 cm; paper speed = 50 mm/sec.

ment (P-wave duration greater than 0.04 second) is often present unless atrial fibrillation or sustained ventricular tachycardia occurs. Sudden arrhythmias usually are accompanied by acute cardiac decompensation. (Tables 23-2 and 23-3)

Radiographs display characteristic generalized cardiomegaly.[6,8–13,15,16,21,22,26,29,30,52] The heart may appear rounded and globoid, especially if pericardial effusion is present. Some breeds, such as the Doberman pinscher, may display only left atrial enlargement. An interstitial and alveolar pulmonary pattern consistent with pulmonary edema may be seen in the perihilar region (i.e., dorsally and caudally). If severe left-sided heart failure occurs (especially in Doberman pinschers and English cocker spaniels), this distribution may be diffuse. Pleural effusion may obscure the cardiac silhouette. Hydroperitoneum and hepatosplenomegaly may be present.

Echocardiography verifies the diagnosis of dilated cardiomyopathy. Classic findings are severe left ventricular dilation, markedly diminished contractility (i.e., fractional shortening), reduced ventricular septal and left ventricular free wall thickness, excursion and systolic thickening, left atrial and right ventricular dilation, reduced systolic aortic root excursion, prominent mitral valve b shoulder, and increased mitral valve E-point septal separation.[8,9,11–13,17,21,22,25,31–33] (Figs. 23-2 through 23-4). Increased E-point septal separation is a sensitive indicator of left ventricular enlargement, even when internal ventricular dimensions appear within nor-

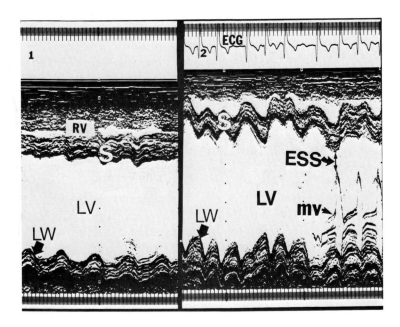

Fig. 23-2 M-mode echocardiograms recorded from two large-breed dogs with dilated cardiomyopathy. *Frame 1* was recorded below the mitral valve and shows a dilated left ventricle (LV) with greatly reduced interventricular septal (S) motion and decreased fractional shortening (contractility). *Frame 2* is a sweep from the left ventricular apex upward to the mitral valve (mv). The LV is greatly dilated and there is notable E-point-septal separation (ESS) - (that is, the distance between the E point of the anterior mitral valve leaflet and the interventricular septum). The septal and left ventricular posterior wall (LW) motion is erratic due to atrial fibrillation. RV, right ventricle; ECG, electrocardiogram. (Courtesy of Dr. N. Sydney Moise.)

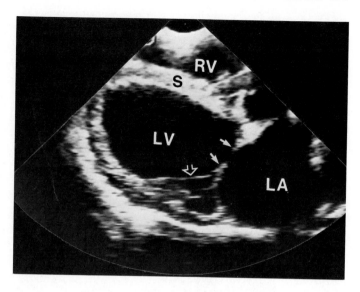

Fig. 23-3 Two-dimensional echocardiogram, long-axis view, recorded at the right intercostal position from a 4-year-old Doberman pinscher with dilated cardiomyopathy. Severe dilation of the left atrium (LA) and left ventricle (LV) is evident. S, interventricular septum; closed arrows, mitral valves; open arrow, chordae tendineae; RV, right ventricle.

mal published limits.[8,25] Segmental wall abnormalities may also be observed.

Clinical laboratory abnormalities include prerenal azotemia, elevated serum ALT (SGPT), and reduced serum protein levels.

BREED VARIABILITIES

Clinical features of classic dilated cardiomyopathy observed in large and giant breeds include weight loss, generalized severe cardiomegaly, biventricular heart failure, and atrial fibrillation as described above. Several breeds, however, display different but consistent variations (Table 23-2). While these breeds may display features typical of the classic category, they frequently exhibit changes characteristic of their breed.

Doberman Pinscher Cardiomyopathy

Dilated cardiomyopathy in Doberman pinschers may resemble the classic giant-breed idiopathic cardiomyopathy. This includes reduced left ventricular contractility, increased left ventricular end-systolic dimensions, and typical historical and physical examination abnormalities. However, a large subset differs consistently with respect to radiographic changes, electrocardiographic (ECG) findings, and prognosis.[8,11–13,21–25] Radiography often shows severe left atrial enlargement rather than generalized cardiomegaly (Fig. 23-5). Alveolar pulmonary edema and enlargement of the right cranial lobar pulmonary vein are the most common extracardiac signs of heart failure. Pulmonary edema may be diffuse rather than confined to dorsal and caudal lung regions. Pleural effusion, when present, is usually mild. ECG changes typically include sinus rhythm with left ventricular enlargement or left bundle branch block pattern (QRS duration greater than 0.07 second) (Fig. 23-6) and ventricular arrhythmias. Ventricular arrhythmias usually persist throughout the course of treatment. Less frequently, these dogs present with or develop atrial fibrillation. Pathologic findings include atrial and ventricular dilation, reduced left ventricular wall thickness, myocyte degeneration, fatty infiltration, and myocardial fibrosis. Prognosis is grave, with most Doberman pinschers dying within 6 weeks of diagnosis.[7–13,20–25]

Occasionally, clinically normal Doberman pinschers are encountered. They may display radiographic mild to moderate left atrial enlargement and echocardiographic moderate to slightly reduced left ventricular contractility. Echocardiographic E-point septal separation is excessive, however, even if ventricular internal dimensions are normal. These dogs may develop acute left-sided congestive heart failue 1 to 15 months after initial detection and respond poorly to therapy. M-mode echocardiography is helpful in diagnosing cardiomyopathy in clinically normal Doberman pinschers or in those

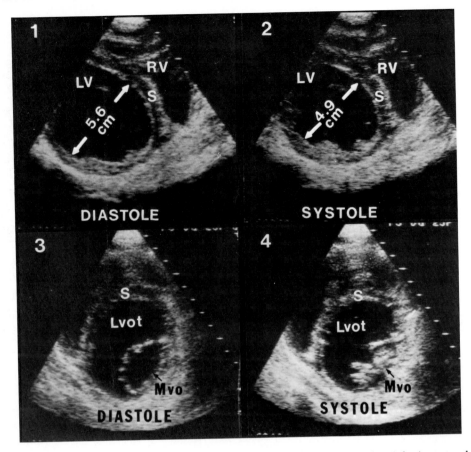

Fig. 23-4 Two-dimensional echocardiograms. *Frames 1* and *2* recorded from the right intercostal position demonstrate the short-axis view at the papillary muscle level of a Doberman pinscher with dilated cardiomyopathy. There is little change in the diastolic and systolic dimensions (fractional shortening is approximately 12.5 percent). *Frames 3* and *4* are short-axis views recorded from the right intercostal position at the level of the mitral valve from a golden retriever with dilated cardiomyopathy. The transducer is turned 180 degrees compared to frames 1 and 2, which causes different positional relationships of the right and left ventricles. A dilated left ventricular outflow tract (LVOT) and a small mitral valve orifice (Mvo) are evident. LV, left ventricle; RV, right ventricle; s, septum. (Courtesy of Dr. N. Syndney Moise.)

experiencing episodic weakness without signs of congestive heart failure or arrhythmias.[25]

Boxer Cardiomyopathy

Boxer cardiomyopathy describes a primary myocardial disorder distinguished by extensive histologic myocardial changes, absence of severe atrial or ventricular dilation, and usually ventricular arrhythmias.[26] Affected boxers range from 6 months to 15 years of age (average: 8.0 to 8.2 years; median: 8.5 years). Males are slightly more represented, and there has been a greater prevalence in some breeding lines.[26,57] Clinical features may be divided into three nearly equal categories: (1) asymptomatic with arrhythmias; (2) syncope or episodic weakness with congestive heart failure; (3) congestive heart failure (left sided or sometimes biventricular failure) with arrhythmias. Murmurs of mitral insufficiency are recorded in about one-half of cases. Thoracic radiographic findings are variable. In most asymptomatic dogs and in about one-half of syncopal animals without heart failure, no significant radiographic abnormalities are present. Cardiomeg-

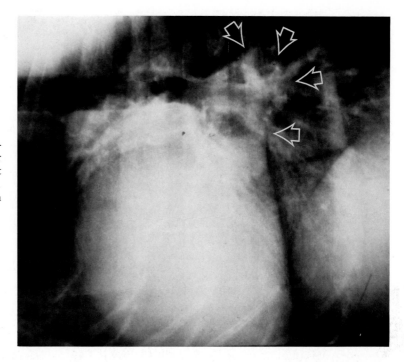

Fig. 23-5 Right lateral thoracic radiograph from a Doberman pinscher with dilated cardiomyopathy. The left atrium is greatly enlarged (arrows). There is slight pulmonary congestion in the perihilar region.

aly and pulmonary edema accompany cases of advanced heart failure. Pleural effusion is uncommon.[26] ECG changes are quite characteristic for boxer cardiomyopathy. Ventricular premature complexes occurring singly, in pairs, or in runs are most common, followed by paroxysmal ventricular tachycardia. Ventricular ectopia characteristically arises from the right ventricle and demonstrates a left bundle branch pattern (i.e., wide, bizarre, upright QRS complexes in leads I, II, III, and aVF) (Fig. 23-7). Supraventricular arrhythmias are occasionally recorded. During normal sinus rhythm, P, QRS, and T complexes are usually unremarkable[26,57] (Table 23-3).

Postmortem findings may indicate mild left ventricular hypertrophy and dilation, left atrial dilation, and thickened nodular mitral (and occasionally, aortic or tricuspid) valves. Histologically, active myocardial changes (e.g., focal myocytolysis, myofiber degeneration, and mild mononuclear cellular infiltration) and chronic alterations (e.g., myofiber atrophy, fibrosis, and fatty change) are routinely present. The chronic changes are more common.[26]

The prognosis for long-term survival in boxers with ventricular arrhythmias and heart failure is usually less than 6 months. Sudden death is common. Boxers in the other categories without congestive heart failure may survive up to 2 years

Fig. 23-6 Lead II electrocardiogram from a 5-year-old male Doberman pinscher with dilated cardiomyopathy. The heart rate exceeds 170 beats/min (sinus tachycardia). QRS complex width equals or exceeds 0.07 seconds, suggesting left ventricular enlargement or left bundle branch block. Ventricular premature complexes (VPC) are present. 1 cm = 1 mV; paper speed = 50 mm/sec.

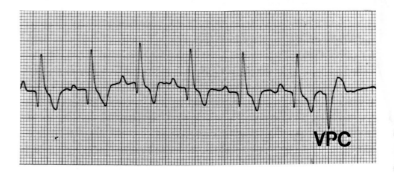

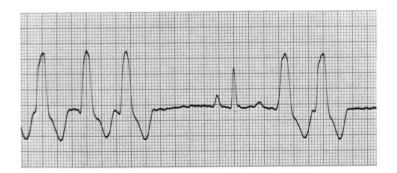

Fig. 23-7 Lead II electrocardiogram from an adult boxer with cardiomyopathy. Paroxysmal ventricular tachycardia is present. Ventricular ectopia (complexes 1 to 3, 5, and 6) arise from the right ventricle and demonstrate a left bundle branch block pattern (wide, bizarre, upright QRS complexes).

in some cases. Arrhythmias, especially ventricular, are often refractory to therapy.[26]

English Cocker Spaniel Cardiomyopathy

In small-breed dogs, dilated cardiomyopathy has been described most consistently in the English cocker spaniel.[15–18] Affected dogs range from 2 to 9 years of age (mean: 5.8 years). Sex distribution has been reportedly equal or displayed male predominance. A familial predisposition has been suggested. Clinical signs most commonly include cough, exercise intolerance, acute dyspnea, and sudden death. Physical examination typically discloses auscultatory abnormalities (e.g., rales, murmurs). The most notable ECG changes included left ventricular enlargement (e.g., tall R waves in lead II and ST-segment slurring) with sinus rhythm. Deep Q waves may be commonly recorded. Radiographic changes include pulmonary edema and biventricular enlargement.[16] Supraventricular arrhythmias (atrial premature complexes) were common in one study.[15] Echocardiographic abnormalities include increased end-systolic and usually end-diastolic dimensions, but depressed myocardial function was recorded in only three-fourths of affected dogs[17] (Table 23-2).

On the basis of a limited number of animal studied, dilated cardiomyopathy in English cocker spaniels may differ from that in large- and giant-breed dogs in several ways: (1) the disease is often typified by a long asymptomatic period, (2) early ECG abnormalities (especially left ventricular enlargement) may be recorded during the asymptomatic period, (3) myocardial function may be less depressed than in other breeds with dilated cardiomyopathy, and

(4) congestive heart failure usually results from progressive systolic dysfunction.[17] English cocker spaniels, like other small-breed dogs, may be concurrently affected with chronic acquired valvular disease.

ENDOCARDIAL FIBROELASTOSIS

Diffuse endocardial thickening by fibrous and elastic tissues has been reported for a few unrelated dogs.[19] Structural and functional features are similar to those observed with dilated cardiomyopathy. The clinical, pathologic, and diagnostic distinction between this syndrome and dilated cardiomyopathy is often unclear. Treatment is therefore similar to that described for systolic dysfunction.

TREATMENT OF HEART FAILURE DUE TO SYSTOLIC DYSFUNCTION

Ideally, management of heart failure due to systolic dysfunction (dilated cardiomyopathy) is directed to (1) treat causative or associated factors and avoid cardiotoxic or cardiosuppressive agents, (2) increase myocardial contractility, (3) reduce or eliminate congestive signs, and (4) manage arrhythmias. Since etiology or contributory factors are usually obscure, standard therapy relies on inotropic agents to augment contractility, diuretics to reduce congestive signs, vasodilators to promote ventricular unloading, as well antiarrhythmic drugs, exercise restriction, and dietary modification[1–3,5,8–13,15–19,21–26,34,37,42–43,58–68] (Table 23-4). Therapy is directed to optimize cardiac output by pharmacologic manipulation of the four major determinants

Table 23-4 Drugs Used in the Management of Canine Dilated Cardiomyopathy

Drug	Use	Dose
Immediate Therapy		
Diuretics		
Furosemide (Lasix)	Reduce's congestion, effusions	2.2–4.4 mg/kg IV, IM bid to qid
Positive inotropes		
Digoxin (Lanoxin)	Life-threatening supraventricular arrhythmias	Rapid IV: 0.01–0.02 mg/kg in 2–4 divided doses
	Inotropic support	0.01–0.015 mg/kg PO bid (max, 0.75 mg divided)
Dobutamine (Dobutrex)	Short-term inotropic support	2–10 µg/kg/min IV CRI
Dopamine (Intropin)	Same	2–5 µg/kg/min IV CRI
Amrinone (Inocor)	Same	1–3 mg/kg IV bolus, 10–100 µg/kg/min CRI
Vasodilators	Ventricular unloading	
Captopril (Capoten)	Balanced vasodilator	0.5–1.0 mg/kg PO bid to tid
Hydralazine (Apresoline)	Arterial dilation	1–2 mg/kg PO bid
Prazosin (Minipress)	Balanced vasodilator	1–2 mg PO bid to tid
2% nitroglycerin ointment (Nitro-Bid)	Venous vasodilator	$\frac{1}{4}$–1 inch cutaneously q4–6 h
Isosorbide dinitrate (Isordril)	Venous vasodilator	0.5–2.0 mg/kg PO bid to tid)
Ventricular antiarrhythmics	Control Ventricular arrhythmias	
Lidocaine (Xylocaine)		2–4 mg/kg IV bolus (max, 8 mg/kg) over 10 min; 25–75 µg/kg IV CRI
Procainamide (Pronestyl, Procan SR)		6–8 mg/kg IV over 5 min (beware of hypotension); 8–20 mg/kg PO, IM tid to qid
Quinidine (Quiniglute Duratabs, Cardioquin)		6–20 mg/kg IM qid (gluconate) or PO (many preparations)
Propranolol (Inderal)		0.02–0.06 mg/kg IV slowly; 0.2–1.0 mg/kg PO tid
Tocainide (Tonocard)		25 mg/kg PO tid
Maintenance Therapy		
Digoxin	Maintenance inotropic support	Same as oral dose above
Ventricular antiarrhythmic drugs	As needed	Same as above

(Continued)

Table 23-4 Drugs Used in the Management of Canine Dilated Cardiomyopathy (*continued*)

Drug	Use	Dose
Maintenance Therapy		
β-*Adrenergic blockers*	Slow ventricular rate below 150 beats/min after digitalized	
Propranolol (Inderal)	Same	0.2–1.0 mg/kg PO tid
Atenolol (Tenormin)	Same Cardioselective	0.25–1.0 mg/kg PO sid to bid
Nadolol (Corgard)	Same	0.5–1.0 mg/kg PO bid
Metoprolol (Lopressor)	Same Cardioselective	12.5–25 mg PO bid to tid
Diuretics	Reduce congestion, effusions	
Furosemide (Lasix)		2.2–4.4 mg/kg PO (or lowest effective dose)
Hydrochlorthiazide (Hydrodiuril)	Combine with furosemide for refractory congestion	2–4 mg/kg PO bid
Spironolactone (Aldactone)	Potassium-sparing diuretic	2–4 mg/kg/day PO
Triamterene (Dyrenium)	Potassium-sparing diuretic	2–4 mg/kg/day PO

CRI, constant-rate infusion.

of left ventricular performance: (1) preload (i.e., ventricular filling pressure); (2) afterload (i.e., arterial pressure and resistance to ventricular emptying); (3) myocardial contractility; and (4) heart rate and rhythm.[58]

Immediate Therapy

Initial treatment depends on the severity, progression, and type of congestive heart failure (Table 23-4). Rapid and fatal decompensation and disease progression are possible, especially when arrhythmias are present. Stressful diagnostic procedures should be temporarily postponed pending aggressive emergency treatment (e.g., intravenous furosemide, vasodilators, supplemental oxygen administration).

Therapeutic thoracocentesis is performed in dyspneic animals when heart and lung sounds are muffled and thoracic percussion indicates effusion. Occasionally, severe ascites must be drained because it impairs respiration. Mechanical fluid removal causes no untoward effects.

Diuretics are intially given to control edema and mobilize effusion. Furosemide is used for its quick onset of action, marked potency, and steep dose-response curve, even in the presence of impaired renal function.[63] The intravenous onset of action and peak effect of furosemide are rapid (5 and 30 minutes, respectively).[67,68] Furosemide may also cause venodilation and preload reduction even before its diuretic effects,[69,70] which helps relieve dyspnea from pulmonary edema. Therefore, in severely dyspneic states, furosemide is administered intravenously or intramuscularly (2.2 to 4.4 mg/kg tid to qid).

If additional preload reduction is necessary due to life-threatening pulmonary edema, topical cutaneous application of 2 percent nitroglycerin ointment (Nitro-Bid) can be beneficial. Some afterload reduction may result as well.[68] Dosage is ¼ to 1 inch applied to the axilla, ear pinna, or a shaved skin region every 4 to 6 hours. Care should be taken to avoid contact with human skin.

Inotropic support is required to stimulate the depressed myocardium, since congestive heart failure is caused by systolic impairment. Digoxin (Lanoxin) has been used most commonly. Maintenance oral digitalization is usually sufficient (0.01 to 0.015 mg/kg PO of lean body weight divided bid, not to exceed 0.75 mg/day in giant-breed dogs). Some animals, especially the Doberman pinscher breed and dogs with impaired renal function, are sensitive to the effects of digitalis. In these situations, the dose is reduced (e.g., 0.25 to 0.375 mg divided bid). Occasionally, a loading dose (i.e., twice the oral maintenance dose in two divided doses) is suggested during the first day to achieve digoxin blood levels more quickly.[9–13] However, this increases the likelihood of digoxin toxicity and should generally be avoided. Intravenous digitalization (0.01 to 0.02 mg/kg in two to four divided doses, given over 4 hours) has been suggested by some investigators when heart rates due to atrial fibrillation exceeds 230 beats/min.[13]

Clinical response to digoxin is unpredictable and inconsistent, and serum blood levels are variable. For example, when digoxin was administered to 10 dogs with dilated cardiomyopathy (0.22 mg/m^2 body surface area bid), it was efficacious in only four cases. Positive inotropic effects could not be predicted by clinical criteria, echocardiographic baseline shortening fraction, heart rate, or jugular venous oxygen tension.[71] Another study, of 81 dogs with atrial fibrillation, showed only a weak correlation between serum digoxin dosage and serum digoxin concentration.[72] Heart failure-related alterations in renal function, volume of distribution, and drug absorbtion may cause variations in efficacy.

Digitalization must be individualized and guided by serum digoxin concentrations when lack of expected response or toxicity is suspected. Electrolytes, blood urea nitrogen, and creatinine should be periodically monitored because azotemia and hypokalemia predispose to digoxin toxicity. Biologic half-life of digoxin is normally 20 to 35 hours. Therapeutic levels after 5 to 7 days of therapy fall between 1.0 and 2.5 ng/ml when assessed 8 to 12 hours after the last oral dose.[13,73–76]

The ECG should be monitored regularly, if isolated ventricular premature complexes (VPCs) are detected during digitalization. Digoxin may be temporarily withdrawn and antiarrhythmic treatment initiated (e.g., lidocaine) if more than 25 VPCs/min or ventricular tachycardia occur. Lidocaine has minimal adverse hemodynamic effects. It is administered as an IV bolus, 2 to 4 mg/kg, repeated to a maximum of 8 mg/kg; alternatively, it may be administered as a constant-rate infusion, 25 to 75 µg/kg/min. Quinidine should be avoided because it may increase the serum digoxin level (by decreasing renal digoxin clearance) and predispose to digoxin toxicity.[77] In addition, the vagolytic effect of quinidine may also accelerate AV conduction and increase the ventricular rate in atrial fibrillation. Procainamide can be used instead, 6 to 20 mg/kg qid to tid IM or PO.

If significant renal disease or renal insufficiency is present, digitoxin may be substituted for digoxin. Digitoxin is rapidly cleared by the liver (rather than by the kidney, as with digoxin) and is highly protein bound. It has a lesser parasympathomimetic effect than digoxin and, therefore, may be less effective in controlling supraventricular arrhythmias.[75,76,78] Its half-life is approximately 8 to 12 hours. The recommended dose of digitoxin (Crystodigin) is 0.04 to 0.08 mg/kg divided bid to tid. Therapeutic serum concentration is 15 to 35 ng/ml when measured 6 to 8 hours after the last oral dose.[73–76]

A more potent inotropic drug may be desired for acute, short-term management when systolic function (contractility) is extremely poor, if cardiogenic shock is present, or if the patient is a Doberman pinscher. Two sympathomimetic amines have been used for this purpose. Dopamine (Intropin) (2 to 5 µg/kg/min) produces intropic effects partly by direct myocardial stimulation and partly by release of myocardial stores of norepinephrine. At higher doses (5 to 15 µg/kg/min), it may cause vasoconstriction (α-adrenergic stimulation), increase heart rate and myocardial oxygen demand, and cause ventricular arrhythmias.[79–81] Dobutamine (Dobutrex) (2 to 10 µg/kg/min) causes direct myocardial stimulation with minimum affect on heart rate or inducement of α-adrenergic vasoconstriction. Therefore, it may be more useful in the management of severe heart failure.[82–85] In addition, long-term hemodynamic benefits have resulted in humans with even brief infusion intervals of this inotrope.[86,87]

Interest has recently focused on a new class of inotropic agents having both positive inotropic and vasodilatory effects. These nonglycoside, nonsympathomimetic positive inotropes selectively inhibit cyclic adenosine (cAMP)-specific cardiac phosphodiesterase F-III.[62] Amrinone can substantially augment performance of the failing heart,[88] although reports of limited efficacy and side effects in humans have surfaced.[89] In dogs with induced myocardial failure, amrinone infusions increased contractility 40 to 200 percent above baseline, increasing cardiac output by 80 percent. This drug is not routinely used except for short-term administration in severe refractory heart failure; the initial dose is 1 to 3 mg/kg (slow IV bolus) followed by 10 to 100 μg/kg/mm constant-rate infusion.[90]

Milrinone, a bipyridine derivative closely related to amrinone, has similar pharmacologic and hemodynamic effects. It is approximately 15 times more potent on a per-milligram basis[91] and is more free of side effects than amrinone.[58] When milrinone was used as the sole therapeutic agent in dogs with myocardial failure, left ventricular function improved in all animals. A small number of dogs experienced worsening of ventricular arrhythmias. An oral dose of 0.5 to 1.0 mg/kg bid is effective in increasing myocardial contractility.[92] The half-life in dogs is 2 to 3 hours, and the positive inotropic effect was 75 percent of maximum 5 to 7 hours after administration. Milrinone may be required every 6 to 8 hours in some dogs.[93] This drug is not yet marketed.

Vasodilator drugs are used to reduce venous congestion and improve cardiac performance by decreasing resistance to left ventricular ejection (i.e., afterload).[60] Elevated afterload is an important consequence in dilated cardiomyopathy in humans. The failing heart may lose the ability to maintain cardiac output in the face of the increased resistance to ventricular outflow. Ventricular performance becomes inversely related to this impedance.[65] An afterload mismatch may develop as a result of increased vascular resistance and an inability to eject an appropriate quantity of blood.[66] In addition, a large percentage of persons with systolic dysfunction have significant mitral regurgitation. Forward cardiac output is enhanced when regurgitation is reduced by vasodilator therapy.[94] Mitral regurgitation is also common with canine dilated cardiomyopathy.[9-13] Various drugs have been used (Table 23-4), including balanced vasodilators such as captopril (Capoten), 0.5 mg/kg bid to tid; prazosin (Minipress), 1 to 2 mg bid to tid); arteriolar dilators such as hydralazine (Apresoline), 1 to 2 mg/kg bid); and venodilators, such as 2 percent nitrolglycerin ointment (Nitro-Bid), ¼ to 1 inch cutaneously every 4 to 6 hours. Potential hazards of vasodilator therapy include the creation or exacerbation of hypotension,

decreased preload and cardiac output, vomiting and diarrhea (especially captopril), and reflex sinus tachycardia (especially hydralazine). Although controlled veterinary clinical trials have not demonstrated long-term benefit, short-term improvement of congestive heart failure have been documented.[95] Moreover, human studies have strongly suggested that some vasodilator drugs improve the prognosis of severely ill patients.[96,97]

Fluid therapy is occasionally required for judicious expansion of the vascular compartment contracted by nonalimentation or overaggressive diuresis or for hypotension caused by vasodilator drug therapy. Fluid dosage and administration rate must be individualized on the basis of phase of heart failure or hydration status or serum protein, electrolyte, creatinine, and blood urea nitrogen concentrations. Submaintenance doses are advocated. Lactated Ringer's solution or a mixture of lactated Ringer's and 5 percent dextrose in water (D_5W) may be cautiously infused at 20 to 40 ml/kg/day divided in two or three doses. Potassium chloride may be added according to serum deficits or empirically supplemented in fluids (5 to 7 mEq/250 ml) if prolonged anorexia or aggressive diuresis occurs. If pulmonary edema occurs, fluid administration should be discontinued.[11] Central venous pressure (CVP) measurements provide a rough estimate of the ability of the heart to pump the fluids being returned to it. Normal CVP is 0 to 5 cm H_2O; measurements within the 15- to 20-cm H_2O range are too high and indicate that fluid administration should be interrupted or stopped.[98]

Maintenance Therapy

Digoxin therapy is continued in order to augment myocardial contractility on the presumption that residual myocardial function or adequate contractile reserve exists.[99,100] Global cardiac performance and systemic perfusion must improve sufficiently if an inotropic drug is to be clinically beneficial.[58]

Atrial fibrillation is often present at or near the time of cardiac decompensation. Because severe atrial enlargement causes or contributes to this arrhythmia,[101,102] conversion to sustained sinus rhythm is usually not possible. Therefore, therapeutic goals focus on reducing the ventricular rate below 150 beats/min to permit sufficient ventricular diastolic filling. Digitalis glycosides are also used for this purpose to slow conduction through the AV node.

The oral maintenance dose of digoxin for large and giant-breed dogs is 0.01 to 0.015 mg/kg divided bid. Therapeutic digoxin levels have been achieved in 2 to 4.5 days using oral maintenance digitalization.[103] When digitalized, some dogs with atrial fibrillation undergo ventricular rate slowing below 150 beats/min, although less than 20 percent may respond in this fashion.[72] Optimal digitalization can be facilitated by serum digoxin evaluations to help verify toxic states or identify subtherapeutic levels. Digoxin dosage must often be reduced if severe weight loss or azotemia develops. Biochemical profiles should be performed to evaluate electrolyte and renal status whenever anorexia or vomiting occurs.

β-Adrenergic blocking agents are usually required to reduce the ventricular rate further in the digitalized patient with atrial fibrillation when digoxin alone has been unsuccessful in controlling the ventricular rate below 150 beats/min. Propranolol, a nonselective β-adrenergic blocker may be administered after the animal has been digitalized for 2 to 3 days.[8–13] Starting dose is 0.5 mg/kg PO divided tid. If needed, daily increments of 10 mg tid are added to this dose (maximum daily dose 1.0 mg/kg tid) until the resting heart rate is 100 to 140 beats/min. Other β-blocking drugs may permit longer dosing intervals such as nadolol (Corgard), 0.5 to 1.0 mg/kg bid, titrated to effect. Drugs with greater β_1-adrenoceptor cardioselectivity include metoprolol (Lopresser), 12.5 to 25 mg bid to tid and atenolol (Tenormin), 0.25 to 1.0 mg/kg PO sid to bid (Table 23-4).

Vasodilators should be continued if adverse effects (e.g., vomiting, diarrhea, hypotension, anorexia) do not occur. Switching to a different agent may avoid the toxicity experienced with an initial drug (Table 23-4).

Boxer and Doberman pinscher breeds usually require a therapeutic approach modified toward management of resistant ventricular arrhythmias. Some dogs respond to procainamide, 8 to 20 mg/kg qid, or to quinidine, 6 to 20 mg/kg tid. Concomitant administration of digoxin and quinidine may predispose to digoxin intoxication; ideally, this combination should be avoided. Propranolol (0.5 to 1.0 mg/kg PO tid) may be added to procainamide in refractory cases. Tocainide (Tonocard) may be used (25 mg/kg PO tid) in lidocaine-responsive patients. Tocainide may have less proarrhythmic and greater antiarrhythmic effects than procainamide or quinidine but has the disadvantage of a brief duration of action (4 hours or less).[104] Prednisolone (1 mg/kg bid) may be given to boxers when arrhythmias are refractory to all antiarrhythmic therapy.

Most dogs may be maintained with digoxin, furosemide, a vasodilator, and a β-blocking drug to control the ventricular rate or arrhythmias. Exercise should be restricted to reduce cardiac work load. Dietary sodium intake should be reduced using either a commercial prescription diet (h/d) or a home preparation. Cardiac cachexia is a common development with dilated cardiomyopathy, and diets should provide adequate protein, vitamins, minerals, and calories.

Diuretic agents must often be increased or modified over time when disease progression and homeoregulatory mechanisms (e.g., aldosterone, antidiuretic hormone) increase renal sodium and water reabsorption and reduce their efficacy.[64] Furosemide may be increased (4.4 to 6.6 mg/kg PO tid), as needed. The addition of another diuretic drug acting at a different site in the nephron or at a similar site by a different mechanism of action may enhance natriuresis and diuresis.[63,105] Diuretic drugs used for this purpose include hydrochlorthiazide (Hydrodiuril), 2 to 4 mg/kg PO bid; hydrochlorthiazide/spironolactone combination product (Aldactazide), 1 to 4 mg/kg/day PO; spironolactone (Aldactone), 2 to 4 mg/kg/day PO; triamterene (Dyrenium), 2 to 4 mg/kg/day PO. The latter two drugs are potassium-sparing agents. They may be selected if hypokalemia has resulted from anorexia or large doses of potent loop diuretics. In general, hypokalemia and metabolic alkalosis are rare. Hyperkalemia is a potential side effect when potassium-sparing diuretics are used in the presence of renal disease, potassium supplementation, or co-therapy with angiotensin-converting enzyme inhibitors (e.g., captopril, enalapril).[2,3,69] A relatively new loop diuretic, bumetanide (Bumex) is 40 to 70 times more potent than furosemide. Potential side effects include ototoxicity and electrolyte imbalance.[106,107] This drug has not yet been carefully evaluated for use in the treatment of canine dilated cardiomyopathy.

Prognosis is guarded. Atrial fibrillation is associated with a poor outcome and a 6-month mortality rate of 74 to 85 percent.[72,108,109] Dogs with atrial fibrillation that demonstrate a positive inotropic response to digoxin (i.e., increased shortening fraction echocardiographically) may live longer than those who do not. Heart rate is probably not a reliable predictor of either digoxin response or life expectancy.[71] Boxers with congestive heart failure and ventricular arrhythmias and Doberman pinschers have the worst prognosis. Sudden death is especially common in these groups. Progressive right-sided heart failure is an ominous sign in any breed.

Many dogs become compensated on medication. Some survive up to 2 years. Overall mean survival is approximately 6 months. Death is associated with congestive heart failure or arrhythmias. Spontaneous resolution has not been reported.

HEART FAILURE DUE TO DIASTOLIC DYSFUNCTION

Ventricular hypertrophy or fibrosis may result from various primary or secondary myocardial disorders.[2,3,6,7,9–14] In humans, these processes decrease left ventricular compliance (i.e., increase myocardial stiffness) and impede diastolic filling. Systolic (pumping) function is usually adequate, but clinical signs result from diastolic impairment. Factors contributing to reduced compliance include impaired ventricular relaxation, myofibrillar architectural disarray, abnormal ventricular cavity shape, endomyocardial fibrosis, myocardial hypertrophy, and ventricular cavity distortion.[2,3,110–112]

Left ventricular hypertrophy is an important compensatory response to chronic left ventricular pressure or volume overload. Therefore, it does not automatically equate with a diagnosis of hypertrophic cardiomyopathy. It may be observed with various systemic, metabolic, or infiltrative diseases, it may occur in athletic individuals, or it may be idiopathic.[9,11–14,112]

Hypertrophic Cardiomyopathy

Hypertrophic cardiomyopathy is rarely clinically diagnosed in dogs. Popularization of cardiac ultrasound, however, may uncover a higher incidence.

The etiology is unknown. Possible causes as well as pathophysiology have been discussed under feline myocardial disease (Ch. 22).

PATHOLOGY

The hallmark pathologic feature of primary (idiopathic) hypertrophic cardiomyopathy is abnormal left ventricular hypertrophy and increased ventricular muscle mass in the absence of a causative systemic or cardiac disease. Disproportionate thickening of the ventricular septum (asymmetric septal hypertrophy) has been recorded more frequently than symmetric hypertrophy in dogs. The ratio of ventricular septal to free wall thickness usually exceeds 1.1. Six of 10 reported cases had ratios greater than or equal to 1.3, although both the septum and free wall were hypertrophied).[113–116] The heart weight to body weight ratio is increased.[116] Ventricular septal disorganization (greater than 5 percent of the tissue section) has been reported in 20 percent of affects dogs.[114,116] Fibrous connective tissue may be present focally or diffusely in the endocardium.[114,115] Decompensated animals may experience congestive heart failure, episodic weakness, syncope, or sudden death.

CLINICAL FINDINGS

Canine idiopathic hypertrophic cardiomyopathy has been insufficiently studied to provide a characteristic clinical description. It has been reported in 13 dogs, ranging from 10 weeks to 13 years of age.[113–117] Various breeds were recorded, with the German shepherd represented four times. Males were predominantly affected.

Clinical history is variable, ranging from asymptomatic to sudden unexplained death. The latter represented causes of mortality in 8 of 10 awake or anesthetized dogs studied retrospectively.[114,115] Evidence of heart failure (e.g., syncope, exercise intolerance, coughing, dyspnea, ascites, hepatomegaly, pleural effusion) were recorded in 4 of 12 dogs.[113–117] Heart murmurs were present in two young asymptomatic dogs, although auscultatory results were not recorded in the larger postmortem retrospective study. In affected humans, a late-onset systolic murmur located between the left apex and base is usually evident when a dynamic subaortic pressure gradient (associated with systolic anterior motion of the mitral valve) is present.[60,118,119] The dynamic obstruction and murmur may be enhanced by factors that increase contractility (e.g., isoproterenol, ventricular premature complexes) or decrease arterial pressure (e.g., sodium nitroprusside). Factors that decrease contractility (e.g., β-adrenergic blocking drugs) or that increase arterial blood pressure (e.g., phenylephrine, methoxamine) may reduce or abolish the dynamic obstruction or associated heart murmur.[113,118]

Electrocardiograms recorded in seven dogs showed a high incidence of conduction abnormalities (e.g., first- and third-degree AV block, bifascicular and right bundle branch block). Depression or slurring of the ST segment was noted in two animals with normal rhythms.[113–115] In humans, characteristic features include increased QRS voltage, left anterior hemiblock, ST- and T-wave abnormalities, prominent abnormal Q waves (suggesting ventricular septal hypertrophy) in leads II, III, aVF, or V_4 to V_6, and ventricular arrhythmias. However, the ECG is often unremarkable.[120,121]

Radiographic findings may be unremarkable. In some cases, moderate left atrial and ventricular enlargement with extracardiac signs of congestive heart failure have been recorded.[113–115]

Echocardiographic characterization is similar to that described for feline hypertrophic cardiomyopathy. Because asymmetric septal hypertrophy was a dominant feature of necropsied cases,[114–116] this may be an expected finding in affected dogs assessed by ultrasound.

Angiographic changes (left ventricular hypertrophy, decreased left ventricular end-systolic volume, mild mitral regurgitation, systolic anterior motion of the mitral valve and variable dynamic subaortic gradient) were demonstrated in one dog.[113]

Differential diagnosis should include congenital aortic stenosis, which causes left ventricular hypertrophy and systolic anterior motion of the mitral valve. Athletic working or hunting dogs may display compensatory left ventricular hypertrophy. Systemic or metabolic disease may cause conduction system abnormalities and should be investigated when AV nodal block or bundle branch blocks are detected.

TREATMENT OF HEART FAILURE ASSOCIATED WITH DIASTOLIC DYSFUNCTION

Therapeutic strategies for heart failure resulting from diastolic dysfunction (hypertrophic or restrictive cardiomyopathy) are directed toward the elimination of pulmonary edema or effusion, the management of arrhythmias, and the modification of factors contributing to diastolic dysfunction.[2,3] Diastolic dysfunction may be reduced by interventions or drugs that decrease ventricular contractility increase left ventricular filling, expand the left ventricular outflow tract, and enhance ventricular distensibility (i.e., compliance).[118,122]

Treatment has not been reported for canine hypertrophic cardiomyopathy. Therapeutic strategies would potentially be modeled after feline and human protocols in which diuretics and β-adrenergic blockers represent the mainstay of medical therapy (Ch. 22).

SECONDARY CARDIOMYOPATHIES

Structural and functional myocardial alterations or injury resulting from known systemic or metabolic abnormalities have been termed secondary cardiomyopathies (Table 23-1). Overlap between categories is common. Identification of causative factors sometimes permits an effective clinical approach toward prevention, treatment, or cure. In most cases, however, underlying causes remain obscure and resultant myocardial injury is nonspecific.[2,3,7,14]

Noninfectious Causes of Myocardial Disease

Noninfectious agents may directly or indirectly damage the myocardium acutely, chronically, transiently, or permanently. Inflammation may not be present. Offending agents include drugs, chemicals, toxins, physical agents (radiation, excessive heat), nutritional disorders, and infectious, systemic, and metabolic diseases.[2,3,7–14]

Hyperthyroidism is uncommon in dogs as compared with cats. Thyroid tumors are usually malignant (adenocarcinoma) rather than benign (adenoma). Clinical canine hyperthyroidism is rare. Thyroid neoplasia represents up to 2 percent of canine neoplasms.[123] There is no sex predilection, but boxers are more commonly affected. In a series of 55 dogs with thyroid tumors, approximately one-third were capable of radioiodine uptake, and about 20 percent exhibited signs of hyperthyroidism.[123,124] Only one-fourth of clinically detected thyroid tumors (generally carcinomas) secrete suficient thyroid hormone to cause hyperthyroidism.[125]

Canine thyrotoxicosis is clinical variable with abrupt or insidious onset. Signs may be mild or severe. Polydipsia and polyurea is one of the most frequent and first abnormalities to develop. Clinical signs occur in proportion to severity and duration of the thyrotoxic state (e.g., excessive panting, restlessness, fatigue and weakness, polyphagia, hyperdefecation, and weight loss in advanced cases). Femoral arterial pulses and precordial apex beats may be hyperkinetic.[123–126] Heart rates seldom exceed the normal range (in contrast to feline hyperthyroidism), although ECG evidence of left ventricular enlargement (tall R waves) may be present.[126] Plasma thyroid hormone levels are elevated.

Prompt surgical thyroidectomy is advocated. Metastasis may occur in 40 percent of dogs with adenocarcinomas by the time of clinical examination and has been detected in up to 80 percent of affected dogs at necropsy. Antithyroid drugs should ideally be used as described in feline hyperthyroidism. Chemotherapy or radiotherapy may be beneficial with inoperable or disseminated disease.

Prognosis is variable. Early detection and resection greatly benefits some animals. With tumors greater than 5 cm in diameter, however, long-term prognosis is poor.[123]

Toxins, chemicals, and *physical agents* may cause cardiotoxicity. Anthracyclines, especially doxorubicin, often cause cardiotoxicity. Arrhythmias (ventricular, supraventricular, and conduction abnormalities), dilated cardiomyopathy, and congestive heart failure have occurred with cumulative doses ranging from greater than 240 mg/m² to 150 mg/m² or less.[126,127] Acute cardiotoxicity may also occur after initial therapy.[128] Characteristic pathologic findings in chronic toxicity include cardiac chamber dilation, systolic (myocardial) failure, myocyte degeneration and atrophy (myofibrillar loss, cytoplasmic vacuolation and myocytolysis), myocardial interstitial fibrosis, and edema.[124,125] Serial ECGs and M-mode echocardiograms are unreliable in predicting doxorubicin-induced cardiomyopathy.[127] Left bundle branch block and ventricular arrhythmias are the most common ECG changes associated with chronic cardiotoxicity and dilated cardiotoxicity and dilated cardiomyopathy with congestive heart failure (Smith G: Personal communication, 1988). Associated heart failure is usually refractory to therapy and may occur over a variable period from the last doxorubicin treatment.

Myocardial injury may also result from other causes, including hydrocarbons, carbon monoxide, mercury, arsenic, selenium deficiency, heat stroke, hypothermia, blunt or penetrating trauma, electric shock, or hypersensitivity reactions.[2,3,7]

Ischemic myocardial injury as a discrete event does not represent a large cause of mortality, as in humans. However, ischemia may result from other diseases and may contribute to arrhythmias and reduced cardiac performance.

Microscopic myocardial infarction is rare but can occur from infective endocarditis-induced coronary embolism[130,131] or from emboli from septic, neoplastic, or thrombotic diseases.[9,13] Microscopic focal myocardial infarction is related to arteriosclerotic vascular lesions (hyalinosis, amyloidosis, thickening of musculoelastic fibers, and microthrombi). This finding is common in older dogs and is often associated with mitral valve myxomatous degeneration and insufficiency (endocardiosis).[132,133] The effects of these lesions are unclear. Myocardial ischemia and necrosis may result from coronary vasoconstriction (secondary to CNS trauma and related increased sympathetic traffic),[134] acute gastric dilation-volvulus,[135] high levels of circulating catecholamines,[136] digitalis toxicity,[137] atherosclerosis (especially with severe hypothyroidism and hypercholesterolemia),[138] and pancreatitis.

Neoplasia may be associated with cardiac infiltration or extracardiac (systemic) abnormalities, depending on whether the heart is affected primarily or secondarily. Cardiac manifestations include disturbances of conduction or rhythm, congestive heart failure, pericardial effusion or tamponade, and syncope. Specific signs are closely related to the anatomic location of the tumor.[139]

Hemangiosarcoma is the most common primary cardiac tumor, although it commonly arises from noncardiac sites. Cardiac origin has been recorded from 3 to 50 percent[140-142] of affected dogs at necropsy. German shepherd dogs aged 2 to 15 years (mean, 10 years) account for one-third of recorded cases.[141-143]

Canine chemodectomas are predominantly aortic body tumors with a predilection for brachycephalic breeds (boxers, Boston terriers) in the 6- to 14-year range. They usually originate at the base of the aorta and/or pulmonary artery. Small tumors are well defined, but large neoplasms may infiltrate the atria, ventricles, and surrounding tissues. Metastasis occurs one-fifth to one-fourth of the time, but local invasion is common.[144]

Myocarditis (inflammation of the interstitium, myocytes or vascular structures) may result from primary or secondary factors. Mild focal inflammation may cause no symptoms, whereas generalized myocarditis may result in fatal arrhythmias and congestive heart failure. Myocarditis or clinical signs may occur from direct invasion and cellular injury or result from toxic, allergic, or hypersensitivity responses by the host to the inciting stimulus.[2,3,145] Diagnosis must often be implied from extracardiac manifestations of the dominant, systemic disease process. ECG changes may be nonspecific (e.g., ST- and T-wave alterations), transient, or sustained or may include atrial and ventricular arrhythmias and conduction disturbances. Arrhythmias may occur during the peak of infection or occur after clinical signs have subsided. Serodiagnostic tests for specific diseases (e.g., trypanosomiasis, toxoplasmosis, parvovirus) may be diagnostically helpful. Therapy is usually directed toward the dominant underlying systemic disease, to alleviation or stabilization of congestive heart failure or management of arrhythmias.[11]

Canine parvovirus became recognized worldwide in 1978.[7,146-152] Myocardial manifestations (usually without concurrent enteritis) included a peracute fatal myocarditis. Robust, healthy pups born into a contaminated environment without sufficient maternal antibody protection were affected during the first 3 to 8 weeks of life. Sudden hyperpnia, dyspnea, crying, cyanosis, and unexpected death from pulmonary edema occurred within minutes to hours. Clinical manifestations included arrhyth-

mias, tachycardia, left apical systolic murmurs, gallop rhythms, pulmonary edema, cardiomegaly, and death before or despite therapy. Postmortem findings included enlarged dilated hearts with pale myocardial streaks. Large basophilic or amphophilic intranuclear inclusion bodies were histologically characteristic (Fig. 23-8). A focal mononuclear cell infiltrate was variably present. This syndrome is now rarely encountered. Widespread development of protective maternal antibody through viral exposure and vaccination is probably responsible.[9,11]

A subclinical form of myocarditis may occur in which nonfatal neonatal parvovirus results in dilated cardiomyopathy and congestive heart failure in young adults, typically 5 or 6 months of age.[7,9-13,151-154] Distinctive diffuse myocardial streaks are diffusely present representing scarring (fibrosis) without histologic evidence of inflammation. Parvovirus myocarditis in adult dogs has been reported but is rare.[155]

Other viruses caused myocarditis in vitro. Canine distemper virus has produced myocarditis in puppies infected experimentally at 5 to 7 days of age but not in those infected at 10 to 21 days of age.[156] Myocardial lesions in the younger group were present by 16 days of age. Lesions consisted of multifocal myonecrosis, minimal inflammatory cell response, mineralization, and fibrosis. Canine herpesvirus has experimentally infected puppies during the second trimester of gestation. This resulted in fetal and perinatal death with associated necrotizing myocarditis and intranuclear inclusion bodies.[157] The role of these viruses in development of myocardial disease has not been established.

Trypanosomiasis (Chagas disease) infects predominantly young, dogs under 2 years of age from the southeastern United States (Louisiana, Texas).[158-161] The protozoan *Trypanosoma cruzi* is enzootic among wild animals and dogs in that region and it is spread by reduvid blood-sucking insects.[159,162] An acute syndrome characterized by cardiac abnormalities (tachycardia, weak arterial pulses, arrhythmias, cardiomegaly, hepatomegaly, pulmonary edema, ascites) and systemic signs (weight loss, diarrhea, lethargy, anorexia, lymphadenopathy, sudden death) results. Granulomatous myocarditis associated with amastigotes of *T. cruzi* (predominantly within myocytes) are the hallmark feature. The right atrium and ventricle become di-

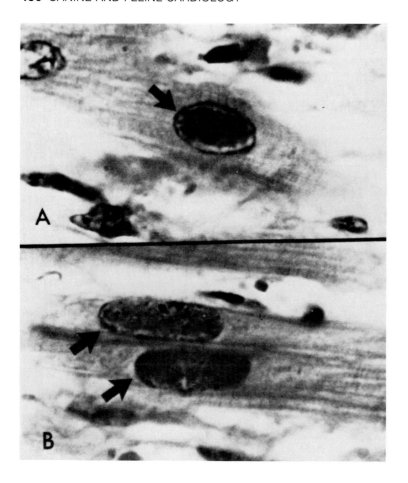

Fig. 23-8 Photomicrographs of myocardium of a 5-week-old German shepherd. (H & E stain, × 1,200.) **(A)** Cardiac myofiber containing a dense intranuclear inclusion body (arrow) surrounded by a clear zone. **(B)** Less dense inclusion bodies completely filling the nuclei (arrows) of cardiac myofibers. (Hayes MA, Russell RG, Babiuk LA: Sudden death in young dogs with myocarditis caused by parvovirus. J Am Vet Med Assoc 174:1197, 1979.)

lated and most severely affected. Lesions also appear in the left heart.[158,161] Antemortem diagnosis is possible using blood culture techniques and serologic testing. Because of public health significance, treatment is generally not undertaken.

Toxoplasmosis caused by the obligate intracellular coccidian parasite, *Toxoplasma gondii* occurs in a wide variety of birds and mammals. Rarely, it can affect the heart as part of a fulminating systemic process. However, myocarditis is overshadowed in most cases by the more dominant systemic effects.

Hepatozoon canis may affect the myocardium during its life cycle (schizogony)[163,164] and has been reported in the Texas gulf coast.[164,165] The brown dog tick, *Rhipicephalus sanguineus,* is the definitive host of *H. canis.* Dogs become infected by ingesting a tick that contains sporulated oocysts. Clinical systemic signs include anorexia, fever, stiffness, neu-

trophilic leukocytosis, and periosteal new bone reaction.[165] Because of the wide distribution of the brown dog tick and mobile pet population, this disease may spread to other locations.

Bacterial myocarditis can result from sepsis, bacterial endocarditis, or pericarditis. Pathologic bacteremia occurs when systemic venous or lymphatic drainage of an infected tissue seeds the bloodstream. Abscessation or focal suppurative myocarditis may result. Fever and arrhythmias provide clinical suspicion, and serial blood cultures should be taken (Ch. 21).

Fungi or algae may affect the heart as a secondary manifestation of disseminated disease. This is often associated with reduced host-defense or immunosuppressive therapy.[11] Aortic valvular endocarditis and endomyocarditis was observed in a dog with generalized cryptococcosis (*Cryptococcus neofor-*

mans).[166] Disseminated *Coccidioides immites* has been reported in the heart[167,168] and aspergillosis (*Aspergillus tereus*) was found in supperative and nonsupperative granulomatous endomyocardial foci.[169,170] *Paecilomyces varioti* was isolated from myocardial granulomas in dogs with systemic paecilomycosis.[171] Algaelike organisms, *Prototheca wickerhamii, P. zopfi,* and *Prototheca* spp have been associated with granulomatous myocarditis and disseminated prototothecosis.[172–175]

Rocky Mountain spotted fever caused by *Rickettsia rickettsii* is transmitted by the bite of the American dog tick, *Dermacentor variabilis*. It causes mild nonspecific signs in many cases. Occasionally, severe systemic diseases results. Fatal ventricular arrhythmias, necrotizing vasculitis, ischemic necrosis, and myocardial thrombosis may result.[176]

Persistent atrial standstill associated with a fascioscapulohumeral–like skeletal muscular dystrophy has been reported in dogs, especially English spaniels.[177,178] The atria of affected dogs are greatly enlarged. Fibrosis and focal myocarditis and necrosis are sometimes evident. Pacemaker therapy has successfully controlled clinical signs due to the bradyarrhythmia in dogs.[179]

Cardiovascular abnormalities may rarely occur as part of polysystemic changes associated with *glycogen storage diseases*. Type II glycogen storage disease (Pompe's disease) was suspected in several Lapland dogs.[180] Cardiomegaly, ECG and radiographic abnormalities, myocardial glycogen infiltration, and biochemical identification of α-glucosidase deficiency were reported.

Inflammatory and degenerative lesions have been demonstrated in the conducting system of dogs. His-bundle stenosis, fibrosis, and degeneration have been described in related pug dogs.[181] Luminal small artery narrowing in the His-bundle region was suggested to be causative of His-bundle degeneration in dogs (mostly Doberman pinschers) with sudden death.[182] AV bundle fibrosis was observed in 12 dogs (10 male, 5 Doberman pinschers) who died unexpectedly.[183] Some displayed sudden viciousness or seizures, and all had hypoxic-type degeneration in the hippocampus and dorsal cerebral cortex. A possible association between arrhythmias and hypoxia was suggested.

REFERENCES

1. Adelman AG, Wigle ED, Felderhof CH, et al: Current concepts of primary cardiomyopathy. Cardiovasc Med 2:495, 1977
2. Wenger NK, Goodwin JF, Roberts WC: Cardiomyopathy and myocardial involvement in systemic disease. p. 1181. In Hurst JW (ed): The Heart. McGraw-Hill, New York, 1986
3. Wynne JW, Braunwald E: The cardiomyopathies and myocarditides. p. 1410. In Braunwald E (ed): Heart Disease. 3rd Ed. WB Saunders, Philadelphia, 1988
4. Report of the WHO/ISFC task force on the definition and classification of cardiomyopathies. Br Heart J 44:672, 1980
5. Goodwin JF: Congestive and hypertrophic cardiomyopathies. A decade of study. Lancet 1:731, 1970
6. Liu SK, Tilley LP: Animal models of primary myocardial diseases. Yale J Biol Med 53:191, 1980
7. Van Vleet JF, Ferrans V: Myocardial diseases of animals. Am J Pathol 124:98, 1986
8. Bonagura JD: Canine myocardial disease: Clinical evaluation and therapy. p. 737. Proceedings of the Fifth Annual Veterinary Medicine Forum. American College of Veterinary Internal Medicine, 1987
9. Thomas WP: Myocardial diseases of the dog. p. 117. In Bonagura JD (ed): Contemporary Issues in Small Animal Practice. Vol. 7: Cardiology. Churchill Livingstone, New York, 1987
10. Tilley LP, Liu SK, Fox PR: Myocardial disease. p. 1029. In Ettinger SJ (ed): Textbook of Veterinary Internal Medicine. 2nd Ed. Vol. I. WB Saunders, Philadelphia, 1983
11. Fox PR: Myocardial disease. In Ettinger SJ (ed): Textbook of Veterinary Internal Medicine. WB Saunders, Philadelphia 1989
12. Wood GL: Canine myocardial diseases. p. 321. In Kirk RW (ed): Current Veterinary Therapy. Vol. VIII. WB Saunders, Philadelphia, 1983
13. Ware WA, Bonagura JD: Canine myocardial diseases. p. 370. In Kirk RW (ed): Current Veterinary Therapy. Vol. IX. WB Saunders, Philadelphia, 1986
14. Fox PR: Cardiovascular disorders in systemic diseases. p. 265. In Tilley LP, Owens JM (eds): Manual of Small Animal Cardiology. Churchill Livingstone, New York, 1985
15. Thomas RE: Congestive cardiac failure in young Cocker Spaniels (a form of cardiomyopathy?): Details of eight cases. J Small Anim Pract 28:265, 1987

16. Staaden RV: Cardiomyopathy of English cocker spaniels. 178:1289, 1981

17. Gooding JP, Robinson WF, Mews GC: Echocardiographic characterization of dilatation cardiomyopathy in the English cocker spaniel. Am J Vet Res 47:1978, 1986

18. Gooding JP, Robinson WF, Wyburn RS, et al: A cardiomyopathy in the English cocker spaniel: A clinico-pathological investigation. J Small Anim Pract 23:133, 1982

19. Lombard CW, Buergielt CD: Endocardial fibroelastosis in four dogs. J Am Anim Hosp Assoc 20:271, 1984

20. Van Vleet JF, Ferrans V, Weirich W: Pathologic alterations in congestive cardiomyopathy of dogs. Am J Vet Res 42:416, 1981

21. Calvert CA, Chapman WL, Toal RL: Congestive cardiomyopathy in Doberman pinscher dogs. J Am Vet Med Assoc 181:598, 1982

22. Calvert CA: Dilated (congestive) cardiomyopathy in Doberman pinschers. Compend Contin Ed 6:417, 1986

23. Hazlett MJ, Maxie MG, Allen DG, et al: A retrospective study of heart disease in Doberman pinscher dogs. Can Vet J 24:205, 1983

24. Hill BL: Canine idiopathic congestive cardiomyopathy. Compend Contin Ed 3:615, 1981

25. Calvert CA, Brown J: Use of M-mode echocardiography in the diagnosis of congestive cardiomyopathy in Doberman pinschers. J Am Vet Med Assoc 189:293, 1986

26. Harpster NK: Boxer cardiomyopathy. p. 329. In Kirk RW (ed): Current Veterinary Therapy. Vol. VIII. WB Saunders, Philadelphia, 1983

27. Tilley LP: Essentials of Canine and Feline Electrocardiography. 2nd Ed. Lea & Febiger, Philadelphia, 1985

28. Edwards NJ: Bolton's Handbook of Canine and Feline Electrocardiography. 2nd Ed. WB Saunders, Philadelphia, 1987

29. Suter PF: Thoracic Radiography. A Text Atlas of Thoracic Diseases of the Dog and Cat. Peter F. Suter, Wettswil, Switzerland, 1984

30. Suter PF: The radiographic diagnosis of canine and feline heart disease. Compend Contin Ed 3:441, 1981

31. Feigenbaum H: Echocardiography. 4th Ed. Lea & Febiger, Philadelphia, 1986

32. Bonagura JD: M-mode echocardiography: Basic principles. Vet Clin North Am 13:299, 1983

33. Bonagura JD, Herring DS: Echocardiography: Acquired heart disease. Vet Clin North Am 15:1209, 1985

34. Keene BW, Panciera DL, Regitz V, et al: Carnitine-linked defects of myocardial metabolism in canine dilated cardiomyopathy. p. 54. Proceedings of the Fourth Annual Veterinary Medicine Forum. Vol. II. American College of Veterinary Internal Medicine, 1986 (abst)

35. Keene BW: Applications of endomyocardial biopsy techniques in the dog. p. 728. Proceedings of the Fifth Annual Veterinary Medicine Forum. American College of Veterinary Internal Medicine, 1987

36. Burk RL, Tilley LP, Henderson BM, et al: Endomyocardial biopsy in the dog. Am J Vet Res 41:2106, 1980

37. Greene HL, Reich SD, Dalen JE: How to minimize doxorubicin toxicity. J Cardiovasc Med 7:306, 1982

38. Ferrans VJ: Overview of cardiac pathology in relation to anthracycline cardiotoxicity. Cancer Treatm Rep 62:955, 1978

39. Gottdiener JS, Appelbaum FR, Ferrans VJ, et al: Cardiotoxicity associated with high dose cyclophosphamide therapy. Arch Intern Med 141:758, 1981

40. Factor SM, Minase T, Cho S, et al: Microvascular spasm in the cardiomyopathic Syrian hamster: A preventative cause of focal myocardial necrosis. Circulation 66:342, 1982

41. Berko B, Swift M: X-linked dilated cardiomyopathy. N Engl J Med 316:1186, 1987

42. Waber LJ, Valle D, Neill C, et al: Carnitine deficiency presenting as familial cardiomyopathy: A treatable defect in carnitine transport. J Pediatr 101:700, 1982

43. Rebouche CJ, Engel AG: Carnitine metabolism and deficiency syndromes. Mayo Clin Proc 58:533, 1983

44. Dec GW, Palacios IF, Fallon JT, et al: Active myocarditis in the spectrum of acute dilated cardiomyopathies. N Engl J Med 312:885, 1985

45. Maisch B, Deeg P, Liebau G, et al: Diagnostic relevance of humoral and cytotoxic immune reactions in primary and secondary dilated cardiomyopathy. Am J Cardiol 52:1072, 1983

46. Unverferth DV: The etiology of idiopathic dilated cardiomyopathy. p. 213. In Unverferth DV (ed): Dilated Cardiomyopathy. Futura, Mount Kisco, NY, 1985

47. Editorial: Selenium in the heart of China. Lancet 2:889, 1979

48. Johnson RA, Baker SS, Fallon JT, et al: An occidental case of cardiomyopathy and selenium deficiency. N Engl J Med 304:1210, 1981

49. Hsu FS, Du SJ: Cardiac diseases in swine. In Roberts HR, Dodds WJ (eds): p. 134. Pig Model for Biomedical Research. Pig Research Institute, Taiwan, Republic of China, 1982

50. Pion PD, Kittleson MD, Rogers QR, et al: Myocardial failure in cats associated with low plasma taurine: A reversible cardiomyopathy. Science 237:697, 1987

51. Grossman W, McLaurin LP, Rolett EL: Alterations in left ventricular relaxation and diastolic compliance in congestive cardiomyopathy. Cardiovasc Res 13:514, 1979

52. Lord PF: Left ventricular diastolic stiffness in dogs with congestive cardiomyopathy and volume overload. Am J Vet Res 37:953, 1976

53. Lord PF, Wood A, Tilley LP, et al: Radiographic and hemodynamic evaluation of cardiomyopathy and thromboembolism in the cat. J Am Vet Med Assoc 164:154, 1974

54. Boyden PA, Tilley LP, Pham TD, et al: Effects of left atrial enlargement on atrial transmembrane potentials and structure in dogs with mitral valve fibrosis. Am J Cardiol 49:1896, 1982

55. Boyden PA, Tilley LP, Albala A, et al: Mechanisms for atrial arrhythmias associated with cardiomyopathy: A study of feline hearts with primary myocardial disease. Circulation 69:1036, 1984

56. Benjamin IJ, Schuster EH, Bulkey BH: Cardiac hypertrophy in idiopathic dilated congestive cardiomyopathy: A clinicopathologic study. Circulation 64:422, 1981

57. Fox PR: Unpublished data—103 consecutive transtelephonic boxer electrocardiograms. Cardiopet, Div Animed, 1988

58. Maskin CS, Le Jemtel MD, Sonnenblick EH: Inotropic drugs for treatment of the failing heart. Cardiovasc Clin 14:1, 1984

59. Goodwin JF: The frontiers of cardiomyopathy. Br Heart J 48:1, 1982

60. Spodick DH: Effective management of congestive cardiomyopathy. Arch Intern Med 142:689, 1982

61. Colucci WS, Wright RF, Braunwald E: New positive inotropic agents in the treatment of congestive heart failure. Mechanisms of action and recent clinical developments. Part 1. N Engl J Med 314:290, 1986

62. Colucci WS, Wright RF, Braunwald E: New positive inotropic agents in the treatment of congestive heart failure. Mechanisms of action and recent clinical developments. Part 2. N Engl J Med 314:349, 1986

63. Opie LH, Kaplan NM: Diuretic therapy. p. 111. In Opie LH (ed): Drugs for the Heart. Grune & Stratton, Orlando, FL, 1987

64. Brest AN: Clinical pharmacology of diuretic drugs. Cardiovasc Clin 14:31, 1984

65. Cohn JN: Vasodilator therapy for heart failure: The influence of impedance on left ventricular performance. Circulation 48:5, 1973

66. Hirota Y, Shimizu G, Kaku K, et al: Mechanisms of compensation and decompensation in dilated cardiomyopathy. Am J Cardiol 54:1033, 1984

67. Frazier HS, Yager H: Drug therapy: The clinical use of diuretics. N Engl J Med 288:246, 1973

68. Smith TW, Braunwald E: The management of heart failure. p. 503. In Braunwald E (ed): Heart Disease. WB Saunders, Philadelphia, 1984

69. Biddle TL, Yu PN: Effect of furosemide on hemodynamics and lung water in acute pulmonary edema secondary to myocardial infarction. Am J Cardiol 43:86, 1979

70. Bourland WA, Day DK, Williamson HE: The role of the kidney in the early nondiuretic action of furosemide to reduce elevated left atrial pressure in the hypervolemic dog. J Pharmacol Exp Ther 282:222, 1977

71. Kittleson MD, Eyster GE, Knowlen GG, et al: Efficacy of digoxin administration in dogs with idiopathic congestive cardiomyopathy. J Am Vet Med Assoc 186:162, 1985

72. Bonagura JD, Ware WA: Atrial fibrillation in the dog: Clinical findings in 81 cases. J Am Anim Hosp Assoc 22:111, 1986

73. Kittleson ME: Drugs used in the management of heart failure. p. 285. In Kirk RW (ed): Current Veterinary Therapy. Vol. VIII. WB Saunders, Philadelphia, 1983

74. Breznock EM: Application of canine plasma kinetics of digoxin and digitoxin to therapeutic digitalization in the dog. Am J Vet Res 34:993, 1973

75. Hamlin RL: Basis for selection of a cardiac glycoside for dogs. p. 241. Proceedings of the First Symposium on Veterinary Pharmacological Therapy, 1978

76. DeRick A, Belpaire FM, Bogeert MG, et al: Plasma concentrations of digoxin and digitoxin during digitalization of healthy dogs and dogs with cardiac failure. Am J Vet Res 39:811, 1978

77. Rameis H: Quinidine-digoxin interaction: Are the pharmacokinetics of both drugs altered? Int J Clin Pharmacol Ther Toxicol 23:145, 1985

78. Runge TM: Clinical implications of differences in pharmacodynamic action of polar and nonpolar cardiac glycosides. Am Heart J 93:248, 1977

79. Goldberg LI: Cardiovascular and renal actions of dopamine: Potential clinical implications. Pharm Rev 24:1, 1972

80. Beregovich J, Bianchi C, Rubler S, et al: Dose-related hemodynamic and renal effects of dopamine in congestive heart failure. Am Heart J 87:550, 1974

81. Goldberg LI: Dopamine-clinical uses of endogenous catecholamine. N Engl J Med 291:707, 1984

82. Kenakin TP: An in vitro quantitative analysis of the alpha adrenoceptor partial agonist activity of dobutamine and its relevance to inotropic selectivity. J Pharmacol Exp Ther 216:210, 1981

83. Ruffolo RR Jr, Spradlin TA, Pollock GD, et al: Alpha and beta adrenergic effects of the stereoisomers of dobutamine. J Pharmacol Exp Ther 219:447, 1981

84. Kittleson MD: Dobutamine. J Am Vet Med Assoc 177:642, 1980

85. Unverferth DV, Blanford M, Kates RE, et al: Tolerance to dobutamine after a 72 hour continuous infusion. Am J Med 69:262, 1980

86. Unverferth DV, Magorien RD, Altshuld R, et al: The hemodynamic and metabolic advantages gained by a three-day infusion of dobutamine in patients with congestive cardiomyopathy. Am Heart J 106:29, 1983

87. Liang C, Sherman LG, Wellington K, et al: Sustained improvement of cardiac function in patients with congestive heart failure after short-term infusion of dobutamine. Circulation 69:113, 1984

88. Benotti JR, Grossman W, Braunwald E, et al: Effects of amrinone on myocardial energy metabolism and hemodynamics in patients with severe heart failure. Circulation 62:29, 1980

89. Franciosa JA: Intravenous amrinone: An advance or a wrong step? Ann Intern Med 102:399, 1985

90. A summary of laboratory and clinical data or Inocor (brand of amrinone). Sterling Winthrop Research Institute, Rensselaer, NY, 1980

91. Alousi AA, Canter JM, Montenaro MJ, et al: Cardiotonic activity of milrinone, a new and potent bipyridine, on the normal and failing heart of experimental animals. J Cardiovasc Pharmacol 5:792, 1983

92. Kittleson MD, Pipers FS, Knauer, KW; et al: Echocardiographic and clinical effects of milrinone in dogs with myocardial failure. Am J Vet Res 46:1659, 1985

93. Kittleson MD, Knowlen GG: Positive inotropic drugs in heart failure. p. 323. In Kirk RW (ed): Current Veterinary Therapy. Vol. IX. WB Saunders, Philadelphia, 1986

94. Weiland DS, Konstam MA, Salem DN, et al: Contribution of reduced mitral regurgitant volume to vasodilator effect in severe left ventricular failure secondary to coronary artery disease or idiopathic dilated cardiomyopathy. Am J Cardiol 58:1046, 1986

95. Kittleson MD, Eyster GE, Olivier NB, et al: Oral hydralazine therapy for chronic mitral regurgitation in the dog. J Am Vet Med Assoc 182:1205, 1983

96. Cohn JN, Archibald DG, Ziesche S, et al: Effect of vasodilator therapy on mortality in chronic congestive heart failure: Results of a Veterans Administration Cooperative Study. N Engl J Med 314:1547, 1986

97. The Consensus Trial Study Group Effects of enalapril on mortality in severe congestive heart failure: Results of the Cooperative North Scandinavian Enalapril Survival Study (Consensus). N Engl J Med 316:1429, 1987

98. Haskins SC: Shock (the pathophysiology and management of the circulatory collapse states). p. 2. In Kirk RW (ed): Current Veterinary Therapy. Vol. VIII. WB Saunders, Philadelphia, 1983

99. Sonnenblick EH: Force-velocity relations in mammalian heart muscle. Am J Physiol 202:931, 1962

100. Dyke SE, Urschel CW, Sonnenblick EH, et al: Detection of latent function in acutely ischemic myocardium in dogs: Comparison of pharmacologic inotropic stimulation and post extrasystolic potentiation (PESP). Circ Res 36:490, 1975

101. Trautwein W, Kassebaum DB, Nelson RM, et al: Electrophysiologic study of human heart muscle. Circ Res 10:306, 1962

102. Garber EB, Morgan MG, Glasser SP: Left atrial size in patients with atrial fibrillation: An echocardiographic study. Am J Med Sci 272:57, 1976

103. Pedersoli WM: Serum digoxin concentrations in healthy dogs treated without a loading dose. J Vet Pharmacol Ther 1:279, 1978

104. Hamlin R: Antiarrhythmic (anti) and proarrhythmic (pro) effects of antiarrhythmics (A) on spontaneous ventricular premature beats (VPB) in dogs. p. 924. Proceedings of the Fifth Annual Veterinary Med Forum. American College of Veterinary Internal Medicine, 1987 (abst 70)

105. Wollam GL, Tarazi RC, Bravo EL, et al: Diuretic potency of combined hydrochlorthiazide and furosemide therapy in patients with azotemia. Am J Med 72:929, 1982

106. Asbury MJ, Gatenby PBB, O'Sullivan S, et al: Bumetanide: Potent new "loop" diuretic. Br Med J 1:211, 1972

107. Brater DC, Chennavasin P, Day B, et al: Bumetanide and furosemide. Clin Pharmacol Ther 34:207, 1983

108. Bohn FK, Patterson DF, Pyle RL: Atrial fibrillation in dogs. Br Vet J 127:485, 1971

109. Thomas RE: Atrial fibrillation in the dog: A review of eight cases. J Small Anim Pract 25:421, 1984

110. Braunwald E, Lambrew CT, Morrow AG, et al: Idiopathic hypertrophic subaortic stenosis. Arc 29/30(suppl 4):1, 1964

111. Sanderson JE, Gibson DG, Brown DJ et al: Left ventricular filling in hypertrophic cardiomyopathy: An angiographic study. Br Heart J 39:661, 1977

112. Panidis IP, Kotter MN, Facc JF, et al: Development and regression of left ventricular hypertrophy. J Am Coll Cardiol 3:1309, 1984

113. Thomas WP, Mathewson JW, Suter PF, et al: Hypertrophic obstructive cardiomyopathy in a dog: Clinical, hemodynamic, angiographic and pathologic studies. J Am Anim Hosp Assoc 20:253, 1984

114. Liu SK, Maron BJ, Tilley LP: Hypertrophic cardiomyopathy in the dog. Am J Pathol 94:497, 1979

115. Liu SK, Maron BJ, Tilley LP: Canine hypertrophic cardiomyopathy. J Am Vet Med Assoc 174:708, 1979

116. Maron BJ, Liu SK, Tilley LP: Spontaneously occurring hypertrophic cardiomyopathy in dogs and cats: A potential animal model of a human disease. p. 73. In Kaltenbach M, Epstein SE (eds): Hypertrophic Cardiomyopathy. Springer-Verlag, Berlin, 1982

117. Swindle MM, Huber AC, Kan JS, et al: Mitral valve prolapse and hypertrophic cardiomyopathy in a pup. J Am Vet Med Assoc 184:1515, 1984

118. Maron BJ, Bonow RO, Cannon RO, et al: Hypertrophic cardiomyopathy. Interrelations of clinical manifestations, pathophysiology and therapy. Part 1. N Engl J Med 316:780, 1987

119. Wiggle ED, Sasson Z, Henderson MA, et al: Hypertrophic cardiomyopathy: The importance of the site and extent of hypertrophy: A review. Prog Cardiovasc Dis 28:1, 1985

120. Savage DD, Serdes SF, Clark CE, et al: Electrocardiographic findings in patients with obstructive and nonobstructive hypertrophic cardiomyopathy. Circulation 58:402, 1978

121. Frank S, Braunwald E: Idiopathic hypertrophic subaortic stenosis: Clinical analysis of 126 patients with emphasis on natural history. Circulation 37:759, 1968

122. Maron BJ, Bonow RO, Cannon RO, et al: Hypertrophic cardiomyopathy. Interrelations of clinical manifestations, pathophysiology, and therapy. Part 2. N Engl J Med 316:844, 1987

123. Loar AS: Canine thyroid tumors. p. 1033. In Kirk RW (ed): Current Veterinary Therapy. Vol. IX. WB Saunders, Philadelphia, 1986

124. Rijnberk A: Iodine metabolism and thyroid disease in the dog. Drukkerij Elinkwijk, Utrecht, The Netherlands, 1971

125. Belshaw BE: Thyroid diseases. p. 1592. In Ettinger SJ (ed): Textbook of Veterinary Internal Medicine. Vol. II. 2nd Ed. WB Saunders, Philadelphia, 1983

126. Rijnberk A, Leav I: Thyroid tumors. p. 1020. In Kirk RW (ed): Current Veterinary Therapy. Vol. VI. WB Saunders, Philadelphia, 1977

127. Van Vleet JF, Ferrans VJ, Weirich WE: Cardiac disease induced by chronic adriamycin administration in dogs and an evaluation of vitamin E and selenium as cardioprotectants. Am J Pathol 99:13, 1980

128. Loar AS, Susaneck SJ: Doxorubicin-induced cardiotoxicity in five dogs. Semin Vet Med Surg 1:68, 1986

129. Kehoe R, Singer DH, Trapani A, et al: Adriamycin induced cardiac dysrhythmias in an experimental dog model. Cancer Treatm Rep 62:963, 1978

130. Nielson SW, Nielson LB: Coronary embolism in valvular bacterial endocarditis in two dogs. J Am Vet Med Assoc 125:376, 1954

131. Sisson D, Thomas WP: Endocarditis of the aortic valve in the dog. J Am Vet Med Assoc 184:570, 1984

132. Detweiler DK, Luginbuhl H, Buchanan JW, et al: The natural history of acquired cardiac disability of the dog. Ann NY Acad Sci 147:318, 1968

133. Johnsson L: Coronary arterial lesions and myocardial infarcts in the dog. A pathologic and microangiopathic study. Acta Vet Scand 38(suppl):1, 1972

134. King JM, Roth L, Haschek WN: Myocardial necrosis secondary to neural lesions in domestic animals. J Am Vet Med Assoc 180:144, 1982

135. Muir WW, Weisbrode SE: Myocardial ischemia in dogs with gastric dilatation-volvulus. J Am Vet Med Assoc 181:363, 1982

136. Van Vleet PD, Burchell HB, Titus JL: Focal myocarditis associated with pheochromocytomas. E Engl J Med 274:1102, 1966

137. Bourdios PS, Dancla JL, Faccini JM, et al: The subacute toxicology of digoxin in dogs: Clinical chemistry and histopathology of heart and kidneys. Arch Toxicol 51:273, 1982

138. Liu SK, Tilley LP, Tappe JP, et al: Clinical and pathologic findings in dogs with atherosclerosis: 21 cases (1970–1983). J Am Vet Med Assoc 189:227, 1986

139. Colucci WS, Braunwald E: Primary tumors of the heart. p. 1457. In Braunwald E (ed): Heart Disease. WB Saunders, Philadelphia, 1984

140. Brown NO, Patnaik AK, MacEwen EG: Canine hemangiosarcoma. J Am Vet Med Assoc 186:56, 1985

141. Pearson CR, Head KW: Malignant hemangioendothelioma (angiosarcoma) in the dog. J Small Anim Pract 17:737, 1976

142. Klein LJ, Zook BC, Munson TO: Primary cardiac hemangiosarcoma in dogs. J Am Vet Med Assoc 157:326, 1970

143. Aronsohn M: Cardiac hemangiosarcoma in the dog: A review of 38 cases. J Am Vet Med Assoc 187:922, 1985

144. Patnaik AK, Liu SK, Hurvitz AI, et al: Canine chemodectoma (extra-adrenal paragangliomas)—A comparative study. J Small Anim Pract 16:785, 1975

145. Wenger NK, Abelman WH, Roberts WC: Myocarditis. p. 1158. In Hurst JW (ed): The Heart. Vol. II. 6th Ed. McGraw-Hill, New York, 1986

146. Hayes MA, Russell RG, Babiuk LA: Sudden death in young dogs with myocarditis caused by parvovirus. J Am Vet Med Assoc 174:1197, 1979

147. Jezyk PF, Haskins ME, Jones CL: Myocarditis of probable viral origin in pups of weaning age. J Am Vet Med Assoc 174:1204, 1979

148. Carpenter JL, Roberts RM, Harpster NK, et al: Intestinal and cardiopulmonary forms of parvovirus infection in a litter of pups. J Am Vet Med Assoc 176:1269, 1980

149. Robinsin WF, Huxtable CR, Pass DA: Canine parvoviral myocarditis: A morphologic description of the natural disease. Vet Pathol 17:282, 1980

150. Lenghans C, Studdert MJ: Generalized parvovirus disease in neonatal pups. J Am Vet Med Assoc 181:41, 1982

151. Kramer JM, Meunier PC, Pollock RVH: Canine parvovirus: Update. Vet Med Small Anim Clin 75:1541, 1980

152. Atwell RB, Kelly WR: Canine parvovirus: A cause of chronic myocardial fibrosis and adolescent congestive heart failure. J Small Anim Pract 21:609, 1980

153. Liu SK: Myocarditis and cardiomyopathy in the dog and cat. Heart Vessels 1(suppl 1):122, 1985

154. Lenghaus C, Studdert MJ: Animal model of human disease: Acute and chronic viral myocarditis; acute diffuse nonsuppurative myocarditis and residual myocardial scarring following infection with canine parvovirus. Am J Pathol 115:316, 1984

155. Ilgen BE, Conroy JD: Fatal cardiomyopathy in an adult dog resembling parvovirus-induced myocarditis: A case report. J Am Vet Med Assoc 18:613, 1982

156. Higgens RJ, Krakowka S, Metzler AE, et al: Canine distemper virus-associated cardiac necrosis in the dog. Vet Pathol 18:472, 1981

157. Hashimoto A, Hirai K, Suzuki Y, et al: Experimental transplacental transmission of canine herpes virus in pregnant bitches during the second trimester of gestation. Am J Vet Res 44:610, 1983

158. Williams GD, Adams LG, Yaeger RG, et al: Naturally occurring trypanosomiasis (Chagas' disease) in dogs. J Am Vet Med Assoc 171:171, 1977

159. Tomlinson MJ, Chapman WL Jr, Hanson WL, et al: Occurrence of antibody to *Trypanosoma cruzi* in dogs in the southeastern United States. Am J Vet Res 42:1444, 1981

160. Tippit TS: Canine trypanosomiasis. Southwest Vet 31:97, 1978

161. Snider TG III: Myocarditis caused by *Trypanosoma cruzi* in a native Lousiana dog. J Am Vet Med Assoc 173:247, 1980

162. Woody NC, Woody HB: American trypanosomiasis. I. Clinical and epidemiologic background of Chagas' disease in the United States. J Pediatr 58:568, 1961

163. McCully RM, Basson PA, Bigalke RD, et al: Observations on naturally acquired hepatozoonosis of wild carnivores and dogs in the Republic of South Africa. Onderstepoort J Vet Res 42:117, 1975

164. Craig TM, Jones LP, Nordgren RM: Diagnosis of *Hepatozoon canis* by muscle biopsy. J Am Anim Hosp Assoc 20:301, 1984

165. Craig TM, Smallwood JE, Knauer KW, et al: *Hepatozoon canis* infection in dogs: Clinical, radiographic and hematologic findings. J Am Vet Med Assoc 173:967, 1978

166. Edwards NJ, Rebhum WC: Generalized cryptococcosis: A case report. J Am Anim Hosp Assoc 15:439, 1979

167. Maddy KT: Disseminated coccidioidomycosis of the dog. J Am Vet Med Assoc 132:483, 1958

168. Reed RE: Diagnosis of disseminated canine coccidioidomycosis. J Am Vet Med Assoc 128:196, 1956

169. Wood GH, Hirsch DC, Selcer RR, et al: Disseminated aspergillosis in a dog. J Am Vet Med Assoc 172:704, 1978

170. Mullaney TP, Levin S, Indrieri RJ: Disseminated aspergillosis in a dog. J Am Vet Med Assoc 182:516, 1983

171. Patnaik AK, Liu SK, Wilkins RJ, et al: Paecilomycosis in a dog. J Am Vet Med Assoc 161:806, 1972

172. Tyler DE, Lorenz MD, Blue JL, et al: Disseminated prototheosis with central nervous system involvement in a dog. J Am Vet Med Assoc 176:987, 1980

173. Moor FM, Schmidt GM, Desai D, et al: Unsuccessful treatment of disseminated prototheosis in a dog. J Am Vet Med Assoc 186:705, 1985

174. Gaunt SD, McGrath RK, Cox HU: Disseminated prototheosis in a dog. J Am Vet Med Assoc 8:906, 1984

175. Merideth RE, Gwin RM, Samuelson DA, et al: Systemic prototheosis with ocular manifestations in a dog. J Am Anim Hosp Assoc 20:153, 1984

176. Rutgers C, Kowalski J, Cole CR, et al: Severe Rocky Mountain spotted fever in five dogs. J Am Hosp Assoc 21:361, 1985

177. Jeraj K, Ogburn PN, Edwards WD, et al: Atrial standstill, myocarditis and destruction of cardiac

conduction system: clinicopathologic correlation in a dog. Am Heart J 99:185, 1980

178. Tilley LP, Liu SK: Persistent atrial standstill in the dog and cat. Proceedings of the American College of Veterinary Internal Medicine, 1983. p. 43 (abst)

179. Tilley LP: Essentials of Canine and Feline Electrocardiography. 2nd Ed. Lea & Febiger, Philadelphia, 1985

180. Walvoort HC, van Nes JJ, Stokhof AA, et al: Canine glycogen storage disease type II: A clinical study of four affected Lapland dogs. J Am Anim Hosp Assoc 20:279, 1984

181. James TN, Robertson BT, Waldo AL, et al: Hereditary stenosis of the His bundle in pug dogs. Circulation 52:1152, 1975

182. James TN, Drake EA: Sudden death in Doberman pinschers. Ann Intern Med 68:821, 1968

183. Meierhenry EF, Liu SK: Atrioventricular bundle degeneration associated with sudden death in the dog. J Am Vet Med Assoc 172:1418, 1978

24

Pericardial Diseases

John R. Reed

Early observations about the pericardium date from antiquity. Hippocrates accurately described the normal pericardium as "a smooth mantle surrounding the heart and containing a small amount of fluid resembling urine." Galen (131 to 201 AD) named the pericardium and its protective function.[1,2] The twentieth century has yielded great advances in physiologic and clinical understanding of the normal and diseased pericardium.

Normal cardiac function may be maintained without the pericardium (e.g., in congenital absence of the pericardium or with surgically removed parietal pericardium). By contrast, life-threatening restriction of ventricular filling and compromised ventricular function may result from advanced pericardial disease.[3] Clinically significant pericardial disease occurs in an estimated 1 percent of dogs with cardiovascular disease and pericardial effusion comprises the most common category.[4,5] In cats, reports of pericardial disease are uncommon.

ANATOMY AND FUNCTION OF THE PERICARDIUM

The pericardium envelops the heart and is composed of two layers. The outer layer, or fibrous pericardium, is continued at its base on the great arteries and veins that enter and leave the heart. The pericardial apex forms the sternopericardiac ligament, which continues to the ventral muscular diaphragmatic periphery. The inner serous pericardium is invaginated by the heart. It forms a parietal layer that is firmly attached to the fibrous pericardium and a visceral layer, the epicardium. The latter is firmly attached to the myocardium, except where coronary vessels, their branches, and fat intervene in the coronary grooves.[6]

Located between the two layers of serous pericardium is the pericardial cavity. In the dog, it contains 0.5 to 15 ml of a serous fluid, which is an ultrafiltrate of serum.[7,8] In health, the optimal quantity and composition of pericardial fluid is maintained and regulated through osmosis, diffusion, and lymphatic drainage across the serosal surface.[9] Pericardial blood supply in the dog is from the pericardial branch of the internal thoracic and pericardiacophrenic arteries.[6]

Functions of the pericardium include prevention of cardiac overdilation, myocardial surface lubrication, protection of the heart from infections or adhesions, maintenance of the heart in a fixed geometric position within the chest, regulation of stroke volume between the two ventricles, and prevention of right ventricular regurgitation when ventricular diastolic pressures are increased.[2,7,10]

495

CONGENITAL PERICARDIAL DISEASES

Congenital pericardial defects in the dog and cat are rare. Most have been found incidently during necropsy examinations.[11] Defects are usually incomplete, occurring predominantly on the left side.[4] I have observed one dog with an incidental partial pericardial defect on the right side. Complete absence of the pericardium has been reported.[4] A potential hazard of partial pericardial defects is herniation of a portion or all of the heart.

PERITONEOPERICARDIAL DIAPHRAGMATIC HERNIA

Peritoneopericardial diaphragmatic hernia (PDH) is the most frequently recognized congenital defect of the pericardium in the dog and cat. Theories on the embryonic development of this congenital defect include (1) failure of the lateral pleuroperitoneal folds and the ventromedial pars sternalis to unite during division of the coelom into abdominal and thoracic cavities,[12] (2) faulty development of the dorsolateral septum transversum or rupture of a thin tissue membrane in this area permitting peritoneal and pericardial communication,[13,14] and (3) prenatal injury to the septum transversum or to the fusion site of the septum transversum and pleuroperitoneal folds.[15]

Whichever the mechanism causing PDH, the end result of embryogenesis is a persistent communication between the pericardial and peritoneal cavities. This permits cranial displacement of abdominal viscera into the pericardial sac while the pleural space remains intact. PDH is never an acquired traumatic defect because there is no natural direct communication between the peritoneal and pericardial cavities after birth. However, traumatic events may cause abdominal contents to move into the pericardial cavity through a PDH and initiate acute clinical signs.

The degree of herniation is variable, ranging from asymptomatic minor herniation to major organ herniation with clinical signs. The liver and gallbladder tend to be herniated most frequently, followed by the small intestines, spleen, stomach, and fatty tissues (e.g., omentum, falciform ligament, mesentery).[16]

Peritoneopericardial diaphragmatic hernia may be associated with other congenital abnormalities. Umbilical hernias are a frequent finding, especially in the Weimaraner breed. Other accompanying congenital anomalies include cardiac defects, such as pectus excavatum and sternebral abnormalities.[16]

Some PDH cases remain undiagnosed for years or are discovered at necropsy. The onset of reported clinical signs of PDH has been from 4 weeks to 15 years of age. Of 48 reported cases (9 cats, 39 dogs), 48 percent were diagnosed within the first year of life, 36 percent from 1 year to 4 years, 10 percent from 4 years to 8 years, and 6 percent after 8 years of life. Fifty-eight percent of these cases occurred in males. Eighteen percent of PDH occurred in the Weimaraner breed.[16]

Clinical signs are most often gastrointestinal (GI) (e.g., vomiting, diarrhea, anorexia, weight loss), followed by respiratory (e.g., dyspnea, cough, wheeze). Abdominal discomfort or swelling, shock, and collapse may occur less frequently.

Physical examination often indicates a diminished or displaced precordial cardiac impulse and muffled heart sounds. With large hernias, the abdomen may be small and devoid of palpable organs. Cardiac tamponade and signs of right-sided congestive heart failure can occur but are rare.[4]

Electrocardiograms (ECGs) may show decreased QRS voltage due to the dampening effect of effusion or herniated abdominal contents. There may also be an axis deviation if cardiac displacement results. Diagnosis is usually confirmed by plain radiographs, which characteristically display an enlarged cardiac silhouette with dorsal tracheal displacement (Fig. 24-1). The diaphragmatic and caudal heart borders consistently overlap.[16] The cardiac silhouettes may display an abnormal overlying radiographic gas or fat density. Plain abdominal radiographs may indicate absence of cranial or mid-abdominal organs or their cranial displacement into the pericardial cavity. Diagnostic confirmation can be facilitated using fluoroscopy, nonselective angiocardiography, pericardiocentesis, upper GI barium series, pneumopericardiography, and peritoneography.[4] Ultrasonography is the preferable diagnostic technique because of its noninvasiveness, safety, and accuracy.

Surgical correction is the recommended treatment. If other congenital defects are present, careful consideration should be given to the surgical risks

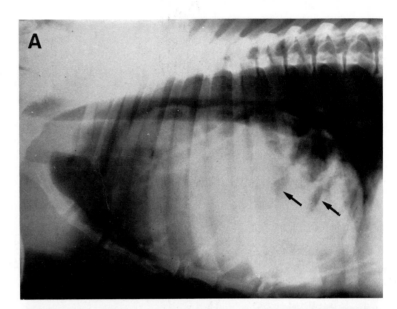

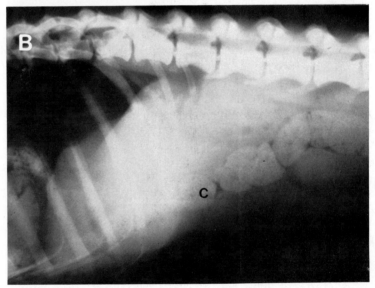

Fig. 24-1 Peritoneopericardial diaphragmatic hernia in a 3-year-old dog. (**A**) Right lateral thoracic radiograph demonstrates a markedly enlarged, globular cardiac silhouette. Gas-filled bowel loops can be seen overlying the cardiac shadow (arrows), and there is silhouetting between the cardiac shadow and the diaphragm. (**B**) Lateral abdominal radiograph reveals the colon (C) extending forward to the heart.

compared with perceived benefits. Prognosis following successful surgery of a noncomplicated PDH is excellent.

PERICARDIAL CYSTS

Pericardial cysts are uncommon. They have been described in the right or left costophrenic angle[17,18] and may be caused by incarcerated omentum from a PDH or from abnormal development of mesenchymal tissues during fetal life.[19–21]

The history, clinical signs, pathophysiology, and diagnosis of pericardial cysts are similar to those of pericardial effusion. The diagnosis can be made using pneumopericardiography (Fig. 24-2) or echocardiography. The origin of cyst attachment is usually at the parietal pericardial apex with most of the cyst lying free within the pericardial space adjacent to the heart. Surgical removal of the cyst coupled

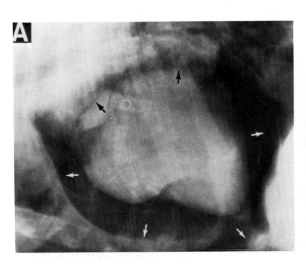

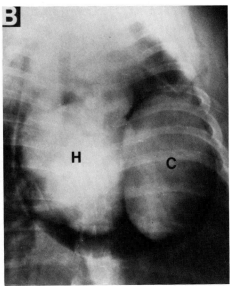

Fig. 24-2 Large pericardial cyst in an 8-month-old male English bulldog. (**A**) Right lateral radiograph shows the cyst (arrows) outlined adjacent to and overlapping the cardiac silhouette. (**B**) Dorsoventral radiograph shows the cyst (C) clearly outlined on the left side of the pericardial space, displacing the heart (H) to the right. (Thomas WP, Reed JR, Gomez JA: Diagnostic pneumopericardiography in dogs with spontaneous pericardial effusion. Vet Radiol 25:2, 1984.)

with parietal pericardiectomy below the phrenic nerves often yields an excellent prognosis.

ACQUIRED PERICARDIAL DISEASES

Pericardial Effusion

Pericardial effusion may be mild and clinically silent or severe enough to cause pericardial tamponade. The latter is a commonly acquired pericardial disorder in dogs and frequently results in right-sided congestive heart failure.[5] Clinically apparent pericardial disease in the cat is rare[22–24] (Table 24-1). However, the principles of diagnosis and treatment in the dog and cat are similar.

The development of increased pericardial pressures from pericardial effusion depends on several factors. These include the rate of fluid accumulation, absolute fluid volume, and the physical characteristics of the pericardium itself.[2]

ETIOLOGY

Pericardial effusions may be categorized etiologically on the basis of fluid characteristics (Table 24-2). These include transudates (or pseudotransudates), exudates (e.g., inflammatory and noninflammatory), and hemorrhagic (e.g., sanguinous and serosanguinous) effusions. In the dog[4,5,25–30] and cat,[24,31,32] clinically significant pericardial effusions are most often hemorrhagic, sterile, and noninflammatory.

The most common causes of hemorrhagic pericardial effusion in the dog are intrapericardial neoplasia[25,28,33] and idiopathic.[30] Hemorrhagic effusion is most common in large-breed, mature (i.e., over 6 years of age), predominantly male dogs. The German shepherd breed may be predisposed to neoplastic (e.g., hemangiosarcoma) and idiopathic hemorrhagic pericardial effusions.[4,31–35]

Neoplasia-induced pericardial effusions are predominantly hemangiosarcoma and heart-base tumors in dogs. Various tumors may uncommonly metastasize to the heart or pericardium in the cat (e.g., hemangiosarcoma, lymphosarcoma).

Table 24-1 Incidence of Feline Pericardial Disease with Various Disorders[a]

Predominant Disease Process (Diagnosis)	Rush et al. (1987)[b]		Harpster (1987)[c]	
	No. of Cats Affected[a]	Percent of Total	No. of Cats Affected[b]	Percent of Total
Feline infectious peritonitis	11	17	5	28
Hypertrophic cardiomyopathy	9	13		
Renal failure	7	11	2	11
Systemic infections	7	11	5	28
Coagulopathy	7	11		
Dilated cardiomyopathy	6	9	1	5.5
Metastatic neoplasia	6	9		
Lymphosarcoma	6	9	1	5.5
Mitral valve malformation	2	3		
Restrictive cardiomyopathy	2	3		
Iatrogenic	2	3		
Unknown/miscellaneous	1	1	4	22
Total	66	100	18	100

[a] Criteria for pericardial disease included findings of pericardial effusion or gross pericardial thickening with microscopic evidence of pericarditis or neoplasia.

[b] Data from Rush J, Keene BW, Fox PR: Retrospective study of pericardial disease in cats. Proceedings of the American College of Veterinary Internal Medicine, 1987 (abst).

[c] Data from Harpster NK: The cardiovascular system. p. 820. In Holzworth J (ed): Diseases of the Cat. Medicine and Surgery. Vol. 1. WB Saunders, Philadelphia, 1987.

Hemangiosarcoma (hemangioendothelioma, angiosarcoma) often originates as a primary tumor in the right atrial or auricular wall.[33,34] It readily metastasizes, especially if it penetrates the right atrial endocardium.[5] Resultant clinical signs are due to metastatic lesions, acute blood loss, pericardial tamponade, or tachyarrhythmias.

Heart-base tumors designate neoplasms originating in the region of the ascending aorta.[36,37] The chemodectoma (chemoreceptor cell tumor, paraganglioma, aortic body tumor) is the most common histologic type and arises from chemodectoma cells.[37–39] It has a reported predilection for brachycephalic breeds (e.g., boxer, bulldog, Boston terrier)[37,40] but has also been identified in numerous breeds. Heart-base tumors tend to be locally invasive and rarely metastasize. Clinical signs are related to their space occupation or secondary pericardial effusion and tamponade.

Other neoplasms may arise from the heart base and include tumors of thyroid, parathyroid, lymphoid, and connective tissue origin.[25,41] However, the various tumor types are clinically indistinguishable.

Mesothelioma is an uncommon tumor that causes pericardial effusion in the dog[42,43] and cat.[24,31] It arises in the mesothelial layer of thoracic and abdominal cavity serous membranes. When it effects the pericardium, hemorrhagic effusions and cardiac tamponade often result.

Idiopathic (benign) pericardial effusion is a common canine disease of uncertain etiology. The Golden retriever, Great Dane, and Saint Bernard breeds may be predisposed,[26,27,29] but it also occurs in most medium- to large-breed dogs ranging from 1 to 14 years (average, 6 years).[25–27,29] Histologically, epicardial and pericardial thickening and fibrosis are common and active inflammation is usually mild.[4,27,29]

Left atrial perforation secondary to advanced chronic acquired atrioventricular (AV) valvular disease is an uncommon cause of hemorrhagic effusion.[44] Acute pericardial hemorrhage, hypotension, and shock may result. Traumatic right ventricular perforation during cardiac catheterization has been reported as a cause of iatrogenic pericardial hemorrhage.[45] All cardiac chambers and great vessels can similarly be punctured during catheterization.

Table 24-2 Pericardial Diseases of the Dog and Cat

Congenital disorders

    Pericardial defects[a]
    Peritoneopericardial hernia[a]
    Pericardial cyst

Acquired disorders

    Pericardial effusion
        Transudate (hydropericardium)[a]
            Congestive heart failure
            Hypoalbuminemia
            Peritoneopericardial hernia
        Exudate (pericarditis)
            Infection—bacterial, fungal
            Sterile—idiopathic, uremic, other
                infectious diseases (FIP)
        Hemorrhage (hemopericardium)
            Neoplasia—hemangiosarcoma, heart-base
                tumor, mesothelioma, lymphosarcoma,
                carcinoma, other
            Trauma—iatrogenic, external
            Cardiac rupture, especially left atrium
            Idiopatic

    Constrictive pericardial disease
        Idiopathic
        Infection—bacterial, fungal
        Pericardial foreign body
        Neoplasia

    Pericardial mass lesions (± effusion/fibrosis)
        Pericardial cyst
        Pericardial abscess
        Neoplasm
        Granuloma—actinomycosis,
            coccidioidomycosis

[a] Conditions that rarely compromise cardiac function (Thomas WP, Reed JR: Pericardial Disease. p. 364. In Kirk RW (ed): Current Veterinary Therapy. Vol. IX. WB Saunders, Philadelphia, 1986. Reprinted with permission from WB Saunders Co.)

Other penetrating cardiac injuries that cause pericardial hemorrhage include gunshot[46] and coronary artery laceration during pericardiocentesis.[4]

Exudative inflammatory pericardial effusion occurs infrequently in the dog and cat. Infectious exudates are usually purulent, serofibrinous, or serosanguinous, and the cytology shows a predominant number of neutrophils along with variable numbers of reactive mesothelial cells.[47] The etiologic agent can be visible in the fluid or identified by aerobic or anaerobic culture. Some bacterial and fungal agents (e.g., *Coccidiodis immitis*) may be particularly difficult to culture. Serologic tests may be necessary for diagnosis. Infectious canine pericarditis has been caused by disseminated tuberculosis,[48] coccidioidomycosis, and actinomycosis, as well as by other bacteria, including *Pasteurella multocida*.[28,49,50] Feline pericarditis has been associated with *Escherichia coli, Staphylococcus aureus, Streptococcus, Enterococcus,* and *Actinomyces* infections.[22]

Sterile inflammatory effusions have been associated with other infectious diseases, including feline infectious peritonitis and toxoplasmosis in cats and leptospirosis and canine distemper in dogs.[40] Chronic uremia can produce a sterile serofibrinous effusion,[40,51] although a hemorrhagic effusion is more common (Tables 24-1 and 24-2). In humans, there are many other causes of inflammatory effusions that could potentially cause disease in the dog and cat.[2,52]

PATHOPHYSIOLOGY

Normally, pericardial pressure equals intrapleural pressure and varies from −3.8 to 3.8 mmHg during respiration.[53] Right and left ventricular diastolic pressures are several millimeters of mercury higher than the pericardial pressure.[54,55]

An increase in pericardial pressure due to fluid accumulation within the pericardial space may result in *cardiac tamponade*. This is characterized by (1) elevated intracardiac pressure, (2) progressive limitation of ventricular diastolic filling, and (3) reduced stroke volume.[2] When pericardial fluid causes intrapericardial pressure to rise to the level of right atrial and ventricular diastolic pressure, the transmural pressure (i.e., the difference between intracardiac diastolic pressure and pericardial pressure) that distends these chambers declines and cardiac tamponade will result.[56] With progressive pericardial fluid accumulation, both pericardial and right ventricular diastolic pressures rise together to the level of left ventricular diastolic pressure (Fig. 24-3). This elevation of all three pressures become associated with a marked decline in cardiac output,

Fig. 24-3 Intracardiac pressures from a dog with cardiac tamponade due to pericardial effusion. Simultaneous pressures are recorded from the left ventricle (LV), pulmonary artery (PA), right ventricle (RV), and right atrium (RA). These pressures demonstrate superposition of the diastolic portions of the atrial and ventricular tracings, equilibration, and elevation (i.e., 20 to 25 mmHg) of end-diastolic pressure. The pulmonary artery and right ventricular systolic pressures are mildly elevated (40 mmHg), while the left ventricular systolic pressure is normal (110 mmHg). (Thomas WP: Pericardial disease. p. 1080. In Ettinger SJ (ed): Textbook of Veterinary Internal Medicine. 2nd Ed. WB Saunders, Philadelphia, 1983. Reprinted with permission from WB Saunders Co.)

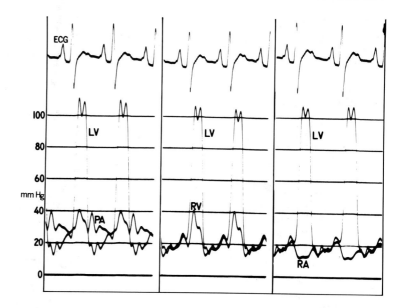

stroke volume, and systemic arterial pressure (cardiogenic shock).[55,56]

Compensatory mechanisms are temporarily effective during cardiac tamponade. Reflex increases in sympathetic tone compensate for reduction in forward stroke volume. Tachycardia and increases in ejection fraction initially help to maintain cardiac output.[55,56] Systemic vascular resistance increases and results in maintenance of systemic arterial pressure. With severe cardiac tamponade, however, compensatory mechanisms are no longer sufficient to maintain systemic arterial pressure. Cardiac output and perfusion of vital organs (including the heart) become impaired.[55-58] Myocardial ischemia may further compromise left ventricular stroke volume.

Pulsus paradoxus is an exaggeration of arterial pulse pressure variation in which the arterial pressure falls more than 10 mmHg with normal inspiration. In the setting of cardiac tamponade, pulsus paradoxus is critically dependent on inspiratory augmentation of systemic venous return and right ventricular filling.[4,59] Inspiration is associated with a reduction in intrapericardial and right atrial pressures. This augments filling from the vena cava into the right atrium and right ventricle as well as pulmonary artery flow and systolic pressure. Increased inspiratory venous return causes marked increase in right ventricular dimensions, accompanied by a re-

duction in left ventricular dimensions, flattening, and displacement of the septum toward the left ventricle. Left atrial and left ventricular diastolic pressures fall and are accompanied by reduced aortic flow and systolic arterial pressure.[60-63] A markedly decreased pulse pressure during inspiration results (Fig. 24-4).

Clinical signs of cardiac tamponade are determined by the rate of pericardial fluid accumulation and ability of the pericardium to stretch. In acute cardiac tamponade, even small volumes of pericardial effusion (50 to 100 ml in the dog) can cause extremes in pericardial pressure. Alternately, the pericardium can stretch to accommodate large fluid volumes, if effusion develops gradually (Fig. 24-5). Pericardial effusions as large as 3L have been reported in the dog.[26] Pericardial fibrosis and thickening is an important limiting factor in the ability of the pericardium to stretch.

Unlike other types of cardiac disease, most causes of pericardial effusion do not significantly affect cardiac contractility or systolic function.

CLINICAL AND DIAGNOSTIC FINDINGS

History

Typically, historical findings in animals with pericardial disease include lethargy, fatigue, weakness, tachypnea, abdominal enlargement, syncope,

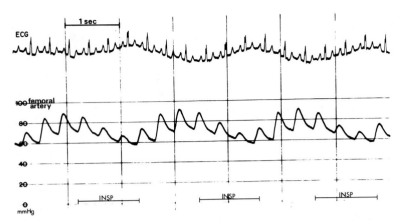

Fig. 24-4 Pulsus paradoxus due to cardiac tamponade. The femoral artery pressure (directly measured) shows an exaggerated fall in mean pressure of 15 to 20 mmHg and a markedly decreased pulse pressure during normal inspiration (INSP). (Thomas WP: Pericardial disease. p. 1080. In Ettinger SJ (ed): Textbook of Veterinary Internal Medicine. 2nd Ed. WB Saunders, Philadelphia, 1983. Reprinted with permission from WB Saunders Co.)

and cough (cats rarely exhibit coughing).[4,25-29] Large pericardial effusions may cause compression of adjacent structures and associated clinical signs (e.g., dyspnea and cough from tracheal compression, dyspnea due to reduced pulmonary expansibility).[2]

Most pericardial effusions develop gradually and, if severe, cardiac tamponade may occur over a period of several days to weeks. Acute tamponade may result from pericardial hemorrhage. Characteristic changes include a decline in systemic arterial blood pressure, elevation of systemic venous pressure and a radiographically small heart.[2]

Physical Examination

In most dogs and cats with cardiac tamponade, physical examination abnormalities are present, although they may be subtle. Larger effusions most often result in diminished audible heart sounds and a less palpable precordial impulse.[26,28] These findings are not specific and may occur with pleural

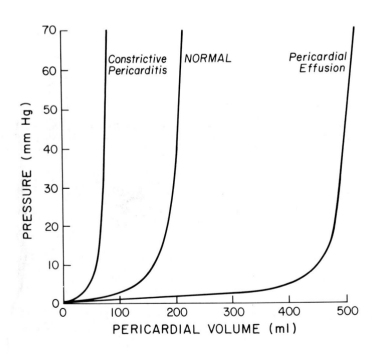

Fig. 24-5 Pericardial pressure-volume curves. Each curve has a relatively flat initial portion, followed by a steep portion at pressures above 10 to 15 mmHg when the elastic limit of the pericardium is reached. When cardiac tamponade is present, removal of a relatively small volume of fluid can cause a rapid reduction in pericardial pressure and relief of clinical signs. (Thomas WP: Pericardial Disease. p. 1080. In Ettinger SJ (ed): Textbook of Veterinary Internal Medicine. 2nd Ed. WB Saunders, Philadelphia, 1983. Reprinted with permission from WB Saunders Co.)

effusions, intrathoracic masses, or obesity. In most cases, other auscultable cardiac abnormalities (murmurs, gallops, arrhythmias) are absent. Patients with left atrial perforation continue to have a systolic murmur of mitral regurgitation, but it may be significantly reduced in intensity from previous examinations.[44] Diminished heart sounds are most meaningful when accompanied by physical examination findings suggesting cardiac compression (e.g., resting sinus tachycardia, peripheral venous hypertension with distention, arterial hypotension, or palpably diminished arterial pulse amplitudes, right heart failure).[4,26,28] The most common physical abnormality in a series of affected human patients was jugular venous distention.[64] To determine venous distention in the dog and cat, hair must be clipped on the neck. Central venous pressure (CVP) can be measured by means of an 18- to 20-gauge jugular vein catheter connected to a water manometer. The CVP often exceeds 9 mmHg with cardiac tamponade.[5]

DIAGNOSTIC FINDINGS

Clinicopathology

There is little published information concerning hematologic and biochemical alterations associated with pericardial diseases. In idiopathic canine peri-

cardial effusion, mild hypoproteinemia was seen in 5 of 27 cases.[26,27,29] In 15 cardiac hemangiosarcoma dogs, the common findings were leukocytosis (neutrophilia) and anemia.[33] In another report, nucleated red blood cells and schistocytes were seen in 5 of 14 cases of cardiac hemangiosarcomas.[28] In my experience, dogs that present with signs of right heart failure (ascites) will have mild elevation in serum alanine aminotransferase and mild hypoproteinemia.

Electrocardiography

There are no pathognomonic ECG features of pericardial disease. However, several findings support the clinical diagnosis of pericardial effusion, including diminished QRS voltages, ST-segment deviation, and electric alternans.

In the dog, QRS complex amplitudes less than 1.0 mV in all limb and thoracic leads are considered diminished.[25,65] The normally low-voltage ECG complexes in cats make detection of diminished complexes nearly impossible. In addition to pericardial effusion, other causes for diminished QRS complex size include pleural effusion, thoracic masses, and obesity.[25] It can also occur in otherwise normal animals.

Electrical alternans is not sensitive or specific for pericardial diseases, but its occurrence is strongly

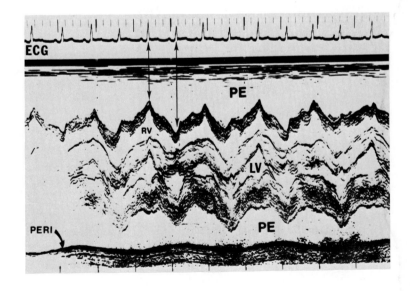

Fig. 24-6 M-mode echocardiogram of a dog with pericardial effusion (PE). Electrical alternans (i.e., alternating R-wave amplitude) is seen on the ECG. Arrows demonstrate the alternating displacement of the heart within the fluid-filled pericardium. Peri, pericardium; RV, right ventricle; LV, left ventricle.

suggestive of moderate to severe pericardial effusion, especially in the appropriate clinical setting.[65,66] Alternation of QRS complex amplitudes is most common and results from oscillation of the heart suspended by the great vessels in the fluid-filled pericardial sac[66] (Fig. 24-6).

The usual rhythm accompanying cardiac tamponade is sinus tachycardia or normal sinus rhythm, with arrhythmias occurring infrequently.[4,28,33] Left atrial enlargement is a common finding.[28] ST-segment alteration is occasionally present in pericardial diseases.[65,66]

Thoracic Radiography

As pericardial effusion volume accumulates, the cardiac silhouette becomes spherically enlarged and loses definition of chamber contour. In most cases of cardiac tamponade, the cardiac silhouette is rounded in both views[25] (Fig. 24-7). With acute pericardial effusion (left atrial rupture), the heart appears rounded, but left atrial enlargement is still evident.[44] Other findings, such as widening of the caudal vena cava, are variable and nonspecific. Pleural effusion from congestive heart failure frequently obscures the cardiac silhouette, and prevents recognition of the typical spherical cardiac shadow. Thoracentesis or diuretic therapy may be needed to evaluate the spherical heart radiographically. Occasionally, a heart-base tumor may cause a visible soft tissue shadow or tracheal displacement over the cranial heartbase.[5] Frequently, primary myocardial disease or certain congenital cardiac defects may impart a globular appearance to the cardiac silhouette. Therefore, these disorders should be considered in the differential diagnoses.

Contrast Angiography

Angiography is rarely required to diagnose pericardial effusion with cardiac tamponade. When performed, venous angiography can outline dorsal displacement of the cardiac chambers and an increased distance between the ventricular endocardium and pericardial surface. Angiography is useful, however, to outline intracardiac portions of atrial or

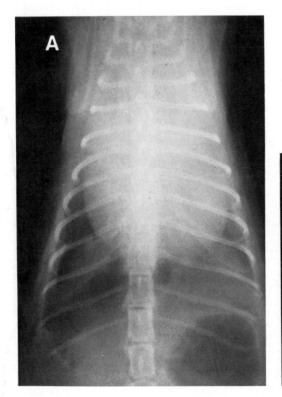

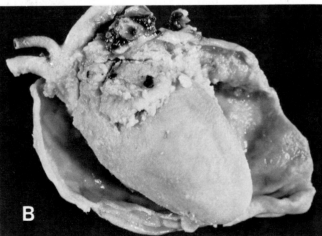

Fig. 24-7 Radiographic features and necropsy correlation of chronic pericardial effusion in a 6-month-old cat. (**A**) The dorsoventral plain radiograph shows a characteristically enlarged globular cardiac silhouette. A small amount of pleural effusion is present. (**B**) At necropsy, the effects of pericarditis have resulted in pericardial fibrosis and thickening. The epicardium is covered with a layer of fibrin.

heartbase tumors, displacement or distortion of normal structures by pericardial masses, or vascular blushing of heart-base tumors.[4,67,68]

Magnetic Resonance Imaging

Magnetic resonance imaging (MRI) is a new non-invasive imaging technique that does not require ionizing radiation. Instead, fluctuating radiofrequency (RF) impulses are applied across a static magnetic field to cause atomic nuclei to align against the field, return to their resting state, and emit specific RF signals. Resolution for detail is far greater than for computed tomography (CT). Cardiac tummors can be imaged as small as 1 mm. The technique is costly and complex but has intrinsic high contrast, especially for cardiovascular structures (Fig. 24-8).

Echocardiography

Echocardiography is the most sensitive and specific technique for detecting pericardial effusion, even in subclinical cases.[28,69] M-mode or two-dimensional echocardiographic techniques display

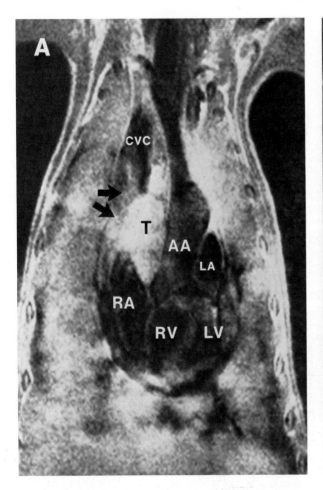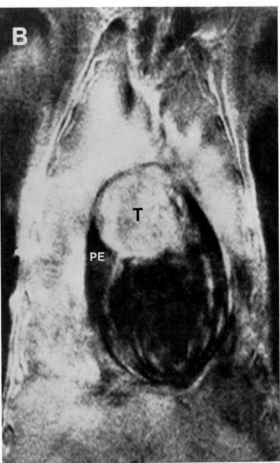

Fig. 24-8 Magnetic resonance imaging (MRI) of a 9-year-old male dog with pericardial effusion and a heart-base tumor. Two coronal views are shown. (**A**) The dorsal portion of the heart-base tumor (T) is elongated and lies between the aortic arch (AA) and cranial vena cava (CVC). The tumor compresses the vena cava, causing reduced blood flow and turbulence (arrows). (**B**) A more ventral coronal view. The tumor and pericardial effusion (PE) are clearly seen, but cardiac chambers are not easily identified. RA, right atrium; LA, left atrium; RV, right ventricle; LV, left ventricle.

pericardial effusion as an echo-free space on both sides of the heart between the pericardium and the right and left ventricular walls.[5] It may demonstrate the alternating displacement (swinging) of the heart within the distended pericardial sac, which is the usual cause for the ECG finding of electric alternans[70] (Fig. 24-6).

The two-dimensional echocardiographic technique displays familiar cardiac tomograms in real time. It can detect and localize cardiac and pericardial masses in most cases and can usually distinguish soft tissue masses arising from the right atrium (e.g., hemangiosarcoma) versus those originating in the region of the ascending aorta (e.g., heart-base tumors)[5,71] (Figs. 24-9 and 24-10). It is the preferred method for distinguishing neoplastic from nonneoplastic effusions and for making recommendations regarding therapy.[5]

Pericardiocentesis

Pericardiocentesis provides definitive diagnosis for pericardial effusion and is relatively safe and simple.[4,5,72–75] Depending on the animal's clinical sta-

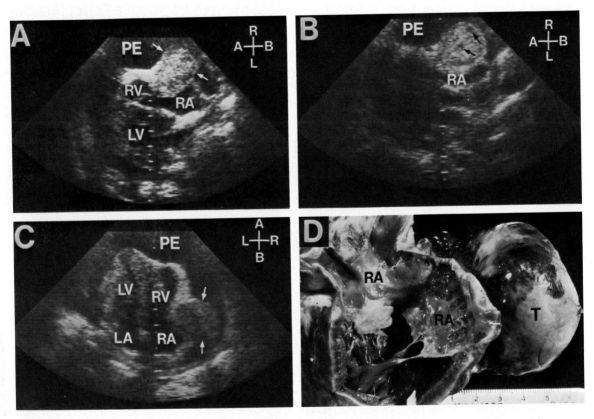

Fig. 24-9 Hemangiosarcoma and pericardial effusion. (**A**) Right intercostal long-axis view. The ovoid tumor mass (arrows) arises from the right atrial wall near the atrioventricular junction. (**B**) Similar view with slight clockwise beam rotation. The mass appears more circular in this view, and two small echolucent (i.e., black) areas are visible within it (arrows). (**C**) Left intercostal four-chamber view. The mass (arrows), which is mainly extracardiac, indents the right heart near the atrioventricular junction. (**D**) Necropsy specimen obtained 1 month after this study shows the large smooth tumor mass (T) protruding from the epicardial surface of the right atrium. A, apex; B, base; R, right; L, left; PE, pericardial effusion; RV, right ventricle; RA, right atrium; LV, left ventricle; LA, left atrium. (Thomas WP, Sisson D, Bauer TG, Reed JR: Detection of cardiac masses in dogs by two-dimensional echocardiography. Vet Radiol 25:65, 1984.)

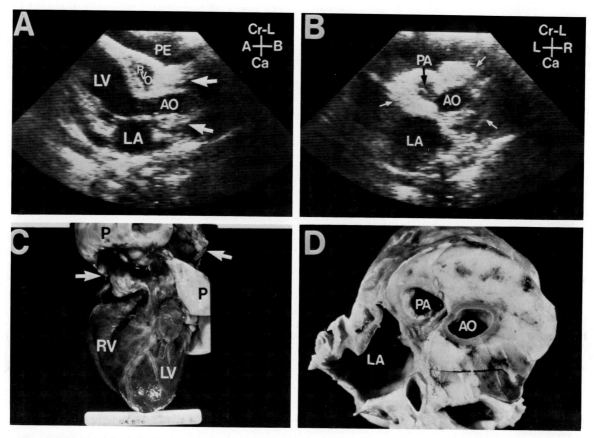

Fig. 24-10 Heart-base tumor (chemodectoma) and pericardial effusion. (**A**) Left intercostal long-axis view. A soft tissue mass (arrows) is visible on both sides of the ascending aorta. (**B**) Short-axis view from the same location obtained by counterclockwise beam rotation. Tumor infiltration (white arrows) surrounds the aorta and pulmonary artery. (**C**) Necropsy specimen viewed from cranial left aspect shows intra- and extrapericardial portions of the tumor (arrows). (**D**) Transverse section through the heart base illustrates the tumor invasion around both great vessels, as seen in **B**. A, apex; B, base; L, left; R, right; Ca, caudal; Cr, cranial; PE, pericardial effusion; RVO, right ventricular outflow tract; LV, left ventricle; AO, aorta; LA, left atrium; PA, pulmonary artery; P, pericardium; RV, right ventricle. (Thomas WP, Sisson D, Bauer TG, Reed JR: Detection of cardiac masses in dogs by two-dimensional echocardiography. Vet Radiol 25:65, 1984.)

tus, light sedation may be required; for example, in dogs, acepromazine, 0.25 to 1.0 mg IV, is used; in cats, ketamine hydrocloride, 4 to 10 mg IV, is given. The patient is then placed in left lateral recumbency, ECG leads are attached, and the area over the right third to seventh intercostal spaces from the sternum to the costochondral junctions are clipped and surgically prepared. The right side is preferred to avoid the lungs and minimize the risk of puncturing a large extramural coronary artery. A 16-gauge, 15- to 20-cm over-the-needle intravascular catheter is prepared by cutting two or three smooth side holes near

the tip with a scalpel blade. A syringe is then attached to the needle. Lidocaine is infiltrated into the intercostal muscles at the puncture site, and a small stab incision is made through the skin. The exact site of entry is best determined by the point of maximum intensity of the cardiac impulse via palpation or auscultation. This is usually between the fourth and sixth ribs just lateral to the sternum and near the cranial border of a rib. During ECG monitoring, the needle-catheter is slowly inserted straight through the chest wall toward the heart while applying intermittent suction to the syringe. When pericardial fluid is obtained, the catheter is carefully advanced over the needle into the pericardial sac. When the epicardium is encountered, a scratching sensation is felt through the catheter.

Once the catheter is in place in the pericardial sac, syringe suction is used to remove as much pericardial fluid as possible. Sterile fluid samples are collected for chemical and cytologic analysis. Bacteriologic culture is performed if cytology indicates possible infection. In dogs and cats, the fluid is usually hemorrhagic or serosanguinous. If there is any doubt about the origin of a hemorrhagic fluid (pericardial versus intracardiac), samples of fluid and peripheral blood are centrifuged in microhematocrit tubes. In most cases, pericardial fluid rarely clots, has a packed cell volume different from that of blood, and has a xanthochromic supernatant. If necessary, the patient's position should be altered to facilitate complete drainage. However, care must be taken to prevent catheter dislodgement. The most common complication of pericardiocentesis is ventricular arrhythmias when the epicardium is contracted by the needle. This readily subsides upon needle retraction.

Pneumopericardiography

Following pericardial drainage, pneumopericardiography can be performed to attempt to identify the source of the effusion.[76] Positive-contrast pericardiography does not yield as much detail as pneumopericardiography and is not recommended. Pneumopericardiography is performed by injecting CO_2 or room air equivalent to two-thirds to three-fourths of the pericardial fluid volume removed. Radiographs are then immediately obtained in the right lateral, left lateral, and dorsoventral positions. The lateral views are the most informative, and it is essntial that both be obtained. The dorsoventral view is less useful than the lateral views but is superior to the ventrodorsal view for assessing atrial and heart-base lesions.[17,77] While two-dimensional echocardiography is the superior technique for identification and localization of cardiac and pericardial masses, pneumopericardiography accurately outlines most cardiac masses and allows differentiation of neoplastic from idiopathic hemorrhagic effusions in approximately 75 to 80 percent of cases[17] (Figs. 24-11 and 24-12). Diagnostic accuracy requires

good technique (complete pericardial drainage, adequate gas volume, multiple views) and knowledge of the appearance of normal cardiac structures in each view.[76] When the study is completed, residual gas is removed, and the pericardial catheter is withdrawn.

Cytology

Laboratory analysis of pericardial fluid will identify chylous and infectious effusions. Heart-base tumors tend to produce effusions that are more serous than those caused by hemangiosarcoma and idiopathic pericarditis. However, wide variability and overlapping ranges for protein content and red cell and nucleated cell counts usually prevent reliable differentiation of these disorders.[28,30] Difficulty in identifying neoplastic cells versus reactive mesothelial cells also prevents reliable diagnosis. In short, hemorrhagic pericardial effusions are etiologically indistinguishable by visual or laboratory analysis. The diagnosis, prognosis, and therapeutic recommendations are based on the results of echocardiography and/or pneumopericardiography.

TREATMENT AND PROGNOSIS

In most patients with pericardial effusion, myocardial contractility is unaffected, and cardiac output is limited by the decreased diastolic ventricular volume. Therefore, inotropic therapy with digitalis glycosides is of little benefit and is not indicated in most cases. Drugs that decrease ventricular afterload (arteriolar vasodilators) or preload (venous vasodilators and diuretics) are also of limited benefit if the pericardial disorder is not corrected. These drugs can cause further reduction of ventricular fillings, decrease cardiac output, and hypotension. They should therefore be used with caution or avoided in patients with cardiac tamponade.

The most effective initial therapeutic technique in patients with clinically significant pericardial effusion is pericardiocentesis. Most effusions that are secondary to other diseases (e.g., heart failure, hypoalbuminemia, pericardial hernia, uremia, infectious diseases) will respond if the cause is eliminated or if medical or surgical treatment is instituted.

Based on the results of culture and sensitivity, infectious pericarditis should be treated aggressively

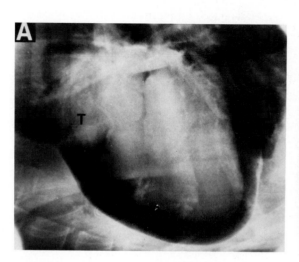

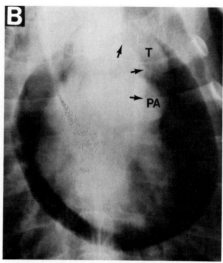

Fig. 24-11 Pneumopericardiogram demonstrating a heart-base tumor in a 9-year old dog. (**A**) In the Right lateral position, the circular tumor mass (T) prevents gas from outlining the ascending aorta at the cranial heart base. (**B**) In the Dorsoventral position the tumor mass (T) outlined cranial and to the left of the aortic arch (arrows) and pulmonary artery (PA). (Thomas WP, Reed JR, Gomez JA: Diagnostic pneumopericardiography in dogs with spontaneous pericardial effusion. Vet Radiol 25:2, 1984.)

with antimicrobial agents. Continuous drainage using an indwelling pericardial catheter for surgical intervention may be indicated.[50,77] A potential major complication of infectious pericarditis is deposition of fibrin on the pericardium and epicardium with development of constrictive pericarditis. This disease responds poorly to therapy. Therefore, the presence of infectious pericarditis should confer a poor prognosis.

With left atrial rupture, pericardiocentesis should be performed in those patients showing signs of cardiac tamponade. Only enough blood should be removed to relieve the patient of clinical signs.[25] Animals with left atrial rupture have a poor prognosis. The tear may heal, and clinical signs of cardiac tamponade may resolve. However, these animals are predisposed to further atrial tears and cardiac tamponade. Surgical exploration should be considered in recurrent hemorrhage from trauma or left atrial rupture.

If a mass lesion is identified as the cause of pericardial effusion, three options are available. The most aggressive approach includes thoracotomy, parietal pericardiectomy, and attempted removal of the mass.

The surgical success with hemangiosarcoma is

unsatisfactory.[28,33,35,78] At surgery, advanced metastatic spread is often noted and survival time short. The use of pericardiocentesis for symptomatic treatment is of limited value. In my experience, acute cardiac tamponade often returns in 24 to 48 hours. Because of their metastatic nature and the potential for sudden bleeding, a conservative approach should be taken and a poor prognosis expected.

Pericardial effusions in heart-base tumor patients usually develop gradually enough that a diagnosis can be made prior to the development of life-threatening cardiac tamponade. Heart-base tumors tend to grow slowly, to be locally invasive, and to be slow to metastasize to other sites. If the heart-base tumor is small, every attempt should be made for total surgical resection. The prognosis is good following excision of well-defined heart-base tumors.[5,79] In some patients with nonresectable heart-base tumors, subtotal parietal pericardiectomy ventral to the phrenic nerve has offered favorable results. Comfortable survival for up to 3 years has been achieved.[5] In patients in which the heart-base tumor has already infiltrated the myocardium, parietal pericardiectomy may be of little benefit.

For animals in which no mass lesions are identified, a conservative approach is recommended.

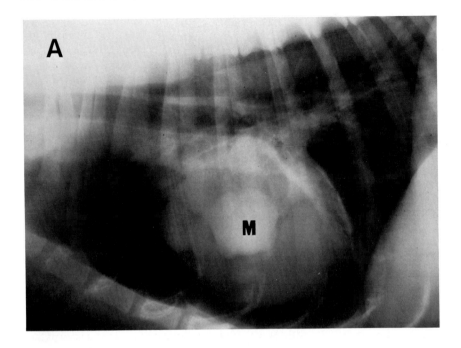

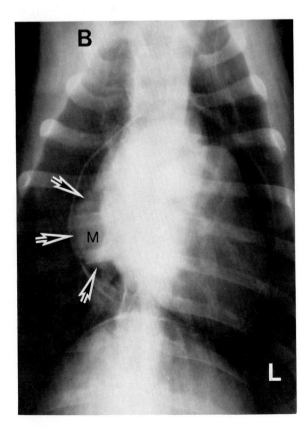

Fig. 24-12 Pneumopericardiogram from an 8-year-old German shepherd with hemangiosarcoma. (**A**) Left lateral and (**B**) Dorsoventral views. An irregular, round mass (M) is outlined (arrows) protruding from the cardiac silhouette on the right side. (Thomas WP: Pericardial Disease. p. 1080. In Ettinger SJ (ed): Textbook of Veterinary Internal Medicine. 2nd Ed. WB Saunders, Philadelphia, 1983. Reprinted with permission from WB Saunders Co.)

Follow-up examination for effusion recurrence using either radiography or echocardiography, or both, is important. In the event of a recurrence, one or two additional pericardiocenteses should be performed. Approximately 50 percent of dogs with idiopathic hemorrhagic pericardial effusions will recover after one or two pericardioceteses.[5] In the remaining half, pericardial effusion may recur within a few days, a few weeks, or as long as 5 years later. For those recurrent cases, subtotal parietal pericardiectomy is recommended and provides favorable clinical results.[27,29,79] Partial pericardiectomy (i.e., pericardial window technique) yields poor results and is not recommended. The use of antiinflammatory drugs such as aspirin and corticosteroids have been beneficial in some cases of pericardial disease in humans. However, the efficacy of these drugs has not been documented in veterinary recurrent idiopathic pericardial effusion.

Constrictive Pericarditis

Constrictive pericarditis is present when a fibrotic, thickened, and adherent pericardium restricts diastolic cardiac filling. Pericardial fibrosis with constriction is considered rare in the dog, and antemortem characterization has not been described in the cat.[80–82] Constrictive pericarditis is usually a symmetric scarring process that produces a uniform restriction of heart-chamber filling. The visceral and parietal pericardial layers can become completely fused, or the constricting process can be produced primarily by the visceral pericardium (epicardium). In rare cases reported in humans and dogs, constricting bands are present over a portion of the heart rather than over the entire heart.[2,80]

Etiology

The etiology of constrictive pericarditis in dogs, as in humans, is often unknown. The primary cause in the dog is idiopathic.[80] In some cases, there is a history of idiopathic or viral pericarditis.[83] Metallic foreign bodies can incite pericardial inflammation and fibrosis.[84] Metallic pellets having direct pericardial contact have been associated with constrictive pericarditis in dogs.[80,81] Actinomycosis and coccidioidomycosis have been implicated in endemic regions.[80,85,86] Other infrequent causes of constrictive pericarditis include chronic renal failure treated with hemodialysis, rheumatoid immunologic disease, neoplastic pericardial infiltration, irradiation, trauma, pacemaker implantation, pyogenic infection, neoplasms (e.g., heart-base tumor, mesothelioma), and drugs that may cause pericarditis followed by constrictive pericarditis (e.g., methysergide, hydralazine, procainamide).[2,80]

Pathophysiology

The hallmark of physiologically significant pericardial constriction is restriction of diastolic ventricular volume. This limitation of diastolic expansion caused by pathologic pericardial changes is responsible for the major hemodynamic consequences that constitute the syndrome of compressive pericardial disease. Invasive hemodynamic studies provide the most reliable evidence of pericardial constriction. They include elevation, superimposition, and equilibration of atrial and ventricular diastolic pressures[57,84,87,88] (Fig. 24-13).

Pericardial fibrosis compromises ventricular wall compliance and limits ventricular filling to early diastole with abrupt cessation of filling by mid-diastole. The result is a sharp, negative, early diastolic atrial and ventricular pulse wave followed by an audible early diastolic "pericardial knock" as ventricular filling suddenly decelerates.[57,88] The waveform of the venous or atrial pulse is dominated by prominent negative x and y waves. These may be of equal amplitude, resulting in an M or W pattern to the pressure tracings (Fig. 24-13). Ventricular pressure tracings typically show a prominent early diastolic descent and a midsystolic plateau, often referred to as the square root ($\sqrt{}$) sign.[87]

By contrast, pericardial effusion interferes with ventricular filling throughout diastole. The result is absence of the early diastolic dip on the ventricular pressure tracing.

Many hemodynamic changes observed in human patients with pericardial constriction have been found in dogs, although the characteristic dip-plateau configuration is not present in every canine case.[80] This makes differentiation from pericardial effusion difficult. The absence of the dip-plateau configuration may reflect the presence of small pericardial effusions and relative lack of epicardial involvement in those dogs.

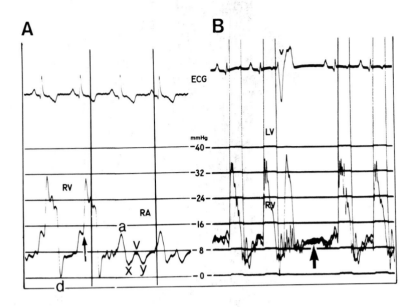

Fig. 24-13 Hemodynamic alterations caused by pericardial constriction in two dogs. (**A**) Right ventricular (RV) and right atrial (RA) pressures. There is a characteristic early diastolic dip (d) and mid-diastolic plateau on the right ventricular tracing. End-diastolic pressure is elevated to 14 mmHg (arrow). On the right atrial tracing, the atrial *a* wave and x and y descents are prominent. (**B**) Simultaneous right ventricular (RV) and left ventricular (LV) pressures. The early diastolic descent is prominent and end-diastolic pressures are elevated and nearly equal (i.e., 12 mmHg). A mid-diastolic plateau (arrow) is seen during the compensatory pause following a premature ventricular beat (v). All tracings recorded at a paper speed of 50 mm/sec. (Thomas WP, Reed JR, Bauer TG, Breznock EM: Constrictive pericardial disease in the dog. J Am Vet Med Assoc 184:546, 1984.)

In patients with constrictive pericarditis as well as cardiac tamponade, restriction of diastolic filling ultimately results in compensatory renal retention of sodium and water. This further contributes to increased systemic venous pressure and initially maintains diastolic ventricular filling despite cardiac compression. However, compression may be so great that diastolic ventricular volumes are decreased. When right and left ventricular preload are reduced, stroke volume and cardiac output fall despite compensatory tachycardia.[2] In severe cases of constrictive pericarditis, myocardial systolic function may be depressed.[89] However, it must be emphasized that systolic function and intrinsic myocardial contractility are usually normal.[90]

PATHOLOGY

On gross examination, the pericardium appears thick, fibrous, and opaque. The parietal pericardium may vary in thickness from 2 to 8 mm.[80–82] Epicardial adhesions are consistent findings but vary in severity. The epicardium appears slightly fibrotic and is usually opaque. Occasionally, it is more seriously effected. Granulomatous masses adherent to and compressing the right ventricular outflow tract

have been seen in dogs with coccidioidomycosis. Pulmonary extension of the fibrotic disease process was reported in one dog that required pneumonectomy in addition to pericardectomy.[80]

In most cases, histologic examination of the pericardium fails to suggest a cause. Histologic abnormalities are nonspecific and include increased, dense fibrous connective tissue, variable amounts of mesothelial proliferation, and reactive or inflammatory cellular infiltrate. In most cases, mild inflammatory infiltrates are present.[80] Degenerating neutrophils and organisms may be seen in an actinomycotic pericardium. Granulomatous inflammation with lymphocytes, plasma cells, and macrophages are found in dogs with coccidioidomycosis.

CLINICAL AND DIAGNOSTIC FINDINGS

History

Dog breeds of medium to large size ranging from 2.5 to 9.5 (mean 6.2) years of age are most commonly affected with males overrepresented.[80–82] Clinical signs are usually associated with right-sided congestive heart failure; abdominal enlargement is common. Less frequently, dyspnea, tachypnea, weakness, syncope, exertional fatigue, and weight loss are reported. The duration of illness varies from weeks to months.

Physical Examination

The most common abnormalities are ascites and jugular venous distention.[80] The femoral arterial pulse pressure may be diminished. Pulsus paradoxus, although not reported in affected dogs, occasionally accompanies human constrictive pericarditis.[2] Heart sounds are frequently diminished, although pleural effusion may mask this finding. Diastolic gallop rhythms, systolic clicks, and murmurs of mitral regurgitation (probably representing concurrent mitral valve disease) may be present, although diastolic pericardial knock is uncommon.[81]

Clinical Pathology

In 16 cases of canine constrictive pericarditis,[80–82] serum biochemical values were essentially normal, and serum protein concentrations were usually decreased (less than 5.5 g/dl); mild anemia (packed cell volume less than 36) and slight leukocytosis (18,000 to 20,000/ml) was occasionally present. Cytology showed modified transudate for thoracic and abdominal effusions and hemorrhagic, chylous, septic pericardial effusions. Bacterial cultures were generally negative.

Electrocardiography

Pericardial fibrosis causes diminished QRS amplitudes (less than 1.0 mV) in standard limb leads (Fig. 24-14). This is similar to pericardial effusion. A more consistent ECG change in constrictive pericarditis in dogs is P-mitrale (left atrial enlargement).[80] These two findings are commonly recorded in affected humans.[84] An ECG pattern resembling right ventricular enlargement has occasionally been demonstrated in humans with granulomatous constrictive pericarditis[91] and has been reported in the dog.[80] Sinus rhythm is normally present but there is increased susceptibility to supraventricular tachycardia or atrial fibrillation during cardiac catheterization.[80]

Thoracic Radiography

Most dogs display mild to moderate cardiomegaly, pleural effusion, lack of pericardial calcification, caudal vena caval widening, and positional distortion.[80–82] Angiocardiography may show atrial and vena caval enlargement or increased endocardial-pericardial distance along the border of the opacified right atrium or ventricle, or it may be normal. In two dogs with coccidioidal pericarditis, angiography demonstrated compression of the right ventricular outflow region (Fig. 24-15).

Echocardiography

Published documentation of canine or feline echocardiographic features is lacking. In humans, ultrasonic diagnosis is difficult. Specific echocardi-

Fig. 24-14 Electrocardiographic abnormalities in dogs with constrictive pericardial disease. (**A**) The P wave is prolonged to 60 msec. QRS amplitudes are diminished in all leads except V₄. (**B**) The P wave is prolonged to 60 msec. QRS amplitudes are not diminished. Simultaneous small S waves in leads I, II, and III and an S wave in V₄ nearly equal to the R wave are suggestive of right ventricular enlargement. Calibration 1 cm = 1 mV; paper speed = 50 mm/sec. (Thomas WP, Reed JR, Bauer TG, Breznock EM: Constrictive pericardial disease in the dog. J Am Vet Med Assoc 184:546, 1984.)

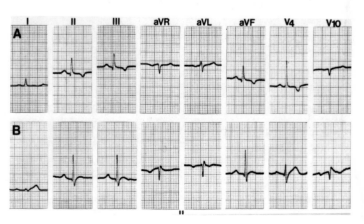

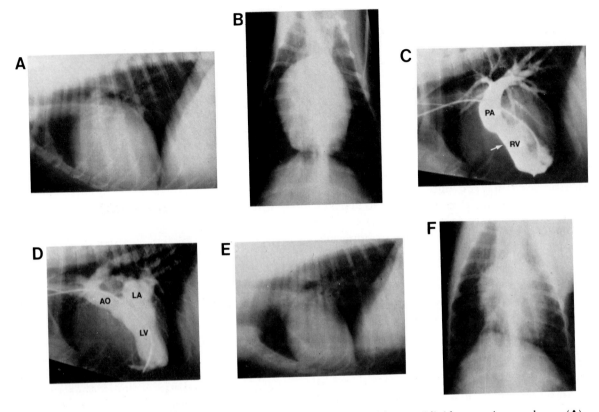

Fig. 24-15 Pre- and postoperative radiographic studies from a dog with a coccidioidomycosis granuloma. (**A**) Preoperative lateral survey radiograph shows moderate cardiomegaly and rounding of cranial and caudal heart borders. (**B**) Dorsoventral view shows moderate cardiomegaly, some rounding, and prominence in the area of the right atrium. (**C**) Right ventricular angiocardiogram (lateral view) shows a large soft tissue density cranial to the right ventricle (RV) and pulmonary artery (PA). The right ventricular outflow region appears indented and flattened (arrow). (**D**) Recirculation phase of the right ventriculogram showing the left side of the heart. The left atrium (LA), left ventricle (LV), and aorta (AO) appear normal. (**E, F**) Lateral and dorsoventral radiographs, respectively, obtained 4 months after pericardectomy. The heart size and shape appear normal. (Thomas WP, Reed JR, Bauer TG, Breznock EM: Constrictive pericardial disease in the dog. J Am Vet Med Assoc 184:546, 1984.)

ographic criteria of human constrictive pericarditis has been reported.[68,92,93]

Hemodynamic Studies

Cardiac catheterization provides the best diagnostic evidence of pericardial constriction. Consistent elevations in CVP (15 to 20 mmHg; normal = 8 mmHg) and high mean atrial and ventricular diastolic pressures are seen. Simultaneous recordings of atrial and ventricular pressures show diastolic equilibration and pressure superimposition (Fig. 24-13).

A prominent, early diastolic dip and mid-diastolic plateau on the ventricular tracings may be seen. When granulomas overlie the right ventricular outflow tract, a systolic pressure gradient may be recorded. Hemodynamic findings in dogs[80] parallel changes reported in human patients.

THERAPY AND PROGNOSIS

Constrictive pericarditis is a progressive disease. Spontaneous reversal of pericardial thickening, abnormal symptoms, or hemodynamic alterations do not occur. A few patients may survive briefly with modest signs of right-sided heart failure treated by diuretics. Most, however, become progressively more disabled despite diuretics; the only treatment is complete pericardial resection.

Fibrosis is limited to the parietal pericardium in most cases, permitting adequate surgical treatment by simple subtotal parietal pericardiectomy. In some, the visceral pericardium is affected. This necessitates epicardial stripping, which is technically more difficult and associated with higher operative and postoperative complications.[79,80] A median sternotomy approach is recommended to maximize surgical exposure and facilitate examination of both sides of the heart, if dessection of epicardial adhesions or epicardial stripping is required. The most common postoperative complication is pulmonary thrombosis 1 day to 7 weeks after surgery.[80] Medical management postoperatively is directed toward the cause of the disorder. Vasodilators and inotropic agents are not indicated, but diuretics may be necessary on a temporary basis. The prognosis is favorable.

In summary, constrictive pericardial disease should be considered in a dog or cat with signs of right heart failure (i.e., jugular distention, ascites, pleural effusion), mild cardiomegaly, and small ECG complexes with increased P-wave duration. Reliable diagnosis requires hemodynamic documentation by cardiac catheterization.

Pericardial Mass Lesions

Most masses within the pericardial sac, including neoplasms, granulomas, cysts, abscesses, and peritoneopericardial hernias cause some degree of pericardial or pleural effusion. They are diagnosed by echocardiography, pneumopericardiography, or angiocardiography. Occasionally, mass lesions are suspected from abnormalities on survey thoracic radiographs, because of abnormalities detected during physical examination (e.g., muffled or displaced heart sounds) or from ECG changes (e.g., diminished QRS voltages). If pleural effusion is present, special diagnostic studies are usually necessary. Two-dimensional echocardiography is the most sensitive and specific technique for imaging neoplasms, cysts, abscesses, and hernias involving the pericardial sac.[71] Angiocardiography will usually outline intracardiac masses or pericardial masses that displace the wall of an opacified chamber. Pneumopericardiography may be useful if sufficient pericardial effusion is present to permit insertion of a pericardial catheter.

A guarded prognosis is warranted in patients with intrapericardial tumors and infectious granulomas. On the other hand, most pericardial cysts and pericardial abscesses can be resected with a favorable long-term prognosis.

REFERENCES

1. Spodick DH: Chronology of pericardial disease. p. 9. In Reddy PS, Leon DF, Shaver JA (eds): Pericardial Disease. Raven Press, New York, 1982
2. Lorell DH, Braunwald E: Pericardial disease. p. 1484. In Braunwald E (ed): Heart Disease. 3rd Ed. WB Saunders, Philadelphia, 1988
3. Moore TC, Shumacker HB: Congenital and experimentally produced pericardial defects. Angiology 4:1, 1953
4. Thomas WP: Pericardial disease. p. 1080. In Ettinger SJ (ed): Textbook of Veterinary Internal Medicine. 2nd Ed. WB Saunders, Philadelphia, 1983
5. Thomas WP, Reed JR: Pericardial disease. p. 364. In Kirk RW (ed): Current Veterinary Therapy. Vol. IX. WB Saunders, Philadelphia, 1986
6. Evans HE, Christensen GC: The heart and arteries. p. 267. In Evans HE, Christensen GC (eds): Miller's Anatomy of The Dog. 2nd Ed. WB Saunders, Philadelphia, 1979
7. Holt JP: The normal pericardium. Am J Cardiol 26:455, 1970
8. Maurer FW, Warren MF, Drinker CK: The composition of mammalian pericardial and peritoneal fluids. Studies of their protein and chloride contents, and the passage of foreign substances from the blood stream into these fluids. Am J Physiol 129:635, 1940
9. Bhargava K, Powers TE, Rudy RL: Pleural and pericardial fluid dynamics in dogs. Indian Vet 49:496, 1972
10. Shabetal R; The pericardium: An essay on some recent developments. Am J Cardiol 42:1036, 1978
11. van der Gaag I, van der Luer RJT: Eight cases of pericardial defects in the dog. Vet Pathol 14:14, 1977
12. Baker GJ, Williams CSF: Diaphragmatic pericardial hernia in the dog. Vet Rec 78:578, 1966
13. Bolton GR, Ettinger S, Rousch JC: Congenital peritoneopericardial diaphragmatic hernia in a dog. J Am Vet Med Assoc 155:723, 1969

14. Finn JP, Martin CL: Diaphragmatic pericardial hernia. J Small Anim Pract 10:295, 1969

15. Clinton JM: A case of congenital pericardio-peritoneal communication in a dog. J Am Vet Rad Soc 8:57, 1967

16. Evans SM, Biery DN: Congenital peritoneopericardial diaphragmatic hernia in the dog and cat: A literature review and 17 additional case histories. Vet Radiol 21:108, 1980

17. Thomas WP, Reed JR, Gomez JA: Diagnostic pneumopercardiography in dogs with spontaneous pericardial effusion. Vet Radiol 25:2, 1984

18. Feigin DS, Fenoglio JJ, McAllister HA, et al: Pericardial cysts: A radiologic-pathologic correlation and review. Radiology 125:15, 1977

19. Marion J, Schwartz A, Ettinger S, et al: Pericardial effusion in a young dog. J Am Vet Med Assoc 157:1055, 1970

20. Nasser WK: Congenital disease of the pericardium. Cardiovasc Clin 7:271, 1976

21. Weitz J, Tilley LP, Moldoff D: Pericardiodiaphragmatic hernia in a dog. J Am Vet Med Assoc 173:1336, 1978

22. Harpster NK: The cardiovascular system. p. 820. In Holzworth J (ed): Diseases of the Cat. Medicine and Surgery. Vol. 1. WB Saunders, Philadelphia, 1987

23. Liu SK: Pathology of feline heart disease. p. 341. In Kirk RW (ed): Current Veterinary Therapy. Vol. V. WB Saunders, Philadelphia, 1974

24. Owens JM: Pericardial effusion in the cat. Vet Clin North Am 7:373, 1977

25. Ettinger SJ, Suter PF: Canine Cardiology. WB Saunders, Philadelphia, 1970

26. Gibbs C, Gaskell CJ, Darke PGG, Wotton PR: Idiopathic pericardial hemorrhage in dogs: A review of fourteen cases. J Small Anim Pract 23:483, 1982

27. Berg RJ, Wingfield WE, Hoopes PJ: Idiopathic hemorrhagic pericardial effusion in eight dogs. J Am Vet Med Assoc 185:988, 1984

28. Berg RJ, Wingfield WE: Pericardial effusion in the dog: A review of 42 cases. J Am Anim Hosp Assoc 20:721, 1984

29. Matthiesen DT, Lammerding J: Partial pericardiectomy for idiopathic hemorrhagic pericardial effusion in the dog. J Am Anim Hosp Assoc 21:41, 1985

30. Sisson D, Thomas WP, Ruehl WW, Zinkl JG: Diagnostic value of pericardial fluid analysis in the dog. J Am Vet Med Assoc 184:51, 1984

31. Tilley LP, Owens JM, Wilkins RJ, Patnaik AK: Pericardial mesothelioma with effusion in a cat. J Am Anim Hosp Assoc 11:60, 1975

32. Bunch SE, Boulton GR, Hornbuckle WE: Pericardial effusion with restrictive pericarditis associated with congestive cardiomyopathy in a cat. J Am Vet Med Assoc 149:1056, 1966

33. Kleine LJ, Zook BC, Munson TO: Primary cardiac hemangiosarcomas in dogs. J Am Vet Med Assoc 174:501, 1979

34. Waller T, Rubarth S: Haemangioendothelioma in domestic animals. Acta Vet Scand 8:234, 1967

35. Aronsohn M: Cardiac hemangiosarcoma in the dog: A review of 38 cases. J Am Vet Med Assoc 164:1201, 1974

36. Nilsson T: Heart-base tumours in the dog. Acta Pathol 37:385, 1955

37. Johnson KH: Aortic body tumors in the dog. J Am Anim Hosp Assoc 21:725, 1985

38. Hayes HM Jr: An hypothesis for the aetiology of canine chemoreceptor system neoplasms, based upon an epidemiological study of 73 cases among hospital patients. J Small Anim Pract 16:337, 1975

39. Patnaik AK, Liu SK, Hurvitz AI, McClelland AJ: Canine chemodectoma (extra-adrenal paragangliomas)—A comparative study. J Small Anim Pract 16:785, 1975

40. Jubb KVF, Kennedy PC: Pathology of Domestic Animals. 2nd Ed. Academic Press, New York, 1974

41. von Bomhard D, Luderer M, Hänichen T, von Sandersleben J: Zur histogenese der herzbasistumoren beim hund. Eine histologische, histochemische und electronenmikroskopisch studie. Zentralbl Vet Med A21:208, 1974

42. Ikede BO, Zubaidy A, Gill CQ: Pericardial mesothelioma with cardiac tamponade in a dog. Vet Pathol 17:496, 1980

43. Thrall DE, Goldschmidt HM: Mesothelioma in the dog: Six case reports. J Am Vet Radiol Soc 19:107, 1978

44. Buchanan JW: Spontaneous left atrial rupture in dogs. In Bloor CM (ed): Comparative Pathophysiology of Circulating Disturbances. Adv Exp Med Biol 223:315, 1972

45. Buchanan JW, Pyle RL: Cardiac tamponade during catheterization of a dog with congenital heart disease. J Am Vet Med Assoc 149:1056, 1966

46. Straw BE, Ogburn P, Wilson JW: Traumatic pericarditis in a dog. J Am Vet Med Assoc 174:501, 1979

47. Perman V, Alsaker RD, Riis RC: Cytology of the dog and cat. American Animal Hospital Association Monograph, South Bend, IN, 1979

48. Fisher EW, Thompson H: Congestive cardiac failure as a result of tuberculous pericarditis. J Small Anim Pract 12:629, 1971

49. Chastain CB, Greve JH, Riedesel DH: Pericardial effusion from granulomatous pleuritis and pericarditis in a dog. J Am Vet Med Assoc 164:1201, 1974

50. Lorenzana R, Richter K, Ettinger SJ, et al: Infectious pericardial effusion in a dog. J Am Anim Hosp Assoc 21:725, 1985

51. Madewell BR, Norrdin RW: Renal failure associated with pericardial effusion in a dog. J Am Vet Med Assoc 167:1091, 1975

52. Spodick DH: Infective pericarditis: Etiologic and clinical spectra. p. 307. In Reddy PS, Leon DF, Shaver JA (eds): Pericardial Disease. Raven Press, New York, 1982

53. Morgan BC, Buntheroth WG, Dillard DH: Relationship of pericardial to pleural pressure during quiet respiration and cardiac tamponade. Circ Res 16:493, 1965

54. Holt JP, Rhode EA, Kines H: Pericardial and Ventricular Pressure. Circ Res 8:1171, 1960

55. Reed JR, Thomas WP: Hemodynamics of progressive pneumopericardium in the dog. Am J Vet Res 45:301, 1984

56. Fowler NO: The physiology of cardiac tamponade. p. 149. In Reddy PS, Leon DF, Shaver JA (eds): Pericardial Disease. Raven Press, New York, 1982

57. Shabetai, R, Fowler, NO. Guntheroth WG: The hemodynamics of cardiac tamponade and constrictive pericarditis. Am J Cardiol 26:480, 1970

58. Wechsler AS, Auerbach BJ, Graham TC, Sabiston DC: Distribution of intramyocardial blood flow during pericardial tamponade: correlation with microscopic anatomy and intrinsic myocardial contractility. J Thorac Cardiovasc Surg 86:847, 1974

59. Fowler NO: Physiology of cardiac tamponade and pulsus paradoxus. Physiological, circulatory, and phramacologic responses in cardiac tamponade. Mod Conc Cardiovasc Dis 47:115, 1978

60. Ruskin J, Bache RJ, Rembert JC, Greenfield JC Jr: Pressure-flow studies in man: Effect of respiration on left ventricular stroke volume. Circulation 48:79, 1973

61. Gabe IT, Mason DT, Gault JH, et al: Effect of respiration on venous return and stroke volume in cardiac tamponade. Br Heart J 32:592, 1970

62. Settle HP, Adolph RJ, Fowler NO, et al: Echocardiographic study of cardiac tamponade. Circulation 56:951, 1977

63. D'Cruz IA, Cohen HC, Prabhu R, Glick G: Diagnosis of cardiac tamponade by echocardiography: Changes in mitral valve motion and ventricular dimension with special reference to paradoxical pulse. Circulation 52:460, 1975

64. Guberman BA, Fowler NO, Engel PJ, et al: Cardiac tamponade in medical patients. Circulation 64:633, 1981

65. Tilley LP: Essentials of Canine and Feline Electrocardiography. 2nd Ed. CV Mosby, St. Louis, 1985

66. Bonagura JD: Electrical alternans associated with pericardial effusion in the dog. J Am Vet Med Assoc 178:574, 1981

67. Buchanan JW: Selective angiography and angiocardiography in dogs with acquired cardiovascular disease. J Am Vet Radiol Soc 6:5, 1965

68. Bohn FK, Rhodes WH: Angiograms and angiocardiograms in dogs and cats: some unusual filling defects. J Am Vet Radiol Soc 11:21, 1970

69. Feigenbaum H: Echocardiography. 3rd Ed. Lea & Febiger, Philadelphia, 1981

70. Bonagura JD, Pipers FS: Echocardiographic features of pericardial effusion in the dog. J Am Vet Med Assoc 179:49, 1981

71. Thomas WP, Sisson D, Bauer TG, Reed JR: Detection of cardiac masses in dogs by two-dimensional echocardiography. Vet Radiol 25:65, 1984

72. Ettinger SJ: Pericardiocentesis. Vet Clin North Am 4:403, 1974

73. Summer-Smith G, Archibald J: Surgical approaches to the treatment of cardiac tamponade. J Am Vet Med Assoc 159:1414, 1971

74. Tilley LP, Wilkins RJ: Pericardial disease. p. 295. In Kirk RW (ed): Current Veterinary Therapy. Vol. V. WB Saunders, Philadelphia, 1974

75. Gompf RE: Pericardial disease. p. 321. In Kirk RW (ed): Current Veterinary Therapy. Vol. VII. WB Saunders, Philadelphia, 1980

76. Reed JR, Thomas WP: Pneumopericardiography in the normal dog. Vet Radiol 24:112, 1983

77. Glancy DL, Richter MA: Catheter drainage of pericardial space. Cathet Cardiovasc Diagn 1:311, 1975

78. Brown NO, Patnaik AK, MacEwen EG: Canine hemangiosarcoma: Retrospective analysis of 104 cases. J Am Vet Med Assoc 186:56, 1985

79. Wagner SD, Breznock EM: Surgical management of pericardial and intramyocardial disease including chemodectomas. p. 470. In Bojrab MJ (ed): Current Techniques in Small Animal Surgery. 2nd Ed. Lea & Febiger, Philadelphia, 1983

80. Thomas WP, Reed JR, Bauer TG, Breznock EM: Constrictive pericardial disease in the dog. J Am Vet Med Assoc 184:546, 1984

81. Schwartz A, Wilson GP, Hamlin RL, et al: Constrictive pericarditis in two dogs. J Am Vet Med Assoc 159:763, 1971

82. Neer TM: Chronic constrictive pericarditis in an American Staffordshire. J Am Anim Hosp Assoc 18:595, 1982

83. Howard EJ, Maier H: Constrictive pericarditis following acute Coxsackie viral pericarditis. Am Heart J 75:247, 1968

84. Spodick DH: Chronic and Constrictive Pericarditis. Grune & Stratton, Orlando, FL, 1964

85. Chapman MG: Cardiac involvement in coccidioi-domycosis. Am J Med 23:87, 1957

86. Smith DM: Canine coccidioidomycosis: A review. Am J Vet Clin Pathol 2:171, 1968

87. Shabetai R: The pathophysiology of constrictive per-icarditis. p. 267. In Reddy PS, Leon DF, Shaver JA (eds): Pericardial Disease. Raven Press, New York, 1982

88. Fowler NO: Constrictive pericarditis: New aspects. Am J Cardiol 50:1014, 1982

89. Harvey RM, Ferrer MI, Cathcart RT, et al: Me-chanical and myocardial factors in chronic constric-tive pericarditis. Circulation 8:695, 1953

90. Lewis BS, Gotsman MS: Left ventricular function in systole and diastole in constrictive pericarditis. Am Heart J 86:23, 1973

91. Chesler E, Mitha AS, Matisonn RE: The ECG of constrictive pericarditis-pattern resembling right ventricular hypertrophy. Am Heart J 91:420, 1976

92. Schnittger I, Bowden RE, Abrams J, Popp R: Echo-cardiography: Pericardial thickening and constrictive pericarditis. Am J Cardiol 42:388, 1978

93. Engel PJ, Fowler NO, Chuwa T, et al: M-mode echocardiography in constrictive pericarditis. J Am Coll Cardiol 6:471, 1985

25

Canine Heartworm Disease

Clay A. Calvert
Clarence A. Rawlings

EPIZOOTIOLOGY

Canine heartworm disease has been considered endemic along the coast of the southeastern United States for as long as the disease has been recognized by the veterinary profession. The American Heartworm Society prepares incidence maps of the United States for the proceedings of its triannual symposium (Fig. 25-1). According to the 1986 map, the prevalence of heartworm infection in adult dogs ranges from 1 to 45 percent, approximately 150 miles inward along the Atlantic coast, from Texas to New Jersey. A similar infection rate is present along the Mississippi river and its major tributaries. An infection rate of less than 1 to 5 percent is present throughout the remainder of the United States and southern Canada, except for Washington, Utah, Idaho, Nevada, and Montana.[1] Even in these states and in Canada there are local areas in which heartworm infection is diagnosed in native dogs. Heartworm disease is also endemic throughout much of the tropical world, especially Japan and Australia.

The prevalence of heartworm infection among various epidemiologic classifications (e.g., breed, sex, dog size, and daily habits) has been reported in several studies. The male to female ratio of infection is 2 to 4:1, which is higher than the population at risk.[2] Although most infections are diagnosed in dogs aged between 3 and 15 years, many cases have been seen in dogs less than 1 year old.[3] Most infected dogs are 4 to 8 years of age. Large dogs are generally more frequently infected than small dogs, and outdoor dogs are four to five times more likely to be infected than are dogs that remain indoors. Hair coat length does not appear to affect infection rate.[2] The breeds in which heartworm infection are most commonly diagnosed at the University of Georgia Veterinary Teaching Hospital are the German shepherd, English pointer, setters, retrievers, and beagles. The boxer was reported as having an unusually high incidence in another survey.[4] Regardless of frequencies reported in epidemiologic studies, individual dogs that are small, have long hair, and live indoors are at risk in endemic regions. We encourage testing and preventive programs for all dogs in regions in which heartworm infection is frequent.

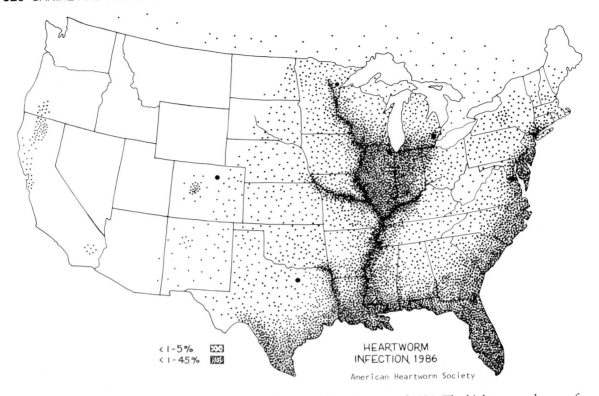

Fig. 25-1 Concentrations of heartworm infection in the United States as of 1986. The highest prevalences of infection are along the Atlantic and Gulf Coasts and in the Midwestern river valleys. (Courtesy of American Heartworm Society, Proceedings of the Heartworm Symposium, Washington, DC, 1986.)

LIFE CYCLE

The life cycle is initiated when gravid females release microfilaria into the vascular system of their canine host. Female heartworms are gravid within 5 months after inoculation of host dogs with infective larvae. Microfilaremia may occur within 5 months, and most experimental infections become patent by 6 months postinoculation.

Microfilaremia implies the presence of adult heartworms, unless the dog has recently been transfused with blood containing microfilaria or has been born to a dog with many microfilaria. *Dirofilaria immitis* microfilaria must be differentiated from those of *Dipetalonema reconditum*. The microfilaria produce minimal, if any, disease in the host. They must go through two molts within a mosquito before becoming capable of developing into an adult heartworm. Approximately 2 to $2\frac{1}{2}$ weeks are required for the microfilaria to undergo two molts and become capable of infecting a naive dog.[5,6] Many species of mosquitoes can transmit heartworm in-fection. The incidence of infection in dogs appears to be related to the population of susceptible mosquitoes. Mosquitoes in colder areas such as Canada have been reported as being successful intermediate hosts, although the development of infective larvae is prolonged.[7]

Within 9 to 12 days of entering the dog via a mosquito-induced wound, the infective larvae develop into fourth-stage larvae (L_4) within the subcutis. At approximately 100 days, the young adult (L_5) enters the vascular system. Young adults are found in the peripheral pulmonary arteries of the caudal lung lobes during the initial months of their residence within the right heart and pulmonary arteries.

PATHOPHYSIOLOGY

Disease responses start at the site of the heartworms within the right heart and pulmonary arteries. Initial changes on the pulmonary arterial surfaces lead to the clinical signs of coughing, dyspnea, hemoptysis, decreased excercise tolerance, congestive heart failure, and poor body condition.

Disease severity and onset are partially a reflection of heartworm number that may vary from 1 to more than 250 per dog.[8] Until the heartworm number exceeds 25 in a 25-kg dog, nearly all the heartworms reside in the caudal pulmonary arteries. As heartworm numbers increase, they move to the right ventricle. The right atrium frequently contains heartworms when the worm burden exceeds 50. Higher numbers of heartworms result in extension into the posterior vena cava.[9]

The pathognomonic lesion for infected dogs is villous myointimal proliferation on the endothelial surface of pulmonary arteries large enough to contain heartworms[10] (Fig. 25-2). Within a few days after arrival of heartworms in the pulmonary arter-

ies, the endothelial surfaces become damaged. This is evidenced by endothelial swelling, widened intercellular junctions, sloughing of longitudinal strips of endothelium, and adhesion of many activated leukocytes and platelets to the damaged areas (Fig. 25-3). The activated cells, particularly platelets, release trophic factors that stimulate migration and multiplication of smooth muscle cells within the tunica media. Smooth muscle cells soon migrate from the media to the intima. These rapidly dividing smooth muscle cells and the collagen produced by them form the villi by 3 to 4 weeks after heartworms arrive in the pulmonary arteries (Fig. 25-4). An endothelial type of cell covers the villi, ranging from a few microns to a few millimeters in size. Some villi become complex in shape and develop areas of endothelial damage, cellular swelling, widened intercellular junctions, sloughing, and adhesion of ac-

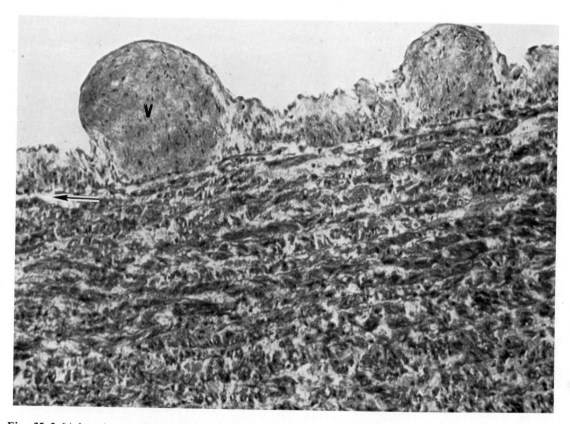

Fig. 25-2 Light micrograph of villi (V) projecting from the surface of a heartworm-injured pulmonary artery into its lumen. The villi are composed of rapidly dividing smooth muscle cells and fibrous connective tissue. The base of the villi appear to arise from the tunica media. The luminal surface, when viewed by scanning electron microscopy, is covered by endothelial-like cells. Arrow points to the junction between the tunica intima and media.

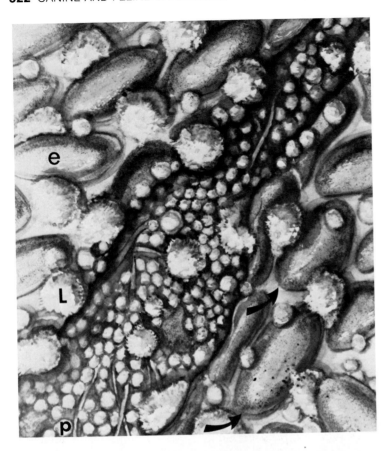

Fig. 25-3 Drawing of the surface of the pulmonary artery as it appears by scanning electron microscopy. This type of injury is produced by heartworms and can be seen within 3 days after heartworms arrive within the pulmonary circulation. The endothelial cells (e) are rounded (arrows) and disoriented as compared to normal endothelial surfaces. Leukocytes (L) that are ruffled are adhered to a strip of arterial wall, which has been denuded of endothelium. The adhesion and activation of platelets and leukocytes result in release of trophic factor(s) that stimulates the smooth muscle cells to form the villi. (Rawlings CA, Keith JC Jr, Schaub RG: Development and resolution of pulmonary disease in heartworm infection: Illustrated review. J Am Anim Hosp Assoc 17:711, 1981.)

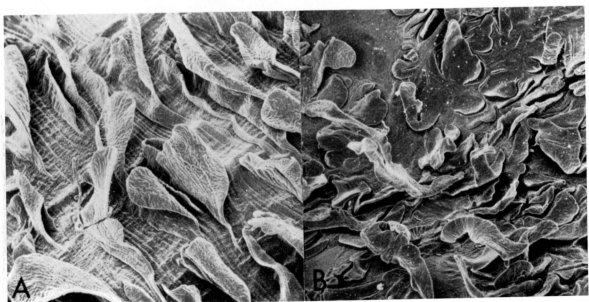

Fig 25-4 Scanning electron micrographs of the surface of the right caudal pulmonary artery from a dog infected with 28 heartworms for 1 year. The surface is extensively involved with rugous and villous proliferations.

tivated leukocyte and platelets similar to those seen initially after heartworm infection. Villous distribution parallels that of heartworm enlodgement in pulmonary arteries and is most severe in the caudal and accessory lung lobes. Permeability of the pulmonary arterial endothelium to serum proteins and water is high when the surface is damaged.[6,8,11–13]

Diseased pulmonary arteries dilate, become tortuous, develop aneurysms, and lose their normal tapering arborization (Fig. 25-5). Abrupt pruning of the arteries can been seen arteriographically where blood flow is obstructed beyond the level at which heartworms reside. Blood flow is frequently diverted to nonaffected lung lobes.[14] Increased permeability produces periarterial edema. This can be seen radiographically as areas of interstitial and alveolar lung disease. The degree of parenchymal lung involvement is proportional to the degree of pulmonary arterial damage but is most severe in proximity to the arteries (Fig. 25-6). Areas of partial lung lobe consolidation may develop.[15] Lung consolidation can produce acute coughing and dyspnea. Disease within the pulmonary arteries impedes arterial flow and increases the work of the right ventricle.[16] Severe disease restricts collateral recruitment of pulmonary arteries necessary to transport the high blood flow during exercise.[17] This in-

creased work produces a sequence of right ventricular dilation, hypertrophy, and failure. A common sign associated with decreased pulmonary compliance, pulmonary hypertension, and increased right ventricular afterload is decreased ability to exercise.

Progression of pulmonary arterial disease has been blocked in studies using platelet-inhibiting drugs such as aspirin, 5 mg/kg/day. Nonsteroid antiinflammatory drugs (e.g., aspirin) reduce platelet adhesion, increase platelet life-span, decrease villous proliferation, and decrease arterial dilation. Aspirin has arrested this disease sequence so successfully that pulmonary arterial pathologic changes have resolved despite persistence of the heartworms.[18] We have observed several dogs in which the clinical signs of disease resolved after aspirin treatment. Aspirin and cage confinement have also markedly improved the success rate in the treatment of dogs with heartworm-induced congestive heart failure.[19]

The killing of adult heartworms by thiacetarsamide treatment leads to two ensuing pathologic stages. The initial response is a clinical exacerbation of the disease. When heartworms die, they disintegrate and lose their molecular mimicry. Fragments move distally and initiate clotting and damage to the luminal endothelium. This endothelial

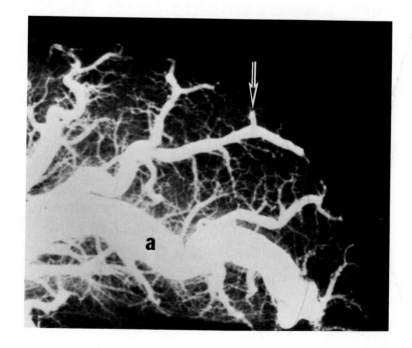

Fig. 25-5 Postmortem pulmonary arteriogram from a dog with heartworm infection. The right caudal lobar artery (a) is the main artery in this photograph and is dilated and severely tortuous. Branches from the lobar artery are also dilated and tortuous, whereas their branches appear to be abruptly pruned (arrow). The dilated arteries are large enough to contain heartworms. These arteries sustain the most severe villous proliferation.

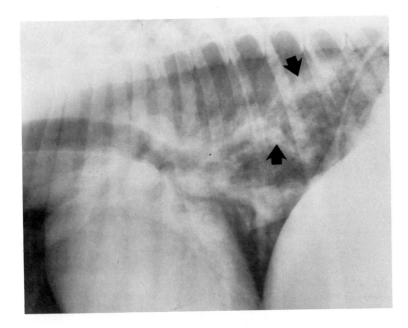

Fig. 25-6 Lateral thoracic radiograph illustrating increased parenchymal lung densities (arrows) in a dog prior to heartworm treatment. The infiltrates are most severe adjacent to the caudal lobar arteries.

damage exacerbates villus production (the initial response to live heartworms) (Fig. 25-4). Blood flow becomes severely impaired, and complete obstruction of pulmonary arterial flow to the caudal lung lobes may occur[20] (Figs. 25-7 and 25-8). Lobes containing dead heartworms develop severe consolidation and do not accommodate either blood-gas exchange or blood flow. Alveolar hypoxia increases pulmonary vascular resistance (hypertension), further impeding arterial blood flow. Severe coughing, dyspnea, and even hemoptysis may develop. Right-sided heart failure can develop acutely in this manner, when blood flow from a compromised right heart is severely impeded.[21] Aspirin administered concurrently with thiacetarsamide treatment reduces the severity of arterial disease markedly and improves pulmonary blood flow. By contrast, anti-inflammatory dosages of corticosteroids increase arterial disease and prolong the presence of heartworm fragments within the pulmonary arteries.[22] Corticosteroids are effective in reducing the acute parenchymal pulmonary disease produced by heartworm death and arterial damage. However, they should be prescribed only in the presence of significant pulmonary disease accompanied by signs such as coughing, hemoptysis, and dyspnea.[21,23]

A second pathologic stage follows this initial response to adult heartworm death. Within 4 to 6 weeks after adulticide treatment, the movement of heartworms away from the large pulmonary arteries permits resolution of previously described arterial surface changes.[20] Arterial disease, pulmonary hypertension, and radiographic changes improve in several months.[17,22,23] While some residual fibrosis may remain about distal arteries, proximal arteries return toward normal as evaluated by hemodynamic function, scanning electron microscopy (SEM), and arteriography.[21,22]

CLINICAL EVALUATION

The diagnosis of heartworm infection should be made before the development of clinical signs. In most geographic regions, 75 to 90 percent of all infected dogs are microfilaremic.[24] Therefore, routine annual testing for the presence of microfilariae will afford a diagnosis relatively early in the course of infection. Dogs not examined annually and those with occult infections are more likely to have more severe pulmonary arterial pathology and clinical signs at the time of diagnosis.

History

The history concerning habitus, use of prophylactic medications, and frequency of microfilaria concentration tests are often informative. Cough-

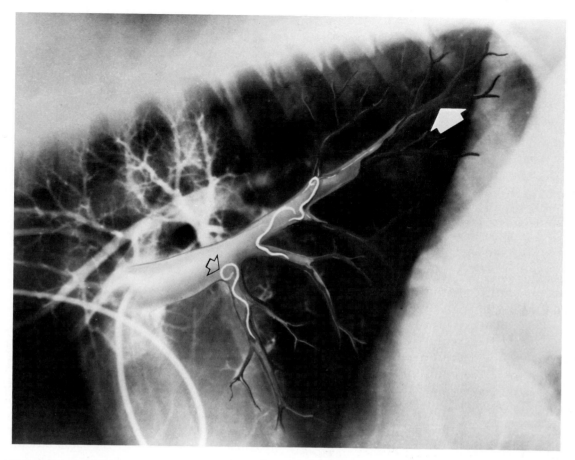

Fig. 25-7 Right pulmonary arteriogram, enhanced by an illustrator, to demonstrate obstruction of flow to the right caudal lung lobe following adulticide treatment. The distal arteries (large white arrow) do not fill, probably due to either intraluminal thrombosis, exuberant villous proliferations, or dead heartworm fragments with surrounding granulomatous inflammation. Dead and dying heartworms (open arrow) are characterized radiographically by a crumpled silhouette in the area of sluggish flow. Despite the severe obstruction of arterial flow, this dog did not have clinical evidence of reduced cardiopulmonary function. This lack of clinical signs was probably the result of strict confinement following thiacetarsamide treatment. (Rawlings CA, Keith JC Jr, Schaub RG: Development and resolution of pulmonary disease in heartworm infection: Illustrated review. J Am Anim Hosp Assoc 17:711, 1981.)

ing, lethargy, poor condition, tachypnea, and dyspnea are common clinical signs consistent with heartworm disease.

Physical Examination

Physical examination findings vary with the severity of pulmonary arterial disease and the presence or absence of associated sequelae. At the University of Georgia Veterinary Teaching Hospital, approximately 55 to 60 percent of heartworm-infected dogs exhibit no or mild clinical signs, such as an occasional cough or subtle lethargy. Approximately one-third of infected dogs have a history of frequent coughing and lethargy. About 10 percent exhibit clinical signs consistent with severe pulmonary arterial disease such as in severe coughing, tachypnea, dyspnea, exercise intolerance, weight loss, hemoptysis, and abdominal distention. In the private practice setting, the proportion of infected dogs with no or minimal clinical signs is greater than that seen at a hospital to which many patients are referred.

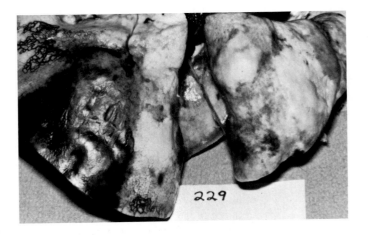

Fig. 25-8 Perfusion-fixed lung removed from a dog 2 weeks after thiacetarsemide treatment. The dog had been pretreated with heparin and Evan's blue dye prior to euthanasia and flushing of residual blood from the pulmonary vasculature with Tyrode's solution for this study. The white areas were perfused; the solid, dark areas indicate lung parenchyma that was not perfused due to obstructed arteries, edema, and inflammation. Thoracic radiographs showed this dark area to have increased density with an alveolar pattern.

Clinical signs may occur with or without severe pulmonary arterial disease during heartworm infection. Occult heartworm disease may cause associated allergic pneumonitis in 10 to 15 percent of affected dogs.[25] This syndrome develops early in the disease course, shortly after microfilariae are produced. Affected dogs exhibit severe coughing, dyspnea, and abnormal pulmonary auscultatory changes (crackles). Severe pulmonary arterial disease, however, is absent.

Pulmonary eosinophilic granulomatosis is a syndrome that has been associated with heartworm disease, especially occult infections.[21,26,27] Coughing, dyspnea, crackles, cyanosis, and muffled heart and lung sounds are usually present. Associated pulmonary arterial disease is of variable severity.

Pulmonary arterial thromboembolic complications are associated with underlying severe arterial disease and may occur before or after adulticide therapy. These complications are characterized variably by coughing, dyspnea, fever, crackles, reduced lung sounds, and hemoptysis.

Epistaxis, associated with thrombocytopenia, may occur in dogs with severe pulmonary arterial disease and thromboembolic complications. Epistaxis may develop prior to adulticide therapy but is more common 2 to 3 weeks afterward.

Hemoglobinuria is associated with either the vena cava syndrome or hemolysis resulting from severe pulmonary arterial disease and thromboembolism. In the latter, thrombocytopenia occurs concomitantly.

DIAGNOSIS

The recommended *minimum data base* for heartworm-infected dogs varies with the clinical circumstances. Dogs that are asymptomatic and that are examined annually for heartworm infection seldom have radiographic or hematologic abnormalities that influence treatment. Dogs with obvious clinical signs, that are middle aged and older, and dogs with suspected occult infections require a more extensive data base. A reasonable minimum data base includes a complete blood count, (CBC), blood urea nitrogen (BUN), and urinalysis.

An *extended data base* is recommended for dogs with clinical signs, older dogs, and dogs with suspected occult infections. This includes a CBC, serum biochemistry profile, urinalysis, and thoracic radiographs. If severe pulmonary artery disease is indicated radiographically, a platelet count is recommended. Dogs with hypoalbuminemia and/or severe proteinuria often have a severe glomerulopathy, occasionally renal amyloidosis. In these cases, 24-hour urine protein determinations and a renal biopsy may be indicated.

CLINICAL PATHOLOGY

Abnormalities in the CBC, serum biochemistry profile, and urinalysis occur in dogs with heartworm disease but are not as consistent or as significant as radiographic changes. Even when present, clinical pathology changes are not diagnostic of heartworm infection. Their greatest value is to identify the unusual dog with significant heartworm-related complications or additional concomitant systemic problems.[21]

The most consistent changes involve the leukogram. Eosinophilia and basophilia have commonly been associated with heartworm infection. The incidence of eosinophilia is probably higher in association with *Dipetalonema reconditum* infection than with *Dirofilaria immitis* infection.[28] Eosinophilia (greater than 1,500 cells/mm^3) and basophilia are supportive evidence of heartworm infection but do not represent the primary basis for diagnosis. In endemic areas, ectoparasitic and endoparasitic infestations limit the value of eosinophilia and basophilia as diagnostic aids. A neutrophilic left shift of the leukogram is commonly seen following adulticide treatment when moderate to severe pulmonary arterial disease is present. The segmented neutrophil and monocyte concentrations in these cases frequently increases. Approximately 10 percent of our patients have a mild regenerative anemia (hematocrit, 27 to 36 percent), probably resulting from hemolysis. Dogs with severe heartworm infection are more likely to demonstrate nonregenerative anemia.

Platelet counts are commonly reduced, since platelet activation and adhesion to damaged endothelium increases their consumption and shortens their life-span.[3,21] Severe thrombocytopenia may occur in association with severe pulmonary arterial disease, particularly following adulticide treatment.

Serum globulin concentrations are frequently increased in heartworm-infected dogs. This may produce an increased total protein concentration, although severely affected dogs may have hypoalbuminemia.

At least 10 percent of our patients have increased serum liver enzyme elevations. These abnormalities seldom alter the treatment approach and usually return to normal within 6 weeks of adulticide treatment. Some dogs have biochemical evidence of decreased liver function, that is, increased retention of bromsulphthalein dye (BSP), especially those with congestive heart failure. However, BSP retention of 8 to 15 percent has not been associated with an increased incidence of acute thiacetarsamide toxicity. Furthermore, BSP excretion is improved within 6 weeks following thiacetarsamide treatment.[3,21]

Some dogs have abnormalities of the urinalysis that are usually the result of heartworm infection. Proteinuria occurs in 20 to 30 percent of heartworm infections and in most cases of severe disease. Amyloidosis and renal tubular insufficiency (the latter resulting in an inability to concentrate the urine) are uncommon complications of heartworm disease. Azotemia may occur but is uncommon.

RADIOLOGY

Since radiographic abnormalities develop early and are characteristic of heartworm infection, they are most useful for indicating the presence and severity of heartworm disease. Typical changes include right ventricular enlargement, increased prominence of the main pulmonary artery, enlarged lobar pulmonary arteries, enlargement (and later, obstruction) of the peripheral pulmonary arteries, and perivascular parenchymal disease. Peripheral lesions tend to be more severe in the caudal lung lobes[21] (Figs. 25-6 and 25-9).

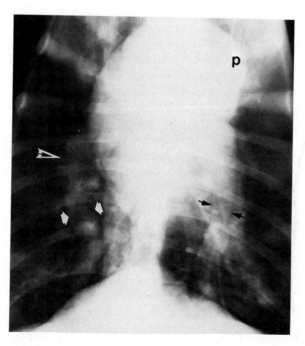

Fig. 25-9 Dorsoventral radiograph of a heartworm-infected dog demonstrating enlargement of the main pulmonary artery segment (p) and caudal lobar arteries (arrows). The right ventricle is also prominent.

Proper positioning and radiographic exposure are critical to the attainment of diagnostic thoracic radiographs. We prefer the ventrodorsal projection over the dorsoventral to assess right ventricular and main pulmonary arterial size. The ventrodorsal position is also easier to align correctly. Assessment of right ventricular and main pulmonary artery segment enlargement is subjective and must be made considering breed variabilities and different thoracic confirmations. Dogs with narrow upright chests (e.g., Irish setters, sight hounds, and Doberman pinschers) tend to have a more upright heart and a smaller cardiac silhouette. Conversely, dogs with a rounder thorax (e.g., beagles) normally have a more prominent right heart and main pulmonary artery. Care must be taken to avoid overinterpretation of these changes in round-chested breeds as indicative of heartworm infection.

By contrast, the dorsoventral projection is more useful in assessing the caudal lobar pulmonary arteries. The diameter of the caudal lobar arteries at their intersection with the ninth ribs should be no larger than the diameters of the ninth ribs.[21] The lateral radiograph is used to measure the right cranial lobar artery and to characterize the parenchymal pattern in the caudal lung lobes. The diameter of the right cranial lobar artery at its intersection with the right fourth rib should not exceed the narrowest diameter of the fourth rib.

Several reports have characterized the frequency of radiographic abnormalities in dogs with heartworm infection. In one study, 85 percent of 200 microfilaria-positive dogs had radiographic changes typical of heartworm infection. Approximately 60 percent demonstrated right ventricular enlargement.[30] Another study identified 72 percent as having enlarged right ventricles.[31] Approximately 75 percent of infected dogs also have enlargement of the main pulmonary artery. Enlargement and/or tortuosity of the lobar arteries is present in approximately 50 percent of cases. When either the cranial or caudal lobar arteries have a measurable increase in diameter, the likelihood of heartworm infection is high.[21] The absence of cranial lobar arterial enlargement does not exclude the possibility of heartworm infection.

Adulticide treatment produces marked radiographic parenchymal changes in response to dying heartworms. Similar but usually less severe signs may be seen in dogs prior to adulticide treatment. Alveolar changes may occur that have ill-defined fluffy margins, coalescence of densities, air bronchograms, lobar distribution of infiltrates, and central localization of the infiltrate. Peribronchiolar nodules may occur as well. Abnormalities are most commonly present in the caudal and the intermediate lung lobes.[20] Parenchymal signs may be predominantly interstitial and indicate fibrosis associated with chronic disease. The alveolar changes may regress rapidly without treatment. When clinical signs are also present, alveolar changes can be reduced rapidly with corticosteroid administration.[23]

ECHOCARDIOGRAPHY

Heartworm disease may cause cardiac changes detectable by echocardiographic evaluation. These include right ventricular and atrial dilation, paradoxic septal motion, reduced left atrial and ventricular dimensions, pulmonary artery enlargement, and pericardial, pleural, and abdominal effusions. Heartworms may sometimes be imaged individually or as a mass when they are incorporated as part of a thrombus (Fig. 25-10; see also Fig. 6-48).

ELECTROCARDIOGRAPHY

The electrocardiogram (ECG) of most dogs infected with adult heartworms is normal. The incidence of chamber enlargement and arrhythmia is low and is associated with severe pulmonary arterial disease and pulmonary hypertension.[31,32]

The most common ECG abnormality is right ventricular hypertrophy,[31–36] which is associated with chronic severe pulmonary arterial disease.[31,32] Chronic pulmonary hypertension (peak systolic pressure of 50 mmHg or mean pressure of 30 mmHg) produces increased right ventricular afterload (pressure overload) leading to right ventricular hypertrophy.[37,38]

The actue right ventricular response to adult heartworms in the pulmonary arteries does not include increased right ventricular pressure or increased force of contraction.[39] The right ventricle appears to dilate initially, a change to which the ECG is relatively insensitive.[40,41] The ECG criteria

Fig. 25-10 M-mode echocardiograms of four dogs with heartworm disease. In *frame 1,* the right ventricle is markedly dilated. The left ventricular cavity is reduced due to poor pulmonary venous return. Paradoxic septal motion is present. Adult heartworms (W) are evident in the right ventricle. S, interventricular septum; LW, left ventricular posterior wall. In *frame 2,* paradoxic septal motion is present (open arrows). Heartworms are visible in the right ventricle, which is dilated. In *frame 3,* a large mass of worms is evident. In *frame 4,* heartworms are entangled within a thrombus in the right ventricle. A, aortic root; La, left atrium. (Courtesy of Dr. N. Syndney Moise.)

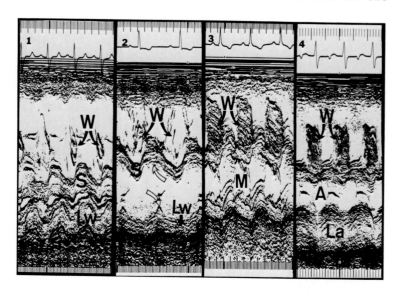

of early or acute cor pulmonale are not well documented in the dog. Many dogs with heartworm disease have radiographic evidence of moderate to severe pulmonary arterial changes and right ventricular enlargement without ECG evidence of right ventricular hypertrophy.[31] In such dogs, however, exercise may incite dyspnea, tachypnea, tachycardia, weakness, or collapse. Telemetric ECG data in these instances demonstrate S-wave and ST-segment changes consistent with acute cor pulmonale.

Some dogs with radiographic evidence of severe pulmonary arterial disease and most dogs with clinically evident heartworm disease-induced right-sided congestive heart failure have definitive ECG evidence of right ventricular hypertrophy. If ascites occurs in a dog with heartworm disease and ECG evidence of right ventricular hypertrophy is absent, the cause of the ascites is seldom right-sided congestive heart failure. When heartworm disease-associated right-sided congestive heart failure is present, radiographic evidence of severe pulmonary arterial disease and right ventricular enlargement are always present. If either the thoracic radiographs or the ECG indicate that severe right ventricular enlargement is absent, right-sided congestive heart failure is seldom present or imminent.[31]

The most accurate ECG correlation of right ventricular hypertrophy with radiographic evidence of severe right ventricular enlargement is made when three or more ECG criteria of right ventricular hypertrophy are present[31,37,42] (Table 25-1). When right ventricular hypertrophy is absent, abnormalities of leads I, II, V_{10}, and mean electrical axis (MEA) (frontal plane) occur in fewer than 10 percent of all instances.[31] Deep S waves in lead V_2 (CV_6LL) are occasionally recorded in dogs without right ventricular hypertrophy.[31,37] When right ventricular

Table 25-1 Detected ECG Criteria of Right Ventricular Hypertrophy in 137 Dogs with Heartworm Disease

ECG Criteria	Dogs with Criteria	
	N	%
$S_{V2} > 0.8$ mV	59	36.5
$S_{V4} > 0.7$ mV	45	33
$MEA_f > 103°$	42	31
$S_1 > 0.05$ mV	39	28
$MEA_x > 90°$	22	16
$S_{II} > 0.35$ mV	21	15
$R/S_{V4} < 0.87$	7	5
Positive T_{V10}	6	4
1 or 2 of the above criteria	19	14
3 or more of the above criteria	47	34

MEA_f, mean electrical axis in the frontal plane; MEA_x, mean electrical axis in the transverse plane; V_2, CV_6LL; V_4, CV_6LU.

hypertrophy is present, abnormalities occur in leads V_2 and V_4 (CV_6LU) with three or more ECG criteria of right ventricular hypertrophy in greater than 75 percent of all instances.[31]

Right atrial enlargement occasionally occurs in dogs with heartworm disease-associated cor pulmonale. P-pulmonale (P_{II} or P_{aVF} greater than 0.4 mV) has been observed in less than 1 percent of all heartworm-infected dogs and a fewer than 5 percent of dogs with severe pulmonary arterial disease in our experience.

Although numerous arrhythmias have been observed with heartworm disease, they are uncommon.[43] In our experience, fewer than 5 percent of infected dogs have cardiac rhythm disturbances, although the incidence may be greater than suspected because of the short monitoring periods routinely employed. Atrial premature contractions and atrial fibrillation are the most commonly recorded arrhythmias.

In summary, the ECG is not an essential component of the data base for dogs with heartworm disease. ECG abnormalities are seldom evident unless severe pulmonary arterial disease is present. If ECG evidence of right ventricular hypertrophy is present, clinical right-sided congestive heart failure is usually present or imminent. If ECG evidence of right ventricular hypertrophy is absent, ascites due to right-sided congestive heart failure is not impending, provided vigorous physical exertion is prevented.

DIAGNOSTIC TESTS

Detection and Identification of Microfilaria

Detection of microfilaria is possible by either concentration or nonconcentration tests. The latter are associated with a higher incidence of false-negative results because a smaller blood volume is examined. These tests may not be specific for differentiating *Dirofilaria immitis* from *Dipetalonema reconditum*.

The most commonly used nonconcentration procedure is the wet smear using a drop of freshly drawn venous blood in which the microfilaria can be seen moving among the red blood cells. The primary criteria for differentiating these microfilaria in

a wet smear is that (1) *Dipetalonema* microfilaria undulate across the slide and *Dirofilaria* tend to gyrate in place; and (2) *Dirofilaria* microfilaria are larger, being at least as wide as the red blood cells. However, size criteria are difficult to assess when microfilaria are active. A less commonly used nonconcentration test is the examination of the buffy coat within the microhematocrit tube.[21]

The concentration tests, using either filters (Difil Test, Evsco, Buena, NJ, and Filarassay-F, Pitman-Moore, Washington Crossing, NJ) or the Knott's technique, should be done when conducting annual or semiannual health maintenance tests, examining dogs with signs of heartworm infection, and determining the efficacy of microfilaricides. Since the volume of blood is greater (1 ml versus 1 drop), the concentration techniques are more sensitive. These tests are similar in their accuracy, and preference is largely subjective. The modified Knott's test is cheaper but requires more time to perform than the filter techniques. Both types of tests lyse the red blood cells and fix the microfilaria. Microfilaria are concentrated by centrifugation with the modified Knott's test and by filtration with the filter tests. With the Knott's test, differentiation of *Dirofilaria immitis* microfilaria (greater than 290 μm in length and 6 μm in width) from *Dipetalonema reconditum* (less than 275 μm in length and les than 6 μm in width) is based on measurements in 2 percent formalin. Size criteria are different when microfilaria are placed in the lysate used in filter tests wherein microfilaria are smaller than when preserved in 2 percent formalin. Morphologic differentiation includes the presence of a tapered head shape, lack of a posterior extremity hook, and straight body shape of *Dirofilaria immitis* microfilaria.[21]

Serodiagnostic Tests

Microfilaria are absent in peripheral blood in 10 to 67 percent of dogs with adult heartworm infection. These so-called occult infections usually account for 10 to 20 percent of infections within a geographic region. True occult infection is often the result of an immune-mediated response that entraps and destroys microfilaria in the lung. Occult heartworm disease is associated with an increased incidence of obvious, sometimes severe, clinical signs. Heartworm infection in the absence of microfilaremia may also result from unisex heartworm populations, sterile heartworms, and immature or pre-patent adult infections. In order to diagnose microfilaria-negative infections, immunodiagnostic tests have been developed. Three tests are being used and have documented value for detecting heartworm infection. Several other tests have been used but have been found to have limited accuracy.[21]

Antibody Tests

The indirect fluorescent antibody (IFA) absorption test has proved useful in the diagnosis of occult heartworm disease in which antibodies to microfilarial cuticular antigen are circulating. Microfilaria are incubated in serum from a dog with suspected heartworm infection. The microfilaria are then washed, placed with rabbit antidog IgG fluorescein isocyanate, and then examined with an ultraviolet microscope. Fluorescence on the microfilarial surface represents a positive test result. This test gives a positive result in about 90 percent of the dogs with true occult heartworm disease. False-positive test results should not occur. However, a positive test result may persist for up to 1 year following effective adulticide treatment. Cross-reactivity with *Dipetalonema* and intestinal parasites has been researched and has not been detected. This test is limited in application to those dogs with immune-mediated disease. The need for sophisticated laboratory technique and equipment limits the use of this test to commercial and state laboratories.

Various other tests, employing enzyme-linked immunosorbent assay (ELISA) methodology, for the detection of adult antibodies were used during the late 1970s and early 1980s, but they have proved unsatisfactory. Their primary problems were associated with false-positive test results, due to either cross-reactivity to other parasites or to being too sensitive. A negative adult antibody ELISA test is strong evidence for the absence of occult heartworm infection.

Adult Antigen Tests

Current tests use monoclonal culture-produced antibodies to circulating adult antigens. These techniques appear to be much more specific than the tests for the detection of adult antibodies. ELISA for adult antigen (Ag-ELISA) (Filarochek, Mallinckrodt, Bohemia, NY; Dirochek, Synbiotics Corp., San Diego, CA; CITE, Agritech Systems, Portland, ME) has been widely tested and is commonly used.

These tests are marketed as kits designed for use in the private practice laboratory. Fresh patient serum is tested and compared with positive and negative tests controls. The reagents include the monoclonal-derived antibody to adult antigens. The presence of heartworm antigen within the serum is indicated by a color reaction. Initial data have shown the tests to be both sensitive and specific. Cross-reactivity with *Dipetalonema* and intestinal parasites has not been detected. False-positive test results appear to be infrequent.

Latex agglutination methodology has also been applied to the detection of adult heartworm antigens in the sera (Difil Test II, EVSCO, Buena, NJ). Latex agglutination is less complicated and is slightly less sensitive than that of ELISA methodology. Other tests are probably forthcoming; with each, the clinician should request documentation of its specificity and sensitivity. Test results must be interpreted with respect to other clinical data.[21]

COMPLICATIONS OF HEARTWORM DISEASE (PREADULTICIDE)

Pulmonary Infiltrates with Eosinophilia

Eosinophilic lung diseases are poorly defined and represent diverse and often unknown etiologies. These disorders are often termed pulmonary eosinophilia, eosinophilic pneumonia, or pulmonary infiltrates with eosinophilia (PIE).[44-48] The term PIE has been recommended as the appropriate designation of these disorders in dogs.[49] PIE is a generic term that should be further defined by other clinical pathology data when possible. It is generally assumed that PIE is an allergic or hypersensitivity reaction to some antigen or chemical.[49]

Pneumonitis Associated with Occult Heartworm Disease

Immune-mediated occult heartworm disease is relatively common.[24,50-52] In heartworm infections, if microfilarial antigen is present in excess quanitites, antibodies are consumed and microfilaremia persists.[50,53,54] In a state of antibody excess, however, with the aid of antibody-dependent leukocyte adhesion, microfilariae become entrapped in the pulmonary circulation.[24,51,52] A predominantly neutrophilic inflammation surrounds the entrapped microfilariae. In some instances, a hypersensitivity reaction occurs and a high concentration of eosinophils dominate the inflammatory reaction.[51,52]

Approximately 10 to 15 percent of dogs with occult heartworm infections develop an allergic or eosinophilic pneumonitis.[25] Clinical signs include progressive coughing, tachypnea, dyspnea, and auscultable crackles. Cyanosis, anorexia, and mild weight loss occasionally develop. Clinical pathologic findings are variable and may include eosinophilia, basophilia, and hyperglobulinemia. Tracheal lavage cytology is usually characterized by a sterile

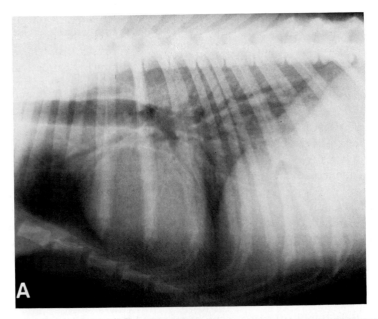

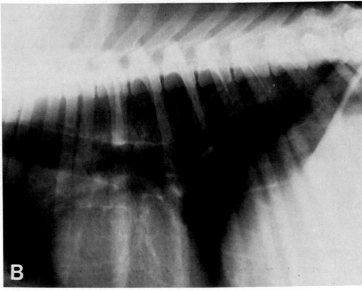

Fig. 25-11 Lateral radiographs illustrating diffuse, mixed, interstitial, and alveolar infiltrates in the caudal lung lobe of a dog with occult heartworm disease-associated allergic pneumonitis before (**A**) and after (**B**) treatment with prednisone.

eosinophilic exudate, with some nondegenerative neutrophils and macrophages. The IFA test for microfilarial cuticular antigen and ELISA and IFA tests for *D. immitis* adult antigens are usually positive.

The thoracic radiographic features of this syndrome include diffuse linear interstitial infiltrates with concomitant diffuse alveolar lung disease (Fig. 25-11). The infiltrate is most prominent in the caudal lung lobes and is characterized cytologically by predominantly eosinophils. In most instances, neither the cranial nor caudal lobar pulmonary arteries are dramatically enlarged. Following resolution of the pneumonitis, there is usually little or no radiographic evidence of vascular or cardiac changes indicative of heartworm disease. The pulmonary infiltrates of eosinophilic pneumonitis may be mistaken for pulmonary edema or pulmonary blastomycosis.

Most dogs respond dramatically to corticosteroid treatment, even though the clinical signs are usually severe. Prednisone (1 to 2 mg/kg/day) usually brings about subjective clinical improvement within 24 to 36 hours. Within 48 hours, radiographic evidence of significant improvement is usual. Corticosteroid treatment is continued for 3 to 5 days and is then stopped 24 hours prior to adulticide therapy. Relapse during or after adulticide therapy has not been reported.

Pulmonary Nodular Eosinophilic Granulomatosis

Pulmonary eosinophilic granulomatosis is a PIE syndrome of unknown etiology, which has been associated with canine heartworm disease.[27,55] We have seen eleven dogs with heartworm disease and this syndrome during the past 8 years. Nine of the dogs lacked circulating microfilariae, but two were Knott's test positive. IFA tests for antibodies against microfilarial cuticular antigen and ELISA test results for adult heartworm antigens were positive in most cases.

Clinical signs associated with pulmonary eosinophilic granulomatosis are similar to those of allergic (eosinophilic) pneumonitis. Coughing, tachypnea, and dyspnea are the predominant physical findings. Clinical pathologic findings are variable and include leukocytosis, neutrophilia, eosinophilia, basophilia, monocytosis, and hyperglobulinemia.

Pleural effusion occurs occasionally and consists of a high protein exudate, with eosinophils predominating.

The thoracic radiographic features usually consist of mixed alveolar and interstitial infiltrates. Multiple pulmonary nodules of diverse sizes and locations are always present (Fig. 25-12). Hilar and mediastinal lymphadenopathy and pleural effusion are inconsistent findings.

Pulmonary granulomas are characterized by a mixed mononuclear and neutrophilic inflammation with an abundance of eosinophils and macrophages. Increased numbers of alveolar cells surround the granulomas. Bronchial smooth muscle proliferation within the granulomas is common. Focal perivascular lymphocytic and eosinophilic cellular infiltration occurs in some granulomas.

Some dogs also have eosinophilic granulomatous lymphadenitis, tracheitis, tonsilitis, splenitis, enteritis, and gastritis. Eosinophilic pericholangitis and eosinophilic infiltration of the liver and kidneys are occasionally detected.

Pulmonary eosinophilic granulomatosis initially responds partially or completely to immunosuppressive dosages of corticosteroids or combinations of corticosteroids and cyclophosphamide or azathioprine. Unfortunately, relapse usually occurs following withdrawal or reduction of corticosteroid hormone treatment or even in the face of continued aggressive treatment. Following relapse, immunosuppressive treatment is of little or no benefit.

Surgical intervention is not recommended. Subsequent granulomas develop in several lobes, and multiple nodules are usually present at the time of diagnosis, even though the extent of lobar involvement is not readily evident on thoracic radiographs.

Prednisone, 2 mg/kg bid, plus azathioprine, 50 mg/m^2/day, for 1 week, then daily for 4 days weekly, is the current recommended treatment for pulmonary eosinophilic granulomatosis in association with heartworm disease. Following improvement of the clinical and pulmonary disease, adulticide and microfilaricide therapy is administered. Immunosuppressive therapy, when effective, is continued for an indefinite period.

Although not all cases of pulmonary eosinophilic granulomatosis may be associated with *D. immitis* infection, the high incidence of heartworm infection with this syndrome suggests a causal relationship in

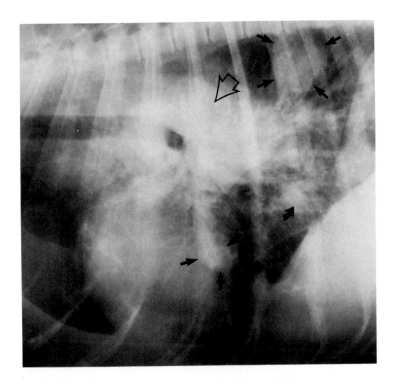

Fig. 25-12 Left lateral radiograph demonstrating pulmonary eosinophilic granulomas (arrows) in a dog with occult heartworm disease.

some dogs. Hypersensitivity reactions to microfilaria are characterized by granulocytic inflammation with a high concentration of eosinophils. Small granulomas consisting of eosinophils and mononuclear and giant cells ensue. In some instances, it may be that the granulomatous reaction becomes unusually severe and progressive. Adult and/or microfilarial antigens in the lungs could trigger such a reaction. However, because of the eosinophilic and granulomatous inflammation seen in various organs and tissues in some dogs, soluble antigens or immune complexes are probably important in the pathogenesis of pulmonary eosinophilic granulomatosis.

Vena Caval Syndrome

The vena caval syndrome is an acute shocklike phenomenon associated with large numbers of heartworms that obstruct venous blood return to the right ventricle. The vena caval syndrome is uncommon outside of highly endemic regions.[56,57] The vast majority of affected dogs, usually 3 to 5 years of age (range, 1.5 to 11 years), do not exhibit clinical signs of heartworm disease prior to the onset

of acute illness. Typical physical examination findings include weakness, pallor, tachypnea, anorexia, hemoglobinuria, and bilirubinuria. Acute collapse with an inability to stand is a common presenting sign.[58,59]

Dogs with vena caval syndrome have an average worm burden of approximately 100 adult worms, with 60 percent present in the right atrium and caudal vena cava. In comparison, nonsymptomatic dogs with heartworm disease may harbor approximately 25 worms with none or only a few located caudal in the vena cava. Heartworm-infected dogs with some exercise intolerance and coughing often have a burden of 45 to 50 worms. Those with approximately 60 worms may have up to 10 to 12 worms in the right atrium and posterior vena cava.[58] The numbers of adult heartworms found in the right ventricle and pulmonary arteries are similar in dogs with the vena caval syndrome, in dogs with moderately severe clinical signs without vena caval syndrome, and in dogs with chronic heartworm disease.[58]

Numerous clinical pathologic abnormalities are associated with the vena caval syndrome. Hemolytic anemia, prerenal azotemia, elevated serum liver enzyme concentrations (e.g., alanine aminotransferase), and abnormal liver function tests (e.g., BSP clearance) are the major findings.[57,59] Hemolytic anemia is predominantly the result of erythrocyte trauma. Direct Coombs' test results are negative, and the concentration of circulating immune complexes is not different from that associated with heartworm disease.[60,61] Hemoglobinemia and hemoglobinuria result from erythrocyte lysis. Microfilaremia is present in most dogs (15 of 17 in one report[3]), but occult infections have been observed.[57]

Most dogs with the vena caval syndrome have ECG evidence of right ventricular hypertrophy.[43] Radiographic evidence of right ventricular and main pulmonary artery segment enlargement is also present.[60]

The diagnosis of the vena caval syndrome should be strongly suspected on the basis of geographic region (i.e., prevalence of the syndrome in the particular locale) and associated clinical signs. Death usually occurs within 24 to 48 hours after the onset of acute signs.[56]

The only effective treatment of vena caval syndrome is surgical removal of some or all of the worms from the vena cava and right atrium. Surgery is performed under local anesthesia (and occasionally mild sedation) through a right jugular venotomy. If intravenous fluids are administered, caution should be taken not to administer an excessive fluid volume. A detailed account of the surgical procedure has been described.[57] Supportive care, such as fluid administration and cardiac rhythm monitoring, should be provided following surgery. Aspirin is recommended for 2 weeks after surgery, at which time thiacetarsamide sodium is administered.

The vena caval syndrome is associated with nearly 100 percent mortality, unless surgical removal of some of the worms is accomplished. A survival rate of greater than 50 percent following surgery has been reported.[57] The success rate of the surgical procedure varies with the skill and experience of the surgeon; results generally improve as more experience is gained.

Severe Pulmonary Arterial Disease

The cardiopulmonary signs of heartworm disease are related to disease of the pulmonary arteries. Heartworm infections of long duration, those associated with high numbers of adult worms, and those associated with occult infections produce the most severe pulmonary arterial disease.[39-41, 62-64]

Approximately 10 percent of heartworm-infected dogs we have seen have clinical and radiographic evidence of severe pulmonary artery disease. Associated clinical signs include severe coughing, tachypnea, dyspnea, exercise intolerance, episodic weakness or syncope, weight loss, and ascites. The mean age of 113 dogs with severe pulmonary arterial disease was 6 years. Only a few were over 10 years of age. Approximately 65 percent of affected dogs lacked detectable microfilaremia.

The cranial and/or caudal lobar arteries of affected dogs are severely enlarged. The caudal lobar arteries are tortuous and have abnormal tapering (Fig. 25-9). The diameters of affected caudal lobar arteries are usually 2.5 to 3.5 times as wide as the ninth rib at their points of intersection and may be 4.5 to 5.0 times as wide. More proximally, the caudal lobar arteries may be six to eight times the diameter of adjacent ribs.

If clinical and radiographic evidence of significant parenchymal lung disease is present prior to adulticide treatment, prednisone, 1 to 2 mg/kg sid to bid, should be administered and continued until these abnormalities resolve. This usually occurs within 5 to 7 days. Corticosteroid therapy is stopped prior to the administration of thiacetarsamide sodium.

The platelet count and packed cell volume should be determined at the time of diagnosis and monitored periodically during the 4 to 6 weeks of hospitalization. Gastrointestinal bleeding occurs occasionally. Pulmonary arterial disease and thromboembolism may be severe enough, particularly following adulticide treatment, to cause thrombocytopenia due to platelet consumption.

Digoxin is not recommended. It does not improve survival rates and may cause digoxin intoxication.[26,64] Decreased volume of distribution due to cachexia and overestimation of lean body weight due to the effect of ascites probably account for the relatively common occurrence of digoxin toxicity.

Since platelet adhesion and activation are involved in the pathogenesis of pulmonary arterial disease, drugs that modify platelet function should be beneficial.[41,65-68] Dogs treated with aspirin have less platelet adhesion, vascular damage, and villus proliferation than do dogs not given aspirin.[66,67,69,70]

The recommended treatment for dogs with severe pulmonary arterial disease is strict cage confinement and aspirin, 5 mg/kg sid. Cage confinement and aspirin must be continued for 1 week (preferably 2 to 3 weeks) prior to adulticide, during adulticide treatment, and for 3 to 4 weeks post-treatment.

Dogs with severe pulmonary arterial disease that we have treated with aspirin and protracted cage confinement survived longer than dogs in which this therapy was omitted. In a series of 74 affected dogs, 34 of 40 (85 percent) which were treated with aspirin and cage confinement survived in contrast to 18 out of 34 (53 percent) that were not given this therapy. The presence of ascites due to right-sided congestive heart failure in these dogs was of no prognostic significance; 43 (58 percent) of 74 dogs with severe pulmonary artery disease had overt clinical evidence of right-sided congestive heart failure (ascites, jugular pulses, distended jugular veins, elevated central venous pressure). Dogs with clinical right-sided congestive heart failure were treated with aspirin, cage confinement, furosemide (1 to 2 mg/kg/day), and a low-sodium diet. There was no difference in the survival rates of dogs with or without right-sided congestive heart failure.

Thromboembolic Complications

Pulmonary arterial thromboembolic complications, although most common following adulticide treatment, may occur prior to thiacetarsamide administration. Such pulmonary arterial disease results from platelet adhesion and activation, inflammation, severe myointimal proliferation, and increased vascular permeability.[41,63] Clinically apparent preadulticide thromboembolic complications are associated with severe pulmonary arterial disease (Figs. 25-4 and 25-7). Severe enlargement and tortuosity of the caudal lobar pulmonary arteries are radiographically apparent in these cases.

Coughing, tachypnea, dyspnea, fever, hemoptysis, auscultatory crackles, and areas of decreased lung sounds are variably present in dogs with thromboembolic lung disease. Such clinical signs may be acute or subacute. Acute thromboembolic lung disease is often associated with tachycardia, pale mucous membranes, and weak or thready femoral pulses.

Increased vascular permeability leads to the interstitial and alveolar inflammation and accumulation of plasma[65] (Fig. 25-8). This results in decreased pulmonary compliance and increased work of breathing. Crackles may be auscultated. Air bronchograms are visible on thoracic radiographs, particularly adjacent to the caudal lobar arteries.

Dyspnea results form hypoxemia caused by ventilation-perfusion mismatching as well as parenchymal fluid accumulation in some instances. Coughing results from similar fluid accumulation and inflammation. Hemoptysis is more commonly, but not exclusively, associated with postadulticide thromboembolic disease. Areas of lung consolidation produced by thromboembolism may be manifested as areas of dullness during auscultation or percussion.

Complete blood count, platelet count, activated clotting times, and thoracic radiographs should be performed in dogs with symptomatic thromboembolic disease. A biochemical profile and urine analysis may be added for a complete data base.

Recommended therapy is strict cage confinement. In addition, if there is clinical and radiographic evidence of secondary parenchymal lung disease, corticosteroid hormones, such as prednisone, 1 to 2 mg/kg/day, are indicated. Judicious intravenous fluid therapy is administered to dogs exhibiting signs consistent with cardiovascular shock (tachycardia, pale mucous membranes, weak; thready pulses, excessive toe-web to rectal temperature differential). Corticosteroid therapy should be continued until there is both clinical and radiographic evidence of significant improvement. This usually occurs in 5 to 7 days. Cage confinement is continued until the clinical signs associated with thromboembolism resolve. Antibiotics and bronchodilators are often prescribed empirically, although in most instances they do not alter the course of the disease.

Since thromboembolic disease of this nature is associated with severe pulmonary arterial disease, aspirin treatment is indicated. Aspirin therapy, 5 mg/kg sid, is begun immediately or after resolution of hemoptysis. It should be continued for 2 to 4 weeks postadulticide.

Azotemia and Proteinuria

Azotemia will be detected if an appropriate minimum database is procured prior to adulticide therapy. Fortunately, primary renal failure is uncommon with heartworm disease. Mild to moderate azotemia (BUN, 30 to 120 mg percent) associated with a concentrated urine (specific gravity, greater than 1.035) is common and often of prerenal origin. Affected dogs are commonly dehydrated. Concomitant problems should be treated prior to thiacetarsamide treatment. Prerenal azotemia is corrected by fluid replacement therapy.

Heartworm disease-induced glomerulopathy may result or contribute to azotemia in association with a relatively concentrated urine. Proteinuria is present in such circumstances. If severe hypoalbuminemia or the nephrotic syndrome are present, irreversible glomerular disease has occurred. Adulticide therapy is not indicated in dogs with the nephrotic syndrome or in dogs with severe azotemia and proteinuria. Conversely, if the BUN is 30 to 120 mg percent with proteinuria, but hypoalbuminemia and the nephrotic syndrome are absent, successful adulticide therapy can be accomplished. Fluid therapy is given to improve renal function to correct the prerenal azotemia. If the BUN is reduced by fluid therapy to less than 50 mg percent, thiacetarsamide therapy can be initiated and fluid therapy should be continued during and for several days following thiacetarsamide administration. In our experience, most dogs with correctable azotemia and proteinuria without hypoalbuminemia, ascites or dependent edema tolerate heartworm treatment. Renal function and proteinuria usually improve following treatment. Long-term follow-up studies have not been conducted.

Glomerulonephritis, Amyloidosis, and the Nephrotic Syndrome

Heartworm-infected dogs occasionally develop a glomerulopathy, sometimes due to renal amyloidosis. Severe proteinuria with hypoalbuminemia, ascites, peripheral edema (nephrotic syndrome), and azotemia eventually occur. Renal biopsy is necessary in order to qualitate and quantitate the extent of glomerular disease. Thiacetarsamide therapy is not indicated in dogs with symptomatic amyloidosis and nephrotic syndrome.

Liver Disease

The most common indication of hepatic disease in heartworm infected dogs is increased serum alkaline phosphatase or serum alanine aminotrans-

ferase, formerly SGPT. These abnormalities are nonspecific and up to 10-fold pretreatment elevations of serum alkaline phosphatase or alanine aminotransferase have not been associated with acute thiacetarsamide toxicity. Likewise, increased bromsulphthalein (BSP) retention up to 15 percent prior to treatment has not been associated with treatment complications. We believe that too much emphasis has been placed on the significance of increased serum liver enzyme concentrations.

Icterus and/or hemoglobinuria occasionally occur in association with severe pulmonary arterial disease or the vena caval syndrome. The prognosis for dogs with concomitant severe pulmonary arterial disease and icterus is poor. In these situations, hypoalbuminemia and an abnormal ammonia tolerance test are usually present, and right-sided congestive heart failure may coexist. Dogs with icterus and evidence of severe hepatic insufficiency are not candidates for thiacetarsamide treatment.

POSTADULTICIDE COMPLICATIONS

Acute Thiacetarsamide Sodium Toxicity

Toxic reaction signs to thiacetarsamide treatment include anorexia, vomiting, depression, fever, diarrhea, tubular casts in the urine sediment, increased serum liver enzyme concentrations, icterus, and bilirubinuria, as well as death. These abnormalities occur in a wide variety of diseases, and none are helpful in predicting dogs destined to have an adverse thiacetarsamide reaction.[70]

Dogs receiving thiacetarsamide should be hospitalized throughout adulticide treatment and monitored closely. One-half to 1 hour before each thiacetarsemide injection, the dog is fed and rectal temperature measured. In addition, urine is examined prior to each injection for the presence of bilirubin and tubular casts.

To determine whether adulticide treatment should be continued, the dog's attitude, appetite, rectal temperature, mucous membrane color, hydration status, and urinalysis are assessed, and the dog is checked for the presence of absence of vomiting. Serum liver enzyme concentrations are not used as indications of toxicity. Icterus and persistent vomiting are always indications for stopping adulticide treatment. If, following initial treatment, a dog vomits only once or twice, has a normal appetite and temperature, and is not depressed, treatment is continued. A combination of any two signs, such as vomiting, depression, anorexia, fever, and diarrhea, are usually sufficient to discontinue treatment.[71] Most adverse reactions occur following the first injection.

Treatment of adverse reactions is nonspecific and consists primarily of intravenous fluid therapy. Dogs with a fever of greater than 103°F (39.4°C) frequently respond to antiinflammatory dosages of corticosteroids. A high-carbohydrate, low-fat diet should be provided, and re-evaluation in 3 to 4 weeks is suggested. When clinical signs have resolved, these dogs should then be given the complete thiacetarsamide sodium treatment and most do not develop further complications.[21]

Microfilaricide Toxicity

Adulticide treatment is followed by microfilaricide treatment in 4 to 6 weeks. Dogs that were healthy prior to adulticide treatment and that did not have complications during arsenical treatment can usually be treated for microfilariae in 4 weeks without complications. Dithiazanine produces blue feces and occasionally vomiting. When vomiting is persistent and does not respond to anticholinergic drugs, the microfilaricide should be changed. Levamisole can cause both vomiting and central nervous system (CNS) toxicity. Neurologic signs frequently begin as nervousness, apprehension, and shaking but may progress to dementia and seizures if therapy is not curtailed. Toxicity tends to resolve, but levamasole treatment should be stopped if CNS toxicity occurs. The side effects of fenthion, when applied topically, are those of organophosphate toxicity. Although these complications are uncommon, we do not recommend fenthion.

Ivermectin toxicity may be manifested as hypersensitivity, idiosyncratic and delayed reactions. Hypersensitivity and delayed reactions are usually associated with high microfilarial counts when more than 90 percent of the microfilaria are killed within 24 hours.[72] Idiosyncratic reactions occur in the collie breed. The incidence of hypersensitivity and delayed reactions is less than 5 percent when the dosage of ivermectin is 50 µg/kg.[72] At a dosage of 200 µg/kg, the incidence of reactions is 15 to 20 percent. The incidence of adverse reactions could be reduced by withholding ivermectin treatment for dogs with high concentrations of microfilariae (greater than 1,000/ml).

Hypersensitivity reactions may be indicated by vomiting, diarrhea, depression, tachypnea, tachycardia, pale mucous membranes, weakness, and shock. Most reactions are mild. Severe reactions can be curtailed if the patient is closely observed and intravenous fluid and soluble corticosteroid hormone treatment is initiated as soon as signs of cardiovascular involvement are detected. Death is likely only when shock is not detected early.

Delayed reactions are occasionally observed 1 to 2 days following ivermectin administration. These reactions are characterized by mild lethargy, partial anorexia, and persist for approximately 24 hours. Collies and collie-mix breeds are at a high risk of developing severe reactions characterized by mydriasis, ataxia, dementia, seizures, and coma. Ivermectin should therefore be avoided in these dogs.[72]

Thromboembolic Lung Disease

Followng thiacetarsamide sodium treatment, pulmonary arterial disease is exacerbated. Extensive endothelial damage results in massive platelet adhesion, myointimal proliferation, and villus hypertrophy.[73] Significant complications occur most frequently in dogs with pre-existing severe pulmonary arterial disease (Figs. 25-4 and 25-7). Thoracic radiographs may be useful to provide a practical estimate of pulmonary arterial disease prior to adulticide treatment.

Dead heartworms produce pulmonary thrombosis, granulomatous arteritis, perivascular edema (due to increased vascular permeability), and hemorrhage. The caudal and accessory lobes are most severely affected.[74] Exacerbated pulmonary disease occurs from 5 to 30 days postadulticide, with the greatest risk of severe thromboembolism occurring from 7 to 17 days after treatment. Associated clinical signs include coughing, fever, dyspnea, auscultatory crackles and/or dullness, hemoptysis, pale mucous membranes, tachycardia, and weak pulses. A regenerative left shift may be indicated from the leukogram, and thrombocytopenia is usually present.

The recommended therapeutic steps for thromboembolic lung disease include cage confinement and corticosteroid hormone administration (prednisone, 1 to 2 mg/kg/day). Bronchodilator drugs and antibiotics are often prescribed empirically. Antibiotics are of questionable benefit, unless results of transtracheal lavage cytology and microbial culture suggest a bacterial infection. Strict cage confinement is the most important aspect of therapy and should be continued until there is clinical and radiographic evidence of resolution of parenchymal lung disease. Judicious fluid administration is indicated if there is evidence of decreased cardiac output (e.g., weak pulses), hypothermia, and increased toe-web to rectal temperature differential. Aspirin, 5 mg/kg sid, may be prescribed and should be continued for 2 to 3 weeks.

Thrombocytopenia

Thrombocytopenia is associated with severe pulmonary arterial disease and may develop before, or more commonly, after adulticide treatment. Pulmonary arterial disease and thromboembolism are exacerbated following adulticide treatment.[65,73] Increased platelet consumption occurs due to accelerated endothelial damage, platelet involvement in the coagulation cascade, and adherence to dead heartworms.[73,75,76]

Thrombocytopenia is most severe from 7 to 17 days following thiacetarsamide sodium administration. Platelet counts below 50,000/mm^3 are associated with severe pulmonary arterial disease and clinical signs of thromboembolic disease, possibly including hemoptysis and epistaxis.

Thrombocytopenia caused by heartworm disease is usually associated with a normal or near-normal activated clotting time; normal prothrombin time, activated partial thromboplastin time, and thrombin time; and the absence of fibrin degradation products. These findings, sometimes referred to as chronic or low-grade disseminated intravascular coagulation (DIC),[77] may be associated with epistaxis, hemoptysis, or radiographic evidence consistent with pulmonary hemorrhage. Treatment is indicated if the platelet count decreases rapidly or is less than 50,000/mm.^{3}

Heparin, 150 to 250 units/kg SC tid, is the recommended treatment for chronic or low-grade DIC. The platelet count usually rises in 1 to 2 days and evidence of bleeding, hemolysis, and hemoglobinuria subside. Heparin therapy should be continued until the platelet count exceeds 100,000/mm^3 and must be administered with caution to patients receiving aspirin.

Severe thrombocytopenia may be averted if the platelet count is monitored by administration of a single intravenous dose of vincristine, 0.4 mg/m^2. This causes the platelet count to increase within 2 to 3 days and usually persists for 7 to 14 days, at which time the risk of thromboembolic complications is lowered.

Hemoglobinuria

Hemoglobinuria, in addition to its association with the vena caval syndrome, is occasionally seen with severe pulmonary arterial disease. It may occur before or after adulticide therapy. Hemoglobinuria results from erythrocyte lysis in diseased pulmonary arteries. Fibrin production associated with local coagulation and thromboemboli is a major cause of erythrocyte trauma.

Hemoglobinuria is associated with thrombocytopenia and low-grade (chronic) DIC. Heparin, 150 to 250 units/kg SC tid, is the recommended treatment. Hemoglobinuria usually improves within 24 to 48 hours as the platelet count increases.

INDICATIONS FOR ASPIRIN TREATMENT

Aspirin is indicated for the treatment of severe pulmonary arterial disease.[18,22,68] The severity of pulmonary arterial disease can be estimated on the basis of thoracic radiographs.[12,62] Aspirin is indicated to ameliorate pulmonary arterial myointimal proliferation and thromboembolic complications before and after thiacetarsamide treatment.[19,22,26] Pulmonary arterial disease is initiated by the presence of adult heartworms and arterial damage is followed by platelet and leukocyte activation. Platelet-derived growth factor (PDGF) stimulates migration and multiplication of smooth muscle cells within the tunica media. These smooth muscle cells and the collagen that they produce form the villi.[3,6,14,17] Diseased arteries dilate, become tortuous, develop aneurysms, and lose compliance. Blood flow is partially or totally obstructed and diverted to noninfected lung lobes.[15] Aspirin inhibits platelet function and release of growth factor. After a period of at least 1 week of treatment, pulmonary endothelial damage begins to improve.

Aspirin is not indicated for the treatment of most dogs with heartworm disease. Severe pulmonary artery disease is indicated when the caudal lobar arteries are at least 1½ times the diameter of the ninth ribs at their points of superimposition on the ventrodorsal or dorsoventral projection. Likewise, severe disease is indicated when the cranial lobar arteries are at least 1.2 times the diameter of the corresponding veins on the lateral projection. Aspirin dosages of 5 to 10 mg/kg/day have been shown to be effective in experimental and spontaneous infections.[18,19]

INDICATIONS FOR CORTICOSTEROID HORMONE TREATMENT

Corticosteroid hormones are indicated for the treatment of pulmonary parenchymal disease that occurs secondary to severe arterial disease and for the treatment of allergic pneumonitis.[22,25] Corticosteroids are usually prescribed after the onset of clinical signs associated with parenchymal lung disease.

Severe pulmonary arterial disease leads to increased permeability of smaller vessels to water, plasma, and inflammatory cells.[6,14,17,18] Periarterial edema and inflammation occur and are characterized radiographically by interstitial and alveolar infiltrates. The degree of lung involvement is proportional to the severity of arterial disease. Parenchymal disease is most severe proximal to diseased lobar arteries but may involve portions of or an entire lung lobe.

The clinical signs associated with parenchymal lung disease include coughing, dyspnea, fever, crackles, and hemoptysis. Vascular damage and coughing can lead to alveolar hemorrhage. Hemoptysis is a sign of severe disease and is exacerbated by exercise. Associated hemorrhage may reach life-threatening severity.

Corticosteroid hormones, such as prednisone, 2 mg/kg/day, are indicated for the treatment of significant parenchymal disease. Affected dogs usually have radiographic evidence of severe arterial disease as well as parenchymal changes. Corticosteroids are not recommended either as prophylactic treatment or for clinical signs of mild parenchymal disease, such as occasional coughing or low-grade fever. Corticosteroid hormones are also indicated for the treatment of occult heartworm disease-associated allergic pneumonitis.[25]

Corticosteroid hormones exacerbate the degree of pulmonary arterial disease and thereby promote further thromboembolisms and reduced pulmonary arterial blood flow.[22,23] Corticosteroids should be employed only when necessary and until there is radiographic and clinical evidence of the resolution of parenchymal disease (usually 5 to 7 days).

THERAPY FOR HEARTWORM DISEASE

Indications for Delayed Treatment

Numerous complications or sequelae of heartworm disease warrant delay of treatment until further evaluation or ancillary treatment can be provided.

PULMONARY DISEASE

Dogs with severe pulmonary artery disease, as assessed radiographically, are at increased risk of developing severe thromboembolic complications. Cage confinement and aspirin are recommended for at least 1 week, (preferably 2 to 3 weeks) prior to adulticide treatment. In some instances, parenchymal lung injury occurs secondary to pulmonary arterial disease. In addition to cage confinement and aspirin treatment, corticosteroid hormones are indicated in these cases. Corticosteroid hormones should be used only when clinical and/or radiographic evidence of significant parenchymal lung disease exists and continued until resolution of these signs occurs (usually in 5 to 7 days).

Right-sided congestive heart failure is a complication of severe pulmonary arterial disease and hypertension. In addition to cage confinement and aspirin treatment, diuretics and a low-sodium diet are recommended.

Occult heartworm associated allergic pneumonitis is a parenchymal lung complication that is usually not associated with severe pulmonary arterial disease. It usually occurs early in the course of adult heartworm infection. Corticosteroid hormone treatment is indicated and usually results in complete remission of the clinical and radiographic signs within 3 to 5 days. Subsequently, corticosteroids are stopped and adulticide therapy initiated.

CAVAL SYNDROME

Adulticide treatment is delayed until some adult worms have been surgically removed and appropriate supportive care has improved the patient's condition.

RENAL DISEASE

The most common renal disorder associated with heartworm disease is glomerulonephritis. Heartworm disease-associated glomerulopathy is characterized by proteinuria, azotemia, and hypoproteinemia. Heartworm treatment should be delayed until the severity of the glomerular disease has been determined and azotemia, if present, corrected.

Prerenal azotemia is another complication that warrants delayed heartworm treatment. It is usually due to dehydration, resulting from either severe pulmonary disease or other disorders. Appropriate supportive care should be provided and fluid therapy instituted in order to correct dehydration.

HYPOPROTEINEMIA

Hypoproteinemia associated with heartworm disease is usually attributable to a glomerulopathy. Adulticide treatment may need to be delayed until further patient assessment and stabilization can be completed.

ICTERUS

Icterus is an uncommon complication prior to adulticide treatment. Where present, it is usually associated with severe chronic heartworm disease. Anemia, hepatic insufficiency, and right-sided congestive heart failure often coexist. In such cases, heartworm treatment is not indicated.

Hemoglobinuria

Hemoglobinuria is associated with either the vena caval syndrome or hemolysis due to severe pulmonary arterial disease and thromboembolism. Adulticide therapy is delayed until successful ancillary treatments have been provided.

ADULTICIDE THERAPY

Thiacetarsamide is the only drug approved for the treatment of adult heartworm infection. Elimination of adult worms results in resolution of pulmonary arterial disease, except for occasional cases of severe disease with extensive chronic fibrosis. Pulmonary arterial disease is the direct result of adult heartworms.

Microfilaricide Preceding Adulticide

It has been proposed, and is the custom of some veterinarians, to employ a microfilaricide (dithiazanine) first, followed in 3 weeks by thiacetarsamide.[78,79] Theoretically, microfilariae, by impeding microcirculation of the liver and kidney, result in biochemical alterations that predispose to acute thiacetarsamide toxicity. Ultrastructural studies have not supported this theory,[80-82] although mild kidney changes have been observed. However, more severe liver and kidney pathology has been observed after microfilaricide treatment.[80,83] Hepatic granulomas develop around dead microfilariae and glomeruli filtering dead microfilariae degenerate and are replaced by fibrous tissue. Acute thiacetarsamide toxicity is not associated with high microfilarial concentrations, and the incidence of toxicity between dogs receiving adulticide or microfilaricide first is not different.[84] Furthermore, it is difficult to clear microfilariae for more than a few days when gravid female worms are present.

Additional Adulticide Drugs

Although drugs such as levamisole (L-tetramisole) and stibophen have been used as adulticide agents, only thiacetarsamide sodium is approved, well tested, and efficacious. The efficacy of levamisole as an adulticide varies widely.[79,85-88] From 0 to 100 percent of adult worms are killed; young female worms are the most resistant. Levamisole, therefore, is not a dependable adulticidal drug.[89]

Thiacetarsamide Sodium Treatment

When stored under refrigeration (2 to 8°C) in amber-colored sealed vials, the expiration time of 1 percent thiacetarsamide is 15 months. However, when not refrigerated, the drug deteriorates rapidly and develops precipitates and a yellow-orange discoloration. Air entering the vials also contributes to more rapid deterioration.

Thiacetarsamide should be injected at intervals of not less than six to eight hours and not more than 15 hours. The recommended dosage is 2.2 mg/kg (0.22 ml/kg) IV. Increased dosages, although possibly increasing adulticide activity, are associated with increased toxicity. The current regimen of two daily injections for 2 days has been recommended for almost a quarter of a century.[89] It has been determined that six injections over a 3-day period are no more efficacious than four injections and result in more severe postadulticide lung complications.[90]

It should not be expected that thiacetarsemide will kill every heartworm in every treated dog. There is variation in efficacy from dog to dog. Immature worms, especially female worms, are more resistant. When prednisolone is administered during and immediately after adulticide treatment, fewer female heartworms are killed.[74,91]

Most male heartworms are killed by thiacetarsamide. Female worms that are 4 to 12 months old and male worms that are 4 months old are resistant to thiacetarsamide.[91] It is not necessary, however, to kill 100 percent of adult heartworms initially. Significant improvement of pulmonary arterial disease occurs following thiacetarsamide treatment, even when some adult worms survive.

Each thiacetarsamide dose should be administered after the patient is observed and examined. It is recommended that infected dogs be fed $\frac{1}{2}$ to 1 hour prior to each injection. A urine sample should be collected and examined for bilirubinuria prior to each treatment. Injections are administered in a peripheral vein as distally as feasible. Venipunctures

should not be repeated at the same site and indwelling catheters are not recommended. Under no circumstances should thiacetarsamide be injected, unless there is 100 percent certainty that the vein has been appropriately cannulated. A butterfly needle facilitates the testing of venipuncture integrity. Sterile saline is first injected to ensure proper needle placement.

DRUG EXTRAVASATION

If any thiacetarsamide is extravasated, the venipuncture area should be treated with topical DMSO twice daily for several days. This treatment appears to be effective in reducing inflammation, swelling, and tissue necrosis. In fact, if only a small volume of drug has been extravasated, tissue necrosis does not occur when topical DMSO is applied. If extravasation is not recognized immediately, the affected area will become swollen, painful, and inflamed within 30 minutes to 2 hours. Topical DMSO should then be applied as soon as the problem is discovered.

MICROFILARICIDE TREATMENT

Although dithiazanine, levamisole, fenthion, and ivermectin are variably effective against microfilariae, only dithiazanine is approved by the Food and Drug Administration (FDA). Microfilaricide treatment is started four to 6 weeks after thiacetarsamide administration. Although microfilarial numbers are quickly reduced, microfilariae are often difficult to eliminate. All microfilaricide drugs are given to effect. Extension of the treatment schedule may therefore be required in some cases.

Dithiazanine

Dithiazanine should be administered at a dosage range of 7 to 11 mg/kg for 7 to 10 days. After 5 to 7 days, microfilarial counts are usually reduced by 90 percent. Low concentrations (less than 10/ml) often persist, even though all adult worms are eliminated. After 7 days, a microfilariae concentration test is performed. If microfilariae are detected and adverse reactions absent, the same dose may be continued or increased to 11 to 15 mg/kg/day for an additional week. If adverse reactions have occurred, an alternate drug is selected.

Adverse reactions caused by dithiazanine include vomiting, diarrhea, anorexia, and occasionally weakness. Reactions are more commonly associated with higher drug dosages. Vomiting may be prevented by dividing the dosage and administering the drug after a small meal or by concurrent administration of an antiemetic drug. Vomitus and feces of dogs receiving dithiazanine are purple colored and will stain fabrics irreversibly.

Levamisole

Levamisole is not FDA approved for use in dogs but is nonetheless a commonly employed microfilaricide. Levamisole eliminates microfilariae in approximately 90 percent of affected dogs when administered at a dosage of 10 to 11 mg/kg/day for 7 to 14 days. Each levamasole dosage should be administered after a small meal. A concentration test is performed after 7 days. If positive, the treatment is continued for 5 to 7 additional days.

The therapeutic index of levamisole is narrow, and variation from the recommended dosage is to be avoided. Vomiting is the most common adverse reaction, but its incidence can be diminished by administering levamisole after a small meal. Levamisole should never be given to a dog that has not recently eaten. Vomiting can also be diminished by prophylactic antiemetic drug treatment. Dividing the daily dosage also diminishes the incidence of adverse reactions, while efficacy seems to be maintained. Lethargy, diarrhea, nervousness, and muscle stiffness or tremors occur less commonly but represent more serious adverse reactions that necessitate the withdrawal of levamisole treatment. If microfilariae persists after 2 weeks of treatment, an alternate drug is chosen.

Levamisole eliminates microfilariae, kills some male adult heartworms, and may sterilize adult female worms. Thus, it is possible that adult heartworms can survive thiacetarsamide and levamisole treatment, even though circulating microfilariae are absent.[73,87] Such an eventuality can be detected if an adult antigen test remains postive several months following completion of levamisole treatment.

Fenthion

Fenthion has been employed as a microfilaricide even though it is not FDA approved for that purpose in dogs. Fenthion (13.8 percent or 20 percent solution) is administered topically, once weekly, at a dosage of 15 mg/kg beginning 4 to 6 weeks after thiacetarsamide treatment. Microfilariae are usually cleared after two to three treatments. If microfilaremia persists, an alternate drug is chosen.

Although fenthion is effective when injected subcutaneously,[92] this method is not recommended. Uncommonly, clinical signs of organophosphate toxicity may occur following fenthion administration.

Ivermectin

Ivermectin is an effective microfilaricide but is not FDA approved for this purpose. A single oral dose (0.05 mg/kg), administered 4 weeks after thiacetarsamide is safe and effective. Ivermectin also blocks reinfection by third-stage larvae, which may have occurred during the previous month. One ml of Ivomec (Merk & Co, Inc, Rahway, NJ) can be diluted in 9 ml propylene glycol, USP, and administered orally at a dosage of 1 ml/20 kg.[93,94] When using this regimen, Ivermectin is administered in the morning and the dog observed throughout the day for evidence of adverse reactions. A microfilaria concentration test is performed 3 to 4 weeks later and, if positive, the protocol is repeated. Microfilaremia persisting after two treatments with ivermectin is indicative of a continued adult heartworm infection. Until further information and testing is available, ivermectin should not be administered to collie and collie-mix dogs.

PREVENTION OF HEARTWORM INFECTION

When microfilaremia has been eliminated by any of the aforementioned drugs, prophylactic therapy should be initiated immediately if reinfection is a potential problem. Several weeks following apparent elimination of microfilariae, after prophylactic therapy has been instituted, another concentration test should be performed in order to detect recrudescence resulting from persisting adult heartworms. This is particularly recommended when dithiazanine or levamisole has been used as a microfilaricide. Concentration tests are then recommended at 6- or 12-month intervals.

Heartworm infection has been effectively prevented by daily treatment with diethylcarbamazine since its introduction during the early 1960s. Ivermectin is also effective in preventing infection and has the advantage of requiring only once a month administration. Thiacetarsemide is effective against some tissue-migrating larvae and may therefore prevent adult heartworm infection when administered at 6-month intervals.

Diethylcarbamazine dosed at 2.5 to 3.0 mg/kg has been tested by many investigators and consistently found to prevent adult heartworms in dogs experimentally infected with larvae. Several products are available and seem to be equally efficacious. Occasional development of one or two adult heartworms has occurred in individual dogs during experimental infections. In addition, some clients apparently forget to give a daily preventative dose and these dogs can develop infections. If a dog develops microfilaremia while on a preventive program, the diethylcarbamazine should be continued while the dog is being treated with the adulticide and subsequent microfilarcide. Diethylcarbamazine probably affects *D. immitis* at the L_3-L_4 molting stage at 9 to 12 days postinfection. Therefore, it should be started prior to the mosquito season.[21]

All dogs in endemic areas should be on a heartworm-preventive program. It is recommended that this be started at the time that puppy immunizations are initiated. In areas that have colder winters and in which *D. immitis* is not endemic, the diethylcarbamazine may be stopped 1 month after the final frost and resumed 1 month prior to the spring mosquito season. A microfilaria concentration test should be performed on puppies at 6 months of age. Prior to the initiation of prophylaxis, dogs must test negative for microfilaremia. During the diethylcarbamazine preventative program, microfilaria concentration tests should be done at least annually and in endemic areas, semiannually.[21]

Diethylcarbamazine has proved a safe drug when given to heartworm negative dogs. Although there have been field reports of induced sterility in male dogs, repeated studies have failed to document decreased reproductive function. In humans and dogs, diethylcarbamazine has been given continuously over several generations without any untoward reproductive effect. Some dogs vomit and appear to be depressed after starting diethylcarbamazine treatment. This subtle reaction, however, seems to be rare.

Microfilaria-positive dogs should not be given diethylcarbamazine, as it may cause adverse reactions of variable severity, including death. Dogs with fewer than 50 microfilariae per milliliter seldom develop reactions.[95] In dogs with a higher concentration of microfilariae, the incidence of adverse reactions ranges from 15 to 86 percent and are usually detected within the first hour after drug administration. During the initial phase of the reaction, dogs become depressed, lethargic, and less responsive to stimuli. Vomiting, defecation, and diarrhea may develop. During the next phase, cardiovascular signs such as bradycardia, decreased heart sounds, and a weak femoral pulse may occur. In the third phase, shock is present, characterized by pale, cool, and tacky mucous membranes, prolonged capillary refill time, decreased arterial pulse, tachycardia, and tachypnea. The dogs salivate, become recumbent, develop hepatomegaly, and die.[96–98] Other typical findings include increased serum liver enzyme concentrations, thrombocytopenia, and leukocytosis. Treatment involves administration of shock dosages of corticosteroids and intravenous fluids.

Ivermectin has proved effective in preventing natural and experimental infection.[99,100] The recommended oral monthly dosage is 6 μg/kg. Its advantages over diethylcarbamazine are that dogs do not need to be free of microfilaria for a preventive program to be started, and even infectious larvae contracted up to 2 months prior to administration should be eliminated. The manufacturer of Heartgard-30 (Merk & Co, Inc, Rahway, NJ), the commercially approved canine prophylactic product, recommends it be given to microfilaria-negative dogs.

SPECIAL PROBLEMS

Diethylcarbamazine and Dogs with Occult Infections

Diethylcarbamazine may be administered to or continued in dogs that have occult heartworm infections. In the absence of circulating microfilariae, adverse reactions will not occur. The use of diethylcarbamazine in these situations will eliminate the possibility of reinfection that exists during and immediately after adulticide treatment.

Diethylcarbamazine in Microfilaremic Dogs

If microfilaremia is discovered in dogs receiving diethylcarbamazine, the drug should be continued during adulticide and microfilaricide treatment. Thus, a possible reinfection during adulticide and microfilaricide treatment is eliminated.

Microfilaria Recurrence Postadulticide and During Microfilaricide Treatment

Following adulticide and microfilaricide treatment, microfilaremia will reoccur if gravid female worms persist. When dithiazanine or levamasole are used as the microfilaricide, a concentration test is recommended at the completion of treatment. Since these drugs usually greatly reduce the microfilaria concentration, a negative test result can occur. If adult gravid female worms persist, microfilarial counts will rapidly increase. This recrudescence will not be detected quickly unless a second microfilariae concentration test is repeated 2 to 6 weeks after microfilaricide treatment.

Young Female Adult Heartworms

Young female *D. immitis* are resistant to thiacetarsamide sodium. These worms may continue to produce microfilariae for weeks or even months after all adult male worms are killed. Immediate retreatment with thiacetarsamide sodium is unlikely to be effective. Retreatment after 6 to 12 months, when the female worms are older, is usually effective.

Prophylaxis in the Face of Microfilaremia

When resistant adult heartworms and microfilariae are present, diethylcarbamazine cannot be administered. As a result, further infection can occur.

This problem can be prevented by the administration of ivermectin at a dosage of 6 mg/kg/month.

REFERENCES

1. Otto GF: Heartworm infection 1986. In Otto GF (ed): Proceedings of the Heartworm Symposium, 1986, American Heartworm Society, Washington DC, 1986
2. Lewis RE, Losonsky JM: Sex and age distribution of dogs with heartworm disease. p. 8. In Otto GF (ed): Proceedings of the Heartworm Symposium, 1977. Veterinary Medicine Publishing Company, Bonner Springs, KS, 1977
3. Calvert CA, Rawlings CA: Diagnosis and management of canine heartworm disease. p. 348. In Kirk RW (ed): Current Veterinary Therapy. Vol. VIII. WB Saunders, Philadelphia, 1983
4. Wallenstein WL, Tibola BJ: Survey of canine filariasis in Maryland area. Incidence of *Dirofilaria immitis* and *Dipetalonema*. J Am Vet Med Assoc 137:712, 1960
5. Orihel TC: Morphology of the larval stages of *Dirofilaria immitis* in the dog. J Parasitol 47:251, 1961
6. Rawlings CA, McCall JW, Lewis RE: The response of the canine's heart and lungs to *Dirofilaria immitis*. J Am Anim Hosp Assoc 14:17, 1978
7. Fortin JF, Slocombe JOD: Survival of *Dirofilaria immitis* in *Aedes triseriatus*. p. 13. In Otto GF (ed): Proceedings of the Heartworm Symposium. Veterinary Medicine Publishing Company, Bonner Springs, KS, 1980
8. Rawlings CA, Keith JC Jr, Schaub RG: Development and resolution of pulmonary disease in heartworm infection: Illustrated review. J Am Anim Hosp Assoc 17:711, 1981
9. Jackson RF, Otto GF, Bauman PM, et al: Distribution of heartworms in the right side of the heart and adjacent vessels of the dog. J Am Vet Med Assoc 149:515, 1966
10. Adcock JL: Pulmonary arterial lesions in canine dirofilariasis. Am J Vet Res 22:655, 1961
11. Schaub RG, Rawlings CA: Pulmonary vascular responses during phases of canine heartworm disease: A scanning electron microscopic study. Am J Vet Res 41:1081, 1980
12. Schaub RG, Rawlings CA, Keith JC Jr: Platelet adhesion and myointimal proliferation in canine pulmonary arteries. Am J Pathol 104:13, 1981
13. Keith JC Jr, Schaub RG, Rawlings CA: Early arterial injury-induced myointimal proliferation in canine pulmonary arteries. Am J Vet Res 44:181, 1983

14. Rawlings CA, Lewis RE, McCall JW: Development and resolution of pulmonary arteriographic lesions in heartworm disease. J Am Anim Hosp Assoc 16:17, 1980
15. Rawlings CA, Losonsky JM, Lewis, McCall JW: Development and resolution of radiographic lesions in canine heartworm disease. J Am Vet Med Assoc 178:1172, 1981
16. Rawlings CA: Acute response of pulmonary blood flow and right ventricular function to *Dirofilaria immitis* adults and microfilaria. Am J Vet Res 41:244, 1980
17. Rawlings CA: Cardiopulmonary function in the dog with *Dirofilaria immitis:* During infection and after treatment. Am J Vet Res 41:319, 1980
18. Rawlings CA, Keith JC Jr, Schaub RG: Effect of acetylsalicylic acid on pulmonary arteriosclerosis induced by a one year *Dirofilaria immitis* infection. Arteriosclerosis 5:355, 1985
19. Calvert CA, Thrall DE: Treatment of canine heartworm disease coexisting with right-side heart failure. Am Vet Med Assoc 180:1201, 1982
20. Rawlings CA, Losonsky JM, Schaub RG, et al: Postadulticide changes in *Dirofilaria immitis* infected beagles. Am J Vet Res 44:8, 1983
21. Rawlings CA: Heartworm Disease in Dogs and Cats. WB Saunders, Philadelphia, 1986
22. Rawlings CA, Keith JC Jr, Losonsky JM, et al: Aspirin and prednisolone modification of post-adulticide pulmonary arterial diseae in heartworm infection: Arteriographic study. Am J Vet Res 44:821, 1983
23. Rawlings CA, Keith JC Jr, Lewis RE, et al: Aspirin and prenisolone modification of radiographic changes caused by adulticide treatment in dogs with heartworm infection. J Am Vet Med Assoc 182:131, 1983
24. Otto GF: The significance of microfilaremia in the diagnosis of heartworm infection. p. 20. In Otto GF (ed): Proceedings of the Heartworm Symposium, 1977. Veterinary Medical Publishing Company, Bonner Springs, KS, 1978
25. Calvert CA, Losonsky JM: Occult heartworm disease associated allergic pneumonitis. J Am Vet Med Assoc 186:1097, 1985
26. Calvert CA, Rawlings CA: Pulmonary manifestations of heartworm disease. Vet Clin North Am 15:991, 1985
27. Confer AW, Qualls CW, MacWilliams RS, et al: Four cases of pulmonary nodular eosinophilic granulomatosis in dogs. Cornell Vet 73:41, 1983
28. Rawlings CA, Prestwood AK, Beck BB: Eosinophilia and basophilia in *Dirofilaria immitis* and *Di-petalonemia reconditum* infections. J Am Anim Hosp Assoc 16:699, 1980
29. Rawlings CA, Prestwood AK, Beck BB: Eosinophilia and basophilia in *Dirofilaria immitis* and *Dipetalonema reconditum* infections. J Am Anim Hosp Assoc 16:699, 1980
30. Lewis RE, Losonsky JM: The frequency of roentgen signs in heartworm disease. p. 73. In Otto GF (ed): Proceedings of the Heartworm Symposium, 1977. Veterinary Medical Publishing Company, Bonner Springs, KS, 1978
31. Calvert CA, Losonsky JM, Brown J, et al: Comparison of radiographic and electrocardiographic abnormalities in canine heartworm disease. Vet Radiol 27:2, 1986
32. Knight DH: Heartworm disease. p. 1097. In Ettinger SJ (ed): Textbook of Veterinary Internal Medicine. 2nd Ed. WB Saunders, Philadelphia, 1983
33. Knight DH, Allen HL, Dietsch GE: Clinical pathology conference. J Am Vet Med Assoc 165:921, 1974
34. Morgan HC: Electrocardiogram of the patient with heartworm disease. J Am Vet Med Assoc 154:375, 1969
35. Beasley JN, Jacques WE: A physiologic and anatomical study of *Dirofilaria immitis* infection in the dog. Fed Proc 22:667, 1963
36. Blackberg SN, Ashman R: Electrocardiographic studies of dogs infected with *Dirofilaria immitis*. J Am Vet Med Assoc 77:204, 1930
37. Hill JD: Electrocardiographic diagnosis of right ventricular enlargement in dogs. J Electrocardiol 4:347, 1971
38. Knight DH: Heartworm heart disease. Adv Vet Sci Comp Med 21:107, 1977
39. Rawlings CA: Acute response to pulmonary blood flow and right ventricular function to *Dirofilaria immitis* adults and microfilaria. Am J Vet Res 41:244, 1980
40. Rawlings CA: Cardiopulmonary function in the dog with *Dirofilaria immitis* during infection and after treatment. Am J Vet Res 41:319, 1980
41. Rawlings CA, McCall JW, Lewis RE: The response of the canine's heart and lungs to *Dirofilaria immitis*. J Am Anim Hosp Assoc 14:17, 1978
42. Wallace CR, Hamilton WF: Study of spontaneous congestive heart failure in the dog. Circ Res 11:301, 1962
43. Ogburn PN, Jackson RF, Seymour WG, et al: Electrocardiographic and phonocardiographic alterations in canine heartworm disease. p. 67. In Otto GF (ed): Proceedings of the Heartworm Symposium, 1977. Veterinary Medicine Publishing Company, Bonner Springs, KS, 1978

44. Carrington CB, Addington WW, Goff AM, et al: Chronic eosinophilic pneumonia. N Engl J Med 25:466, 1964

45. Lindesmith L: Prolonged pulmonary infiltration with eosinophilia NC Med J 25:566, 1964

46. Liebow AA, Carrington CB: The eosinophilic pneumonias. Medicine (Baltimore) 48:251, 1969

47. Morrissey WL, Gaensler EA, Carrington CB, et al: Chronic eosinophilic pneumonia. Respiration 32:453, 1975

48. Pearson DJ, Rosenow EC: Chronic eosinophilic pneumonia. Mayo Clin Proc 53:73, 1978

49. Head JR, Suter PF, Ettinger SJ: Lower respiratory tract diseases. p. 661. In Ettinger SJ (ed): Textbook of Veterinary Internal Medicine. 1st Ed. WB Saunders, Philadelphia, 1975

50. Wong MM: Studies on microfilaremia in dogs. II. Levels of microfilaremia in relation to immunologic responses of the host. Am J Trop Med Hyg 13:66, 1964

51. Wong MM: Experimental occult dirofilariasis in dogs with special reference to immunological responses and its relationship to "eosinophilic lung" in man. SE Asian J Trop Med Public Health 5:480, 1974

52. Wong MM, Suter PF, Rhode EA, et al: Dirofilariasis without circulating microfilariae: A problem in diagnosis. J Am Vet Med Assoc 163:133, 1973

53. Pacheco G: Progressive changes in certain serological responses to *Dirofilaria immitis* infection in the dog. J Parasitol 52:311, 1966

54. Weiner DJ, Bradley RE: Serologic changes in primary and secondary infections of beagle dogs with *Dirofilaria immitis*. p. 77. In Bradley RE, Pacheco G (eds): Canine Heartworm Disease: The Current Knowledge. University of Florida Press, Gainesville, FL, 1972

55. Carroll JM, Simon J: Eosinophilic granuloma in a dog. J Am Vet Med Assoc 150:526, 1967

56. Jackson RF: The vena cavae syndrome. p. 48. In Otto GF (ed): Proceedings of the Heartworm Symposium, 1974. Veterinary Medicine Publishing Company, Bonner Springs, KS, 1974

57. Jackson RF: The vena cavae or liver failure syndrome of heartworm disease. J Am Vet Med Assoc 194:384, 1969

58. Jackson RF, Otto GF, Bauman PM, et al: Distribution of heartworms in the right side of the heart and adjacent vessels. J Am Vet Med Assoc 149:515, 1966

59. Atwell RB, Farmer TS: Clinical pathology of the caval syndrome in canine dirofilariasis in northern Australia. J Small Anim Pract 23:675, 1982

60. Atwell RB: Possible mechanisms of the caval syndrome in dogs with *Dirofilaria immitis*. Aust Vet J 59:161, 1982

61. Buoro IBJ, Atwell RB: Intravascular hemolytic syndrome in dogs. Vet Rec 112:573, 1983

62. Knight DH: Evolution of pulmonary arterial disease in canine dirofilariasis: Evaluation by blood pressure measurements and angiography. p. 55. Proceedings of the Heartworm Symposium, 1980. Veterinary Medicine Publishing Company, Edwardsville, KS, 1980

63. Rawlings CA, Keith JC, Schaub RG: Development and resolution of pulmonary disease in heartworm infection. J Am Anim Hosp Assoc 17:711, 1981

64. Thrall DE, Calvert CA: Radiographic evaluation of canine heartworm disease coexisting with right heart failure. Vet Radiol 24:124, 1983

65. Schaub RG, Rawlings CA: Pulmonary vascular response during phases of canine heartworm disease. Am J Vet Res 41:1081, 1980

66. Schaub RG, Rawlings CA, Keith JC: Platelet adhesion and myointimal proliferation in canine pulmonary arteries. Am J Pathol 104:13, 1981

67. Schaub RG, Keith JC, Rawlings CA: Effect of long term aspirin treatment on platelet adhesion to chronically damaged canine pulmonary arteries. Thromb Haemost 46:680, 1981

68. Schaub RG, Keith JC, Rawlings CA: The effect of acetylsalicylic acid on vascular damage and myointimal proliferation in canine pulmonary arteries subjected to chronic injury by *Dirofilaria immitis* infection. Am J Vet Res 44:449, 1983

69. Rawlings CA, Schaub RG, Keith JC: Aspirin reduces pulmonary arterial arteriosclerosis due to chronic vascular injury. In the Sixty-eighth Annual Meeting of the Federation Proceedings, St. Louis, MO, 1984 (abst 4040)

70. Rawlings CA, Keith JC, Losonsky JM, et al: An aspirin prednisolone combination to modify postadulticide lung disease in heartworm infected dogs. Am J Vet Res 45:2371, 1984

71. Hoskins JD, Hagstad HV, Hribernik TN: Effects of thiacetarsamide sodium in Louisiana dogs with naturally-occurring canine heartworm disease. p. 134. In Otto GF (ed): Proceedings of the Heartworm Symposium, 1983. Veterinary Medicine Publishing Company, Edwardsville, KS, 1983

72. Seward RL, Brokken ES, Plue RE: Ivemectin vs. Heartworm—A status update. p. 1. In Otto GF (ed). Proceedings of the Heartworm Symposium, 1986. American Heartworm Society, Washington, DC, 1986

73. Rawlings CA, Losonsky JM, Schaub RG, et al: Pos-

tadulticide changes in *Dirofilaria immitis* infected beagles. Am J Vet Res 44:8, 1983

74. Rawlings CA, Keith JC, McCall JW, et al: Thiacetarsamide efficacy. p. 141. In Otto GF (ed): Proceedings of the Heartworm Symposium, 1983. Veterinary Medicine Publishing Company, Edwardsville, KS, 1983

75. Ishahara K, Kitagawa H, Ojuma J, et al: Clinicopathological studies in canine dirofilarial hemoglobinuria. Jpn J Vet Sci 40:525, 1978

76. Clemmons RM, Yamaguchi RA, Fleming TL, et al: The interaction between heartworms and platelets. p. 15. In Otto GF (ed): Proceedings of the Heartworm Symposium, 1983. Veterinary Medicine Publishing Company, Edwardsville, KS, 1983

77. Greene CE: Management of DIC and thrombosis. p. 401. In Kirk RW (ed): Current Veterinary Therapy. Vol. VIII. WB Saunders, Philadelphia, 1983

78. Garlick NL: The management of canine dirofilariasis. Canine Pract 2:22, 1975

79. Garlick NL: Canine dirofilariasis: Levamisole treatment. Canine Pract 3:64, 1976

80. Simpson CF, Jackson RF: Fate of microfilariae of *Dirofilaria immitis* following use of levamasole as a microfilaricide. Z Parasitenkd 68:93, 1982

81. Klei TR, Crowell WA, Thompson PE: Ultrastructural glomerular changes associated with filariasis. Am J Trop Med Hyg 23:608, 1974

82. Casey HW, Splitter GA: Membranous glomerulonephritis in dogs infected with *Dirofilaria immitis*. Vet Pathol 12:111, 1975

83. Wallace CR, Screws R: Preliminary study of microfilaria embolization after filaricidal therapy. p. 42. In Bradley RE, Pacheco G (eds): Canine Heartworm Disease: The Current Knowledge. University of Florida Press, Gainesville, FL, 1972

84. Courtney CH, Boring JG: A comparison of the reaction of thiacetarsamide before and after the use of a microfilaricide. p. 89. In Otto GF (ed): Proceedings of the Heartworm Symposium, 1977. Veterinary Medicine Publishing Company, Bonner Springs, KS, 1978

85. Carr SH, Besmer RR: A clinical study, heartworm treatment with levamisole. Canine Pract 2:13, 1975

86. Bradley RE, Alfort BT: Efficacy of levamisole resinate against *Dirofilaria immitis* in dogs. Mod Vet Pract 58:518, 1977

87. Chaikin RJ: Levamisole as a simultaneous microfilaricide/adulticide in canine heartworm disease. Canine Pract 6:32, 1979

88. Atwell RB, Carlisle C, Robinson S: The effectiveness of levamisole hydrochloride in the treatment of adult *Dirofilaria immitis*. Aust Vet J 55:531, 1972

89. Jackson RF: The activity of levamisole against the various stages of *Dirofilaria immitis* in the dog. p. 111. In Otto GF (ed): Proceedings of the Heartworm Symposium, 1977. Veterinary Medicine Publishing Company, Bonner Springs, KS, 1978

90. Jackson RF, Otto GF: Thiacetarsamide reevaluation. p. 137. In Otto GF (ed): Proceedings of the Heartworm Symposium, 1980. Veterinary Medicine Publishing Company, Bonner Springs, KS, 1981

91. McCall JW, Lewis RE, Rawlings CA, et al: Reevaluation of thiacetarsamide as an adulticidal agent against *Dirofilaria immitis* in dogs. p. 141. In Otto GF (ed): Proceedings of the Heartworm Symposium, 1980. Veterinary Medicine Publishing Company, Bonner Springs, KS, 1981

92. Rawlings CA, Dawe DL, McCall JW, et al: Four types of occult *Dirofilaria immitis* infection in dogs. J Am Vet Med Assoc 180:1323, 1982

93. Lambert G, Mierritt FR, Fuller DA, et al: Evaluation of a new microfilaricide in dogs. Vet Med Small Anim Clinic 65:676, 1970

94. Jackson RF: Ivermectin again. Am Heartworm Soc Bull 10:9, 1984

95. Rawlings CA, Greene CE, Dawe DL, et al: Diethylcarbamazine adverse reaction and relationship to microfilaremia. p. 143. In Otto GF (ed): Proceedings of the American Heartworm Symposium, 1986. American Heartworm Society, Washington, DC, 1986

96. Palumbo NE, Perri SF, Desowitz RS, et al: Preliminary observations on adverse reactions to diethylcarbamazine (DEC) in dogs infected with *Dirofilaria immitis*. p. 97. In Otto GF (ed): Proceedings of the Heartworm Symposium, 1977. Veterinary Medicine Publishing Company, Edwardsville, KS, 1978

97. Powers DG, Parbuoni EL, Furrow RD: *Dirofilaria immitis* I. Adverse reactions associated with diethylcarbamazine therapy in microfilaremic dogs. p. 108. In Otto GF (ed): Proceedings of the Heartworm Symposium, 1980. Veterinary Medicine Publishing Company, 1980

98. Atwell RB, Boreham PFL: Studies on the adverse reactions following diethylcarbamazine to microfilaria-positive (*D. immitis*) dogs. p. 105. Proceedings of the Heartworm Symposium, 1983. Veterinary Medicine Publishing Company, Edwardsville, KS, 1983

99. Campbell WC, Blair LS, Seward RL: Ivermectin vs. heartworm: The present status. p. 146. In Otto GF (ed): Proceedings of the Heartworm Symposium, 1983. Veterinary Medicine Publishing Company, Edwardsville, KS, 1983

100. McCall JW, Cowgill LM, Plue RE, Evans T, et al: Prevention of natural acquisition of heartworm infection in dogs by monthly treatment with ivermectin. p. 150. In Otto GF (ed): Proceedings of the Heartworm Symposium, 1983. Veterinary Medicine Publishing Company, Edwardsville, KS, 1983

26

Feline Heartworm Disease

Clay A. Calvert

The importance of *Dirofilaria immitis* as a feline pathogen is uncertain but probably underestimated. Until recently, heartworm infection in cats was difficult to diagnose, with most reports based on necropsy findings.[1-9] Increased awareness of the potential for heartworm infection in cats coupled with newer diagnostic techniques has increased the frequency of antemortem diagnoses.[10-14] Whether the incidence of *D. immitis* infection in cats is greater than in the past remains uncertain. However, with the advent of readily available practical and accurate serologic tests, the incidence of feline heartworm disease will be easier to determine.

EPIZOOTIOLOGY

Feline heartworm disease has been reported worldwide, and its prevalence is generally believed to parallel that of the dog, but at a lower rate for comparable geographic regions.[11] The prevalence of feline heartworm disease, based on necropsy surveys, has varied from 0 to 8.5 percent of examined cats (mean, 1.9 percent) as compared with a 5.4 to 59.1 percent prevalence among comparable dog populations (mean, 34.6 percent).[1-16]

The difficulty in determining the incidence of feline heartworm disease is related to host-parasite interactions. In comparison with *D. immitis* infection of the dog, the cat is affected by a lower adult worm burden. In natural infections, fewer numbers of infective larvae mature to adult worms. In experimental infections, the maturation period is longer, the prepatent period is prolonged, microfilaremia is more likely to be absent or of short duration, and the adult worm life-span is shorter.[1,17-23] The lack of circulating microfilariae in most infections and aberrant worm migration are the two factors that contribute most to the difficulty in making an antemortem diagnosis.

Cats may become infected with *D. immitis* at almost any age, the most common ages at the time of diagnosis being 3 to 6 years.[11,23] There have been no recognized breed predilections and no specific predisposing factors. Although cats dwelling mostly indoors have been infected, it is apparent that outdoors habitation in endemic areas increases the risk of exposure. Most infected cats are male, which may be a reflection of increased outside habitation.

Cats infected with *D. immitis* may harbor none to nine adult worms in their hearts. Two to four adult worms are typically found in the right ventricle and

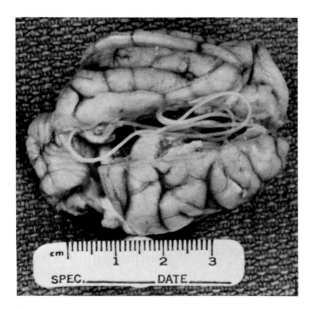

Fig. 26-1 Partially dissected brain of a cat that exhibited seizures, dementia, eosinophilia, and hyperglobulinemia. Two adult heartworms were present in the lateral ventricle inside a cerebral hemisphere.

pulmonary arteries of infected cats.[1–9] The incidence of aberrant larval migration in cats is unknown (although it is greater than in the dog), and the lateral ventricles of the brain are the most common extra-cardiopulmonary site[4,7,13,14,17,20,24–26] (Fig. 26-1). Following experimental larval inoculation, the percentage of cats that develop adult worms varies from less than 10 percent to more than 75 percent. Fewer than 15 percent of infective larvae survive,[1–9] whereas 36 to 65 percent of the infective larvae inoculated into dogs reach adulthood[18,27] (Rawlings CA: Personal communication, 1985). Likewise, the survival of adult *D. immitis* after transplantation into cats is more variable than in the dog.[28,29]

PATHOPHYSIOLOGY

The cardiopulmonary disease resulting from adult *D. immitis* infection in cats is generally comparable to that of the dog.[30–34] As in the dog, pulmonary arterial disease is initiated by the presence of adult worms. The reader is referred to the section on canine heartworm disease for details (Ch. 25). The smaller pulmonary arteries develop more severe muscular hypertrophy than that seen in dogs, and

these smaller arteries tend to lack villous proliferations.[22] As in the dog, vascular damage leads to thromboembolic disease, leakage of plasma into the perivascular tissues, partial or complete lobar lung consolidation, and on occasion predominantly allergic lung disease. The branches of the lobar pulmonary arteries may be completely occluded. Whereas myointimal proliferation and muscle hypertrophy are the major pathologic changes in the dog contributing to pulmonary arterial occlusion, adult heartworms in the cat can obstruct the branches of the pulmonary arteries.

The beginning of pulmonary arterial damage can be detected soon after adult worm transplantation.[23] Pulmonary artery enlargement can be detected within 1 week of adult heartworm transplantation.[23] Adventitial and perivascular infiltration of inflammatory cells, predominantly eosinophils and neutrophils, follows endothelial damage and platelet adhesion to the subendothelium.[22,30] As in the dog, the caudal lung lobes are most severely affected.

Within 3 to 5 months of innoculation with infective larvae and within 2 weeks from transplantation of adult heartworms, radiographic changes typical of heartworm disease are present. These changes include pulmonary artery enlargement, right ventricular enlargement, and both diffuse and focal parenchymal lung disease.[15,35] In the cat, the main pulmonary artery segment is not visible on dorsoventral or ventrodorsal radiographic projections. The caudal lobar pulmonary arteries enlarge to the greatest extent and earliest in the course of the disease (best delineated in the dorsoventral radiographic view). The lobar arteries may become tortuous, and their branches are frequently thrombosed, producing a pruning effect as visualized by plain or contrast radiography (Figs. 26-2 and 26-3).

Chronic effects of feline heartworm infection have not been well documented. However, one study demonstrated live adult worms 30 months after experimental inoculation of infective third-stage larvae.[36] This finding demonstrates that chronic heartworm disease can develop in the cat.

CLINICAL MANIFESTATIONS

History

The historical complaints associated with feline heartworm disease are either nonspecific or referable to either the cardiopulmonary or nervous system.

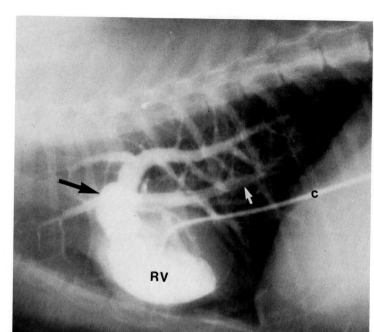

A

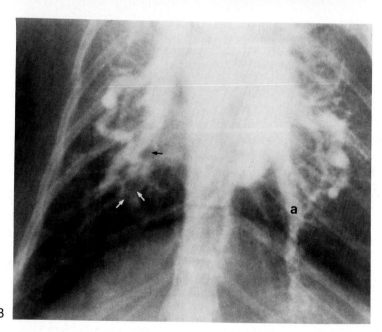

B

Fig. 26-2 Selective right ventriculogram of a cat infected with heartworms. (**A**) Enlargement of the main pulmonary artery segment (black arrow) and caudal lobar artery (white arrow) is evident. Right ventricular enlargement is present. Linear filling defects produced by adult worms occur within this caudal lobar artery. RV, right ventricle; C, catheter. (**B**) Ventrodorsal thoracic radiograph displaying enlargement and tortuosity of lobar pulmonary arteries. Flow of contrast agent is obstructed (arrows) in the right caudal lobar artery (compare with the left caudal lobar artery). a, left caudal lobar artery.

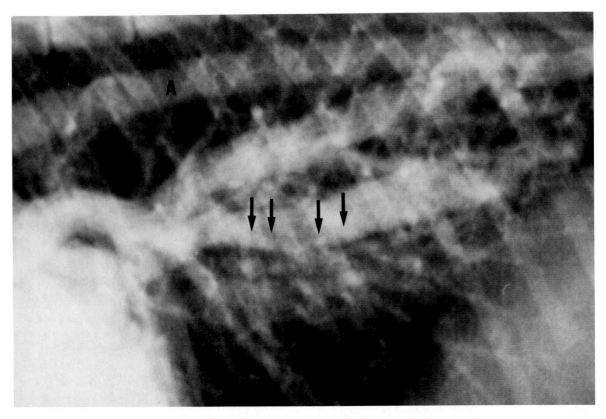

Fig. 26-3 Nonselective angiocardiogram (right-lateral view) of a cat with clinical heartworm infection. Caudal lobar pulmonary artery tortuosity and pruning are evident. Linear filling defects are visualized in the pulmonary arteries (arrows) caused by adult heartworms. A, aorta. (Courtesy of Dr. Philip Fox.)

In some instances, the primary presenting complaints are lethargy, anorexia, and vomiting. Vomiting is often the primary presenting complaint, especially with cardiopulmonary-associated disease. In other instances, a history referable to specific systems can be subsequently elicited.

A history consistent with an acute or subacute onset of neurologic disease is common and may be associated with lethargy and anorexia. Seizures, dementia, ataxia, circling, mydriasis, apparent blindness, and salivation are variably reported.

The most common specific historical complaints are associated with cardiopulmonary disease. Coughing is the most frequent sign described, tends to be paroxysmal, and may coexist with dyspnea. Its chronicity depends on client awareness and the stage of disease when the patient is examined. Sedentary behavior may be related to respiratory signs, especially when the disease is advanced.

Syncope and signs consistent with right-sided congestive heart failure occur less commonly than in the dog and are associated with severe pulmonary artery disease and presumed pulmonary hypertension. Syncope is usually manifested during physical exertion.

Physical Examination

Physical examination abnormalities in heartworm-infected cats may be absent or nonspecific or may indicate disease of either the central nervous or cardiopulmonary system. Some heartworm-infected cats do not manifest clinical signs, and the infection may be self-limiting. In others, only a nonspecific generalized depression is detected. Occasionally, evidence of neurologic disease such as dementia, ataxia, abnormal pupillary light responses,

Table 26-1 Classification of Clinical Signs Associated with Feline Heartworm Disease

Acute Clinical Signs	Chronic Clinical Signs
Sudden death[a]	PIE syndrome[b]
Pulmonary embolism	Coughing
Dyspnea, cough	Dyspnea
Hemoptysis	Cardiopulmonary
Shock	Lethargy
Neurologic	Exercise intolerance
Seizures	Right CHF[c]
Coma	Anorexia
Blindness	Gastrointestinal
Dementia	Vomiting
Ataxia	Anorexia
Circling	
Head tilt	
Salivation	

[a] Probably from severe pulmonary thromboembolism or heartworm occlusion of the main pulmonary artery.
[b] Pulmonary infiltrates of eosinophilia.
[c] Right-sided congestive heart failure.

abnormal oculocephalic reflexes, or blindness may be apparent.

Cardiopulmonary disease comprises the most common specific physical examination abnormality. Tachycardia, tachypnea, dyspnea, respiratory crackles, gallop heart rhythm, systolic heart murmur, muffled heart-lung sounds, and ascites may be variably detected. As a general rule, signs referable to both the nervous and cardiopulmonary systems seldom coexist.

Historical and physical findings may be classified basically into acute and chronic categories (Table 26-1). Although acute cardiopulmonary distress from pulmonary arterial obstruction may be the initial clinical abnormality, chronic signs such as coughing, paroxysmal dyspnea, vomiting, and anorexia are more commonly observed.

DIAGNOSTIC TECHNIQUES

Special Considerations

The diagnosis of heartworm infection in cats is complicated by variable and often nonspecific historical complaints and clinical signs, inconsistent clinical pathology findings, and a usual lack of circulating microfilariae. In endemic regions, the index of suspicion of heartworm disease is increased in cats exhibiting coughing. Radiographic evidence of pulmonary infiltrates consistent with vascular or intersitial lung disease is often present. Eosinophilia is usually absent. Vomiting, due to unexplained mechanisms, is a surprisingly common manifestation of heartworm infection in cats. Acute onset of neurologic signs must include aberrant heartworm larval migration as a differential diagnosis in endemic regions. Other diseases that cause clinical signs consistent with heartworm infection are listed in Table 26-2. The most common cardiopulmonary diseases that may produce clinical signs similar to those of heartworm disease are *Aelurostrongylus abs-*

Table 26-2 Diseases That May Produce Clinical Signs Similar to Those of Heartworm Disease

Major Sign	Diseases
Cough	PIE syndromes[a]
	Feline asthma
	Lungworms (*Aelurostronglyus abstrusus*)
	Lung flukes (*Paragonimus kellicotti*)
	Pneumonia (e.g., bacterial; *Toxoplasma*)
	Mediastinal lymphosarcoma
Dyspnea	All of the above
	Cardiomyopathy
	Feline infectious peritonitis
	Pyothorax
	Chylothorax
	Diaphragmatic hernia
Pleural effusion (muffled heart-lung sounds)	Feline infectious peritonitis
	Pyothorax
	Mediastinal lymphosarcoma
	Chylothorax
	Diaphragmatic hernia
	Cardiomyopathy
Neurologic disease	Feline infectious peritonitis
	Feline leukemia virus-related diseases
	Brain tumor (e.g., meningioma)
	Thiamine deficiency
	Idiopathic seizure disorders

[a] Pulmonary infiltrate with eosinophilia.

trusus (lungworm) infection, feline asthma, and cardiomyopathies.

All cats exhibiting clinical signs consistent with heartworm disease should be thoroughly evaluated. A minimum data base is recommended to include a complete blood count, serum biochemical profile, urinalysis, microfilaria concentration test, immunodiagnostic tests, thoracic radiographs, and an electrocardiogram (ECG).

Thoracic Radiography

Radiographic abnormalities in feline heartworm disease are often less obvious than in dogs infected with heartworms. Enlargement of the main pulmonary artery segment is not well visualized in the cat.[15,35] Both lateral and ventrodorsal projections must be closely examined. Caudal lobar pulmonary artery enlargement is better visualized by the dorsoventral projection[15,35,37] (Fig. 26-4). However, caudal lobar arteries of the normal cat are often prominent, and misinterpretation of these arteries for pathologic changes is possible.

Right ventricular enlargement is an inconsistent finding. When ECG evidence of right ventricular enlargement and pleural effusion occurs, radiographic evidence of right ventricular enlargement is usually present. Thoracocentesis is often necessary before the cardiac silhouette can be visualized.

Radiographic evidence of parenchymal lung disease may be associated with allergic pneumonitis due to heartworm infection (Fig. 26-5) or thromboembolic disease (Fig. 26-6). These cats usually cough and exhibit acute respiratory distress. Thromboembolism most often affects the caudal lobar arteries. It may be a consequence of natural heartworm infection or may result from adulticide therapy. Perivascular and parenchymal radiographic changes are usually focal, but diffuse patterns may occur with advanced disease or heartworm death following thiacetarsamide administration.

Clinical Pathology

Hematologic abnormalities are not consistently found in heartworm-infected cats. A normocytic, normochromic, nonregenerative anemia consistent with chronic disease eventually occurs. Approximately 25 to 35 percent of infected cats are anemic at the time of diagnosis. Eosinophilia and basophilia are inconsistent findings. In experimental infections, eosinophilia is present from 3 to 7 months after innoculation with infective larvae in association with adult worms in the heart.[15,21,22] Within a few months of the arrival of adult worms in the heart and pulmonary arteries, eosinophil counts decrease, and only approximately one-third of infected cats have eosinophilia at the time of diagnosis.[11,38] All four experimentally infected cats in one long-term study had approximately 4,000 eosinophils/μl when checked 30 months postinfection.[36] Basophilia, although suggestive of heartworm disease, is less common than eosinophilia. A neutrophilic leukocytosis tends to occur with advanced disease states. Thromboembolic lung disease is associated with marked leukocytosis, usually with a left shift and monocytosis. Thrombocytopenia may also be associated with severe thromboembolic complications.

Serum biochemical abnormalities are usually associated only with advanced cardiopulmonary disease. Prerenal azotemia commonly occurs with right-sided congestive heart failure. Increased serum alkaline phosphatase may accompany passive hepatic congestion from heart failure. Occasionally, severe right-sided congestive heart failure may result in dilutional hyponatremia and mild hyperkalemia. The latter results from decreased glomerular filtration and is associated with mild to moderate azotemia.

Hyperglobulinemia, although inconsistently present, is the most common serum chemistry abnormality. If recorded in a cat with clinical or radiographic cardiopulmonary signs in endemic areas, the index of suspicion of heartworm disease should increase. Hyperglobulinemia is presumed to be related to chronic antigenic stimulation. Lungworm infection, feline asthma, and lung fluke (*Paragonimus kellicotti*) infection are not associated with hyperglobulinemia.

Mild proteinuria detected by urinalysis may result from heartworm disease. The incidence of heartworm-induced glomerulopathy, including amyloidosis, is unknown, but clinical experience apparently suggests that it is not high.

Transtracheal lavage may yield an eosinophilic exudate suggesting allergic or parasitic respiratory disease. Evidence of bacterial infection is usually ab-

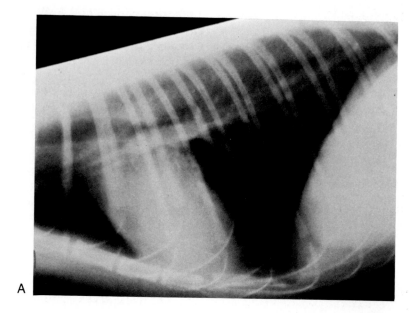

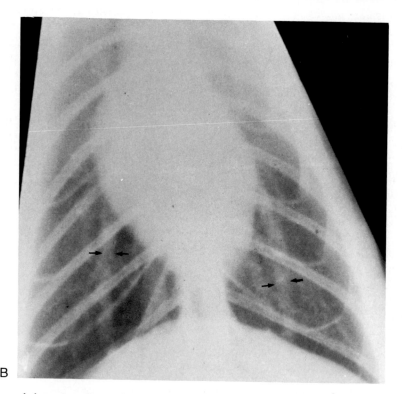

Fig. 26-4 (**A**) Lateral thoracic radiograph of a heartworm-infected cat exhibiting coughing, eosinophilia, and hyperglobulinemia. Pulmonary arteries appear normal. (**B**) Ventrodorsal thoracic radiograph of the same cat. Caudal lobar arteries are enlarged (arrows). An indirect fluorescent antibody test for microfilarial cuticular antigen and an adult antigen test were positive.

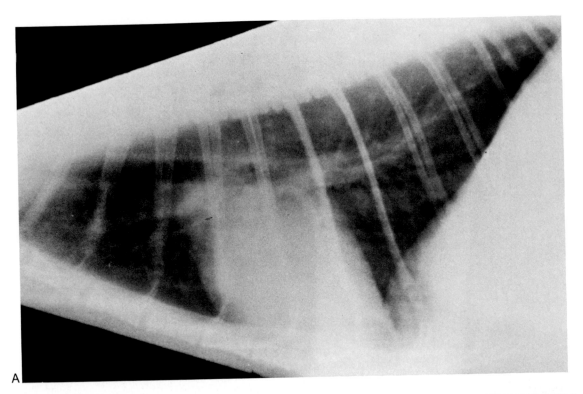

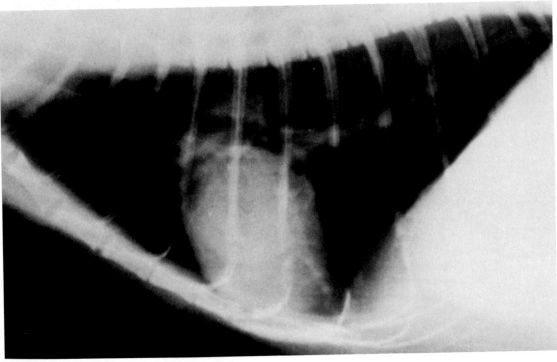

Fig. 26-5 (**A**) Lateral thoracic radiograph showing moderate right-sided cardiomegaly, mild tortuosity of the pulmonary arteries, and a generalized nonspecific interstitial pattern infiltrate throughout the lung. Dyspnea, coughing, eosinophilia, and hyperglobulinemia were present. These findings are consistent with dirofilariasis and allergic pneumonitis. The indirect fluorescent antibody test for microfilarial cuticular antigen was positive. (**B**) Lateral thoracic radiograph of the same cat taken after 3 days of prednisolone therapy (5 mg bid). The cardiac size is slightly reduced, and there is a dramatic clearing of the previously noted pulmonary infiltrate.

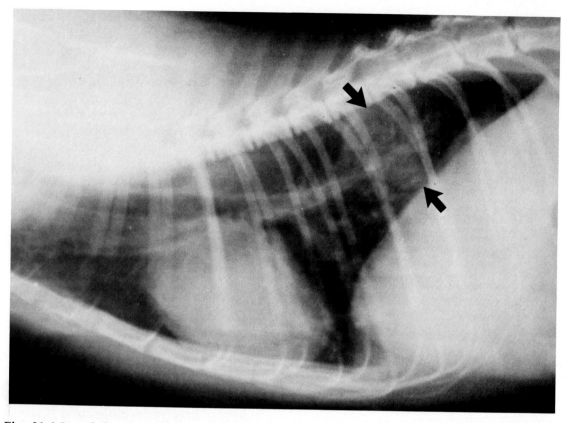

Fig. 26-6 Lateral thoracic radiograph showing right-sided cardiomegaly as evidenced by increased contact between the heart and the sternum as well as an increased cranial-to-caudal cardiac dimension. There is a generalized nonspecific interstitial pattern infiltrate throughout the entire lung. In the caudal lung lobe region, there is a patch of dense alveolar-pattern infiltrate (black arrows). A smaller patch is present just ventral to the caudal vena cava. The ventrodorsal radiograph (not pictured) showed caudal lung lobe infiltrates. These findings were consistent with a diagnosis of dirofilariasis and pulmonary infarcts.

sent. The presence of eosinophilic pneumonitis observed on cytologic evaluation of tracheal aspirates correlated with the anticipated patency period (average, 242 days after experimental infection).[21] However, another study demonstrated that eosinophilic pneumonitis was noted from tracheal aspirate cytology before patency was possible but at the expected time of larval arrival in the pulmonary arteries.[36] This suggests that tracheal aspirates may be a sensitive early indicator of heartworm-related pulmonary disease. Feline asthma, lungworm, and lung fluke infection may also be associated with similar eosinophilic infiltrates.

Pleural effusion may result from right-sided congestive heart failure caused by heartworm dis-

ease. It is also a common manifestation of various diseases, including feline infectious peritonitis, mediastinal lymphosarcoma, pyothorax, true chylothorax, diaphragmatic hernia, and cardiomyopathy. An effusion characterized as a high-protein modified transudate is produced by diaphragmatic hernias, cardiomyopathy, and heartworm disease. Cytologic evaluation of effusions should help in differentiating heartworm-associated effusion from that caused by other disorders.

In addition, congestive heart failure due to heartworm disease is usually associated with both pleural effusion and ascites, while heart failure due to cardiomyopathies seldom results in measurable ascites.

Microfilaria Concentration Tests

Most cats with heartworm disease are not microfilaremic. Only 11 of 25 cats (44 percent) inoculated with third stage (infective) larvae developed microfilaremia,[21,22] and this incidence was greater than that associated with natural infections.[1-14] The prepatent period in experimentally infected cats in which microfilariae were detected was approximately 8 months.[21] This exceeds that of the dog (5 to 6.5 months). Furthermore, microfilariae counts tend to be low. In one study, 6 of 8 cats had less than 2 microfilariae/ml of venous blood and the duration of microfilaremia was brief.[21] Only 1 percent of susceptible mosquitoes feeding on cats with this concentration of microfilaremia developed infective larvae.[15,21] This fact alone probably explains the lower prevalence of heartworm infection in cats.

Increasing the frequency of blood sampling and using large volumes of blood for diagnostic testing may increase the sensitivity of concentration tests (e.g., modified Knott technique). However, the accuracy is always low. Furthermore, considering that few adult worms are usually present, unisex infections are much more likely to occur in the cat than in the dog. Although a concentration test should be a component of the minimum data base for cats with suspected infections, repeated sampling is neither necessary nor recommended.

Immunodiagnostic Tests

Serologic tests have greatly facilitated the diagnosis of feline heartworm disease. Currently, two commercial tests (Filarocheck, Mallinckrodt Inc., Bohemia, NY; Dirocheck, Synbiotics, San Diego, CA) identify adult *D. immitis* antigens in the serum of infected cats using enzyme-linked immunosorbent assay (ELISA). They are sensitive and specific and modifications are not required for use with feline serum. Adult *D. immitis* antigens may be detected 2 weeks after transplantation of adult worms. By 4 weeks after transplantation, 10 of 10 cats (100 percent) tested positive using ELISA methodology. Uninfected cats did not test positive (McCall J: Personal communication, 1985).

The indirect fluorescent antibody (IFA) test for the detection of antibodies to microfilarial cuticular antigen is clinically useful. Antibodies may be detected 7 months after innoculation of larvae in cats that developed gravid female worms.[22] False-positive results do not occur. However, if unisex infections are present, the IFA tests would be negative, since it depends on the production of microfilariae with a subsequent antibody response. Because of the clinical possibility of unisex infections, the requirement for antifeline antiserum, and the sparcity of laboratories performing this test, it has not been widely used.

Serologic tests, such as the ELISA and IFA test, that attempt to identify antibodies directed against adult *D. immitis* antigens are of limited value. Such tests are associated with an unacceptably high rate of false-positive test results. False-negative results are uncommon and are therefore useful to help exclude the possibility of heartworm infection. Immunodiagnostic tests are most relevant when results are combined with the history, physical examination, and other diagnostic tests. A high titer in the absence of supporting clinical or diagnostic findings should prompt reconsideration of the diagnosis.

Electrocardiography

The incidence of abnormal electrocardiographic findings in heartworm-infected cats is unknown. Many infected cats have normal electrocardiograms. Severe pulmonary hypertension increases right ventricular afterload which results in right ventricular hypertrophy (RVH), which may be detected by the ECG. Most cats that exhibit clinical signs of right sided congestive heart failure have ECG abnormalities consistent with RVH. The ECG criteria of RVH in the cat, although not as well documented, are similar to those in the dog.[11,39,40] The frontal plane mean electrical axis in the cat is greater than in the dog,[39] particularly when the ECG is recorded with the cat in right lateral recumbancy. A frontal plane axis exceeding +120 degrees is frequently the result of a prominent Q wave in lead I and does not necessarily indicate RVH. An S wave in lead I, a deep S wave in leads II, III, aVF, V_2, or V_4, and a frontal plane mean electrical axis exceeding +150 degrees are consistent with RVH (see Ch. 4). The diagnostic accuracy of ECG in cases of RVH is probably increased by requiring that three or more ECG criteria be present.[40]

Although the ECGs of many cats with heartworm disease do not reflect RVH, when RVH is detected, heartworm disease should be suspected. This is true because other diseases producing RVH are rare in the cat. The most common heart diseases of the adult cat—cardiomyopathies—rarely produce RVH. Right bundle branch block may occur in association with cardiomyopathies and may be confused with RVH. An ECG pattern consistent with left anterior fascicular block (hemiblock) resembles that of RVH, but the former produces a left axis deviation (-30 to -90 degrees) in the frontal plane.[41]

Disturbances of cardiac rhythm are uncommonly associated with heartworm disease. When present, tachyarrhythmias are more often ventricular in origin, are associated with advanced pulmonary artery disease, and are most often detected in cats with right-sided congestive heart failure.

THERAPY

Whether treatment of heartworm-infected cats is efficacious is unknown. In general, infected cats exhibiting clinical signs should probably be treated. In the absence of clinical signs, adulticide therapy may be delayed and the patient's clinical progression monitored. The recommended treatment is thiacetarsamide sodium (Carparsolate, Abbott Laboratories, N. Chicago, IL), 2.2 mg/kg IV bid for 2 days. Because circulating microfilariae are usually absent, evaluation of adulticide treatment is difficult. As in the dog, it should not be expected that thiacetarsemide will kill every adult worm in every infected cat. In some microfilaremic cats, repeated adulticide treatments have been required.[12,13,38] As in the dog, young adult female worms may be difficult to eradicate.[42] If clinical and radiographic signs of thromboembolic disease occur following adulticide administration, a degree of efficacy may be implied. Serologic tests that detect adult heartworm antigens are useful to monitor success of adulticide therapy. These antigens disappear from the serum within 3 months of effective therapy.

COMPLICATIONS OF THIACETARSAMIDE TREATMENT

Some cats experience anorexia and vomiting following the first or second dosage of thiacetarsamide. The incidence of such reactions is undocumented but is probably no greater than in the dog. These side effects usually warrant temporary cessation of treatment. A second attempt at thiacetarsamide administration is recommended in 2 to 4 weeks.

Acute fulminant pulmonary edema and death have been observed after intravenous carparsolate injection in some infected cats. This was not associated with pulmonary thromboembolism and may represent an idiosyncratic drug reaction. Because of the seriousness of this potential reaction. I recommend premedication with an antihistamine and soluble corticosteroid.

Thromboembolic complications are unpredictable and may occur 5 to 14 days after adulticide treatment. They are observed most commonly in cats with radiographic evidence of severe pulmonary arterial changes (e.g., enlargement, tortuosity). Acute thromboembolism in the cat is associated with an increased risk of death as compared with such reactions in dogs. Furthermore, sudden death or peracute respiratory distress may develop in cats that apparently tolerate adulticide treatment well. Aspirin administration has not been effective in reducing or preventing pulmonary arterial disease and hypertension or improving blood flow[42,43] (Rawlings CA: Personal communication, 1985).

Perivascular extravasation of thiacetarsamide is to be avoided at all costs. It is recommended that an indwelling intravenous catheter be used for adulticide administration. If a jugular catheter is in place, all administered doses may be given by this route. Because of local phlebitis produced by thiacetarsamide and peripheral indwelling catheters, it is recommended that only two intravenous doses be administered through one catheter. A second catheter should be placed in a different vein through which the remaining treatments are to be administered. Even though a catheter is used, its patency and integrity must be confirmed before each injection to avoid perivascular thiacetarsamide injection.

TREATMENT OF CLINICAL MANIFESTATIONS FROM HEARTWORM DISEASE

Under certain circumstances it is necessary to delay adulticide treatment so that concomitant disorders may be evaluated and treated. These include allergic pneumonitis, pulmonary thromboembolism, and right-sided congestive heart failure.

Allergic pneumonitis (Fig. 26-5) associated with heartworm infection occurs in some infected cats and resembles that reported in dogs.[44] The incidence of this syndrome in infected cats is unknown. Allergic pneumonitis is a syndrome of pulmonary infiltrate with eosinophilia that has certain clinical and radiographic traits in common with feline asthma or lungworm infection. Affected cats should be treated first with corticosteroids. Prednisolone at 5 mg od to bid usually causes dramatic improvement. After 3 to 5 days, this drug may be stopped and adulticide treatment begun. The radiographic resolution of vascular-interstitial lung disease often facilitates subsequent radiographic assessment of lobar pulmonary arterial disease.

Because of the possibility that corticosteroids may interfere with the action of thiacetarsamide, it is recommended that prednisolone be withdrawn prior to adulticide therapy. If necessary, prednisolone may be reintroduced five days after adulticide treatment.[43]

Pulmonary thromboembolic disease may be already present when heartworm disease is diagnosed. Coughing, fever, abnormal auscultatory lung sounds (e.g., crackles), and sometimes hemoptysis are associated clinical findings. This complication should be confirmed by thoracic radiography. The minimum data base in such instances should include a platelet count and activated clotting time. Affected cats should be hospitalized in cage confinement to eliminate physical activity. Supplemental oxygen is administered to cats experiencing severe respiratory distress or cyanosis. If there is no hemoptysis or other evidence of bleeding, and severe thrombocytopenia (less than 50,000/mm^3) is present, heparin sodium (50 U/kg, SQ tid) may be administered for several days. The platelet count will usually increase dramatically during this time. Adulticide therapy is initiated after 1 to 2 weeks of hospitalization when both clinical and radiographic evidence suggests significant improvement.

Some cats with severe pulmonary arterial disease are presented for signs of right-sided congestive heart failure (e.g., pleural effusion often accompanied by ascites). Dyspnea is usually proportional to the volume of pleural effusion. Coughing or radiographic evidence of thromboembolism-associated parenchymal lung disease may or may not be present. Distention of the jugular veins, jugular venous pulses, and central venous pressure elevation are typically present. The ECG is usually suggestive of right ventricular enlargement.

Cats with right-sided congestive heart failure should be treated with cage confinement for 1 to 2 weeks prior to adulticide therapy. In cases of severe pleural effusion, it may be necessary initially to perform therapeutic thoracocentesis. Paracentesis is usually not necessary unless ascites inhibits respiration. Furosemide is recommended at low dosages (1 mg/kg od to bid). Overzealous diuresis must be avoided since affected cats are usually dehydrated. Digoxin is not recommended in these patients because of the risk of toxicity and lack of proven efficacy. In heartworm-infected dogs, digoxin does not improve survival and is frequently associated with toxic side effects.

Successful treatment of advanced heartworm disease with congestive heart failure is dependent upon cage confinement and careful fluid and electrolyte management prior to adulticide treatment. These tactics must be continued for at least 6 weeks after adulticide therapy. Corticosteroids are indicated before or after adulticide treatment when there is clinical and radiographic evidence of parenchymal lung disease caused by severe pulmonary arterial thromboembolism.

Pulmonary arterial thromboembolic disease may occur after adulticide treatment. Its consequences in the cat are worse than the dog. This is because the bronchoesophageal artery provides significant collateral circulation to the lungs in the dog but not in the cat. Pulmonary thromboembolism is most likely to occur 5 to 14 days after adulticide administration, but may occur up to 4 weeks after treatment. It may occur acutely or peracutely and can result in sudden death. Observed clinical signs may include fever, coughing, dyspnea, auscultatory pulmonary crackles, hemoptysis, sinus tachycardia, pale mucous membranes, and hypotension. Severely affected cats should be treated with a shock protocol of intravenous corticosteroids, aminophylline, oxygen, and intravenous fluids. Less severely affected patients may be treated with anti-inflammatory dosages of corticosteroids and aminophylline.

Microfilaricide treatment is indicated only in those patients in which microfilaremia has been detected. Both levamasole and dithiazanine have been used.[13,14]

Diethylcarbamazine citrate is seldom recommended for chemoprophylaxis. This is because of the difficulty encountered with daily administration of medicaments to cats and the relatively low risk of reinfection.

REFERENCES

1. Soifer FK: Dirofilariasis in a cat. Vet Med Small Anim Clin 71:484, 1976
2. Lillis WG: *D. immitis* in dogs and cats from south central New Jersey. J Parasitol 50:802, 1964
3. Benard MA: Acute dirofilarial death. Can Vet J 11:190, 1970
4. Mandelker L, Brutus RL: Feline and canine dirofilarial encephalitis. J Am Vet Med Assoc 159:776, 1971
5. Stackhouse LL, Claugh E: Clinical report: Five cases of feline dirofilariasis. Vet Med Small Anim Clin 67:1309, 1972
6. Sherman WA, Wechster SJ: Unusual case of heartworm disease in a cat. Vet Med Small Anim Clin 70:1320, 1975
7. Cusick PK, Todd KS, Blake JA, et al: *D. immitis* in the brain and heart of a cat from Massachusetts. J Am Anim Hosp Assoc 12:490, 1976
8. Noyes JD: Illinois State Veterinary Medical Association yearly heartworm survey. p. 1. In Otto GF (ed): Proceedings of the Heartworm Symposium. Veterinary Medicine Publishing Co, Bonner Springs, KS, 1978
9. Seymore DN: Dirofilariasis in a cat. Mod Vet Pract 61:251, 1980
10. Dillon AR, Sakas PS, Buxton BAQ, et al: Indirect immunofluorescence testing for diagnosis of occult *Dirofilaria immitis* infection in three cats. J Am Vet Med Assoc 180.80, 1982
11. Calvert CA, Mandell CP: Diagnosis and management of feline heartworm disease. J Am Vet Med Assoc 180:550, 1982
12. Harlton BW: Treatment of dirofilariais in a domestic cat. Vet Med Small Anim Clin 69:1440, 1974
13. Schwartz A: Two cases of feline heartworm disease. Feline Pract 5:20, 1975
14. Hawe RS: The diagnosis and treatment of occult dirofilariasis in a cat. J Am Anim Hosp Assoc 14:577, 1979
15. Donahoe JM, Kneller SK, Lewis RE: Hematologic and radiographic changes in cats after innoculation with infective larvae of *Dirofilaria immitis*. J Am Vet Med Assoc 168:413, 1976
16. Otto GF: Epizootiology of canine heartworm disease. p. 1. In Bradley R (ed): Canine Heartworm Disease: Current Knowledge. University of Florida Press, Gainesville, FL, 1972
17. Otto GF: Occurrence of heartworm in unusual locations and unusual hosts. p. 6. In Otto GF (ed): Proceedings of the Heartworm Symposium. Veterinary Medicine Publishing Co, Bonner Springs, KS, 1974
18. Pacheco G: Synopsis of Dr. Kume's report at the first international symposium on canine heartworm disease. p. 137. In Bradley R (ed): Canine Heartworm Disease: Current Knowledge. University of Florida Press, Gainesville, FL, 1972
19. Mann FH, Fratta I: Transplantation of adult heartworms into dogs and cats. J Parasitol 39:139, 1953
20. Fowler JL, Matsuda K, Fernan RC: Experimental infection of the domestic cat with *D. immitis*. J Am Vet Med Assoc 8:79, 1972
21. Donahoe JM: Experimental infection of cats with *D. immitis*. J Parasitol 61:599, 1975
22. Wong MM, Pederson NC, Cullen J: Dirofilariasis in cats. J Am Anim Hosp Assoc 19:855, 1983
23. Dillon R: Feline dirofilariasis. Vet Clin North Am 14:1185, 1984
24. Donahoe JM, Holzinger EA: *D. immitis* in the brains of a dog and a cat. J Am Vet Med Assoc 164:518, 1974
25. Otto GF: Abnormal host-abnormal location. Am Heartworm Soc Bull 4:14, 1978
26. Griffiths HJ, Schlotthauer JC, Gehrman FW: Feline dirofilariasis. J Am Vet Med Assoc 140:61, 1962
27. Donahoe JM: Clinical aspects of feline dirofilariasis. p. 59. In Otto GF (ed): Proceedings of the Heartworm Symposium. Veterinary Medicine Publishing Co, Bonner Springs, KS, 1974
28. Mann PH, Fratta I: Transplantation of adult heartworms, *Dirofilaria immitis* into dogs and cats. J Parasitol 39:139, 1953
29. Dzimianski MT, McCall JW, Perry Ed, Rawlings CA: *Dirofilaria immitis* infections in cats following transplantation of adult heartworms. In Proceedings of the American Association of Veterinary Parasitology, New Orleans, LA, 1984 (abst 42)

30. Byerly CS, Donahoe MR, Todd KS: Histopathologic changes in cats experimentally infected with *Dirofilaria immitis*. p. 79. In Otto FG (ed): Proceedings of the Heartworm Symposium. Veterinary Medicine Publishing Co, Bonner Springs, KS, 1974

31. Schaub RG, Rawlings CA, Keith JC: Platelet adhesion and myointimal proliferation in canine pulmonary arteries. Am J Pathol 104:13, 1981

32. Schaub RG, Rawlings CA: Pulmonary vascular response during phases of canine heartworm disease. Am J Vet Res 41:1082, 1980

33. Schaub RG, Rawlings CA, Stewart GJ: Scanning electron microscopy of canine arteries and veins. Am J Vet Res 41:1441, 1980

34. Keith JC, Schaub RG, Rawlings, CA: Early arterial injury induced myointimal proliferation in canine pulmonary arteries. Am J Vet Res 44:181, 1983

35. Donahoe JM, Kneller SK, Lewis RE: In vivo pulmonary arteriography in cats infected with *D. immitis*. J Am Vet Radiol Soc 17:147, 1976

36. Dillon AR, Brawner WR, Grieve RB, et al: The chronic effects of experimental *D. immitis* infection in cats. Semin Vet Med Surg Small Anim 11:72, 1987

37. Losonsky JM, Thrall DE, Lewis RE: Thoracic radiographic abnormalities in 200 dogs with sponta-neous heartworm infestation. Vet Radiol 24:120, 1983

38. Dillon R: Feline heartworm disease: Clinical evaluation. p. 31. In Otto GF (ed): Proceedings of the Heartworm Symposium. Veterinary Medicine Publishing Co, Edwardsville, KS, 1983

39. Calvert CA, Coulter DB: Electrocardiographic values for anesthetized cats in lateral and sternal recumbencies. Am J Vet Res 42:1453, 1981

40. Hill JD: Electrocardiographic diagnosis of right ventricular enlargement. J Electrocardiol 4:347, 1971

41. Tilley LP: Essentials of canine and feline electrocardiography. 2nd Ed. Lea & Febiger, Philadelphia, 1985

42. Rawlings CA, Keith JC, McCall JW: Thiacetarsamide efficiency. p. 141. In Otto GF (ed): Proceedings of the Heartworm Symposium. Veterinary Medicine Publishing Co, Edwardsville, KS, 1983

43. Rawlings CA, Keith JC, Losonsky JM, et al: Aspirin and prednisolone modification of post-adulticide pulmonary arterial disease in heartworm infection. Am J Vet Res 44:821, 1983

44. Calvert CA: Pneumonitis associated with occult heartworm disease in dogs. J Am Vet Med Assoc 186:1097, 1985

27

Cardiac Involvement in Systemic Disease

Philip R. Fox
C. E. Rhett Nichols

Many conditions and diseases affecting the heart and blood vessels originate not in these structures but in other organs.[1-3] Secondary cardiovascular abnormalities may sometimes constitute the predominant clinical finding or principal medical concern.[3] In other instances, cardiovascular changes may be overshadowed by dominant systemic manifestations of the disease. A classification of important disorders affecting the heart is listed in Table 27-1. Many of these diseases have been previously discussed (Chs. 10 through 12, 21 through 24).

Endocrine and metabolic disorders affecting the heart are common in the dog and cat. Cardiac abnormalities are often reversible after appropriate diagnostic and therapeutic intervention.

THYROTOXICOSIS (HYPERTHYROIDISM)

The clinical syndrome resulting from excessive thyroid hormone secretion is one of the most common feline endocrine disorders,[4,5] with an approximate incidence of 1 out of every 300 cats.[5] By contrast, it is rare in the dog.[6] Cardiovascular hemodynamics are altered by both direct effects of thyroid hormone on the heart and increased adrenergic stimulation. A hyperkinetic high output heart failure state may result. This condition is discussed in detail in Chapter 12.

HYPOTHYROIDISM

Spontaneous hypothyroidism is one of the most common endocrinopathies in the dog. Most cases are related to plasmacytic-lymphocytic infiltration of the thyroid gland or idiopathic thyroid gland atrophy.[7] In the cat, bilateral thyroidectomy and overdose of either radioactive iodine or antithyroid drugs in the treatment of hyperthyroidism are the most common causes.

Primary hypothyroidism usually occurs in middle-aged and older dogs. Predisposed breeds include golden retrievers, Doberman pinschers, dachshunds, Irish setters, and miniature schnauzers.[8] No sex predisposition exists.[9] Spontaneous hypothyroidism in the cat is rare.[7]

Table 27-1 Classification of Systemic and Metabolic Disorders Affecting the Cardiovascular System

Endocrine
    Thyrotoxicosis
    Hypothyroidism
    Hypoadrenocorticism (Addison's disease)
    Hyperadrenocorticism (Cushing's disease)
    Acromegaly
    Renal disease
    Atherosclerosis
Metabolic
    Hyperkalemia
    Hypokalemia
    Hypercalcemia
    Hypocalcemia
    Uremia
Hypertensive cardiovascular disease
Anemia
Neoplasia
Infectious diseases
Chemical and drug toxicities
Obesity
Cor pulmonale
Nutritional disorders
Micellaneous

Clinical Abnormalities

The onset of clinical abnormalities is usually gradual. The most consistent clinical signs include fatigue, exercise intolerance, obesity, and dermatologic abnormalities, such as dry hair coat, alopecia, and hyperpigmentation.[10]

Abnormal laboratory findings include a high incidence of hypercholesterolemia[9] and elevated serum creatinine phosphokinase levels. A moderate normochromic, normocytic anemia is not unusual in longstanding cases.

Cardiovascular signs associated with severe hypothyroidism include bradycardia, weak cardiac apex beat, decreased QRS complex amplitude, and rarely cardiac arrhythmias associated with cardiomyopathy.[9,11] Atherosclerosis of coronary vessels with impaired circulation may be an inciting factor in the development of heart dysfunction.[12] In humans, there are many reports of electrocardiographic (ECG) changes with hypothyroidism, including sinus bradycardia conduction disturbances (e.g., first-degree heart block), low QRS voltage, axis deviations, prolongation of the QRS interval, and flattened or inverted T waves.[13–15]

In a study of 19 dogs with primary hypothyroidism, the most frequently observed abnormalities were low QRS voltage, inverted T waves, and sinus bradycardia.[16] Many ECG changes were reversed with thyroid replacement therapy and there appeared to be a correlation between ECG changes and the severity of the clinical signs of hypothyroidism. Experimental findings in dogs suggest that thyroid hormone influences the atrioventricular (AV) conduction system of the heart, since AV conduction time is prolonged in hypothyroid dogs.[14]

The mechanism by which thyroid hormones affect the heart is not clearly understood. Several authorities have suggested a direct effect of thyroid hormones, perhaps causing ultrastructural changes in the cell membrane resulting in a decreased number of β-adrenergic receptors.[17] In addition, thyroid hormone sensitizes the heart to catecholamines. A deficiency of thyroid hormone may cause bradycardia secondary to a lack of this sensitization.[18]

In hypothyroid humans, a reversible type of cardiomyopathy has been documented. Cardiac failure is a rare consequence of hypothyroidism in the absence of underlying cardiac disease.[19] Similarly, impaired myocardial contractility has clearly been demonstrated in dogs with experimentally induced hypothyroidism.[15,20] Echocardiographic studies of dogs with induced hypothyroidism have demonstrated impaired myocardial function, as shown by thinning of the left ventricular posterior wall and interventricular septum, decreased shortening fraction, and decreased left ventricular posterior wall excursion.[21] Despite myocardial impairment associated with severe canine hypothyroidism, hemodynamic, echocardiographic, or pathologic findings suggestive of congestive heart failure have not been found.

Although hypothyroidism has been suspected to induce dilated cardiomyopathy in some dogs, the relationship between hypothyroidism and overt congestive heart failure has yet to be documented convincingly. In a recent study of thyroid function in dogs with congestive cardiomyopathy, resting serum thyroid hormone concentrations were subnormal in 5 of the 13 dogs evaluated, but only one dog had concurrent hypothyroidism based on the results of thyroid-stimulating hormone (TSH) response testing.[22] Care must be taken not to misdiagnose hypothyroidism in dogs with heart failure, since any severe illness can falsely lower basal thyroid hormone levels when thyroid function is actually normal.

Diagnosis

The diagnosis of hypothyroidism is made by measuring basal serum thyroxine (T_4) and triiodothyronine (T_3) concentrations by radioimmunoassay. Subnormal thyroid hormone levels are suggestive but not definitive for a diagnosis of hypothyroidism. Current drug therapy (glucocorticoids, phenylbutazone, diazepam) or concurrent illness may artificially lower basal serum T_4 and T_3 levels.[17] Therefore, to establish a definitive diagnosis, a TSH response test may have to be performed. Unfortunately, a number of different protocols for the TSH stimulation test have been advocated in the literature,[23-26] emphasizing the importance of following the procedure recommended by the specific laboratory being used.

Therapy

Treatment for hypothyroidism simply involves thyroid hormone replacement. Synthetic levothyronine (T_4) is the initial therapy of choice (20 μg/kg every 12 hours).[24] Some dogs may require only once daily administration.

The required dose of levothyroxine may correlate better with metabolic rate than with body weight.[25] Metabolic rate, in turn, is related more closely to body surface area than to body weight. The recommended dosage of levothyroxine based on body surface area is 0.5 mg/m².

Thyroid supplementation increases basal metabolism, oxygen consumption, and heart rate. In dogs with congestive heart failure, a sudden increase in demand for oxygen delivery to peripheral tissue may place undue stress on a poorly functioning heart. Thus, some authorities suggest that if hypothyroidism is suspected in a patient with heart failure, the initial replacement dosage of thyroid hormone should be 50 percent of the standard recommended dosage.[26]

HYPOADRENOCORTICISM

Hypoadrenocorticism (Addison's disease) is an uncommon endocrine disorder in the dog and is extremely rare in the cat.[27-31] The disorder most often develops in young to middle-aged female dogs and shows no breed predilection.

Adrenocortical insufficiency results from a deficiency of glucocorticoid and/or mineralocorticoid secretion from the adrenal cortex. Either destruction of the adrenal cortex (primary adrenocortical insufficiency) or deficient pituitary adrenocorticotrophic hormone (ACTH) production (secondary adrenocortical insufficiency) may impair adrenocortical function and produce hypoadrenocorticism.

Primary adrenocortical insufficiency is the most common cause of hypoadrenocorticism and is thought to be an immune-mediated process whereby the adrenal cortex is destroyed by a plasmacytic-lymphocytic infiltrate.[32,33] A common iatrogenic cause of adrenal insufficiency involves o,p'-DDD (Lysodren) adminstration in the treatment of canine Cushing's disease.[34]

Clinical Findings

Historical signs with hypoadrenocorticism include depression, lethargy, anorexia, weakness, vomiting, diarrhea, and a waxing-waning course of disease.[35] Abnormalities noted on physical examination include depression, weakness, dehydration, and malaise. Cardiac signs may include bradycardia and weak femoral arterial pulses.[35]

Most clinical manifestations are attributable to deficiencies of both mineralocorticoids (aldosterone) and cortisol. Aldosterone acts to control sodium, potassium, and water homeostasis. Its main site of action is the renal tubule, where it promotes sodium and chloride absorption and potassium secretion.[32,33] Lack of aldosterone results in impaired ability to conserve sodium and excrete potassium, with resultant hyponatremia and hyperkalemia. Continued sodium loss results in hypovolemia, hypotension, reduced cardiac output, and decreased perfusion of the kidneys and other tissues. The decreased glomerular filtration rate causes prerenal azotemia and mild metabolic acidosis.

In the heart, hyperkalemia decreases cellular excitability, increases the refractory period, and slows conduction velocity. As a result of hypovolemia and poor tissue perfusion, hypoxia contributes to increased myocardial irritability. Ventricular fibrillation or sinoatrial (SA) standstill may eventually occur in severe hyperkalemic states.[35]

Cortisol is required to maintain normal cardiovascular function.[27] Cardiac contractility deteriorates rapidly in acute adrenal insufficiency.[36-39] Although the cause of the contractile failure is unknown, it is closely related to the actual plasma cortisol concentration. Chronic adrenal insufficiency is also associated with impaired cardiac performance. Cardiac output, heart rate, and peak left ventricular work become decreased. The affected heart is smaller than normal, has decreased metabolism, and shows an abnormally low rate of oxygen utilization.[38,39] With stress, the chronically adrenalectimized animal may develop vascular collapse, leading to death. These cardiovascular abnormalities can be prevented or reversed by appropriate replacement of corticosteroids.[36]

Typical laboratory abnormalities include hyponatremia, hyperkalemia, and azotemia. Mild to moderate hypercalcemia occurs in about one-third of dogs with untreated hypoadrenocorticism. The hemogram may reveal a normocytic, normochromic anemia and increased eosinophil and lymphocyte counts.[35]

Decreased heart size is a nonspecific radiographic finding concomitant with acute adrenocortical insufficiency and its associated hypovolemia.[40] This is usually accompanied by a flattening and decreased diameter of the descending aortic arch and a small posterior vena cava. Esophageal dilation may occur rarely, but the cause is unclear. This sometimes resolves with treatment of adrenocortical insufficiency and may be a reflection of generalized muscle weakness.

Electrocardiographic changes are frequently seen with adrenocortical insufficiency.[27] Cardiac tissues are especially susceptible to changes in membrane potential induced by hyperkalemia. Classically, progressive effects of hyperkalemia on the P-QRS-T complex include peaking of the T wave, shortening and widening of the P wave, prolongation of the PR interval, flattening and eventual disappearance of the P wave, widening of the QRS complex, irregular R-R intervals, and sine-wave pattern of the QRS-T complex.[27,30]

When serum potassium levels exceed 8 to 9 mEq/L, severe cardiac conduction abnormalities may occur, including AV junction delay, slowed conduction in the His-Purkinje system, and delays in ventricular muscle conduction. Electrocardiographically, these defects appear as AV heart block, idioventricular and escape complexes and rhythms.[27,30] Eventually, severe hyperkalemia results in ventricular fibrillation or asystole.

In a study of 100 dogs with adrenocortical insufficiency, characteristic hyperkalemic ECG changes (e.g., high peaked T waves, prolonged QRS duration, dampened R waves, bradycardia, persistent atrial standstill) were noted in 46 cases (Peterson ME, Nichols R: Unpublished data). There was poor correlation between specific ECG abnormalities and serum potassium levels. While the effects of elevated K^+ on the heart are usually unimportant below 7 mEq/L, six dogs in this study with persistent atrial standstill had K^+ values below 6 mEq/L. Atrial fibrillation and paroxysmal atrial tachycardia were present in two hyperkalemic dogs.

Experimentally, known ECG features of hyperkalemia have been produced by raising only serum potassium levels.[35] Clinically, virtually any arrhythmia or conduction disturbance may arise in the setting of hyperkalemia, depending on the rate of increase in serum potassium levels, associated electrolyte and acid-base abnormalities, or underlying heart disease. For example, ECG changes or hyperkalemia are exaggerated by hyponatremia and acidosis as well as by hypocalcemia. Therefore, while the ECG is useful in detecting and estimating the severity of hyperkalemia, there may be poor correlation between the serum potassium concentration and ECG changes due to above mentioned factors.

Diagnosis

Measurement of plasma cortisol before and after stimulation with exogenous ACTH is the best means to confirm adrenocortical insufficiency. A sluggish or absent response to ACTH administration suggests lack of adrenal reserve and a diagnosis of hypoadrenocorticism.[35] The use of serum sodium and potassium concentrations alone is sometimes unreliable, since these electrolytes may be normal in some affected dogs.

Treatment

The treatment of acute adrenocortical insufficiency is directed toward correcting hypotension and hypovolemia, improving vascular integrity by providing an immediate source of glucocorticoid, and correcting electrolyte imbalance and acidosis.

Normal saline is the fluid of choice because it will aid in correcting hypovolemia, hyponatremia, and hypochloremia. Hyperkalemia is reduced by simple dilution and by improved renal perfusion and glomerular filtration. The vast majority of dogs in hypoadrenal crisis with hyperkalemia can be treated successfully by rapid intravenous administration of normal saline. Some dogs may require the addition of glucose if hypoglycemia is suspected or known to be present.

In the unusual circumstance in which rapid saline administration fails to alter life-threatening cardiac arrhythmias, other emergency measures may be undertaken to alter cell membrane abnormalities or restore the transcellular gradient. Membrane excitability is defined as the difference between the resting and the threshold potentials. When the resting potential is reduced in the presence of hyperkalemia, increasing the extracellular calcium concentration reduces the membrane threshold potential and restores normal membrane excitability. In the presence of a severe, life-threatening conduction disturbance, calcium gluconate (1.0 ml/kg of a 10% solution) may be given intravenously over 3 to 4 minutes.[41] Continuous ECG monitoring is necessary, and conduction abnormalities usually improve during administration of this solution. The effect is transient, since the serum potassium concentration is unchanged and the calcium is rapidly excreted or taken up by other tissues.

In the hyperkalemic patient, movement of potassium into cells restores the transcellular gradient without altering total-body potassium. This may be accomplished by the administration of either glucose and regular insulin or of sodium bicarbonate. Insulin has been shown to decrease serum potassium levels by causing an intracellular shift of potassium from the extracellular fluid space. Because insulin lowers blood glucose levels, it is mandatory to give glucose during the insulin infusion. A safe and effective IV dose of regular insulin is 0.5 unit/kg with 2 g glucose administered intravenously per unit of insulin.[30,41] The serum potassium level should decline within 30 minutes. The effect lasts 4 hours. This administration of insulin and dextrose can be repeated if necessary.

Since acidosis promotes the transfer of potassium out of cells, the use of sodium bicarbonate to reverse the movement of potassium in a severely acidotic patient is a logical therapeutic measure. The recommended dose of sodium bicarbonate is 1 to 2 mEq/kg administered by slow IV infusion over a 15-minute period.[41]

In addition to these various rapid-acting treatment options, mineralocorticoids should be given to maintain electrolyte balance. Desoxycorticosterone acetate (DOCA) in oil is the initial mineralocorticoid of choice. The initial dose is 0.2 to 0.4 mg/kg IM (up to a maximum of 5 mg).[35]

Once the patient is stabilized and eating without vomiting, oral mineralocorticoid therapy (fludrocortisone acetate) can be initiated. Fludrocortisone acetate (Florinef) must be administered daily for the control of hypoadrenocorticism. The average dose in most dogs is about 20 µg/kg/day.[35]

In dogs with secondary hypoadrenocorticism, mineralocorticoid therapy is usually not required. Daily maintenance doses of glucocorticoids (e.g., prednisone, 0.2 mg/kg/day) are usually sufficient to control the clinical signs associated with this disease.

HYPERADRENOCORTICISM

Spontaneous canine hyperadrenocorticism (Cushing's syndrome) is a disorder caused by excessive production of cortisol by the adrenal cortex.[42–44] In 85 to 90 percent of affected dogs, the sustained hypercortisolism is caused by excessive pituitary gland ACTH secretion, which results in bilateral adrenocortical hyperplasia (pituitary-dependent hyperadrenocorticism). In the remaining dogs, unilateral tumors of the adrenal cortex secrete cortisol independent of endogenous ACTH control and are responsible for cortisol overproduction.[42,45,46]

Clinical Abnormalities

Spontaneous canine hyperadrenocorticism usually develops in middle-aged to older dogs. However, pituitary-dependent hyperadrenocorticism may occur as young as 1 year.[42] Pituitary-dependent hyperadrenocorticism develops most frequently in poodles, dachshunds, and boxers but can affect any breed. Although functional adrenal tumors show no breed predilection in dogs, large animals are affected more often than the toy breeds. Both sexes are equally affected by PDH, whereas 70 to 75 percent of dogs with adrenal tumors are female.[42,47]

Common abnormalities observed in dogs with naturally occurring hyperadrenocorticism include polyuria, polydipsia, pendulous abdomen, hepatomegaly, hair loss, lethargy, muscle weakness and atrophy, and increased panting.[42–44] Because of the multisystemic effects of long-term glucocorticoid excess, dogs with hyperadrenocorticism usually develop clinical signs reflecting dysfunction of many organ systems. In addition to cortisol excess, the compressive effects of a pituitary or adrenal neoplasm (and its metastases) may also contribute to the clinical signs in some dogs with hyperadrenocorticism.

Clinical manifestations of hyperadrenocorticism may be mild to severe and can be modified by the duration and etiology of the disorder. The disease course is usually insidious and slowly progressive. In a few cases, clinical signs may be intermittent, with periods of remission and relapse.[48] Others, however, especially with adrenocortical carcinoma, may have rapid onset and disease progression. These dogs may fail to develop dermatologic signs commonly observed in hyperadrenocorticism.

The hemogram may show mature leukocytosis, eosinopenia, and lymphopenia, although these changes are inconsistent. The most common serum biochemical abnormality is elevated serum alkaline phosphatase levels. Other findings may include hypercholesterolemia, elevated ALT (SGPT), hyperglycemia, and hypophosphatemia. Occasionally, mild hypokalemia has occurred.[49]

Abdominal radiographs may reveal abdominal distention, hepatomegaly, and vertebral osteopenia. Unilateral calcification in the area of the adrenal gland suggests an adrenocortical tumor.[50]

Cardiovascular Manifestations

Hypertension, a classic feature of human Cushing's disease, has been reported in dogs with hyperadrenocorticism.[44,51] Cortisol excess appears to elevate plasma renin substrate, the circulating protein upon which renin acts to release angiotensin I.[52] In addition, cortisol potentiates the effects of vasoconstrictive agents on vascular smooth muscle.[53] Therefore, it is likely that the hypertension associated with hyperadrenocorticism is produced by angiotensin-mediated vasoconstriction and increased sensitivity of vascular smooth muscle to vasoactive agents. Such elevations in blood pressure may contribute to the left ventricular hypertrophy and congestive heart failure that sometimes develop in dogs with hyperadrenocorticism.

Thoracic radiographs often show cardiomegaly associated with a prominent left heart and, occasionally, pulmonary edema. Mineralization of upper airways is common. Electrocardiographically, tall R waves indicative of left ventricular enlargement are a frequent finding. Hyperadrenocorticism frequently affects older breeds that have chronic acquired AV valvular insufficiency. The combined effect of valvular insufficiency and hyperadrenocorticism may increase the risk of cardiac decompensation.

Thromboembolism is a well-recognized complication in human patients with Cushing's syndrome.[54] Similarly, pulmonary thrombosis has been documented in dogs with hyperadrenocorticism.[55] Most of these affected dogs were undergoing therapy for hyperadrenocorticism when the embolic event occurred. Affected dogs develop acute respiratory distress. There may be no radiographic abnormalities. Alternatively, pleural effusion, increased diameter and blunting of the pulmonary arteries, lack of perfusion of obstructed pulmonary vasculature, and overperfusion of the unobstructed pulmonary vasculature may be evident. Thrombosis may be confirmed with pulmonary angiography or with a radionuclide lung scan.[55,56] Although the pathogenesis is unclear, elevations in coagulation factors have been reported in both humans and dogs and may contribute to a hypercoagulable state.[54]

Approximately one-third of dogs with hyperadrenocorticism exhibit increased panting and hyperventilation at rest.[49] Although the precise cause of the rapid respiratory rate is unclear, it may be due to stimulatory effects of cortisol on the respiratory center. In some cases, severe dyspnea may develop secondary to congestive heart failure or pulmonary thrombosis.

Diagnosis

Once hyperadrenocorticism is suspected, additional laboratory testing should proceed through two stages. The objective of the first stage is to confirm the diagnosis of hyperadrenocorticism. Either the ACTH stimulation test or the low-dose dexamethasone suppression test may be used to separate dogs with Cushing's disease from normal dogs. An exaggerated cortisol response to exogenous ACTH above the upper limits of normal suggests hyperadrenocorticism. More than 85 percent of dogs with pituitary-dependent hyperadrenocorticism have an exaggerated response to ACTH stimulation.[57] More than one-half of dogs with adrenocortical tumors also hyperrespond.[47,58,59] With the low-dose dexamethasone suppression test for diagnostic evaluation, lack of serum cortisol suppression to less than 1 μg/dl suggests Cushing's disease.[49] Further differentiation may require high-dose dexamethasone testing, measurement of baseline ACTH levels, pituitary or adrenal computed tomography scanning, or exploratory laparotomy.

Treatment

Most dogs with PDH are placed on a loading dose of o,p'-DDD (Lysodren) for 7 to 10 days. The daily dose may vary from 30 to 50 mg/kg. In addition, prednisone (0.2 mg/kg/day) is added to combat the cortisol-lowering side effects of o,p'-DDD.[49,60]

After the initial loading period, adrenal reserve is evaluated with the ACTH stimulation. Once basal and post-ACTH levels are within the basal cortisol range (1 to 4 μg/dl), patients are placed on maintenance o,p'-DDD therapy (30 to 50 mg/kg weekly in divided doses).[49] Animals that display exaggerated ACTH responses above the basal cortisol range are reloaded with o,p'-DDD for 5 days and then reevaluated. If possible, adrenocortical tumors should be surgically removed[61]. However, dogs with increased surgical risk (e.g., congestive heart failure, pyelonephritis, renal failure) may be treated effectively with o,p'-DDD.

In general, dogs with hyperadrenocorticism and congestive heart failure appear to respond poorly to therapy consisting of only digitalization and low-salt diet. Management of congestive heart failure and hypertension is best accomplished with the judicious use of diuretics and vasodilators and treatment of the underlying cause of the hyperadrenocorticism.

Therapy for pulmonary thromboembolism consists of general medical support, oxygen, anticoagulants (e.g., heparin), and time. The prognosis for this condition is guarded to grave.

ACROMEGALY

Acromegaly is a disorder of chronic excessive growth hormone (GH) secretion characterized by overgrowth of connective tissue, bone, and viscera. In humans, this is usually caused by a pituitary tumor or hyperplasia of pituitary acidophils.[62–66] GH exhibits both anabolic and catabolic activity. Its catabolic action (enhanced lipolysis and restricted glucose transport caused by insulin resistance) is mediated by the GH peptide. Anabolic effects appear to be mediated by insulin-like GH factors (somatomedins).[67]

Acromegaly has been reported in dogs and cats.[68–71] Most canine cases have been reported in intact older females (mean age: 10 years, range: 8 to 11 years).[69] In the dog, acromegaly is most commonly induced by progesterone. It may develop following prolonged administration of progestogens or during the diestrual phase of the estrous cycle in the intact older bitch.[70] Stimulation of GH secretion by exogenous progestogens appears to be dose related, with larger dosages producing higher basal GH concentrations.[72] Progestogen therapy in the dog results in hyperplasia and hypertrophy of pituitary somatotrophs.[73] In cats as in humans, acromegaly is most often associated with a somatotroph tumor of the pars distalis.[63,64,74] Administration of progestational compounds or the presence of increased serum progesterone levels during diestrus has not been reported to cause feline acromegaly. The mean age of affected cats is 10 years, with a range of 8 to 14 years. Reported cases are too few to determine a breed or sex predisposition (Peterson ME, unpublished data).

Clinical Abnormalities

The most consistent clinical sign in dogs is inspiratory stridor resulting from excessive soft tissue overgrowth of the orolingual, oropharyngeal, or orolaryngeal region. In some, impaired respiration results in exercise intolerance, fatigue, and frequent panting. Other signs include enlargement of the feet, head, and abdomen, as well as palpably thickened skin with excessive folds (especially about the head, neck, and distal extremities), polyuria, polydipsia, and polyplasia.[67]

In cats, the most common clinical manifestation is insulin resistant diabetes mellitus with associated polyuria, polydipsia, polyphagia and cardiomyopathy. Thick, coarse hair coats, thickened skin about the face and neck, arthropathies, organomegaly, and weight gain are other signs (Peterson ME: Unpublished data).

Clinicopathologic features in dogs include hyperglycemia (but not overt diabetes mellitus) and mild serum alkaline phosphatase elevation.[67] In cats, severe glucose intolerance with hyperglycemia and glycosuria, mild increases in alkaline phosphatase, alanine aminotransferase and aspartase aminotransferase, and hyperphosphatemia (probably from the effects of GH on renal tubular phosphate clearance) may occur (Peterson ME: Unpublished data).

Radiographic change in both dogs and cats may include soft tissue swelling of the head and neck, visceromegaly, cardiomegaly, hyperostosis of the bony calvarium, thickened and elongated mandibles, widened joint space between the long bones of the limbs, thickened epiphyseal trabeculae, and narrowed medullary cavity with long bone diaphyseal thickening.[62,67,75] (Peterson ME: Unpublished data)

Cardiovascular Manifestations

In humans, cardiomegaly, hypertension, atherosclerosis, and cardiomyopathy are associated with acromegaly.[76] While cardiomegaly may be related to the generalized effect of GH and/or somatomedin on protein synthesis, other factors may be important as well. These include hypertension, atherosclerosis, and acromegaly-induced cardiomyopathy.

Hypertension occurs in 15 to 20 percent of human acromegalics.[76] The underlying pathophysiology is unclear, but studies suggest that GH may directly stimulate sodium retention, with the resultant expansion of extracellular fluid volume.[77]

Many human acromegalics without evidence of hypertension or atherosclerosis have significant cardiac dysfunction.[78] Echocardiographic evidence of left ventricular hypertrophy, ECG abnormalities, and a 10 to 20 percent incidence of overt congestive heart failure occur. Acromegalic cardiomyopathy may be a specific entity. Microscopic examination of the heart reveals moderate to marked interstitial fibrosis, increased collagen content of the cardiac muscle, and hypertrophy of individual cardiac fibers.[76]

In a study of six acromegalic cats, cardiomyopathy was evident in five and resulted in the death of three cats. One was diagnosed as having congestive cardiomyopathy at necropsy. Two others died of left-sided congestive heart failure. Serial thoracic radiographs demonstrated progressive generalized cardiomegaly followed by development of pulmonary edema in these cats (Peterson ME: Unpublished data).

Disproportionate cardiomegaly (concentric hypertrophy of the left ventricle) occurs in approximately 50 to 75 percent of humans with acromegaly; its severity is related to the duration of the disease.[76] Likewise, two cats included in this study exhibited profound left ventricular hypertrophy and increased septal wall thickness, as seen echocardiographically. Hypertension, common in persons with acromegaly, was not investigated in these cats.

Diagnosis

A tentative diagnosis of acromegaly is based on history, clinical signs, and laboratory and radiographic findings. Dog owners should be questioned about the reproductive cycle and possible progestogen treatment.

A definitive diagnosis of acromegaly requires documentation of elevated, nonsuppressible basal serum GH elevations.[67] Most acromegalic cats have high basal GH levels (Peterson ME: Unpublished data). In humans and dogs with mild acromegaly, GH secretion is episodic, and basal concentrations may fall into the normal range. Therefore, confirmation of presumed acromegaly may require evaluation of pituitary somatotroph responsiveness to a glucose suppression test. Administration of a glucose load either orally or intravenously results in suppression of GH levels in normal dogs, but not in dogs with acromegaly.[67]

The most sensitive method to demonstrate a pituitary mass is through the use of computed tomography (CT). It has been possible with this technique to demonstrate a large expanding mass in the area of the sella turcica following administration of a radiographic contrast agent in two acromeg.lic cats (Peterson ME: Unpublished data). CT can be used to document the presence of a pituitary tumor, to help establish a mode of therapy (i.e., surgery, medical, radiotherapy), and to monitor response to treatment.

Treatment

In humans, primary therapy involves selective surgical extirpation of the somatotroph tumor by a transphenoid approach.[62-66] Similar surgical techniques have met with little success in dogs or cats (Peterson ME: Unpublished data). Cobalt radiation therapy has proved ineffective or only transiently effective in veterinary medicine (Peterson ME: Unpublished data). Medical treatment in people (e.g., bromocriptine and long-acting somatostatin analogues, both of which inhibit GH secretion) has been equally ineffective in animals. Nevertheless, the short-term prognosis for feline acromegaly appears to be good simply with symptomatic therapy. In general, cats with cardiomyopathy have responded well to furosemide (2.2 mg/kg/day). Hyperglycemia may be controlled using large doses of NPH insulin in divided daily doses. The survival time of the six acromegalic cats in this series has ranged from 8 to 30 months. Two cats are still alive.

In acromegalic dogs, withdrawal of exogenous progestogen therapy or ovariohysterectomy is the therapy of choice. In general, clinical signs will resolve over a period of 1 to 3 months.

RENAL DISEASE

Renal disease (uremia) may have deleterious effects on cardiovascular structure and function. There is a strong relationship among heart function, vascular volume regulation, and electrolyte homeostasis. A number of systemic alterations may result from renal disease, including fluid and electrolyte imbalances, acidosis, anemia, uremia, endocrine disorders (renin-angiotensin system), nutritional deficiences, and hypertension.[79]

Exercise capacity may be impaired in persons with chronic renal failure.[79,80] Metabolic acidosis resulting from renal inability to excrete H^+ ions may decrease myocardial performance and reduce myocardial response to catecholamines.[81] Hyperkalemia may occur when renal potassium excretion is impaired. Hypocalcemia may result from reduced intestinal calcium absorbtion and metastatic calcification due to high plasma phosphate levels. Uremic toxins may accumulate,[82] although the reported effects of uremia on myocardial performance are variable and conflicting. Chronic anemia due to erythropoietin deficiency and uremic toxins may decrease systemic vascular resistance and result in a hyperkinetic state.[83] Hyperparathyroidism secondary to chronic renal failure may depress cardiac function.[84]

Hypertension commonly occurs with chronic renal disease and has been recorded in 50 to 93 percent of affected animals.[85] Hypertension resulting from chronic renal failure increases cardiac worklod and predisposes to structural cardiovascular alterations. Causes of renal hypertension are many and include alterations in the renin-angiotensin and sympathetic pressor systems and in extracellular fluid volume and sodium levels, and subsequent derangement of hemodynamic autoregulation.[85-87]

Treatment

Therapeutic strategies are directed toward correcting the underlying renal disorders, if possible (e.g., antibiotics, dietary changes), reducing myocardial work (e.g., vasodilators to reduce afterload), and generalized medical patient support for renal failure. This includes judicious fluid therapy, treatment of hyperkalemia and hypercalcemia if present, and dietary sodium restriction and diuretics to reduce salt retention.

HYPERKALEMIA

The effects of progressive hyperkalemia are to decrease the resting membrane potential (i.e., becomes less negative). Initially, this makes the cells more excitable but at less negative levels of resting membrane potential fibers become less excitable.[88,89] Different cardiac tissues vary widely in sensitivities to potassium. The sinus node and His bundle are more resistant than ventricular myocardium, which is more resistant than atrial tissue.

An important clinical manifestation of hyperkalemia is its effect on cardiac conduction. The sequence of ECG changes associated with high serum potassium levels correlates loosely with the degree of hyperkalemia in the following order: peaking of the T wave, shortening and widening of the p wave, prolongation of the PR interval, eventual disappearance of the P wave, widening of the QRS complex, irregular R-R intervals, and sine-wave-type QRS-T complexes.[90] AV block, idioventricular rhythms, escape beats, ventricular fibrillation, and asystole may occur.[91,92] Neuromuscular symptoms include weakness and even flaccid paralysis, but cardiotoxicity usually precedes these manifestations in severe cases.

Therapy

Hyperkalemia should be considered a potential complication when oliguria or serious renal dysfunction is present. The most common occurrence is in association with feline urethral obstruction syndrome. Other causes of hyperkalemia in dogs and cats include adrenocortical insufficiency (dogs), iatrogenic overzealous administration of potassium chloride infusions, and severe metabolic and respiratory acidosis.

The treatment of hyperkalemia is clinically directed by the level of serum potassium, ECG findings, and clinical signs. If the ECG reflects changes attributable to hyperkalemia other than peaked T waves, or if the serum potassium level exceeds 6.5 mEq/L, aggressive and prompt therapy should be instituted. The acute treatment of hyperkalemia is intended to reverse cellular membrane abnormalities, restore the transcellular gradient by moving potassium into cells, and remove excess potassium from the body.[93] Administration of calcium gluconate, sodium bicarbonate, and glucose with regular insulin has been detailed under the section hypoadrenocorticism.

Most adrenocortical insuffiency patients can be treated with saline diuresis and cortisone adminis-

tration alone. However, hyperkalemic urethral obstruction cats, especially those with severe ECG abnormalities, appear to respond best to insulin-dextrose infusions followed by saline diuresis.[94] In the absence of cardiac abnormalities and serum potassium levels in the range of 6.0 to 8.0 mEq/L, the administration of normal saline will usually lower the serum potassium level as long as urine output is normal.

HYPOKALEMIA

Hypokalemia in dogs and cats is seldom of clinical importance until serum potassium levels fall below 3.5 mEq/L.[95] Hypokalemia occurs as a result of factors that influence the transcellular distrubution of potassium and/or total body potassium. Common causes of include (1) overzealous administration of fluids devoid of or low in potassium (dilutional hypokalemia); (2) potassium loss from the gastrointestinal tract during severe vomiting or diarrhea (e.g., parvovirus gastroenteritis); (3) urinary loss, especially during treatment of polyuric renal failure in the face of anorexia or secondary to excessive use of diuretic agents such as furosemide; (4) alkalosis, both respiratory and metabolic; (5) side effect of treatment of the diabetic ketoacidotic patient.[96] In the latter, most are total-body potassium deficient because of decreased potassium intake from anorexia and excessive urinary potassium wasting from prolonged osmotic diuresis. This potassium-deficient state is worsened by fluid therapy (which causes diuresis and dilutional hypokalemia) and by insulin administration (which shifts potassium from the extracellular to intracellular fluid compartment).

Clinical Abnormalities

Clinical manifestations of hypokalemia result from skeletal muscle weakness and paralytic ileus.[97] Potassium depletion and the associated hypokalemia produce muscle weakness and paralysis by a number of effects on muscle and its blood supply.[98] Although the degree of hypokalemia does not always correlate with the degree of total-body potassium depletion, serum potassium levels usually correlate well with onset and severity of weakness. Generally, patients with serum potassium levels of 3 to 3.5

mEq/L rarely show detectable clinical weakness. Weakness is usually observed when serum potassium is at or below 2.5 mEq/L.[99] In humans, serum potassium levels below 2 mEq/L are associated with exercise-induced rhabomyolysis and muscle paralysis.[98]

Hypokalemia and potassium depletion are recognized but not well-documented causes of clinical hypomotility and paralytic ileus. Abdominal distention, vomiting, and constipation can accompany the hypomotile state. Experimental studies in potassium depleted rats and dogs have demonstrated normal muscle tone in the bowel. However, as potassium stores are further depleted, muscle tone also decreases, leading to dilation of bowel segments.[100] These animal studies explain in part why gastric atony and megacolon occur in severely potassium-depleated patients.[101]

In dogs, hypokalemia can cause ECG changes, including progressive ST-segment sagging and decreased T-wave amplitude.[102] Other reported canine ECG abnormalities include prominent U waves, increased amplitude and duration of the QRS complex, slightly prolonged PR interval, and increased P-wave amplitude and duration.[103] In addition, atrial and ventricular premature contractions are frequently seen in hypokalemic animals.[102]

The interaction of digitalis and potassium is clinically important. Hypokalemia may intensify the tendency of digitalis to produce ectopic beats and arrhythmias and augment the digitalis-induced depression of AV conduction.[104] For this reason, potassium balance must be carefully monitored and controlled in patients receiving digitalis preparations.

Treatment

The treatment of established or anticipated potassium deficiency requires evaluation of several factors, including the type of potassium salt to be supplemented, the route of replacement, the quantity and rate of potassium administration, and correction of the primary disease process that caused this electrolyte disturbance.

Potassium should be supplemented orally whenever possible since this is the safest route of administration. For example, mild hypokalemia may be treated conservatively with foods having high po-

Table 27-2 Intravenous Potassium Supplementation

Serum Potassium (mEq/L)	mEq Potassium Added per 250 ml Fluids
<2.0	20
2.0–2.5	15
2.6–3.0	10
3.1–3.5	7

tassium content, such as meats, nuts, bananas, citrus juice, or vegetables.[105]

The anorexic or vomiting patient with moderate or severe hypokalemia (up to 3.0 mEq/L) usually requires parenteral administration of potassium chloride. The ketoacidotic diabetic may be phosphate as well as potassium depleted. Parental potassium phosphate is the most rational therapy in these cases. Potassium can be administered subcutaneously or slowly intravenously after being diluted in parental fluids. The maximum rate of parenteral potassium administration should not exceed 0.5 mEq/kg/hr.[106] The hypokalemic dog or cat often requires 3 to 5 mEq/kg of potassium per day to correct existing deficits.[103] Table 27-2 presents a convenient outline of guidelines for potassium supplementation.[107]

Adjustments in the dose of potassium administration are based on serial ECGs and frequent monitoring of serum electrolyte concentrations. Potassium supplementation should never be given to an anuric animal.

HYPERCALCEMIA

Hypercalcemia is defined as serum calcium that consistently exceeds 12 mg/dl in mature dogs and 11 mg/dl in cats. The recognition of hypercalcemia has become more common with routine determination of serum calcium as part of biochemical profiles. The causes of hypercalcemia can be divided into two basic categories: those due to increased gut absorption, and those resulting from increased bone resorption. Several conditions are commonly associated with or are causes of hypercalcemia in dogs and cats: (1) young growing animals (nonpathologic),[108] (2) paraneoplastic syndromes associated with cancer (e.g., lymphosarcoma, multiple myeloma and anal sac apocrine gland adenocarcinoma),[109-113] (3) hypoadrenocorticism,[114] and (4) primary renal failure.[108] Primary hyperparathyroidism, a common cause of hypercalcemia in persons is uncommon in veterinary medicine.[109,114]

Hypercalcemia in mature animals is often an indication of underlying malignant neoplasia. Metastasis to bone can cause local dissolution and release of calcium.[109] In myeloma and lymphoma (and perhaps others) osteoclast-activating factor may mediate bone dissolution. Although ectopic secretion of parathormone in malignancy has been suspected for many years, recent evidence suggests that this mechanism occurs rarely, if ever. Rather, a substance that is immunologically distinct from parathormone but that shares certain physiologic actions (hypercalcemia, decreased renal tubular phosphate absorption) may account for so-called humoral hypercalcemia of malignancy. Other humoral mediators of hypercalcemia include prostaglandins and vitamin D.[115]

Primary renal disease can cause hypercalcemia. In many instances it is difficult to determine if hypercalcemia is the cause of the renal disease or the result of renal dysfunction. Most cases of primary renal failure are associated with low or normal serum calcium levels. Postulated mechanisms for hypercalcemia associated with primary renal failure include decreased renal calcium excretion, increased concentrations of parathormone (due to increased secretion and decreased renal tubular degradation), and autonomous parathyroid activity.[116-118]

Mild to moderate hypercalcemia occurs in about one-third of dogs with untreated hypoadrenocorticism and develops most frequently in extremely ill hypoadrenal dogs.[113] The severity of the hypercalcemia is usually in direct proportion to the severity of dehydration or electrolyte abnormality. The mechanism for this hypercalcemia is unclear. Normocalcemia is rapidly restored in clinical patients following appropriate therapy for adrenal insufficiency.

Clinical Abnormalities

Hypercalcemia may produce a complex of signs characterized by anorexia, nausea and vomiting, constipation, polyuria, polydipsia, and CNS disturbances, including lethargy, stupor, and coma.[108]

As ionized serum calcium (the active form of calcium) rises above normal, cell membranes become less excitable. Decreased neuromuscular excitability of smooth muscle for example, results in anorexia, vomiting and constipation. Generalized muscle weakness occurs with similar involvement of skeletal muscles. Decreased neuromuscular excitability of the brain results in depression, one of the most noticeable clinical signs.[119] Excessive bone resorption leads to nonspecific lameness, loss of teeth, and long bone fractures accompanying even mild trauma. Hypercalcemia causes polyuria and compensatory polydipsia by inhibiting the action of antidiuretic hormone at the level of the distal tubule and collecting ducts.

Cardiovascular Manifestation

Dramatic calcium fluctuation alters the duration of transmembrane action potential. Experimentally, marked elevation of plasma calcium levels may depress intraventricular conduction and induce ventricular premature systoles and fibrillation.[120] These effects are secondary to prolongation of the transmembrane action potential. In persons with extreme serum calcium elevation, PR-interval prolongation, AV block, and QRS complex prolongation have been reported.[121] Generally, however, arrhythmias do not accompany clinical hypercalcemia.[114]

Hypercalcemia speeds the rate of ventricular repolarization and is therefore associated most often with a shortened QT interval. However, there is a lack of a predictable correlation between the QR interval and serum calcium concentration, largely because other factors in addition to calcium levels affect the QT interval. These include drugs, myocardial disease, and other electrolyte disturbances. Other ECG changes associated with hypercalcemia include a shortened and occasionally depressed ST segment.[121]

Calcium and Blood Pressure

Hypercalcemia increases smooth muscle tension,[122] producing vasoconstriction, increased vascular resistance, and occasionally increased blood pressure.[123] Decreased glomerular filtration rate and renal blood flow result from vasoconstriction induced by hypercalcemia.[124,125] Sustained vasoconstriction may result in ischemic renal injury and further deterioration of renal function.

Diagnosis

Before implementing a diagnostic plan to identify the cause of hypercalcemia, it is important to exclude laboratory error and spurious elevation from hemoconcentration or lipemia. Moreover, because serum calcium determinations are measures of total calcium and approximately one-half of serum calcium is bound to albumin, patients with hypoalbumenia may have falsely lowered calcium values.

A standard diagnostic evaluation may include a complete blood count, biochemical profile, urinalysis, chest and abdominal radiographs, lymph node aspirate and/or biopsy, serum electrophoresis, radiographic bone survey, and a careful rectal examination. In some cases of hypercalcemia due to occult neoplasia, a cortisone response test may be performed. Hypercalcemia associated with primary hyperparathyroidism will not respond to high-dose cortisone therapy, whereas with some types of neoplasia (especially lymphoma), transient reduction of the hypercalcemic state will result.

Therapy

The decision for aggressive medical therapy is based on the severity of clinical signs, renal function, ECG changes, and neurologic abnormalities. When the $Ca^{2+} \times PO_4^{2-}$ product is less than 60, there is usually no urgent requirement for lowering the serum calcium level as the risk for soft tissue mineralization is low.[125] However, when dehydration, renal dysfunction, cardiac arrhythmias, or severe neurologic disease exists, the need for medical therapy is imperative. A serum calcium above 15 mg/dl in association with stupor or coma and renal insufficiency (hypercalcemic crisis) requires immediate treatment.

Therapy of acute symptomatic hypercalcemia begins with volume expansion, which alone may be adequate in mild-to-moderate hypercalcemia.[108,125] Saline (0.9 percent sodium chloride) increases urinary calcium excretion by inhibiton of tubular sodium reabsorption at those sites where sodium and calcium transport appear to be linked. However, rapid expansion of the extracellular volume may produce volume overload, particularly in older pa-

tients or those with underlying heart disease. An adjunct to this therapy, once hydration has been re-established, is a diuretic such as furosemide that acts at the loop of Henle. This serves to potentiate calciuria by inhibiting sodium and calcium transport. Furosemide is dosed at 2 to 4 mg/kg in the dog and 1 to 2 mg/kg in the cat once to twice daily.[126] In addition, glucocorticoids may be given (prednisolone, 1 to 1.5 mg/kg PO bid) in those cases of suspected lymphoproliferative disease or multiple myeloma. Glucocorticoids have a direct steroid toxic effect on some cancer cells, limit bone resorption, decrease intestinal calcium absorption, and enhance renal excretion of calcium.[127]

Additional therapy depends on the severity of clinical signs. Severe hypercalcemia (greater than or equal to 15 mg/dl) with acute neurologic, cardiovascular, or renal dysfunction constitutes hypercalcemic crisis and is a medical emergency. In most instances, the addition of mithramycin or calcitonin (both agents decrease bone resorption by inhibiting osteoclasts) to saline-furosemide infusion enhances therapy for emergency situations.[125] Rarely is the immediate reduction of serum ionized calcium levels by infusion of sodium EDTA required.

HYPOCALCEMIA

The most common causes of hypocalcemia in veterinary medicine include puerperal tetany in the lactating bitch, idiopathic and iatrogenic hypoparathyroidism, hypoalbumenia of any cause, chronic renal failure in association with phosphorus retention, and acute pancreatitis.[128,129]

The functional disturbances and clinical manifestations of hypocalcemia are primarily the result of increased neuromuscular excitability and tetany.[130,131] Tremors, twitching, cramps, and muscle spasms occur as well as gait changes due to stiffness and ataxia. Focal, psychomotor, and generalized seizures and behavioral changes may occur as well. Death due to severe hypocalcemia can result from status epilepticus or muscular paralysis with respiratory arrest. Clinical signs of hypocalcemia tend to be episodic, and the degree of hypocalcemia does not always correlate with the severity of clinical signs.

Cardiac Manifestation of Hypocalcemia

Many hypocalcemic animals exhibit ECG abnormalities. These may include tachycardias, deep wide T waves, prolongation of the QT interval, and tall R waves.[131,132] There appears to be a good correlation between the severity of the hypocalcemia and the duration of the ST segment.

Experimental studies have documented the importance of calcium ions in the contraction of cardiac muscle. Acute elevations of calcium augment cardiac contractility, while acute reductions of calcium decrease cardiac contractility. However, at least in humans, hypocalcemia is usually not associated with clinical heart failure.[133]

Treatment

Not all animals require therapy to restore normocalcemia, particularly when there are no clinical signs. For example, animals with hypocalcemia secondary to hypoproteinemia will not require therapy, since the serum ionized calcium fraction remains normal and they exhibit no clinical signs.

The ionized fraction of serum calcium must be low for the hypocalcemia to be of clinical importance. However, a notable exception to treating hypocalcemia without clinical signs is the post-surgical thyroidectomy patient. If serum calcium levels are 6 mg/dl or less after surgery, hypoparathyroidism must be assumed until proved otherwise, and therapy for hypocalcemia should be started immediately.[134]

Hypocalcemic tetany or convulsions are indications for the immediate intravenous administration of calcium. A commonly used preparation for parenteral use is calcium gluconate; a dose of 1 to 1.5 mg/kg of body weight should be slowly infused over a 10- to 20-minute period.[134] ECG monitoring is advisable during infusion; if bradycardia or shortening of the Q-T interval occurs, administration should be slowed or temporarily discontinued.

Once the life-threatening signs of hypocalcemia have been controlled, calcium can be added to maintenance intravenous fluids and admininstered by slow infusion. Oral calcium and vitamin D supplementation should be initiated as soon as oral medication can be tolerated.[134]

When animals are stabilized, the chronic treatment of hypoparathyroidism requires a maintenance dosage of a vitamin D preparation together with an adequate dietary and/or supplemental calcium. If puerperal tetany is suspected, puppies should be removed from the bitch for 24 hours to reduce the lactational drain of calcium. Supplemental dietary calcium and vitamin D have proven useful in preventing relapses in certain bitches with this disorder.

HYPERTENSIVE CARDIOVASCULAR DISEASE

Hypertension is a clinical state in which systemic arterial pressure is abnormally high due to a disease or secondary systemic process. Prolonged hypertension may result in cardiovascular changes unrelated to the inciting mechanism.

Hypertensive cardiovascular disease may be associated with various conditions: (1) essential hypertension, an idiopathic process; (2) hypertension as the predominant manifestation of pheochromocytoma or renovascular disease; or (3) hypertension comprising one of several known problems due to pyelonephritis, glomerulonephritis, collagen vascular disease, polycystic kidneys, Cushing's syndrome, diabetes mellitus, polycythemia, hyperthyroidism, and hypothyroidism.[85–87,135–140]

Factors implicated in the pathogenesis of hypertension include disorders of hemodynamics and vasomotor regulation, autonomic nervous system function, and humeral control of pressure, volume and renal sodium handling.[135–137] Increase in total peripheral vascuar resistance elevate both systolic and diastolic pressure.[138]

Pathologic changes result from the disease causing hypertension. Target organs altered as a consequence of hypertension. The heart, for example, becomes hypertrophied due to the increased pressure overload on the left ventricle. Atherosclerosis and myointimal proliferation of arteries and arterioles may occur. Hypertensive retinopathy (retinal hemorrhage, straightening of renal vessels, papilledema, retinal detachment), cerebrovascular accidents, and renal lesions (e.g., glomerulosclerosis, renal capillary occlusion, arteriosclerosis, ischemia) may result.[85,139,140]

Diagnosis

Hypertension is not a disease but a clinical sign. Accurate reproducible blood pressure measurements are essential for its diagnosis. The arterial pressure of any animal may vary depending on multiple variables, including sympathetic activity (fright, excitement, pain), state of hydration, and skeletal muscle tone. Clinical signs of acute blindness, ocular hemorrhage, epistaxis, or abnormal mentation are particularly suggestive of hypertension.[85,140]

Blood pressure may be measured directly by percutaneous femoral artery puncture or assessed indirectly and noninvasively by ultrasonic doppler or oscillometric techniques utilizing inflatable cuffs.[141–143] Normal values for conscious dogs using a direct technique is 148 ± 16 mmHg, systolic; 87 ± 8 mmHg, diastolic; 102 ± 9 mmHg, mean. Arterial hypertension occurs when sustained systolic or diastolic pressures exceed 180 and 95 mmHg, respectively.[85]

In cats, normal values have been reported for unanesthetized animals using femoral arterial puncture (171 ± 22 mmHg, systolic; 123 ± 17 mmHg, diastolic; 149 ± 24 mmHg, mean).[143] In other feline studies hypertension was defined as sustained systolic pressure greater than 170 mmHg and diastolic pressure greater than 100 mmHg.[144]

When hypertension is verified, a diagnostic search for treatable or reversible causes should be initiated. In addition to the standard data base (chest and abdominal radiographs, complete blood count, biochemical profile, urinalysis), other diagnostic modalities must be considered: ultrasonography, excretory urography, renal biopsy, and tests for hyperadrenocorticism, hyperthyroidism, hypothyroidism, and pheochromocytoma.

Treatment

Therapy is directed both at the primary inciting disease causing arterial hypertension and at alleviating injury to end organs affected by the hypertensive state. Management includes dietary sodium restriction and pharmacologic therapy in relationship to the severity and responsiveness of the hypertensive state.

Dietary sodium should be reduced to constitute 0.1 to 0.3 percent of the diet on a dry matter basis for dogs and 0.4 percent for cats. Dietary sodium intake should be gradually reduced over 3 to 4 weeks while renal function is monitored. Altered renal function may occur in animals with renal insufficiency as sodium balance is re-established.[85,140]

Drug strategies employ diuretics for initial pharmacologic management, β-adrenergic antagonists as second-stage antihypertensive medications, and vasodilators for cases refractory to other measures. Current pharmacologic therapies are generally empirical and require more extensive clinical testing.

ANEMIA

Acute anemia results in tissue hypoxia due to reduced oxygen-carrying capactiy. Vascular dilation, decreased peripheral vascular resistance, and lower blood viscosity cause cardiac output to increase, thereby restoring normal tissue oxygen supply.[145–147] With chronic anemia of moderate severity, increased cardiac work is not usually required for compensatory adjustments in oxygen flow. Decreased oxygen affinity results from a shift in the oxygen dissociation curve to the right by increased synthesis of 2,3-diphosphoglycerate, which decreases hemoglobin affinity for oxygen and enhances oxygen unloading.[148] In addition, blood redistribution among tissues improves oxygen flow.[145]

It is believed that anemia may cause congestive heart failure mainly when underlying cardiac disease is present.[149] The anemia causes a high cardiac output state, which increases cardiac work. In humans, cardiac enlargement and congestive heart failure from chronic blood loss anemia is unlikely unless hemoglobin concentration is below 5 g/dl blood.[150]

NEOPLASIA

The heart may be affected by cancer by direct tumor infiltration or indirectly by systemic or paraneoplastic syndromes. Cardiac neoplasms may be classifed by location or histologic type. Possible mechanisms for metastasis include direct extension, implantation, hematogenous spread, and lymphatic transfer.[151,152]

Table 27-3 Clinical Features Suggestive of
Cardiac Neoplasia

Syncope
General or episodic weakness
Dyspnea
Weight loss
Arrhythmias[a]
Radiographic findings
    Normal cardiac silhouette (cardiac metastases)
    Abnormal cardiac silhouette
        Some heart-base tumors
        Pericardial effusion
    Abnormal anterior mediastinum
Hemopericardium/hemothorax
Obstructive effusions (pericardial, thoracic, abdominal)
Congestive heart failure
Cardiac tamponade
Heart murmur
Jugular venous distention
Multiorgan neoplastic metastases[b]

[a] Especially with a radiographically normal cardiac silhouette in older animals with myocardial metastasis.
[b] Diagnostic ultrasound useful in this assessment.

Clinical recognition of cardiac neoplasia is often difficult (Table 27-3). Since dyspnea is a common finding associated with cardiopulmonary metastasis, differential diagnosis must include pre-existing chronic lung disease, pleural effusion, pneumonia, heartworm disease, pulmonary emboli, congestive heart failure, and pericardial disease. A diagnostic workup includes the standard laboratory data base, ECG, chest and abdominal radiographs, and cytologic evaluation of pericardial, pleural, or abdominal effusions. Specialized tests are often necessary, such as echocardiography or pneumopericardiography.

During evaluation of the heart and pericardium, nonneoplastic lesions may appear grossly, clinically, or echocardiographically as tumors. Examples include mural thrombi, excessive moderator band networks, diaphragmatic hernias, infectious endocarditis, myocardial abscesses, and Chiari's network (remnants of the right-sided valve of the sinus venosus).[151]

In order to diagnose cardiac neoplasia, one must maintain a high index of suspicion. Hemodynamic abnormalities secondary to arrhythmias, pericardial effusion, space-occupying lesions, or systemic em-

bolism may result from cancer involving the heart or pericardium.

Hemangiosarcoma is the most common canine tumor. Heart-base tumors (chemodectomas) occur less frequently (Ch. 23). Lymphosarcoma occasionally infiltrates the myocardium (Ch. 22). Various other tumors may affect the heart.

Therapy is usually unrewarding. There has been little benefit from chemotherapy in malignant cardiac tumors.[153]

INFECTIOUS DISEASES

Myocarditis is an inflammatory process involving myocytes or interstitium; it may result from bacterial, mycotic, viral, rickettsial, and parasitic organisms. Clinical manifestation vary widely from asymptomatic to fatal arrhythmias and congestive heart failure. Often, the underlying systemic infection overshadows cardiac manifestations. The ECG may be normal or may display atrial or ventricular arrhythmias, conduction defects, or ST-T abnormalities.[1-3] Specific forms of myocarditis and infective agents are discussed in Chapters 21, 22, and 23.

CHEMICAL AND DRUG TOXICITIES

Myocardial cellular injury from toxins may result from microvascular spasm, highly reactive oxygen radicals, calcium ion excess, metabolic abnormalities, vasoactive hormones, or cellular hormone receptor abnormalities.[1-3] Doxorubicin, an antineoplastic agent, has as its major limiting factor cardiac toxicity (Chs. 22 and 23). Free radical generation and peroxidation of subcellular membranes may cause myocardial injury. Other toxins affecting the heart include fluorinated hydrocarbons, spider and snake venom, digitalis glycosides, other heavy metals, and hypersensitivity reactions to various drugs and agents.

OBESITY

Obesity may predispose to a number of cardiovascular abnormalities that increase morbidity and mortality. An association between obesity and hypertension has been established.[154] Weight reduction reduces arterial pressure in both normotensive and hypertensive persons.[155] The obesity hypoventilation syndrome (pickwickian syndrome) is thought to be caused by hypoventilation due to reduced respiratory center activity.[156] This usually accompanies older small breed dogs with chronic obstructive pulmonary disease and collapsed trachea. Many of these dogs have increased vagal tone with associated sinus arrhythmia and occasionally, second-degree AV block.

COR PULMONALE

Pulmonary heart disease refers to a cardiac disorder resulting from abnormalities in pulmonary circulation. It describes cor pulmonale, a form of secondary right heart disease and potentially, right ventricular failure, precipitated by acute or chronic pressure overload from pulmonary hypertension. Cor pulmonale may refer to (1) increased pulmonary vascular resistance or pulmonary arterial pressure due to primary lung disease; or (2) right ventricular hypertrophy secondary to longstanding pulmonary mechanical vascular obstruction (e.g., pulmonary emboli) or to pulmonary arterial vasoconstriction with subsequent muscular hyperplasia.[157–159] Pulmonary arterial vasoconstriction is mediated by some combination of alveolar hypoxia, low mixed-venous oxygen tension, respiratory acidosis, and possibly hypercapnia.[160,161] A diagnosis of cor pulmonale is excluded if pulmonary hypertension results from congenital heart disease or left-sided heart disorders.[157–159]

Pathophysiology

The cause of pulmonary arterial hypertension resulting in cor pulmonale depends on the specific underlying disease process. Basically, it is due to loss of effective pulmonary vascular units. Pulmonary vascular resistance increases and pulmonary hypertension develops. Eventually, the right ventricle may fail. Resting and exercise cardiac output may fall.[161] A reduction of more than 50 percent of the cross-sectional pulmonary vasculature must occur before pulmonary hypertension will result.[158]

Various disorders may be associated with cor pul-

monale. In older dogs, chronic obstructive pulmonary disease is common. It is a term applied to the clinical syndrome produced by multiple pathologic conditions, including bronchitis, bronchiolitis, and emphysema. Obesity (pickwickian syndrome) is a frequent contributing factor that adversely affects mechanical respiration. Alveolar hypoventilation and hypoxemia may result causing pulmonary arteriolar vasoconstriction.[157] Heartworm infection can cause pulmonary artery disease (intimal proliferation) and cor pulmonale.[162,163] Decreased pulmonary vascular patency may occur by mechanical obstruction from thromboembolism with hyperadrenocorticism, endocarditis, renal amyloidosis, and nephrotic syndrome.[164,165]

Diagnosis

Acute cor pulmonale may have acute or gradual cardiopulmonary signs, including anorexia, weakness, depression, or panting. Severe cases display orthopnea, cyanosis, and sudden death. Coughing is uncommon. Chronic cor pulmonale is associated with more gradual development of respiratory signs (dyspnea, wheezing, chronic cough). Dogs and cats with chronic obstructive pulmonary disease may exhibit a chronic cough, expiratory effort or prolongation, expiratory wheeze, and air trapping evident on thoracic radiographs. The latter often shows enlargement of the right heart and pulmonary artery segment. Auscultation may reveal a prominent or split second heart sound, a soft systolic murmur of tricuspid insufficiency, or abnormal lung sounds. If right-sided congestive heart failure is present, there may be jugular venous distention with jugular pulses, muffled heart and lung sounds due to pleural or pericardial effusions, hepatosplenomegaly, or peripheral edema. Electrocardiographic changes are inconsistent and variable with cor pulmonale. Sensitivity and specificity of the ECG for right-axis deviation (greater than 105 degrees in the frontal plane) is low. Increased P-wave amplitude (P-pulmonale) may occur in dogs with chronic cor pulmonale.[157–161]

Treatment

Theraputic strategies should strive to relieve arterial hypoxemia and thereby reverse pulmonary vasoconstriction. This decreases right ventricular workload by reducing pulmonary hypertension. Treatment must be individualized to alleviate respiratory failure with respect to the cause and severity of the underlying disorders.[157,158,160,166] Improvement of respiratory gas exchange with supplemental oxygen (35 to 50 percent oxygen enriched mixture) helps reverse hypoxemia and respiratory acidosis.[167] Bronchodilators may improve reversible airway obstruction and improve pulmonary gas exchange. Antibiotics should be considered if a bacterial infectious component is suspected.[168] Corticosteroid use must be carefully assessed as to its likely effect on underlying abnormalities. Pulmonary thromboembolism may be treated with strict cage rest, oxygen, and anticoagulation therapy (e.g., heparin and vitamin K antagonists and/or antiplatelet drugs such as aspirin).[158] Cardiac measures for right ventricular failure include strict cage rest and furosemide. Digitalization is controversial, and vasodilators should be used cautiously, if at all. Weight reduction is encouraged in obese animals. Other specific therapy (e.g., sodium thiacetarsemide) is directed at specific underlying disorders. Prognosis is linked to the underlying pulmonary disorder.

NUTRITIONAL DISORDERS

One of the most striking nutritional disorders affecting the heart is myocardial failure in cats associated with taurine deficiency[169] (Chs. 10 and 22). Carnitine deficiency has been demonstrated using endomyocardial biopsy in some dogs (especially boxers) with dilated cardiomyopathy.[170] Nutritional abnormalities and heart disease is a growing topic of clinical investigation.

MISCELLANEOUS DISORDERS

Pheochromocytomas are tumors of the adrenal cortex or paraganglia. They are rare in the dog (6 to 10 percent are malignant) and are not reported in the cat. They may secrete catecholamines causing tachycardia, arrhythmias, and myocardial injury. Alternatively, they may secrete peptide hormones such as vasoactive intestinal peptide, adrenocortical hormone, calcitonin, or parathyroid hormone. Clinical signs result from compression, invasion of

surrounding tissues (especially the caudal vena cava), or secretory products. Excision is the only satisfactory treatment.[171,172]

Cardiac glycogenosis (glycogen storage disease of the heart, Pompe's disease) has been diagnosed in Lapland dogs[173] (Ch. 23). Mucopolysaccharidosis has been reported in cats, but cardiac involvement has not been significant.[174,175] Persistent atrial standstill has been associated with a fascioscapulohumeral-like skeletal muscular dystrophy in dogs, especially English spaniels.[176]

REFERENCES

1. Wenger NK, Goodwin JF, Roberts WC: Cardiomyopathy and myocardial involvement in systemic disease. p. 1181. In Hurst JW (ed): The Heart. McGraw-Hill, New York, 1986
2. Wynne JW, Braunwald E: The cardiomyopathies and myocarditides. p. 1399. In Braunwald E (ed): Heart Disease. 2nd Ed. WB Saunders, Philadelphia, 1984
3. Fox PR: Cardiovascular disorders in system diseases. p. 265. In Tilley LP, Owens JM (eds): Manual of Small Animal Cardiology. Churchill Livingstone, New York, 1985
4. Peterson ME, Kintzer PP, Cavanagh PG, et al: Feline hyperthyroidism: Pre-treatment clinical and laboratory evaluation of 131 cases. J Am Vet Med Assoc 183:103, 1983
5. Peterson ME: Feline hyperthyroidism. Vet Clin North Am 14:809, 1984
6. Loar AS: Canine thyroid tumors. p. 1033. In Kirk RW (ed): Current Veterinary Therapy. Vol. IX. WB Saunders, Philadelphia, 1986
7. Feldman EC, Melson RW: Hypothyroidism. In Canine and Feline Endocrinology and Reproduction. WB Saunders, Philadelphia, 1987
8. Milne KL, Hayes HM: Epidemiologic features of canine hypothyroidism. Cornell Vet 71:3, 1981
9. Muller GH, Kirk RW, Scott DW: Small Animal Dermatology. 3rd Ed. WB Saunders, Philadelphia, 1983
10. Nesbitt GH, Izzo J, Peterson ME, et al: Canine hypothyroidism: A retrospective study of 108 cases. J Am Vet Med Assoc 177:1117, 1980
11. Manning PJ: Thyroid gland and arterial lesions in Beagles with familial hypothyroidism and hyperlipoprotienemia. J Am Vet Med Assoc 40:820, 1979
12. Patterson JS, Pusley MS, Zachary JF: Neurological manifestations of cerebrovascular atherosclerosis as-

sociated with primary hypothyroidism in a dog. J Am Vet Med Assoc 186:499, 1985

13. Braunwald E, Sonnenblick EH, Spann JF, et al: Effects of heart failure, ventricular hypertrophy and alterations in the thyroid state on the contractility of isolated cardiac muscle. Ann NY Acad Sci 156:379, 1969

14. Goel BG, Hanson CS, Han BS: Atrioventricular conduction in hyper and hypothyroid dogs. Am Heart J 83:504, 1972

15. Skelton CL, Sonnenblick EH: The cardiovascular system. p. 1140. In Ingbar SH, Braverman LE (eds): The Thyroid. 5th Ed. JB Lippincott, Philadelphia, 1986

16. Nijhuis AH, Stokhuf AA, Huisman GH, et al: ECG changes in dogs with hypothyroidism. Tijdschr Diergeneesk 103:736, 1985

17. Stiles GL, Stadel JM, DeLean A, et al: Hypothyroidism modulates beta-adrenergic receptor-adenylate cyclase interaction in rat reticulocyles. J Clin Invest 68:1450, 1981

18. Ganong WF: The thyroid gland. p. 250. In Ganong WF (ed): Review of Medical Physiology. 10th Ed. Lange Medical Publications, Los Altos, CA, 1981

19. Santos AD, Miller RP, Mathew PK: Echocardiographic characterization of the reversible cardiomyopathy of hypothyroidism. Am J Med 68:675, 1980

20. Taylor RR, Covell JW, Ross J: Influence of the thyroid state on left ventricular tension-velocity relations in the intact, sedated dog. J Clin Invest 48:775, 1969

21. Miller CW, Boone JA, Soderberg SA, et al: Echocardiographic assessment of cardiac function in beagles with experimentally produced hypothyroidism. J Ultrasound Med 3(suppl):157, 1984

22. Calvert CA, Chapman WL, Toal RL: Congestive cardiomyopathy in Doberman pinscher dogs. J Am Vet Med Assoc 181:598, 1982

23. Ferguson DC: Thyroid function tests in the dog. Recent concepts. Vet Clin North Am 14:783, 1984

24. Rosychuk RA: Management of hypothyroidism. p. 869. In Kirk RW (ed): Current Veterinary Therapy. Vol. VIII. WB Saunders, Philadelphia, 1983

25. Chastain CB: Canine hypothyroidism. J Am Vet Med Assoc 181:345, 1982

26. Rijnberk A: Hypothyroidism. p. 791. In Kirk RW (ed): Current Veterinary Therapy. Vol. V. WB Saunders, Philadelphia, 1974

27. Feldman EL, Tyrrell JB: Hypoadrenocorticism. Vet Clin North Am 7:555, 1977

28. Johnessee JS, Peterson ME, Gilbertson SR: Primary hypoadrenocorticism in a cat. J Am Vet Med Assoc 183:881, 1983

29. Mulnix JA: Hypoadrenocorticism in the dog. J Am Anim Hosp Assoc 7:220, 1971

30. Schaer M: Hypoadrenocorticism. In Kirk RW (ed): p. 983. Current Veterinary Therapy. Vol. VII. WB Saunders, Philadelphia, 1980

31. Willard MD, Schall WD, McCaw DE, et al: Canine hypoadrenocorticism: Report of 37 cases and review of 39 previously reported cases. J Am Vet Med Assoc 180:59, 1982

32. Liddle GW: The adrenals. p. 249. In Williams RA (ed): Textbook of Endocrinology. 6th Ed. WB Saunders, Philadelphia, 1981

33. Liddle GW: The adrenals. p. 249. In Williams RH (ed): Textbook of Endocrinology. WB Saunders, Philadelphia, 1981

34. Capen CC, Martin SL: Endocrine disorders. p. 1351. In Ettinger SJ (ed): Textbook of Veterinary Internal Medicine. WB Saunders, Philadelphia, 1978

35. Feldman EL, Peterson ME: Hypoadrenocorticism. Vet Clin North Am 14:751, 1984

36. Fruhman LA, Baxter JD, Tyrrell JB: The adrenal cortex. p. 385. In Felix P (ed): Endocrinology and Metabolism. McGraw-Hill, New York, 1981

37. Christy NP: Adrenal cortical steroids in various types of hypertension. p. 169. In Manger MW (ed): Hormones and Hypertension. Charles C Thomas, Springfield, IL, 1966

38. Lefer AM: Corticosteroids and circulatory function. p. 191. In Greep RO, Astwood EB (eds): Handbook of Physiology. Sect 7: Endocrinology. Vol. VI: Adrenal Gland. American Physiological Society, Washington, DC, 1975

39. Baxter TD: Glucocorticoid hormone action. p. 67. In Gill GW (ed): Pharmacology of Adrenal Cortical Hormones. Pergamon, Oxford, 1979

40. Rendano OJ, Alexander JE: Heart size changes in experimentally-induced adrenal insufficiency in the dog: A radiographic study. J Am Vet Radiol Soc 17:57, 1976

41. Kanis CL, Lowenstein JL: The emergency treatment of hyperkalemia. Med Clin North Am 65:165, 1981

42. Feldman EC: The adrenal cortex. p. 1650. In Ettinger SJ (ed): Textbook of Veterinary Internal Medicine. 2nd Ed. WB Saunders, Philadelphia, 1983

43. Owens JM, Drucker WD: Hyperadrenocorticism in the dog: Canine Cushing's syndrome. Vet Clin North Am 7:583, 1977

44. Scott DW: Hyperadrenocorticism (hyperadrenocorticism, hyperadrenocorticalism, Cushing's Disease, Cushing's syndrome). Vet Clin North Am 9:3, 1979

45. Feldman EC: Distinguishing dogs with functioning adrenocortical tumors from dogs with pituitary-dependent hyperadrenocorticism. J Am Vet Med Assoc 183:195, 1983

46. Peterson ME, Drucker WD: Advances in the diagnosis and treatment of canine Cushing's syndrome. p. 17. In Proceedings of the Gaines Veterinary Symposium, 1981

47. Peterson ME, Gilbertson SR, Drucker WD: Plasma cortisol responses to exogenous ACTH in 22 dogs with hyperadrenocorticism caused by adrenocortical neoplasia. J Am Vet Med Assoc 180:542, 1982

48. Peterson ME, Cavanagh PG, Willard M, et al: Pituitary-dependent canine hyperadrenocorticism with spontaneous remission. p. 19. In Proceedings of the American College of Veterinary Internal Medicine, 1982

49. Peterson ME: Hyperadrenocorticism. Vet Clin North Am 14:731, 1984

50. Huntlegy K, Frazer J, Gibbs C, et al: The radiological features of canine Cushing's syndrome. A review of forty-eight cases. J Small Anim Pract 23:369, 1982

51. Kallett A, Cowgill LD: Hypertensive states in the dog. p. 79. In Proceedings of the American College of Veterinary Internal Medicine, 1982

52. Krakoff L, Nicolis G, Amsel B: Pathogenesis of hypertension in Cushing's syndrome. Am J Med 58:216, 1975

53. Kalsner S: Mechanism of hydrocortisone potentiation of response to epinephrine and norepinephrine in rat aorta. Circ Res 24:383, 1969

54. Sjoberg HE, Blomback M, Granberg PO: Thromboembolic complications, heparin treatment and increased coagulation factors in Cushing's syndrome. Acta Med Scand 199:95, 1976

55. Burns MS, Kelley AB, Hornof WJ, et al: Pulmonary artery thrombosis in three dogs with hyperadrenocorticism. J Am Vet Med Assoc 178:388, 1981

56. King RR, Mauderly JL, Hahn FF, et al: Pulmonary function studies in a dog with pulmonary thromboembolism associated with Cushing's disease. J Am Anim Hosp Assoc 21:555, 1985

57. Feldman EC: Comparison of ACTH response and dexamethasone suppression as screening tests in canine hyperadrenocorticism. J Am Vet Med Assoc 182:506, 1983

58. Feldman EC: The effect of functional adrenocortical tumors on plasma cortisol and corticotropin concentrations in dogs. J Am Vet Med Assoc 178:823, 1981

59. Meijer MC, Lubberink AAME, Rijnberk A, et al: Adrenocortical function tests in dogs with hyperfunctioning adrenocortical tumors. J Endocrinol 80:315, 1979

60. Peterson ME: o,p'-DDD (mitotane) treatment of canine pituitary-dependent hyperadrenocorticism. J Am Vet Med Assoc 182:527, 1983

61. Eigenmann JE, Lubberink ME: The adrenals. p. 1851. In Slatter DH (ed): Textbook of Small Animal Surgery. Vol. II. WB Saunders, Philadelphia, 1985

62. Daugheday WH: The anterior pituitary. p. 600. In Wilson JD, Foster DN (eds): Williams Textbook of Endocrinology. 7th Ed. WB Saunders, Philadelphia, 1985

63. Jackson IMD: Growth-hormone-secreting pituitary adenomas. p. 109. In Post KD, Jackson IMD, Richlins S (eds): The Pituitary Adenoma. Plenum Medical Book Co, New York, 1980

64. Melmed S, Braunstein D, Horvath E, et al: Pathophysiology of acromegly. Endocrinol Rev 4:271, 1983

65. Jadresic A, Banks LM, Child DF, et al: The acromegaly syndrome. Q J Med 202:189, 1982

66. Rabin D, McKenna TJ: The pituitary gland. p. 13. In Rabin D, McKenna TJ (eds): Clinical Endocrinology and Metabolism. Grune & Stratton, Orlando, FL, 1982

67. Eigenmann, JE: Acromegaly in the dog. Vet Clin North Am 14:827, 1984

68. Rijnberk A, Eigenmann JE, Belshaw BE, et al: Acromegaly associated with transient overproduction of growth hormone in a dog. J Am Vet Med Assoc 177:534, 1980

69. Eigenmann JE, Venker-van Haagen AJ: Progestogen-induced and spontaneous canine acromegaly due to reversible growth hormone overproduction: Clinical picture and pathogenesis. J Am Anim Hosp Assoc 17:813, 1981

70. Eigenmann JE, Eigenmann RY, Rijnberk A, et al: Progesterone-controlled growth hormone overproduction and naturally occurring canine diabetes and acromegaly. Acta Endocrinol (Copenh) 104:167, 1983

71. Eigenmann JE, Wortman JA, Haskins ME: Elevated growth hormone levels and diabetes mellitus in a cat with acromegalic features. J Am Anim Hosp Assoc 20:747, 1984

72. Scott DW, Concannon PW: Gross and microscopic changes in the skin of dogs with progestagen-induced acromegaly and elevated growth hormone levels. J Am Anim Hosp Assoc 19:523, 1983

73. Graf KJ, El Etreby MF: The role of the anterior pituitary gland in progestogen-induced mammary gland changes in the beagle. Drug Res 28:54, 1978

74. Eigenmann JE, Wortman JA, Haskins ME: Elevated growth hormone levels and diabetes mellitus in a cat with acromegalic features. J Am Anim Hosp Assoc 20:747, 1984

75. Kellgren JH, Ball J, Tuttan GK: The articular and other limb changes in acromegaly. Q J Med 21:405, 1952

76. Williams GH, Braunwald E: Endocrine and nutritional disorders and heart disease. p. 1825. In Braunwald E (ed): Heart Disease: A Textbook of Cardiovascular Medicine. WB Saunders, Philadelphia, 1980

77. Strauch G, Vallotton MB, Tomton Y: The renin-angiotensin-aldosterone system in normotensive and hypertensive patients with acromegaly. N Engl J Med 287:795, 1972

78. Pepine CJ, Aloia J: Heart muscle disease in acromegaly. Am J Med 48:530, 1970

79. Jahn HA, Schohn DC, Schmitt RL: The heart in renal disease. p. 988. In Cheng TO (ed): The International Textbook of Cardiology. Pergamon Press, New York, 1986

80. Pehrson SK, Jonasson R, Lins LE: Cardiac performance in various stages of renal failure. Br Heart J 52:667, 1984

81. Beierholm EA, Grantham RN, O'Keefe DD, et al: Effects of acid-base changes, hypoxia and catecholamines on ventricular performance. Am J Physiol 228:1555, 1975

82. Scheuer J, Stezoski SW: The effects of uremic compounds on cardiac function and metabolism. J Mol Cell Cardiol 5:287, 1973

83. Varat MA, Adolph RJ, Fowler NO: Cardiovascular effects of anemia. Am Heart J 83:415, 1972

84. Massry SG: Parathyroid hormone and uremic myocardiopathy. Contrib Nephrol 41:231, 1984

85. Cowgill LD, Kallet AJ: Systemic hypertension. p. 360. In Kirk RW (ed): Current Veterinary Therapy. Vol. IX. WB Saunders, Philadelphia, 1986

86. Weidmann P, Maxwell MH, Tuper AN, et al: Plasma renin activity and blood pressure in terminal renal failure. N Engl J Med 285:757, 1971

87. Davies DL, Schalekamp MA, Beevers DG, et al: Abnormal relation between exchangeable sodium and the renin-angiotension system in malignant hypertension and in hypertension with chronic renal failure. Lancet 1:683, 1973

88. Fisch C: Relation of electrolyte disturbances to cardiac arrhythmias. Circulation 47:408, 1973

89. Hodgkin AL, Horowitz P: The influence of potassium and chloride ions on the membrane potential of single muscle fibers. J Physiol (Lond) 148:127, 1959

90. Tilley LP: Essentials of Canine and Feline Electrocardiology. 2nd Ed. Lea & Febiger, Philadelphia, 1985

91. Ettinger PO, Regan TJ, Oldewurtel HA: Hyperkalemia, cardiac conduction and the electrocardiogram: A review. Am Heart J 88:360, 1974

92. Surawicz B: Electrolytes and the electrocardiogram. Postgrad Med 55:123, 1974

93. Kanis CL, Lowenstein J: The emergency treatment of hyperkalemia. Med Clin North Am 65:165, 1981

94. Schaer M: Hyperkalemia in cats with urethral obstruction: Electrocardiographic abnormalities and treatment. Vet Clin North Am 7:407, 1977

95. Schaer M: Disorders of sodium and potassium homeostasis. p. 211. In Proceedings of the American Animal Hospital Association, 1977

96. Cox M: Potassium homeostasis. Med Clin North Am 65:363, 1981

97. Lowenstein J: Hypokalemia and hyperkalemia. Med Clin North Am 57:1435, 1973

98. Knochel JP: Neuromuscular manifestations of electrolyte disorders. Am J Med 72:521, 1982

99. Epstein FH: Signs and symptoms of electrolyte disorders. In Maxwell MH, Kleenan CR (eds): Clinical Disorders of Fluid and Electrolyte Metabolism. 3rd Ed. McGraw-Hill, New York, 1980

100. Henrikson HW: Effect of potassium deficiency in gastrointestinal motility in rats. Am J Physiol 164:263, 1951

101. Schuster MM: Megacolon in adults. p. 1812. In Sleisenger MH, Fordtran IS (eds): Gastrointestional Disease. 2nd Ed. WB Saunders, Philadelphia, 1978

102. Feldman EC: Influence of non-cardiac disease on the heart. p. 340. In Kirk RW (ed): Current Veterinary Therapy. Vol. VII. WB Saunders, Philadelphia, 1980

103. Schaer M: Disorders of potassium metabolism. Vet Clin North Am 12:399, 1982

104. Dubois GD, Arieff AI: Clinical manifestations of electrolyte disorders. p. 1087. In Arief AI, Detrinto RA (eds): Fluid, Electrolytes and Acid-Base Disorders. Churchill Livingstone, New York, 1985

105. Lindeman D, Papper S: Therapy of fluid and electrolyte disorders. Ann Intern Med 82:64, 1975

106. Hammond PB: Drugs altering the fluid balance. p. 829. In Jones LM (ed): Veterinary Pharmacology and Therapeutics. Iowa State University Press, Ames, 1965

107. Greene RW, Scott RC: Lower Urinary Tract Disease. p. 1572. In Ettinger SJ (ed): Textbook of Veterinary Internal Medicine. WB Saunders, Philadelphia, 1975

108. Chew DJ, Meuten DJ: Disorders of calcium and phophorous metabolism. Vet Clin North Am 12:411, 1982

109. MacEwen EG, Siegel SD: Hypercalcemia: A paraneoplastic disease. Vet Clin North Am 7:187, 1977

110. Osborne CA, Stevens JB: Pseudohyperparathyroidism in the dog. J Am Vet Med Assoc 162:125, 1973

111. Hause WR, Stevenson S, Meuten DJ, et al: Pseudohyperparathyroidism associated with adenocarci-

noma of anal sac origin in four dogs. J Am Anim Hosp Assoc 17:373, 1981

112. Meuten DJ, Cooper BJ, Capen CC, et al: Hypercalcemia associated with an adenocarcinoma derived form the apocrine glands of the anal sac. Vet Pathol 18:454, 1981

113. Peterson ME, Feinman JM: Hypercalcemia associated with hypoadrenocorticism in sixteen dogs. J Am Vet Med Assoc 181:802, 1982

114. Berger B, Feldman EC: Primary hyperparathyroidism in dogs: 21 cases (1976–1986). J Am Vet Med Assoc 191:350, 1987

115. Skrabanen JB, McPartlin J, Purvell D: Tumor hypercalcemia and ectopic hyperparathyroidism. Medicine (Baltimore) 59:262, 1980

116. Meuten DJ: Hypercalcemia. Vet Clin North Am 14:891, 1984

117. Finco PR, Rawland GW: Hypercalcemia secondary to chronic renal failure in the dog: A report of four cases. J Am Vet Med Assoc 173:990, 1978

118. Watson ADJ, Canfield PJ: Renal failure, hyperparathyroidism and hypercalcemia in a dog. Aust Vet J 55:177, 1979

119. Peterson P: Psychiatric disorders in primary hyperparathyroidism. J Clin Endocrinol Metab 28:1491, 1968

120. Sarawitz B, Geltes LS: Effect of electrolyte disorders on the heart and circulation. p. 539. In Conn HL, Jr, Horowitz O (eds): Cardiac and Vascular Disease. Lea & Febiger, Philadelphia, 1971

121. Bronsky D, Dubin A, Walstein SJ, et al: Calcium and the electrocardiogram: The electrocardiographic manifestation of marked hypercalcemia. Am J Cardiol 1:833, 1961

122. Altura BJ: Influence of calcium ions on microvascular permeability, contractibility and reactivity. Adv Microcirc 11:62, 1982

123. Local effect of sodium, calcium and magnesium upon small and large blood vessels of the dog forelimb. Circ Res 8:57, 1960

124. Lins BE: Renal function in hypercalcemic dogs during hydropenia and during saline infusions. Acta Physiol Scand 106:177, 1979

125. Parfitt AM, Kleere Kuper M: Clinical disorders of calcium, phosphorus and magnesium metabolism. In Maxwell MH, Kleeman CK (eds): Clinical Disorders of Fluid and Electrolyte Metabolism. McGraw-Hill, New York, 1980

126. Ong SC, Shalitone RJ, Gallagher P, et al: Effect of furosemide in experimental hypercalcemia in dogs. Proc Soc Exp Biol Med 145:227, 1974

127. Strumpf M, Dowalski MA, Mandy GR: Effects of glucocorticoids on osteoclast-activating factor. J Lab Clin Med 92:772, 1978

128. Chew DJ, Meuten DJ: Disorders of calcium and phosphorus metabolism. Vet Clin North Am 12:411, 1982

129. Capen CC, Martin SL: Calcium metabolism and disorder of the parathyroid glands. Vet Clin North Am 7:513, 1977

130. Schaer M, Cavanagh P, Hause W, et al: Iatrogenic hyperphosphatemia, hypocalcemia and hypernatremia in a cat. J Am Anim Hosp Assoc 13:39, 1977

131. Sherding RG, Meuten DJ, Chew DJ, et al: Primary hypoparathyroidism in the dog. J Am Vet Med Assoc 176:439, 1980

132. Dubois GD, Ariett AI: Clinical manifestations of electrolyte disorders. p. 1087. In Ariet AI, Detrinto RA (eds): Fluid, Electrolytes and Acid-Base Disorders. Churchill Livingstone, New York, 1985

133. Shiner PT, Harris WS, Weissler AM: Effects of acute changes in serum calcium levels in the systolic time intervals in man. Am J Cardiol 24:42, 1969

134. Peterson ME: Hypoparathyroidism. p. 1039. In Kirk RW (ed): Current Veterinary Therapy. Vol. IX. WB Saunders, Philadelphia, 1986

135. Schohn D, Weidman P, Jahn H, et al: Norepinephrine related mechanism in hypertension accompanying renal failure. Kidney Int 28:814, 1985

136. Liard JF, Tarazi RC, Ferrario CM, et al: Hemodynamic and humeral characteristics of hypertension induced by prolonged stellate ganglion stimulation in conscious dogs. Circ Res 36:455, 1975

137. Oparil S, Haber E: The renin-angiotension system. N Engl J Med 291:389, 446, 1974

138. Guyton AC, Coleman TG, Cowley AW Jr, et al: Arterial pressure regulation: Overriding dominance of the kidneys in long-term regulation and in hypertension. Am J Med 52:584, 1972

139. Koch-Weser J: The therapeutic challenge of systolic hypertension. N Engl J Med 289:481, 1973

140. Ross LA: Hypertension—Pathophysiology and management. Proc Am Anim Hosp Assoc 54:350, 1987

141. Kittleson MD, Olivier NB: Measurement of systemic arterial blood pressure. Vet Clin North Am 13:321, 1983

142. Weiser MG, Spangler WL, Gribble DH: Blood pressure measurement in the dog. J Am Vet Med Assoc 171:364, 1977

143. Gordon DB, Goldblatt H: Direct percutaneous determination of systemic blood pressure and production of renal hypertension in the cat. Proc Soc Exp Biol Med 125:177, 1967

144. Morgan RV: Systemic hypertension in four cats: Ocular and medical findings. J Am Anim Hosp Assoc 22:615, 1986

145. Erslev AJ, Caro J: Anemia of cancer and its cardiovascular effects. p. 185. In Kappor AS, Reynolds RD (eds): Cancer and the Heart. Springer-Verlag, New York, 1986

146. Fowler NO, Holmes JC: Blood viscosity and cardiac output in acute experimental anemia. J Appl Physiol 39:453, 1975

147. Fowler NO, Holmes JC: Ventricular function in anemia. J Appl Physiol 31:260, 1971

148. Bellingham AJ, Grimes AJ: Red cell 2,3-diphosphoglycerate. Br J Haematol 25:555, 1973

149. Varat MA, Adolph RJ, Fowler NO: Cardiovascular effects of anemia. Am Heart J 83:415, 1972

150. Fowler NO: High cardiac output states. p. 395. In Hurst JW (ed): The Heart. 6th Ed. McGraw-Hill, New York, 1986

151. Lammers RJ, Bloor CM: Pathology of cardiac tumors. p. 1. In Kapoor AS, Reynolds RD (eds): Cancer and the Heart. Springer-Verlag, New York, 1986

152. Smith LH: Secondary tumors of the heart. Rev Surg 33:223, 1976

153. Reynolds RD: Medical management of cardiac tumors. In Kapoor AS, Reynolds RD (eds): Cancer and the Heart. Springer-Verlag, New York, 1986

154. Berchtold P, Jorgen SV, Kemmer M, et al: Obesity and hypertension: Cardiovascular response to weight reduction—A review. Hypertension 4:50, 1982

155. Reisin E, Abel R, Modan M, et al: Effect of weight loss without salt restriction on the reduction of blood pressure in overweight hypertensive patients. N Engl J Med 298:1, 1978

156. Rochester DF, Enson Y: Current concepts in the pathogenesis of the obesity-hypoventilation syndrome: Mechanical and circulatory factors. Am J Med 57:402, 1972

157. Fox PR: Cor pulmonale. p. 313. In Kirk RW (ed): Current Veterinary Therapy. Vol. VIII. WB Saunders, Philadelphia, 1983

158. Spaulding GL, Owens JM: Cor pulmonale. p. 167. In Tilley LP, Owens JM (eds): Manual of Small Animal Cardiology. Churchill Livingstone, New York, 1985

159. Ferrer MI: Cor pulmonale (pulmonary heart disease): Present day status. Am Heart J 89:657, 1975

160. Welch MH: Obstructive diseases. p. 663. In Guenther CA, Welch MH (eds): Pulmonary Medicine. 2nd Ed. JB Lippincott, Philadelphia, 1982

161. Fishman AP: Chronic cor pulmonale. p. 355. In Lung Diseases: State of the Art, 1976–1977. American Lung Association, New York, 1978

162. Knight DH: Heartworm disease. p. 1097. In Ettinger SJ (ed): Textbook of Veterinary Internal Medicine. 2nd Ed. WB Saunders, Philadelphia, 1983

163. Dillon R: Feline dirofilariasis. Vet Clin North Am 14:1185, 1984

164. Burns MG, Kelly AB, Hornoff WJ, et al: Pulmonary artery thrombosis in three dogs with hyperadrenocorticism. J Am Vet Med Assoc 178:388, 1981

165. Burns MG: Pulmonary thromboembolism. p. 257. In Kirk RW (ed): Current Veterinary Therapy. Vol. VIII. WB Saunders, Philadelphia, 1983

166. Spence TH: Acute respiratory failure in chronic obstructive lung disease. p. 260. In Kirby RR, Taylor RW (eds): Respiratory Failure. Year Book Medical Publishers, Chicago, 1986

167. Eldridge F, Gherman C: Studies of oxygen administration in respiratory failure. Ann Intern Med 68:569, 1968

168. Petty TL: Management of acute and chronic bronchitis. p. 149. In Sande MA, Root RK (eds): Respiratory Infections. Vol. 5. Churchill Livingstone, New York, 1986

169. Pion PD, Kittleson MD, Rogers QR, et al: Myocardial failure in cats associated with low plasma taurine: A reversible cardiomyopathy. Science 237:697, 1987

170. Keene BW, Panciera DL, Regitz V, et al: Carnitine-linked defects of myocardial metabolism in canine dilated cardiomyopathy. Proceedings of the Fourth Annual Veterinary Medicine Forum, American College of Veterinary Internal Medicine. Vol. II. p.14–54, 1986 (abst)

171. Twedt DC, Wheeler SL: Pheochromocytoma in the dog. Vet Clin North Am 14:766, 1984

172. Chastain CB, Ganjam VK (eds): Clinical Endocrinology of Companion Animals. Lea & Febiger, Philadelphia, 1986

173. Walvoort HC, van Nes JJ, Stokhof AA, et al: Canine glycogen storage disease type II: A clinical study of four affected Lapland dogs. J Am Anim Hosp Assoc 20:279, 1984

174. Haskins ME, Jezyk PF, Desnick RJ: Mucopolysaccharidosis in a domestic short-haired cat: A disease distinct from that seen in the Siamese cat. J Am Vet Med Assoc 175:384, 1979

175. Haskins ME, Aguirre GD, Jezyk PF, et al: The pathology of feline arylsulfatase-B deficient mucopolysaccharidosis. Am J Pathol 101:657, 1980

176. Tilley LP, Liu SK: Persistent atrial standstill in the dog and cat. Proceedings of the American College of Veterinary Internal Medicine, p. 43, 1983 (abst)

Section 5

CARDIOVASCULAR SURGERY

28

Anesthesia and the Heart

Diane E. Mason
John A. E. Hubbell

Current trends in animal health care have given veterinarians the opportunity to practice medical and surgical treatment of increasing sophistication. This expanded service often involves the anesthetic management of dogs and cats at relatively high anesthetic risk due to congenital or acquired cardiovascular disorders or systemic diseases.

Most frequently, animals with cardiovascular disease are presented for noncardiovascular surgery. The presence of heart disease may be incidental but is often the major factor to contend with when inducing and maintaining anesthesia. For example, a tooth extraction represents a high-risk procedure in a geriatric dog or cat with congestive heart failure. Similarly, open reduction of a femoral fracture involves more than just orthopedic skills in a dog with ventricular arrhythmias from traumatic myocarditis.

Less commonly, the patient will present for cardiovascular surgery (e.g., correction of patent ductus arteriosus or persistent right aortic arch, palliative surgery for ventricular septal defect or tetralogy of Fallot, or correction of pulmonic stenosis). In addition, older patients may require anesthesia for pacemaker implantation, pericardectomy, or removal of heart-base tumors.

No single ideal anesthetic regimen is appropriate for all patients with cardiac disease. The clinician must approach each case on an individual basis and must assess the interaction of a variety of factors. These include the pathophysiology of the cardiac lesion, the presence of coexisting systemic or metabolic diseases, the surgical procedure and its physiologic effects on the patient, the anesthetic drug effects on the cardiovascular system, and the interaction between the anesthetic agents and concurrent patient medication.[1,2]

Thorough assessment of the animal's cardiovascular disease combined with patient stabilization is necessary prior to anesthetic induction. The basis for choosing appropriate drugs and drug techniques is knowledge of their effects on cardiovascular hemodynamics. For successful management of anesthesia in animals with cardiovascular disease, one must be able to predict the effect of a drug, anticipate potential complications, recognize changes early, and treat problems as they arise.

PREOPERATIVE PATIENT ASSESSMENT

The presence of heart disease in a patient scheduled for anesthesia dictates the need for a more specific preoperative workup than that routinely performed. A beneficial starting point with every patient is a complete medical history. The rate of progression of the disease and the degree of systemic, metabolic, or cardiovascular compromise needs to be established. Knowledge of current drug therapy and associated patient response is important. Specific questions should be directed toward the common signs of cardiac disease, such as coughing, dyspnea, weight loss, edema, exercise intolerance, or syncopal episodes.

Physical examination can help in judging myocardial performance and systemic output. This can be facilitated by observation for pallor or prolonged capillary refill time, mental depression, or abnormal venous pulses. Palpation of femoral arteries for pulse pressure and pulse deficits and auscultation for murmurs, arrhythmias, rales, or increased bronchovesicular sounds are helpful. Physical abnormalities detected that are unrelated to the cardiac disease but that potentially affect anesthesia (e.g., abnormal lung sounds or trachaeal collapse) should be noted.

The *minimum data base* for any animal with cardiac disease being prepared for anesthesia should consist of a complete blood count (CBC) differential, biochemical profile, electrocardiogram (ECG), and thoracic radiograph.

The hemogram may provide useful information. For example, it may indicate anemia, which can impair oxygenation during anesthesia. Polycythemia increases blood viscosity, may decrease tissue oxygenation, and often indicates significant right-to-left shunting of blood (e.g., tetralogy of Fallot). Assessment of packed cell volume and total protein give an indication of the patient's hydration status. Differential white blood cell counts may indicate stress, infection, or inflammatory diseases not readily apparent during the physical examination. Cellular atypia may suggest systemic disorders, such as leukemia, heartworm infection (e.g., eosinophilia and basophilia) or lead toxicity (e.g., basophilic stippling of reticulocytes and nucleated red blood cells).

Specific values of interest in a biochemical profile include serum electrolytes (Na^+, K^+, Cl^-, Ca^{2+}), renal indices (BUN and creatinine), serum albumin, liver enzymes (SGPT, SGOT, serum alkaline phosphatase), and serum glucose. Cardiac dysrhythmias and poor myocardial performance may be associated with an inappropriate balance of serum sodium, potassium, or calcium.[2,3] Hypercalcemia may indicate paraneoplastic syndromes secondary to tumors. Increased renal parameters may suggest low cardiac output, especially in cats with systolic dysfunction. They may also suggest concomitant renal disease. Prerenal azotemia is a frequent finding in decompensated cardiac patients. Irreversible kidney damage can be induced by prolonged hypotension due to anesthesia if renal dysfunction is already present.[4] Anesthetic agents should be selected that minimally decrease systemic blood pressure, and should be combined with volume expansion to maintain renal perfusion. Elevations of liver enzymes may occur from chronic passive liver congestion due to heart failure and with feline hyperthyroidism. Decreased serum albumin may indicate liver dysfunction or protein-losing disease. With heart failure, it may contribute to peripheral and pulmonary edema formation. Moreover, the dosage of highly protein-bound drugs may need to be reduced due to an increase in the unbound active drug fraction.[5]

Arterial and venous blood gases can provide valuable information concerning the metabolic status and ventilatory capacity of the patient. They may also provide evidence for the presence of shunts. Metabolic acidosis may be seen with severe cardiovascular compromise due to poor tissue perfusion and warrant measures to improve cardiac output. Calculated base deficits can be corrected more accurately with sodium bicarbonate administration. Ventilatory support, either before or immediately after induction, may help maintain normocapnia if respiratory acidosis is present. Metabolic alkalosis, often accompanied by hypokalemia, is a potential complication of chronic diuretic therapy.[6]

The ECG gives information concerning cardiac size, specific chamber enlargement, and electrolyte balance as well as indicating stability of cardiac rhythm. Certain rhythm disturbances confer a poor risk for anesthesia. These include persistent ventricular arrhythmias (especially those nonresponsive to antiarrhythmic therapy), heart rates of less than 60 in dogs and 80 in cats that do not increase in response to anticholinergics, or right bundle branch block development as a manifestation of progressive heart disease. When combined with the depressant effects of anesthetics, these rhythm disturbances are potentiators of cardiac arrest. Preanesthetic placement of a temporary intravenous pacemaker is necessary to maintain cardiac output in bradycardic dogs undergoing anesthesia for permanent pacemaker implantation.[7]

Thoracic radiographs will confirm and define heart enlargement; indicate the degree of lung perfusion; and disclose the presence of pulmonary edema, pleural effusion, or other cardiopulmonary disorders. Cardiopulmonary diseases that could predispose to anesthetic complications can be detected by radiographic evaluation. Additional information can be provided by angiography, echocardiography, and cardiac catheterization.

Dogs above 6 months of age, living in or having traveled in areas endemic for heartworms, and not treated with heartworm preventive medicine, and cats with appropriate histories and clinical signs should be tested for microfilaria. Direct and serologic tests may be employed for diagnosis.

PREOPERATIVE PATIENT PREPARATION

Having established the minimum data base, the next step is to address pertinent aspects of the cardiac disorder that may adversely affect anesthetic induction, maintenance, monitoring, and recovery. The patient should be stabilized before induction of anesthesia.

Dysrhythmias should be corrected whenever possible. It is important to establish a stable rhythm that maximizes cardiac output and minimizes the possible development of malignant arrhythmias. Before administering antiarrhythmic drugs, either systemic or metabolic abnormalities or concurrent medication responsible for the rhythm disturbance should be discovered and corrected. For example, an irregular cardiac rhythm developed while receiving cardiac glycosides should prompt evaluation for digitalis toxicity. Persistent tachycardia or bradycardia requires evaluation of serum potassium prior to anesthesia. The choice of appropriate fluid therapy will decrease the patient's risk for cardiac conducting system abnormalities resulting from inappropriate sodium and potassium balance. Correct administration rates and volumes will help avoid pulmonary edema in cardiac patients and maintain adequate preload in volume-depleted animals.

Patient stability should be reviewed in relation-ship to dependence on current drug therapy and potential interactions between these medications and anesthetic agents. The concurrent use of drugs with significant protein binding may decrease the dose required of certain anesthetic drugs, such as barbiturates or diazepam.[5] A rule of thumb for assessing the necessity for concurrent drug therapy is to continue if it has improved the patient's condition or stabilized the hemodynamic or metabolic status or if discontinuation could be associated with adverse side effects or patient instability.

If digitalis is controlling supraventricular arrhythmias or helping maintain a state of cardiac compensation, it should not be discontinued prior to anesthesia. It is important to maintain potassium levels within a normal range in the digitalized patient, to avoid exacerbation of toxicity. For enhanced preoperative or intraoperative inotropic support, an intravenous constant infusion of a sympathomimetic agent (e.g., dopamine or dobutamine) can be administered. These drugs are more potent than digitalis, and their effects are more easily controlled.[8]

Propranolol is sometimes used in the treatment of hypertrophic cardiomyopathy and tachyarrhythmias, as palliative therapy for tetralogy of Fallot, and in feline hyperthyroidism. Because of its antiadrenergic effects, propranolol can add to the negative inotropic effects of inhalation agents. Bronchoconstriction may be exacerbated in asthmatics or in patients with chronic obstructive pulmonary disease because bronchodilation, a response to β_2-adrenergic stimulation, is blocked by propranolol. However, sudden withdrawal of propranolol therapy can result in tachycardia, arrhythmias, and hypertension.[9] It should therefore be continued prior to anesthesia, but the patient must be monitored for these potential adverse reactions. If necessary, the β-blockade of propranolol may be overcome intraoperatively with β-adrenergic agonists, such as dopamine or dobutamine.[8]

Cardiogenic pulmonary edema should be treated preoperatively with diuretics (especially furosemide), positive inotropic agents, and/or vasodilators.[6] Intraoperative measures to improve gas exchange after endotracheal intubation may be beneficial and include supplemental oxygen administration, bronchodilators, and suction. Positive end-expiratory pressure (PEEP) and positive-pressure ventilation

(PPV) after intubation may also help increase the arterial oxygen content by reducing alveolar flooding by edema.[10]

Circulatory shunts have a direct effect on the induction of anesthesia in animals with congenital heart disease. Left-to-right shunts cause pulmonary hyperperfusion. Rapid uptake of inhalation agents and induction may result causing acute central nervous system (CNS) depression.[5] A left-to-right shunt may cause a delay in anesthetic effect after administration of an intravenous induction agent. This is because a portion of the bolus is recirculated through the pulmonary vasculature before making its way to the CNS. Fatal overdosage could result if the initial bolus is promptly followed by additional drug administration before adequate time for induction has elapsed.

Right-to-left shunts produce pulmonary hypoperfusion. Decreased pulmonary blood flow may result in slow induction, when using inhalation agents.[5] By contrast, intravenous induction agents produce rapid onset of action, because drug boluses partially bypass the pulmonary circuit, traveling immediately to the systemic circulation and the CNS. Moreover, anesthesia may exacerbate a right-to-left shunt by lowering the systemic blood pressure.[11] Maintaining a stable and adequate mean systemic blood pressure in these patients is essential in order to avoid this problem.

Pericardiocentesis is recommended prior to anesthetic induction in any animal in which significant pericardial effusion has been documented. Pericardial effusion may cause severe ventricular underfilling, decreased cardiac output, lowered systemic blood pressure, alterations in coronary blood flow, and myocardial ischemia.[12] The introduction of an anesthetic agent under these conditions could lead to ventricular fibrillation. Moreover, the cardiac output of patients with pericardial effusion is often highly dependent on heart rate, since stroke volume is limited by an underfilled left ventricle. Therefore, avoidance of drugs that result in bradycardia and prevention of deep anesthetic levels are essential for these patients.

Ascites can be detrimental to the anesthetized animal. Secondary diaphragmatic pressure may interfere with thoracic expansion and ventilation. Preoperative drainage of a portion of the ascitic fluid will reduce respiratory distress in these situations.

ESTABLISHING ANESTHETIC RISK

Once the patient has been medically evaluated and stabilized, it is useful to classify the severity or stage of cardiac disease and the relative risk of the surgical procedure. The American Society of Anesthesiologists (ASA) has develped a classification of patient risk category to decide the individual risk of anesthesia and appropriate drug strategy (Table 28-1).

A classification scheme for functional phases of heart failure in humans devised by the New York Heart Association has been modified and adapted for dogs[13] (Ch. 8). Phase I heart failure characterizes an animal with normal exercise tolerance without overt signs of pulmonary or systemic disease related to its heart problem. Animals with compensated phase I heart failure would be placed in ASA category 2. Virtually any drug among the list of premedicants or induction agents (Tables 28-2 and 28-3) would be suitable, including potent inhalation agents and nitrous oxide. The choice of anesthetic technique should be based on the particular anesthetic needs.

Phase II heart failure is characterized by occasional coughing and dyspnea after strenuous exercise. The animal is usually comfortable at rest. These patients can be placed in ASA category 3. The clinician should confine premedication to the use of diazepam, narcotics, or ketamine. Induction can be carried out with intravenous diazepam/ketamine, narcotics, low dosages of thiobarbiturates, thiamylal/lidocaine, or etomidate. Any of the potent agents are acceptable, but it may be safer to supplement anesthesia with narcotics rather than to maintain anesthesia solely with inhalation agents.

Phase III heart failure patients cough or become dyspneic after minimal exercise and at night. Phase IV heart failure describes fulminant congestive heart failure that is clinically obvious at rest. Phase III and early phase IV heart disease patients become grouped under ASA category 4. Great care must be taken for successful anesthesia in these patients. Diazepam premedication in dogs and low doses of ketamine in cats could be used if necessary. Narcotic induction is recommended, but etomidate can be used as well. If inhalant anesthesia is selected, isoflurane is the preferred agent. Narcotic supplementation with lower doses of inhalation agents will

Table 28-1 American Society of Anesthesiologists Risk Categories for Anesthesia

ASA Category	Patient Description
1	Normal patient with no organic disease
2	Patient with mild systemic disease
3	Patient with severe systemic disease limiting activity but not incapacitating
4	Patient with incapacitating systemic disease that is a constant threat to life
5	Moribund patient not expected to live 24 hours with or without surgery
E	Emergency operation, designated by placing E after appropriate category

Table 28-2 Premedicants for the Cardiovascular Patient

Drug	Dosage (mg/kg)	Dog/Cat	Route	Class of Heart Failure	ASA Category
Atropine	0.02–0.06	Both	IM/IV	I–III	II–IV
Glycopyrrolate	0.005–0.01	Both	IM/IV	I–III	II–IV
Lenperone	0.2–1.0	Both	IM	I	II
Diazepam	0.2–0.5	Both	IV	I–IV	II–V
Ketamine	5–10	Cat	IM	I–IV	II–V
Innovar-Vet	0.1 ml/kg	Dog	IM	I–IV	II–V
Morphine	0.2–0.5	Dog	IM	I–IV	II–V
Oxymorphone	0.05–0.1	Both	IM	I–IV	II–V

IM, intramuscular; IV, intravenous.

Table 28-3 Intravenous Agents for the Cardiovascular Patient

Drug	Dosage (mg/kg)	Dog/Cat	Class of Heart Failure	ASA Category
Thiamylal	6–12	Both	I–II	II
Thiopental	8–15	Both	I–II	II
Thiamylal/lidocaine	4 mg/kg of each drug	Dog	I–III	II–III
Etomidate	1–2	Both	I–IV	II–IV
Diazepam (2.5 mg/ml) + Ketamine (50 mg/ml)	0.1–0.15 ml/kg*	Both	I–IV	II–IV
Oxymorphone	0.025–0.05	Both	I–IV	II–V
Fentanyl	0.002–0.006	Dog	I–IV	II–V
Innovar-Vet	0.05 ml/kg	Dog	I–IV	II–V
Pancuronium	0.04	Both	I–IV	II–V
Atracurium	0.15–0.50	Both	I–IV	II–V
Vecuronium	0.05–0.25	Both	I–IV	II–V

* Dose in ml of 1:1 Diazepam: Ketamine mixture

maintain an adequate depth of anesthesia in dogs or cats.

Late-phase IV heart failure animals are at very high risk and are placed in ASA category 5. The potential benefit to be derived from surgery must be weighed carefully against the risk of anesthesia. In dogs, narcotic agents are the safest, combined with neuromuscular blocking drugs and local anesthesia, when possible. Lower dosages are necessary when heart failure becomes more advanced.

ANESTHETIC AGENTS

Anesthetic agents may directly affect the myocardial, mechanical, or electric activity of the heart or may indirectly influence cardiac function through their action on the nervous system or vasculature (Tables 28-4 and 28-5). Normally, animals have a large cardiovascular reserve that allows the stress of anesthesia to be well tolerated. However, patients with cardiovascular compromise may have exhausted much of this reserve and are often unable to compensate for the effects of anesthetic agents. In these cases, drug dosages must be carefully titrated to the minimal amount required to obtain a desired effect.

There are many ways to induce and maintain anesthesia in the compromised high-risk cardiac patient. Balanced anesthesia employing a combination of several drugs may be the best approach. It permits

Table 28-4 Clinical Effects of Common Premedicants

Drug	Rate and Rhythm Changes	Contractility	Blood Pressure	Myocardial Oxygen Consumption	Cardiac Output
Anticholinergics	Transient AV block; sinus tachycardia	↑	NC	↑	↑
Phenothiazines	Reflex tachycardia; antiarrhythmic	↓	↓	↑	↑
Butyrophenones	Reflex tachycardia; antiarrhythmic		Slight ↓	NC	NC
Benzodiazepines	NC	NC	NC	↓	NC
Xylazine	Bradycardia; first- and second-degree AV block; arrhythmogenic	↓	Initial ↑, then ↓	↓	↓
Ketamine	Sinus tachycardia	↑	↑	↑	↑
Morphine	Bradycardia; first- and second-degree AV block	NC	May ↓ (histamine)	NC	May ↓ (bradycardia)
Meperidine	Bradycardia; first- and second-degree AV block; reflex tachycardia	↓	↓	NC	↓
Oxymorphone	Bradycardia; first- and second-degree AV block	NC	NC	NC	May ↓ (bradycardia)
Fentanyl	Bradycardia; first- and second-degree AV block	NC	NC	NC	May ↓ (bradycardia)
Innovar-Vet	Bradycardia; first- and second-degree AV block	NC	NC	NC	May ↓ (bradycardia)

↑, increase; ↓, decrease; NC, no change.

Table 28-5 Clinical Effects of Common Intravenous Agents

Drug	Rate and Rhythm Changes	Contractility	Blood Pressure	Myocardial Oxygen Consumption	Cardiac Output
Thiobarbiturates	Reflex tachycardia; bigeminy; ventricular ectopia	↓	↓	↑	↓
Thiamylal/lidocaine	Reflex tachycardia; antiarrhythmic	↓	Slight ↓	↑	↓
Etomidate	No change	NC	Slight ↓	NC	NC
Innovar-Vet	Bradycardia; first- and second-degree AV block	↑	NC	NC	May ↓ (bradycardia)
Diazepam/ketamine	Rate increase	↑	↑	↑	↑
Pancuronium	Rate increase; ventricular arrhythmias	NC	↑	↑	↑
Atracurium	Rate increase at high dose due to histamine release	NC	May ↓ (histamine)	NC	NC
Vecuronium	NC	NC	NC	NC	NC

↑, increase; ↓, decrease; NC, no change.

the use of lower doses, minimizes cardiovascular depression, and allows for adjustment of variables, such as analgesia, muscle relaxation, and hypnosis. Clinical evaluation of anesthetic drug effects on cardiovascular function should focus on changes in heart rate and rhythm (ECG monitoring), blood pressure, and cardiac output (e.g., capillary refill time, mucous membrane color, urine output), and contractility (inferred by apex beat, heart sounds). Indirect blood pressure measurement is becoming increasingly available through the use of various commercial instruments.

PREANESTHETIC DRUGS

Anticholinergics (e.g., atropine and glycopyrolate) are used for premedication mainly to increase heart rate and reduce salivation (Table 28-2). These agents have a peripheral antivagal effect at the sinoatrial (SA) node and decrease atrioventricular (AV) conduction time. Heart rate increases and, as a result, cardiac output and blood pressure may increase secondarily.

Anticholinergics are arrhythmogenic because of their effect on the AV conduction system. Intravenous atropine may transiently slow the heart rate and cause first- or second-degree AV block due to initial central nervous system (CNS) vagomimetic activity.[15] It is therefore advisable to use an anticholinergic only if bradycardia develops during the anesthetic period. One must weigh the advantages of an increased stable heart rate resulting from atropine administration against the inability to detect early anesthetic-induced reduction in the heart rate (indicating deepening anesthesia) due to vagolytic action of the drug. Furthermore, excessive increases in heart rate from anticholinergics may critically elevate myocardial oxygen consumption and predispose to arrhythmias in patients with heart disease.

Phenothiazine tranquilizers, while providing excellent tranquilization, should be used with great caution in the cardiovascularly compromised patient. Phenothiazines are potent α-adrenergic and dopaminergic-blocking drugs.[14] They have a direct negative inotropic effect, and their action on α-adrenergic receptors in vascular smooth muscle results in vasodilation and hypotension. Hypotension is often followed by reflex tachycardia, which secondarily increases myocardial oxygen consumption. Rarely, acepromazine causes profound brady-cardia with first- or second-degree AV block. Phenothiazines are antiarrhythmic and protect the myocardium against both barbiturate- and epineph-rine-induced arrhythmias.[16] This property must be weighed against the deleterious effects mentioned above.

The cardiovascular depressant properties of bu-tyrophenones are similar to the phenothiazine tran-quilizers but are less severe.[17] Like phenothiazines, they are α-adrenergic blocking drugs and can confer protection to the myocardium from catecholamine-induced arrhythmias.[18] Although the butyrophen-one tranquilizers have less deleterious side effects than the phenothiazines, they should be used with caution and the dose titrated to produce the desired effect. Droperidol is a butyrophenone tranquilizer that is most commonly used in dogs in combination with fentanyl (Innovar-Vet). Lenperone is another potentially useful butyrophenone agent.

Diazepam is a benzodiazepine derivative that can be safely used in the cardiac patient. It produces minimal depressant effects on the cardiovascular system, resulting in little change in heart rate, con-tractility, blood pressure, or cardiac output.[19] Di-azepam may improve coronary blood flow and at the same time decrease myocardial oxygen con-sumption.[20] It has an antiarrhythmic effect because of its ability to decrease sympathetic tone centrally, and it is compatible with most other anesthetic agents. However, when used in combination with high doses of fentanyl, diazepam significantly de-creases stroke volume, cardiac output, and systemic blood pressure.[21] Owing to the solubility charac-teristics of diazepam, it is formulated in a 40 percent propylene glycol base. Rapid intravenous admin-istration of propylene glycol can be cardiotoxic and can induce hypotension and bradycardia.

Xylazine is a poor choice for use as a sedative in a compromised cardiac patient. An α₂-agonist, xy-lazine causes central reduction in sympathetic tone. Vagally mediated bradycardia and reduction in con-tractility occur after xylazine administration. Its α-agonistic effects result in transient hypertension due to increased peripheral vascular resistance. This is followed by prolonged hypotension. Cardiac out-put is adversely affected through negative inotropy, bradycardia, and increased afterload.[22] In addition, xylazine potentiates arrhythmias and increases myo-cardial sensitivity to catecholamines.[16]

Ketamine is an excellent drug for use in most car-diac patients, particularly cats. Because of its ability to cause excitement, delirium, and convulsions, ke-tamine should not be used in the dog unless in com-bination with a CNS sedative. An intravenous com-bination of diazepam and ketamine is an excellent induction agent in canine and feline cardiac patients. The direct effect of ketamine on the myocardium is to decrease contractility. However, it often acts as a positive inotrope through its sympathetic nervous system effects, which override its direct myocardial depressant property.[24] An increase in heart rate, myocardial oxygen consumption, cardiac output, and systemic blood pressure can result. Ketamine may exert myocardial depressant effects on the car-diac patient whose sympathetic tone is already high due to cardiac decompensation.

Narcotics are useful in dogs for premedication, induction, and maintenance of anesthesia. Narcotics have predictable but minimal hemodynamic effects in the critically ill patient. Analgesia is excellent and, in most instances, the sedation-hypnosis provided is good. Arousal of the severely depressed animal or reversal of respiratory depression postoperatively may be accomplished with a narcotic antagonist (e.g., naloxone).

Morphine may cause bradycardia by inducing central vagal stimulation. This effect can be pre-vented with administration of anticholinergics, if necessary. Myocardial performance is maintained with morphine, although histamine release may be stimulated. This can decrease peripheral vascular re-sistance and potentially contribute to hypoten-sion.[25,26]

Meperidine has one-tenth the analgesic potency of morphine but is a much greater cardiovascular depressant.[27] It decreases myocardial contractility directly, causes peripheral vasodilation, and me-diates hypotension.

Oxymorphone is commonly used in combination with tranquilizers as a neuroleptanalgesic agent in the dog or cat. Although 10 times more potent an analgesic than morphine, oxymorphone may not produce enough CNS depression when used alone. Its use does, however, reduce the dosage of other agents necessary for induction. Oxymorphone is excellent intraoperatively in the dog or cat for supplementing a light plane of anesthesia, provided the animal is monitored for bradycardia.

Fentanyl is also a useful narcotic for intraoperative anesthetic supplementation. Its rapid onset of action is advantageous in this circumstance. Fentanyl may cause dysphoria and muscle rigidity, when used in the conscious dog. Therefore, it is most often given in combination with droperidol in the neuroleptanalgesic combination, Innovar-Vet. Fentanyl with droperidol provides excellent cardiovascular stability, whether administered intramuscularly for sedation or given intravenously as an induction agent. Bradycardia is a consistent feature when this combination is administered intravenously but can be prevented or alleviated by the administration of anticholinergics (e.g., atropine). Innovar-Vet has been shown to increase peripheral vascular resistance, result in an acute increase in systemic blood pressure, and cause a significant increase in left ventricular contractility and coronary blood flow.[28]

DRUGS USED FOR ANESTHETIC INDUCTION

A number of drugs or drug combinations may be used to induce anesthesia successfuly in the cardiac patient (Tables 28-2 through 28-5). Intravenous Innovar-Vet and diazepam with ketamine have already been mentioned.

Thiobarbiturates are the most frequently administered intravenous induction agents in veterinary medicine. They may be used safely in many instances in the compromised patient, but cardiac depressant effects may occur.[29] For example, thiobarbiturate boluses may cause impaired myocardial contractility and vasodilation. This effect leads to peripheral pooling of venous blood, resulting in decreased ventricular filling pressures and an overall decrease in cardiac output. The hypotension and decreased cardiac output that result cause a reflex tachycardia through sympathetic nervous system stimulation, increasing myocardial oxygen consumption. Development of arrhythmias, especially ventricular bigemini or other ectopia, can occur.[30] The patient that has poor ventricular function preoperatively (e.g., myocardial or systolic dysfunction) or unstable cardiac rhythm is not a good candidate for thiopental or thiamylal induction.

Because the severity of the aforementioned side effects is directly correlated with the dose, small doses of thiobarbiturates may be tolerated and may be adequate for induction in the depressed or well-sedated animal.

The intravenous use of a thiobarbiturate with lidocaine may offer a safe alternative to induction with thiobarbiturates alone in the canine cardiac patient.[31] Lidocaine reduces by approximately 50 percent the amount of thiobarbiturate required for induction. In addition, lidocaine has antiarrhythmic properties and the ability to diminish reflex responses to endotracheal intubation (i.e., laryngospasm and tachycardia). The two drugs should not be mixed in the same syringe, because precipitation will occur.

Etomidate is an intravenous hypnotic agent that has potential value for anesthetic induction in dogs or cats with cardiovascular compromise. Bolus administration produces a clinical effect similar to that of the thiobarbiturates, with little or no change in hemodynamics. Contractility is not adversely affected. Only a small reduction of arterial blood pressure occurs, while mean coronary blood flow is preserved.[32]

DRUGS USED FOR ANESTHETIC MAINTENANCE

Maintenance of anesthesia in canine and feline cardiac patients can be achieved using inhalation agents, or in dogs with a combination of high-dose narcotics with skeletal muscle relaxants.

Maintenance with inhalation agents is advantageous because of their ease of administration and the ability to control the level of anesthesia. Inhalation agents are compatible with essentially all other anesthetic drugs, and their cardiovascular depressant effects are dose related. Thus, if analgesia is supplemented with the concurrent use of narcotics, low doses of inhalation agents may be highly effective, even in the high-risk small animal patient. All potent inhalation agents cause depression in myocardial function and decreased systemic blood pressure in direct proportion to the depth of anesthesia.[33]

Halothane should be used with caution in the cardiac patient because of its arrhythmogenicity and marked cardiac depressant quality. Cardiac output and myocardial oxygen consumption are decreased.[34] Halothane sensitizes the myocardium to catecholamines, an effect that does not appear to be dose related.[35] In fact, light planes of halothane anesthesia may exacerbate its arrhythmogenic properties due to endogenous catecholamine release in response to surgical stress.

Methoxyflurane depresses cardiac output and decreases total peripheral resistance, resulting in hypotension.[34] It is an excellent analgesic even in light planes of anesthesia. Since its cardiac depressant effects are dose related, methoxyflurane can be used successfully at reduced doses in the cardiac patient. Because of its high tissue solubility, it is associated with prolonged induction, recovery, and slow change in anesthetic depth. This can be a distinct disadvantage in the critically ill patient.

Enflurane causes a decrease in systemic blood pressure due to its cardiac depressant properties; it also reduces total peripheral resistance. Its potency is less than that of other inhalation agents. The need to maintain animals at higher alveolar concentrations in order to achieve adequate anesthesia may increase the direct cardiodepressant effects.[34] The ability of enflurane to increase myocardial sensitivity to catecholamines is less than that of halothane.

Isoflurane mediates hypotension through its action of decreasing total peripheral resistance. At surgical planes of anesthesia, it does not alter myocardial contractility.[34] Cardiac output is well maintained at anesthetic dosages. The margin between the lethal dose and anesthetic dose of isoflurane is the widest of any of the modern potent inhalation agents. It does not sensitize the heart to catecholamine-induced arrhythmias and is the safest inhalation agent for use in the compromised animal.[34]

Nitrous oxide is beneficial for use in the cardiac patient. It does not alter blood pressure by itself and, when used in combination with other potent inhalation agents, reduces the concentration of inhalation agent required. Nitrous oxide slightly increases sympathetic cardiac activity and provides hemodynamic stability.[34] In combination with fentanyl, it causes a marked decrease in cardiac output and systemic blood pressure.[36] Nitrous oxide should be avoided or at least discontinued 10 to 15 minutes before chest closure begins to prevent exacerbation of a pneumothorax after thoracotomy. It should be avoided in an animal with poor oxygenation preoperatively and discontinued if hypoxemia develops during the anesthetic period.

The advantages of classic balanced anesthesia in dogs (narcotics plus tranquilization and neuromuscular blocking agents) include decreased myocardial depression, maintenance of more adequate levels of systemic blood pressure, and easy reversibility. However, this technique using drug combinations is complex and requires careful patient monitoring well into the postoperative period. Narcotics have been discussed in relationship to their minimal cardiovascular effects.

The preferred neuromuscular blocking agents in the cardiac patient are the nondepolarizing muscle relaxants, such as atracurium, vecuronium, or pancuronium (Table 28-3). Nondepolarizing agents do not alter serum potassium levels as might occur with a depolarizing neuromuscular blocker. Neither pancuronium or vecuronium causes significant histamine release, and both are reversible postoperatively. Their cardiovascular effects include an increase in heart rate, blood pressure, and cardiac output.[37]

INTRAOPERATIVE PATIENT MONITORING

Careful patient monitoring is essential to permit early recognition and correction of anesthetic problems. An ECG monitor should be used throughout the anesthetic period. Pharmacologic intervention is not always required in the presence of intraoperative arrhythmias. Some etiologic factors associated with arrhythmias that may be reversible without the use of antiarrhythmic drugs include hypoxia or hypercarbia, acid-base disturbances, excess endogenous catecholamines, electrolyte abnormalities, autonomic reflexes, and anesthetic agents.[38]

It is beneficial to have two intravenous access sites in any high-risk patient undergoing anesthesia. This approach facilitates rapid intravenous infusion of fluid through one catheter and drug administration through the other; it also allows for simultaneous fluid, blood, or plasma administration as necessary.

Attention to fluid therapy is of utmost importance

in the cardiac patient. A fluid administration rate of 10 ml/kg/hr can be used as a basic intraoperative guideline. If hypotension and poor cardiac output are evident, volume expansion may be accomplished by increasing the rate of fluid administration. Continued fluid therapy into the postoperative period is advised until hemodynamic stability and adequate urine production are achieved.

Measurement of urine output can be a useful indicator of fluid therapy. Renal perfusion is sensitive to changes in autonomic tone and is dependent on maintaining a mean arterial blood pressure greater than 60 mmHg.[39] Reduced urinary output results from decreased renal perfusion if renal function is adequate. Inadequate urine production should prompt measures to improve renal perfusion (e.g., decreasing anesthetic depth, volume expansion to correct hypotension, positive inotropic agents to improve cardiac output). Dopamine has been shown to act as a renal vasodilator at low dosages, improving renal perfusion and urine production.[14]

Monitoring central venous pressure (CVP) can provide valuable information to guide fluid administration during surgery. Normal CVP is 0 to 5 cm H_2O. If the cardiac output appears adequate (i.e., normal peripheral perfusion, strong arterial pulses, and cardiac apex beat suggesting normal arterial blood pressure), a satisfactory cardiovascular state may exist. If fluid administration increases CVP more than 10 cm H_2O, fluid overload or cardiac failure may be evident. Measurements in the range of 15 to 20 cm H_2O are too high. Fluid administration may need to be reduced or discontinued. Measures to improve cardiac function include decreasing anesthetic depth and positive inotrope infusion (e.g., dopamine or dobutamine). Administration of colloid rather than crystalloid fluids may decrease the likelihood of pulmonary edema formation, provided that the alveolar-capillary membrane is intact. Furosemide should be given intravenously if pulmonary edema develops. Low CVP generally indicates hypovolemia. Fluid administration should be increased to elevate CVP to the upper limit of normal.[40,41]

Blood pressure monitoring is beneficial in the anesthetized cardiac patient and is the most accurate way of assessing whether adequate tissue perfusion pressures are being maintained. Heart rate and pulse pressure have been shown to correlate poorly with actual arterial blood pressures and could be misleading when relied on solely as a perfusion estimate.[41,42] It should also be remembered that arterial pressure alone is not an indicator of cardiac output. Oscillometric devices are available for indirect blood pressure measurement. The Dinamap (Criticon, Tampa, FL) automated blood pressure recorder is based on detection of blood pressure pulse changes within a cuff bladder caused by diameter changes in the underlying artery.[43] The device works best on medium and large dogs. Readings are more difficult to obtain in small dogs and usually cannot be obtained in cats.[44] Commercial devices using ultrasonic kinetoarteriography (Doppler ultrasound) are also available (Arteriosonde, Hoffman-La Roche, Cranberry, NJ). Their use has been demonstrated in cats.[45,46]

Controlled ventilation is necessary during thoracotomy and prolonged surgical procedures. If available, blood-gas monitoring to assess the effectiveness of ventilation is beneficial. Ventilation should be improved by increasing the number of breaths per minute or tidal volume (i.e., the amount of air moving into the lungs with each inspiration) if hypercapnia occurs. Inadequate oxygenation with normal arterial PCO_2 ($PaCO_2$) can be caused by certain cardiac shunts. Inadequate oxygenation could also indicate a ventilation-perfusion mismatch as occurs with low cardiac output states or lung pathology (e.g., pulmonary edema).[47]

When controlling ventilation, it is important to maintain a proper inspiratory-to-expiratory time ratio. Prolonged inspiratory times cause extended periods of positive pressure within the thoracic cavity, decreasing cardiac venous return. An inspiratory-expiratory ratio of 1:2 to 1:4 is therefore recommended to avoid adverse effects on cardiac output.

Surgical blood loss can become a critical factor during anesthetic management of cardiac patients. Whole blood for transfusion should be obtained prior to the anesthetic period whenever significant blood loss is anticipated. Fresh plasma transfusion alone may be sufficient in the patient with hypoproteinemia, thrombocytopenia, or clotting disorders.

POSTOPERATIVE PATIENT MONITORING

Hypothermia is a deleterious consequence of anesthesia in many cats and dogs, and may occur during or after surgical completion. Animals should be kept warm postoperatively with externally applied heat and warmed fluids. Shivering uses a great deal of metabolic energy. Lactic acidosis can result from tissue hypoxia in animals with poor cardiac output due to heart disease.

Electrocardiographic monitoring may need to be continued for some animals postoperatively. Emergency resuscitative equipment and drugs should be on hand at all times during and after anesthesia. Intrathoracic and extrathoracic paddles and a direct-current defibrillator should be in good working order in the surgery room to avoid needless loss of time during resuscitative efforts. Progressive intraoperative or postoperative decline in physical status should signal a need to decrease anesthestic depth, provide ventilatory support, and expand circulating volume with intravenous fluids. Positive inotropic agents (e.g., dopamine, dobutamine) may be needed to improve myocardial function.

Thus, successful anesthesia in the small animal cardiac patient depends on a number of factors. The veterinarian must take time to understand the patient's disease, be able to anticipate problems that might arise in the compromised animal, and be prepared to intervene at the earliest signs of a downward trend in the animal's condition.

REFERENCES

1. Bull AP: The anesthetic evaluation and management of the surgical patient with heart disease. Surg Clin North Am 63:1035, 1983
2. Stark DCC, Silvay G: Anesthetic management for cardiac surgery not requiring cardiopulmonary bypass. Int Anesthesiol Clin 17:71, 1979
3. Vaughan RS, Lunn JN: Potassium and the anaesthetist. Anaesthesia 28:118, 1973
4. Maddern PJ: Anaesthesia for the patient with impaired renal function. Anaesth Intensive Care 11:321, 1983
5. Eger EI: Anesthetic uptake and action. Waverly Press, Baltimore, 1974
6. Bonagura JD: Fluid and electrolyte management of the cardiac patient. Vet Clin North Am Small Anim Pract 12:501, 1982
7. Bonagura JD, Helphrey ML, Muir WW: Complications associated with permanent pacemaker implantation in the dog. J Am Vet Med Assoc 182:149, 1983
8. Pennock JL: Perioperative management of drug therapy. Surg Clin North Am 63:1049, 1983
9. Muir WW, Sams R: Clinical pharmacodynamics and pharmacokinetics of beta-adrenoceptor blocking drugs in veterinary medicine. Compend Cont Ed 6:156, 1984
10. Sibbald WJ, Calvin JE, Holliday RL, et al: Concepts in the pharmacologic and nonpharmacologic support of cardiovascular function in critically ill surgical patients. Surg Clin North Am 63:455, 1983
11. Kaplan JA: Cardiac Anesthesia. Grune & Stratton, New York, 1979
12. Shabetai R, Fowler NO, Guntheroth WG: The hemodynamics of cardiac tamponade and constrictive pericarditis. Am J Cardiol 26:480, 1970
13. Ettinger SJ, Suter PF: Canine Cardiology. WB Saunders, Philadelphia, 1970
14. Gilman AG, Goodman LS, Rall TW, et al (eds): Goodman and Gilman's The Pharmacologic Basis of Therapeutics. 7th Ed. Macmillan, New York, 1985
15. Muir WW: Effects of atropine on cardiac rates and rhythms in dogs. J Am Vet Med Assoc 172:917, 1978
16. Muir WW, Werner LL, Hamlin RL: Effects of xylazine and acetylpromazine upon induced ventricular fibrillation in dogs anesthetized with thiamylal and halothane. Am J Vet Res 36:1299, 1975
17. Hall LW, Clarke KW: Veterinary Anesthesia. 8th Ed. Bailliere Tindall, London, 1983
18. Bertolo L, Novakovic L, Penna M: Antiarrhythmic effects of droperidol. Anesthesiology 37:529, 1972
19. Abel RM, Staroscik RN, Reis RL: The effects of diazepam (Valium) on left ventricular function and systemic vascular resistance. J Pharmacol Exp Ther 173:364, 1970
20. Abel RM, Reis RL, Staroscik RN: Coronary vasodilatation following diazepam (Valium). Br J Pharmacol 38:620, 1970
21. Reves JG, Kissin I, Fournier SE: Additive negative inotropic effect of a combination of diazepam and fentanyl. Anesth Analg 63:97, 1984
22. Klide AM, Calderwood HW, Soma LR: Cardiopulmonary effect of xylazine in dogs. Am J Vet Res 36:931, 1975
23. Wright M: Pharmacologic effects of ketamine and its use in veterinary medicine. J Am Vet Med Assoc 180:1462, 1982
24. Haskins SC, Farver TB, Patz JD: Ketamine in dogs. Am J Vet Res 46:1855, 1985

25. Vatner SF, March JD, Swain JF: Effects of morphine on coronary and left ventricle dynamics in conscious dogs. J Clin Invest 55:207, 1975

26. Roscow CE, Moss J, Philbin DM, et al: Histamine release during morphine and fentanyl anesthesia. Anesthesiology 56:93, 1982

27. DeCastro J, Van de Water A, Wouters L, et al: Comparative study of cardiovascular, neurologic, and metabolic side effects of eight narcotics in dogs. Acta Anaesthesiol Belg 30:5, 1979

28. Buckhold DK, Erickson HH, Lumb WV: Cardiovascular response to fentanyl-droperidol and atropine in the dog. Am J Vet Res 38:479, 1977

29. Conway CM, Ellis DB: Hemodynamic effects of short-acting barbiturates. Br J Anaesth 41:534, 1969

30. Muir WW: Electrocardiographic interpretation of thiobarbiturate-induced dysrhythmias in dogs. J Am Vet Med Assoc 170:1419, 1977

31. Bjorling DE, Rawlings CA: Induction of anesthesia with thiopental-lidocaine combination in dogs with cardiopulmonary disease. J Am Anim Hosp Assoc 20:445, 1984

32. Gooding JM, Weng JT, Smith RA, et al: Cardiovascular and pulmonary responses following etomidate induction of anesthesia in patients with demonstrated cardiac disease. Anesth Analg 58:40, 1979

33. Hickey RF, Eger EI: Circulatory effects of inhaled anaesthetics. p. 441. In Prys-Roberts C (ed): The Circulation in Anaesthesia. Blackwell Scientific Publications, London, 1980

34. Stevens WC: From ether to isoflurane: Comparison of general anesthetics. Lecture 120. In ASA Annual Refresher Course Lectures, 1983

35. Bednarski RM, Muir WW: Arrhythmogenicity of dopamine, dobutamine and epinephrine in thiamylal-halothane anesthetized dogs. Am J Vet Res 44:2341, 1983

36. Bovill JG, Sebel PS, Stanley TH: Opioid analgesics in anesthesia: With special reference to their use in cardiovascular anesthesia. Anesthesiology 61:731, 1984

37. Savarese JJ, Philbin DM: Cardiovascular effects of neuromuscular blocking agents. Int Anesthesiol Clin 17:13, 1979

38. Philbin DM, Hutter AM Jr: Intraoperative cardiac arrhythmias. Int Anesthesiol Clin 17:55, 1979

39. Pitts RF: Physiology of the Kidney and Body Fluids. Yearbook Medical Publishers, Chicago, 1964

40. Kelman GR: Interpretation of CVP measurements. Anaesthesia 26:209, 1971

41. Haskins SC: Shock. p. 2. In Kirk RW (ed): Current Veterinary Therapy. Vol. VIII. WB Saunders, Philadelphia, 1983

42. Cullen DJ: Interpretation of blood-pressure measurements in anesthesia. Anesthesiology 40:6, 1974

43. Meldrum SJ: The principles underlying Dinamap—A microprocessor based instrument for the automatic determination of mean arterial pressure. J Med Eng Technol 2:243, 1978

44. Kittleson MD, Olivier NB: Measurement of systemic arterial blood pressure. Vet Clin North Am 13:321, 1983

45. Klevans LR, Hirhaler G, Kovacs JL: Indirect blood pressure determination by Doppler technique in renal hypertensive cats. Am J Physiol 237:H720, 1979

46. Morgan RV: Systemic hypertension in four cats: Ocular and medical findings. J Am Anim Hosp Assoc 22:615, 1986

47. Shapiro BA, Harrison RA, Walton JR: Clinical Application of Blood Gases. 3rd Ed. Yearbook Medical Publishers, Chicago, 1982

29

Basic Cardiovascular Surgery and Procedures

George E. Eyster
Maralyn R. Probst

PREREQUISITES FOR SUCCESSFUL SURGERY

The success of cardiovascular surgery procedures depends on a thorough understanding of anatomy and physiology. A high level of technical surgical skill and experience is required and must be supplemented with good anesthesia support. No other area of surgery requires such close teamwork between the surgeon and the anesthesiologist. In addition, the anesthesiologist must also be knowledgeable in cardiovascular physiology and must be particularly aware of anesthetic effects on the cardiovascular system (Ch. 28). Likewise, both the surgeon and the anesthesiologist must be familiar with the pathophysiology of the cardiovascular disease in which the surgery and anesthesia is to be performed. For example, left-sided backward heart failure may decrease perfusion and ventilation and thereby alter the uptake of anesthetic gases. The cyanotic disease tetralogy of Fallot causes poor lung perfusion but speeds the delivery of injectable anesthetics to the brain. The cardiac intervention of slowing or stopping blood flow would be more deleterious in a patient with poor perfusion or myocardial ischemia. For these and many other reasons, the cardiac surgeon and anesthesiologist must work to plan the anesthesia and surgical procedure together and relate well at the surgical table, if success is to be attained.

SURGICAL MONITORING

Fortunately, many of the cardiovascular variables are easily monitored with relatively inexpensive, very reliable, and readily available equipment. Some method of monitoring cardiac electric activity is mandatory for cardiac surgery. In addition, either direct or indirect measurement of arterial blood pressure can be helpful; a simple central venous pressure (CVP) monitoring system is frequently useful, particularly in right-sided heart disease. If available, blood-gas determinations can predict the development of conditions that could cause difficulties in anesthesia and monitor the effectiveness of intraoperative cardiac and pulmonary performance.

During open chest surgical procedures, the sur-

605

geon has the ability to monitor both blood pressure and ventilation by direct palpation or observation of various cardiac structures. The pink appearance of the heart, particularly the left atrium, indicates good ventilation and adequate oxygenation. In patients developing cyanosis or in whom ventilation is inadequate, the heart appears darker; this appearance may precede electrocardiographic (ECG) or blood pressure abnormalities. The blood pressure can be determined approximately by palpating the aortic arch or descending aorta. Digital pressure on the aorta should cause the vessel to move away from the pressure point if the arterial pressure exceeds 120 mmHg. If the vessel wall indents and the whole artery moves as it is pressed, pressure is approximately 80 to 120 mmHg. If, with digital pressure, the artery indents easily and almost occludes before it is moved, arterial pressure is below 80 mmHg, and the animal is too deeply anesthetized or is in a severely low cardiac output state.

The presence of bradycardia should be avoided at all costs during cardiac surgery. Bradycardia is usually an indication of an anesthetic level that is far deeper than necessary. In our experience, bradyarrhythmias are more troublesome and potentially more severe than tachyarrhythmias. For these reasons, we believe that maintaining an artificially elevated heart rate with atropine is helpful and reduces the frequency of difficult-to-manage arrhythmias. Atropine should always be administered in patients requiring manipulation at the base of the heart. This is particularly true with patent ductus arteriosus surgery, since vagal nerve irritation at that area produces profound bradycardia unless a vagolytic drug is used.

SURGICAL APPROACHES

Pericardiocentesis

Pericardiocentesis is accomplished by introducing a needle into the pericardial sac. This may be done safely only in the area of the cardiac notch. The cardiac notch is the portion on the right chest wall where no lung overlies the heart. It is found at approximately the level bordered by the costochondral junction, ventral from the fourth to the sixth ribs.

Use of the cardiac notch area (1) avoids laceration of lung or coronary vessels, (2) avoids puncturing a high-pressure chamber, and (3) allows the needle to be introduced far from the thin-walled atrial chambers. Consequently, the tap is made into the pericardial sac over the right ventricular chamber. If the ventricle is inadvertently touched, or even if the needle is introduced into the ventricular chamber, no major bleeding will occur.

The technique for pericardiocentesis requires clipping and surgically scrubbing the right ventral midthorax. The needle is inserted at the level of the costochondral junction at the posterior third of the rib space to avoid the intercostal artery, vein, and nerve. Negative pressure is applied and the needle is advanced until heart is touched or until the desired fluid is withdrawn. Local anesthesia may be applied at the skin site, but this is frequently more painful than the process of pericardiocentesis.

Median Sternotomy

The median sternotomy approach to the heart is most popular in humans but has not been used extensively in the dog or cat. It is our opinion that the medium sternotomy is an ideal technique for some procedures such as tumor removal, pericardectomy, or exploratory surgery. Procedures such as right ventriculotomy can be accomplished through the median sternotomy, and the approach may be considered. The advantages of median sternotomy over a lateral thoracotomy are (1) visualization of both sides of the thorax (2) proximity to the right ventricular outflow tract, (3) visualization of all heart chambers, and (4) reduced hemorrhage for some procedures requiring heparin therapy.

Median sternotomy can be accomplished by placing the animal in dorsal recumbency and incising the skin just cranial to the manubrium to just caudal to the xiphoid. The procedure need not extend along the full length of the sternum, if wide exposure of the thorax is not required. The approach to the cranial heart may require only the median sternotomy from the manubrium to the mid-sternal area, while procedures on the caudal portion of the heart may be accomplished with incisions only from mid-sternum to xiphoid. In any case, the approach is made strictly on the midline, so that no muscles need be transected. The incision continues between the pectoral muscles and the sternebrae, and the sternebrae are divided by saw, chisel, or heavy scissors. Closure of median sternotomy usually requires wiring of the sternebrae and at least three layers of tissue closure. Healing is facilitated if the sternebrae have not been cut from manubrium to xiphoid, so that several sternebrae may be left to stabilize the sternum. A disadvantage of median sternotomy is delayed healing if pleural effusion continues postoperatively. Because of the patient's preference for sternal positioning, the pleural effusion will seep into the surgical site. This will delay and occasionally prohibit healing.

Lateral Thoracotomy

By far the most common surgical approach to the heart in domestic animals is by lateral thoracotomy. A left lateral thoracotomy at the fourth intercostal space can be used for nearly all clinical surgical procedures involving the heart and can be applied for thoracotomies at most other intercostal spaces.

With the animal in right lateral recumbency, the fourth intercostal space is identified at the posterior border of the scapula. The skin incision is made from the level of the ventral portion of the vertebrae to just proximal to the ventral midline of the animal. The cutaneous trunci and subcutaneous tissues are divided using scissors. Most thoracotomy bleeding will occur at this layer. The latissimus dorsi muscle is the first major structure to be cut and is partially transected from its ventral border, approximately halfway to its dorsal border. The latissimus dorsi does not need to be transected but requires constant dorsal retraction throughout the procedure if the partial transection is not performed. The scalenus muscle inserts as an aponeurosis beginning at the fifth rib. The fibrous aponeurosis should be transected and the scalenus reflected anteriorly. At this point, the intercostal space should be verified. This can be done by palpating beneath the latissimus dorsi to the thoracic inlet and counting the ribs. In extremely small animals, a curved hemostat may be passed to the thoracic inlet and reflected off each rib to identify the fourth intercostal space. The serratus ventralis muscle is divided between its heads at the appropriate rib space. The fascia and connective tis-

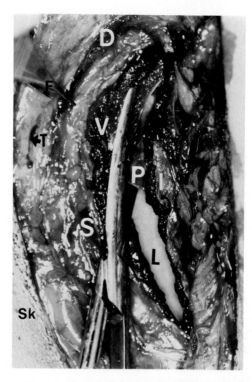

Fig. 29-1 Left lateral thoracotomy at the fourth intercostal space. Craniad is to the left. Visible, from left to right, are skin (Sk), cutaneous trunci (T), latissimus dorsi (D) at the forceps (F), the anteriorly reflected scalenus (S), serratus ventralis (V), and the intercostal muscles (I). The pleura (P) is being cut and the lung (L) is seen through the thoracic opening.

sue is divided over the fourth intercostal space, revealing the intercostal muscles. The external and internal intercostal muscles are divided in the posterior one-third of the rib space, thereby protecting the intercostal artery, vein, and nerve. The pleura is then visualized.

The anesthesiologist should permit the lungs to collapse as a small hole is made in the pleura. The pleural incision is then extended dorsally and ventrally (Fig. 29-1). At the ventral end of the incision, care should be taken not to interrupt the internal thoracic artery as it courses within 1 cm of the lateral border of the sternum. Rib retractors are placed. The left anterior lung is then rotated at its base and packed posteriorly. This completes the lateral thoracotomy in the left fourth intercostal space. It reveals the structures of the heart appropriate for most of the surgical procedures discussed below.

SURGICAL PROCEDURES FOR CARDIOVASCULAR DISEASE

Atrial Septal Defect

Atrial septal defect is a very rare cardiac lesion in the dog and is seen only occasionally in the cat. Septum primum defects are more commonly seen in the cat (part of the endocardial cushion defect) and may cause clinical symptoms.[1] However, solitary atrial septal defect of the secundum type rarely produces symptomatology in the dog or cat. Consequently, surgical repair for atrial septal defect is infrequently accomplished[2] and usually requires open heart surgery. The techniques for open heart surgery is not described in this text; however, with cardiopulmonary bypass, the right atrium may be opened and the defect closed either with direct suture or by patch. Cardiac bypass for atrial septal defect is perhaps the most easily accomplished of the open heart surgical procedures.

Tricuspid Valve Disease

Surgery of the tricuspid valve for tricuspid regurgitation is currently not done in veterinary medicine. Surgery for tricuspid dysplasia or Ebstein's anomaly has been performed[3]; however, results are poor and cannot be recommended at this time. Valve replacement requires open heart surgery and tricuspid valve replacement requires long-term anticoagulation. These techniques are not reliable in the dog.

Pulmonic Stenosis

Pulmonic stenosis is one of the most common congenital heart defects seen in the dog but is rare in the cat. In the dog, the condition may occur in any of five distinct areas. Peripheral pulmonic stenosis has been seen only very rarely in domestic animals. Supravalvular pulmonic stenosis, valvular pulmonic stenosis, discrete subvalvular pulmonic stenosis, and muscular infundibular pulmonic stenosis are more frequently found. Pulmonary valve dysplasia may present as a malformed valve, including the immediate subvalvular tissue. It appears as part of a combination of valvular and subvalvular pulmonic stenosis. Muscular infundibular pulmonic stenosis may occur singularly or secondary to any of the other types. Identification of the precise type and location of pulmonic stenosis is important, since surgical techniques vary depending on the type and site of the pulmonic stenosis.

It is therefore imperative that definitive diagnosis and characterization be ascertained before surgery. Venous angiography alone may be used to identify the area of stenosis. The severity of the disease may be indicated by the thickness of the right ventricular wall. When coupled with a right ventricular hypertrophy pattern on the ECG, these tests may imply the necessity for surgery. However, if facilities are available, the superior technique to determine the severity of pulmonic stenosis and thereby provide surgical criteria is measurement of the right ventricular to pulmonary artery pressure gradient. This can only be accomplished by cardiac catheterization and is best performed with a catheter placed in the pulmonary artery and a separate catheter in the right ventricle. More frequently, a catheter placed in the pulmonary artery is withdrawn to the right ventricle. The pressures are thus recorded. These techniques permit assessment of the gradient and the pullout technique identifies the area of gradient change. In severe pulmonic stenosis, it may not be advisable to introduce the catheter into the pulmonary artery, since the additional size of the catheter may compromise cardiac output through a small pulmonary valve opening. A right ventricular systolic pressure of 120 mmHg is critically elevated and is always associated with the need for surgery. With right ventricular pressures of 120 mmHg and pulmonary artery pressures of 20 mmHg, for example, the gradient is 100 mmHg. Surgery is not recommended with right ventricular pressures of 70 mmHg or less or gradients of 50 mmHg or less. Surgical intervention may be indicated with right ventricular pressures of 70 to 120 mmHg or gradients of 50 to 100 mmHg. Equivocal pressures must be associated with clinical signs to indicate if surgery should be performed. If the lower to medium pressure ranges are found in mature animals, the condition most likely does not require surgery. However, if the lower to middle pressure ranges are associated with growing animals, it can be anticipated that the disease will become more severe and that the animal will become a surgical candidate.

The surgical techniques for pulmonic stenosis may vary from relatively simple (e.g., bistoury or Brock technique), to moderately complicated (e.g., pulmonary arteriotomy or patch-graft technique), reasonably complicated (e.g., grafting procedures) or technically difficult (e.g., open heart surgery). The techniques are described and their advantages and disadvantages explained below.

BISTOURY TECHNIQUE

The most simple procedure for pulmonic stenosis is the bistoury technique. This has been used in veterinary medicine since 1961,[4] and the value of the procedure is related to its simplicity. The bistoury technique is appropriate for only valvular pulmonic stenosis.

The bistoury technique for pulmonic stenosis is accomplished through a left lateral thoracotomy in the fourth intercostal space or by median sternotomy. The right ventricular outflow tract is visualized and a pursestring suture placed in the relatively avascular portion. A stab incision is made into the right ventricle, a bistoury (frequently a teat bis-

toury) is introduced into the right ventricular outflow tract across the stenotic valve, and the valve is cut (Fig. 29-2). It is probably advantageous to make several cuts. The bistoury is removed, the purse string is tightened down, and closure is routine.

The bistoury technique for pulmonic stenosis requires little to no aftercare, and the results are excellent in pure valvular pulmonic stenosis. The technique is of no advantage in supravalvular or muscular pulmonic stenosis and has little value in subvalvular pulmonic stenosis or in cases of severely dysplastic pulmonary valves. Another disadvantage of bistoury repair for pulmonic stenosis is lack of visualization of the obstructed area, but in valvular pulmonic stenosis this is not a major fault.

MODIFIED BROCK PROCEDURE

The modified Brock procedure used for muscular pulmonic stenosis is very similar to the bistoury technique except that the instrument introduced is an infundibular rongeur. The offending tissue is excised with the rongeur. Closure and postoperative management are identical to the bistoury technique.[5]

The Brock procedure is used effectively for only solitary muscular or infundibular pulmonic stenosis

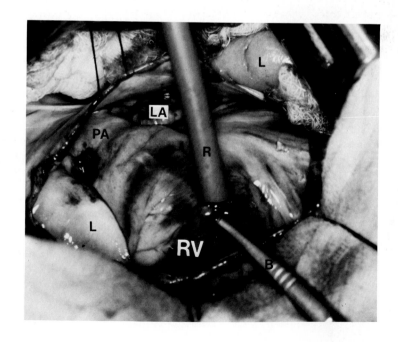

Fig. 29-2 Left lateral thoracotomy at the fourth intercostal space. A bistoury (B) is introduced through a pursestring suture in a Rommel tourniquet (R) (to control bleeding) and into the right ventricle (RV). It is passed through the obstruction where cuts are then made in the vascular or fibrous subvalvular ring. L, lung; PA, pulmonary artery; LA, left auricle.

and is of no value for the other types. A major disadvantage of the technique is the inability to visualize the muscle tissue being removed.

VALVULOTOME VALVOTOMY

Valve dilation using a valvulotome is similar to the previously described techniques. In using a valvulotome, both valvular and fibrous subvalvular stenoses and most dysplastic pulmonary valve obstructions can be opened. The technique is identical to the previously described procedures; however, in this case the valvulotome is introduced into the right ventricle and is passed into the obstructed area. The valvulotome is then opened, and cuts are made in either the valve or subvalvular tissue, or both. Closure and postoperative management is identical to the previously described techniques.

Valvulotome valvotomy for pulmonic stenosis is effective in valvular, subvalvular, and dysplastic pulmonic stenosis. The disadvantages in the technique include the lack of visualization of the offending area as the valvulotome cuts are made. However, if the patient is correctly selected for the appropriate type of pulmonic stenosis, valvotomy using a valvulotome is very effective.

INFLOW OCCLUSION AND PULMONARY ARTERIOTOMY

Perhaps the most efficient technique for valvular, immediate subvalvular, or pulmonary valve dysplasia pulmonic stenosis is inflow occlusion and pulmonary arteriotomy (Swan procedure).[6] Originally, the techniques used mild hypothermia, but this is not necessary in the dog.

The inflow occlusion pulmonary arteriotomy repair for pulmonic stenosis is accomplished through a left lateral thoracotomy in the fourth intercostal space. The lungs are reflected and umbilical tapes placed around the anterior and posterior vena cavae. The anterior vena cava is identified by careful blunt dissection cranial to the heart across the mediastinum and ventral to the brachiocephalic artery. Once the vena cava is identified, umbilical tape is passed around the vessel, and a Rommel tourniquet is loosely positioned over the umbilical tape. The posterior vena cava is poorly identified from a fourth intercostal space. The heart must be rotated cranially. This necessitates breaking down the mediastinum caudal to the heart. Once visualization of the vena cava has been accomplished, the tourniquet is placed in a similar manner. The pericardium is opened dorsal and parallel to the phrenic nerve. Pericardial basket sutures are placed on both edges of the cut pericardium, and the heart is elevated using the basket sutures. The pulmonary artery is identified, and a double row of 4-0 vascular stay sutures is placed in the post-stenotic dilatation or slightly toward the heart from the post-stenotic dilation. The animal is ventilated well; the Rommel tourniquets are then positioned to occlude the vena cava. Approximately 15 seconds is required for the right side of the heart to empty, and an incision is made in the pulmonary artery between the stay sutures. The pulmonary artery is opened (Fig. 29-3), suction is applied to permit visualization, and the stenotic pulmonary valve or subvalvular tissue can be cut by scalpel, scissors, or valve dilator. The valve is re-formed to approximate a normal valve or is excised, depending on the type of disease. When the corrective procedures have been completed, the stay sutures are elevated, a partially occluding clamp is placed on the pulmonary artery closing the opening, and the tourniquets are removed from the vena cava to re-establish the circulation. Throughout the occlusion procedure, some hemorrhage will occur, since the azygos vein and coronary sinus blood flow continues, necessitating the need for suction. The occlusion time should be kept to less than 3 minutes, preferably less than 2 minutes, which is almost always adequate for the repair (if not, a second occlusion can be done after 5 minutes). After circulation is re-established, the pulmonary artery is closed with a 4-0 continuous suture pattern. Closure and postoperative management in these patients is routine. The patients tend to have a slight, 1- to 2-hour delay in recovery from anesthesia which is probably associated with the short period of anoxia sustained during the inflow occlusion.

Pulmonary arteriotomy is effective in valvular and subvalvular dysplastic valves. It is not effective in muscular infundibular stenosis, nor is it effective in supravalvular pulmonic stenosis. The technique has the significant advantage of permitting visualization of the offending obstructive tissue. Therefore, a satisfactory correction can be observed. The

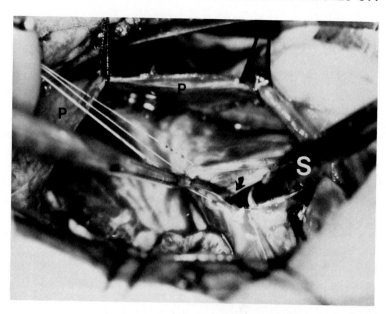

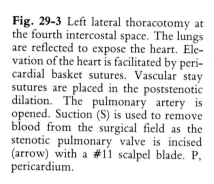

Fig. 29-3 Left lateral thoracotomy at the fourth intercostal space. The lungs are reflected to expose the heart. Elevation of the heart is facilitated by pericardial basket sutures. Vascular stay sutures are placed in the poststenotic dilation. The pulmonary artery is opened. Suction (S) is used to remove blood from the surgical field as the stenotic pulmonary valve is incised (arrow) with a #11 scalpel blade. P, pericardium.

disadvantages of inflow occlusion for pulmonic stenosis are (1) the slightly more difficult surgical technique, and (2) the fact that in immature animals the fibrosis associated with the surgery will become permanent. This technique is therefore not recommended in animals under 6 months of age.

PATCH-GRAFT TECHNIQUE

Recently, a technique that is effective for valvular and subvalvular dysplastic valves and muscular pulmonic stenosis has been used in veterinary medicine.[7] The patch-graft technique is usually performed with a cutting wire positioned under a patch in such a way that when the wire is pulled, the ventricular wall is cut, opening the ventricle and pulmonary artery to the patch. The technique of patch graft and cutting wire is relatively simple. In severe pulmonic stenosis, particularly with right ventricular hypertrophy or dysplastic or very fibrous valves, the procedure is not always aesthetically pleasing and is difficult to perform successfully.

The patch-graft technique is accomplished through a left lateral thoracotomy in the fourth intercostal space or by median sternotomy. The right ventricular outflow tract to the pulmonary valve is identified. A cutting wire is placed into the ventricle and pushed out the main pulmonary artery. This approach is facilitated by passing the wire through an over-the-needle catheter. The difficulty in identifying the ventricular chamber inside the thickened right ventricular wall is aided by the catheter as blood will flow through the catheter when the ventricular chamber is penetrated. A small urinary catheter or large 14- to 16-gauge over-the-needle injection catheter can be used. The ventricular chamber is identified, and the catheter is passed into the pulmonary artery. A stylet is then placed into the catheter to facilitate exiting the catheter from the pulmonary artery through the arterial wall. A Gigli wire is passed through the catheter, and the catheter is withdrawn. We have found it advantageous to put a small 6-0 pursestring suture in the pulmonary artery around the catheter at its exit point to eliminate continual bleeding while the patch is being sutured into place. A Dacron or pericardial patch is then placed over the wire from the pulmonary artery to the right ventricle. The patch is secured by continuous suture with the last one or two sutures not drawn down (Fig. 29-4). When the patch is in place, the cutting wire is then pulled out and the right ventricle, proximal pulmonary artery, and the obstructed area of pulmonic stenosis are opened into the patch. Digital pressure controls the bleeding at the last two sutures as the wire is removed at the

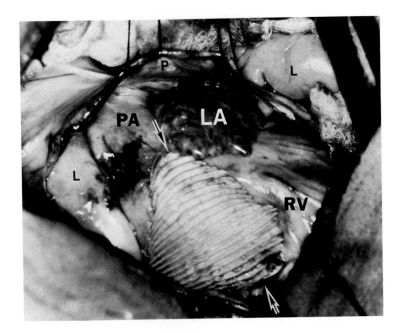

Fig. 29-4 Left lateral thoracotomy at the fourth intercostal space. The lungs (L) are reflected. The pericardium (P) is incised parallel and ventral to the phrenic nerve. Pericardial basket sutures are placed to assist in elevating the heart. A patch graft of woven Dacron is in place from the pulmonary artery (top arrow) to the body of the right ventricle (bottom arrow). PA, pulmonary artery; LA, left auricle; RV, right ventricle.

ventral portion of the patch. The last sutures are then secured.

A chest drain tube should be placed and should remain for 24 hours after completion of the patch-graft technique. The effusion that may occur as a result of foreign material (i.e., Dacron) may cause continuous pleural effusion and drainage for 2 to 3 days. After 12 hours without effusion, the drain tube can be removed. Animals undergoing patch-graft technique with foreign material should be placed on antibiotics preoperatively and maintained on antibiotics for approximately 1 week. After the chest drain tube is removed, the patient management can be similar to the previously described techniques.

The great advantage of the patch-graft repair for pulmonic stenosis is that it permits expansion and decompression of the right ventricular chamber. The other advantage of this technique is that the patch can be made very large to facilitate growth in the young patient that would otherwise require multiple surgeries because of severe pulmonic stenosis at a young age. Disadvantages of the technique are related to the difficulty of entering the right ventricular lumen when severe hypertrophy is present, the brutal manipulation involved in cutting the right ventricle, and the difficulty in some cases of cutting

through the fibrous, thickened pulmonic stenosis with the cutting wire.

L. K. Anderson (East Lansing, MI, 1985) recently suggested a modification of the patch-graft technique. In the Anderson revision, no cutting wire is used. Thus, blood loss and trauma to the right ventricular wall are reduced. After placing the patch graft, inflow occlusion is used as above and a pulmonary arteriotomy is performed distal to the patch graft. Using scissors or scalpel, the right ventricle, stenotic valve area and proximal pulmonary artery are cut and opened into the patch. This technique permits direct visualization of the outflow into the patch and eliminates the risk associated with the occasional unwanted tear by the cutting suture. This modification has become our preferred patch-graft technique.

CONDUIT REPAIR

A variety of types of pulmonic stenosis can be repaired by conduits. In the case of supravalvular pulmonic stenosis, a conduit for the proximal pulmonary artery to distal pulmonary artery around the obstruction can be used.[8] In some types of severe dysplasia, conduits from the right ventricle to the pulmonary artery can be used to bypass the obstruction. In the rare involvement with tricuspid atresia, conduits from the right atrium to the pulmonary artery (Fontan procedure) can be used to bypass the obstruction. To date the only successful use of conduits in veterinary medicine have been from proximal pulmonary artery to distal pulmonary artery or from the right ventricle to the pulmonary artery.

The surgical procedure for conduit repair is accomplished by a left lateral thoracotomy in the fourth intercostal space or, depending on the type of repair, by a median sternotomy. The conduit is attached distally to the pulmonary artery by end-to-side anastomosis after the distal pulmonary artery has been partially occluded. The proximal attachment of the conduit depends on the amount of tissue and on the structures to be bypassed. Attachment to the proximal pulmonary artery for supravalvular pulmonic stenosis is identical to the attachment distally. The attachment to the right ventricle is made with difficulty and sometimes requires removal of a right ventricular plug and a cage dilation of the right ventricular cavity to prevent occlusion of the conduit inflow. In the Fontan procedure, the valved conduit is usually attached to the right atrial appendage. Because of the technically difficult aspects of conduit repair, they can be recommended only for major institutions at this time. The future for use of conduits in pulmonic stenosis, however, appears to be bright.

OPEN HEART SURGERY

The final technique for repair of pulmonic stenosis used in veterinary medicine is open-heart surgery. Although these techniques have been worked out, they are currently too expensive and require a major commitment of both equipment and personnel. The techniques are effective for all types of pulmonic stenosis but cannot be recommended for clinical practice at this time.

Ventricular Septal Defect

Ventricular septal defect is the most common congenital cardiac defect of the cat and is one of the most common lesions found in the dog. Fortunately, most animals with ventricular septal defect that survive to 6 weeks of age (the time at which a veterinarian usually first becomes acquainted with

them) have a defect so small that surgical or medical intervention is unnecessary. The diagnosis of ventricular septal defect is described elsewhere, but it must be remembered that the presence of a loud ventricular septal defect murmur does not necessarily mean that the lesion is severe. A clinical indication of severe ventricular septal defect can be made by the presence of a secondary functional pulmonic stenosis murmur, main pulmonary artery enlargement on the dorsoventral radiograph, or radiographic evidence of overcirculated lungs. If these are present or if the animal is symptomatic, surgical treatment of ventricular septal defect can be considered. In extremely young animals, the management of ventricular septal defect using diuretics and perhaps digitalization might be considered in an attempt to improve the patient for surgery or delay surgery in the hope that spontaneous closure of the defect might occur.

Three methods of repair for ventricular septal defect have been used in veterinary medicine. Open-heart surgical repair[9] is curative but carries a high risk and is expensive. Deep hypothermic circulatory arrest[10] is curative, extremely time consuming, carries a high risk, and requires extensive familiarity with hypothermia surgery. Pulmonary artery banding is palliative, relatively simple, carries a very low risk, but cannot be performed in immature animals.[11]

PULMONARY ARTERY BANDING

In pulmonary artery banding, an umbilical tape band is placed on the pulmonary artery to increase right ventricular pressure and therefore decrease the left-to-right ventricular shunt. This palliative technique can be easily and successfully performed in mature dogs or cats with ventricular septal defect. Surgery is performed through a left lateral thoracotomy in the fourth intercostal space in the routine manner. The pulmonary artery is visualized in its usual position and is usually distended. By careful blunt dissection using a right-angle forceps, the main pulmonary artery is circled, preferably cranially to caudally, on the medial side. By dissecting around the artery from cranial to caudal, inadvertent tearing of the right pulmonary artery is less likely. The dissection should be carried out close to the heart since the main pulmonary artery in the dog is quite short. Once the instrument has circled behind the main pulmonary artery, an umbilical tape is passed around the vessel.

The pulmonary artery can then be compressed with the umbilical tape until the pulmonary artery is one-third its original diameter or, if distended, one-third the apparent diameter at the pulmonary valve (Fig. 29-5). The umbilical tape is then sutured at that position to maintain the pulmonary artery at the one-third normal diameter. If desired, a knot can then be placed in the umbilical tape. Pulmonary artery size should decrease, and the color of the pulmonary artery should darken with reduction of the shunt. If the band is placed too loosely, right ventricular pressure will not be elevated sufficiently to reduce shunt flow from the left ventricle. If the band is placed too tightly, potential right-to-left shunting through the ventricular septal defect can produce

severe cyanotic heart disease. If pressure measurements can be made, the pulmonary artery pressure should be reduced to one-half the prebanding pressure, or the right ventricular pressure should be increased to twice the prebanding pressure. These pressures can be measured by a small needle inserted directly into the pulmonary artery distal to the band or into the right ventricular lumen. Closure and postoperative management are routine. Animals with pulmonary artery banding recover quickly and can usually be discharged the following day.

Animals with pulmonary artery banding should be monitored over the following week to 10 days to ensure that no cyanosis develops. If cyanosis occurs, right-to-left shunting has developed and the band must be removed or loosened. Animals with pulmonary artery bands can be expected to have normal longevity; however, they may have reduced

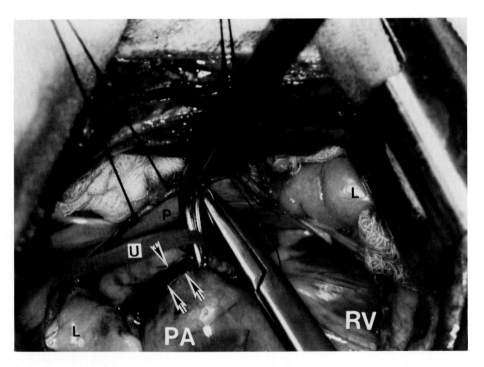

Fig. 29-5 Left lateral thoracotomy at the fourth intercostal space. The lungs (L) are reflected and the pericardium is incised parallel and dorsal to the phrenic nerve. Pericardial basket sutures assist in elevating the heart. An umbilical tape is positioned around the pulmonary artery (arrows), tightened, and held in position with right-angle forceps. The pulmonary artery diameter is reduced to one-third the diameter of the pulmonary artery at its origin, the pulmonary valve annulus. Sutures are then placed (e.g., needle holder) and tied in the umbilical tape to maintain this tape diameter. P, pericardium; U, umbilical tape; PA, pulmonary artery (labeled at the approximate level of the pulmonary valve annulus); RV, right ventricle.

activity. In the human, pulmonary artery banding is used to support patients with overcirculated lungs until definitive curative procedures can be accomplished, usually by 6 years of age. In the dog, the technique is the definitive procedure and with animals, can be considered an effective technique. Long-term results with pulmonary artery banding (in excess of 10 years) have been good.

Tetralogy of Fallot

The surgical treatment of tetralogy of Fallot should be instituted only when medical therapy fails. Approximately 50 percent of animals with tetralogy can be expected to have significant reduction of clinical signs by medical management using β-adrenergic blockade. Animals with medical therapy have slightly compromised life-styles but can be quite comfortable as household pets.

In dogs or cats with tetralogy that are not responsive to medical management, surgical palliation or correction can be considered. A few successful surgical corrections for tetralogy of Fallot using open heart surgery have been reported. The procedure is costly and carries a high mortality. It cannot be advised at this time.

Palliative procedures for tetralogy of Fallot using systemic to pulmonary artery shunts appear to be effective and can be recommended in dogs not responsive to medical therapy. These shunts include the classic Blalock-Taussig anastomosis, Pott's anastomosis, or graft or conduit connections.[12,13] The Blalock anastomosis is described here as a typical procedure.

BLALOCK ANASTOMOSIS

The purpose of shunt surgery is to return a large portion of the partially oxygenated systemic blood to the lung, to then be oxygenated and returned to the left side of the heart. The Blalock anastomosis has been used successfully in humans since 1947; first, as a final repair and currently as a palliative technique.

Blalock anastomosis is accomplished through a left thoracotomy at the fourth intercostal space. The darkened pulmonary artery can be visualized. The left subclavian artery is identified and ligated as far distally as possible. The artery is then clamped using a bulldog clamp and transected distally. The left subclavian artery is then mobilized toward the pulmonary artery. If the arc for the left subclavian artery is smooth, a direct end-to-side anastomosis of the left subclavian to pulmonary artery can be accomplished. The pulmonary artery is partially occluded with a Satinsky-type clamp and, with the continuous suture pattern, the anastomosis can be made. The pulmonary artery clamp is removed, the suture holes are allowed to fill with blood, and 1 or 2 minutes later the bulldog clamp on the subclavian artery can be removed (Fig. 29-6).

If the animal is small or the left subclavian artery appears to kink at the origin from the aorta when rotated toward the pulmonary artery, a revision of the left subclavian artery origin should be considered. The aorta, at the point where the subclavian artery exists, should be clamped with a partially occluding clamp. A diamond-shaped incision, partially including the aorta and partially including the left subclavian artery, can be made at the junction of the subclavian artery and aorta. The subclavian artery is then rotated toward the pulmonary artery, and the two angles of the diamond are sutured together. This makes a more direct outflow from the aorta to the left subclavian artery and removes the shelf of tissue produced by kinking of the vessel as it is rotated ventrally and posteriorly. The final portion of the anastomosis to the pulmonary artery is carried out in the routine manner.

POTT'S ANASTOMOSIS AND CONDUIT SHUNTS

Pott's anastomosis is a simple side-to-side pulmonary artery to aorta anastomosis. The surgery requires the use of expensive Pott's clamps, which are used to partially occlude the aorta. Techniques of anastomosis are similar to other vascular anastomoses, but the size and length of the fistula developed must be carefully monitored lest extreme pulmonary recirculation and left-sided heart failure develop. For those reasons Pott's anastomosis is not recommended at this time for small animals.

Conduit shunt from aorta to pulmonary artery has been described in veterinary medicine for tetralogy. The techniques require microsurgical skills and are probably limited to large institutions at this time.

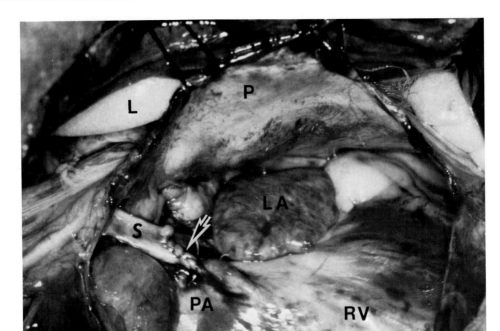

Fig. 29-6 Left lateral thoracotomy at the fourth intercostal space. The lungs (L) and left subclavian artery (S) are reflected to expose the main pulmonary artery (PA). These two arteries have been anastomosed in an end-to-side pattern (arrow) completing the Blalock anastomosis as a palliative procedure for tetralogy of Fallot. P, pericardium; LA, left auricle; RV, right ventricle.

Patent Ductus Arteriosus

Fortunately, the most common congenital heart defect in the dog is readily amenable to surgical correction. Patent ductus arteriosus, nearly always fatal if left untreated, can be *cured* surgically with a success rate of greater than 95 percent. Animals with surgically corrected patent ductus arteriosus can be expected to live a normal life.

Surgery should be performed at the earliest possible date. Young age or small size are not contraindications for therapy; however, large older dogs have a significantly lower success rate.[14] This may be attributable to the increased difficulty of surgery, their large size, the development of left-sided heart failure, or myocardial disease. Smaller breeds with patent ductus arteriosus tend to develop left-sided

backward heart failure and pulmonary edema at an earlier age and over a shorter time period than larger breeds. If patent ductus arteriosus is identified early, the animal is usually operated on in a compensated state without clinical signs of heart failure. However, 50 percent of dogs presented for patent ductus arteriosus surgery will have mitral regurgitation secondary to left ventricular dilation and subsequent dilation of the mitral annulus. These animals with secondary mitral regurgitation may have pulmonary edema due to left-sided heart failure. Large breeds that are permitted to persist with the disease may develop atrial fibrillation, at which time successful surgical therapy for patent ductus arteriosus is less than 50 percent.

Occasionally, dogs with patent ductus arteriosus

may develop pulmonary hypertension and secondary right-to-left shunt. More frequently, right-to-left shunt in dogs is a result of persistence of the fetal circulation, so that the embryologic right-to-left pulmonary to aortic flow persists into the neonatal period. Dogs with right-to-left shunting patent ductus arteriosus, regardless of cause, are inoperable, and the disease can be considered fatal.

Surgery for patent ductus arteriosus is relatively simple. Animals with evidence of pulmonary edema, mitral valve regurgitation, or left-sided heart failure should have profound diuresis induced 12 hours before surgery. Digitalization and other heart failure medications are not as effective as inducing diuresis, and in many critical patients the delay incurred for digitalization increases the risk of surgery.

STANDARD DISSECTION TECHNIQUE

Surgery for patent ductus arteriosus is carried out through left lateral thoracotomy at the fourth intercostal space in the routine manner after high-dose atropinization. The atropine is administered preoperatively, since manipulation of the vagus nerve must be accomplished to visualize the ductus. The left cranial lung lobe is rotated posteriorly, revealing the right ventricular outflow tract and descending aorta. An incision is made into the pericardium parallel to and between the vagus and phrenic nerves. The vagus nerve is identified, looped with umbilical tape, and elevated along with the pericardium off the heart and the aorta. By means of right-angle forceps, the normal cleavage plane between the cranial dorsal aorta and posterior ventral pulmonary artery is opened. This plane is just cranial to the ductus. The ductus can now be visualized beneath the elevated vagus nerve, ventral to the aorta and dorsal to the pulmonary artery (Fig. 29-7). The right-angle forceps is passed beneath the aorta, posterior to the ductus, and around and down to the previously opened cleavage plane. With the right-angle forceps beneath the ductus, two double 0 silk sutures are carried behind the ductus, positioned, and tied. The aortic side of the ductus is tied first. Closure is routine.

In dogs heavier than 7 kg, safety ties may be placed on the arch vessels in an effort to control

bleeding if bleeding occurs. These are simply accomplished with umbilical tape by looping the left subclavian and brachiocephalic arteries and placing a Blalock tourniquet around the descending aorta. An additional incision is made in the pericardium ventral to the phrenic nerve. With the availability of these safety measures, bleeding produced by a tear in the ductus can be controlled. The umbilical tapes are tightened on the subclavian and brachiocephalic arteries and on the aorta to control all systemic arterial backflow to the ductus. A large vascular clamp is placed across the pulmonary artery and aorta through the opening made in the pericardium at the transverse sinus of the pericardium. This stops all forward bleeding from the aorta and the pulmonary artery. Once back-bleeding from the pulmonary artery is stopped, all blood flow in the circulatory system is stopped and a clamp or suture can be placed on the torn ductus. Duration of occlusion must be kept less than 2 minutes. Animals weighing less than 7 kg would probably exsanguinate before the safety sutures and clamps could be applied; therefore, the safety technique is generally not recommended in these small animals.

JACKSON TECHNIQUE

An additional technique for suture placement around the ductus eliminates dissection posterior to the friable ductus. This Jackson technique[15] requires passing one end of the sutures beneath the aorta cranial to the ductus and out the prepared cleavage point between the aorta and pulmonary artery. The other end of the sutures is carried under the aorta from dorsal to ventral posterior to the ductus (Fig. 29-8). When the ends of the sutures are pulled together and tied, the suture is pulled beneath the ductus, thereby occluding it. This technique eliminates the risk of dissection to the right of the ductus, a friable and dangerous area, but precludes the positioning of double sutures on the ductus.

Postoperative management of patent ductus arteriosus patients is extremely simple. Most animals are awake and moving within 1 hour after completion of surgery and usually can be discharged the following day. The owner should be cautioned that the animal should not engage in strenuous exercise during the ensuing 3 weeks, but no other restrictions are required. Animals with corrected patent ductus

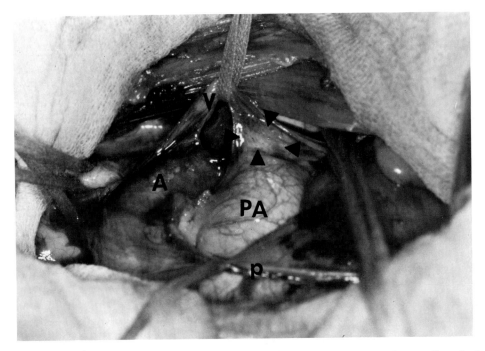

Fig. 29-7 Left lateral thoracotomy at the fourth intercostal space. The lungs have been reflected, the vagus nerve (V) has been elevated (top), and the phrenic nerve (P) is visualized at the bottom. The patent ductus arteriosus is exposed and is barely visible (within arrows) between the aorta (dorsal) and the pulmonary artery (ventral). The patent ductus arteriosus is medial to the vagus nerve.

arteriosus should not be used for breeding since approximately one-half of their offspring will develop the disease.

Approximately 1.5 percent of ductus ligations will recanalize. The cause of recanalization is frequently unknown; however, infection at the time of surgery may precipitate it. In patients in which recanalization occurs, the problem will usually recur within 2 months of the original surgery. When recanalization has occurred, the animal should be reoperated. This technique requires difficult dissection and the placement of expensive patent ductus clamps. The ductus is then divided between the clamps and sutured with 6-0 vascular suture. This technique is extremely difficult, carries a high risk, and should be considered only by surgeons experienced in vascular surgery.

Mitral Valve Disease

After heartworm disease, mitral valve regurgitation is the most common acquired heart disease in dogs. The incidence may be as high as 8 percent of dogs over 5 years of age.[16] Although clinical signs may develop that are referable to the regurgitation, most animals do not develop congestive heart failure. The disease is usually progressive. The signs associated with mitral regurgitation are primarily due to compression of the left main bronchus and may be severe. Medical therapy (e.g., vasodilators) may reduce the size of the left atrium and associated compression of the left main bronchus. In a small percentage of dogs with mitral regurgitation, left-sided backward heart failure occurs. Appropriate medical management should be instituted (Chs. 8 and 20).

In a few animals with mitral regurgitation, surgical treatment has been performed.[17,18] Patients selected for surgery must be in otherwise good health. This precludes dogs exhibiting signs of mitral regurgitation secondary to cardiomyopathy. These procedures are primarily of academic interest at this time. The cost of valve conduits, extensive surgery, or of cardiopulmonary bypass and valve replace-

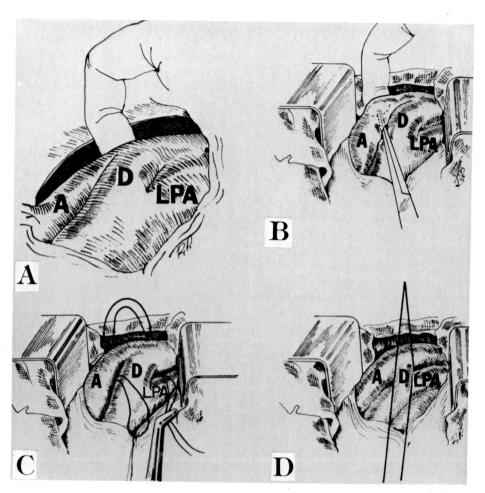

Fig. 29-8 (**A**) Dissection prior to ligature placement for patent ductus arteriosus. Following incision of the mediastinum dorsal to the aorta, the dissection to the medial aspect of the aorta (**A**) is performed digitally. Between the left subclavian and first intercostal vessels (at the fifth space) there are no vessels, nor are there fragile structures medial to the aorta in the mediastinum. The aorta is thoroughly mobilized on its medial aspect. D, patent ductus; LPA, left pulmonary artery. (**B**) Ligature placement for patent ductus arteriosus. A pair of blunt, smooth hemostats are passed ventral to the aortic arch (**A**) aided by the index finger. The tips of the instrument should be kept close to the aorta. The instrument should be thin enough to insure that stretching of the patent ductus and pulmonary artery is minimal. Once passed, the instrument grasps the midpoint of a suture, which is drawn to the lateral aortic aspect. (**C**) The maneuver used in **B** is repeated caudal to the ductus (**D**) around the descending aorta (**A**), and the two free ends of the looped ligature are pulled laterally. Care is taken to prevent the ligatures from becoming entwined. LPA, left pulmonary artery. (**D**) The suture is placed under tension, and the medial aortic lengths are gently placed by traction medial to the ductus (**D**). The looped cranial suture is cut in two, forming two separate ligatures encircling the ductus that are carefully and slowly tied. (Henderson RA, Jackson WF: Patent ductus arteriosus. p. 455. In Bojrab MJ (ed): Current Techniques in Small Animal Surgery. 2nd Ed. Lea & Febiger, Philadelphia, 1983.)

ment eliminates these techniques for all but a few patients at several selective institutions.

Mitral valve stenosis is rare in small animal veterinary medicine. Surgical considerations are therefore not addressed here.

Aortic Stenosis

Aortic stenosis is one of the most common canine congenital anomalies and presents a significant management problem. Although medical management has been suggested, it cannot resolve or hemodynamically stabilize the typical candidate with subvalvular fibrous obstruction. Mildly affected dogs with subvalvular aortic stenosis exhibit no clinical signs and can be expected to live a normal life. Evaluation requires demonstration of left ventricular hypertrophy and obstruction by echocardiography or by angiography. These diagnostic tests associated with physical findings are confirmatory. Final classic diagnosis of severity depends on cardiac catheterization and left ventricular pressure measurement. The severity of aortic stenosis is generally considered either mild with left ventricular to aortic gradients of less than 50 mmHg, moderate when left ventricular to aortic gradients are 50 to 90 mmHg, or severe with left ventricular to aortic gradients greater than 90 mmHg. In the human, critical aortic stenosis is thought to be present when the left ventricular to aortic gradient exceeds 100 mmHg. In veterinary medicine, we can safely assume that animals affected with mild aortic stenosis will have no signs; we believe that these animals will live normal lives. Unfortunately, we must assume that animals with severe aortic stenosis will have signs associated with the disease or that their lives will be shortened considerably. Animals with moderate aortic stenosis—a clinical gray zone—have variable signs and life expectancies. If surgical intervention is to be considered, it should be attempted only in animals with severe aortic stenosis, since the mortality and morbidity associated with the current surgical techniques are high.

VALVE CONDUITS

Left ventricle to aortic valve conduits have been used for the past several years[19] for aortic stenosis. The conduit is attached proximally to the apex of the left ventricle and to the descending aorta distally. The valve in the conduit protects against aortic regurgitation. The device permits decompression of the left ventricle and provides an alternate exit for blood from the left ventricle, reducing the critical hypertrophy that occurs with the disease. To date, results have been variable and the cost of valve conduits high.

OPEN HEART SURGERY

Open heart surgical excision of the subvalvular aortic ring has been described in veterinary medicine. Although this technique appears to be effective, the intraoperative mortality of 20 percent plus the cost of open heart surgical repair greatly reduces the use of this procedure.

We recently developed a technique of incising the subvalvular aortic ring using a Garbodi valvulotome. The procedure is accomplished through a left lateral thoracotomy at the fifth intercostal space. The apex of the left ventricle is identified and a large deep, pursestring suture placed there. A stab incision is then made into the left ventricular cavity and the valvulotome introduced into the left ventricle. The left index finger is placed around the base of the heart at the aortic valve to act as a guide to direct the valvulotome toward the aortic valve. When the tip of the valvulotome is palpated, the valvulotome is advanced through the obstruction on through the aortic valve, and the valvulotome is opened. Multiple cuts are then made as the valvulotome is retracted through the subvalvular area, incising the obstructive ring. When the valvulotome can be opened fully and the subvalvular area dilated, the valvulotome is removed from the left ventricle, and the pursestring suture is tied. Closure is routine. Results of surgery using the valvulotome appear to be good to date. Recent surgical successes have improved the survival rate to greater than 75 percent. Postoperative management is simple. Care usually requires only about 72 hours for observation and management of dysrhythmias if present. Long-term 5-year results are not available at this time.

With our present knowledge of aortic stenosis, some questions regarding the advisability of surgery should be addressed:

Question 1: When is the appropriate time to operate? If the symptoms associated with aortic stenosis, syncope, and sudden death are related to dysrhythmias secondary to hypertrophy, the surgery should be accomplished before severe hypertrophy occurs.

Question 2: How severe a gradient should be present before surgery is instituted? With a high surgical mortality (25 percent), the disease must be much worse than the surgery if the surgery is to be advised. This eliminates mild and asymptomatic moderate aortic stenosis patients from surgical consideration.

Question 3: What are the long-term results with surgical therapy? Long-term results with valve dilation and left ventricular to aortic conduit are not available. Long-term results (at least 5 years) with open heart surgical techniques are becoming available. Unfortunately, approximately 50 percent of these dogs develop signs of congestive cardiomyopathy at 5 or more years of age. Whether this is related to cardioplegia used during surgery, myocardial damage that occurred before the surgical therapy or to other factors, is not known at this time. The long-term results with surgical treatment of severe aortic stenosis are therefore still unknown.

Vascular Ring Anomalies

Vascular ring anomalies are seen in small dogs and cats and are associated with gastrointestinal signs, particularly regurgitation. For the purposes of this discussion, anomalies are divided into two groups: persistent right aortic arch and others (including double aortic arch and arch branch anomalies).

Patients with vascular ring anomalies are usually presented to the veterinarian at an early age when these animals are first fed solid food. These animals exhibit regurgitation either immediately or shortly after eating. If allowed to persist, the animals develop emaciation, starvation, and aspiration pneumonia and may die of pneumonia or malnutrition. Occasionally, mild forms of the vascular ring anomalies will present with infrequent and minimal signs.

The diagnosis of a vascular ring anomaly is made by contrast radiography from a barium swallow (see Fig. 19-12). The dilated esophagus will be identified just cranial to the heart. Occasionally, the precise area of constriction may be seen. The differential diagnosis of persistent right aortic arch or other vascular ring anomaly usually cannot be made without specific angiographic techniques. However, because of the high incidence of persistent right aortic arch (95 percent of anomalies), the cause of the obstruction is assumed to be persistent right aortic arch.[20] Since the surgical exposure is similar in all types of obstructions, further diagnostic workup is not recommended. The treatment of vascular ring anomalies is surgical division of one of the obstructing tissues.

Surgery for persistent right aortic arch as in other vascular ring anomalies is performed through a lateral thoracotomy in the left fourth intercostal space. The dilated esophagus is readily identified, and the obstructive vascular structure can be seen just caudal to the dilation of the esophagus (see Fig. 19-13). In persistent right aortic arch, the rightward aorta is usually not visualized, since it is to the right of the dilated esophagus. The tight white glistening band of the ligamentum arteriosum or patent ductus arteriosus may be identified as it obstructs the esophagus. With blunt dissection, the obstructing band is isolated, double ligated, and divided. Approximately 10 percent of the bands are patent. At the dorsal rightward end of the band, the aorta may be just visualized. The ventral, leftward pulmonary artery is easily visualized. After the ligamentum arteriosum is divided, the esophagus is bluntly freed from surrounding mediastinal tissue, which might act as a continuing constriction. At this time, the esophageal stethoscope should be passed from the distended esophagus through the constricted area into the caudal esophagus. If the esophagus is still somewhat constricted, bougienage should be instituted. This can be accomplished using a Foley catheter with the balloon placed at the constricted area. After freeing the esophagus and dilating it internally, the chest is closed in a routine manner.

Postoperatively, the patient should be fed small amounts of liquid diet frequently, preferably elevated until normal esophageal activity can return. The animals can be slowly returned to a normal feeding plan in a period of 2 to 6 weeks. In severely affected animals, esophageal motility may never return.

The prognosis for persistent right aortic arch surgery depends on the severity of the distention and the damage incurred to the distended esophagus. Consequently, immediately after the diagnosis has been established, the diet should be returned to liquid. Surgery should be performed as soon as feasible in an effort to eliminate permanent disruption of esophageal musculature and nerve supply as a result of distention. If surgery is performed before severe distention and pocketing occur, the results can be excellent. If the esophagus has distended to greater than twice normal, results are guarded.

Other vascular ring anomalies, including double aortic arch and arch vessel anomalies, are approached similarly to persistent right aortic arch. If, at the time of surgery, additional vessels are seen or aberrant subclavian arteries are visualized, they can be divided. In cases of double aortic arch, a decision must be made as to which arch to sacrifice. Preferably, the one without branches or the least prominent branch should be chosen. If the left aortic arch appears to be the largest, the patient's chest should be closed. Later, at an early convenient time, a right thoracotomy should be performed and the right aortic arch divided. Postoperative management of other vascular ring anomalies is similar to that of persistent right aortic arch. The prognosis for treatment of aberrant arch vessels is very good. Prognosis for success with double aortic arch is very poor. Fortunately, double aortic arches are only rarely recognized.

Heartworm Disease

Although rarely needed and uncommonly performed today, surgical removal of heartworms has been a successful and valuable treatment for patients with severe heartworm disease. Surgical removal of adult worms is the only successful therapeutic modality for severe postcaval heartworm syndrome.[21]

This technique is performed in the critical terminal postcaval heartworm patient. These dogs can be managed successfully by right jugular venotomy and removal of the heartworms by alligator forceps. Local anesthetic infiltration over the right jugular vein is usually all that is necessary, since such patients are prostrate and require little, if any, sedation. If available, fluoroscopy can permit visualization during manipulation.

An incision is made over the right jugular furrow.

The jugular vein is identified, occluded distally, and opened. Alligator forceps are introduced into the jugular vein and advanced into the heart, and worms are grasped and removed. At completion, the jugular vein is ligated and the skin closed. The technique is effective in approximately 85 percent of dogs with postcaval heartworm syndrome, which would otherwise be fatal. This technique can be used to reduce the worm load prior to medical treatment.

Canine heartworm disease with worms located in the right ventricle, or more frequently in the pulmonary artery, may represent a surgical disease in two situations. One includes dogs that have concurrent renal or hepatic dysfunction, restricting the use of arsenical compounds; the other involves the rare valuable field dog with severe heartworms that would be compromised by pulmonary embolization due to routine arsenical treatment. The surgeries that are effective for this type of heartworm disease were previously described for pulmonic stenosis and involve right ventriculotomy using alligator forceps rather than the bistoury, and worm removal by the forceps. Pulmonary arteriotomy after inflow occlusion and direct removal of the worms is a preferable procedure. The surgical techniques are relatively simple and have a lower morbidity in critical heartworm patients than does routine medical therapy.

Pericardial Disease

Pericardectomy for chronic pericardial disease in the dog is technically a simple procedure. However, in severe pericardial disease, the pericardium may be up to 1 cm thick, with extensive vascularization and granulomatous change, and the surgery is very difficult. Pericardial windows are not effective in this disease and should not be recommended. This is because pericardial adhesions form and adhere to the heart postoperatively. Since the disease process does not stop, the procedure is therefore no more effective than pericardiocentesis.

Since removal of most or all pericardium is required for successful pericardectomy, median sternotomy is necessary for an effective surgical exposure. Because of the granulomatous, vascular nature of the affected pericardium, electrocautery is advised for this dissection. The owner must be advised that with median sternotomy, if the procedure is not curative, persistent postoperative bleeding or effusion may be life-threatening, since it will interfere with healing of the median sternotomy incision. However, untreated chronic pericardial disease is eventually fatal, and effective surgical intervention is indicated.

Median sternotomy is performed as described previously, incising approximately the posterior two-thirds to three-fourths of the sternum. The phrenic nerves are carefully dissected free of the pericardium, and the pericardium is removed using electrosurgical techniques as close to the heart base as can safely be accomplished. Strict control of hemorrhage must be maintained. Routine chest closure is performed. Postoperative chest drainage should be maintained for at least 24 hours, or until little additional pleural effusion is collected.

If adequate removal of the pericardium is accomplished and postoperative effusion is limited, pericardectomy is a very effective procedure for chronic pericardial effusion and tamponade. Excessive postoperative effusion or inadequate removal of pericardium may produce unacceptable results, including heart failure and death.

Cardiac Tumors

The most common cardiac tumors, right atrial hemangiosarcoma and heart-base tumor, are generally not amenable to surgery. However, there have been recent reports of surgical removal of both neoplasms.[22]

Hemangiosarcoma, a primary or secondary tumor, affects the right atrium. If the tumor is primary and is identified early, it could be surgically removed. The signs associated with right atrial hemangiosarcoma are those of pericardial effusion and tamponade due to tumor erosion and bleeding into the pericardium. The procedure in cases of early disease involves isolating the tumor with a vascular clamp beneath the base of the tumor, excision, and closure of the atrium. Results of right atrial hemangiosarcoma surgery have been poor to date. The nature of the tumor, the advanced stage before symptoms, and the surgical difficulties with advanced tumors have contributed to this poor result.

Heart-base tumor, long recognized as a common neoplasm of the cardiovascular system, is a relatively slow-growing locally invading cancer. Unlike the comparable tumor in humans, it is nonse-

creting. Consequently, the signs of heart-base tumor are associated with the structures compromised by the growth of the mass. These tumors are located between the aorta and pulmonary artery and can reach enormous size before clinical signs are recognized. The usual signs of heart-base tumor are associated with hemorrhage into the pericardial sac producing effusion and pericardial tamponade.

Heart-base tumor has not been treated until recently; however, nonpublished reports of surgical excision and chemotherapy suggest a more favorable outcome for those tumors that are diagnosed and treated early.

REFERENCES

1. Tashjian RJ, Das KM, Palich WE, et al: Studies on cardiovascular disease in the cat. Ann NY Acad Sci 127:581, 1965
2. Eyster GE, Anderson LK, Krehbiel JD, et al: Surgical repair of atrial septal defect in a dog. J Am Vet Med Assoc 169:1081, 1976
3. Eyster GE, Anderson LK, Evans AT, et al: Ebstein's anomaly: A report of three cases in the dog. J Am Vet Med Assoc 170:709, 1977
4. Custer MA, Kantor AF, Gilman RA, DeRiemer RH: Correction of pulmonic stenosis. J Am Vet Med Assoc 139:565, 1961
5. Brock RC: Pulmonary valvotomy for the relief of congenital pulmonary stenosis. Br Med J 1:1121, 1948
6. Swan H, Zeavin J, Blount SG Jr, Virtue RW: Surgery by direct vision in the open heart during hypothermia. JAMA 153:1081, 1953
7. Breznock EM, Wood GL: A patch-graft technique for correction of pulmonic stenosis in dogs. J Am Vet Med Assoc 169:1090, 1970
8. Ford RF, Spaulding GL, Eyster GE: Use of an extracardiac conduit in the repair of supravalvular pulmonic stenosis in a dog. J Am Vet Med Assoc 172:922, 1978
9. Braden TD, Appleford MD, Hartsfield SM: Correction of a ventricular septal defect in a dog. J Am Vet Med Assoc 161:507, 1972
10. Weirich WE, Blevins WE: Ventricular septal defect repair. Vet Surg 7:2, 1978
11. Eyster GE, Whipple RD, Anderson LK, et al: Pulmonary artery banding for ventricular septal defect in dogs and cats. J Am Vet Med Assoc 170:434, 1977

12. Eyster GE, Braden TD, Appleford MD, et al: Surgical management of tetralogy of Fallot. J Small Anim Pract 18:387, 1977

13. Miller CW, Holmberg DL, Bowen V, et al: Microsurgical management of tetralogy of Fallot in a cat. J Am Vet Med Assoc 186:708, 1985

14. Eyster GE, Eyster JT, Cords GB, et al: Patent ductus arteriosus in the dog: Characteristics of occurrence and results of surgery in one hundred consecutive cases. J Am Vet Med Assoc 168:435, 1976

15. Jackson WF, Henderson RA: Ligature placement in closure of patent ductus arteriosus. J Am Anim Hosp Assoc 15:55, 1979

16. Detweiler DK, Hubben K, Patterson FD: Survey of cardiovascular disease in dogs—Preliminary report on the first 1000 dogs surveyed. Am J Vet Res 21:329, 1960

17. Breznock EM, Bauer T, Strack D, et al: Prosthetic mitral and tricuspid valve implantation in dogs using deep surface hypothermia. Am Coll Vet Surg 1983 (abstr)

18. Eyster GE, Weber W, Chi S, et al: Mitral valve prosthesis for correction of mitral regurgitation in a dog. J Am Vet Med Assoc 168:1115, 1976

19. Breznock EM, Whiting P, Pendrays D, et al: Valved apico-aortic conduit for relief of left ventricular hypertension caused by discrete subaortic stenosis in dogs. J Am Vet Med Assoc 182:51, 1983

20. van den Ingh TSAM, van der Linde-Sipman JS: Vascular rings in dogs. J Am Vet Med Assoc 164:939, 1974

21. Jackson WF, Seymour WG, Growney PG, Otto GF: Surgical treatment of the caval syndrome of canine heartworm disease. J Am Vet Med Assoc 171:1065, 1977

22. Aronsohn M: Cardiac hemangiosarcoma in the dog: A review of 38 cases. J Am Vet Med Assoc 187:922, 1985

30

Pacemaker Therapy

Michael Schollmeyer

HISTORICAL PERSPECTIVES

The use of electrical impulses to stimulate and control the heart rate in human patients with an external pacemaker was reported by Zoll[1] in 1952. Chardack et al.[2] reported in 1960 the first successful clinical implant of an internal pacemaker in humans. The earliest report of an implanted pacemaker in the veterinary literature was in 1968 by Buchanan et al.[3]

Early pacemakers were large, bulky devices that lasted less than 18 months. Advances in electronic circuitry, battery, materials technology, and manufacturing techniques permitted miniaturation of pacemakers and increased their life-span.[4–6] A modern pacemaker can weigh less than 30 g and have a useful life of more than 12 years. New surgical techniques, diagnostic procedures, and simpler easy-to-use auxiliary equipment have made pacemaker therapy routine in human medicine. The worldwide annual estimate of human pacemaker implants is more than 200,000, with approximately 115,000 occurring in the United States.[7]

The therapeutic use of pacemakers in veterinary medicine has been uncommon because of the high costs of pacemakers and their accessory equipment. During the past 5 years, some manufacturers have offered pacemakers to veterinarians for a small fee, which has made implants more economical. Pacemakers explanted from deceased humans have also been resterilized and used in veterinary patients. These two programs are estimated to account for 125 to 150 implants of artificial pacemakers per yer in veterinary patients. Virtually all are implanted in dogs,[8–17] although internal pacemaker therapy has been reported in a cat (Moise NS: Personal communication, 1986) and horse[18] with symptomatic bradycardia.

INDICATIONS

Artificial pacing of the heart may be indicated for any animal that has bradycardia with symptoms of insufficient cardiac output that cannot be maintained with drug therapy. Symptoms of fatigue, dyspnea, or cough at rest or with minimum exercise as well as syncope could be indicative of low cardiac output. Electrocardiographic (ECG) documentation of conduction defects or supraventricular arrhythmias (Table 30-1), coupled with clinical symptoms, can clearly demonstrate the need for artificial pacing. The most common indications encountered in clinical practice involve long-term treatment of symptomatic bradycardia due to high-grade second-degree atrioventricular (AV) block (Mobitz type II); complete AV block; sick sinus syndrome, including sinus bradycardia, sinus arrest, sinoatrial (SA)

Table 30-1 Indications for the Use of Artificial Cardiac Pacing

Supraventricular arrhythmias
    Atrial fibrillation with slow ventricular response
    Atrial flutter with slow ventricular response
    Sick sinus syndrome[a]
        Sinus arrest
        Sinus brachycardia
        SA block
        Bradycardia-tachycardia syndrome
    Persistent atrial standstill

Conduction defects
    Second-degree AV block, Mobitz type II (high grade)[a]
    Third-degree AV block[a]

[a] Most commonly encountered clinical indications for pacemaker therapy in dogs.

block, and the bradycardia-tachycardia syndrome; and persistent atrial standstill.[8-17] Pacemaker therapy when successful can dramatically reduce or eliminate clinical signs attributable to these arrhythmias (Fig. 30-1).

EQUIPMENT

An artificial pacemaker has two major components: the pulse generator and the lead. The *pulse generator* contains the battery and circuits, producing the electric impulse to stimulate the heart.

Pulse generators are classified by a five-letter code established by the Intersociety Commission for Heart Disease to describe pulse generator function[19] (Table 30-2). Commonly, only the first three letters of the code are used. The first digit indicates which chamber is being paced (e.g., V, ventricle, A, atrium, D, both chambers). The second digit represents the chamber in which sensing occurs. The third digit identifies the mode of response, once the pacemaker system has sensed the event (e.g., I indicates that the pacemaker system is inhibited, T indicates that a spontaneous event will trigger a pacemaker discharge in the chamber that has been sensed or in a lower chamber, and D designates a double response). The fourth and fifth digits relate to special options. The fourth digit describes the degree of programmability (0 indicates that the pulse generator is nonprogrammable, P indicates that the pacemaker has one or two programmable parameters, and M indicates three or more programmable features). The fifth digit indicates whether the pacemaker has a unique function used to control tachycardia. Currently VOOOO (ventricular paced, asynchronous, fixed-rate, nonprogrammable) and VVIPO (ventricular paced, sensed, inhibited, rate, and output programmable) pulse generators are routinely implanted in clinical settings for dogs.

The *pacemaker lead* is an insulated wire that conducts the electric impulse emitted from the pulse generator to the heart. The lead is composed of a connector pin on one end (that fits into the connector port of the pulse generator), the conductor wire, and the electrode. The conductor wire is covered with an insulating material of silicone or polyurethane. Leads that have electrodes implanted

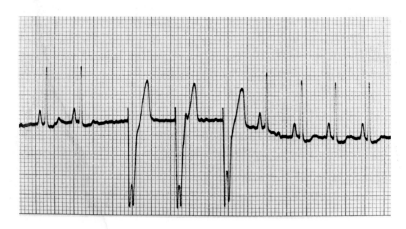

Fig. 30-1 ECG from a 15-year-old dachshund treated with a VVI demand pacemaker for syncope due to sick-sinus syndrome. The first and second complexes from the left are normal SA nodal initiated beats. When ventricular asystole occurs, the pulse generator discharges after sensing a heart rate below which it is programmed to discharge. The third, fourth, and fifth beats are pacemaker-initiated complexes. When the dog's innate sinus node activity recurred (sixth complex), pacemaker discharge was inhibited. (Courtesy of Dr. Philip R. Fox.)

Table 30-2 Pacemaker Identification Code

First letter	→	Chamber paced	A, Atrium
			V, Ventricle
			D, Both
Second Letter	→	Chamber sensed	A, atrium
			V, Ventricle
			D, Both
			O, None
Third letter	→	Mode of response	I, Inhibited
			T, Triggered
			D, Both
			O, None

Example: A pacemaker classified as a VVI would pace the ventricle, sense the ventricle, and be inhibited by spontaneous ventricular activity.

(Parsonnet V, Furman S, Smyth NPD: A revised code for pacemaker identification. Pacemaker Study Group. Circulation 64:60A, 1981. By permission of the American Heart Association, Inc.)

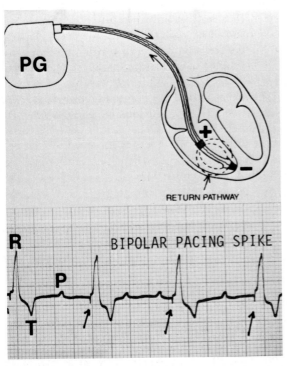

Fig. 30-2 Illustration of a bipolar pacing system consisting of a pulse generator (PG) and lead. Both the positive and negative electrodes are located at the distal end of the lead. Since the current travels only a short distance between electrodes, the pacing spike amplitude (arrows) is smaller than that generated by a unipolar system. The paced rhythm displays these spikes preceding each QRS-T complex. Complete AV block is evidenced by lack of correlation between P waves and QRS-T complexes. (Courtesy of Medtronic, Minneapolis, MN.)

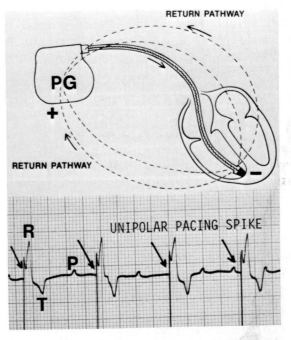

Fig. 30-3 Illustration of a unipolar pacing system consisting of a pulse generator (PG) and lead. A single negative electrode is located at the distal end of the lead. The positive electrode is the pulse generator. Because electric current from the generator travels a long distance from the negative electrode through the body to the positive electrode, a large pacing spike (arrows) is transcribed just preceding each QRS-T complex. (Courtesy of Medtronic, Minneapolis, MN.)

into the myocardium from the surface of the heart are called epicardial leads. Leads implanted transvenously having electrodes against the inside surface of the heart chambers are called endocardial leads (Figs. 30-2 through 30-5).

Endocardial leads are implanted in the right ventricle from a vein in the upper chest or neck in humans. This is the most widely used method of pacing in humans because of the ease of lead implantation using local anesthesia. Although this technique has been evaluated in dogs with clinical disease,[17] implantation requires fluoroscopic guidance, and lead dislodgement is a common complication.

Epicardial leads are most commonly used. They require a thoracotomy or ventral midline celiotomy and diaphragm incision to expose the left ventricular myocardium for insertion.[8-13,15,16] Lead dislodgement is uncommon, but morbidity and mortality are greater.

Leads are also classified as either bipolar or unipolar, depending on the electrode placement on the lead. A bipolar lead has both the anode and cathode electrodes at or near the tip of the pacemaker lead. Current travels from the pulse generator, through the lead to the cathode and then to the anode (Fig. 30-2). Because the electrodes are very close together near the lead tip, the distance that the current travels is short and bipolar leads have greater resistance to electromagnetic interference. However, the sensing characteristics are not as good as with unipolar leads.[20,23] A unipolar lead has the cathode electrode (−) at the distal lead tip. The anode electrode (+) is the outside of the pulse generator. Pacing current travels from the pulse generator, through the lead, to the cathode electrode, and through body tissues to the anode electrode (pulse generator case) (Fig. 30-3). Thus, the resistance to electromagnetic and myopotential interference is less than with a bipolar electrode but sensing characteristics are superior.[20,23]

Additional equipment required to aid in the implant of a pulse generator are a *pacing systems analyzer* (PSA) and a programmer. A PSA is a device connected to a lead during implant to determine the pacing and sensing thresholds of the patient. These thresholds are used to determine the most optimal lead placement and margin of safety for the patient.[20,23]

The *programmer* is the device used to program the pulse generator to meet the patient's needs. By means of a radiofrequency (RF) signal, the pro-

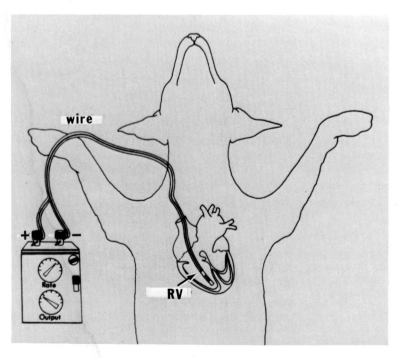

Fig. 30-4 Illustration of a temporary pacemaker attached to a transvenous bipolar lead (wire) inserted through the jugular vein into the right ventricle (RV). (Tilley LP: Essentials of Canine and Feline Cardiology. 2nd Ed. Lea & Febiger, Philadelphia, 1985.)

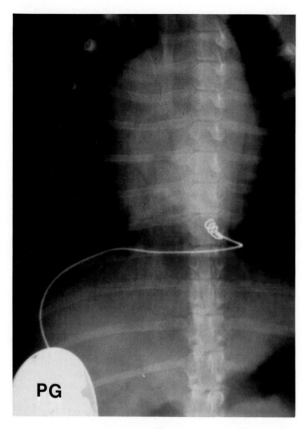

Fig. 30-5 Postoperative ventrodorsal thoracic radiograph of a dog, illustrating the location of the pulse generator (PG) and epicardial lead placement. A ventral abdominal transdiaphragmatic approach was used for surgical implantation. The corkscrew epicardial lead is within the left ventricular apex. (Courtesy of Dr. Philip Fox.)

grammer can noninvasively reprogram the pulse generator before, during, or after implant. Programmers work only with pulse generators from the same manufacturer. Various pacemaker models have different programmable features. The most basic features are rate, pulse width, and sensing sensitivity.[20,23]

An *external pacemaker* (models 5840, 5880A, Demand Pacemaker, Medtronic, Minneapolis, MN) and disposable bipolar lead are required for temporary pacing prior to surgery. The lead is introduced into the external jugular vein and directed to the right ventricle under fluoroscopic guidance or in conjunction with ECG monitoring. Intraoperatively, the temporary pacing rate should be set in the demand (synchronous) mode below the rate programmed into the pulse generator to avoid competing rhythms.

SURGERY

Preoperative Evaluation

A nine-lead ECG, thoracic radiographs, serum biochemical profiles, hemogram, urine analysis, and heartworm test (where appropriate) should be obtained prior to surgery. These data are essential to ensure proper patient pre- and post-operative management. Any corrective fluid replacement or medications for stabilizing the patients should also be supplied. Congestive heart failure will sometimes be present concomitantly with rhythm or conduction disturbances and needs to be treated with cage rest, diuretics, digoxin, vasodilators, or transvenous pacing prior to surgical implantation.[8-13]

Patient Preparation

Whatever surgical approach is used to implant the pacing system, the hair must be clipped and the skin shaved and scrubbed with an antiseptic surgical scrub solution. Strict aseptic techniques must be adhered to. If any postsurgical infection occurs at the lead or pulse generator sites, the devices may have to be removed to treat the infections adequately.

Anesthesia

The most critical phase of anesthesia is the induction phase. Most patients are high anesthetic risk cardiac cases and should be made as stable as possible before surgery. It is highly recommended to pace the patient with a temporary pacemaker for 1 to 3 days prior to surgery to determine that pacing will benefit the patient and to increase cardiac output. There is no single ideal anesthetic regimen for all patients (Chap. 28). The following protocol has been generally safe and effective. Anesthesia is accomplished by preanesthetizing with diazepam (0.1 to 0.25 mg/kg IM) or morphine (0.2 to 0.5 mg/kg IM) and atropine sulfate (0.05 mg/kg SC). Induction is accomplished by giving thiamylal sodium (4 to 6 mg/kg IV) and is maintained with enflurane or isoflurane with oxygen or halathone with oxygen as a second choice. The patient should be monitored electrocardiographically[8–13,20] during induction and surgery.

Surgical Approaches for Permanent Pacemaker Implantation

The surgical approach depends on the type of lead to be implanted. Insertion of a transvenous pacing electrode through the jugular vein into the right ventricle powered by a temporary pacemaker is recommended for epicardial lead placement and when endocardial lead implantation requires general anesthesia[10–16] (Fig. 30-4). This greatly reduces the risk of anesthesia.

ENDOCARDIAL LEAD PLACEMENT

Transvenous Technique

Endocardial lead placement requires an approach through a vein large enough to accept the pacemaker lead.[17] The right or left external jugular vein is used near the thoracic inlet. A 2- to 3-cm incision is made in the skin over the vein at this site, the vein is ligated cranial to the site of introduction, and a small incision is made in the vessel. The lead is introduced and directed under fluoroscopic guidance into the cranial vena cava and into the right atrium. The lead is manipulated by a wire stylet within the lumen of the lead. The tip of the lead is guided through the tricuspid valve orifice and positioned at the right ventricular apex. The lead is fixed in the external jugular vein by a double ligature of nonabsorbable suture. After the pacemaker is connected to the wire, the pulse generator is placed in a subcutaneous pocket created anteriorly (by a separate incision) at the dorsolateral aspect of the neck. It is secured to underlying muscle and fascia by nonabsorbable suture. Because of the need for fluoroscopy, this technique is not commonly used in clinical practice. The rate of endocardial lead dislodgement is high. The lower neck region does not have enough surface area to facilitate a subcutaneous pocket for the pulse generator in small dogs.

EPICARDIAL LEAD PLACEMENT

Implantation of epicardial leads requires a visual approach to the left ventricular apex to ensure proper insertion of the lead. These pacemaker leads are the most commonly used in veterinary practice. Three basic surgical approaches have been advocated: (1) intercostal or lateral thoracotomy, (2) midline celiotomy with caudal one-third median sternotomy, and (3) ventral abdominal transdiaphragmatic.

Intercostal or Lateral Thoracotomy Approach

The intercostal approach is made through the fifth intercostal space from either the right or left side of the thorax.[8,9,11,16] The lungs are packed anteriorly to expose the heart. The pericardial sac near the apex of the heart is incised, and a left ventricular epicardial site is located that is avascular and preferably apical. The epicardial lead (6917 Epicardial Lead with Applicator, Medtronic, Minneapolis, MN) is implanted by using an insertion tool that has the lead preloaded on it. The corkscrew of the lead is placed against the epicardium, and the lead is screwed $2\frac{1}{2}$ turns into the myocardium, using the tool. The lead is dislodged from the tool, and the electrode tip is checked for proper placement. The Dacron pad on the lead tip should rest firmly against the epicardium. If not, the insertion tool is reapplied using the opposite end of the tool, and the lead is given an additional turn until the Dacron pad is against the surface of the heart. If available, the lead is connected to a PSA device, and pacing and sensing thresholds are taken. If the thresholds are within acceptable limits (Table 30-3), the lead is brought out of the incision, connected to the inner tunneling tool (part of the pacemaker lead insertion tool assembly), and tunneled subcutaneously to an area behind the last rib. An incision (large enough to accept the generator) is made to the level of the subcutaneous tissue (below the cutaneous trunci muscles). A pocket is made in the subcutaneous space using blunt dissection. The lead is pulled through the subcutaneous tunnel to the pocket. The pulse generator is connected to the lead, the set screw tightened, and the generator placed in the pocket. If a bipolar system is used, successful pacing would be evident by

Table 30-3 Acceptable Thresholds for Artificial Cardiac Pacing at a Pulse Width of 0.5 msec[a,b]

Type of Threshold	Ventricle	Atrial
Stimulation	≤1.0 V	≤ 1.5 V
	≤1.0 mA	≤1.5 mA
Sensing	≥4.0 mV	≥4.0 mV

[a] A 6917 lead is not recommended for atrial application.

[b] Medtronic Sutureless Myocardial Pacing Lead for Implantable Pulse Generators, model 6917A–T, Medtronic, Minneapolis, Minnesota.

the ECG trace or by observing the increased rate of the paced heart. The heart rate should equal the set rate of the generator. If a unipolar system is used, pacing will start when the circuit is completed (i.e., when the pulse generator makes contact with the body). The pocket containing the generator is closed with a three-layer closure: one layer using 2-0 or 3-0 absorbable suture near the generator to reduce any potential spaces, a second absorbable suture to close the subcuticular tissue, and finally a nonabsorbable skin suture. The chest incision is closed in the standard manner.

Midline Celiotomy, Caudal One-Third Median Sternotomy Approach

The midline celiotomy technique has been used for both small and large dogs.[10,11,16] Starting at the midline, an incision is made from the anterior one-third of the abdomen to the caudal one-third of the sternum. If the pulse generator is to be placed in the abdomen, the caudal end of the incision should be extended to the umbilicus. The incision is carried through the midline of the xiphoid cartilage and xiphoid process to the level of the sixth sternebra. A retractor is used to spread the incision to visualize the cardiac apex. The pericardium is excised, and the epicardial lead is implanted using the implant tool on the left ventricular apex. Care should be taken to screw in the lead so that the Dacron pad is flush against the epicardium.

The lead is passed around the diaphragm, through the peritoneum caudal to the left lobe of the liver. The lead is connected to the pulse generator and the

set screw tightened to secure the lead to the generator. The unipolar system is activated by placing the generator against the peritoneal wall, and the ECG is observed for capture. A sufficient loop of lead wire is placed in the thoracic cavity to prevent any strain on the implanted lead tip. The pulse generator may be placed outside the abdomen in medium and large dogs but not in small dogs (weighing less than 10 kg), which have insufficient room for flank placement of the pacemaker. Subcutaneous insertion facilitates replacing or changing the pulse generator or reprogramming it, if necessary. Generators placed in the abdominal cavity may be inserted in a Dacron mesh pouch (Parsonnet Pulse Generator Pouch, USCI, Billerica, MA). This is sutured to the inner abdominal wall with 2-0 nonabsorbable suture. Excellent results have also been achieved without the Parsonnet Pouch by simply allowing the pulse generator to lie in the abdominal cavity. Incisions in the sternum, diaphragm, and abdomen are closed in routine fashion.

Ventral Abdominal Transdiaphragmatic Approach

A ventral midline abdominal incision is made from the umbilicus to the xiphoid.[12,13] The incision is retracted, and a 3- to 5-cm longitudinal incision is made in the left lateral muscular portion of the diaphragm from the xiphoid to the central tendon to expose the apex of the heart. The pericardium is incised and the edges stabilized with Allis tissue forceps or temporary stay sutures. The epicardial screw-in lead is implanted in the myocardium of the left ventricular apex with the aid of the insertion tool as previously described. The lead is then passed from the thoracic cavity into the abdominal cavity through the diaphragmatic incision and lateral to the liver. A small length of redundant lead cable is left in the thoracic cavity to prevent tension on the wire. A double pursestring suture is placed in the diaphragm, surrounding the wire to help stabilize it. The lead is connected to the generator and placed between the liver and diaphragm or permitted to float free. The diaphragmatic and abdominal incisions are closed in the standard manner.

This surgical approach and technique is technically simple, quick, and efficient. It causes minimal tissue trauma compared with thoracotomy, has been associated with a low incidence of complications postoperatively, and has been used successfully in dogs without untoward effects for several years. In large dogs, however, a pulse generator in the abdomen may be too deep to be reached by a magnetic programming instrument. This may alter or prevent postoperative pulse-generator reprogramming and interrogation.[12]

POSTOPERATIVE CARE

If the generator is placed in a subcutaneous pocket, a firm but nonconstricting bandage should be placed around the abdomen to stabilize the generator. Postoperative radiographs are taken to confirm the location of the lead and generator (Fig. 30-5). Pulse rates are taken frequently to compare heart rate with the set pacemaker rate. If there is any discrepancy of more than 5 beats/min between the set rate of the generator and the pulse rate, an ECG should be taken and evaluated for pacemaker capture. If ventricular tachycardia should occur, intravenous bolus of lidocaine (2 to 4 mg/kg) may be needed. Broad-spectrum antibiotics should be given for 7 days postoperatively. The bandages should be changed daily and the incision sites and pockets checked for redness and swelling. If fluid distends the pulse-generator pocket, aseptic drainage with a 16- or 18-gauge needle and syringe may be required.

Care must be taken to avoid introducing bacteria or hitting the lead with the needle. Bandages are removed 5 days postoperatively, unless complications due to seroma formation occur. The animal should have its activity restricted for 10 to 14 days. Occasionally, excitable animals are lightly tranquilized to help prevent postoperative seroma formation as a result of excessive activity.

SURGICAL CONSIDERATIONS FOR REPLACING THE PULSE GENERATOR

Depending on the energy requirements needed to pace the heart, pulse generators can have a useful battery life of 5 to 10 years.[21,22] Therefore,

during the normal clinical course of a pacemaker implant, the pulse generator may have to be replaced if the battery is depleted. Malfunctions of the pulse generator circuitry can also be a reason for pulse generator replacement. Considerations should there-fore be made during the initial implant to place the generator in a position that would permit access to the generator without performing a surgical procedure that is more complicated than the initial implant. Replacement of the pulse generator is simpler and less risky if the generator is implanted subcutaneously. The surgical procedure would be relatively minor compared with the initial implant.

If any excessive lead is present, it should be placed under the generator during the initial implant. This will reduce the chance of inadvertent damage to the lead by surgical instruments during the replacement procedure.

FOLLOW-UP PROCEDURES

Patients can be released in 3 to 5 days, depending on recovery and clinical course. In noncomplicated procedures (i.e., no heart failure, ascites, or underlying disease states), the patients can be sent home under exercise restriction and close client monitoring for recurrence of clinical signs similar to those it presented with (e.g., exercise intolerence, dyspnea, coughing, ascites, syncope, weakness) until reexamined during suture removal. More complicated cases, especially any involving heart failure, postoperative complications, or disorders of other systems, should be rechecked frequently as the condition indicates. Follow-up procedures should include a full history, physical examination, and ECG, conducted as often as weekly for the first month and every 3 months thereafter (if battery depletion is a concern), or 1 month postoperatively followed by visits every 6 months (for new pulse generators).

Pacing rates should be checked during each follow-up examination and adjusted to the proper rate for the patient. Pacemaker rates should be set at the lowest rate necessary to prevent recurrence of clinical signs. Small dogs and cats can be set at 100 beats/

min, while larger breeds do well at 75 to 80 beats/min. If it is necessary to change rates, a programmer can be used (if the pulse generator is of the programmable type). Only programmers manufactured by the pulse generator manufacturer will be able to reprogram the pacemaker.

COMPLICATIONS

Complications related to pacemaker implants are divided into two categories[8-17] (Table 30-4). Complications that are the result of poor implant procedures are classified as surgical complications; those related to device failures are classified in the device failure category. Complications can be many and varied. However, the most significant in our experience are those related to the surgical implant. Device failure, except normal battery depletion, are less common.

Evaluation of clinical and ECG abnormalities is necessary for diagnosis of complications and successful management. After a thorough history, physical examination, and ECG, chest and abdominal radiographs are taken. Many causes of cardiac pacing failure may be suggested radiographically[14] (Table 30-5). Complications with pacemaker im-

Table 30-4 Complications Associated with Pacemaker Implants

Complication Type	Cause	Treatment
Surgical		
Lead dislodgement	Improper implant technique	Reimplant.
Postsurgical infections	Contamination of surgical site or device	Remove device, give antibiotics, reimplant at another site.
Serum pocket in PG pocket	Pocket too large for generator, failure to stabilize P.G. in pocket.	Bandage and/or drain serum.
Skin erosion over PG (implanted subcutaneously)	P.G. too large, infected pocket, sutures too tight, allergic reactions to P.G.	Treat underlying cause. May have to remove device and reimplant at another site.
Pacemaker not capturing the heart	Stimulation thresholds exceed output of generator; set screw not properly tightened.	Determine thresholds and reimplant lead at another site; check set screws on pacer.
Device related		
No PG output	Battery depleted.	Replace PG.
PG output but failure to capture heart	Insulation damage on lead; exit block.	Replace lead.
Oversensing of pacemaker causing inhibition, no output from PG	Component failure in lead and/or P.G., cardiac signals inadequate, electromagnetic interference (EMI).	Determine cause. Replace PG; reimplant lead at another site. Reprogram PG. If possible, remove from source of EMI.

PG, pulse generator.

Table 30-5 Causes of Cardiac Pacemaker Failure as Detected from Radiographs

Type of Failure	Cause of Failure
Lead dislodgement	
Epicardial lead	Screw-in electrode disconnected from myocardium
Endocardial lead	Dislodged from right ventricular apex
Lead fracture	Commonly at distal electrode tip, junction at lead and pulse generator, thoracotomy exit site, other stress points
Ventricular perforation	By endocardial electrode
Lead-pulse generator disconnection	Can occur with epicardial or endocardial leads

plantation should not be unexpected but often may be successfully managed.

REFERENCES

1. Zoll PM: Resuscitation of the heart in ventricular standstill by external electrical stimulation. N Engl J Med 247:768, 1952
2. Chardack WM, Gage AA, Greatbatch W: A transistorized, self-contained, implantable pacemaker for the long-term correction of complete heart block. Surgery 48:643, 1960
3. Buchanan JW, Dear MG, Pyle RL, et al: Medical and pacemaker therapy of complete heart block and congestive heart failure in a dog. J Am Vet Med Assoc 158:1099, 1968
4. Parsonnet V, Zucker IR, Gilbert L, et al: Clinical use of an implantable standby pacemaker. JAMA 196:784, 1966
5. Symth NPD, Citron P, Keshishian J, et al: Permanent perverous atrial sensing and pacing with a new J-shaped lead. J Thorac Cardiovasc Surg 72:565, 1976
6. Parsonnet V, Furman S, Smyth NPD: Implantable cardiac pacemakers: Status report and resource guideline. Report of the International Society Commission for Heart Disease Resources. Am J Cardiol 34:487, 1974
7. Lasche PA: Cardiac pacing, technology and follow-up. Focus on Crit Care 10:28, 1983
8. Lombard CW, Tilley LP, Yoshioka M: Pacemaker implantation in the dog: Survey and literature review. J Am Anim Hosp Assoc 17:751, 1981
9. Yoshioka M, Tilley LP, Harvey HJ, et al: Permanent pacemaker implantation in the dog. J Am Anim Hosp Assoc 17:746, 1981
10. Helphrey M, Schollmeyer M: Pacemaker therapy. p. 373. In Kirk RW (ed): Current Veterinary Therapy. Vol. VIII. WB Saunders, Philadelphia, 1983
11. Bonagura JD, Helphrey M, Muir W: Complications associated with permanent pacemaker implantation in the dog. J Am Vet Med Assoc 182:149, 1983
12. Fox PR, Matthiesen DT, Purse D, et al: Ventral abdominal, transdiaphragmatic approach for implantation of cardiac pacemakers in the dog. J Am Vet Med Assoc 189:1303, 1986
13. Fingeroth JM, Birchard SJ: Transdiaphragmatic approach for permanent cardiac pacemaker implantation in the dog. Vet Surg 15:329, 1986
14. Tilley LP, Miller MS, Owens JM: Radiographic aspects of cardiac pacemakers. Semin Vet Med Surg Small Anim 1:165, 1986
15. Klement P, Del-Nido P, Wilson J: The use of cardiac pacemakers in veterinary medicine. Compend Contin Ed 6:893, 1984
16. Tilley LP: Essentials of Canine and Feline Electrocardiography. Lea & Febiger, Philadelphia, 1985
17. Sisson D: Permanent transvenous pacemaker implantation in the dog. Proceedings of the Fourth Annual Veterinary Medicine Forum, Vol. 2, 1986
18. Reef VB, Clark ES, Oliver JA, et al: Implantation of a permanent transvenous pacing catheter in a horse with complete heart block. J Am Vet Med Assoc 189:449, 1986
19. Parsonnet V, Furman S, Smyth NPD: A revised code for pacemaker identification. Pacemaker Study Group. Circulation 64:60A, 1981
20. Zipes DP, Duffin EG: Cardiac pacemakers. p. 744. In Braunwald E (ed): Heart Disease. WB Saunders, Philadelphia, 1984
21. An overview of pacing. Medtronic Currents 7251C, 1979
22. Winner JA, Bell W: Stimulation thresholds and permanent pacing. Medtronic Currents 77-EM-0410, 1977
23. Spectrax-SX, HT, UL, UM, SXT. Technical Manual. Medtronic, Minneapolis, MN.

Section 6

PATHOLOGY OF THE CARDIOVASCULAR SYSTEM

31

Necropsy Techniques for the Heart and Great Vessels

Sanford P. Bishop

Before postmortem examination of the heart, the examiner should be thoroughly familiar with the clinical history and any procedures performed during life. A thorough external examination should be conducted, and all organs should be inspected, with particular attention to abnormal fluid accumulations.[1] The left thoracic cavity should be opened by cutting the ribs at the sternal border and near their vertebral connection, and reflecting the rib cage dorsally. The thoracic arteries and veins should be carefully dissected, and the heart and lungs then removed in one piece from the thorax. Methods for dissecting the heart and great vessels have been described for the dog and cat.[1-5] Techniques and nomenclature for postmortem examination of the human heart[2,6] have been modified for veterinary medicine and are described below (Fig. 31-1).

DISSECTION OF THE HEART

The aorta and pulmonary artery should be transected several centimeters distal to the valves, and the pulmonary veins severed as close to the lungs as possible. The pericardium is opened and any fluid noted, and the surface of the heart is examined.

The heart is opened by making an initial incision into the main pulmonary artery. This incision is then extended into the right ventricle along the junction of the right ventricular free wall and the interventricular septum, downward to the apex of the heart following the septal wall, and finally up the posterior heart border into the right atrium. In the right atrium, the incision is made approximately 1 cm dorsal and parallel to the coronary groove into the right auricle. The cranial vena cava is not incised, since this cut would destroy the sinus node for histologic examination (Fig. 31-1A,B).

The left atrium is then opened by inserting scissors into one of the pulmonary veins and extending the incision into the left auricle. The endocardial surface of the left atrium is examined for the presence of any lesions, particularly focal endocardial thickenings or jet lesions indicating mitral valve insufficiency. The mitral valve is carefully inspected from the left atrium before incising the mitral annulus, taking careful note of the valve surface and

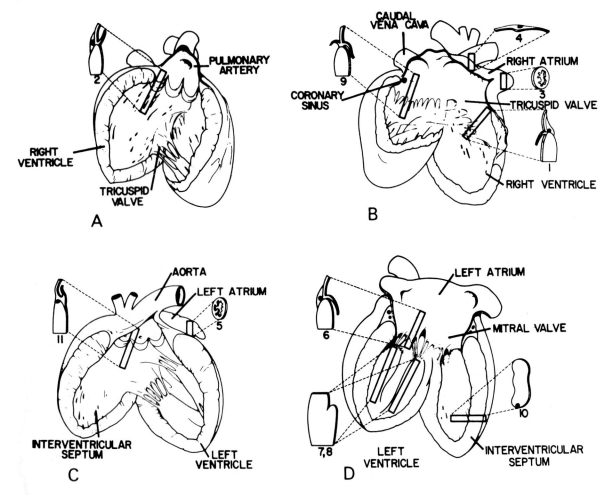

Fig. 31-1 Diagram of heart opened along lines of blood flow as described in text. Numbered drawings illustrate the shape of tissues as removed for histologic section. (**A**) Right ventricular cavity and pulmonary outflow tract. (**B**) Right ventricle and right atrium. (**C**) Left ventricle and aortic outflow tract. (**D**) Left ventricle and left atrium.

the chordae tendineae. Ruptured chordae tendineae, which occur mainly in the dog, will be apparent by this inspection.

The left ventricle is then opened by an incision made down its posterior wall between the posterior papillary muscle of the left ventricle and the interventricular septum. To make this incision, it is necessary to cut some of the chordae tendineae of the mitral valve. If it is desired not to cut the chordae tendineae of the mitral valve, the incision should be made directly through the middle of the posterior papillary muscle, so that the left ventricle is opened with a vertical incision from the atrium to the apex

of the left ventricle, bisecting the posterior papillary muscle. The incision in the left ventricle is then continued from the apex toward the base along the anterior wall of the heart and into the outflow tract of the ventricle to the aorta. In the cat, care should be taken in this step to avoid inadvertent cutting of excessive, abnormal left ventricular moderator bands, if present. They may bridge the left ventricular septum and free wall.[7] Ultimately, they may need to be severed to permit reflection of the left ventricular wall. The heart is now completely opened and all of the valvular complexes and endocardium may be examined (Fig. 31-1).

Table 31-1 Heart Weight, Body Weight, and Associated Ratios in Normal Dogs and Cats

		BW (kg)	HW/BW (g/kg)	RV/BW (g/kg)	LV+S/BW (g/kg)	RV/ HW	LV+S/HW	LV+S/RV
Normal beagles	Mean	10.22	6.69	1.37	4.25	0.207	0.650	3.13
(N = 26)	SD	1.23	0.68	0.17	0.42	0.014	0.034	0.23
Normal mixed-	Mean	13.49	7.41	1.67	4.71	0.225	0.635	2.82
breed dogs	SD	5.18	1.02	0.26	0.67	0.020	0.028	0.23
(N = 47)								
Normal cats	Mean	3.08	3.68	0.67	2.41	0.184	0.659	3.56
(N = 33)	SD	0.57	0.60	0.15	0.37	0.025	0.025	0.23

BW, body weight; HW, total heart weight; LV+S, left ventricle plus septum; RV, right ventricular free wall; SD, standard deviation.

The opened left and right atrioventricular (AV) valve rings should be measured with a flexible ruler and expressed as a ratio of left to right AV ring circumference. The normal ratio for the dog is 0.90 ± 0.07 (SD) and for the cat, 0.82 ± 0.07. Deviations from this ratio are useful indicators of AV ring dilation.

The heart is weighed after completely trimming extraneous tissue at the base. The ratio of heart weight to body weight is useful to evaluate the extent of cardiac hypertrophy in various conditions, such as feline myocardial disease. To quantitate the degree of left or right ventricular hypertrophy, ventricular weights should be obtained, although this dissection will destroy the specimen. The dissection is made by completing the separation of the right ventricular free wall from the right atrium at the coronary groove, continuing through the crista supraventricularis to the pulmonic valve. The left atrium is separated completely from the left ventricle at the AV ring. The right ventricular free wall weight and the combined left ventricle and interventricular septal weight are obtained. In my experience, measurement of wall thickness is not useful for comparison between animals. Postmortem rigor and subsequent relaxation of rigor cause ventricular wall thickness to be considerably different from that during life, and may provide very mis-

Table 31-2 Heart Weight, Body Weight, and Associated Ratios in Normal and Cardiomyopathic Cats[a]

Myocardial Disease	No. of Cats	Body weight (kg)	Heart weight (g)	Ratio of Heart weight to Body weight
Hyperthyroid related	23	3.3 ± 0.3	22.6 ± 2.1	7.0 ± 0.3
Restrictive	15	4.6 ± 0.2	30.6 ± 1.7	6.4 ± 0.3
Symmetric hypertrophic	35	4.5 ± 0.2	27.5 ± 0.8	6.3 ± 0.1
Asymmetric hypertrophic	16	4.4 ± 0.1	27.5 ± 0.8	6.3 ± 0.3
Dilated (congestive)	21	4.5 ± 0.1	24.1 ± 0.9	5.4 ± 0.3
Excessive moderator bands	21	4.5 ± 0.2	21.6 ± 0.8	4.5 ± 0.2
Control (normal)	36	4.8 ± 0.2	18.4 ± 0.6	3.83 ± 0.2

[a] Mean ± SEM.
(Liu SK, Peterson ME, Fox PR: Hypertrophic cardiomyopathy and hyperthyroidism in the cat. J Am Vet Med Assoc 185:52, 1984.)

leading information. Normal total cardiac and regional weight ratios for a group of colony-raised beagles, a group of mixed-breed dogs, and normal cats are given (Table 31-1). Heart weight to body weight ratios in various feline myocardial diseases and for normal cats are also listed[8] (Table 31-2).

FIXATION AND HISTOPATHOLOGIC EVALUATION OF THE HEART

Heart tissue to be studied histopathologically should be fixed in 10 percent phosphate-buffered formalin for a minimum of 24 hours. All clotted blood should be removed from the chambers and the tissue rinsed with formalin. If the heart is to be fixed prior to dissection, the chambers should be loosely packed with cotton to retain the chamber shape and permit adequate penetration of fixative. Perfusion fixation, special fixatives, and other specialized procedures are required for specific and experimental studies, but their description is beyond the scope of this chapter.

Histopathologic sections should be taken as blocks of tissue not more than 3 mm thick to evaluate the various anatomic components of the heart. Figure 31-1 illustrates the location and shape of tissue blocks, which will include all major anatomic regions of the heart.

REFERENCES

1. Liu SK: Postmortem examination of the heart. Vet Clin North Am 13:379, 1983
2. Layman TE, Edwards JE: A method of dissection of the heart and major pulmonary vessels. Arch Pathol Lab Med 82:314, 1966
3. Coffin DL: Necropsy procedure for the dog and cat. In Jones TC, Gleiser CA (eds): Veterinary Necropsy Procedures. JB Lippincott, Philadelphia, 1954
4. Harrison BM: Dissection of the Cat. 5th Ed. CV Mosby, St. Louis, 1966
5. Evans, HE, deLahunta A: Miller's Guide to the Dissection of the Dog. 2nd Ed. WB Saunders, Philadelphia, 1980
6. Edwards WD, Tajik AJ, Seward JB: Standardized nomenclature and anatomic basis for regional tomographic analysis of the heart. Mayo Clin Proc 56:479, 1981
7. Liu SK, Fox PR, Tilley LP: Excessive moderator bands in the left ventricles of 21 cats. J Am Vet Med Assoc 180:1215, 1982
8. Liu Sk, Peterson ME, Fox PR: Hypertrophic cardiomyopathy and hyperthyroidism in the cat. J Am Vet Med Assoc 185:52, 1984

32

Cardiovascular Pathology

Si-Kwang Liu

Clinical interest in veterinary cardiology began in the 1960s. Congenital cardiac disorders have since been widely described in cats and dogs. A partial list of reported canine and feline congenital anomalies includes mitral valve complex malformation, tricuspid valve dysplasia, tetralogy of Fallot, patent ductus arteriosus, aortic and pulmonic stenosis, atrial and ventricular septal defects, persistent right aortic arch, truncus arteriosus, double-outlet right ventricle, left ventricular aneurysm, persistent common atrioventricular (AV) canal, endocardial fibrosis with cardiomegaly, excessive left ventricular moderator bands, and cor triatriatum.[1-13] A variety of vascular anomalies have been described in both species.

Numerous cardiac disorders may be acquired. In dogs, they include chronic AV valvular disease (e.g., endocardiosis),[14] parvovirus myocarditis,[11,15] ruptured chordae tendineae,[16] atherosclerosis,[11,17] and persistent atrial standstill.[11] Hypertrophic and dilated cardiomyopathy, conduction-system abnormalities, and atrial standstill are reported in dogs and cats.[11,18-22] Endocarditis of unknown etiology and restrictive cardiomyopathy are described in the cat.[3,11,15] Vegetative endocarditis is reported in the dog and cat but is rare in felines.[23]

CONGENITAL CARDIAC DISORDERS

Mitral Valve Complex Malformation

In dogs, malformation of the mitral valve complex is most often observed in large-breed males (e.g., Great Dane, German shepherd). Clinical signs are usually evident before 10 months of age in severely affected dogs. These animals suffer left-sided volume overload due to mitral insufficiency. An associated heart murmur is usually present. Pulmonary edema due to left-sided heart failure results.

Gross pathologic findings include greater than normal heart weights, left ventricular dilation, and marked left atrial enlargement and hypertrophy. Mitral valve complex alterations include enlarged annulus, short and thick leaflets, short and stout horizontally arranged chordae tendineae, upward malposition of atrophic or hypertrophic papillary muscles, insertion of one papillary muscle directly into one or both valve leaflets, and left ventricular hypertrophy or dilatation (Fig. 32-1). This anomaly is often associated with dysplasia of the tricuspid

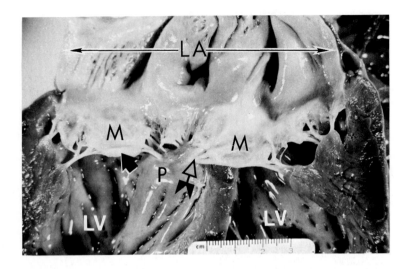

Fig. 32-1 Left heart from an 8-month-old male English bulldog with malformation of the mitral valve complex. Note severe dilatation and hypertrophy of the left atrium (LA) and hypertrophy of the left ventricle (LV). Mitral valve leaflets (M) are thickened (closed black arrow). Chordae tendineae are short and stout. Upward malposition of the papillary muscles is evident. The mitral valve septal leaflet inserts directly (open arrow) onto the anterior papillary muscle (P). There is mild diffuse endocardial fibrosis.

valve, patent ductus arteriosus, aortic stenosis, and ventricular septal defect.[4,7]

In cats, mitral complex malformation is the most common congenital cardiac anomaly. Severely affected animals display clinical signs before 1 year of age.[2,3,5,11] Clinical and pathologic findings are similar to those in the dog.

Mitral regurgitation results from several factors in affected animals. Enlargement of the mitral valve annulus is a cause of insufficiency.[24,25] Abnormally short, thick valve leaflets or restricted leaflet movement by shortened, thickened chordae tendineae is contributory. Papillary muscle malalignment is frequently present in these animals. Insertion of mitral leaflets directly onto a papillary muscle also distorts leaflet mobility by anatomically pulling them into the ventricle, preventing firm systolic leaflet apposition.

Tricuspid Valve Dysplasia

In dogs, tricuspid valve dysplasia occurs fairly commonly in large-breed males.[6] Clinical signs usually occur before 1 year of age. Affected animals display evidence of right-sided heart failure (e.g., pleural effusion, ascites, hepatosplenomegaly, jugular venous pulse) and have heart murmurs of tricuspid regurgitation.

In the cat, dysplasia of the tricuspid valve is common, especially in the domestic short-hair breed.[2,3,6,11] It is often present in association with

malformation of the mitral valve. Right-sided heart failure occurs in severely affected animals. Biventricular failure may result when both AV valves are involved.

Gross pathologic changes include focal and diffuse thickening of tricuspid valve leaflets, faulty development of chordae tendineae and papillary muscles, improper separation of tricuspid valve components from the right ventricular wall, and inappropriate insertion of valve leaflets into papillary muscles (Fig. 32-2). These changes are identical to those found in similarly affected humans.[26]

Aortic Stenosis

The lesion causing aortic stenosis can occur below the valve (subvalvular), at the valve (valvular), or above the valve (supravalvular). It constitutes a fibrous stenosis, causing a fixed outflow obstruction to left ventricular emptying.

In dogs, most cases involve a subvalvular fibrous ring originating from the cranioventral mitral valve leaflet obstructing the left ventricular outflow tract.[27,28] It is most commonly detected in the boxer, golden retriever, German shepherd, and Newfoundland breeds. A mode of inheritance in Newfoundlands has been reported as polygenic or autosomal-dominant (with modifiers) for discrete subaortic stenosis.[28]

Affected puppies are usually asymptomatic. A systolic murmur heard loudest at the aortic region

Fig. 32-2 Right heart from a 2-year-old female domestic short-hair cat with tricuspid valve dysplasia. The right atrium (RA) and ventricle (RV) are severely dilated. Tricuspid valve leaflets attach abnormally to the interventricular septum (black arrow) and directly onto fused, distorted papillary muscles (open arrow). Trabeculae carneae (T) project from the inner surface of the lateral right ventricular wall, forming characteristic muscular columns. P, papillary muscles.

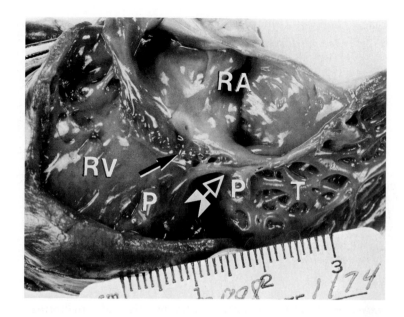

of the left third to fourth intercostal space, radiating rightward, and hypokinetic femoral arterial pulses are typically present. Severe stenosis may cause sudden death in young adults or predispose to secondary mitral insufficiency, aortic insufficiency, atrial fibrillation, and congestive heart failure.

In the cat, congenital aortic stenosis is usually supravalvular, but the aortic valve leaflets are also malformed. Affected cats are often stunted, and acute heart failure usually develops before 18 months of age.[3]

Pathologic changes include concentric left ventricular hypertrophy due to left ventricular pressure overload; left atrial enlargement and hypertrophy (especially if secondary mitral insufficiency has occurred); a fibrous ring at the subvalvular, valvular, or supraventricular location; and post-stenotic dilatation of the ascending aorta (Fig. 32-3). Endocarditis and focal myocarditis may be associated with this condition due to endothelial damage, which results from blood traversing through a discrete stenosis under high pressure and velocity.

Pulmonic Stenosis

Obstruction of right ventricular ejection may occur at several sites due to congenital pulmonic stenosis. Lesions include fusion or thickening of pulmonic valve leaflets (valvular stenosis), stricture of

the main pulmonary artery above the valve (supraventricular stenosis), or narrowing of the right ventricular outflow tract proximal to the pulmonic valve (subvalvular stenosis).

In dogs this is a relatively common anomaly. The

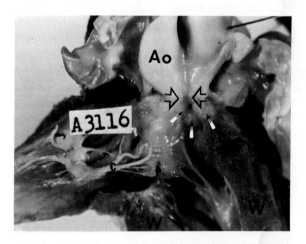

Fig. 32-3 Left heart from a young cat with aortic stenosis. The aortic valve is fibrotic and dysplastic (three small arrows), causing valvular stenosis. In addition, a discrete supravalvular stenosis is evident (open arrows). Note post-stenotic dilatation of the proximal ascending aorta (Ao). Other abnormalities include mitral valve malformation (note long, wide chordae tendineae), extensive fibrosis of the posterior papillary muscle, and left ventricular hypertrophy. W, left ventricular wall; C, chordae tendineae.

beagle, bulldog, Samoyed, Chihuahua, miniature schnauzer, keeshond, and wire-haired fox terrier are predisposed.[29-31] It has been demonstrated to be inherited in the beagle.[32] Dogs with mild stenosis may have a left basilar ejection murmur without symptoms. Severely affected animals develop right-sided heart failure, exercise intolerance, or exertional syncope (due to low cardiac output).

In cats, pulmonic stenosis is rare. Affected felines are usually stunted, display intermittent episodes of dyspnea and cyanosis, and ultimately die by 7 months of age.[3,33,34] Dysplasia of the pulmonic valve is usually the rule (valvular stenosis); infundibular hypertrophy is generally present as well. When pulmonic stenosis occurs it is usually associated with tetralogy of Fallot (Fig. 32-4). Isolated pulmonic stenosis is rare in felines.

Pathologic findings relate in part to the pulmonic stenosis-induced right ventricular pressure overload (i.e., severe right ventricular hypertrophy). Post-stenotic dilation of the main pulmonary artery results from turbulence caused by blood crossing the stenotic valve at high velocity. Valvular pulmonic stenosis is due to dysplasia of the pulmonic valve cusps and/or thickened, partially fused or eccentric cusps with hypoplasia of the valve annulus[29,32] (Fig. 32-4). Changes secondary to severe valvular stenosis include tricuspid insufficiency with associated right atrial enlargement. Hypertrophy of the infundibular portion of the right ventricular outflow tract and supraventricular crest are typically present.[29] In the dog, supraventricular stenosis is rare and subvalvular stenosis uncommon.[29,31]

Tetralogy of Fallot

This anomaly is characterized by four major components: (1) high ventricular septal defect, (2) obstruction to right ventricular outflow (i.e., pulmonic stenosis), (3) biventricular origin (i.e., dextroposition) of the aorta, and (4) right ventricular hypertrophy (Fig. 32-4). The principal cause of right ventricular outflow tract obstruction in the cat is marked hypertrophy of the crista supraventricularis and infundibular portion of the right ventricular free wall,[3,33] whereas valvular pulmonic stenosis is causative in dogs.

In dogs, tetralogy of Fallot is often detected in the English bulldog and keeshond breeds. It is inherited as a polygenetic trait in the keeshond and is attributable to maldevelopment of the conotruncal septum.[8] Most animals with this defect have exercise intolerance, exertional syncope, cyanosis, polycythemia, stunted growth, a systolic left basilar murmur of pulmonic stenosis, and sometimes a systolic right sternal border murmur due to the ventricular septal defect. Sudden death may occur at a young age, but right-sided congestive heart failure is uncommon.

Affected felines usually undergo a more rapid demise with death occuring by eight months of age.[3,33,35,36] Occasionally, cats may live into adulthood and survival times of 2 to 5 years have been reported.[37,38]

Patent Ductus Arteriosus

Normally the ductus arteriosus closes during the first few days of life. If it remains patent, it generally causes a volume overload to the pulmonary circulation and left heart due to the left-to-right shunt.

Patent ductus arteriosus is the most common canine congenital cardiac anomaly. It is most frequently identified in females. Poodles, collies, Shetland sheepdogs, German shepherds, cocker spaniels, Pomeranians, and Irsh setters are predisposed.[8,9,39] The defect is transmitted as a polygenic trait in poodles.[40] Severely affected puppies may die in the early neonatal period by 8 weeks of age. Thereafter, they may survive into early adulthood and die of left-sided heart failure.[41]

Classic findings of a left-to-right-shunting patent ductus arteriosus include a "machinery" murmur heard loudest at the left base, and hyperkinetic ("waterhammer") femoral arterial pulses. Rarely, right-to-left shunting causes loss of the diastolic murmur, exercise intolerance, and differential cyanosis. In cats, this anomaly is occasionally detected. Most reported cases have been in the domestic short-hair breed with a predisposition for females.[42-44]

Pathologic findings reveal the patent ductus arteriosus opening into the main pulmonary trunk just proximal to the bifurcation of the left and right pulmonary arteries. In right-to-left shunting patent ductus arteriosus, a large-diameter ductus may be present with pulmonary arterial medical hyperplasia, right ventricular hypertrophy, and hypoplasia of the left ventricle, left atrium, and ascending aorta.

Fig. 32-4 Heart from a 5-month-old male domestic short-hair cat with tetralogy of Fallot. (**A**) Right ventricular outflow tract and pulmonic valve are exposed. Hypertrophy of the infundibular portion of right ventricular outflow tract and supraventricular crest (open arrow) and pulmonary valve fibrosis (dysplasia) (three black arrows) narrow the pulmonary outflow tract. Severe hypertrophy of the right ventricular wall (W) is evident. (**B**) Left ventricle and aortic root of same cat. A large ventricular septal defect (curved arrow) is present. The arotic root (Ao) and aortic semilunar valves (small arrows) are illustrated. The left ventricle is hypertrophied. Severe right ventricular hypertrophy is evident. Mitral valve malformation and endocardial fibrosis are present. MPA, main pulmonary artery; RW, right ventricular wall; p, papillary muscle.

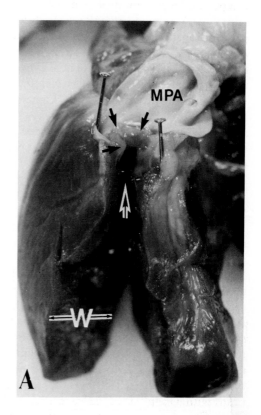

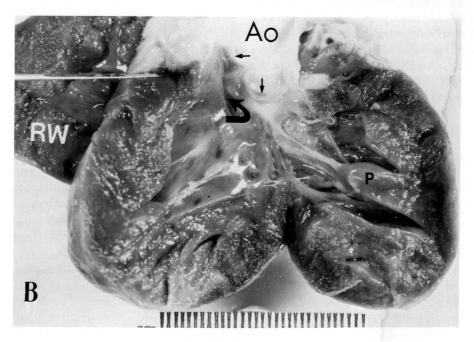

With left-to-right shunting patent ductus arteriosus, a smaller ductus is usually present with marked left atrial and ventricular enlargement.[40,45,46] Owing to chronic volume overload, left atrial and ventricular dilation can become marked. The main pulmonary artery may be dilated and display intimal fibrosis (i.e., jet lesions) near the ductus. Occasionally, an aorticopulmonary septal defect (i.e., aorticopulmonary "window") occurs between the ascending aorta and pulmonary trunk rather than a patent ductus arteriosus.

Atrial Septal Defects

Uncommon as isolated defects in the dog and cat, these lesions represent a through-and-through communication between the atria at the septal level.[3,41,48,50] They are often present with other congenital heart anomalies (Fig. 32-5). Isolated atrial septal defects create a conduit for blood to shunt from the left to right atrium, thereby causing a diastolic volume overload on the right heart. Several types of interatrial defects may be recognized during necropsy. Pathologic findings vary, depending on the type of atrial septal defect, amount and direction of shunting, and degree of pulmonary hypertension.

Ostium secundum defects involve the region of the fossa ovalis forming the dorsal and middle portions of the interatrial septum. Remnants of the right venous valve (Chiari's network) have been identified.[51] Ostium primum defects lie in the ventral portion of the interatrial septum and are very uncommon. They may involve the dorsal interventricular septum and medial mitral valve cusp.[50] Left-to-right shunting may cause enlargement of the right atrium, right ventricle, and main pulmonary artery.

A patent foramen ovale is occasionally detected but rarely in conjunction with cardiac chamber pathology. This is because its flaplike valve only permits bloodflow from the right to left atrium. This normally does not occur due to dominant left atrial pressure.

Persistent Common Atrioventricular Canal

In the cat, persistent common AV canal (endocardial cushion defect) is one of the more common congenital cardiac anomalies. It is formed by a lower interatrial septal defect and a defect of the uppermost ventricular septum at the level of the coronary sinus with malformation of the AV valves (Fig. 32-5). Affected cats usually display massive, generalized cardiomegaly, are stunted, and die of congestive heart failure by 7 to 10 months of age.[3,11,33,52]

Ventricular Septal Defects

Ventricular septal defects are typically located high in the membranous portion of the interventricular septum. The dominant left ventricular pressures usually cause blood to shunt from the left to the right ventricle. The location of ventricular septal defects usually directs blood into the right ventricular outflow tract which essentially spares the right ventricular cavity. This causes pulmonary overcirculation and increased venous return to the left atrium and left ventricle.[39]

In dogs, breeding experiments have suggested a genetic pattern of inheritance.[53] It has been reported in many purebreds and mixed breeds and English bulldogs may be predisposed.[54]

In cats, this is a common defect and may occur alone or in combination with other anomalies. Approximately one-third of ventricular septal defects detected at necropsy were associated with tricuspid valve dysplasia.[3]

Pathologic changes usually include a high membranous septal defect just below the aortic valve with dilatation of the left atrium and ventricle (Fig. 32-6). In a series of 12 dogs and one cat in which corrective surgery was performed, anatomic defects were reported in three general areas. Viewed from the right ventricle, the most common location was below the crista ventricularis at the junction of the anterior and septal tricuspid leaflets. When viewed from the left ventricle, the defect was under the commissure of the right and noncoronary aortic valve cusp. The second most common location was above the crista ventricularis, just below the pulmonary valve in the right ventricular outflow tract, or below the left coronary aortic valve cusp when viewed from the left ventricle. The third most common location was at various or multiple sites.[55]

Right ventricular hypertrophy may develop if right-to-left shunting has occurred, especially if large septal defects and pulmonary hypertension are

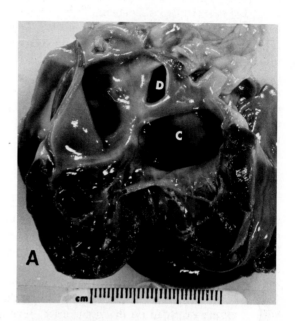

Fig. 32-5 Heart of a 3-year-old female domestic short-hair cat with ostium secundum atrial septal defect (D) and endocardial cushion defect (C), causing a common atrioventricular canal. (**A**) Left heart displays severe left atrial enlargement and moderate left ventricular dilatation. (**B**) Right heart shows severe right atrial and ventricular dilatation. Tricuspid valve dysplasia is evidenced by thickened irregular valve leaflets (arrows) and direct insertion of tricuspid valves onto a fused papillary muscle (P).

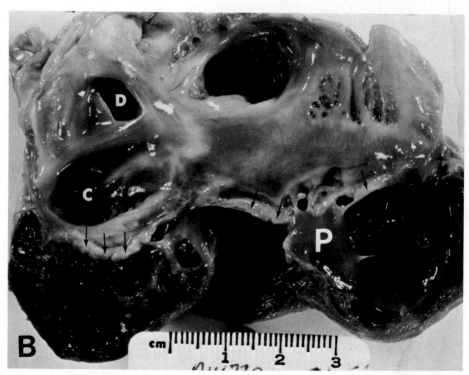

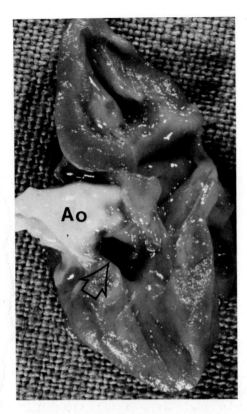

Fig. 32-6 Left side of the heart from a 12-day-old male Tibetan terrier. A high ventricular septal defect is situated in the membranous portion of the ventricular septum just below the aortic valve cusps (arrow). Ao, aorta.

present. Large ventricular septal defects are also associated with tetralogy of Fallot (Fig. 32-4B).

In cats, ventricular septal defects may contribute to complex malformations including AV valvular dysplasia and low atrial septal defect (i.e., common AV canal). Congestive heart failure may occur with severe lesions in both species.

Neonatal Cardiac Failure Associated with Atrioventricular Valvular Malformation in Kittens

Neonatal cardiac failure associated with AV valvular malformation (endocardial fibroelastosis with cardiomegaly) in kittens was previously described as neonatal endocardial fibroelastosis,[2] endocardial fibrosis with cardiomegaly[3] and possibly, kitten mortality complex.[56] On the basis of new evidence,

however, it is more accurately characterized as neonatal cardiac failure due to AV valvular malformation with secondary endocardial fibroplasia.

Typically, this anomaly results in a syndrome of early neonatal death. In a series of 26 affected kittens from 16 litters necropsied at the Animal Medical Center, the mean age was 32 days (range: 2 to 70 days). Breeds represented included domestic shorthair, Siamese, Abyssinian, and Burmese. Litter size was usually small (two or three kittens). Most died suddenly or were depressed, anorectic, and dyspneic for only a few hours before death.

Gross pathologic findings included a globular, enlarged heart. Both atria are enlarged and hypertrophied with opaque endocardial surfaces. Ventricles are dilated and upward malposition of the papillary muscles is noted. Pronounced mitral valve malformation, tricuspid valve dysplasia, endocardial fibrosis, excessive and abnormal moderator bands, pulmonary edema, pleural effusion, and ascites comprise the principal gross changes. Ventricular free walls tend to be thinner than normal in older kittens.

Microscopically, myocytes are thin and may display sarcoplasmic coagulation, granulation, vacuolation and fragmentation. They are separated by extracellular edematous ground substance. Myocytolysis is often severe. In kittens under 2 weeks of age, degenerated cellular debris and edematous exudate are observed in the endocardium and in and around moderator bands. In kittens aged 3 to 6 weeks, thin, elongated myocytes are separated by delicate fibers and extracellular edematous ground substance. Endocardium is thickened by fibroplasia, elastosis, proliferation of myofibrocytes, and Anitschkow's cells. Extensive endocardial fibroplasia and elastosis may occur in kittens that are more than 7 weeks of age. Pulmonary alveolar septae are thickened by proliferation of epithelial cells and histiocytes. The alveolar lumens are filled with proteinaceous fluid and active macrophages.

These kittens clinically resemble cats with acute systolic dysfunction. Acute congestive cardiomyopathy with muscle fiber degeneration and associated endocardial fibroelastosis has been reported as a postulated cause of kittens mortality complex.[56] Endocardial fibrosis and elastosis in the Animal Medical Center series displayed similarities to certain features described in humans[57] and cats.[58] These lesions may be secondary to severe mitral regurgitation and overload, since diffuse ventricular endocardial fibrosis occurs in association with congenital valvular defects,[3,4] mitral regurgitation,[59] and following mitral valve replacement in humans.[60] Alternatively, given the number of feline viral diseases, it is possible that prenatal viral myocarditis or associated immune-mediated reaction is causitive or contributory. Endocardial fibroelastosis has also been reported in the Burmese breed as an inherited anomaly.[58]

Excessive Left Ventricular Moderator Bands

Excessive numbers of left ventricular moderator bands bridging the left ventricular septum and free wall and entangling papillary muscles have been associated with heart failure and death in cats[12] (Fig. 32-7). This ubiquitous abnormality is associated with many morphologic variations. Older cats to

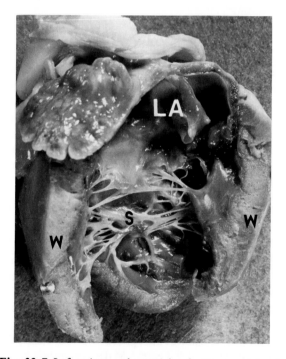

Fig. 32-7 Left atrium and ventricle of a 10-year-old male domestic short-hair cat. Extensive abnormal networks of left ventricular moderator bands are present connecting the ventricular septum (S) and left ventricular free wall (W). LA, left atrium.

week-old kittens are affected. The presence of dense abnormal moderator band networks in neonatal kittens suggests that at one extreme it may represent a congenital anomaly responsible for acute cardiac decompensation and heart failure. They are more commonly detected in older cats with cardiomyopathy. Their contribution to cardiomyopathies or congestive heart failure has not been clearly established. The variability in number, pattern, density, and severity of moderator band networks suggests various phenotypic expressions of this abnormality. It is not known whether this disorder is inherited.

ACQUIRED CARDIAC DISEASES

Chronic Atrioventricular Valvular Diseases

Chronic AV valvular disease (endocardiosis) is a degenerative disorder of the mitral and tricuspid valves. Also termed AV valvular endocardiosis, fibrosis, or myxomatous transformation, this disease may result in significant valvular incompetency, insufficiency, and volume overload.

In dogs, chronic valvular disease is the most common acquired cardiac disorder.[61–63] Its reported incidence at necropsy varies from 34 percent in one study of 404 dogs,[64] to 64 percent in another series of 550 dogs.[65] While virtually all breeds are affected, it occurs much more frequently in small and toy breeds. Males may be slightly more frequently affected than females.

Necropsy findings show that the mitral valve is abnormal in approximately two-thirds of cases, while both the mitral and tricuspid valves are abnormal less frequently. Occasionally, the tricuspid valve alone is affected.[66]

Valvular leaflets are grossly thickened, and lesions vary in intensity and severity. Valve edges are nodular and the leaflets are contracted and shrunken. Chordae tendineae may be short and stout, or long and thin. Ruptured chordae are often observed in the septal mitral leaflet (see Fig. 20-1).

As a result of AV valvular insufficiency, the corresponding atria and ventricles are often dilated and thickened (i.e., eccentric hypertrophy). The AV annulus is generally enlarged. Jet lesions (focal, thickened, fibrotic endocardial lesions) may be present and related to forceful regurgitation of blood from

Histologic examination reveals myocardial cellular hypertrophy. Myocardial cellular disorganization, however, is present in the ventricular septum only 20 percent of the time[21,22] (Fig. 32-10). In human hypertrophic cardiomyopathy, asymmetric septal hypertrophy and disorganization of cardiac muscle cells are more common and predominate in the ventricular septum.[76,80-83]

A secondary cause of left ventricular hypertrophy (i.e., secondary cardiomyopathy) is common in older cats (average age, 13 years) and is caused by thyrotoxicosis. There is no breed or sex predilection.[84,85] The ratio of heart weight to body weight is greatest for these cats compared with all other primary myocardial diseases. Most display symmetric left ventricular hypertrophy. Pleural effusion and pulmonary edema are present in one quarter of decompensated, untreated cases.[79,84,85] Functional thyroid gland adenoma (adenomatous hyperplasia) involving one or both thyroids is the usual cause of excessive serum thyroid hormone production.

Histologic cardiac abnormalities include large, hyperchromatic nuclei, interstitial fibrosis, endocardial fibroplasia, fibrosis of the AV node, and marked disorganization of cardiac muscle cells.[84]

Dilated (Congestive) Cardiomyopathy

Dilated (congestive) cardiomyopathy may be caused by many different factors or denote an end-stage pathway for myocardial injury.[86] Predominant features include generalized severe dilation of all four heart chambers, increased end-diastolic and end-systolic volumes, and systolic (pump) failure.

In cats there is an increased incidence in Siamese, Abyssinian, and Burmese breeds. Middle-aged cats are usually affected, although dilated cardiomyopathy has been observed in cats of all ages.[3,74,75,78,79,87] There is an equal sex distribution.

In dogs dilated cardiomyopathy affects predominantly large and giant breeds, especially dobermans, great Danes, Irish wolfhounds, Saint Bernards, and German shepherds. Cocker spaniels (especially English) and other smaller breeds can occasionally be affected. This disorder occurs in males four times more commonly than females, typically from 2 to 5 years of age (average, 5 years).[11,75,88,89] Gross pathologic findings in cats show an en-

larged and globular heart due to extreme dilation of the ventricles and atria (Fig. 32-11). Papillary muscles and ventricular trabeculae are flattened and atrophied. Alterations of the mitral valve complex are commonly identified in one-half of affected cases. They include short and thick leaflets; short, stout, long, or thin chordae tendineae; and upward malposition of papillary muscles. Alternations of the tricuspid valve complex include adhesion of the septal leaflet to the ventricular septum and direct insertion of the lateral leaflet into the papillary muscles. These gross valvular complex changes are similar to those observed in kittens with mitral malformation and tricuspid dysplasia. Thus, differentiating between primary myocardial disease and valvular malformation may be difficult. The heart weight of cats with dilated cardiomyopathy is greater than normal but less than that of hearts with hypertrophic cardiomyopathy. Aortic thromboembolism is present in about one-third of these animals. Most cats with dilated cardiomyopathy have pleural effusion. Occasionally, ascites and pulmonary edema are present.[11,87]

Histologically, myocardial cells appear thinner than normal and are separated by edematous extracellular ground substances or connective tissue. Myocytolysis is common.

Pathologic changes in dogs are generally similar to those described in cats. However, with canine dilated cardiomyopathy there is less severe alteration in AV valve morphology and aortic thromboembolism does not occur.

Doberman pinschers often display acute fulminant pulmonary edema if necropsied during the initial onset of clinical signs. Severe right heart failure (e.g., pericardial, pleural, or abdominal effusion) is common later in the disease.

Boxers may display only mild left atrial and ventricular dilatation. One-half of affected dogs have thickened AV valves or occasionally, immobile, thickened aortic valves. Histologic changes recorded in hearts involve both chronic and active inflammatory lesions. Active changes include focal myocytolysis, myonecrosis, hemorrhage and mild mononuclear cell infiltration (e.g., macrophages, lymphocytes, plasma cells). Chronic changes are more common and are shown by myofiber atrophy, fibrosis, fatty infiltration, and fatty change.[88]

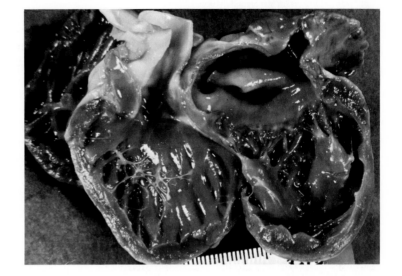

Fig. 32-11 Left heart from a 12-year-old, male domestic short-hair cat with systolic failure and severe dilatation of the left atrium and ventricle. Upward malposition of the papillary muscles, shortened chordae tendineae, and a small network of aberrant moderator bands are also present.

Feline Restrictive Cardiomyopathy and Myocarditis

Restrictive Cardiomopathy has been reported in cats 8 months to 19 years old; it is the rarest feline primary myocardial disease.[3,11,15,20,78,79] The dominant functional characteristic is abnormal myocardial stiffness causing diastolic dysfunction. Although most present clinically with left ventricular hypertrophy and endomyocardial fibrosis, others display apparently earlier stages in which microscopic evidence of myocarditis is evident. This may suggest that restrictive cardiomyopathy is an end-stage process resulting from a previous inflammatory process.

Gross pathologic findings include a heart weight greater than that of normal cats due to left ventricular hypertrophy. Dilation of the right atrium and ventricle is common. Extreme left atrial enlargement occurs and this chamber may become larger than the left ventricle. Pronounced diffuse endocardial thickening with whitish-gray, opaque, fibrous material is a pathologic hallmark. It is observed in the left ventricular outflow and inflow tracts, over the papillary muscles, chordae tendineae, and left ventricular free wall. Endocardial fibrosis may cause adhesions between papillary muscle and myocardium, distortion and fusion of chordae tendineae, distortion of mitral leaflets, and occasionally obliteration of the left ventricular cavity. Mural, left atrial, or distal aortic thromboembolism is very common[20] (Fig. 32-12).

Histologic features include extreme endocardial thickening by hyaline, fibrous, and granulation tissue. The surface is covered by a layer of hyaline tissue and collagenous fibers, occasionally displaying chondroid metaplasia. Underneath is loose, cellular, fibrous tissue. Adjacent to the myocardium is granulation tissue made up of histiocytes, lymphocytes, and plasma cells. Hypertrophy of myocytes and interstitial fibroplasia is common. Myocytolysis and arteriosclerosis in left ventricular free wall and septal intramural coronary arteries may accompany severe endomyocardial fibrosis in advanced cases.[3,20] These changes are similar but not identical to those in humans with restrictive cardiomyopathy.[90,91]

Heart Failure Associated with Excessive, Abnormal Left Ventricular Moderator Bands

Moderator bands (trabeculae septomarginalis) are normally present in the feline right ventricle[92] and in both canine ventricles.[93] In cats, abnormal diffuse networks of left ventricular moderator bands have been reported in association with congestive heart failure, ventricular dilatation, and hypertrophy without breed or sex predisposition.[12] Since then, abnormal moderator band networks have been

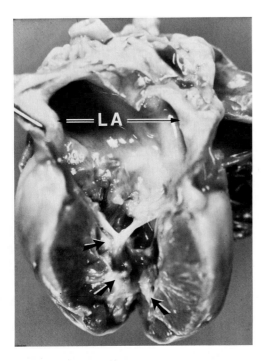

Fig. 32-12 Left heart from a 13-year-old male domestic short-hair cat with restrictive cardiomyopathy. The left atrium (LA) is greatly enlarged, and left ventricular hypertrophy is pronounced. There is diffuse endocardial fibrosis of the atrium. Severe endomyocardial fibrosis of the left ventricle causes fibrous adhesions and partial obliteration (arrows) of the ventricular chamber. (Courtesy of Dr. Philip Fox.)

identified in kittens as young as 1 day old. This finding suggests that in some cats at least, they represent congenital lesions.

The age range is wide (1.5 to 13 years; average: 6.5 years). There is extreme variation in excessive moderator band structure and density (e.g., from one small band to a "spiderweb" effect). These observations suggest that their pathologic role or significance might vary.

Gross pathologic findings show that affected hearts are small with irregular-shaped contours, rounded apexes, and occasionally indentation of the mid-left ventricular epicardial surface. Heart weight is significantly lower than for hypertrophic, dilated, or restrictive cardiomyopathic hearts but not significantly less than that of clinically normal hearts. The left ventricular cavity is irregularly narrowed in one-fourth to one-half of affected hearts because

of excessive abnormal moderator band networks. They connect papillary muscles, free wall, or both to the ventricular septum and may be adhered to these structures (Fig. 32-7). Left ventricular hypertrophy was generally noted in younger cats and dilation in older cats, although this was not always so. Pulmonary edema and/or pleural effusion may be present.[12] Aortic thromboembolism has been detected in up to one-third of necropsied cases.

Histologically, the moderator bands consisted of central Purkinje's fibers and dense, parallel collagenous fibers covered by endothelium. There is loose, fibrous connective tissue between the endothelium and the collagenous fibers. Some moderator bands are composed of Purkinje fibers surrounded by loose fibrous connective tissue, adipose tissue, lymphocytes, and blood vessels and are covered by endothelium.

Myocarditis

Many infectious agents can injure myocardial tissue and induce degeneration or inflammation (Fig. 32-13). Most often the myocardium is affected secondary to a generalized systemic infection.[73,75]

Viral myocarditis due to canine parvovirus has been widely described in puppies.[15,75,89,94] Acute myocarditis from parvovirus occurs in pups under 12 weeks of age, while fatal chronic myocarditis can manifest signs of heart failure in dogs up to 6 months old.

Gross pathologic findings may include cardiac dilation, ventricular hypertrophy, pale areas throughout the ventricles with some foci of petechia, pulmonary edema, and pleural effusion. The left atrium and ventricle are most severely affected.[15,94]

Histologically, 4- to 7-week-old pups affected acutely demonstrate thin myocytes separated by extracellular, edematous ground substance, histiocytes, fibroblasts, and delicate fibrous tissue. Inflammatory reaction is usually absent. Nuclei of monocytes may contain single, large, distinct, homogeneous intranuclear inclusion bodies. Myocytes may display granulation, coagulation, and cytoplasmic fragmentation. In slightly older puppies (6 to 9 weeks), extensive inflammatory reaction may occur, consisting of lymphocytes and plasma cells. Adjacent myocytes display cytoplasmic coagulation, granulation, fragmentation, and lysis. Inflam-

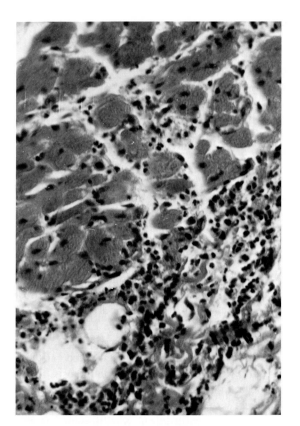

Fig. 32-13 Histologic section of myocardium from an 18-month-old male domestic short-hair cat with myocarditis. Note focal infiltration of lymphocytes, plasma cells, and neutrophils within and adjacent to myocytes. Myocyte degeneration and necrosis is evident, especially toward the bottom right of the photomicrograph. (H & E stain, ×80.)

mation subsides in juveniles (14 to 24 weeks of age) and histiocytes, fibroblasts, granulation, and fibrous connective tissue predominate. Myofibrocytes are increased in and around intramural coronary arteries. Sarcoplasmic granulation, coagulation, fragmentation, and lysis occur in myocytes within and surrounding areas of fibrosis. Microscopic changes are most severe in the left ventricular free wall and interventricular septum.[15]

Other infectious agents (e.g., canine distemper virus), trypanosomiasis, toxoplasmosis, fungi, algae, and rickettsiae) may affect the myocardium. Infiltrative diseases (e.g., neoplasia), toxic substances (e.g., myocardial depressant factors, heavy metals, ethyl alcohol), metabolic diseases (e.g.,

chronic uremia, hypothyroidism), chemicals (e.g., doxorubicin), and physical agents (e.g., heat stroke) can cause myocardial degeneration or inflammation.[73-75,89]

Conduction-System Lesions

Arrhythmias, syncope, and sudden death may result from a variety of acquired lesions of the conduction system. Various factors may be causative or contributory, including infections or inflammatory diseases and cardiomyopathies.[2,3,18,73-75] Terminal narrowing of small arteries in the region of the conducting system may cause degenerative changes, and hereditary factors may be involved in some cases.[95]

Doberman pinschers may have a higher reported incidence of sudden death with AV nodal degeneration. Affected animals range from 7 months to 5 years (average, 4 years). Syncope and unexpected viciousness are associated with the syndrome.[96]

Conduction system abnormalities have been reported in cats from 6 months to 16 years of age

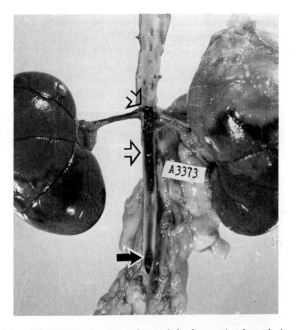

Fig. 32-14 Distal aorta of an adult domestic short-hair cat with hypertrophic cardiomyopathy, congestive heart failure, and thromboembolic disease. Emboli are present near the renal arteries (open arrows) and at the distal aortic trifurcation (closed arrow).

22. Liu SK, Maron BJ, Tilley LP: Hypertrophic cardiomyopathy in the dog. Am J Pathol 94:497, 1979

23. Shouse CL, Meier H: Acute vegetative endocarditis in the dog and cat. J Am Vet Med Assoc 129:278, 1956

24. Dear MG: Mitral incompetence in dogs of 0–5 years of age. J Small Anim Pract 12:1, 1971

25. Hamlin RL, Harris SG: Mitral incompetence in Great Dane pups. J Am Vet Med Assoc 154:790, 1969

26. Becker AE, Beacker MJ, Edwards JE: Pathologic spectrum of dysplasia of the tricuspid valve. Arch Pathol Lab Med 91:167, 1971

27. Muna WFT, Ferrans VJ, Pierce JE, Roberts WC: Discrete subaortic stenosis in Newfoundland dogs: Association of infective endocarditis. Am J Cardiol 41:746, 1978

28. Pyle RL, Peterson DF, Chacko S: The genetics and pathology of discrete subaortic stenosis in the Newfoundland dog. Am Heart J 92:324, 1976

29. Fingland RB, Bonagura JD, Myer CW: Pulmonic stenosis in the dog: 29 cases (1975–1984). J Am Anim Hosp Assoc 189:218, 1986

30. McCaw D, Aronson E: Congenital cardiac disease in dogs. Mod Vet Pract 65:509, 1984

31. Eyster GE: Pulmonic stenosis. p. 462. In Bojrab MJ (ed): Current Techniques in Small Animal Surgery. 2nd Ed. WB Saunders, Philadelphia, 1983

32. Patterson DF, Haskins ME, Schnarr WR: Hereditary dysplasia of the pulmonary valve in beagle dogs. Pediatr Cardiol 47:631, 1981

33. Bolton GR, Liu SK: Congenital heart disease in the cat. Vet Clin North Am 7:341, 1977

34. Hawe RS: Pulmonic stenosis in a cat. J Am Anim Hosp Assoc 17:777, 1981

35. Bolton GR, Ettinger SJ, Liu SK: Tetralogy of Fallot in three cats. J Am Vet Med Assoc 160:1622, 1972

36. Eyster GE, Weber W, McQuillan W: Tetralogy of Fallot in a cat. J Am Vet Med Assoc 171:280, 1977

37. van Heerden J, Lourens DC: Tetralogy of Fallot in a two-and-one-half-year old cat. J Am Anim Hosp Assoc 17:129, 1981

38. Hawe RS, Witter WR, Wilson JB: Tetralogy of Fallot in a five-year old cat. J Am Anim Hosp Assoc 15:329, 1979

39. Bonagura JD: Congenital heart disease. p. 3. American College of Veterinary Internal Medicine. Proceedings of the Fourth Annual Veterinary Medical Forum. Vol. 1. 1986

40. Patterson DF, Pyle RL, Buchanan JW, et al: Hereditary patent ductus arteriosis and its sequelae in the dog. Circ Res 29:1, 1971

41. Pyle RL: Congenital heart disease. p. 933. In Ettinger SJ (ed): Textbook of Veterinary Internal Medicine. 2nd Ed. WB Saunders, Philadelphia, 1983

42. Jones CL, Buchanan JW: Patent ductus arteriosis: Anatomy and surgery in a cat. J Am Vet Med Assoc 179:364, 1981

43. Jeraj K, Ogburn P, Lord P, Wilson JW: Patent ductus arteriosis with pulmonary hypertension in a cat. J Am Vet Med Assoc 172:1432, 1978

44. Cohen JS, Tilley LP, Liu SK, DeHoff WD: Patent ductus arteriosis in five cats. J Am Anim Hosp Assoc 11:95, 1975

45. Detweiler DK, Patterson DF: Prevalence and types of cardiovascular disease in dogs. Ann NY Acad Sci 127:481, 1965

46. Zook BC: Some spontaneous cardiovascular lesions in dogs and cats. Adv Cardiol 13:148, 1974

47. Jeraj K, Ogburn P, Johnston GR, et al: Atrial septal defect (sinus venosus type) in a dog. J Am Vet Med Assoc 177:342, 1980

48. Troy GC, Turnwald GH: Atrial fibrillation and abnormal ventricular conduction presented as right bundle branch block in a dog with an atrial septum primum defect. J Am Anim Hosp Assoc 15:417, 1979

49. Eyster GE, Anderson LK, Krehbeil JD, et al: Surgical repair of atrial septal defect in the dog. J Am Vet Med Assoc 169:1081, 1976

50. Hamlin RL, Smith CR, Smetzer DL: Ostium secundum type interatrial septal defects in the dog. J Am Vet Med Assoc 143:149, 1963

51. Pyle RL, Patterson DF: Multiple cardiovascular malformations in a family of Boxer dogs. J Am Vet Med Assoc 160:965, 1972

52. Liu SK, Ettinger SJ: Persistent common atrioventricular canal in two cats. J Am Vet Med Assoc 153:556, 1968

53. Patterson DF, Pyle RL, van Mierop LHS, et al: Hereditary defects of the conotruncal septum in keeshond dogs: Pathologic and genetic studies. Am J Cardiol 34:187, 1974

54. Mulvihill JJ, Priester WA: Congenital heart disease in dogs: Epidemiologic similarities to man. Teratology 7:73, 1973

55. Weirich WE, Blevins WE: Ventricular septal defect repair. Vet Surg 7:2, 1978

56. Scott FW, Weiss RC, Post JE, et al: Kitten mortality complex (neonatal FIP?). Feline Pract 9:44, 1979

57. Bryan CS, Oppenheimer EH: Ventricular endocardial fibroelastosis: Basis for its presence or absence in cases of pulmonic and aortic atresia. Arch Pathol Lab Med 87:82, 1969

58. Paaseh LH, Zook BC: The pathogenesis of endocardial fibroelastosis in the Burmese cat. Lab Invest 42:197, 1980

59. Moller JH, Lucas RV, Adams P, et al. Endocardial fibroelastosis: A clinical and anatomic study of 47 patients with emphasis on its relationship to mitral insufficiency. Circulation 30:759, 1964

60. Roberts WC, Morrow AG: Secondary left ventricular endocardial fibroelastosis following mitral valve replacement—Cause of cardiac failure in late postoperative period. Circulation 37(suppl II): 101, 1968

61. Ettinger SJ, Suter PF: Canine Cardiology. WB Saunders, Philadelphia, 1970

62. Keene BW, Bonagura JD: Valvular heart disease. p. 311. In Kirk RW (ed): Current Veterinary Therapy. Vol. VIII. WB Saunders, Philadelphia, 1983

63. Zook BC: Some spontaneous cardiovascular lesions in dogs and cats. Comparative pathology of the heart. Adv Cardiol 13:148, 1974

64. Janes TC, Zook BC: Aging changes in the vascular system of animals. Ann NY Acad Sci 127:671, 1965

65. Das KM, Tashjian RJ: Chronic mitral valve disease in the dog. Vet Med 60:1209, 1965

66. Buchanan JW: Chronic valvular disease (endocardiosis) in dogs. Adv Vet Sci Comp Med 21:75, 1977

67. King BD, Clark MA, Baba N, et al: "Myxomatous" mitral valves: Collagen dissolution as the primary defect. Circulation 66:288, 1982

68. Yamaguchi RA, Pipers FA, Gamble DA: Echocardiographic evaluation of a cat with bacterial vegetative endocarditis. J Am Vet Med Assoc 183:118, 1983

69. Calvert CA: Valvular bacterial endocarditis in the dog. J Am Vet Med Assoc 180:1080, 1982

70. Anderson CA, Dubielzig RR: Vegetative endocarditis in dogs. J Am Anim Hosp Assoc 20:149, 1984

71. Sisson D, Thomas WP: Endocarditis of the aortic valve in the dog. J Am Vet Med Assoc 184:570, 1984

72. Murdoch DB, Baker JR: Bacterial endocarditis in the dog. J Small Anim Pract 18:687, 1977

73. Wynne J, Braunwald E: The cardiomyopathies and myocarditides. p. 1410. In Braunwald E (ed): Heart Disease. 3rd Ed. WB Saunders, Philadelphia, 1988

74. Fox PR, Tilley LP, Liu SK: The cardiovascular system. p. 249. In Pratt PW (ed): Feline Medicine. American Veterinary Publications, Santa Barbara, 1983

75. Tilley LP, Liu SK, Fox PR: Myocardial disease. p. 1029. In Ettinger SJ (ed): Textbook of Veterinary Internal Medicine. Vol. 1. 2nd Ed. WB Saunders, Philadelphia, 1983

76. Tilley LP, Liu SK: The striking similarity between myocardial disease in cats and man. Med Times 106:2, 1978

77. Tilley LP, LIU SK, Gilbertson SR, et al: Primary myocardial disease in the cat: A model for human cardiomyopathy. Am J Pathol 87:493, 1977

78. Fox PR: Feline myocardial diseases. p. 337. In Kirk RW (ed): Current Veterinary Therapy. Vol. VIII. WB Saunders, Philadelphia, 1983

79. Bond BR, Fox PR: Advances in feline cardiomyopathy. Vet Clin North Am 14:1021, 1984

80. Fowler NP: Diagnosis of myocardial disease. Cardiovasc Clin 4:77, 1972

81. Goodwin JF, Oakley CW: The cardiomyopathies. Br Heart J 34:545, 1972

82. Maron BJ, Epstein SE: Hypertrophic cardiomyopathy: A discussion of nomenclature. Am J Cardiol 43:1242, 1979

83. Roberts WC, Ferrans V: Pathologic aspects of certain cardiomyopathies. Circ Res 35(suppl II):128, 1974

84. Liu SK, Peterson ME, Fox PR: Hypertrophic cardiomyopathy and hyperthyroidism in the cat. J Am Vet Med Assoc 185:52, 1984

85. Peterson ME, Kintzer PP, Cavanagh PG, et al: Feline hyperthyroidism: Pretreatment clinical and laboratory evaluation of 131 cases. J Am Vet Med Assoc 183:103, 1983

86. Fuster VF, Gersh BJ, Guiliani ER, et al: The natural history of idiopathic dilated cardiomyopathies. Am J Cardiol 47:525, 1981

87. Fox PR: Feline myocardial diseases: A clinical approach. p. 57. Proceedings of the Ninth Annual Kal Kan Symposium, Cardiology, 1985

88. Harpster NK: Boxer cardiomyopathy. p. 329. In Kirk RW (ed): Current Veterinary Therapy. Vol. VIII. WB Saunders, Philadelphia, 1983

89. Ware WA, Bonagura JD: Canine myocardial diseases. p. 370. In Kirk RW (ed): Current Veterinary Therapy. Vol. IX. WB Saunders, Philadelphia, 1986

90. Olsen EGJ: Cardiomyopathies. Cardiovasc Clin 4:240, 1972

91. Olsen EGJ: The pathology of cardiomyopathies. A critical analysis. Am Heart J 98:384, 1979

92. Truex RC, Warshow LJ: The incidence and size of the moderator band in man and in mammals. Anat Rec 82:361, 1942

93. Miller ME, Christensen GC, Evans HE: Anatomy of the Dog. 2nd Ed. WB Saunders, Philadelphia, 1964

94. Carpenter JL, Roberts RM, Harpster NK, King NW: Intestinal and cardiopulmonary forms of parvovirus infection in a litter of pups. J Am Vet Med Assoc 176:1269, 1980

95. James TN, Robertson BT, Malds AL, et al: Hereditary stenosis of the His bundle in the pug dog. Circulation 52:1152, 1975

96. Meierhenry EF, Liu SK: Atrioventricular bundle degeneration associated with sudden death in the dog. J Am Vet Med Assoc 172:1418, 1978

97. Hirsch J: Hypercoagulability. Semin Hematol 14:409, 1977

98. Furster V, Chesebro JH: Antithrombotic therapy: Role of platelet-inhibitor drugs. I. Current concepts of thrombogenesis: Role of platelets. Mayo Clin Proc 56:102, 1981

99. Griffiths I, Duncan ID: Ischaemic neuromyopathy in cats. Vet Rec 104:518, 1979

100. Suter PF: Diseases of the peripheral vessels. p. 1062. In Ettinger SJ (ed): Textbook of Veterinary Internal Medicine. Vol. 1. 2nd Ed. WB Saunders, Philadelphia, 1983

101. Green RA, Russo EA, Greene RT, et al: Hypoalbuminemia-related platelet hypersensitivity in two dogs with nephrotic syndrome. J Am Vet Med Assoc 186:485, 1985

102. DeBartola SP, Meuten DJ: Renal amyloidosis in two dogs presented for thromboembolic phenomena. J Am Anim Hosp Assoc 16:129, 1980

103. Burns MG, Kelly AB, Hornof WJ, et al: Pulmonary artery thrombosis in three dogs with hyperadrenocorticism. J Am Vet Med Assoc 178:388, 1981

104. Tilley LP, Liu SK: Persistent atrial standstill in the dog and cat. Proc Am Coll Vet Intern Med 43, 1983 (abst)

105. Bloomfield MB, Sinclair-Smith BC: Persistent atrial standstill. Am J Med 39:335, 1965

Index

Page numbers followed by *f* represent figures; those followed by *t* represent tables